ICD-10-PCS 2020

The Complete Official Codebook

AMA
AMERICAN MEDICAL
ASSOCIATION

AMA publications fund initiatives that drive improvements
in patient health, practice innovation and medical education.

AMAstore.com

Notice

ICD-10-PCS: The Complete Official Codebook is designed to be an accurate and authoritative source regarding coding and every reasonable effort has been made to ensure accuracy and completeness of the content. However, the American Medical Association (AMA) makes no guarantee, warranty, or representation that this publication is accurate, complete, or without errors. It is understood that the AMA is not rendering any legal or other professional services or advice in this publication and that the AMA bears no liability for any results or consequences that may arise from the use of this book.

Our Commitment to Accuracy

The AMA is committed to producing accurate and reliable materials. To report corrections, please call the AMA Unified Service Center at (800) 621-8335. AMA product updates, errata, and addendum can be found at amaproductupdates.org.

To purchase additional copies, contact the AMA at (800) 621-8335 or visit the AMA store at amastore.com. Refer to product number OP201120.

Copyright

Acknowledgments

Marianne Randall, CPC, *Product Manager*

Karen Schmidt, BSN, *Technical Director*

Anita Schmidt, BS, RHIA, AHIMA-approved ICD-10-CM/PCS Trainer, *Clinical Technical Editor*

Peggy Willard, CCS, AHIMA-approved ICD-10-CM/PCS Trainer, *Clinical Technical Editor*

Stacy Perry, *Manager, Desktop Publishing*

Tracy Betzler, *Senior Desktop Publishing Specialist*

Hope M. Dunn, *Senior Desktop Publishing Specialist*

Katie Russell, *Desktop Publishing Specialist*

Kate Holden, *Editor*

Anita Schmidt, BS, RHIA, AHIMA-approved ICD-10-CM/PCS Trainer

Ms. Schmidt has expertise in ICD-10-CM/PCS, DRG, and CPT with more than 15 years' experience in coding in multiple settings, including inpatient, observation, and same-day surgery. Her experience includes analysis of medical record documentation, assignment of ICD-10-CM and PCS codes, and DRG validation. She has conducted training for ICD-10-CM/PCS and electronic health record. She has also collaborated with clinical documentation specialists to identify documentation needs and potential areas for physician education. Most recently she has been developing content for resource and educational products related to ICD-10-CM, ICD-10-PCS, DRG, and CPT. Ms. Schmidt is an AHIMA-approved ICD-10-CM/PCS trainer and is an active member of the American Health Information Management Association (AHIMA) and the Minnesota Health Information Management Association (MHIMA).

Peggy Willard, CCS, AHIMA-approved ICD-10-CM/PCS Trainer

Ms. Willard has 18 years of experience in the healthcare field. Her expertise is in ICD-10-CM and ICD-10-PCS, including in-depth analysis of medical record documentation, ICD-10-CM/PCS code and DRG assignment, as well as clinical documentation improvement (CDI). In recent years Ms. Willard has been responsible for the creation and development of several products for Optum360 Coding Solutions that are designed to assist with appropriate application of the ICD-10-CM and ICD-10-PCS coding systems. She has several years of prior experience in Level I adult and pediatric trauma hospital and inpatient rehabilitation facility (IRF) coding, specializing in ICD-9-CM diagnosis and procedural coding, with emphasis in conducting coding audits, and conducting coding training for coding staff and clinical documentation specialists. Ms. Willard is an AHIMA-approved ICD-10 CM/PCS trainer and is an active member of the American Health Information Management Association (AHIMA) and the Minnesota Health Information Management Association (MHIMA).

Contents

What's New for 2020

The Centers for Medicare and Medicaid Services is the agency charged with maintaining and updating ICD-10-PCS. CMS released the most current revisions, a summary of which may be found on the CMS website at: https://www.cms.gov/Medicare/Coding/ICD10/2020-ICD-10-PCS.html

Due to the unique structure of ICD-10-PCS, a change in a character value may affect individual codes and several code tables.

Change Summary Table

2019 Total	New Codes	Revised Titles	Deleted Codes	2020 Total
78,881	734	2	2,056	77,559

ICD-10-PCS Code FY 2020 Totals, By Section

Medical and Surgical	67,257
Obstetrics	302
Placement	861
Administration	1,332
Measurement and Monitoring	418
Extracorporeal or Systemic Assistance and Performance	48
Extracorporeal or Systemic Therapies	46
Osteopathic	100
Other Procedures	77
Chiropractic	90
Imaging	2,941
Nuclear Medicine	463
Radiation Therapy	2,019
Physical Rehabilitation and Diagnostic Audiology	1,380
Mental Health	30
Substance Abuse Treatment	59
New Technology	136
Total	77,559

ICD-10-PCS Table Changes Highlights

- The Bifurcation qualifier was removed from the root operation tables of Dilation and Extirpation in the Upper Arteries body system and from Dilation, Extirpation and Restriction in the Lower Arteries body system.
- Intraluminal device, flow diverter device value was added to the root operation table Restriction in the Upper Arteries body system.
- The Coronary Artery body parts were added to the Insertion and Supplement root operation tables in the Heart and Great Vessels body system.
- Approach values were added to the body part Gastric Vein in the Occlusion root operation table of the Lower Veins body system.
- Sinus body parts added to the root operation Supplement in the Ear, Nose, Sinus body system.
- Vagina was added as a qualifier to the Large Intestine body part in the Transfer root operation table in the Gastrointestinal body system.
- External removed as an approach value for the Breast body parts in several of the root operation tables of Skin and Breast body system.

- Device value, Subcutaneous Defibrillator Lead, added to the root operations Insertion, in the Subcutaneous Tissue and Fascia, Chest body part and Removal and Revision to use with Subcutaneous Tissue and Fascia, Trunk body part.
- Internal Fixation Device, Intramedullary Limb Lengthening was added as a device to the Humeral Shaft body parts in the Insertion root operation table of Upper Bones body system.
- Internal Fixation Device, Intramedullary Limb Lengthening was added as a device to the Femoral Shaft and Tibia body parts in the Insertion root operation table of Lower Bones body system.
- Upper and Lower Jaw body parts were added to the Extirpation root operation table in the Anatomical Regions, General body system.
- Stem Cells, T-cell Depleted Hematopoietic substance added to the Transfusion root operation table for the Circulatory body system in the Administration section.
- Intraoperative was added to Circulatory, Oxygenation in the Extracorporeal or Systemic Assistance and Performance section.
- Fluorescence Guided Procedure was added to the Other Procedures section.
- Unidirectional Source qualifier added to all low dose rate palladium 103 isotope rows, in the Brachytherapy table in the Radiation Therapy section.
- Many new substances and devices were added to the New Technology tables – see New Definitions Addenda – Device and Substance Definitions for more information.
- New qualifiers added to the Bypass root operation tables in several body systems including:
  - Central Nervous System and Cranial Nerves
  - Heart and Great Vessels
  - Upper Arteries
  - Gastrointestinal (also added body parts to Bypass table)

New Definitions Addenda

Section 0 - Medical and Surgical Root Operations

ICD-10-PCS Value	Definition	
Control	Delete	Explanation: The site of the bleeding is coded as an anatomical region and not to a specific body part.

Section 0 - Medical and Surgical Body Part Definitions

ICD-10-PCS Value	Definition	
Popliteal Artery, Left Popliteal Artery, Right	Add	Tibioperoneal trunk
Add Skin, Chest	Add	Breast procedures, skin only
Subcutaneous Tissue and Fascia, Face	Add	Submandibular space

Section 0 - Medical and Surgical Device Definitions

ICD-10-PCS Value		Definition	
Add	Internal Fixation Device, Intramedullary Limb Lengthening for Insertion in Lower Bones	Add	PRECICE intramedullary limb lengthening system
Add	Internal Fixation Device, Intramedullary Limb Lengthening for Insertion in Upper Bones	Add	PRECICE intramedullary limb lengthening system
Intraluminal Device		Delete	Pipeline™ Embolization device (PED)
Add	Intraluminal Device, Flow Diverter for Restriction in Upper Arteries	Add	Flow Diverter embolization device
		Add	Pipeline™ (Flex) embolization device
		Add	Surpass Streamline™ Flow Diverter
Monitoring Device		Delete	Reveal (DX)(XT)
		Add	Reveal (LINQ)(DX)(XT)
Radioactive Element		Add	CivaSheet®
Add	Subcutaneous Defibrillator Lead in Subcutaneous Tissue and Fascia	Add	S-ICD™ lead

Section 0 - Medical and Surgical Device Aggregation Table

Specific Device		for Operation		in Body System		General Device	
Add	Internal Fixation Device, Intra-medullary Limb Lengthening	Add	Insertion	Add	Lower Bones	Add 6	Internal Fixation Device, Intra-medullary
				Add	Upper Bones		
Add	Intraluminal Device, Flow Diverter	Add	Restriction	Add	Upper Arteries	Add D	Intra-luminal Device

Section 3 - Administration Substance Definitions

ICD-10-PCS Value	Definition	
Anti-Infective Envelope	Add	Antibacterial Envelope (TYRX) (AIGISRx)
	Add	TYRX Antibacterial Envelope

Section X - New Technology Root Operation

ICD-10-PCS Value		Definition	
Add	Dilation	Add	Definition: Expanding an orifice or the lumen of a tubular body part.
		Add	Explanation: The orifice can be a natural orifice or an artificially created orifice. Accomplished by stretching a tubular body part using intraluminal pressure or by cutting part of the orifice or wall of the tubular body part.
Add	Measurement	Add	Definition: Determining the level of a physiological or physical function at a point in time.

Section X - New Technology Device/Substance/Technology

ICD-10-PCS Value		Definition	
Delete	Andexanet Alfa, Factor Xa Inhibitor Reversal Agent	Delete	Factor Xa Inhibitor Reversal Agent, Andexanet Alfa
Add	Apalutamide Antineoplastic	Add	ERLEAD™
Add	Coagulation Factor Xa, Inactivated	Add	Andexanet Alfa, Factor Xa Inhibitor Reversal Agent
		Add	Andexxa
		Add	Coagulation Factor Xa (Recombinant), Inactivated
		Add	Factor Xa Inhibitor Reversal Agent, Andexanet Alfa
Add	Fosfomycin Anti-infective	Add	CONTEPO™
		Add	Fosfomycin injection
Add	Gilteritinib Antineoplastic	Add	XOSPATA®
Add	Imipenem-cilastatin-relebactam Anti-infective	Add	IMI/REL
Add	Intraluminal Device, Sustained Release Drug-Eluting in New Technology	Add	Eluvia™ Drug-eluting Vascular Stent System
		Add	SAVAL Below-the-Knee (BTK) Drug-eluting Stent System
Add	Intraluminal Device, Sustained Release Drug-eluting, Four or More in New Technology	Add	Eluvia™ Drug-eluting Vascular Stent System
		Add	SAVAL Below-the-Knee (BTK) Drug-eluting Stent System
Add	Intraluminal Device, Sustained Release Drug-eluting, Three in New Technology	Add	Eluvia™ Drug-eluting Vascular Stent System
		Add	SAVAL Below-the-Knee (BTK) Drug-eluting Stent System
Add	Intraluminal Device, Sustained Release Drug-Eluting, Two in New Technology	Add	Eluvia™ Drug-eluting Vascular Stent System
		Add	SAVAL Below-the-Knee (BTK) Drug-eluting Stent System
Add	Iobenguane I-131 Antineoplastic	Add	AZEDRA®
		Add	Iobenguane I-131, High Specific Activity (HSA)

ICD-10-PCS Value		Definition	
Add	Meropenem-vaborbactam Anti-infective	Add	Vabomere™
Add	Ruxolitinib (T)	Add	Jakafi®
Add	Tagraxofusp-erzs Antineoplastic	Add	ELZONRIS™
Add	Ventoclax Antineoplastic	Add	Venclexta®

List of Updated Files

2020 Official ICD-10-PCS Coding Guidelines

- New guidelines D1.a, D1.b, and D1.c added in response to public comment
- Guidelines page 1, paragraph 3, A9, B2.1a, B3.1b, B3.2c, B3.5, B3.9, B4.1b, E1.a, and E1.b revised in response to public comment and internal review
- Downloadable PDF, file name pcs_guidelines_2020.pdf

2020 ICD-10-PCS Code Tables and Index (Zip file)

- Code tables for use beginning October 1, 2019
- Downloadable PDF, file name is pcs_2020.pdf
- Downloadable xml files for developers, file names are icd10pcs_tables_2020.xml, icd10pcs_index_2020.xml, icd10pcs_definitions_2020.xml
- Accompanying schema for developers, file names are icd10pcs_tables.xsd, icd10pcs_index.xsd, icd10pcs_definitions.xsd

2020 ICD-10-PCS Codes File (Zip file)

- ICD-10-PCS Codes file is a simple format for non-technical uses, containing the valid FY 2020 ICD-10-PCS codes and their long titles
- File is in text file format, file name is icd10pcs_codes_2020.txt
- Accompanying documentation for codes file, file name is icd10pcsCodesFile.pdf
- Codes file addenda in text format, file name is codes_addenda_2020.txt

2020 ICD-10-PCS Order File (Long and Abbreviated Titles) (Zip file)

- ICD-10-PCS order file is for developers, provides a unique five-digit "order number" for each ICD-10-PCS table and code, as well as a long and abbreviated code title
- ICD-10-PCS order file name is icd10pcs_order_2020.txt
- Accompanying documentation for tabular order file, file name is icd10pcsOrderFile.pdf
- Tabular order file addenda in text format, file name is order_addenda_2020.txt

2020 ICD-10-PCS Final Addenda (Zip file)

- Addenda files in downloadable PDF, file names are tables_addenda_2020.pdf, index_addenda_2020.pdf, definitions_addenda_2020.pdf
- Addenda files also in machine readable text format for developers, file names are tables_addenda_2020.txt, index_addenda_2020.txt, definitions_addenda_2020.txt

2020 ICD-10-PCS Conversion Table (Zip file)

- ICD-10-PCS code conversion table is provided to assist users in data retrieval, in downloadable Excel spreadsheet, file name is icd10pcs_conversion_table_2020.xlsx
- Conversion table also in machine readable text format for developers, file name is icd10pcs_conversion_table_2020.txt
- Accompanying documentation for code conversion table, file name is icd10pcsConversionTable.pdf

Introduction

History of ICD-10-PCS

The World Health Organization has maintained the International Classification of Diseases (ICD) for recording cause of death since 1893. It has updated the ICD periodically to reflect new discoveries in epidemiology and changes in medical understanding of disease.

The International Classification of Diseases Tenth Revision (ICD-10), published in 1992, is the latest revision of the ICD. The WHO authorized the National Center for Health Statistics (NCHS) to develop a clinical modification of ICD-10 for use in the United States. This version, called ICD-10-CM, is intended to replace the previous U.S. clinical modification, ICD-9-CM, that has been in use since 1979. ICD-9-CM contains a procedure classification; ICD-10-CM does not.

CMS, the agency responsible for maintaining the inpatient procedure code set in the United States, contracted with 3M Health Information Systems in 1993 to design and then develop a procedure classification system to replace volume 3 of ICD-9-CM.

The result, ICD-10-PCS, was initially completed in 1998. The code set has been updated annually since that time to ensure that ICD-10-PCS includes classifications for new procedures, devices, and technologies.

The development of ICD-10-PCS had as its goal the incorporation of the following major attributes:

- **Completeness:** There should be a unique code for all substantially different procedures.

- **Unique definitions:** Because ICD-10-PCS codes are constructed of individual values rather than lists of fixed codes and text descriptions, the unique, stable definition of a code in the system is retained. New values may be added to the system to represent a specific new approach or device or qualifier, but whole codes by design cannot be given new meanings and reused.

- **Expandability:** As new procedures are developed, the structure of ICD-10-PCS should allow them to be easily incorporated as unique codes.

- **Multi-axial codes:** ICD-10-PCS codes should consist of independent characters, with each individual component retaining its meaning across broad ranges of codes to the extent possible.

- **Standardized terminology:** ICD-10-PCS should include definitions of the terminology used. While the meaning of specific words varies in common usage, ICD-10-PCS should not include multiple meanings for the same term, and each term must be assigned a specific meaning. There are no eponyms or common procedure terms in ICD-10-PCS.

- **Structural integrity:** ICD-10-PCS can be easily expanded without disrupting the structure of the system. ICD-10-PCS allows unique new codes to be added to the system because values for the seven characters that make up a code can be combined as needed. The system can evolve as medical technology and clinical practice evolve, without disrupting the ICD-10-PCS structure.

In the development of ICD-10-PCS, several additional general characteristics were added:

- **Diagnostic information is not included in procedure description:** When procedures are performed for specific diseases or disorders, the disease or disorder is not contained in the procedure code. The diagnosis codes, not the procedure codes, specify the disease or disorder.

- **Explicit not otherwise specified (NOS) options are restricted:** Explicit "not otherwise specified," (NOS) options are restricted in ICD-10-PCS. A minimal level of specificity is required for each component of the procedure.

- **Limited use of not elsewhere classified (NEC) option:** Because all significant components of a procedure are specified in ICD-10-PCS, there is generally no need for a "not elsewhere classified" (NEC) code option. However, limited NEC options are incorporated into ICD-10-PCS where necessary. For example, new devices are frequently developed, and therefore it is necessary to provide an "other device" option for use until the new device can be explicitly added to the coding system.

- **Level of specificity:** All procedures currently performed can be specified in ICD-10-PCS. The frequency with which a procedure is performed was not a consideration in the development of the system. A unique code is available for variations of a procedure that can be performed.

ICD-10-PCS code structure results in qualities that optimize the performance of the system in electronic applications, and maximize the usefulness of the coded healthcare data. These qualities include:

- **Optimal search capability:** ICD-10-PCS is designed for maximum versatility in the ability to aggregate coded data. Values belonging to the same character as defined in a section or sections can be easily compared, since they occupy the same position in a code. This provides a high degree of flexibility and functionality for data mining.

- **Consistent characters and values:** Stability of characters and values across vast ranges of codes provides the maximum degree of functionality and flexibility for the collection and analysis of data. Because the character definition is consistent, and only the individual values assigned to that character differ as needed, meaningful comparisons of data over time can be conducted across a virtually infinite range of procedures.

- **Code readability:** ICD-10-PCS resembles a language in the sense that it is made up of semi-independent values combined by following the rules of the system, much the way a sentence is formed by combining words and following the rules of grammar and syntax. As with words in their context, the meaning of any single value is a combination of its position in the code and any preceding values on which it may be dependent.

ICD-10-PCS Code Structure

ICD-10-PCS has a seven-character alphanumeric code structure. Each character contains up to 34 possible values. Each value represents a specific option for the general character definition. The 10 digits Ø–9 and the 24 letters A–H, J–N, and P–Z may be used in each character. The letters O and I are not used so as to avoid confusion with the digits Ø and 1. An ICD-10-PCS code is the result of a process rather than as a single fixed set of digits or alphabetic characters. The process consists of combining semi-independent values from among a selection of values, according to the rules governing the construction of codes.

	Section	Body System	Root Operation	Body Part	Approach	Device	Qualifier
Characters:	1	2	3	4	5	6	7

A code is derived by choosing a specific value for each of the seven characters. Based on details about the procedure performed, values for each character specifying the section, body system, root operation, body part, approach, device, and qualifier are assigned. Because the definition of each character is also a function of its physical position in the code, the same letter or number placed in a different position in the code has a different meaning.

The seven characters that make up a complete code have specific meanings that vary for each of the 17 sections of the manual.

Procedures are then divided into sections that identify the general type of procedure (e.g., Medical and Surgical, Obstetrics, Imaging). The first character of the procedure code always specifies the section. The second through seventh characters have the same meaning within each section, but may mean different things in other sections. In all sections, the third character specifies the general type of procedure performed (e.g., Resection, Transfusion, Fluoroscopy), while the other characters give additional information such as the body part and approach.

In ICD-10-PCS, the term *procedure* refers to the complete specification of the seven characters.

Number of Codes in ICD-10-PCS

The table structure of ICD-10-PCS permits the specification of a large number of codes on a single page. At the time of this publication, there are 77,559 codes in the 2020 ICD-10-PCS.

ICD-10-PCS Manual

Index

Codes may be found in the index based on the general type of procedure (e.g., resection, transfusion, fluoroscopy), or a more commonly used term (e.g., appendectomy). For example, the code for percutaneous intraluminal dilation of the coronary arteries with an intraluminal device can be found in the Index under *Dilation*, or a synonym of *Dilation* (e.g., angioplasty). The Index then specifies the first three or four values of the code or directs the user to see another term.

Example:

> **Dilation**
>> Artery
>>> Coronary
>>>> One Artery Ø27Ø

Based on the first three values of the code provided in the Index, the corresponding table can be located. In the example above, the first three values indicate table Ø27 is to be referenced for code completion.

The tables and characters are arranged first by number and then by letter for each character (tables for ØØ-, Ø1-, Ø2-, etc., are followed by those for ØB-, ØC-, ØD-, etc., followed by ØB1, ØB2, etc., followed by ØBB, ØBC, ØBD, etc.).

Note: The Tables section must be used to construct a complete and valid code by specifying the last three or four values.

Tables

The Tables are composed of rows that specify the valid combinations of code values. In most sections of the system, the upper portion of each table contains a description of the first three characters of the procedure code. In the Medical and Surgical section, for example, the first three characters contain the name of the section, the body system, and the root operation performed.

For instance, the values *Ø27* specify the section *Medical and Surgical* (Ø), the body system *Heart and Great Vessels* (2) and the root operation *Dilation* (7). As shown in table Ø27, the root operation (*Dilation*) is accompanied by its definition.

The lower portion of the table specifies all the valid combinations of characters 4 through 7. The four columns in the table specify the last four characters. In the Medical and Surgical section they are labeled body part, approach, device and qualifier, respectively. Each row in the table specifies the valid combination of values for characters 4 through 7.

Table 1: Row from table Ø27

Ø   **Medical and Surgical**
2   **Heart and Great Vessels**
7   **Dilation**   Definition: Expanding an orifice or the lumen of a tubular body part

                       Explanation: The orifice can be a natural orifice or an artificially created orifice. Accomplished by stretching a tubular body part using intraluminal pressure or by cutting part of the orifice or wall of the tubular body part.

Body Part Character 4	Approach Character 5	Device Character 6	Qualifier Character 7
Ø Coronary Artery, One Artery 1 Coronary Artery, Two Arteries 2 Coronary Artery, Three Arteries 3 Coronary Artery, Four or More Arteries	Ø Open 3 Percutaneous 4 Percutaneous Endoscopic	4 Intraluminal Device, Drug-eluting 5 Intraluminal Device, Drug-eluting, Two 6 Intraluminal Device, Drug-eluting, Three 7 Intraluminal Device, Drug-eluting, Four or More D Intraluminal Device E Intraluminal Device, Two F Intraluminal Device, Three G Intraluminal Device, Four or More T Intraluminal Device, Radioactive Z No Device	6 Bifurcation Z No Qualifier

The rows of this table can be used to construct 240 unique procedure codes. For example, code Ø27Ø3DZ specifies the procedure for dilation of one coronary artery using an intraluminal device via percutaneous approach (i.e., percutaneous transluminal coronary angioplasty with stent).

The valid codes shown in table 2 are constructed using the first body part value in table 1 (i.e., one coronary artery), combined with all the valid approaches and devices listed in the table, and the value "No Qualifier."

Table 2: Code titles for dilation of one coronary artery (Ø27Ø)

Ø27ØØ4Z	Dilation of Coronary Artery, One Artery with Drug-eluting Intraluminal Device, Open Approach
Ø27ØØ5Z	Dilation of Coronary Artery, One Artery with Two Drug-eluting Intraluminal Devices, Open Approach
Ø27ØØ6Z	Dilation of Coronary Artery, One Artery with Three Drug-eluting Intraluminal Devices, Open Approach
Ø27ØØ7Z	Dilation of Coronary Artery, One Artery with Four or More Drug-eluting Intraluminal Devices, Open Approach
Ø27ØØDZ	Dilation of Coronary Artery, One Artery with Intraluminal Device, Open Approach
Ø27ØØEZ	Dilation of Coronary Artery, One Artery with Two Intraluminal Devices, Open Approach
Ø27ØØFZ	Dilation of Coronary Artery, One Artery with Three Intraluminal Devices, Open Approach
Ø27ØØGZ	Dilation of Coronary Artery, One Artery with Four or More Intraluminal Devices, Open Approach
Ø27ØØTZ	Dilation of Coronary Artery, One Artery with Radioactive Intraluminal Device, Open Approach
Ø27ØØZZ	Dilation of Coronary Artery, One Artery, Open Approach
Ø27Ø34Z	Dilation of Coronary Artery, One Artery with Drug-eluting Intraluminal Device, Percutaneous Approach
Ø27Ø35Z	Dilation of Coronary Artery, One Artery with Two Drug-eluting Intraluminal Devices, Percutaneous Approach
Ø27Ø36Z	Dilation of Coronary Artery, One Artery with Three Drug-eluting Intraluminal Devices, Percutaneous Approach
Ø27Ø37Z	Dilation of Coronary Artery, One Artery with Four or More Drug-eluting Intraluminal Devices, Percutaneous Approach
Ø27Ø3DZ	Dilation of Coronary Artery, One Artery with Intraluminal Device, Percutaneous Approach
Ø27Ø3EZ	Dilation of Coronary Artery, One Artery with Two Intraluminal Devices, Percutaneous Approach
Ø27Ø3FZ	Dilation of Coronary Artery, One Artery with Three Intraluminal Devices, Percutaneous Approach
Ø27Ø3GZ	Dilation of Coronary Artery, One Artery with Four or More Intraluminal Devices, Percutaneous Approach
Ø27Ø3TZ	Dilation of Coronary Artery, One Artery with Radioactive Intraluminal Device, Percutaneous Approach
Ø27Ø3ZZ	Dilation of Coronary Artery, One Artery, Percutaneous Approach
Ø27Ø44Z	Dilation of Coronary Artery, One Artery with Drug-eluting Intraluminal Device, Percutaneous Endoscopic Approach
Ø27Ø45Z	Dilation of Coronary Artery, One Artery with Two Drug-eluting Intraluminal Devices, Percutaneous Endoscopic Approach
Ø27Ø46Z	Dilation of Coronary Artery, One Artery with Three Drug-eluting Intraluminal Devices, Percutaneous Endoscopic Approach
Ø27Ø47Z	Dilation of Coronary Artery, One Artery with Four or More Drug-eluting Intraluminal Devices, Percutaneous Endoscopic Approach
Ø27Ø4DZ	Dilation of Coronary Artery, One Artery with Intraluminal Device, Percutaneous Endoscopic Approach
Ø27Ø4EZ	Dilation of Coronary Artery, One Artery with Two Intraluminal Devices, Percutaneous Endoscopic Approach
Ø27Ø4FZ	Dilation of Coronary Artery, One Artery with Three Intraluminal Devices, Percutaneous Endoscopic Approach
Ø27Ø4GZ	Dilation of Coronary Artery, One Artery with Four or More Intraluminal Devices, Percutaneous Endoscopic Approach
Ø27Ø4TZ	Dilation of Coronary Artery, One Artery with Radioactive Intraluminal Device, Percutaneous Endoscopic Approach
Ø27Ø4ZZ	Dilation of Coronary Artery, One Artery, Percutaneous Endoscopic Approach

Table 3: Rows from table 00H

0   **Medical and Surgical**
0   **Central Nervous System and Cranial Nerves**
H   **Insertion**   Definition: Putting in a nonbiological appliance that monitors, assists, performs, or prevents a physiological function but does not physically take the place of a body part
Explanation: None

Body Part Character 4		Approach Character 5	Device Character 6	Qualifier Character 7
0 Brain Cerebrum Corpus callosum Encephalon		**0** Open	**2** Monitoring Device **3** Infusion Device **4** Radioactive Element, Cesium-131 Collagen Implant **M** Neurostimulator Lead **Y** Other Device	**Z** No Qualifier
0 Brain Cerebrum Corpus callosum Encephalon		**3** Percutaneous **4** Percutaneous Endoscopic	**2** Monitoring Device **3** Infusion Device **M** Neurostimulator Lead **Y** Other Device	**Z** No Qualifier
6 Cerebral Ventricle Aqueduct of Sylvius Cerebral aqueduct (Sylvius) Choroid plexus Ependyma Foramen of Monro (intraventricular) Fourth ventricle Interventricular foramen (Monro) Left lateral ventricle Right lateral ventricle Third ventricle	**E** Cranial Nerve **U** Spinal Canal Epidural space, spinal Extradural space, spinal Subarachnoid space, spinal Subdural space, spinal Vertebral canal **V** Spinal Cord	**0** Open **3** Percutaneous **4** Percutaneous Endoscopic	**2** Monitoring Device **3** Infusion Device **M** Neurostimulator Lead **Y** Other Device	**Z** No Qualifier

Table 3, is split into three rows; values of characters must all be selected from within the same row of the table. Row 1 and 2 indicate that the body part (character 4) value 0 and Qualifier value Z may both be used in combination with device values 2, 3, M or Y. However, the approach (character 5) and device (character 6) values are not exactly the same for both rows. As shown in row 1, Body part value Brain (0) with Device value Radioactive Element, Cesium-131 Collagen Implant (4) can only be used with approach value Open (0). In other words, code 00H034Z would be invalid as the approach value 3 is only applicable to row 2 and the device value 4 is only applicable to row 1. It would be inappropriate to build a code for body part 0 if all of the values are not contained in its own row.

Note: In this manual, there are instances in which some tables due to length must be continued on the next page. Each section must be used separately and value selection must be made within the same row of the table.

Character Meanings

In each section, each character has a specific meaning, and this character meaning remains constant within that section. Character meaning tables have been provided at the beginning of each body system in the Medical and Surgical section (0) and the Obstetric section (1) to help the user identify the character members available within that section. These tables have purple headers, unlike the official code tables that have green headers and **SHOULD NOT** be used to build a PCS code. Following is an excerpt of a character meaning table.

Table 4: Rows from Central Nervous System and Cranial Nerves - Character Meanings Table

Operation–Character 3		Body Part–Character 4		Approach–Character 5		Device–Character 6		Qualifier–Character 7	
1	Bypass	0	Brain	0	Open	0	Drainage Device	0	Nasopharynx
2	Change	1	Cerebral Meninges	3	Percutaneous	2	Monitoring Device	1	Mastoid Sinus
5	Destruction	2	Dura Mater	4	Percutaneous Endoscopic	3	Infusion Device	2	Atrium
7	Dilation	3	Epidural Space, Intracranial	X	External	4	Radioactive Element, Cesium-131 Collagen Implant	3	Blood Vessel
8	Division	4	Subdural Space, Intracranial			7	Autologous Tissue Substitute	4	Pleural Cavity
9	Drainage	5	Subarachnoid Space, Intracranial			J	Synthetic Substitute	5	Intestine
B	Excision	6	Cerebral Ventricle			K	Nonautologous Tissue Substitute	6	Peritoneal Cavity
C	Extirpation	7	Cerebral Hemisphere			M	Neurostimulator Lead	7	Urinary Tract
D	Extraction	8	Basal Ganglia			Y	Other Device	8	Bone Marrow
F	Fragmentation	9	Thalamus			Z	No Device	9	Fallopian Tube
H	Insertion	A	Hypothalamus					A	Subgaleal Space
J	Inspection	B	Pons					B	Cerebral Cisterns

Sections

Procedures are divided into sections that identify the general type of procedure (e.g., Medical and Surgical, Obstetrics, Imaging). The first character of the procedure code always specifies the section.

The sections are listed below:

Medical and Surgical section

Ø   Medical and Surgical

Medical and Surgical-related sections

1   Obstetrics

2   Placement

3   Administration

4   Measurement and Monitoring

5   Extracorporeal or Systemic Assistance and Performance

6   Extracorporeal or Systemic Therapies

7   Osteopathic

8   Other Procedures

9   Chiropractic

Ancillary Sections

B   Imaging

C   Nuclear Medicine

D   Radiation Therapy

F   Physical Rehabilitation and Diagnostic Audiology

G   Mental Health

H   Substance Abuse Treatment

New Technology Section

X   New Technology

Medical and Surgical Section (Ø)

Character Meaning

The seven characters for Medical and Surgical procedures have the following meaning:

Character	Meaning
1	Section
2	Body System
3	Root Operation
4	Body Part
5	Approach
6	Device
7	Qualifier

The Medical and Surgical section constitutes the vast majority of procedures reported in an inpatient setting. Medical and Surgical procedure codes all have a first character value of Ø. The second character indicates the general body system (e.g., Mouth and Throat, Gastrointestinal). The third character indicates the root operation, or specific objective, of the procedure (e.g., Excision). The fourth character indicates the specific body part on which the procedure was performed (e.g., Tonsils, Duodenum). The fifth character indicates the approach used to reach the procedure site (e.g., Open). The sixth character indicates whether a device was left in place during the procedure (e.g.,

Synthetic Substitute). The seventh character is qualifier, which has a specific meaning for each root operation. For example, the qualifier can be used to identify the destination site of a *Bypass*. The first through fifth characters are always assigned a specific value, but the device (sixth character) and the qualifier (seventh character) are not applicable to all procedures. The value *Z* is used for the sixth and seventh characters to indicate that a specific device or qualifier does not apply to the procedure.

Section (Character 1)

Medical and Surgical procedure codes all have a first character value of Ø.

Body Systems (Character 2)

Body systems for Medical and Surgical section codes are specified in the second character.

Body Systems

Ø   Central Nervous System and Cranial Nerves

1   Peripheral Nervous System

2   Heart and Great Vessels

3   Upper Arteries

4   Lower Arteries

5   Upper Veins

6   Lower Veins

7   Lymphatic and Hemic Systems

8   Eye

9   Ear, Nose, Sinus

B   Respiratory System

C   Mouth and Throat

D   Gastrointestinal System

F   Hepatobiliary System and Pancreas

G   Endocrine System

H   Skin and Breast

J   Subcutaneous Tissue and Fascia

K   Muscles

L   Tendons

M   Bursae and Ligaments

N   Head and Facial Bones

P   Upper Bones

Q   Lower Bones

R   Upper Joints

S   Lower Joints

T   Urinary System

U   Female Reproductive System

V   Male Reproductive System

W   Anatomical Regions, General

X   Anatomical Regions, Upper Extremities

Y   Anatomical Regions, Lower Extremities

Root Operations (Character 3)

The root operation is specified in the third character. In the Medical and Surgical section there are 31 different root operations. The root operation identifies the objective of the procedure. Each root operation has a precise definition.

- *Alteration:* Modifying the natural anatomic structure of a body part without affecting the function of the body part

- *Bypass:* Altering the route of passage of the contents of a tubular body part

- *Change:* Taking out or off a device from a body part and putting back an identical or similar device in or on the same body part without cutting or puncturing the skin or a mucous membrane

- *Control:* Stopping, or attempting to stop, postprocedural or other acute bleeding

- *Creation:* Putting in or on biological or synthetic material to form a new body part that to the extent possible replicates the anatomic structure or function of an absent body part

- *Destruction:* Physical eradication of all or a portion of a body part by the direct use of energy, force, or a destructive agent

- *Detachment:* Cutting off all or a portion of the upper or lower extremities

- *Dilation:* Expanding an orifice or the lumen of a tubular body part

- *Division:* Cutting into a body part without draining fluids and/or gases from the body part in order to separate or transect a body part

- *Drainage:* Taking or letting out fluids and/or gases from a body part

- *Excision:* Cutting out or off, without replacement, a portion of a body part

- *Extirpation:* Taking or cutting out solid matter from a body part

- *Extraction:* Pulling or stripping out or off all or a portion of a body part by the use of force

- *Fragmentation:* Breaking solid matter in a body part into pieces

- *Fusion:* Joining together portions of an articular body part rendering the articular body part immobile

- *Insertion:* Putting in a nonbiological appliance that monitors, assists, performs, or prevents a physiological function but does not physically take the place of a body part

- *Inspection:* Visually and/or manually exploring a body part

- *Map:* Locating the route of passage of electrical impulses and/or locating functional areas in a body part

- *Occlusion:* Completely closing an orifice or lumen of a tubular body part

- *Reattachment:* Putting back in or on all or a portion of a separated body part to its normal location or other suitable location

- *Release:* Freeing a body part from an abnormal physical constraint by cutting or by use of force

- *Removal:* Taking out or off a device from a body part

- *Repair:* Restoring, to the extent possible, a body part to its normal anatomic structure and function

- *Replacement:* Putting in or on biological or synthetic material that physically takes the place and/or function of all or a portion of a body part

- *Reposition:* Moving to its normal location or other suitable location all or a portion of a body part

- *Resection:* Cutting out or off, without replacement, all of a body part

- *Restriction:* Partially closing an orifice or lumen of a tubular body part

- *Revision:* Correcting, to the extent possible, a portion of a malfunctioning device or the position of a displaced device

- *Supplement:* Putting in or on biological or synthetic material that physically reinforces and/or augments the function of a portion of a body part

- *Transfer:* Moving, without taking out, all or a portion of a body part to another location to take over the function of all or a portion of a body part

- *Transplantation:* Putting in or on all or a portion of a living body part taken from another individual or animal to physically take the place and/or function of all or a portion of a similar body part

The above definitions of root operations illustrate the precision of code values defined in the system. There is a clear distinction between each root operation.

A root operation specifies the objective of the procedure. The term *anastomosis* is not a root operation, because it is a means of joining and is always an integral part of another procedure (e.g., Bypass, Resection) with a specific objective. Similarly, *incision* is not a root operation, since it is always part of the objective of another procedure (e.g., Division, Drainage). The root operation *Repair* in the Medical and Surgical section functions as a "not elsewhere classified" option. *Repair* is used when the procedure performed is not one of the other specific root operations.

Appendix B provides additional explanation and representative examples of the Medical and Surgical root operations. Appendix C groups all root operations in the Medical and Surgical section into subcategories and provides an example of each root operation.

Body Part (Character 4)

The body part is specified in the fourth character. The body part indicates the specific anatomical site of the body system on which the procedure was performed (e.g., Duodenum). Tubular body parts are defined in ICD-10-PCS as those hollow body parts that provide a route of passage for solids, liquids, or gases. They include the cardiovascular system and body parts such as those contained in the gastrointestinal tract, genitourinary tract, biliary tract, and respiratory tract.

Approach (Character 5)

The technique used to reach the site of the procedure is specified in the fifth character. There are seven different approaches:

- *Open*: Cutting through the skin or mucous membrane and any other body layers necessary to expose the site of the procedure

- *Percutaneous*: Entry, by puncture or minor incision, of instrumentation through the skin or mucous membrane and any other body layers necessary to reach the site of the procedure

- *Percutaneous Endoscopic*: Entry, by puncture or minor incision, of instrumentation through the skin or mucous membrane and any other body layers necessary to reach and visualize the site of the procedure

- *Via Natural or Artificial Opening*: Entry of instrumentation through a natural or artificial external opening to reach the site of the procedure

- *Via Natural or Artificial Opening Endoscopic*: Entry of instrumentation through a natural or artificial external opening to reach and visualize the site of the procedure

- *Via Natural or Artificial Opening with Percutaneous Endoscopic Assistance:* Entry of instrumentation through a natural or artificial external opening and entry, by puncture or minor incision, of instrumentation through the skin or mucous membrane and any other body layers necessary to aid in the performance of the procedure

- *External*: Procedures performed directly on the skin or mucous membrane and procedures performed indirectly by the application of external force through the skin or mucous membrane

The approach comprises three components: the access location, method, and type of instrumentation.

Access location: For procedures performed on an internal body part, the access location specifies the external site through which the site of the procedure is reached. There are two general types of access locations: skin or mucous membranes, and external orifices. Every approach value except external includes one of these two access locations. The skin or mucous membrane can be cut or punctured to reach the procedure site. All open and percutaneous approach values use this access location. The site of a procedure can also be reached through an external opening. External openings can be natural (e.g., mouth) or artificial (e.g., colostomy stoma).

Method: For procedures performed on an internal body part, the method specifies how the external access location is entered. An open method specifies cutting through the skin or mucous membrane and any other intervening body layers necessary to expose the site of the procedure. An instrumentation method specifies the entry of instrumentation through the access location to the internal procedure site. Instrumentation can be introduced by puncture or minor incision, or through an external opening. The puncture or minor incision does not constitute an open approach because it does not expose the site of the procedure. An approach can define multiple methods. For example, *Via Natural or Artificial Opening with Percutaneous Endoscopic Assistance* includes both the initial entry of instrumentation to reach the site of the procedure, and the placement of additional percutaneous instrumentation into the body part to visualize and assist in the performance of the procedure.

Type of instrumentation: For procedures performed on an internal body part, instrumentation means that specialized equipment is used to perform the procedure. Instrumentation is used in all internal approaches other than the basic open approach. Instrumentation may or may not include the capacity to visualize the procedure site. For example, the instrumentation used to perform a sigmoidoscopy permits the internal site of the procedure to be visualized, while the instrumentation used to perform a needle biopsy of the liver does not. The term "endoscopic" as used in approach values refers to instrumentation that permits a site to be visualized.

Procedures performed directly on the skin or mucous membrane are identified by the external approach (e.g., skin excision). Procedures performed indirectly by the application of external force are also identified by the external approach (e.g., closed reduction of fracture).

Appendix A compares the components (access location, method, and type of instrumentation) of each approach and provides an example and illustration of each approach.

Device (Character 6)
The device is specified in the sixth character and is used only to specify devices that remain after the procedure is completed. There are four general types of devices:

- Biological or synthetic material that takes the place of all or a portion of a body part (e.g, skin graft, joint prosthesis).

- Biological or synthetic material that assists or prevents a physiological function (e.g., IUD).

- Therapeutic material that is not absorbed by, eliminated by, or incorporated into a body part (e.g., radioactive implant).

- Mechanical or electronic appliances used to assist, monitor, take the place of or prevent a physiological function (e.g., cardiac pacemaker, orthopedic pin).

While all devices can be removed, some cannot be removed without putting in another nonbiological appliance or body-part substitute.

When a specific device value is used to identify the device for a root operation, such as *Insertion* and that same device value is not an option for a more broad range root operation such as *Removal*, select the general device value. For example, in the body system Heart and Great Vessels, the specific device character for Cardiac Lead, Pacemaker in root operation *Insertion* is J. For the root operation *Removal*, the general device character M Cardiac Lead would be selected for the pacemaker lead.

ICD-10-PCS contains a PCS Device Aggregation Table (see appendix F) that crosswalks the *specific* device character values that have been created for specific root operations and specific body part character values to the *general* device character value that would be used for root operations that represent a broad range of procedures and general body part character values, such as Removal and Revision.

Instruments used to visualize the procedure site are specified in the approach, not the device, value.

If the objective of the procedure is to put in the device, then the root operation is *Insertion*. If the device is put in to meet an objective other than *Insertion*, then the root operation defining the underlying objective of the procedure is used, with the device specified in the device character. For example, if a procedure to replace the hip joint is performed, the root operation *Replacement* is coded, and the prosthetic device is specified in the device character. Materials that are incidental to a procedure such as clips, ligatures, and sutures are not specified in the device character. Because new devices can be developed, the value *Other Device* is provided as a temporary option for use until a specific device value is added to the system.

Qualifier (Character 7)
The qualifier is specified in the seventh character. The qualifier contains unique values for individual procedures. For example, the qualifier can be used to identify the destination site in a *Bypass*.

Medical and Surgical Section Principles
In developing the Medical and Surgical procedure codes, several specific principles were followed.

Composite Terms Are Not Root Operations
Composite terms such as colonoscopy, sigmoidectomy, or appendectomy do not describe root operations, but they do specify multiple components of a specific root operation. In ICD-10-PCS, the components of a procedure are defined separately by the characters making up the complete code. The only component of a procedure

specified in the root operation is the objective of the procedure. With each complete code the underlying objective of the procedure is specified by the root operation (third character), the precise part is specified by the body part (fourth character), and the method used to reach and visualize the procedure site is specified by the approach (fifth character). While colonoscopy, sigmoidectomy, and appendectomy are included in the Index, they do not constitute root operations in the Tables section. The objective of colonoscopy is the visualization of the colon and the root operation (character 3) is *Inspection*. Character 4 specifies the body part, which in this case is part of the colon. These composite terms, like colonoscopy or appendectomy, are included as cross-reference only. The index provides the correct root operation reference. Examples of other types of composite terms not representative of root operations are *partial* sigmoidectomy, *total* hysterectomy, and *partial* hip replacement. Always refer to the correct root operation in the Index and Tables section.

Root Operation Based on Objective of Procedure

The root operation is based on the objective of the procedure, such as *Resection* of transverse colon or *Dilation* of an artery. The assignment of the root operation is based on the procedure actually performed, which may or may not have been the intended procedure. If the intended procedure is modified or discontinued (e.g., excision instead of resection is performed), the root operation is determined by the procedure actually performed. If the desired result is not attained after completing the procedure (i.e., the artery does not remain expanded after the dilation procedure), the root operation is still determined by the procedure actually performed.

Examples:

- Dilating the urethra is coded as *Dilation* since the objective of the procedure is to dilate the urethra. If dilation of the urethra includes putting in an intraluminal stent, the root operation remains *Dilation* and not *Insertion* of the intraluminal device because the underlying objective of the procedure is dilation of the urethra. The stent is identified by the intraluminal device value in the sixth character of the dilation procedure code.
- If the objective is solely to put a radioactive element in the urethra, then the procedure is coded to the root operation *Insertion*, with the radioactive element identified in the sixth character of the code.
- If the objective of the procedure is to correct a malfunctioning or displaced device, then the procedure is coded to the root operation *Revision*. In the root operation *Revision*, the original device being revised is identified in the device character. *Revision* is typically performed on mechanical appliances (e.g., pacemaker) or materials used in replacement procedures (e.g., synthetic substitute). Typical revision procedures include adjustment of pacemaker position and correction of malfunctioning knee prosthesis.

Combination Procedures Are Coded Separately

If multiple procedures as defined by distinct objectives are performed during an operative episode, then multiple codes are used. For example, obtaining the vein graft used for coronary bypass surgery is coded as a separate procedure from the bypass itself.

Redo of Procedures

The complete or partial redo of the original procedure is coded to the root operation that identifies the procedure performed rather than *Revision*.

Example:

> A complete redo of a hip replacement procedure that requires putting in a new prosthesis is coded to the root operation *Replacement* rather than *Revision*.

The correction of complications arising from the original procedure, other than device complications, is coded to the procedure performed. Correction of a malfunctioning or displaced device would be coded to the root operation *Revision*.

Example:

> A procedure to control hemorrhage arising from the original procedure is coded to *Control* rather than *Revision*.

Examples of Procedures Coded in the Medical Surgical Section

The following are examples of procedures from the Medical and Surgical section, coded in ICD-10-PCS.

- Suture of skin laceration, left lower arm: ØHQEXZZ

  Medical and Surgical section (Ø), body system *Skin and Breast* (H), root operation *Repair* (Q), body part *Skin, Left Lower Arm* (E), *External* Approach (X) *No device* (Z), and *No qualifier* (Z).

- Laparoscopic appendectomy: ØDTJ4ZZ

  Medical and Surgical section (Ø), body system *Gastrointestinal* (D), root operation *Resection* (T), body part *Appendix* (J), *Percutaneous Endoscopic* approach (4), No Device (Z), and No qualifier (Z).

- Sigmoidoscopy with biopsy: ØDBN8ZX

  Medical and Surgical section (Ø), body system *Gastrointestinal* (D), root operation *Excision* (B), body part *Sigmoid Colon* (N), *Via Natural or Artificial Opening Endoscopic* approach (8), *No Device* (Z), and with qualifier *Diagnostic* (X).

- Tracheostomy with tracheostomy tube: ØB11ØF4

  Medical and Surgical section (Ø), body system *Respiratory* (B), root operation *Bypass* (1), body part *Trachea* (1), *Open* approach (Ø), with *Tracheostomy Device* (F), and qualifier *Cutaneous* (4).

Obstetrics Section (1)

Character Meanings

The seven characters in the Obstetrics section have the same meaning as in the Medical and Surgical section.

Character	Meaning
1	Section
2	Body System
3	Root Operation
4	Body Part
5	Approach
6	Device
7	Qualifier

The Obstetrics section includes procedures performed on the products of conception only. Procedures on the pregnant female are coded in the Medical and Surgical section (e.g., episiotomy). The term "products of conception" refers to all physical components of a pregnancy, including the fetus, amnion, umbilical cord, and placenta. There is no differentiation of the products of conception based on gestational age.

Thus, the specification of the products of conception as a zygote, embryo or fetus, or the trimester of the pregnancy is not part of the procedure code but can be found in the diagnosis code.

Section (Character 1)
Obstetrics procedure codes have a first character value of *1*.

Body System (Character 2)
The second character value for body system is *Pregnancy*.

Root Operation (Character 3)
The root operations *Change, Drainage, Extraction, Insertion, Inspection, Removal, Repair, Reposition, Resection,* and *Transplantation* are used in the obstetrics section and have the same meaning as in the Medical and Surgical section.

The Obstetrics section also includes two additional root operations, *Abortion* and *Delivery*, defined below:

- *Abortion*: Artificially terminating a pregnancy

- *Delivery*: Assisting the passage of the products of conception from the genital canal

A cesarean section is not a separate root operation because the underlying objective is *Extraction* (i.e., pulling out all or a portion of a body part).

Body Part (Character 4)
The body part values in the obstetrics section are:

- *Products of conception*

- *Products of conception, retained*

- *Products of conception, ectopic*

Approach (Character 5)
The fifth character specifies approaches and is defined as are those in the Medical and Surgical section. In the case of an abortion procedure that uses a laminaria or an abortifacient, the approach is *Via Natural or Artificial Opening*.

Device (Character 6)
The sixth character is used for devices such as fetal monitoring electrodes.

Qualifier (Character 7)
Qualifier values are specific to the root operation and are used to capture details of the procedure, such as whether forceps or a vacuum were used during an Extraction, the type of fluid taken out during a Drainage procedure, or the products of conception body system that was repaired.

Placement Section (2)

Character Meanings
The seven characters in the Placement section have the following meaning:

Character	Meaning
1	Section
2	Body System
3	Root Operation
4	Body Region
5	Approach
6	Device
7	Qualifier

Placement section codes represent procedures for putting a device in or on a body region for the purpose of protection, immobilization, stretching, compression, or packing.

Section (Character 1)
Placement procedure codes have a first character value of *2*.

Body System (Character 2)
The second character contains two values specifying either *Anatomical Regions* or *Anatomical Orifices*.

Root Operation (Character 3)
The root operations in the Placement section include only those procedures that are performed without making an incision or a puncture. The root operations *Change* and *Removal* are in the Placement section and have the same meaning as in the Medical and Surgical section.

The Placement section also includes five additional root operations, defined as follows:

- *Compression*: Putting pressure on a body region

- *Dressing*: Putting material on a body region for protection

- *Immobilization*: Limiting or preventing motion of an external body region

- *Packing*: Putting material in a body region or orifice

- *Traction*: Exerting a pulling force on a body region in a distal direction

Body Region (Character 4)
The fourth character values are either body regions (e.g., *Upper Leg*) or natural orifices (e.g., *Ear*).

Approach (Character 5)
Since all placement procedures are performed directly on the skin or mucous membrane, or performed indirectly by applying external force through the skin or mucous membrane, the approach value is always *External*.

Device (Character 6)
The device character is always specified (except in the case of manual traction) and indicates the device placed during the procedure (e.g., cast, splint, bandage, etc.). Except for casts for fractures and dislocations, devices in the Placement section are off the shelf and do not require any extensive design, fabrication, or fitting. Placement of devices that require extensive design, fabrication, or fitting are coded in the Rehabilitation section.

Qualifier (Character 7)

The qualifier character is not specified in the Placement section; the qualifier value is always *No Qualifier*.

Administration Section (3)

Character Meanings

The seven characters in the Administration section have the following meaning:

Character	Meaning
1	Section
2	Body System
3	Root Operation
4	Body System/Region
5	Approach
6	Substance
7	Qualifier

Administration section codes represent procedures for putting in or on a therapeutic, prophylactic, protective, diagnostic, nutritional, or physiological substance. The section includes transfusions, infusions, and injections, along with other similar services such as irrigation and tattooing.

Section (Character 1)

Administration procedure codes have a first character value of *3*.

Body System (Character 2)

The body system character contains only three values: *Indwelling Device, Physiological Systems and Anatomical Regions,* or *Circulatory System*. The *Circulatory System* is used for transfusion procedures.

Root Operation (Character 3)

There are three root operations in the Administration section.

* *Introduction*: Putting in or on a therapeutic, diagnostic, nutritional, physiological, or prophylactic substance except blood or blood products

* *Irrigation*: Putting in or on a cleansing substance

* *Transfusion*: Putting in blood or blood products

Body/System Region (Character 4)

The fourth character specifies the body system/region. The fourth character identifies the site where the substance is administered, not the site where the substance administered takes effect. Sites include *Skin and Mucous Membranes, Subcutaneous Tissue,* and *Muscle*. These differentiate intradermal, subcutaneous, and intramuscular injections, respectively. Other sites include *Eye, Respiratory Tract, Peritoneal Cavity,* and *Epidural Space*.

The body systems/regions for arteries and veins are *Peripheral Artery, Central Artery, Peripheral Vein,* and *Central Vein*. The *Peripheral Artery* or *Vein* is typically used when a substance is introduced locally into an artery or vein. For example, chemotherapy is the introduction of an antineoplastic substance into a peripheral artery or vein by a percutaneous approach. In general, the substance introduced into a peripheral artery or vein has a systemic effect.

The *Central Artery* or *Vein* is typically used when the site where the substance is introduced is distant from the point of entry into the artery or vein. For example, the introduction of a substance directly at the site of a clot within an artery or vein using a catheter is coded as an introduction of a thrombolytic substance into a central artery or vein by a percutaneous approach. In general, the substance introduced into a central artery or vein has a local effect.

Approach (Character 5)

The fifth character specifies approaches as defined in the Medical and Surgical section. The approach for intradermal, subcutaneous, and intramuscular introductions (i.e., injections) is *Percutaneous*. If a catheter is placed to introduce a substance into an internal site within the circulatory system, then the approach is also *Percutaneous*. For example, if a catheter is used to introduce contrast directly into the heart for angiography, then the procedure would be coded as a percutaneous introduction of contrast into the heart.

Substance (Character 6)

The sixth character specifies the substance being introduced. Broad categories of substances are defined, such as anesthetic, contrast, dialysate, and blood products such as platelets.

Qualifier (Character 7)

The seventh character is a qualifier and is used to indicate whether the substance is *Autologous* or *Nonautologous*, or to further specify the substance.

Measurement and Monitoring Section (4)

Character Meanings

The seven characters in the Measurement and Monitoring section have the following meaning:

Character	Meaning
1	Section
2	Body System
3	Root Operation
4	Body System
5	Approach
6	Function/Device
7	Qualifier

Measurement and Monitoring section codes represent procedures for determining the level of a physiological or physical function.

Section (Character 1)

Measurement and Monitoring procedure codes have a first character value of *4*.

Body System (Character 2)

The second character values for body system are A, *Physiological Systems* or B, *Physiological Devices*.

Root Operation (Character 3)

There are two root operations in the Measurement and Monitoring section, as defined below:

* *Measurement*: Determining the level of a physiological or physical function at a point in time

- *Monitoring*: Determining the level of a physiological or physical function repetitively over a period of time

Body System (Character 4)
The fourth character specifies the specific body system measured or monitored.

Approach (Character 5)
The fifth character specifies approaches as defined in the Medical and Surgical section.

Function/Device (Character 6)
The sixth character specifies the physiological or physical function being measured or monitored. Examples of physiological or physical functions are *Conductivity, Metabolism, Pulse, Temperature,* and *Volume.* If a device used to perform the measurement or monitoring is inserted and left in, then insertion of the device is coded as a separate Medical and Surgical procedure.

Qualifier (Character 7)
The seventh character qualifier contains specific values as needed to further specify the body part (e.g., central, portal, pulmonary) or a variation of the procedure performed (e.g., ambulatory, stress). Examples of typical procedures coded in this section are EKG, EEG, and cardiac catheterization. An EKG is the measurement of cardiac electrical activity, while an EEG is the measurement of electrical activity of the central nervous system. A cardiac catheterization performed to measure the pressure in the heart is coded as the measurement of cardiac pressure by percutaneous approach.

Extracorporeal or Systemic Assistance and Performance Section (5)

Character Meanings
The seven characters in the Extracorporeal or Systemic Assistance and Performance section have the following meaning:

Character	Meaning
1	Section
2	Body System
3	Root Operation
4	Body System
5	Duration
6	Function
7	Qualifier

In Extracorporeal or Systemic Assistance and Performance procedures, equipment outside the body is used to assist or perform a physiological function. The section includes procedures performed in a critical care setting, such as mechanical ventilation and cardioversion; it also includes other services such as hyperbaric oxygen treatment and hemodialysis.

Section (Character 1)
Extracorporeal or Systemic Assistance and Performance procedure codes have a first character value of *5.*

Body System (Character 2)
The second character value for body system is A, *Physiological Systems.*

Root Operation (Character 3)
There are three root operations in the Extracorporeal or Systemic Assistance and Performance section, as defined below.

- *Assistance*: Taking over a portion of a physiological function by extracorporeal means

- *Performance*: Completely taking over a physiological function by extracorporeal means

- *Restoration*: Returning, or attempting to return, a physiological function to its natural state by extracorporeal means

The root operation *Restoration* contains a single procedure code that identifies extracorporeal cardioversion.

Body System (Character 4)
The fourth character specifies the body system (e.g., cardiac, respiratory) to which extracorporeal or systemic assistance or performance is applied.

Duration (Character 5)
The fifth character specifies the duration of the procedure—*Single, Intermittent,* or *Continuous.* For respiratory ventilation assistance or performance, the duration is specified in hours— *< 24 Consecutive Hours, 24–96 Consecutive Hours,* or *> 96 Consecutive Hours.* For urinary procedures, duration is specified as *Intermittent, Less than 6 Hours Per Day; Prolonged Intermittent, 6-18 hours Per Day*; or *Continuous, Greater than 18 hours Per Day.* Value 6, *Multiple* identifies serial procedure treatment.

Function (Character 6)
The sixth character specifies the physiological function assisted or performed (e.g., oxygenation, ventilation) during the procedure.

Qualifier (Character 7)
The seventh character qualifier specifies the type of equipment used, if any.

Extracorporeal or Systemic Therapies Section (6)

Character Meanings
The seven characters in the Extracorporeal or Systemic Therapies section have the following meaning:

Character	Meaning
1	Section
2	Body System
3	Root Operation
4	Body System
5	Duration
6	Qualifier
7	Qualifier

In extracorporeal or systemic therapy, equipment outside the body is used for a therapeutic purpose that does not involve the assistance or performance of a physiological function.

Section (Character 1)
Extracorporeal or Systemic Therapy procedure codes have a first character value of 6.

Body System (Character 2)
The second character value for body system is *Physiological Systems*.

Root Operation (Character 3)
There are 11 root operations in the Extracorporeal or Systemic Therapy section, as defined below.

- *Atmospheric Control*: Extracorporeal control of atmospheric pressure and composition

- *Decompression*: Extracorporeal elimination of undissolved gas from body fluids

  Coding note: The root operation *Decompression* involves only one type of procedure: treatment for decompression sickness (the bends) in a hyperbaric chamber.

- *Electromagnetic Therapy*: Extracorporeal treatment by electromagnetic rays

- *Hyperthermia*: Extracorporeal raising of body temperature

  Coding note: The term hyperthermia is used to describe both a temperature imbalance treatment and also as an adjunct radiation treatment for cancer. When treating the temperature imbalance, it is coded to this section; for the cancer treatment, it is coded in section *D Radiation Therapy*.

- *Hypothermia*: Extracorporeal lowering of body temperature

- *Perfusion*: Extracorporeal treatment by diffusion of therapeutic fluid

- *Pheresis*: Extracorporeal separation of blood products

  Coding note: Pheresis may be used for two main purposes: to treat diseases when too much of a blood component is produced (e.g., leukemia) and to remove a blood product such as platelets from a donor, for transfusion into another patient.

- *Phototherapy*: Extracorporeal treatment by light rays

  Coding note: Phototherapy involves using a machine that exposes the blood to light rays outside the body, recirculates it, and then returns it to the body.

- *Shock Wave Therapy*: Extracorporeal treatment by shock waves

- *Ultrasound Therapy*: Extracorporeal treatment by ultrasound

- *Ultraviolet Light Therapy*: Extracorporeal treatment by ultraviolet light

Body System (Character 4)
The fourth character specifies the body system on which the extracorporeal or systemic therapy is performed (e.g., skin, circulatory).

Duration (Character 5)
The fifth character specifies whether the procedure was performed once (single) or multiple times.

Qualifier (Character 6)
The sixth character for Extracorporeal or Systemic Therapies is *No Qualifier*, except for root operation Perfusion which has a sixth character qualifier of *Donor Organ*.

Qualifier (Character 7)
The seventh character qualifier is used in the root operation *Pheresis* to specify the blood component on which pheresis is performed and in the root operation *Ultrasound Therapy* to specify site of treatment.

Osteopathic Section (7)

Character Meanings
The seven characters in the Osteopathic section have the following meaning:

Character	Meaning
1	Section
2	Body System
3	Root Operation
4	Body Region
5	Approach
6	Method
7	Qualifier

Section (Character 1)
Osteopathic procedure codes have a first character value of *7*.

Body System (Character 2)
The body system character contains the value *Anatomical Regions*.

Root Operation (Character 3)
There is only one root operation in the Osteopathic section.

- *Treatment*: Manual treatment to eliminate or alleviate somatic dysfunction and related disorders

Body Region (Character 4)
The fourth character specifies the body region on which the osteopathic treatment is performed.

Approach (Character 5)
The approach for osteopathic treatment is always *External*.

Method (Character 6)
The sixth character specifies the method by which the treatment is accomplished.

Qualifier (Character 7)
The seventh character is not specified in the Osteopathic section and always has the value *None*.

Other Procedures Section (8)

Character Meanings

The seven characters in the Other Procedures section have the following meaning:

Character	Meaning
1	Section
2	Body System
3	Root Operation
4	Body Region
5	Approach
6	Method
7	Qualifier

The Other Procedures section includes acupuncture, suture removal, and in vitro fertilization.

Section (Character 1)

Other Procedure section codes have a first character value of *8*.

Body System (Character 2)

The second character values for body systems are *Physiological Systems and Anatomical Regions* and *Indwelling Device*.

Root Operation (Character 3)

The Other Procedures section has only one root operation, defined as follows:

* *Other Procedures*: Methodologies that attempt to remediate or cure a disorder or disease.

Body Region (Character 4)

The fourth character contains specified body-region values, and also the body-region value *None*.

Approach (Character 5)

The fifth character specifies approaches as defined in the Medical and Surgical section.

Method (Character 6)

The sixth character specifies the method (e.g., *Acupuncture, Therapeutic Massage*).

Qualifier (Character 7)

The seventh character is a qualifier and contains specific values as needed.

Chiropractic Section (9)

Character Meanings

The seven characters in the Chiropractic section have the following meaning:

Character	Meaning
1	Section
2	Body System
3	Root Operation
4	Body Region
5	Approach
6	Method
7	Qualifier

Section (Character 1)

Chiropractic section procedure codes have a first character value of *9*.

Body System (Character 2)

The second character value for body system is *Anatomical Regions*.

Root Operation (Character 3)

There is only one root operation in the *Chiropractic* section.

* *Manipulation:* Manual procedure that involves a directed thrust to move a joint past the physiological range of motion, without exceeding the anatomical limit.

Body Region (Character 4)

The fourth character specifies the body region on which the chiropractic manipulation is performed.

Approach (Character 5)

The approach for chiropractic manipulation is always *External*.

Method (Character 6)

The sixth character is the method by which the manipulation is accomplished.

Qualifier (Character 7)

The seventh character is not specified in the Chiropractic section and always has the value *None*.

Imaging Section (B)

Character Meanings

The seven characters in Imaging procedures have the following meaning:

Character	Meaning
1	Section
2	Body System
3	Type
4	Body Part
5	Contrast
6	Qualifier
7	Qualifier

Imaging procedures include plain radiography, fluoroscopy, CT, MRI, and ultrasound. Nuclear medicine procedures, including PET, uptakes, and scans, are in the nuclear medicine section. Therapeutic radiation procedure codes are in a separate radiation therapy section.

Section (Character 1)
Imaging procedure codes have a first character value of *B*.

Body System (Character 2)
In the Imaging section, the second character defines the body system, such as *Heart* or *Gastrointestinal System*.

Type (Character 3)
The third character defines the type of imaging procedure (e.g., MRI, ultrasound). The following list includes all types in the *Imaging* section with a definition of each type:

- *Computerized Tomography (CT Scan)*: Computer reformatted digital display of multiplanar images developed from the capture of multiple exposures of external ionizing radiation

- *Fluoroscopy*: Single plane or bi-plane real time display of an image developed from the capture of external ionizing radiation on a fluorescent screen. The image may also be stored by either digital or analog means

- *Magnetic Resonance Imaging (MRI)*: Computer reformatted digital display of multiplanar images developed from the capture of radiofrequency signals emitted by nuclei in a body site excited within a magnetic field

- *Plain Radiography*: Planar display of an image developed from the capture of external ionizing radiation on photographic or photoconductive plate

- *Ultrasonography*: Real time display of images of anatomy or flow information developed from the capture of reflected and attenuated high frequency sound waves

Body Part (Character 4)
The fourth character defines the body part with different values for each body system (character 2) value.

Contrast (Character 5)
The fifth character specifies whether the contrast material used in the imaging procedure is *High Osmolar, Low Osmolar,* or *Other Contrast* when applicable.

Qualifier (Character 6)
The sixth character qualifier provides further detail regarding the nature of the substance or technologies used, such as *Unenhanced and Enhanced (contrast), Laser,* or *Intravascular Optical Coherence*.

Qualifier (Character 7)
The seventh character is a qualifier that may be used to specify certain procedural circumstances, the method by which the procedure was performed, or technologies utilized, such as *Intraoperative, Intravascular, or Transesophageal*.

Nuclear Medicine Section (C)
Character Meanings
The seven characters in the Nuclear Medicine section have the following meaning:

Character	Meaning
1	Section
2	Body System
3	Type
4	Body Part
5	Radionuclide
6	Qualifier
7	Qualifier

Nuclear Medicine is the introduction of radioactive material into the body to create an image, to diagnose and treat pathologic conditions, or to assess metabolic functions. The Nuclear Medicine section does not include the introduction of encapsulated radioactive material for the treatment of cancer. These procedures are included in the Radiation Therapy section.

Section (Character 1)
Nuclear Medicine procedure codes have a first character value of *C*.

Body System (Character 2)
The second character specifies the body system on which the nuclear medicine procedure is performed.

Type (Character 3)
The third character indicates the type of nuclear medicine procedure (e.g., planar imaging or nonimaging uptake). The following list includes the types of nuclear medicine procedures with a definition of each type.

- *Nonimaging Nuclear Medicine Assay:* Introduction of radioactive materials into the body for the study of body fluids and blood elements, by the detection of radioactive emissions

- *Nonimaging Nuclear Medicine Probe:* Introduction of radioactive materials into the body for the study of distribution and fate of certain substances by the detection of radioactive emissions; or alternatively, measurement of absorption of radioactive emissions from an external source

- *Nonimaging Nuclear Medicine Uptake:* Introduction of radioactive materials into the body for measurements of organ function, from the detection of radioactive emissions

- *Planar Nuclear Medicine Imaging*: Introduction of radioactive materials into the body for single-plane display of images developed from the capture of radioactive emissions

- *Positron Emission Tomography (PET) Imaging:* Introduction of radioactive materials into the body for three dimensional display of images developed from the simultaneous capture, 180 degrees apart, of radioactive emissions

- *Systemic Nuclear Medicine Therapy:* Introduction of unsealed radioactive materials into the body for treatment

- *Tomographic (Tomo) Nuclear Medicine Imaging*: Introduction of radioactive materials into the body for three dimensional display of images developed from the capture of radioactive emissions

Body Part (Character 4)

The fourth character indicates the body part or body region studied; with regional (e.g., *lower extremity veins*) and combination (e.g., *liver and spleen*) body parts commonly used.

Radionuclide (Character 5)

The fifth character specifies the radionuclide, the radiation source. The option *Other Radionuclide* is provided in the nuclear medicine section for newly approved radionuclides until they can be added to the coding system. If more than one radiopharmaceutical is given to perform the procedure, then more than one code is used.

Qualifier (Character 6 and 7)

The sixth and seventh characters are qualifiers but are not specified in the *Nuclear Medicine* section; the value is always *None*.

Radiation Therapy Section (D)

Character Meanings

The seven characters in the Radiation Therapy section have the following meaning:

Character	Meaning
1	Section
2	Body System
3	Modality
4	Treatment Site
5	Modality Qualifier
6	Isotope
7	Qualifier

Section (Character 1)

Radiation therapy procedure codes have a first character value of *D*.

Body System (Character 2)

The second character specifies the body system (e.g., central nervous system, musculoskeletal) irradiated.

Modality (Character 3)

The third character specifies the general modality used (e.g., beam radiation).

Treatment Site (Character 4)

The fourth character specifies the body part that is the focus of the radiation therapy.

Modality Qualifier (Character 5)

The fifth character further specifies the radiation modality used (e.g., photons, electrons).

Isotope (Character 6)

The sixth character specifies the isotopes introduced into the body, if applicable.

Qualifier (Character 7)

The seventh character may specify whether the procedure was performed intraoperatively.

Physical Rehabilitation and Diagnostic Audiology Section (F)

Character Meanings

The seven characters in the Physical Rehabilitation and Diagnostic Audiology section have the following meaning:

Character	Meaning
1	Section
2	Section Qualifier
3	Type
4	Body System/Region
5	Type Qualifier
6	Equipment
7	Qualifier

Physical rehabilitation procedures include physical therapy, occupational therapy, and speech-language pathology. Osteopathic procedures and chiropractic procedures are in separate sections.

Section (Character 1)

Physical Rehabilitation and Diagnostic Audiology procedure codes have a first character value of *F*.

Section Qualifier (Character 2)

The section qualifier *Rehabilitation* or *Diagnostic Audiology* is specified in the second character.

Type (Character 3)

The third character specifies the type. There are 14 different values, which can be classified into four basic types of rehabilitation and diagnostic audiology procedures, defined as follows:

> *Assessment*: Includes a determination of the patient's diagnosis when appropriate, need for treatment, planning for treatment, periodic assessment, and documentation related to these activities
>
> Assessments are further classified into more than 100 different tests or methods. The majority of these focus on the faculties of hearing and speech, but others focus on various aspects of body function, and on the patient's quality of life, such as muscle performance, neuromotor development, and reintegration skills.
>
> - *Speech Assessment*: Measurement of speech and related functions
> - *Motor and/or Nerve Function Assessment*: Measurement of motor, nerve, and related functions
> - *Activities of Daily Living Assessment*: Measurement of functional level for activities of daily living
> - *Hearing Assessment*: Measurement of hearing and related functions
> - *Hearing Aid Assessment*: Measurement of the appropriateness and/or effectiveness of a hearing device
> - *Vestibular Assessment*: Measurement of the vestibular system and related functions
>
> *Caregiver Training*: Educating caregiver with the skills and knowledge used to interact with and assist the patient

Caregiver Training is divided into 18 different broad subjects taught to help a caregiver provide proper patient care.

- *Caregiver Training*: Training in activities to support patient's optimal level of function

Fitting(s): Design, fabrication, modification, selection, and/or application of splint, orthosis, prosthesis, hearing aids, and/or other rehabilitation device

The fifth character used in *Device Fitting* procedures describes the device being fitted rather than the method used to fit the device. Definitions of devices, when provided, are located in the definitions portion of the ICD-10-PCS tables and index, under section F, character 5.

- *Device Fitting*: Fitting of a device designed to facilitate or support achievement of a higher level of function

Treatment: Use of specific activities or methods to develop, improve, and/or restore the performance of necessary functions, compensate for dysfunction and/or minimize debilitation

Treatment procedures include swallowing dysfunction exercises, bathing and showering techniques, wound management, gait training, and a host of activities typically associated with rehabilitation.

- *Speech Treatment*: Application of techniques to improve, augment, or compensate for speech and related functional impairment

- *Motor Treatment*: Exercise or activities to increase or facilitate motor function

- *Activities of Daily Living Treatment*: Exercise or activities to facilitate functional competence for activities of daily living

- *Hearing Treatment*: Application of techniques to improve, augment, or compensate for hearing and related functional impairment

- *Cochlear Implant Treatment*: Application of techniques to improve the communication abilities of individuals with cochlear implant

- *Vestibular Treatment*: Application of techniques to improve, augment, or compensate for vestibular and related functional impairment

The type of treatment includes training as well as activities that restore function.

Body System/Region (Character 4)
The fourth character specifies the body region and/or system on which the procedure is performed.

Type Qualifier (Character 5)
The fifth character is a type qualifier that further specifies the procedure performed. Examples include therapy to improve the range of motion and training for bathing techniques. Refer to appendix I for definitions of these types of procedures.

Equipment (Character 6)
The sixth character specifies the equipment used. Specific equipment is not defined in the equipment value. Instead, broad categories of equipment are specified (e.g., aerobic endurance and conditioning, assistive/adaptive/supportive, etc.)

Qualifier (Character 7)
The seventh character is not specified in the Physical Rehabilitation and Diagnostic Audiology section and always has the value *None*.

Mental Health Section (G)
Character Meanings
The seven characters in the Mental Health section have the following meaning:

Character	Meaning
1	Section
2	Body System
3	Type
4	Qualifier
5	Qualifier
6	Qualifier
7	Qualifier

Section (Character 1)
Mental health procedure codes have a first character value of *G*.

Body System (Character 2)
The second character is used to identify the body system elsewhere in ICD-10-PCS. In this section it always has the value *None*.

Type (Character 3)
The third character specifies the procedure type, such as crisis intervention or counseling. There are 12 types of mental health procedures.

- *Psychological Tests:* The administration and interpretation of standardized psychological tests and measurement instruments for the assessment of psychological function

- *Crisis Intervention:* Treatment of a traumatized, acutely disturbed, or distressed individual for the purpose of short-term stabilization

- *Medication Management:* Monitoring and adjusting the use of medications for the treatment of a mental health disorder

- *Individual Psychotherapy:* Treatment of an individual with a mental health disorder by behavioral, cognitive, psychoanalytic, psychodynamic, or psychophysiological means to improve functioning or well-being

- *Counseling:* The application of psychological methods to treat an individual with normal developmental issues and psychological problems in order to increase function, improve well-being, alleviate distress, maladjustment, or resolve crises

- *Family Psychotherapy:* Treatment that includes one or more family members of an individual with a mental health disorder by behavioral, cognitive, psychoanalytic, psychodynamic, or psychophysiological means to improve functioning or well-being

- *Electroconvulsive Therapy:* The application of controlled electrical voltages to treat a mental health disorder

- *Biofeedback:* Provision of information from the monitoring and regulating of physiological processes in conjunction with cognitive-behavioral techniques to improve patient functioning or well-being

- *Hypnosis:* Induction of a state of heightened suggestibility by auditory, visual, and tactile techniques to elicit an emotional or behavioral response

- *Narcosynthesis:* Administration of intravenous barbiturates in order to release suppressed or repressed thoughts

- *Group Psychotherapy:* Treatment of two or more individuals with a mental health disorder by behavioral, cognitive, psychoanalytic, psychodynamic, or psychophysiological means to improve functioning or well-being

- *Light Therapy:* Application of specialized light treatments to improve functioning or well-being

Qualifier (Character 4)
The fourth character is a qualifier to indicate that counseling was educational or vocational or to indicate type of test or method of therapy.

Qualifier (Character 5, 6 and 7)
The fifth, sixth, and seventh characters are not specified and always have the value *None*.

Substance Abuse Treatment Section (H)

Character Meanings
The seven characters in the Substance Abuse Treatment section have the following meaning:

Character	Meaning
1	Section
2	Body System
3	Type
4	Qualifier
5	Qualifier
6	Qualifier
7	Qualifier

Section (Character 1)
Substance Abuse Treatment codes have a first character value of *H*.

Body System (Character 2)
The second character is used to identify the body system elsewhere in ICD-10-PCS. In this section, it always has the value *None*.

Type (Character 3)
The third character specifies the type of procedure. There are seven values classified in this section, as listed below:

- *Detoxification Services:* Detoxification from alcohol and/or drugs

- *Individual Counseling:* The application of psychological methods to treat an individual with addictive behavior

- *Group Counseling:* The application of psychological methods to treat two or more individuals with addictive behavior

- *Individual Psychotherapy:* Treatment of an individual with addictive behavior by behavioral, cognitive, psychoanalytic, psychodynamic, or psychophysiological means

- *Family Counseling:* The application of psychological methods that includes one or more family members to treat an individual with addictive behavior

- *Medication Management:* Monitoring and adjusting the use of replacement medications for the treatment of addiction

- *Pharmacotherapy:* The use of replacement medications for the treatment of addiction

Qualifier (Character 4)
The fourth character further specifies the procedure type. These qualifier values vary dependent upon the Root Type procedure (Character 3). Root type 2, *Detoxification Services* contains only the value Z, *None* and Root type 6, *Family Counseling* contains only the value 3, *Other Family Counseling*, whereas the remainder Root Type procedures include multiple possible values.

Qualifier (Character 5, 6 and 7)
The fifth through seventh characters are designated as qualifiers but are never specified, so they always have the value *None*.

New Technology Section (X)

General Information
Section X New Technology is a section added to ICD-10-PCS beginning October 1, 2015. The new section provides a place for codes that uniquely identify procedures requested via the New Technology Application Process or that capture other new technologies not currently classified in ICD-10-PCS.

Section X does not introduce any new coding concepts or unusual guidelines for correct coding. In fact, Section X codes maintain continuity with the other sections in ICD-10-PCS by using the same root operation and body part values as their closest counterparts in other sections of ICD-10-PCS. For example, the codes for the infusion of ceftazidime-avibactam, use the same root operation (Introduction) and body part values (Central Vein and Peripheral Vein) in section X as the infusion codes in section 3 Administration, which are their closest counterparts in the other sections of ICD-10-PCS.

Character Meanings
The seven characters in the new technology section have the following meaning:

Character	Meaning
1	Section
2	Body System
3	Root Operation
4	Body Part
5	Approach
6	Device/Substance/Technology
7	Qualifier

Section (Character 1)
New technology procedure codes have a first character value of *X*.

Body System (Character 2)
The second character values for body system combine the uses of body system, body region, and physiological system as specified in other sections in ICD-10-PCS.

Root Operation (Character 3)

The third character utilizes the same root operation values as their counterparts in other sections of ICD-10-PCS.

Body Part (Character 4)

The fourth character specifies the same body part values as their closest counterparts in other sections of ICD-10-PCS.

Approach (Character 5)

The fifth character specifies approaches as defined in the Medical and Surgical section.

Device/Substance/Technology (Character 6)

The sixth character specifies the key feature of the new technology procedure. It may be specified as a new device, a new substance, or other new technology. Examples of sixth character values are *blinatumomab antineoplastic immunotherapy, orbital atherectomy technology,* and *intraoperative knee replacement sensor.*

Qualifier (Character 7)

The seventh character qualifier is used exclusively to specify the new technology group, a number or letter that changes each year that new technology codes are added to the system. For example, Section X codes added for the first year have the seventh character value 1, *New Technology Group 1*, and the next year that Section X codes are added have the seventh character value 2, *New Technology Group 2*, and so on. Changing the seventh character value to a unique letter or number every year that there are new codes in the new technology section allows the ICD-10-PCS to "recycle" the values in the third, fourth, and sixth characters as needed.

New Technology Coding Instruction

Section X codes are standalone codes. They are not supplemental codes. Section X codes fully represent the specific procedure described in the code title, and do not require any additional codes from other sections of ICD-10-PCS. When section X contains a code title which describes a specific new technology procedure, only that X code is reported for the procedure. There is no need to report a broader, non-specific code in another section of ICD-10-PCS.

For example, code XW04321 Introduction of Ceftazidime-Avibactam Anti-infective into Central Vein, Percutaneous Approach, New Technology Group 1, would be reported to indicate that Ceftazidime-Avibactam Anti-infective was administered via central vein. A separate code from table 3E0 in the Administration section of ICD-10-PCS would not be reported in addition to this code. The X section code fully identifies the administration of the ceftazidime-avibactam antibiotic, and no additional code is needed.

The New Technology section codes are easily found by looking in the ICD-10-PCS Index or the Tables. In the Index, the name of the new technology device, substance or technology for a section X code is included as a main term. In addition, all codes in section X are listed under the main term New Technology. The new technology code index entry for ceftazidime-avibactam is shown below.

Ceftazidime-Avibactam Anti-infective XW0

New Technology
    Ceftazidime-Avibactam Anti-infective XW0

Sources

All material contained in this manual is derived from the ICD-10-PCS Coding System files, revised and distributed by the Centers for Medicare and Medicaid Services, FY 2020.

ICD-10-PCS Index and Tabular Format

The *ICD-10-PCS: The Complete Official Code Set* is based on the official version of the International Classification of Diseases, 10th Revision, Procedure Classification System, issued by the U.S. Department of Health and Human Services, Centers for Medicare and Medicaid Services. This book is consistent with the content of the government's version of ICD-10-PCS and follows their official format.

Index

The Alphabetic Index can be used to locate the appropriate table containing all the information necessary to construct a procedure code, however, the PCS tables should always be consulted to find the most appropriate valid code. Users may choose a valid code directly from the tables—he or she need not consult the index before proceeding to the tables to complete the code.

Main Terms

The Alphabetic Index reflects the structure of the tables. Therefore, the index is organized as an alphabetic listing. The index:

- Is based on the value of the third character
- Contains common procedure terms
- Lists anatomic sites
- Uses device terms

The main terms in the Alphabetic Index are root operations, root procedure types, or common procedure names. In addition, anatomic sites from the Body Part Key and device terms from the Device Key have been added for ease of use.

Examples:

> *Resection* (root operation)
>
> *Fluoroscopy* (root type)
>
> *Prostatectomy* (common procedure name)
>
> *Brachial artery* (body part)
>
> *Bard® Dulex™ mesh* (device)

The index provides at least the first three or four values of the code, and some entries may provide complete valid codes. However, the user should always consult the appropriate table to verify that the most appropriate valid code has been selected.

Root Operation and Procedure Type Main Terms

For the *Medical and Surgical* and related sections, the root operation values are used as main terms in the index. The subterms under the root operation main terms are body parts. For the Ancillary section of the tables, the main terms in the index are the general type of procedure performed.

Examples:

> **Biofeedback** GZC9ZZZ
> **Destruction**
>   Acetabulum
>   Left ØQ55
>   Right ØQ54
>   Adenoids ØC5Q
>   Ampulla of Vater ØF5C
> **Planar Nuclear Medicine Imaging**
>   Abdomen CW1Ø

See Reference

The second type of term in the index uses common procedure names, such as "appendectomy" or "fundoplication." These common terms are listed as main terms with a "see" reference noting the PCS root operations that are possible valid code tables based on the objective of the procedure.

Examples:

> **Tendonectomy**
>   *see* Excision, Tendons ØLB
>   *see* Resection, Tendons ØLT

Use Reference

The index also lists anatomic sites from the Body Part Key and device terms from the Device Key. These terms are listed with a "use" reference. The purpose of these references is to act as an additional reference to the terms located in the Appendix Keys. The term provided is the Body Part value or Device value to be selected when constructing a procedure code using the code tables. This type of index reference is not intended to direct the user to another term in the index, but to provide guidance regarding character value selection. Therefore, "use" references generally do not refer to specific valid code tables.

Examples:

> **CoAxia NeuroFlo catheter**
>   *use* Intraluminal Device
> **Epitrochlear lymph node**
>   *use* Lymphatic, Right Upper Extremity
>   *use* Lymphatic, Left Upper Extremity
> **SynCardia Total Artificial Heart**
>   *use* Synthetic Substitute

Code Tables

ICD-10-PCS contains 17 sections of Code Tables organized by general type of procedure. The first three characters of a procedure code define each table. The tables consist of columns providing the possible last four characters of codes and rows providing valid values for each character. Within a PCS table, valid codes include all combinations of choices in characters 4 through 7 contained in the same row of the table. All seven characters must be specified to form a valid code.

There are three main sections of tables:

- Medical and Surgical section:
  - *Medical and Surgical* (Ø)
- Medical and Surgical-related sections:
  - *Obstetrics* (1)
  - *Placement* (2)
  - *Administration* (3)
  - *Measurement and Monitoring* (4)
  - *Extracorporeal or Systemic Assistance and Performance* (5)
  - *Extracorporeal or Systemic Therapies* (6)
  - *Osteopathic* (7)
  - *Other Procedures* (8)
  - *Chiropractic* (9)

- Ancillary sections:

    — *Imaging* (B)

    — *Nuclear Medicine* (C)

    — *Radiation Therapy* (D)

    — *Physical Rehabilitation and Diagnostic Audiology* (F)

    — *Mental Health* (G)

    — *Substance Abuse Treatment* (H)

- New Technology section:

    — *New Technology* (X)

The first three character values define each table. The root operation or root type designated for each table is accompanied by its official definition.

Example:

Table ØØF provides codes for procedures on the central nervous system that involve breaking up of solid matter into pieces:

Character 1, Section	Ø: Medical and Surgical
Character 2, Body System	Ø: Central Nervous System and Cranial Nerves
Character 3, Root Operation	F: Fragmentation: Breaking solid matter in a body part into pieces

Tables are arranged numerically, then alphabetically.

When reviewing tables, the user should keep in mind that:

- Some tables may cover multiple pages in the code book—to ensure maximum clarity about character choices, valid entries do not split rows between pages. For instance, the entire table of valid characters completing a code beginning with 4A1 is split between two pages, but the split is between, not within, rows. This means that all the valid sixth and seventh characters for, say, body system *Arterial* (3) and approach *External* (X) are contained on one page.

- Individual entries may be listed in several horizontal "selection" lines.

- When a table is continued onto another page, a note to this effect has been added in red.

Body Part Definitions:

An exclusive Optum360 feature in the tables is the incorporation of the body part definitions provided in appendix E into the Medical and Surgical section (Ø) tables under their appropriate body part characters in the fourth column (character 4). This provides the user a direct reference to all anatomical descriptions, terms, and sites that could be coded to that particular body part value.

Paired body parts typically have values for the right and left side and in some cases a value for bilateral. These paired body parts often have the same list of inclusive body part definitions. When there are paired body parts with the same body part definitions, the first listed body part (usually the right side) contains the list of body part definitions while the second listed body part (usually the left side) contains a *See* instruction. This *See* instruction references the body part value that contains the body part definitions. In the table below, body part value P – Upper Eyelid, Left is followed by a *See* instruction that states *See N Upper Eyelid, Right*. All body part descriptions under value N also apply to body part value P.

Example:

Ø **Medical and Surgical**
8 **Eye**
M **Reattachment**   Definition: Putting back in or on all or a portion of a separated body part to its normal location or other suitable location
                    Explanation: Vascular circulation and nervous pathways may or may not be reestablished

Body Part Character 4	Approach Character 5	Device Character 6	Qualifier Character 7

N **Upper Eyelid, Right**
    Lateral canthus
    Levator palpebrae superioris muscle
    Orbicularis oculi muscle
    Superior tarsal plate
P **Upper Eyelid, Left**
    See N Upper Eyelid, Right
Q **Lower Eyelid, Right**
    Inferior tarsal plate
    Medial canthus
R **Lower Eyelid, Left**
    See Q Lower Eyelid, Right
	X External	**Z** No Device	**Z** No Qualifier

ICD-10-PCS Additional Features

Use of Official Sources

The *ICD-10-PCS: The Complete Official Code Set* contains the official U.S. Department of Health and Human Services, Tenth Revision, Procedure Classification System, effective for the current year.

Color-coding, symbol, and other annotations in this manual that identify coding and reimbursement issues are derived from various official federal government sources, including Medicare Code Editor (MCE), version 36, ICD-10 MS-DRG Definitions Manual Files, version 36, and the *Federal Register*, volume 83, number 88, May 7, 2018 ("Hospital Inpatient Prospective Payment Systems for Acute Care Hospitals and the Long Term Care Hospital Prospective Payment System and Proposed Policy Changes and Fiscal Year 2020 Rates; Proposed Rule"). For the most current files related to IPPS, please refer to the following:

https://www.cms.gov/Medicare/Medicare-Fee-for-Service-Payment/AcuteInpatientPPS/IPPS-Regulations-and-Notices.html.

Table Notations

Many tables in ICD-10-PCS contain color or symbol annotations that may aid in code selection, provide clinical or coding information, or alert the coder to reimbursement issues affected by the PCS code assignment. These annotations are most often displayed on or next to a character 4 value. Some character 4 values may have more than one annotation.

Refer to the color/symbol legend at the bottom of each page in the tables section for an abridged description of each color and symbol.

Annotation Box

An annotation box has been appended to all tables that contain color-coding or symbol annotations. The color bar or symbol attached to a character 4 value is provided in the box, as well as a list of the valid PCS code(s) to which that edit applies. The box may also list conditional criteria that must be met to satisfy the edit.

For example, see Table 00F. Four character 4 body part values have a gray color bar. In the annotation box below the table, the gray color bar is defined as "Non-OR," or a nonoperating room procedure edit. Following the Non-OR annotation are the PCS codes that are considered nonoperating room procedures from that row of Table 00F.

Bracketed Code Notation

The use of bracketed codes is an efficient convention to provide all valid character value alternatives for a specific set of circumstances. The character values in the brackets correspond to the valid values for the character in the position the bracket appears.

Examples:

In the annotation box for Table 00F the Noncovered Procedure edit (NC) applies to codes represented in the bracketed code 00F[3,4,5,6]XZZ.

> 00F[3,4,5,6]XZZ   Fragmentation in (Central Nervous System and Cranial Nerves), External Approach

The valid fourth character values (Body Part) that may be selected for this specific circumstance are as follows:

3	Epidural Space, Intracranial
4	Subdural Space, Intracranial
5	Subarachnoid Space, Intracranial
6	Cerebral Ventricle

The fragmentation of matter in the spinal canal, Body Part value U, is not included in the noncovered procedure code edits.

Color-Coding/Symbols

New and Revised Text

To highlight changes to the PCS tables for the current year, the new and revised text is provided in green font.

Medicare Code Edits

Medicare administrative contractors (MACs) and many payers use Medicare code edits to check the coding accuracy on claims. The coding edits in this manual are only those directly related to ICD-10-PCS codes and are used for acute care hospital inpatient admissions.

The PCS related Medicare code edits are listed below:

- Invalid procedure code
- *Sex conflict
- *Questionable obstetric admission
- *Noncovered procedure
- *Limited coverage procedure

Starred edits above that are related to PCS issues are identified in this manual by symbols as described below.

Sex Edit Symbols

The sex edit symbols below are used to detect inconsistencies between the patient's sex and the procedure. The symbols below most often appear to the right of the body part (character 4) value but may also be found to the right of the qualifier (character 7) value:

♂ Male procedure only

♀ Female procedure only

QA **Questionable Obstetric Admission**

An inpatient admission is considered questionable when a vaginal or cesarean delivery code is assigned without a corresponding secondary diagnosis code describing the outcome of delivery. Both a delivery (ICD-10-PCS) code and an outcome-of-delivery (ICD-10-CM) code must be present to avoid errors in MS-DRG assignment. This symbol is found only in the Obstetrics Section, appearing to the right of the body part (character 4) value.

NC **Noncovered Procedure**

Medicare does not cover all procedures. However, some noncovered procedures, due to the presence of certain diagnoses, are reimbursed.

LC **Limited Coverage**

For certain procedures whose medical complexity and serious nature incur extraordinary associated costs, Medicare limits coverage to a portion of the cost. The limited coverage edit indicates the type of limited coverage.

ICD-10 MS-DRG Definitions Manual Edits

An MS-DRG is assigned based on specific patient attributes, such as principal diagnosis, secondary diagnoses, procedures, and discharge status. The attributes (edits) provided in this manual are only those directly related to ICD-10-PCS codes and are used for acute care hospital inpatient admissions.

Non-Operating Room Procedures Not Affecting MS-DRG Assignment

In the Medical and Surgical section (ØØ1-ØYW) and the Obstetric section (1Ø2-1ØY) tables **only,** ICD-10-PCS procedures codes that DO NOT affect MS-DRG assignment are identified by a **gray color bar** over the body part (character 4) value and are considered non-operating room (non-OR) procedures.

NOTE: The majority of the ICD-10-PCS codes in the Medical and Surgical-Related, Ancillary and New Technology section tables are non-operating room procedures that do not typically affect MS-DRG assignment. Only the Valid Operating Room and DRG Non-Operating Room procedures are highlighted in these sections, *see* Non-Operating Room Procedures Affecting MS-DRG Assignment and Valid OR Procedure description below.

Non-Operating Room Procedures Affecting MS-DRG Assignment

Some ICD-10-PCS procedure codes, although considered non-operating room procedures, may still affect MS-DRG assignment. In all sections of the ICD-10-PCS book, these procedures are identified by a **purple color bar** over the body part (character 4) value.

Valid OR Procedure

In the Medical and Surgical-Related (2WØ-9WB), Ancillary (BØØ-HZ9) and New Technology (X2A-XYØ) section tables **only**, any codes that are considered a valid operating room procedure are identified with a **blue color bar** over the body part (character 4) value and will affect MS-DRG assignment. All codes without a color bar (blue or purple) are considered non-operating room procedures.

Hospital-Acquired Condition Related Procedures

Procedures associated with hospital-acquired conditions (HAC) are identified with the **yellow color bar** over the body part (character 4) value.

Combination Only

Some ICD-10-PCS procedure codes that describe non-operating room procedures can group to a specific MS-DRG but only when used in combination with certain other ICD-10-PCS procedure codes. Such codes are designated by a **red color bar** over the body part (character 4) value.

⊞ **Combination Member**

A combination member, which can be either a valid operating room procedure or a non-operating room procedure, is an ICD-10-PCS procedure code that can influence MS-DRG assignment either on its own or in combination with other specific ICD-10-PCS procedure codes. Combination member codes are designated by a plus sign (⊞) to the right of the body part (character 4) value.

Note: In the few instances when a code is both a combination member and a non-operating room procedure affecting the MS-DRG assignment, the body part (character 4) value will have a purple color bar and the combination member icon.

See Appendix L for Procedure Combinations

Under certain circumstances, more than one procedure code is needed in order to group to a specific MS-DRG. When codes within a table have been identified as a Combination Only (**red color bar**) or Combination Member (⊞) code, there is also a footnote instructing the coder to *see Appendix L*. Appendix L contains tables that identify the other procedure codes needed in the combination and the title and number of the MS-DRG to which the combination will group.

Other Table Notations

AHA Coding Clinic:

Official citations from AHA's *Coding Clinic for ICD-10-CM/PCS* have been provided at the beginning of each section, when applicable. Each specific citation is listed below a header identifying the table to which that particular *Coding Clinic* citation applies. The citations appear in purple type with the year, quarter, and page of the reference as well as the title of the question as it appears in that *Coding Clinic's* table of contents. *Coding Clinic* citations included in this edition have been updated through first quarter 2019.

Appendixes

The resources described below have been included as appendixes for *ICD-10-PCS The Complete Official Code Set*. These resources further instruct the coder on the appropriate application of the ICD-10-PCS code set.

Appendix A: Components of the Medical and Surgical Approach Definitions

This resource further defines the approach characters used in the Medical and Surgical (Ø) section. Complementing the detailed definition of the approach, additional information includes whether or not instrumentation is a part of the approach, the typical access location, the method used to initiate the approach, related procedural examples, and illustrations all of which will help the user determine the appropriate approach value.

Appendix B: Root Operation Definitions

This resource is a compilation of all root operations found in the Medical and Surgical-related sections (Ø-9) of this PCS manual. It provides a definition and in some cases a more detailed explanation of the root operation, to better reflect the purpose or objective. Examples of related procedure(s) may also be provided.

Appendix C: Comparison of Medical and Surgical Root Operations

The Medical and Surgical root operations are divided into groups that share similar attributes. These groups, and the root operations in each group, are listed in this resource along with information identifying the target of the root operation, the action used to perform the root operation, any clarification or further explanation on the objective of the root operation, and procedure examples.

Appendix D: Body Part Key

When an anatomical term or description is provided in the documentation but does not have a specific body part character within a table, the user can reference this resource to search for the anatomical description or site noted in the documentation to determine if there is a specific PCS body part character (character 4) to which the anatomical description or site could be coded.

Appendix E: Body Part Definitions

This resource is the reverse look-up of the Body Part Key. Each table in the Medical and Surgical section (Ø) of the PCS manual contains anatomical terms linked to a body part character or value, for example, in Table ØBB the Body Part (character 4) of 1 is Trachea. The body part Trachea may have anatomical structures or descriptions that may be used in procedure documentation instead of the term trachea. The Body Part Definitions list other anatomical structures or synonyms that are included in specific ICD-10-PCS body part values. According to the body part definitions, in the example above, cricoid cartilage is included in the Trachea (character 1) body part.

Appendix F: Device Key and Aggregation Table

The Device Key helps users code the appropriate PCS sixth character for device. Devices are listed alphabetically by brand name or commonly used medical terminology and are translated to the appropriate PCS language or value. The key also reflects the body system where the device is located. For example, a SAPIEN valve used for transaortic valve replacement translates to Zooplastic Tissue in Heart and Great Vessels.

The Aggregation Table crosswalks specific device character value definitions for specific root operations in a specific body system to the more general device character value to be used when the root operation covers a wide range of body parts and the device character represents an entire family of devices.

Appendix G: Device Definitions

This resource is a reverse look-up to the Device Key. The user may reference this resource to see all the specific devices that may be grouped to a particular device character (character 6).

Example:
The operative report states, "An internal fixation device was used to repair a fractured femur. Kirschner wire, bone screws and neutralization plate all used and left in the bone at the end of the procedure. "

Although PCS requires all devices left in the body to be coded and the operative report lists three different devices, a check in the device definitions shows that all of these devices are included in the PCS value "Internal Fixation Device" and require only one code.

Appendix H: Substance Key/Substance Definitions

The Substance Key lists substances by trade name or synonym and relates them to a PCS character in the Administration (3) or New Technology (X) section in the sixth character Substance or seventh character Qualifier column.

The Substance Definitions table is the reverse look-up of the substance key, relating all substance categories, the sixth- or seventh character values, to all trade name or synonyms that may be classified to that particular character.

Appendix I: Sections B-H Character Definitions

In each ancillary section (B-H) the characters in a particular column may have different meanings depending on which section the user is working from. This resource provides the values for the characters in these sections as well as a definition of the character value.

Appendix J: Hospital Acquired Conditions

This comprehensive table displays codes identifying conditions that are considered reasonably preventable when occurring during the hospital admission and may prevent the case from grouping to a higher-paying MS-DRG. Many of these HACs are conditional and are based on reporting of a specific ICD-10-CM diagnosis code in combination with certain ICD-10-PCS procedure codes, all of which are noted in this table.

Appendix K: Coding Exercises and Answers

This resource provides the coding exercises with answers, and in some cases a brief explanation as to the reason that particular code was used.

Appendix L: Procedure Combination Tables

The procedure combination tables provided in this resource illustrate certain procedure combinations that must occur in order to assign a specific MS-DRG.

ICD-10-PCS Official Guidelines for Coding and Reporting 2020

Narrative changes appear in **bold** text.

The Centers for Medicare and Medicaid Services (CMS) and the National Center for Health Statistics (NCHS), two departments within the U.S. Federal Government's Department of Health and Human Services (DHHS) provide the following guidelines for coding and reporting using the International Classification of Diseases, 10th Revision, Procedure Coding System (ICD-10-PCS). These guidelines should be used as a companion document to the official version of the ICD-10-PCS as published on the CMS website. The ICD-10-PCS is a procedure classification published by the United States for classifying procedures performed in hospital inpatient health care settings.

These guidelines have been approved by the four organizations that make up the Cooperating Parties for the ICD-10-PCS: the American Hospital Association (AHA), the American Health Information Management Association (AHIMA), CMS, and NCHS.

These guidelines are a set of rules that have been developed to accompany and complement the official conventions and instructions provided within the ICD-10-PCS itself. **They are intended to provide direction that is applicable in most circumstances. However, there may be unique circumstances where exceptions are applied.** The instructions and conventions of the classification take precedence over guidelines. These guidelines are based on the coding and sequencing instructions in the Tables, Index and Definitions of ICD-10-PCS, but provide additional instruction. Adherence to these guidelines when assigning ICD-10-PCS procedure codes is required under the Health Insurance Portability and Accountability Act (HIPAA). The procedure codes have been adopted under HIPAA for hospital inpatient healthcare settings. A joint effort between the healthcare provider and the coder is essential to achieve complete and accurate documentation, code assignment, and reporting of diagnoses and procedures. These guidelines have been developed to assist both the healthcare provider and the coder in identifying those procedures that are to be reported. The importance of consistent, complete documentation in the medical record cannot be overemphasized. Without such documentation accurate coding cannot be achieved.

Conventions

A1. ICD-10-PCS codes are composed of seven characters. Each character is an axis of classification that specifies information about the procedure performed. Within a defined code range, a character specifies the same type of information in that axis of classification.

Example:
The fifth axis of classification specifies the approach in sections Ø through 4 and 7 through 9 of the system.

A2. One of 34 possible values can be assigned to each axis of classification in the seven-character code: they are the numbers Ø through 9 and the alphabet (except I and O because they are easily confused with the numbers 1 and Ø). The number of unique values used in an axis of classification differs as needed.

Example:
Where the fifth axis of classification specifies the approach, seven different approach values are currently used to specify the approach.

A3. The valid values for an axis of classification can be added to as needed.

Example:
If a significantly distinct type of device is used in a new procedure, a new device value can be added to the system.

A4. As with words in their context, the meaning of any single value is a combination of its axis of classification and any preceding values on which it may be dependent.

Example:
The meaning of a body part value in the Medical and Surgical section is always dependent on the body system value. The body part value Ø in the Central Nervous body system specifies Brain and the body part value Ø in the Peripheral Nervous body system specifies Cervical Plexus.

A5. As the system is expanded to become increasingly detailed, over time more values will depend on preceding values for their meaning.

Example:
In the Lower Joints body system, the device value 3 in the root operation Insertion specifies Infusion Device and the device value 3 in the root operation Replacement specifies Ceramic Synthetic Substitute.

A6. The purpose of the alphabetic index is to locate the appropriate table that contains all information necessary to construct a procedure code. The PCS Tables should always be consulted to find the most appropriate valid code.

A7. It is not required to consult the index first before proceeding to the tables to complete the code. A valid code may be chosen directly from the tables.

A8. All seven characters must be specified to be a valid code. If the documentation is incomplete for coding purposes, the physician should be queried for the necessary information.

A9. Within a PCS table, valid codes include all combinations of choices in characters 4 through 7 contained in the same row of the table. In the example below, ØJHT3VZ is a valid code, and ØJHW3VZ is *not* a valid code.

Section:	Ø	**Medical and Surgical**
Body System:	J	**Subcutaneous Tissue and Fascia**
Operation:	H	**Insertion** Putting in a nonbiological appliance that monitors, assists, performs, or prevents a physiological function but does not physically take the place of a body part

Body Part		Approach		Device		Qualifier	
S Subcutaneous Tissue and Fascia, Head and Neck **V** Subcutaneous Tissue and Fascia, Upper Extremity **W** Subcutaneous Tissue and Fascia, Lower Extremity	**Ø** Open **3** Percutaneous		**1** Radioactive Element **3** Infusion Device **Y** **Other Device**		**Z** No Qualifier	
T Subcutaneous Tissue and Fascia, Trunk	**Ø** Open **3** Percutaneous		**1** Radioactive Element **3** Infusion Device **V** Infusion Pump **Y** **Other Device**		**Z** No Qualifier	

A10. "And," when used in a code description, means "and/or," except when used to describe a combination of multiple body parts for which separate values exist for each body part (e.g., Skin and Subcutaneous Tissue used as a qualifier, where there are separate body part values for "Skin" and "Subcutaneous Tissue").

Example:
Lower Arm and Wrist Muscle means lower arm and/or wrist muscle.

A11. Many of the terms used to construct PCS codes are defined within the system. It is the coder's responsibility to determine what the documentation in the medical record equates to in the PCS definitions. The physician is not expected to use the terms used in PCS code descriptions, nor is the coder required to query the physician when the correlation between the documentation and the defined PCS terms is clear.

Example:
When the physician documents "partial resection" the coder can independently correlate "partial resection" to the root operation Excision without querying the physician for clarification.

Medical and Surgical Section Guidelines (section Ø)

B2. Body System

General guidelines

B2.1a. The procedure codes in **Anatomical Regions, General, Anatomical Regions, Upper Extremities and Anatomical Regions, Lower Extremities** can be used when the procedure is performed on an anatomical region rather than a specific body part, or on the rare occasion when no information is available to support assignment of a code to a specific body part.

Examples:
Chest tube drainage of the pleural cavity is coded to the root operation Drainage found in the **body system Anatomical Regions, General.**

Suture repair of the abdominal wall is coded to the root operation Repair in the **body system Anatomical Regions, General**.

Amputation of the foot is coded to the root operation Detachment in the body system Anatomical Regions, Lower Extremities.

B2.1b. Where the general body part values "upper" and "lower" are provided as an option in the Upper Arteries, Lower Arteries, Upper Veins, Lower Veins, Muscles and Tendons body systems, "upper" or "lower" specifies body parts located above or below the diaphragm respectively.

Example:
Vein body parts above the diaphragm are found in the Upper Veins body system; vein body parts below the diaphragm are found in the Lower Veins body system.

B3. Root Operation

General guidelines

B3.1a. In order to determine the appropriate root operation, the full definition of the root operation as contained in the PCS Tables must be applied.

B3.1b. Components of a procedure specified in the root operation definition **or** explanation **as integral to that root operation** are not coded separately. Procedural steps necessary to reach the operative site and close the operative site, including anastomosis of a tubular body part, are also not coded separately.

Examples:
Resection of a joint as part of a joint replacement procedure is included in the root operation definition of Replacement and is not coded separately.

Laparotomy performed to reach the site of an open liver biopsy is not coded separately.

In a resection of sigmoid colon with anastomosis of descending colon to rectum, the anastomosis is not coded separately.

Exceptions:
Mastectomy followed by breast reconstruction, both resection and replacement of the breast are coded separately.

Multiple procedures

B3.2. During the same operative episode, multiple procedures are coded if:

a. The same root operation is performed on different body parts as defined by distinct values of the body part character.

   Examples:
   Diagnostic excision of liver and pancreas are coded separately.

   Excision of lesion in the ascending colon and excision of lesion in the transverse colon are coded separately.

b. The same root operation is repeated in multiple body parts, and those body parts are separate and distinct body parts classified to a single ICD-10-PCS body part value.

   Examples:
   Excision of the sartorius muscle and excision of the gracilis muscle are both included in the upper leg muscle body part value, and multiple procedures are coded.

   Extraction of multiple toenails are coded separately.

c. Multiple root operations with distinct objectives are performed on the same body part.

   Example:
   Destruction of sigmoid lesion and bypass of sigmoid colon are coded separately.

d. The intended root operation is attempted using one approach but is converted to a different approach.

   Example:
   Laparoscopic cholecystectomy converted to an open cholecystectomy is coded as percutaneous endoscopic Inspection and open Resection.

Discontinued or incomplete procedures

B3.3. If the intended procedure is discontinued or otherwise not completed, code the procedure to the root operation performed. If a procedure is discontinued before any other root operation is performed, code the root operation Inspection of the body part or anatomical region inspected.

Example:
A planned aortic valve replacement procedure is discontinued after the initial thoracotomy and before any incision is made in the heart muscle, when the patient becomes hemodynamically unstable. This procedure is coded as an open Inspection of the mediastinum.

Biopsy procedures

B3.4a. Biopsy procedures are coded using the root operations Excision, Extraction, or Drainage and the qualifier Diagnostic.

Examples:

Fine needle aspiration biopsy of fluid in the lung is coded to the root operation Drainage with the qualifier Diagnostic.

Biopsy of bone marrow is coded to the root operation Extraction with the qualifier Diagnostic.

Lymph node sampling for biopsy is coded to the root operation Excision with the qualifier Diagnostic.

Biopsy followed by more definitive treatment

B3.4b. If a diagnostic Excision, Extraction, or Drainage procedure (biopsy) is followed by a more definitive procedure, such as Destruction, Excision or Resection at the same procedure site, both the biopsy and the more definitive treatment are coded.

Example:

Biopsy of breast followed by partial mastectomy at the same procedure site, both the biopsy and the partial mastectomy procedure are coded.

Overlapping body layers

B3.5. If root operations **such as** Excision, **Extraction,** Repair or Inspection are performed on overlapping layers of the musculoskeletal system, the body part specifying the deepest layer is coded.

Example:

Excisional debridement that includes skin and subcutaneous tissue and muscle is coded to the muscle body part.

Bypass procedures

B3.6a. Bypass procedures are coded by identifying the body part bypassed "from" and the body part bypassed "to." The fourth character body part specifies the body part bypassed from, and the qualifier specifies the body part bypassed to.

Example:

Bypass from stomach to jejunum, stomach is the body part and jejunum is the qualifier.

B3.6b. Coronary artery bypass procedures are coded differently than other bypass procedures as described in the previous guideline. Rather than identifying the body part bypassed from, the body part identifies the number of coronary arteries bypassed to, and the qualifier specifies the vessel bypassed from.

Example:

Aortocoronary artery bypass of the left anterior descending coronary artery and the obtuse marginal coronary artery is classified in the body part axis of classification as two coronary arteries, and the qualifier specifies the aorta as the body part bypassed from.

B3.6c. If multiple coronary arteries are bypassed, a separate procedure is coded for each coronary artery that uses a different device and/or qualifier.

Example:

Aortocoronary artery bypass and internal mammary coronary artery bypass are coded separately.

Control vs. more definitive root operations

B3.7. The root operation Control is defined as, "Stopping, or attempting to stop, postprocedural or other acute bleeding." If an attempt to stop postprocedural or other acute bleeding is unsuccessful, and to stop the bleeding requires performing a more definitive root operation, such as Bypass, Detachment, Excision, Extraction, Reposition, Replacement, or

Resection, then the more definitive root operation is coded instead of Control.

Example:

Resection of spleen to stop bleeding is coded to Resection instead of Control.

Excision vs. Resection

B3.8. PCS contains specific body parts for anatomical subdivisions of a body part, such as lobes of the lungs or liver and regions of the intestine. Resection of the specific body part is coded whenever all of the body part is cut out or off, rather than coding Excision of a less specific body part.

Example:

Left upper lung lobectomy is coded to Resection of Upper Lung Lobe, Left rather than Excision of Lung, Left.

Excision for graft

B3.9. If an autograft is obtained from a different procedure site in order to complete the objective of the procedure, a separate procedure is coded, **except when the seventh character qualifier value in the ICD-10-PCS table fully specifies the site from which the autograf**t **was obtained**.

*Example**s:***

Coronary bypass with excision of saphenous vein graft, excision of saphenous vein is coded separately.

Replacement of breast with autologous deep inferior epigastric artery perforator (DIEP) flap, excision of the DIEP flap is not coded separately. The seventh character qualifier value Deep Inferior Epigastric Artery Perforator Flap in the Replacement table fully specifies the site of the autograft harvest.

Fusion procedures of the spine

B3.10a. The body part coded for a spinal vertebral joint(s) rendered immobile by a spinal fusion procedure is classified by the level of the spine (e.g. thoracic). There are distinct body part values for a single vertebral joint and for multiple vertebral joints at each spinal level.

Example:

Body part values specify Lumbar Vertebral Joint, Lumbar Vertebral Joints, 2 or More and Lumbosacral Vertebral Joint.

B3.10b. If multiple vertebral joints are fused, a separate procedure is coded for each vertebral joint that uses a different device and/or qualifier.

Example:

Fusion of lumbar vertebral joint, posterior approach, anterior column and fusion of lumbar vertebral joint, posterior approach, posterior column are coded separately.

B3.10c. Combinations of devices and materials are often used on a vertebral joint to render the joint immobile. When combinations of devices are used on the same vertebral joint, the device value coded for the procedure is as follows:

- If an interbody fusion device is used to render the joint immobile (alone or containing other material like bone graft), the procedure is coded with the device value Interbody Fusion Device

- If bone graft is the *only* device used to render the joint immobile, the procedure is coded with the device value Nonautologous Tissue Substitute or Autologous Tissue Substitute

- If a mixture of autologous and nonautologous bone graft (with or without biological or synthetic extenders or binders) is used to render the joint immobile, code the procedure with the device value Autologous Tissue Substitute

Examples:

Fusion of a vertebral joint using a cage style interbody fusion device containing morsellized bone graft is coded to the device Interbody Fusion Device.

Fusion of a vertebral joint using a bone dowel interbody fusion device made of cadaver bone and packed with a mixture of local morsellized bone and demineralized bone matrix is coded to the device Interbody Fusion Device.

Fusion of a vertebral joint using both autologous bone graft and bone bank bone graft is coded to the device Autologous Tissue Substitute.

Inspection procedures

B3.11a. Inspection of a body part(s) performed in order to achieve the objective of a procedure is not coded separately.

Example:

Fiberoptic bronchoscopy performed for irrigation of bronchus, only the irrigation procedure is coded.

B3.11b. If multiple tubular body parts are inspected, the most distal body part (the body part furthest from the starting point of the inspection) is coded. If multiple non-tubular body parts in a region are inspected, the body part that specifies the entire area inspected is coded.

Examples:

Cystoureteroscopy with inspection of bladder and ureters is coded to the ureter body part value.

Exploratory laparotomy with general inspection of abdominal contents is coded to the peritoneal cavity body part value.

B3.11c. When both an Inspection procedure and another procedure are performed on the same body part during the same episode, if the Inspection procedure is performed using a different approach than the other procedure, the Inspection procedure is coded separately.

Example:

Endoscopic Inspection of the duodenum is coded separately when open Excision of the duodenum is performed during the same procedural episode.

Occlusion vs. Restriction for vessel embolization procedures

B3.12. If the objective of an embolization procedure is to completely close a vessel, the root operation Occlusion is coded. If the objective of an embolization procedure is to narrow the lumen of a vessel, the root operation Restriction is coded.

Examples:

Tumor embolization is coded to the root operation Occlusion, because the objective of the procedure is to cut off the blood supply to the vessel.

Embolization of a cerebral aneurysm is coded to the root operation Restriction, because the objective of the procedure is not to close off the vessel entirely, but to narrow the lumen of the vessel at the site of the aneurysm where it is abnormally wide.

Release procedures

B3.13. In the root operation Release, the body part value coded is the body part being freed and not the tissue being manipulated or cut to free the body part.

Example:

Lysis of intestinal adhesions is coded to the specific intestine body part value.

Release vs. Division

B3.14. If the sole objective of the procedure is freeing a body part without cutting the body part, the root operation is Release. If the sole objective of the procedure is separating or transecting a body part, the root operation is Division.

Examples:

Freeing a nerve root from surrounding scar tissue to relieve pain is coded to the root operation Release.

Severing a nerve root to relieve pain is coded to the root operation Division.

Reposition for fracture treatment

B3.15. Reduction of a displaced fracture is coded to the root operation Reposition and the application of a cast or splint in conjunction with the Reposition procedure is not coded separately. Treatment of a nondisplaced fracture is coded to the procedure performed.

Examples:

Casting of a nondisplaced fracture is coded to the root operation Immobilization in the Placement section.

Putting a pin in a nondisplaced fracture is coded to the root operation Insertion.

Transplantation vs. Administration

B3.16. Putting in a mature and functioning living body part taken from another individual or animal is coded to the root operation Transplantation. Putting in autologous or nonautologous cells is coded to the Administration section.

Example:

Putting in autologous or nonautologous bone marrow, pancreatic islet cells or stem cells is coded to the Administration section.

Transfer procedures using multiple tissue layers

B3.17. The root operation Transfer contains qualifiers that can be used to specify when a transfer flap is composed of more than one tissue layer, such as a musculocutaneous flap. For procedures involving transfer of multiple tissue layers including skin, subcutaneous tissue, fascia or muscle, the procedure is coded to the body part value that describes the deepest tissue layer in the flap, and the qualifier can be used to describe the other tissue layer(s) in the transfer flap.

Example:

A musculocutaneous flap transfer is coded to the appropriate body part value in the body system Muscles, and the qualifier is used to describe the additional tissue layer(s) in the transfer flap.

B4. Body Part

General guidelines

B4.1a. If a procedure is performed on a portion of a body part that does not have a separate body part value, code the body part value corresponding to the whole body part.

Example:

A procedure performed on the alveolar process of the mandible is coded to the mandible body part.

B4.1b. If the prefix "peri" is combined with a body part to identify the site of the procedure, and the site of the procedure is not further specified, then the procedure is coded to the body part named. This guideline applies only when a more specific body part value is not available.

Examples:

A procedure site identified as perirenal is coded to the kidney body part when the site of the procedure is not further specified.

A procedure site described in the documentation as peri-urethral, and the documentation also indicates that it is the vulvar tissue and not the urethral tissue that is the site of the procedure, then the procedure is coded to the vulva body part.

A procedure site documented as involving the periosteum is coded to the corresponding bone body part.

B4.1c. If a procedure is performed on a continuous section of a tubular body part, code the body part value corresponding to the furthest anatomical site from the point of entry.

Example:
A procedure performed on a continuous section of artery from the femoral artery to the external iliac artery with the point of entry at the femoral artery is coded to the external iliac body part.

Branches of body parts

B4.2. Where a specific branch of a body part does not have its own body part value in PCS, the body part is typically coded to the closest proximal branch that has a specific body part value. In the cardiovascular body systems, if a general body part is available in the correct root operation table, and coding to a proximal branch would require assigning a code in a different body system, the procedure is coded using the general body part value.

Examples:
A procedure performed on the mandibular branch of the trigeminal nerve is coded to the trigeminal nerve body part value.

Occlusion of the bronchial artery is coded to the body part value Upper Artery in the body system Upper Arteries, and not to the body part value Thoracic Aorta, Descending in the body system Heart and Great Vessels.

Bilateral body part values

B4.3. Bilateral body part values are available for a limited number of body parts. If the identical procedure is performed on contralateral body parts, and a bilateral body part value exists for that body part, a single procedure is coded using the bilateral body part value. If no bilateral body part value exists, each procedure is coded separately using the appropriate body part value.

Examples:
The identical procedure performed on both fallopian tubes is coded once using the body part value Fallopian Tube, Bilateral.

The identical procedure performed on both knee joints is coded twice using the body part values Knee Joint, Right and Knee Joint, Left.

Coronary arteries

B4.4. The coronary arteries are classified as a single body part that is further specified by number of arteries treated. One procedure code specifying multiple arteries is used when the same procedure is performed, including the same device and qualifier values.

Examples:
Angioplasty of two distinct coronary arteries with placement of two stents is coded as Dilation of Coronary Artery, Two Arteries with Two Intraluminal Devices.

Angioplasty of two distinct coronary arteries, one with stent placed and one without, is coded separately as Dilation of Coronary Artery, One Artery with Intraluminal Device, and Dilation of Coronary Artery, One Artery with no device.

Tendons, ligaments, bursae and fascia near a joint

B4.5. Procedures performed on tendons, ligaments, bursae and fascia supporting a joint are coded to the body part in the respective body system that is the focus of the procedure. Procedures performed on

joint structures themselves are coded to the body part in the joint body systems.

Examples:
Repair of the anterior cruciate ligament of the knee is coded to the knee bursa and ligament body part in the bursae and ligaments body system.

Knee arthroscopy with shaving of articular cartilage is coded to the knee joint body part in the Lower Joints body system.

Skin, subcutaneous tissue and fascia overlying a joint

B4.6. If a procedure is performed on the skin, subcutaneous tissue or fascia overlying a joint, the procedure is coded to the following body part:

- Shoulder is coded to Upper Arm
- Elbow is coded to Lower Arm
- Wrist is coded to Lower Arm
- Hip is coded to Upper Leg
- Knee is coded to Lower Leg
- Ankle is coded to Foot

Fingers and toes

B4.7. If a body system does not contain a separate body part value for fingers, procedures performed on the fingers are coded to the body part value for the hand. If a body system does not contain a separate body part value for toes, procedures performed on the toes are coded to the body part value for the foot.

Example:
Excision of finger muscle is coded to one of the hand muscle body part values in the Muscles body system.

Upper and lower intestinal tract

B4.8. In the Gastrointestinal body system, the general body part values Upper Intestinal Tract and Lower Intestinal Tract are provided as an option for the root operations Change, Inspection, Removal and Revision. Upper Intestinal Tract includes the portion of the gastrointestinal tract from the esophagus down to and including the duodenum, and Lower Intestinal Tract includes the portion of the gastrointestinal tract from the jejunum down to and including the rectum and anus.

Example:
In the root operation Change table, change of a device in the jejunum is coded using the body part Lower Intestinal Tract.

B5. Approach

Open approach with percutaneous endoscopic assistance

B5.2. Procedures performed using the open approach with percutaneous endoscopic assistance are coded to the approach Open.

Example:
Laparoscopic-assisted sigmoidectomy is coded to the approach Open.

External approach

B5.3a. Procedures performed within an orifice on structures that are visible without the aid of any instrumentation are coded to the approach External.

Example:
Resection of tonsils is coded to the approach External.

B5.3b. Procedures performed indirectly by the application of external force through the intervening body layers are coded to the approach External.

> *Example:*
> Closed reduction of fracture is coded to the approach External.

Percutaneous procedure via device

B5.4. Procedures performed percutaneously via a device placed for the procedure are coded to the approach Percutaneous.

> *Example:*
> Fragmentation of kidney stone performed via percutaneous nephrostomy is coded to the approach Percutaneous.

B6. Device

General guidelines

B6.1a. A device is coded only if a device remains after the procedure is completed. If no device remains, the device value No Device is coded. In limited root operations, the classification provides the qualifier values Temporary and Intraoperative, for specific procedures involving clinically significant devices, where the purpose of the device is to be utilized for a brief duration during the procedure or current inpatient stay. If a device that is intended to remain after the procedure is completed requires removal before the end of the operative episode in which it was inserted (for example, the device size is inadequate or a complication occurs), both the insertion and removal of the device should be coded.

B6.1b. Materials such as sutures, ligatures, radiological markers and temporary post-operative wound drains are considered integral to the performance of a procedure and are not coded as devices.

B6.1c. Procedures performed on a device only and not on a body part are specified in the root operations Change, Irrigation, Removal and Revision, and are coded to the procedure performed.

> *Example:*
> Irrigation of percutaneous nephrostomy tube is coded to the root operation Irrigation of indwelling device in the Administration section.

Drainage device

B6.2. A separate procedure to put in a drainage device is coded to the root operation Drainage with the device value Drainage Device.

Obstetric Section Guidelines (section 1)

C. Obstetrics Section

Products of conception

C1. Procedures performed on the products of conception are coded to the Obstetrics section. Procedures performed on the pregnant female other than the products of conception are coded to the appropriate root operation in the Medical and Surgical section.

> *Examples:*
> Amniocentesis is coded to the products of conception body part in the Obstetrics section.
>
> Repair of obstetric urethral laceration is coded to the urethra body part in the Medical and Surgical section.

Procedures following delivery or abortion

C2. Procedures performed following a delivery or abortion for curettage of the endometrium or evacuation of retained products of conception are all coded in the Obstetrics section, to the root operation Extraction and the body part Products of Conception, Retained.

Diagnostic or therapeutic dilation and curettage performed during times other than the postpartum or post-abortion period are all coded in the Medical and Surgical section, to the root operation Extraction and the body part Endometrium.

Radiation Therapy Section Guidelines (section D)

D. Radiation Therapy Section

Brachytherapy

D1.a. Brachytherapy is coded to the modality Brachytherapy in the Radiation Therapy section. When a radioactive brachytherapy source is left in the body at the end of the procedure, it is coded separately to the root operation Insertion with the device value Radioactive Element.

> *Example:*
> Brachytherapy with implantation of a low dose rate brachytherapy source left in the body at the end of the procedure is coded to the applicable treatment site in section D, Radiation Therapy, with the modality Brachytherapy, the modality qualifier value Low Dose Rate, and the applicable isotope value and qualifier value. The implantation of the brachytherapy source is coded separately to the device value Radioactive Element in the appropriate Insertion table of the Medical and Surgical section. The Radiation Therapy section code identifies the specific modality and isotope of the brachytherapy, and the root operation Insertion code identifies the implantation of the brachytherapy source that remains in the body at the end of the procedure.

> *Exception:*
> Implantation of Cesium-131 brachytherapy seeds embedded in a collagen matrix to the treatment site after resection of brain tumor is coded to the root operation Insertion with the device value Radioactive Element, Cesium-131 Collagen Implant. The procedure is coded to the root operation Insertion only, because the device value identifies both the implantation of the radioactive element and a specific brachytherapy isotope that is not included in the Radiation Therapy section tables.

D1.b. A separate procedure to place a temporary applicator for delivering the brachytherapy is coded to the root operation Insertion and the device value Other Device.

> *Examples:*
> Intrauterine brachytherapy applicator placed as a separate procedure from the brachytherapy procedure is coded to Insertion of Other Device, and the brachytherapy is coded separately using the modality Brachytherapy in the Radiation Therapy section.
>
> Intrauterine brachytherapy applicator placed concomitantly with delivery of the brachytherapy dose is coded with a single code using the modality Brachytherapy in the Radiation Therapy section.

New Technology Section Guidelines (section X)

E. New Technology Section

General guidelines

E1.a. Section X codes fully represent the specific procedure described in the code title, and do not require additional codes from other sections of ICD-10-PCS. When section X contains a code title which **fully** describes a specific new technology procedure, **and it is the** only **procedure performed, only the section** X code is reported for the procedure. **There is no need to report an additional code in another section of ICD-10-PCS.**

Example:
XWØ4321 Introduction of Ceftazidime-Avibactam Anti-infective into Central Vein, Percutaneous Approach, New Technology Group 1, can be coded to indicate that Ceftazidime-Avibactam Anti-infective was administered via a central vein. A separate code from table 3EØ in the Administration section of ICD-10-PCS is not coded in addition to this code.

E1.b. When multiple procedures are performed, New Technology section X codes are coded following the multiple procedures guideline.

Examples:
Dual filter cerebral embolic filtration used during transcatheter aortic valve replacement (TAVR), X2A5312 Cerebral Embolic Filtration, Dual Filter in Innominate Artery and Left Common Carotid Artery, Percutaneous Approach, New Technology Group 2, is coded for the cerebral embolic filtration, along with an ICD-10-PCS code for the TAVR procedure.

Magnetically controlled growth rod (MCGR) placed during a spinal fusion procedure, a code from table XNS, Reposition of the Bones is coded for the MCGR, along with an ICD-10-PCS code for the spinal fusion procedure.

F. Selection of Principal Procedure

The following instructions should be applied in the selection of principal procedure and clarification on the importance of the relation to the principal diagnosis when more than one procedure is performed:

1. Procedure performed for definitive treatment of both principal diagnosis and secondary diagnosis

    a. Sequence procedure performed for definitive treatment most related to principal diagnosis as principal procedure.

2. Procedure performed for definitive treatment and diagnostic procedures performed for both principal diagnosis and secondary diagnosis.

    a. Sequence procedure performed for definitive treatment most related to principal diagnosis as principal procedure

3. A diagnostic procedure was performed for the principal diagnosis and a procedure is performed for definitive treatment of a secondary diagnosis.

    a. Sequence diagnostic procedure as principal procedure, since the procedure most related to the principal diagnosis takes precedence.

4. No procedures performed that are related to principal diagnosis; procedures performed for definitive treatment and diagnostic procedures were performed for secondary diagnosis

    a. Sequence procedure performed for definitive treatment of secondary diagnosis as principal procedure, since there are no procedures (definitive or nondefinitive treatment) related to principal diagnosis.

# #

3f (Aortic) Bioprosthesis valve *use* Zooplastic Tissue in Heart and Great Vessels

A

Abdominal aortic plexus *use* Abdominal Sympathetic Nerve
Abdominal esophagus *use* Esophagus, Lower
Abdominohysterectomy *see* Resection, Uterus ØUT9
Abdominoplasty
  see Alteration, Abdominal Wall ØWØF
  see Repair, Abdominal Wall ØWQF
  see Supplement, Abdominal Wall ØWUF
Abductor hallucis muscle
  use Foot Muscle, Left
  use Foot Muscle, Right
AbioCor® Total Replacement Heart *use* Synthetic Substitute
Ablation
  see Control bleeding in
  see Destruction
Abortion
  Abortifacient 10A07ZX
  Laminaria 10A07ZW
  Products of Conception 10A0
  Vacuum 10A07Z6
Abrasion *see* Extraction
Absolute Pro Vascular (OTW) Self-Expanding Stent System *use* Intraluminal Device
Accessory cephalic vein
  use Cephalic Vein, Left
  use Cephalic Vein, Right
Accessory obturator nerve *use* Lumbar Plexus
Accessory phrenic nerve *use* Phrenic Nerve
Accessory spleen *use* Spleen
Acculink (RX) Carotid Stent System *use* Intraluminal Device
Acellular Hydrated Dermis *use* Nonautologous Tissue Substitute
Acetabular cup *use* Liner in Lower Joints
Acetabulectomy
  see Excision, Lower Bones ØQB
  see Resection, Lower Bones ØQT
Acetabulofemoral joint
  use Hip Joint, Left
  use Hip Joint, Right
Acetabuloplasty
  see Repair, Lower Bones ØQQ
  see Replacement, Lower Bones ØQR
  see Supplement, Lower Bones ØQU
Achilles tendon
  use Lower Leg Tendon, Left
  use Lower Leg Tendon, Right
Achillorrhaphy *see* Repair, Tendons ØLQ
Achillotenotomy, achillotomy
  see Division, Tendons ØL8
  see Drainage, Tendons ØL9
Acromioclavicular ligament
  use Shoulder Bursa and Ligament, Left
  use Shoulder Bursa and Ligament, Right
Acromion (process)
  use Scapula, Left
  use Scapula, Right
Acromionectomy
  see Excision, Upper Joints ØRB
  see Resection, Upper Joints ØRT
Acromioplasty
  see Repair, Upper Joints ØRQ
  see Replacement, Upper Joints ØRR
  see Supplement, Upper Joints ØRU
Activa PC neurostimulator *use* Stimulator Generator, Multiple Array in ØJH
Activa RC neurostimulator *use* Stimulator Generator, Multiple Array Rechargeable in ØJH
Activa SC neurostimulator *use* Stimulator Generator, Single Array in ØJH
Activities of Daily Living Assessment F02
Activities of Daily Living Treatment F08
ACUITY™ Steerable Lead
  use Cardiac Lead, Defibrillator in 02H
  use Cardiac Lead, Pacemaker in 02H

Acupuncture
  Breast
    Anesthesia 8E0H300
    No Qualifier 8E0H30Z
  Integumentary System
    Anesthesia 8E0H300
    No Qualifier 8E0H30Z
Adductor brevis muscle
  use Upper Leg Muscle, Left
  use Upper Leg Muscle, Right
Adductor hallucis muscle
  use Foot Muscle, Left
  use Foot Muscle, Right
Adductor longus muscle
  use Upper Leg Muscle, Left
  use Upper Leg Muscle, Right
Adductor magnus muscle
  use Upper Leg Muscle, Left
  use Upper Leg Muscle, Right
Adenohypophysis *use* Pituitary Gland
Adenoidectomy
  see Excision, Adenoids ØCBQ
  see Resection, Adenoids ØCTQ
Adenoidotomy *see* Drainage, Adenoids ØC9Q
Adhesiolysis *see* Release
Administration
  Blood products *see* Transfusion
  Other substance *see* Introduction of substance in or on
Adrenalectomy
  see Excision, Endocrine System ØGB
  see Resection, Endocrine System ØGT
Adrenalorrhaphy *see* Repair, Endocrine System ØGQ
Adrenalotomy *see* Drainage, Endocrine System ØG9
Advancement
  see Reposition
  see Transfer
Advisa (MRI) *use* Pacemaker, Dual Chamber in ØJH
AFX® Endovascular AAA System *use* Intraluminal Device
AIGISRx Antibacterial Envelope *use* Anti-Infective Envelope
Alar ligament of axis *use* Head and Neck Bursa and Ligament
Alfieri Stitch Valvuloplasty *see* Restriction, Valve, Mitral 02VG
Alimentation *see* Introduction of substance in or on
Alteration
  Abdominal Wall ØWØF
  Ankle Region
    Left ØYØL
    Right ØYØK
  Arm
    Lower
      Left ØXØF
      Right ØXØD
    Upper
      Left ØXØ9
      Right ØXØ8
  Axilla
    Left ØXØ5
    Right ØXØ4
  Back
    Lower ØWØL
    Upper ØWØK
  Breast
    Bilateral ØHØV
    Left ØHØU
    Right ØHØT
  Buttock
    Left ØYØ1
    Right ØYØØ
  Chest Wall ØWØ8
  Ear
    Bilateral Ø9Ø2
    Left Ø9Ø1
    Right Ø9ØØ
  Elbow Region
    Left ØXØC
    Right ØXØB
  Extremity
    Lower
      Left ØYØB
      Right ØYØ9
    Upper
      Left ØXØ7
      Right ØXØ6

Alteration — *continued*
  Eyelid
    Lower
      Left Ø80R
      Right Ø80Q
    Upper
      Left Ø80P
      Right Ø80N
  Face ØWØ2
  Head ØWØØ
  Jaw
    Lower ØWØ5
    Upper ØWØ4
  Knee Region
    Left ØYØG
    Right ØYØF
  Leg
    Lower
      Left ØYØJ
      Right ØYØH
    Upper
      Left ØYØD
      Right ØYØC
  Lip
    Lower ØCØ1X
    Upper ØCØØX
  Nasal Mucosa and Soft Tissue Ø9ØK
  Neck ØWØ6
  Perineum
    Female ØWØN
    Male ØWØM
  Shoulder Region
    Left ØXØ3
    Right ØXØ2
  Subcutaneous Tissue and Fascia
    Abdomen ØJØ8
    Back ØJØ7
    Buttock ØJØ9
    Chest ØJØ6
    Face ØJØ1
    Lower Arm
      Left ØJØH
      Right ØJØG
    Lower Leg
      Left ØJØP
      Right ØJØN
    Neck
      Left ØJØ5
      Right ØJØ4
    Upper Arm
      Left ØJØF
      Right ØJØD
    Upper Leg
      Left ØJØM
      Right ØJØL
  Wrist Region
    Left ØXØH
    Right ØXØG
Alveolar process of mandible
  use Mandible, Left
  use Mandible, Right
Alveolar process of maxilla *use* Maxilla
Alveolectomy
  see Excision, Head and Facial Bones ØNB
  see Resection, Head and Facial Bones ØNT
Alveoloplasty
  see Repair, Head and Facial Bones ØNQ
  see Replacement, Head and Facial Bones ØNR
  see Supplement, Head and Facial Bones ØNU
Alveolotomy
  see Division, Head and Facial Bones ØN8
  see Drainage, Head and Facial Bones ØN9
Ambulatory cardiac monitoring 4A12X45
Amniocentesis *see* Drainage, Products of Conception 1090
Amnioinfusion *see* Introduction of substance in or on, Products of Conception 3E0E
Amnioscopy 10J08ZZ
Amniotomy *see* Drainage, Products of Conception 1090
AMPLATZER® Muscular VSD Occluder *use* Synthetic Substitute
Amputation *see* Detachment
AMS 800® Urinary Control System *use* Artificial Sphincter in Urinary System
Anal orifice *use* Anus
Analog radiography *see* Plain Radiography
Analog radiology *see* Plain Radiography
Anastomosis *see* Bypass

Anatomical snuffbox
  use Lower Arm and Wrist Muscle, Left
  use Lower Arm and Wrist Muscle, Right
Andexanet Alfa, Factor Xa Inhibitor Reversal Agent
  use Coagulation Factor Xa, Inactivated
Andexxa *use* Coagulation Factor Xa, Inactivated
AneuRx® AAA Advantage® *use* Intraluminal Device
Angiectomy
  see Excision, Heart and Great Vessels 02B
  see Excision, Lower Arteries 04B
  see Excision, Lower Veins 06B
  see Excision, Upper Arteries 03B
  see Excision, Upper Veins 05B
Angiocardiography
  Combined right and left heart *see* Fluoroscopy, Heart, Right and Left B216
  Left Heart *see* Fluoroscopy, Heart, Left B215
  Right Heart *see* Fluoroscopy, Heart, Right B214
  SPY system intravascular fluorescence *see* Monitoring, Physiological Systems 4A1
Angiography
  see Fluoroscopy, Heart B21
  see Plain Radiography, Heart B20
Angioplasty
  see Dilation, Heart and Great Vessels 027
  see Dilation, Lower Arteries 047
  see Dilation, Upper Arteries 037
  see Repair, Heart and Great Vessels 02Q
  see Repair, Lower Arteries 04Q
  see Repair, Upper Arteries 03Q
  see Replacement, Heart and Great Vessels 02R
  see Replacement, Lower Arteries 04R
  see Replacement, Upper Arteries 03R
  see Supplement, Heart and Great Vessels 02U
  see Supplement, Lower Arteries 04U
  see Supplement, Upper Arteries 03U
Angiorrhaphy
  see Repair, Heart and Great Vessels 02Q
  see Repair, Lower Arteries 04Q
  see Repair, Upper Arteries 03Q
Angioscopy 02JY4ZZ, 03JY4ZZ, 04JY4ZZ
Angiotensin II *use* Synthetic Human Angiotensin II
Angiotripsy
  see Occlusion, Lower Arteries 04L
  see Occlusion, Upper Arteries 03L
Angular artery *use* Face Artery
Angular vein
  use Face Vein, Left
  use Face Vein, Right
Annular ligament
  use Elbow Bursa and Ligament, Left
  use Elbow Bursa and Ligament, Right
Annuloplasty
  see Repair, Heart and Great Vessels 02Q
  see Supplement, Heart and Great Vessels 02U
Annuloplasty ring *use* Synthetic Substitute
Anoplasty
  see Repair, Anus 0DQQ
  see Supplement, Anus 0DUQ
Anorectal junction *use* Rectum
Anoscopy 0DJD8ZZ
Ansa cervicalis *use* Cervical Plexus
Antabuse therapy HZ93ZZZ
Antebrachial fascia
  use Subcutaneous Tissue and Fascia, Left Lower Arm
  use Subcutaneous Tissue and Fascia, Right Lower Arm
Anterior cerebral artery *use* Intracranial Artery
Anterior cerebral vein *use* Intracranial Vein
Anterior choroidal artery *use* Intracranial Artery
Anterior circumflex humeral artery
  use Axillary Artery, Left
  use Axillary Artery, Right
Anterior communicating artery *use* Intracranial Artery
Anterior cruciate ligament (ACL)
  use Knee Bursa and Ligament, Left
  use Knee Bursa and Ligament, Right
Anterior crural nerve *use* Femoral Nerve
Anterior facial vein
  use Face Vein, Left
  use Face Vein, Right
Anterior intercostal artery
  use Internal Mammary Artery, Left
  use Internal Mammary Artery, Right

Anterior interosseous nerve *use* Median Nerve
Anterior lateral malleolar artery
  use Anterior Tibial Artery, Left
  use Anterior Tibial Artery, Right
Anterior lingual gland *use* Minor Salivary Gland
Anterior (pectoral) lymph node
  use Lymphatic, Left Axillary
  use Lymphatic, Right Axillary
Anterior medial malleolar artery
  use Anterior Tibial Artery, Left
  use Anterior Tibial Artery, Right
Anterior spinal artery
  use Vertebral Artery, Left
  use Vertebral Artery, Right
Anterior tibial recurrent artery
  use Anterior Tibial Artery, Left
  use Anterior Tibial Artery, Right
Anterior ulnar recurrent artery
  use Ulnar Artery, Left
  use Ulnar Artery, Right
Anterior vagal trunk *use* Vagus Nerve
Anterior vertebral muscle
  use Neck Muscle, Left
  use Neck Muscle, Right
Antibacterial Envelope (TYRX) (AIGISRx) *use* Anti-Infective Envelope
Antigen-free air conditioning *see* Atmospheric Control, Physiological Systems 6A0
Antihelix
  use External Ear, Bilateral
  use External Ear, Left
  use External Ear, Right
Antimicrobial envelope *use* Anti-Infective Envelope
Antitragus
  use External Ear, Bilateral
  use External Ear, Left
  use External Ear, Right
Antrostomy *see* Drainage, Ear, Nose, Sinus 099
Antrotomy *see* Drainage, Ear, Nose, Sinus 099
Antrum of Highmore
  use Maxillary Sinus, Left
  use Maxillary Sinus, Right
Aortic annulus *use* Aortic Valve
Aortic arch *use* Thoracic Aorta, Ascending/Arch
Aortic intercostal artery *use* Upper Artery
Aortography
  see Fluoroscopy, Lower Arteries B41
  see Fluoroscopy, Upper Arteries B31
  see Plain Radiography, Lower Arteries B40
  see Plain Radiography, Upper Arteries B30
Aortoplasty
  see Repair, Aorta, Abdominal 04Q0
  see Repair, Aorta, Thoracic, Ascending/Arch 02QX
  see Repair, Aorta, Thoracic, Descending 02QW
  see Replacement, Aorta, Abdominal 04R0
  see Replacement, Aorta, Thoracic, Ascending/Arch 02RX
  see Replacement, Aorta, Thoracic, Descending 02RW
  see Supplement, Aorta, Abdominal 04U0
  see Supplement, Aorta, Thoracic, Ascending/Arch 02UX
  see Supplement, Aorta, Thoracic, Descending 02UW
Apalutamide Antineoplastic XW0DXJ5
Apical (subclavicular) lymph node
  use Lymphatic, Left Axillary
  use Lymphatic, Right Axillary
Apneustic center *use* Pons
Appendectomy
  see Excision, Appendix 0DBJ
  see Resection, Appendix 0DTJ
Appendicolysis *see* Release, Appendix 0DNJ
Appendicotomy *see* Drainage, Appendix 0D9J
Application *see* Introduction of substance in or on
Aquablation therapy, prostate XV508A4
Aquapheresis 6A550Z3
Aqueduct of Sylvius *use* Cerebral Ventricle
Aqueous humour
  use Anterior Chamber, Left
  use Anterior Chamber, Right
Arachnoid mater, intracranial *use* Cerebral Meninges
Arachnoid mater, spinal *use* Spinal Meninges
Arcuate artery
  use Foot Artery, Left
  use Foot Artery, Right

Areola
  use Nipple, Left
  use Nipple, Right
AROM (artificial rupture of membranes) 10907ZC
Arterial canal (duct) *use* Pulmonary Artery, Left
Arterial pulse tracing *see* Measurement, Arterial 4A03
Arteriectomy
  see Excision, Heart and Great Vessels 02B
  see Excision, Lower Arteries 04B
  see Excision, Upper Arteries 03B
Arteriography
  see Fluoroscopy, Heart B21
  see Fluoroscopy, Lower Arteries B41
  see Fluoroscopy, Upper Arteries B31
  see Plain Radiography, Heart B20
  see Plain Radiography, Lower Arteries B40
  see Plain Radiography, Upper Arteries B30
Arterioplasty
  see Repair, Heart and Great Vessels 02Q
  see Repair, Lower Arteries 04Q
  see Repair, Upper Arteries 03Q
  see Replacement, Heart and Great Vessels 02R
  see Replacement, Lower Arteries 04R
  see Replacement, Upper Arteries 03R
  see Supplement, Heart and Great Vessels 02U
  see Supplement, Lower Arteries 04U
  see Supplement, Upper Arteries 03U
Arteriorrhaphy
  see Repair, Heart and Great Vessels 02Q
  see Repair, Lower Arteries 04Q
  see Repair, Upper Arteries 03Q
Arterioscopy
  see Inspection, Artery, Lower 04JY
  see Inspection, Artery, Upper 03JY
  see Inspection, Great Vessel 02JY
Arthrectomy
  see Excision, Lower Joints 0SB
  see Excision, Upper Joints 0RB
  see Resection, Lower Joints 0ST
  see Resection, Upper Joints 0RT
Arthrocentesis
  see Drainage, Lower Joints 0S9
  see Drainage, Upper Joints 0R9
Arthrodesis
  see Fusion, Lower Joints 0SG
  see Fusion, Upper Joints 0RG
Arthrography
  see Plain Radiography, Non-Axial Lower Bones BQ0
  see Plain Radiography, Non-Axial Upper Bones BP0
  see Plain Radiography, Skull and Facial Bones BN0
Arthrolysis
  see Release, Lower Joints 0SN
  see Release, Upper Joints 0RN
Arthropexy
  see Repair, Lower Joints 0SQ
  see Repair, Upper Joints 0RQ
  see Reposition, Lower Joints 0SS
  see Reposition, Upper Joints 0RS
Arthroplasty
  see Repair, Lower Joints 0SQ
  see Repair, Upper Joints 0RQ
  see Replacement, Lower Joints 0SR
  see Replacement, Upper Joints 0RR
  see Supplement, Lower Joints 0SU
  see Supplement, Upper Joints 0RU
Arthroplasty, radial head
  see Replacement, Radius, Left 0PRJ
  see Replacement, Radius, Right 0PRH
Arthroscopy
  see Inspection, Lower Joints 0SJ
  see Inspection, Upper Joints 0RJ
Arthrotomy
  see Drainage, Lower Joints 0S9
  see Drainage, Upper Joints 0R9
Articulating Spacer (Antibiotic) *use* Articulating Spacer in Lower Joints
Artificial anal sphincter (AAS) *use* Artificial Sphincter in Gastrointestinal System
Artificial bowel sphincter (neosphincter) *use* Artificial Sphincter in Gastrointestinal System
Artificial Sphincter
  Insertion of device in
    Anus 0DHQ
    Bladder 0THB
    Bladder Neck 0THC
    Urethra 0THD

Artificial Sphincter — *continued*
  Removal of device from
    Anus ØDPQ
    Bladder ØTPB
    Urethra ØTPD
  Revision of device in
    Anus ØDWQ
    Bladder ØTWB
    Urethra ØTWD
Artificial urinary sphincter (AUS) *use* Artificial Sphincter in Urinary System
Aryepiglottic fold *use* Larynx
Arytenoid cartilage *use* Larynx
Arytenoid muscle
  use Neck Muscle, Left
  use Neck Muscle, Right
Arytenoidectomy *see* Excision, Larynx ØCBS
Arytenoidopexy *see* Repair, Larynx ØCQS
Ascenda Intrathecal Catheter *use* Infusion Device
Ascending aorta *use* Thoracic Aorta, Ascending/Arch
Ascending palatine artery *use* Face Artery
Ascending pharyngeal artery
  use External Carotid Artery, Left
  use External Carotid Artery, Right
Aspiration, fine needle
  Fluid or gas *see* Drainage
  Tissue biopsy
    see Excision
    see Extraction
Assessment
  Activities of daily living *see* Activities of Daily Living Assessment, Rehabilitation F02
  Hearing *see* Hearing Assessment, Diagnostic Audiology F13
  Hearing aid *see* Hearing Aid Assessment, Diagnostic Audiology F14
  Intravascular perfusion, using indocyanine green (ICG) dye *see* Monitoring, Physiological Systems 4A1
  Motor function *see* Motor Function Assessment, Rehabilitation FØ1
  Nerve function *see* Motor Function Assessment, Rehabilitation FØ1
  Speech *see* Speech Assessment, Rehabilitation FØØ
  Vestibular *see* Vestibular Assessment, Diagnostic Audiology F15
  Vocational *see* Activities of Daily Living Treatment, Rehabilitation FØ8
Assistance
  Cardiac
    Continuous
      Balloon Pump 5AØ221Ø
      Impeller Pump 5AØ221D
      Other Pump 5AØ2216
      Pulsatile Compression 5AØ2215
    Intermittent
      Balloon Pump 5AØ211Ø
      Impeller Pump 5AØ211D
      Other Pump 5AØ2116
      Pulsatile Compression 5AØ2115
  Circulatory
    Continuous
      Hyperbaric 5AØ5221
      Supersaturated 5AØ522C
    Intermittent
      Hyperbaric 5AØ5121
      Supersaturated 5AØ512C
  Respiratory
    24-96 Consecutive Hours
      Continuous Negative Airway Pressure 5AØ9459
      Continuous Positive Airway Pressure 5AØ9457
      Intermittent Negative Airway Pressure 5AØ945B
      Intermittent Positive Airway Pressure 5AØ9458
      No Qualifier 5AØ945Z
    Continuous, Filtration 5AØ92ØZ
    Greater than 96 Consecutive Hours
      Continuous Negative Airway Pressure 5AØ9559
      Continuous Positive Airway Pressure 5AØ9557
      Intermittent Negative Airway Pressure 5AØ955B
      Intermittent Positive Airway Pressure 5AØ9558

Assistance — *continued*
  Respiratory — *continued*
    Greater than 96 Consecutive Hours — *continued*
      No Qualifier 5AØ955Z
    Less than 24 Consecutive Hours
      Continuous Negative Airway Pressure 5AØ9359
      Continuous Positive Airway Pressure 5AØ9357
      Intermittent Negative Airway Pressure 5AØ935B
      Intermittent Positive Airway Pressure 5AØ9358
      No Qualifier 5AØ935Z
Assurant (Cobalt) stent *use* Intraluminal Device
Atherectomy
  see Extirpation, Heart and Great Vessels Ø2C
  see Extirpation, Lower Arteries Ø4C
  see Extirpation, Upper Arteries Ø3C
Atlantoaxial joint *use* Cervical Vertebral Joint
Atmospheric Control 6AØZ
AtriClip LAA Exclusion System *use* Extraluminal Device
Atrioseptoplasty
  see Repair, Heart and Great Vessels Ø2Q
  see Replacement, Heart and Great Vessels Ø2R
  see Supplement, Heart and Great Vessels Ø2U
Atrioventricular node *use* Conduction Mechanism
Atrium dextrum cordis *use* Atrium, Right
Atrium pulmonale *use* Atrium, Left
Attain Ability® lead Ø2H
  use Cardiac Lead, Defibrillator in Ø2H
  use Cardiac Lead, Pacemaker in Ø2H
Attain Starfix® (OTW) lead
  use Cardiac Lead, Defibrillator in Ø2H
  use Cardiac Lead, Pacemaker in Ø2H
Audiology, diagnostic
  see Hearing Aid Assessment, Diagnostic Audiology F14
  see Hearing Assessment, Diagnostic Audiology F13
  see Vestibular Assessment, Diagnostic Audiology F15
Audiometry *see* Hearing Assessment, Diagnostic Audiology F13
Auditory tube
  use Eustachian Tube, Left
  use Eustachian Tube, Right
Auerbach's (myenteric) plexus *use* Abdominal Sympathetic Nerve
Auricle
  use External Ear, Bilateral
  use External Ear, Left
  use External Ear, Right
Auricularis muscle *use* Head Muscle
Autograft *use* Autologous Tissue Substitute
Autologous artery graft
  use Autologous Arterial Tissue in Heart and Great Vessels
  use Autologous Arterial Tissue in Lower Arteries
  use Autologous Arterial Tissue in Lower Veins
  use Autologous Arterial Tissue in Upper Arteries
  use Autologous Arterial Tissue in Upper Veins
Autologous vein graft
  use Autologous Venous Tissue in Heart and Great Vessels
  use Autologous Venous Tissue in Lower Arteries
  use Autologous Venous Tissue in Lower Veins
  use Autologous Venous Tissue in Upper Arteries
  use Autologous Venous Tissue in Upper Veins
Autotransfusion *see* Transfusion
Autotransplant
  Adrenal tissue *see* Reposition, Endocrine System ØGS
  Kidney *see* Reposition, Urinary System ØTS
  Pancreatic tissue *see* Reposition, Pancreas ØFSG
  Parathyroid tissue *see* Reposition, Endocrine System ØGS
  Thyroid tissue *see* Reposition, Endocrine System ØGS
  Tooth *see* Reattachment, Mouth and Throat ØCM
Avulsion *see* Extraction
Axial Lumbar Interbody Fusion System *use* Interbody Fusion Device in Lower Joints
AxiaLIF® System *use* Interbody Fusion Device in Lower Joints

Axicabtagene Ciloeucel *use* Engineered Autologous Chimeric Antigen Receptor T-cell Immunotherapy
Axillary fascia
  use Subcutaneous Tissue and Fascia, Left Upper Arm
  use Subcutaneous Tissue and Fascia, Right Upper Arm
Axillary nerve *use* Brachial Plexus
AZEDRA® *use* Iobenguane I-131 Antineoplastic

B

BAK/C® Interbody Cervical Fusion System *use* Interbody Fusion Device in Upper Joints
BAL (bronchial alveolar lavage), diagnostic *see* Drainage, Respiratory System ØB9
Balanoplasty
  see Repair, Penis ØVQS
  see Supplement, Penis ØVUS
Balloon atrial septostomy (BAS) Ø2163Z7
Balloon Pump
  Continuous, Output 5AØ221Ø
  Intermittent, Output 5AØ211Ø
Bandage, Elastic *see* Compression
Banding
  see Occlusion
  see Restriction
Banding, esophageal varices *see* Occlusion, Vein, Esophageal Ø6L3
Banding, laparoscopic (adjustable) gastric
  Initial procedure ØDV64CZ
  Surgical correction *see* Revision of device in, Stomach ØDW6
Bard® Composix® Kugel® patch *use* Synthetic Substitute
Bard® Composix® (E/X) (LP) mesh *use* Synthetic Substitute
Bard® Dulex™ mesh *use* Synthetic Substitute
Bard® Ventralex™ Hernia Patch *use* Synthetic Substitute
Barium swallow *see* Fluoroscopy, Gastrointestinal System BD1
Baroreflex Activation Therapy® (BAT®)
  use Stimulator Generator in Subcutaneous Tissue and Fascia
  use Stimulator Lead in Upper Arteries
Bartholin's (greater vestibular) gland *use* Vestibular Gland
Basal (internal) cerebral vein *use* Intracranial Vein
Basal metabolic rate (BMR) *see* Measurement, Physiological Systems 4AØZ
Basal nuclei *use* Basal Ganglia
Base of Tongue *use* Pharynx
Basilar artery *use* Intracranial Artery
Basis pontis *use* Pons
Beam Radiation
  Abdomen DWØ3
    Intraoperative DWØ33ZØ
  Adrenal Gland DGØ2
    Intraoperative DGØ23ZØ
  Bile Ducts DFØ2
    Intraoperative DFØ23ZØ
  Bladder DTØ2
    Intraoperative DTØ23ZØ
  Bone
    Intraoperative DPØC3ZØ
    Other DPØC
  Bone Marrow D7ØØ
    Intraoperative D7ØØ3ZØ
  Brain DØØØ
    Intraoperative DØØØ3ZØ
  Brain Stem DØØ1
    Intraoperative DØØ13ZØ
  Breast
    Left DMØØ
      Intraoperative DMØØ3ZØ
    Right DMØ1
      Intraoperative DMØ13ZØ
  Bronchus DBØ1
    Intraoperative DBØ13ZØ
  Cervix DUØ1
    Intraoperative DUØ13ZØ
  Chest DWØ2
    Intraoperative DWØ23ZØ
  Chest Wall DBØ7
    Intraoperative DBØ73ZØ
  Colon DDØ5

Beam Radiation — *continued*
 Colon — *continued*
  Intraoperative DD053Z0
 Diaphragm DB08
  Intraoperative DB083Z0
 Duodenum DD02
  Intraoperative DD023Z0
 Ear D900
  Intraoperative D9003Z0
 Esophagus DD00
  Intraoperative DD003Z0
 Eye D800
  Intraoperative D8003Z0
 Femur DP09
  Intraoperative DP093Z0
 Fibula DP0B
  Intraoperative DP0B3Z0
 Gallbladder DF01
  Intraoperative DF013Z0
 Gland
  Adrenal DG02
   Intraoperative DG023Z0
  Parathyroid DG04
   Intraoperative DG043Z0
  Pituitary DG00
   Intraoperative DG003Z0
  Thyroid DG05
   Intraoperative DG053Z0
 Glands
  Intraoperative D9063Z0
  Salivary D906
 Head and Neck DW01
  Intraoperative DW013Z0
 Hemibody DW04
  Intraoperative DW043Z0
 Humerus DP06
  Intraoperative DP063Z0
 Hypopharynx D903
  Intraoperative D9033Z0
 Ileum DD04
  Intraoperative DD043Z0
 Jejunum DD03
  Intraoperative DD033Z0
 Kidney DT00
  Intraoperative DT003Z0
 Larynx D90B
  Intraoperative D90B3Z0
 Liver DF00
  Intraoperative DF003Z0
 Lung DB02
  Intraoperative DB023Z0
 Lymphatics
  Abdomen D706
   Intraoperative D7063Z0
  Axillary D704
   Intraoperative D7043Z0
  Inguinal D708
   Intraoperative D7083Z0
  Neck D703
   Intraoperative D7033Z0
  Pelvis D707
   Intraoperative D7073Z0
  Thorax D705
   Intraoperative D7053Z0
 Mandible DP03
  Intraoperative DP033Z0
 Maxilla DP02
  Intraoperative DP023Z0
 Mediastinum DB06
  Intraoperative DB063Z0
 Mouth D904
  Intraoperative D9043Z0
 Nasopharynx D90D
  Intraoperative D90D3Z0
 Neck and Head DW01
  Intraoperative DW013Z0
 Nerve
  Intraoperative D0073Z0
  Peripheral D007
 Nose D901
  Intraoperative D9013Z0
 Oropharynx D90F
  Intraoperative D90F3Z0
 Ovary DU00
  Intraoperative DU003Z0
 Palate
  Hard D908
   Intraoperative D9083Z0
  Soft D909

Beam Radiation — *continued*
 Palate — *continued*
  Soft — *continued*
   Intraoperative D9093Z0
 Pancreas DF03
  Intraoperative DF033Z0
 Parathyroid Gland DG04
  Intraoperative DG043Z0
 Pelvic Bones DP08
  Intraoperative DP083Z0
 Pelvic Region DW06
  Intraoperative DW063Z0
 Pineal Body DG01
  Intraoperative DG013Z0
 Pituitary Gland DG00
  Intraoperative DG003Z0
 Pleura DB05
  Intraoperative DB053Z0
 Prostate DV00
  Intraoperative DV003Z0
 Radius DP07
  Intraoperative DP073Z0
 Rectum DD07
  Intraoperative DD073Z0
 Rib DP05
  Intraoperative DP053Z0
 Sinuses D907
  Intraoperative D9073Z0
 Skin
  Abdomen DH08
   Intraoperative DH083Z0
  Arm DH04
   Intraoperative DH043Z0
  Back DH07
   Intraoperative DH073Z0
  Buttock DH09
   Intraoperative DH093Z0
  Chest DH06
   Intraoperative DH063Z0
  Face DH02
   Intraoperative DH023Z0
  Leg DH0B
   Intraoperative DH0B3Z0
  Neck DH03
   Intraoperative DH033Z0
 Skull DP00
  Intraoperative DP003Z0
 Spinal Cord D006
  Intraoperative D0063Z0
 Spleen D702
  Intraoperative D7023Z0
 Sternum DP04
  Intraoperative DP043Z0
 Stomach DD01
  Intraoperative DD013Z0
 Testis DV01
  Intraoperative DV013Z0
 Thymus D701
  Intraoperative D7013Z0
 Thyroid Gland DG05
  Intraoperative DG053Z0
 Tibia DP0B
  Intraoperative DP0B3Z0
 Tongue D905
  Intraoperative D9053Z0
 Trachea DB00
  Intraoperative DB003Z0
 Ulna DP07
  Intraoperative DP073Z0
 Ureter DT01
  Intraoperative DT013Z0
 Urethra DT03
  Intraoperative DT033Z0
 Uterus DU02
  Intraoperative DU023Z0
 Whole Body DW05
  Intraoperative DW053Z0
Bedside swallow F00ZJWZ
Berlin Heart Ventricular Assist Device *use* Implantable Heart Assist System in Heart and Great Vessels
Bezlotoxumab Monoclonal Antibody XW0
Biceps brachii muscle
 use Upper Arm Muscle, Left
 use Upper Arm Muscle, Right
Biceps femoris muscle
 use Upper Leg Muscle, Left
 use Upper Leg Muscle, Right

Bicipital aponeurosis
 use Subcutaneous Tissue and Fascia, Left Lower Arm
 use Subcutaneous Tissue and Fascia, Right Lower Arm
Bicuspid valve *use* Mitral Valve
Bili light therapy *see* Phototherapy, Skin 6A60
Bioactive embolization coil(s) *use* Intraluminal Device, Bioactive in Upper Arteries
Biofeedback GZC9ZZZ
Biopsy
 see Drainage with qualifier Diagnostic
 see Excision with qualifier Diagnostic
 see Extraction with qualifier Diagnostic
BiPAP *see* Assistance, Respiratory 5A09
Bisection *see* Division
Biventricular external heart assist system *use* Short-term External Heart Assist System in Heart and Great Vessels
Blepharectomy
 see Excision, Eye 08B
 see Resection, Eye 08T
Blepharoplasty
 see Repair, Eye 08Q
 see Replacement, Eye 08R
 see Reposition, Eye 08S
 see Supplement, Eye 08U
Blepharorrhaphy *see* Repair, Eye 08Q
Blepharotomy *see* Drainage, Eye 089
Blinatumomab Antineoplastic Immunotherapy XW0
Block, Nerve, anesthetic injection 3E0T3BZ
Blood glucose monitoring system *use* Monitoring Device
Blood pressure *see* Measurement, Arterial 4A03
BMR (basal metabolic rate) *see* Measurement, Physiological Systems 4A0Z
Body of femur
 use Femoral Shaft, Left
 use Femoral Shaft, Right
Body of fibula
 use Fibula, Left
 use Fibula, Right
Bone anchored hearing device
 use Hearing Device, Bone Conduction in 09H
 use Hearing Device in Head and Facial Bones
Bone bank bone graft *use* Nonautologous Tissue Substitute
Bone Growth Stimulator
 Insertion of device in
  Bone
   Facial 0NHW
   Lower 0QHY
   Nasal 0NHB
   Upper 0PHY
   Skull 0NH0
 Removal of device from
  Bone
   Facial 0NPW
   Lower 0QPY
   Nasal 0NPB
   Upper 0PPY
   Skull 0NP0
 Revision of device in
  Bone
   Facial 0NWW
   Lower 0QWY
   Nasal 0NWB
   Upper 0PWY
   Skull 0NW0
Bone marrow transplant *see* Transfusion, Circulatory 302
Bone morphogenetic protein 2 (BMP 2) *use* Recombinant Bone Morphogenetic Protein
Bone screw (interlocking) (lag) (pedicle) (recessed)
 use Internal Fixation Device in Head and Facial Bones
 use Internal Fixation Device in Lower Bones
 use Internal Fixation Device in Upper Bones
Bony labyrinth
 use Inner Ear, Left
 use Inner Ear, Right
Bony orbit
 use Orbit, Left
 use Orbit, Right
Bony vestibule
 use Inner Ear, Left

Bony vestibule — *continued*
  use Inner Ear, Right
Botallo's duct *use* Pulmonary Artery, Left
Bovine pericardial valve *use* Zooplastic Tissue in Heart and Great Vessels
Bovine pericardium graft *use* Zooplastic Tissue in Heart and Great Vessels
BP (blood pressure) *see* Measurement, Arterial 4A03
Brachial (lateral) lymph node
  use Lymphatic, Left Axillary
  use Lymphatic, Right Axillary
Brachialis muscle
  use Upper Arm Muscle, Left
  use Upper Arm Muscle, Right
Brachiocephalic artery *use* Innominate Artery
Brachiocephalic trunk *use* Innominate Artery
Brachiocephalic vein
  use Innominate Vein, Left
  use Innominate Vein, Right
Brachioradialis muscle
  use Lower Arm and Wrist Muscle, Left
  use Lower Arm and Wrist Muscle, Right
Brachytherapy
  Abdomen DW13
  Adrenal Gland DG12
  Back
    Lower DW1LBB
    Upper DW1KBB
  Bile Ducts DF12
  Bladder DT12
  Bone Marrow D710
  Brain D010
  Brain Stem D011
  Breast
    Left DM10
    Right DM11
  Bronchus DB11
  Cervix DU11
  Chest DW12
  Chest Wall DB17
  Colon DD15
  Cranial Cavity DW10BB
  Diaphragm DB18
  Duodenum DD12
  Ear D910
  Esophagus DD10
  Extremity
    Lower DW1YBB
    Upper DW1XBB
  Eye D810
  Gallbladder DF11
  Gastrointestinal Tract DW1PBB
  Genitourinary Tract DW1RBB
  Gland
    Adrenal DG12
    Parathyroid DG14
    Pituitary DG10
    Thyroid DG15
  Glands, Salivary D916
  Head and Neck DW11
  Hypopharynx D913
  Ileum DD14
  Jejunum DD13
  Kidney DT10
  Larynx D91B
  Liver DF10
  Lung DB12
  Lymphatics
    Abdomen D716
    Axillary D714
    Inguinal D718
    Neck D713
    Pelvis D717
    Thorax D715
  Mediastinum DB16
  Mouth D914
  Nasopharynx D91D
  Neck and Head DW11
  Nerve, Peripheral D017
  Nose D911
  Oropharynx D91F
  Ovary DU10
  Palate
    Hard D918
    Soft D919
  Pancreas DF13
  Parathyroid Gland DG14
  Pelvic Region DW16

Brachytherapy — *continued*
  Pineal Body DG11
  Pituitary Gland DG10
  Pleura DB15
  Prostate DV10
  Rectum DD17
  Respiratory Tract DW1QBB
  Sinuses D917
  Spinal Cord D016
  Spleen D712
  Stomach DD11
  Testis DV11
  Thymus D711
  Thyroid Gland DG15
  Tongue D915
  Trachea DB10
  Ureter DT11
  Urethra DT13
  Uterus DU12
Brachytherapy, CivaSheet®
  see Brachytherapy with qualifier Unidirectional Source
  see Insertion with device Radioactive Element
Brachytherapy seeds *use* Radioactive Element
Breast procedures, skin only *use* Skin, Chest
Broad ligament *use* Uterine Supporting Structure
Bronchial artery *use* Upper Artery
Bronchography
  see Fluoroscopy, Respiratory System BB1
  see Plain Radiography, Respiratory System BB0
Bronchoplasty
  see Repair, Respiratory System 0BQ
  see Supplement, Respiratory System 0BU
Bronchorrhaphy *see* Repair, Respiratory System 0BQ
Bronchoscopy 0BJ08ZZ
Bronchotomy *see* Drainage, Respiratory System 0B9
Bronchus Intermedius *use* Main Bronchus, Right
BRYAN® Cervical Disc System *use* Synthetic Substitute
Buccal gland *use* Buccal Mucosa
Buccinator lymph node *use* Lymphatic, Head
Buccinator muscle *use* Facial Muscle
Buckling, scleral with implant *see* Supplement, Eye 08U
Bulbospongiosus muscle *use* Perineum Muscle
Bulbourethral (Cowper's) gland *use* Urethra
Bundle of His *use* Conduction Mechanism
Bundle of Kent *use* Conduction Mechanism
Bunionectomy *see* Excision, Lower Bones 0QB
Bursectomy
  see Excision, Bursae and Ligaments 0MB
  see Resection, Bursae and Ligaments 0MT
Bursocentesis *see* Drainage, Bursae and Ligaments 0M9
Bursography
  see Plain Radiography, Non-Axial Lower Bones BQ0
  see Plain Radiography, Non-Axial Upper Bones BP0
Bursotomy
  see Division, Bursae and Ligaments 0M8
  see Drainage, Bursae and Ligaments 0M9
BVS 5000 Ventricular Assist Device *use* Short-term External Heart Assist System in Heart and Great Vessels
Bypass
  Anterior Chamber
    Left 08133
    Right 08123
  Aorta
    Abdominal 0410
    Thoracic
      Ascending/Arch 021X
      Descending 021W
  Artery
    Anterior Tibial
      Left 041Q
      Right 041P
    Axillary
      Left 03160
      Right 03150
    Brachial
      Left 03180
      Right 03170
    Common Carotid
      Left 031J0
      Right 031H0
    Common Iliac
      Left 041D
      Right 041C

Bypass — *continued*
  Artery — *continued*
    Coronary
      Four or More Arteries 0213
      One Artery 0210
      Three Arteries 0212
      Two Arteries 0211
    External Carotid
      Left 031N0
      Right 031M0
    External Iliac
      Left 041J
      Right 041H
    Femoral
      Left 041L
      Right 041K
    Foot
      Left 041W
      Right 041V
    Hepatic 0413
    Innominate 03120
    Internal Carotid
      Left 031L0
      Right 031K0
    Internal Iliac
      Left 041F
      Right 041E
    Intracranial 031G0
    Peroneal
      Left 041U
      Right 041T
    Popliteal
      Left 041N
      Right 041M
    Posterior Tibial
      Left 041S
      Right 041R
    Pulmonary
      Left 021R
      Right 021Q
    Pulmonary Trunk 021P
    Radial
      Left 031C
      Right 031B
    Splenic 0414
    Subclavian
      Left 03140
      Right 03130
    Temporal
      Left 031T0
      Right 031S0
    Ulnar
      Left 031A
      Right 0319
  Atrium
    Left 0217
    Right 0216
  Bladder 0T1B
  Cavity, Cranial 0W110J
  Cecum 0D1H
  Cerebral Ventricle 0016
  Colon
    Ascending 0D1K
    Descending 0D1M
    Sigmoid 0D1N
    Transverse 0D1L
  Duct
    Common Bile 0F19
    Cystic 0F18
    Hepatic
      Common 0F17
      Left 0F16
      Right 0F15
    Lacrimal
      Left 081Y
      Right 081X
    Pancreatic 0F1D
      Accessory 0F1F
  Duodenum 0D19
  Ear
    Left 091E0
    Right 091D0
  Esophagus 0D15
    Lower 0D13
    Middle 0D12
    Upper 0D11
  Fallopian Tube
    Left 0U16
    Right 0U15

Bypass — *continued*
Gallbladder ØF14
Ileum ØD1B
Intestine
  Large ØD1E
  Small ØD18
Jejunum ØD1A
Kidney Pelvis
  Left ØT14
  Right ØT13
Pancreas ØF1G
Pelvic Cavity ØW1J
Peritoneal Cavity ØW1G
Pleural Cavity
  Left ØW1B
  Right ØW19
Spinal Canal ØØ1U
Stomach ØD16
Trachea ØB11
Ureter
  Left ØT17
  Right ØT16
Ureters, Bilateral ØT18
Vas Deferens
  Bilateral ØV1Q
  Left ØV1P
  Right ØV1N
Vein
  Axillary
    Left Ø518
    Right Ø517
  Azygos Ø510
  Basilic
    Left Ø51C
    Right Ø51B
  Brachial
    Left Ø51A
    Right Ø519
  Cephalic
    Left Ø51F
    Right Ø51D
  Colic Ø617
  Common Iliac
    Left Ø61D
    Right Ø61C
  Esophageal Ø613
  External Iliac
    Left Ø61G
    Right Ø61F
  External Jugular
    Left Ø51Q
    Right Ø51P
  Face
    Left Ø51V
    Right Ø51T
  Femoral
    Left Ø61N
    Right Ø61M
  Foot
    Left Ø61V
    Right Ø61T
  Gastric Ø612
  Hand
    Left Ø51H
    Right Ø51G
  Hemiazygos Ø511
  Hepatic Ø614
  Hypogastric
    Left Ø61J
    Right Ø61H
  Inferior Mesenteric Ø616
  Innominate
    Left Ø514
    Right Ø513
  Internal Jugular
    Left Ø51N
    Right Ø51M
  Intracranial Ø51L
  Portal Ø618
  Renal
    Left Ø61B
    Right Ø619
  Saphenous
    Left Ø61Q
    Right Ø61P
  Splenic Ø611
  Subclavian
    Left Ø516
    Right Ø515

Bypass — *continued*
Vein — *continued*
  Superior Mesenteric Ø615
  Vertebral
    Left Ø51S
    Right Ø51R
  Vena Cava
    Inferior Ø610
    Superior Ø21V
  Ventricle
    Left Ø21L
    Right Ø21K
Bypass, cardiopulmonary 5A1221Z

C

Caesarean section *see* Extraction, Products of Conception 10D0
Calcaneocuboid joint
  use Tarsal Joint, Left
  use Tarsal Joint, Right
Calcaneocuboid ligament
  use Foot Bursa and Ligament, Left
  use Foot Bursa and Ligament, Right
Calcaneofibular ligament
  use Ankle Bursa and Ligament, Left
  use Ankle Bursa and Ligament, Right
Calcaneus
  use Tarsal, Left
  use Tarsal, Right
Cannulation
  see Bypass
  see Dilation
  see Drainage
  see Irrigation
Canthorrhaphy *see* Repair, Eye Ø8Q
Canthotomy *see* Release, Eye Ø8N
Capitate bone
  use Carpal, Left
  use Carpal, Right
Caplacizumab XWØ
Capsulectomy, lens *see* Excision, Eye Ø8B
Capsulorrhaphy, joint
  see Repair, Lower Joints ØSQ
  see Repair, Upper Joints ØRQ
Cardia *use* Esophagogastric Junction
Cardiac contractility modulation lead *use* Cardiac Lead in Heart and Great Vessels
Cardiac event recorder *use* Monitoring Device
Cardiac Lead
  Defibrillator
    Atrium
      Left Ø2H7
      Right Ø2H6
    Pericardium Ø2HN
    Vein, Coronary Ø2H4
    Ventricle
      Left Ø2HL
      Right Ø2HK
  Insertion of device in
    Atrium
      Left Ø2H7
      Right Ø2H6
    Pericardium Ø2HN
    Vein, Coronary Ø2H4
    Ventricle
      Left Ø2HL
      Right Ø2HK
  Pacemaker
    Atrium
      Left Ø2H7
      Right Ø2H6
    Pericardium Ø2HN
    Vein, Coronary Ø2H4
    Ventricle
      Left Ø2HL
      Right Ø2HK
  Removal of device from, Heart Ø2PA
  Revision of device in, Heart Ø2WA
Cardiac plexus *use* Thoracic Sympathetic Nerve
Cardiac Resynchronization Defibrillator Pulse Generator
  Abdomen ØJH8
  Chest ØJH6
Cardiac Resynchronization Pacemaker Pulse Generator
  Abdomen ØJH8

Cardiac Resynchronization Pacemaker Pulse Generator — *continued*
  Chest ØJH6
Cardiac resynchronization therapy (CRT) lead
  use Cardiac Lead, Defibrillator in Ø2H
  use Cardiac Lead, Pacemaker in Ø2H
Cardiac Rhythm Related Device
  Insertion of device in
    Abdomen ØJH8
    Chest ØJH6
  Removal of device from, Subcutaneous Tissue and Fascia, Trunk ØJPT
  Revision of device in, Subcutaneous Tissue and Fascia, Trunk ØJWT
Cardiocentesis *see* Drainage, Pericardial Cavity ØW9D
Cardioesophageal junction *use* Esophagogastric Junction
Cardiolysis *see* Release, Heart and Great Vessels Ø2N
CardioMEMS® pressure sensor *use* Monitoring Device, Pressure Sensor in Ø2H
Cardiomyotomy *see* Division, Esophagogastric Junction ØD84
Cardioplegia *see* Introduction of substance in or on, Heart 3E08
Cardiorrhaphy *see* Repair, Heart and Great Vessels Ø2Q
Cardioversion 5A2204Z
Caregiver Training FØFZ
Caroticotympanic artery
  use Internal Carotid Artery, Left
  use Internal Carotid Artery, Right
Carotid glomus
  use Carotid Bodies, Bilateral
  use Carotid Body, Left
  use Carotid Body, Right
Carotid sinus
  use Internal Carotid Artery, Left
  use Internal Carotid Artery, Right
Carotid (artery) sinus (baroreceptor) lead *use* Stimulator Lead in Upper Arteries
Carotid sinus nerve *use* Glossopharyngeal Nerve
Carotid WALLSTENT® Monorail® Endoprosthesis *use* Intraluminal Device
Carpectomy
  see Excision, Upper Bones ØPB
  see Resection, Upper Bones ØPT
Carpometacarpal ligament
  use Hand Bursa and Ligament, Left
  use Hand Bursa and Ligament, Right
Casting *see* Immobilization
CAT scan *see* Computerized Tomography (CT Scan)
Catheterization
  see Dilation
  see Drainage
  see Insertion of device in
  see Irrigation
  Heart *see* Measurement, Cardiac 4A02
  Umbilical vein, for infusion Ø6H033T
Cauda equina *use* Lumbar Spinal Cord
Cauterization
  see Destruction
  see Repair
Cavernous plexus *use* Head and Neck Sympathetic Nerve
CBMA (Concentrated Bone Marrow Aspirate) *use* Concentrated Bone Marrow Aspirate
CBMA (Concentrated Bone Marrow Aspirate) injection, intramuscular XKØ23Ø3
Cecectomy
  see Excision, Cecum ØDBH
  see Resection, Cecum ØDTH
Cecocolostomy
  see Bypass, Gastrointestinal System ØD1
  see Drainage, Gastrointestinal System ØD9
Cecopexy
  see Repair, Cecum ØDQH
  see Reposition, Cecum ØDSH
Cecoplication *see* Restriction, Cecum ØDVH
Cecorrhaphy *see* Repair, Cecum ØDQH
Cecostomy
  see Bypass, Cecum ØD1H
  see Drainage, Cecum ØD9H
Cecotomy *see* Drainage, Cecum ØD9H
Ceftazidime-Avibactam Anti-infective XWØ
Celiac ganglion *use* Abdominal Sympathetic Nerve
Celiac lymph node *use* Lymphatic, Aortic
Celiac (solar) plexus *use* Abdominal Sympathetic Nerve

Choledocholithotomy *see* Extirpation, Duct, Common Bile 0FC9
Choledochoplasty
  see Repair, Hepatobiliary System and Pancreas 0FQ
  see Replacement, Hepatobiliary System and Pancreas 0FR
  see Supplement, Hepatobiliary System and Pancreas 0FU
Choledochoscopy 0FJB8ZZ
Choledochotomy *see* Drainage, Hepatobiliary System and Pancreas 0F9
Cholelithotomy *see* Extirpation, Hepatobiliary System and Pancreas 0FC
Chondrectomy
  see Excision, Lower Joints 0SB
  see Excision, Upper Joints 0RB
  Knee *see* Excision, Lower Joints 0SB
  Semilunar cartilage *see* Excision, Lower Joints 0SB
Chondroglossus muscle *use* Tongue, Palate, Pharynx Muscle
Chorda tympani *use* Facial Nerve
Chordotomy *see* Division, Central Nervous System and Cranial Nerves 008
Choroid plexus *use* Cerebral Ventricle
Choroidectomy
  see Excision, Eye 08B
  see Resection, Eye 08T
Ciliary body
  use Eye, Left
  use Eye, Right
Ciliary ganglion *use* Head and Neck Sympathetic Nerve
Circle of Willis *use* Intracranial Artery
Circumcision 0VTTXZZ
Circumflex iliac artery
  use Femoral Artery, Left
  use Femoral Artery, Right
CivaSheet® *use* Radioactive Element
CivaSheet® Brachytherapy
  see Brachytherapy with qualifier Unidirectional Source
  see Insertion with device Radioactive Element
Clamp and rod internal fixation system (CRIF)
  use Internal Fixation Device in Lower Bones
  use Internal Fixation Device in Upper Bones
Clamping *see* Occlusion
Claustrum *use* Basal Ganglia
Claviculectomy
  see Excision, Upper Bones 0PB
  see Resection, Upper Bones 0PT
Claviculotomy
  see Division, Upper Bones 0P8
  see Drainage, Upper Bones 0P9
Clipping, aneurysm
  see Occlusion using Extraluminal Device
  see Restriction using Extraluminal Device
Clitorectomy, clitoridectomy
  see Excision, Clitoris 0UBJ
  see Resection, Clitoris 0UTJ
Clolar *use* Clofarabine
Closure
  see Occlusion
  see Repair
Clysis *see* Introduction of substance in or on
Coagulation *see* Destruction
Coagulation Factor Xa, Inactivated XW0
Coagulation Factor Xa, (Recombinant) Inactivated
  use Coagulation Factor Xa, Inactivated
COALESCE® radiolucent interbody fusion device *use* Interbody Fusion Device, Radiolucent Porous in New Technology
CoAxia NeuroFlo catheter *use* Intraluminal Device
Cobalt/chromium head and polyethylene socket *use* Synthetic Substitute, Metal on Polyethylene in 0SR
Cobalt/chromium head and socket *use* Synthetic Substitute, Metal in 0SR
Coccygeal body *use* Coccygeal Glomus
Coccygeus muscle
  use Trunk Muscle, Left
  use Trunk Muscle, Right
Cochlea
  use Inner Ear, Left
  use Inner Ear, Right
Cochlear implant (CI), multiple channel (electrode)
  use Hearing Device, Multiple Channel Cochlear Prosthesis in 09H

Cochlear implant (CI), single channel (electrode)
  use Hearing Device, Single Channel Cochlear Prosthesis in 09H
Cochlear Implant Treatment F0BZ0
Cochlear nerve *use* Acoustic Nerve
COGNIS® CRT-D *use* Cardiac Resynchronization Defibrillator Pulse Generator in 0JH
COHERE® radiolucent interbody fusion device *use* Interbody Fusion Device, Radiolucent Porous in New Technology
Colectomy
  see Excision, Gastrointestinal System 0DB
  see Resection, Gastrointestinal System 0DT
Collapse *see* Occlusion
Collection from
  Breast, Breast Milk 8E0HX62
  Indwelling Device
    Circulatory System
      Blood 8C02X6K
      Other Fluid 8C02X6L
    Nervous System
      Cerebrospinal Fluid 8C01X6J
      Other Fluid 8C01X6L
  Integumentary System, Breast Milk 8E0HX62
  Reproductive System, Male, Sperm 8E0VX63
Colocentesis *see* Drainage, Gastrointestinal System 0D9
Colofixation
  see Repair, Gastrointestinal System 0DQ
  see Reposition, Gastrointestinal System 0DS
Cololysis *see* Release, Gastrointestinal System 0DN
Colonic Z-Stent® *use* Intraluminal Device
Colonoscopy 0DJD8ZZ
Colopexy
  see Repair, Gastrointestinal System 0DQ
  see Reposition, Gastrointestinal System 0DS
Coloplication *see* Restriction, Gastrointestinal System 0DV
Coloproctectomy
  see Excision, Gastrointestinal System 0DB
  see Resection, Gastrointestinal System 0DT
Coloproctostomy
  see Bypass, Gastrointestinal System 0D1
  see Drainage, Gastrointestinal System 0D9
Colopuncture *see* Drainage, Gastrointestinal System 0D9
Colorrhaphy *see* Repair, Gastrointestinal System 0DQ
Colostomy
  see Bypass, Gastrointestinal System 0D1
  see Drainage, Gastrointestinal System 0D9
Colpectomy
  see Excision, Vagina 0UBG
  see Resection, Vagina 0UTG
Colpocentesis *see* Drainage, Vagina 0U9G
Colpopexy
  see Repair, Vagina 0UQG
  see Reposition, Vagina 0USG
Colpoplasty
  see Repair, Vagina 0UQG
  see Supplement, Vagina 0UUG
Colporrhaphy *see* Repair, Vagina 0UQG
Colposcopy 0UJH8ZZ
Columella *use* Nasal Mucosa and Soft Tissue
Common digital vein
  use Foot Vein, Left
  use Foot Vein, Right
Common facial vein
  use Face Vein, Left
  use Face Vein, Right
Common fibular nerve *use* Peroneal Nerve
Common hepatic artery *use* Hepatic Artery
Common iliac (subaortic) lymph node *use* Lymphatic, Pelvis
Common interosseous artery
  use Ulnar Artery, Left
  use Ulnar Artery, Right
Common peroneal nerve *use* Peroneal Nerve
Complete (SE) stent *use* Intraluminal Device
Compression
  see Restriction
  Abdominal Wall 2W13X
  Arm
    Lower
      Left 2W1DX
      Right 2W1CX
    Upper
      Left 2W1BX

Compression — *continued*
  Arm — *continued*
    Upper — *continued*
      Right 2W1AX
  Back 2W15X
  Chest Wall 2W14X
  Extremity
    Lower
      Left 2W1MX
      Right 2W1LX
    Upper
      Left 2W19X
      Right 2W18X
  Face 2W11X
  Finger
    Left 2W1KX
    Right 2W1JX
  Foot
    Left 2W1TX
    Right 2W1SX
  Hand
    Left 2W1FX
    Right 2W1EX
  Head 2W10X
  Inguinal Region
    Left 2W17X
    Right 2W16X
  Leg
    Lower
      Left 2W1RX
      Right 2W1QX
    Upper
      Left 2W1PX
      Right 2W1NX
  Neck 2W12X
  Thumb
    Left 2W1HX
    Right 2W1GX
  Toe
    Left 2W1VX
    Right 2W1UX
Computer Assisted Procedure
  Extremity
    Lower
      No Qualifier 8E0YXBZ
      With Computerized Tomography 8E0YXBG
      With Fluoroscopy 8E0YXBF
      With Magnetic Resonance Imaging 8E0YXBH
    Upper
      No Qualifier 8E0XXBZ
      With Computerized Tomography 8E0XXBG
      With Fluoroscopy 8E0XXBF
      With Magnetic Resonance Imaging 8E0XXBH
  Head and Neck Region
    No Qualifier 8E09XBZ
    With Computerized Tomography 8E09XBG
    With Fluoroscopy 8E09XBF
    With Magnetic Resonance Imaging 8E09XBH
  Trunk Region
    No Qualifier 8E0WXBZ
    With Computerized Tomography 8E0WXBG
    With Fluoroscopy 8E0WXBF
    With Magnetic Resonance Imaging 8E0WXBH
Computerized Tomography (CT Scan)
  Abdomen BW20
    Chest and Pelvis BW25
  Abdomen and Chest BW24
  Abdomen and Pelvis BW21
  Airway, Trachea BB2F
  Ankle
    Left BQ2H
    Right BQ2G
  Aorta
    Abdominal B420
      Intravascular Optical Coherence B420Z2Z
    Thoracic B320
      Intravascular Optical Coherence B320Z2Z
  Arm
    Left BP2F
    Right BP2E
  Artery
    Celiac B421

Computerized Tomography (CT Scan) — *continued*
Artery — *continued*
  Celiac — *continued*
    Intravascular Optical Coherence
      B421Z2Z
  Common Carotid
    Bilateral B325
    Intravascular Optical Coherence
      B325Z2Z
  Coronary
    Bypass Graft
      Intravascular Optical Coherence
        B223Z2Z
      Multiple B223
    Multiple B221
      Intravascular Optical Coherence
        B221Z2Z
  Internal Carotid
    Bilateral B328
    Intravascular Optical Coherence
      B328Z2Z
  Intracranial B32R
    Intravascular Optical Coherence
      B32RZ2Z
  Lower Extremity
    Bilateral B42H
      Intravascular Optical Coherence
        B42HZ2Z
    Left B42G
      Intravascular Optical Coherence
        B42GZ2Z
    Right B42F
      Intravascular Optical Coherence
        B42FZ2Z
  Pelvic B42C
    Intravascular Optical Coherence
      B42CZ2Z
  Pulmonary
    Left B32T
      Intravascular Optical Coherence
        B32TZ2Z
    Right B32S
      Intravascular Optical Coherence
        B32SZ2Z
  Renal
    Bilateral B428
      Intravascular Optical Coherence
        B428Z2Z
    Transplant B42M
      Intravascular Optical Coherence
        B42MZ2Z
  Superior Mesenteric B424
    Intravascular Optical Coherence
      B424Z2Z
  Vertebral
    Bilateral B32G
    Intravascular Optical Coherence
      B32GZ2Z
Bladder BT20
Bone
  Facial BN25
  Temporal BN2F
Brain B020
Calcaneus
  Left BQ2K
  Right BQ2J
Cerebral Ventricle B028
Chest, Abdomen and Pelvis BW25
Chest and Abdomen BW24
Cisterna B027
Clavicle
  Left BP25
  Right BP24
Coccyx BR2F
Colon BD24
Ear B920
Elbow
  Left BP2H
  Right BP2G
Extremity
  Lower
    Left BQ2S
    Right BQ2R
  Upper
    Bilateral BP2V
    Left BP2U
    Right BP2T
Eye
  Bilateral B827

Computerized Tomography (CT Scan) — *continued*
Eye — *continued*
  Left B826
  Right B825
Femur
  Left BQ24
  Right BQ23
Fibula
  Left BQ2C
  Right BQ2B
Finger
  Left BP2S
  Right BP2R
Foot
  Left BQ2M
  Right BQ2L
Forearm
  Left BP2K
  Right BP2J
Gland
  Adrenal, Bilateral BG22
  Parathyroid BG23
  Parotid, Bilateral B926
  Salivary, Bilateral B92D
  Submandibular, Bilateral B929
  Thyroid BG24
Hand
  Left BP2P
  Right BP2N
Hands and Wrists, Bilateral BP2Q
Head BW28
Head and Neck BW29
Heart
  Intravascular Optical Coherence B226Z2Z
  Right and Left B226
Hepatobiliary System, All BF2C
Hip
  Left BQ21
  Right BQ20
Humerus
  Left BP2B
  Right BP2A
Intracranial Sinus B522
  Intravascular Optical Coherence B522Z2Z
Joint
  Acromioclavicular, Bilateral BP23
  Finger
    Left BP2DZZZ
    Right BP2CZZZ
  Foot
    Left BQ2Y
    Right BQ2X
  Hand
    Left BP2DZZZ
    Right BP2CZZZ
  Sacroiliac BR2D
  Sternoclavicular
    Bilateral BP22
    Left BP21
    Right BP20
  Temporomandibular, Bilateral BN29
  Toe
    Left BQ2Y
    Right BQ2X
Kidney
  Bilateral BT23
  Left BT22
  Right BT21
  Transplant BT29
Knee
  Left BQ28
  Right BQ27
Larynx B92J
Leg
  Left BQ2F
  Right BQ2D
Liver BF25
Liver and Spleen BF26
Lung, Bilateral BB24
Mandible BN26
Nasopharynx B92F
Neck BW2F
Neck and Head BW29
Orbit, Bilateral BN23
Oropharynx B92F
Pancreas BF27
Patella
  Left BQ2W
  Right BQ2V

Computerized Tomography (CT Scan) — *continued*
Pelvic Region BW2G
Pelvis BR2C
  Chest and Abdomen BW25
Pelvis and Abdomen BW21
Pituitary Gland B029
Prostate BV23
Ribs
  Left BP2Y
  Right BP2X
Sacrum BR2F
Scapula
  Left BP27
  Right BP26
Sella Turcica B029
Shoulder
  Left BP29
  Right BP28
Sinus
  Intracranial B522
    Intravascular Optical Coherence
      B522Z2Z
  Paranasal B922
Skull BN20
Spinal Cord B02B
Spine
  Cervical BR20
  Lumbar BR29
  Thoracic BR27
Spleen and Liver BF26
Thorax BP2W
Tibia
  Left BQ2C
  Right BQ2B
Toe
  Left BQ2Q
  Right BQ2P
Trachea BB2F
Tracheobronchial Tree
  Bilateral BB29
  Left BB28
  Right BB27
Vein
  Pelvic (Iliac)
    Left B52G
      Intravascular Optical Coherence
        B52GZ2Z
    Right B52F
      Intravascular Optical Coherence
        B52FZ2Z
  Pelvic (Iliac) Bilateral B52H
    Intravascular Optical Coherence
      B52HZ2Z
  Portal B52T
    Intravascular Optical Coherence
      B52TZ2Z
  Pulmonary
    Bilateral B52S
      Intravascular Optical Coherence
        B52SZ2Z
    Left B52R
      Intravascular Optical Coherence
        B52RZ2Z
    Right B52Q
      Intravascular Optical Coherence
        B52QZ2Z
  Renal
    Bilateral B52L
      Intravascular Optical Coherence
        B52LZ2Z
    Left B52K
      Intravascular Optical Coherence
        B52KZ2Z
    Right B52J
      Intravascular Optical Coherence
        B52JZ2Z
  Spanchnic B52T
    Intravascular Optical Coherence
      B52TZ2Z
  Vena Cava
    Inferior B529
      Intravascular Optical Coherence
        B529Z2Z
    Superior B528
      Intravascular Optical Coherence
        B528Z2Z
Ventricle, Cerebral B028
Wrist
  Left BP2M

Computerized Tomography (CT Scan) — *continued*
Wrist — *continued*
Right BP2L
Concentrated Bone Marrow Aspirate (CBMA) injection, intramuscular XK02303
Concerto II CRT-D *use* Cardiac Resynchronization Defibrillator Pulse Generator in 0JH
Condylectomy
see Excision, Head and Facial Bones 0NB
see Excision, Lower Bones 0QB
see Excision, Upper Bones 0PB
Condyloid process
use Mandible, Left
use Mandible, Right
Condylotomy
see Division, Head and Facial Bones 0N8
see Division, Lower Bones 0Q8
see Division, Upper Bones 0P8
see Drainage, Head and Facial Bones 0N9
see Drainage, Lower Bones 0Q9
see Drainage, Upper Bones 0P9
Condylysis
see Release, Head and Facial Bones 0NN
see Release, Lower Bones 0QN
see Release, Upper Bones 0PN
Conization, cervix *see* Excision, Cervix 0UBC
Conjunctivoplasty
see Repair, Eye 08Q
see Replacement, Eye 08R
CONSERVE® PLUS Total Resurfacing Hip System
use Resurfacing Device in Lower Joints
Construction
Auricle, ear *see* Replacement, Ear, Nose, Sinus 09R
Ileal conduit *see* Bypass, Urinary System 0T1
Consulta CRT-D *use* Cardiac Resynchronization Defibrillator Pulse Generator in 0JH
Consulta CRT-P *use* Cardiac Resynchronization Pacemaker Pulse Generator in 0JH
Contact Radiation
Abdomen DWY37ZZ
Adrenal Gland DGY27ZZ
Bile Ducts DFY27ZZ
Bladder DTY27ZZ
Bone, Other DPYC7ZZ
Brain D0Y07ZZ
Brain Stem D0Y17ZZ
Breast
Left DMY07ZZ
Right DMY17ZZ
Bronchus DBY17ZZ
Cervix DUY17ZZ
Chest DWY27ZZ
Chest Wall DBY77ZZ
Colon DDY57ZZ
Diaphragm DBY87ZZ
Duodenum DDY27ZZ
Ear D9Y07ZZ
Esophagus DDY07ZZ
Eye D8Y07ZZ
Femur DPY97ZZ
Fibula DPYB7ZZ
Gallbladder DFY17ZZ
Gland
Adrenal DGY27ZZ
Parathyroid DGY47ZZ
Pituitary DGY07ZZ
Thyroid DGY57ZZ
Glands, Salivary D9Y67ZZ
Head and Neck DWY17ZZ
Hemibody DWY47ZZ
Humerus DPY67ZZ
Hypopharynx D9Y37ZZ
Ileum DDY47ZZ
Jejunum DDY37ZZ
Kidney DTY07ZZ
Larynx D9YB7ZZ
Liver DFY07ZZ
Lung DBY27ZZ
Mandible DPY37ZZ
Maxilla DPY27ZZ
Mediastinum DBY67ZZ
Mouth D9Y47ZZ
Nasopharynx D9YD7ZZ
Neck and Head DWY17ZZ
Nerve, Peripheral D0Y77ZZ
Nose D9Y17ZZ
Oropharynx D9YF7ZZ
Ovary DUY07ZZ

Contact Radiation — *continued*
Palate
Hard D9Y87ZZ
Soft D9Y97ZZ
Pancreas DFY37ZZ
Parathyroid Gland DGY47ZZ
Pelvic Bones DPY87ZZ
Pelvic Region DWY67ZZ
Pineal Body DGY17ZZ
Pituitary Gland DGY07ZZ
Pleura DBY57ZZ
Prostate DVY07ZZ
Radius DPY77ZZ
Rectum DDY77ZZ
Rib DPY57ZZ
Sinuses D9Y77ZZ
Skin
Abdomen DHY87ZZ
Arm DHY47ZZ
Back DHY77ZZ
Buttock DHY97ZZ
Chest DHY67ZZ
Face DHY27ZZ
Leg DHYB7ZZ
Neck DHY37ZZ
Skull DPY07ZZ
Spinal Cord D0Y67ZZ
Sternum DPY47ZZ
Stomach DDY17ZZ
Testis DVY17ZZ
Thyroid Gland DGY57ZZ
Tibia DPYB7ZZ
Tongue D9Y57ZZ
Trachea DBY07ZZ
Ulna DPY77ZZ
Ureter DTY17ZZ
Urethra DTY37ZZ
Uterus DUY27ZZ
Whole Body DWY57ZZ
CONTAK RENEWAL® 3 RF (HE) CRT-D *use* Cardiac Resynchronization Defibrillator Pulse Generator in 0JH
Contegra Pulmonary Valved Conduit *use* Zooplastic Tissue in Heart and Great Vessels
CONTEPO™ *use* Fosfomycin Anti-Infective
Continuous Glucose Monitoring (CGM) device *use* Monitoring Device
Continuous Negative Airway Pressure
24-96 Consecutive Hours, Ventilation 5A09459
Greater than 96 Consecutive Hours, Ventilation 5A09559
Less than 24 Consecutive Hours, Ventilation 5A09359
Continuous Positive Airway Pressure
24-96 Consecutive Hours, Ventilation 5A09457
Greater than 96 Consecutive Hours, Ventilation 5A09557
Less than 24 Consecutive Hours, Ventilation 5A09357
Continuous renal replacement therapy (CRRT) 5A1D90Z
Contraceptive Device
Change device in, Uterus and Cervix 0U2DXHZ
Insertion of device in
Cervix 0UHC
Subcutaneous Tissue and Fascia
Abdomen 0JH8
Chest 0JH6
Lower Arm
Left 0JHH
Right 0JHG
Lower Leg
Left 0JHP
Right 0JHN
Upper Arm
Left 0JHF
Right 0JHD
Upper Leg
Left 0JHM
Right 0JHL
Uterus 0UH9
Removal of device from
Subcutaneous Tissue and Fascia
Lower Extremity 0JPW
Trunk 0JPT
Upper Extremity 0JPV
Uterus and Cervix 0UPD

Contraceptive Device — *continued*
Revision of device in
Subcutaneous Tissue and Fascia
Lower Extremity 0JWW
Trunk 0JWT
Upper Extremity 0JWV
Uterus and Cervix 0UWD
Contractility Modulation Device
Abdomen 0JH8
Chest 0JH6
Control bleeding in
Abdominal Wall 0W3F
Ankle Region
Left 0Y3L
Right 0Y3K
Arm
Lower
Left 0X3F
Right 0X3D
Upper
Left 0X39
Right 0X38
Axilla
Left 0X35
Right 0X34
Back
Lower 0W3L
Upper 0W3K
Buttock
Left 0Y31
Right 0Y30
Cavity, Cranial 0W31
Chest Wall 0W38
Elbow Region
Left 0X3C
Right 0X3B
Extremity
Lower
Left 0Y3B
Right 0Y39
Upper
Left 0X37
Right 0X36
Face 0W32
Femoral Region
Left 0Y38
Right 0Y37
Foot
Left 0Y3N
Right 0Y3M
Gastrointestinal Tract 0W3P
Genitourinary Tract 0W3R
Hand
Left 0X3K
Right 0X3J
Head 0W30
Inguinal Region
Left 0Y36
Right 0Y35
Jaw
Lower 0W35
Upper 0W34
Knee Region
Left 0Y3G
Right 0Y3F
Leg
Lower
Left 0Y3J
Right 0Y3H
Upper
Left 0Y3D
Right 0Y3C
Mediastinum 0W3C
Nasal Mucosa and Soft Tissue 093K
Neck 0W36
Oral Cavity and Throat 0W33
Pelvic Cavity 0W3J
Pericardial Cavity 0W3D
Perineum
Female 0W3N
Male 0W3M
Peritoneal Cavity 0W3G
Pleural Cavity
Left 0W3B
Right 0W39
Respiratory Tract 0W3Q
Retroperitoneum 0W3H
Shoulder Region
Left 0X33

Control bleeding in — *continued*
  Shoulder Region — *continued*
    Right ØX32
  Wrist Region
    Left ØX3H
    Right ØX3G
Control, Epistaxis *see* Control bleeding in, Nasal Mucosa and Soft Tissue Ø93K
Conus arteriosus *use* Ventricle, Right
Conus medullaris *use* Lumbar Spinal Cord
Conversion
  Cardiac rhythm 5A2204Z
  Gastrostomy to jejunostomy feeding device *see* Insertion of device in, Jejunum ØDHA
Cook Biodesign® Fistula Plug(s) *use* Nonautologous Tissue Substitute
Cook Biodesign® Hernia Graft(s) *use* Nonautologous Tissue Substitute
Cook Biodesign® Layered Graft(s) *use* Nonautologous Tissue Substitute
Cook Zenaprom™ Layered Graft(s) *use* Nonautologous Tissue Substitute
Cook Zenith AAA Endovascular Graft
  use Intraluminal Device
  use Intraluminal Device, Branched or Fenestrated, One or Two Arteries in Ø4V
  use Intraluminal Device, Branched or Fenestrated, Three or More Arteries in Ø4V
Coracoacromial ligament
  use Shoulder Bursa and Ligament, Left
  use Shoulder Bursa and Ligament, Right
Coracobrachialis muscle
  use Upper Arm Muscle, Left
  use Upper Arm Muscle, Right
Coracoclavicular ligament
  use Shoulder Bursa and Ligament, Left
  use Shoulder Bursa and Ligament, Right
Coracohumeral ligament
  use Shoulder Bursa and Ligament, Left
  use Shoulder Bursa and Ligament, Right
Coracoid process
  use Scapula, Left
  use Scapula, Right
Cordotomy *see* Division, Central Nervous System and Cranial Nerves ØØ8
Core needle biopsy *see* Excision with qualifier Diagnostic
CoreValve transcatheter aortic valve *use* Zooplastic Tissue in Heart and Great Vessels
Cormet Hip Resurfacing System *use* Resurfacing Device in Lower Joints
Corniculate cartilage *use* Larynx
CoRoent® XL *use* Interbody Fusion Device in Lower Joints
Coronary arteriography
  see Fluoroscopy, Heart B21
  see Plain Radiography, Heart B20
Corox (OTW) Bipolar Lead
  use Cardiac Lead, Defibrillator in Ø2H
  use Cardiac Lead, Pacemaker in Ø2H
Corpus callosum *use* Brain
Corpus cavernosum *use* Penis
Corpus spongiosum *use* Penis
Corpus striatum *use* Basal Ganglia
Corrugator supercilii muscle *use* Facial Muscle
Cortical strip neurostimulator lead *use* Neurostimulator Lead in Central Nervous System and Cranial Nerves
Costatectomy
  see Excision, Upper Bones ØPB
  see Resection, Upper Bones ØPT
Costectomy
  see Excision, Upper Bones ØPB
  see Resection, Upper Bones ØPT
Costocervical trunk
  use Subclavian Artery, Left
  use Subclavian Artery, Right
Costochondrectomy
  see Excision, Upper Bones ØPB
  see Resection, Upper Bones ØPT
Costoclavicular ligament
  use Shoulder Bursa and Ligament, Left
  use Shoulder Bursa and Ligament, Right
Costosternoplasty
  see Repair, Upper Bones ØPQ
  see Replacement, Upper Bones ØPR
  see Supplement, Upper Bones ØPU

Costotomy
  see Division, Upper Bones ØP8
  see Drainage, Upper Bones ØP9
Costotransverse joint *use* Thoracic Vertebral Joint
Costotransverse ligament *use* Rib(s) Bursa and Ligament
Costovertebral joint *use* Thoracic Vertebral Joint
Costoxiphoid ligament *use* Sternum Bursa and Ligament
Counseling
  Family, for substance abuse, Other Family Counseling HZ63ZZZ
  Group
    12-Step HZ43ZZZ
    Behavioral HZ41ZZZ
    Cognitive HZ40ZZZ
    Cognitive-Behavioral HZ42ZZZ
    Confrontational HZ48ZZZ
    Continuing Care HZ49ZZZ
    Infectious Disease
      Post-Test HZ4CZZZ
      Pre-Test HZ4CZZZ
    Interpersonal HZ44ZZZ
    Motivational Enhancement HZ47ZZZ
    Psychoeducation HZ46ZZZ
    Spiritual HZ4BZZZ
    Vocational HZ45ZZZ
  Individual
    12-Step HZ33ZZZ
    Behavioral HZ31ZZZ
    Cognitive HZ30ZZZ
    Cognitive-Behavioral HZ32ZZZ
    Confrontational HZ38ZZZ
    Continuing Care HZ39ZZZ
    Infectious Disease
      Post-Test HZ3CZZZ
      Pre-Test HZ3CZZZ
    Interpersonal HZ34ZZZ
    Motivational Enhancement HZ37ZZZ
    Psychoeducation HZ36ZZZ
    Spiritual HZ3BZZZ
    Vocational HZ35ZZZ
  Mental Health Services
    Educational GZ60ZZZ
    Other Counseling GZ63ZZZ
    Vocational GZ61ZZZ
Countershock, cardiac 5A2204Z
Cowper's (bulbourethral) gland *use* Urethra
CPAP (continuous positive airway pressure) *see* Assistance, Respiratory 5A09
Craniectomy
  see Excision, Head and Facial Bones ØNB
  see Resection, Head and Facial Bones ØNT
Cranioplasty
  see Repair, Head and Facial Bones ØNQ
  see Replacement, Head and Facial Bones ØNR
  see Supplement, Head and Facial Bones ØNU
Craniotomy
  see Division, Head and Facial Bones ØN8
  see Drainage, Central Nervous System and Cranial Nerves ØØ9
  see Drainage, Head and Facial Bones ØN9
Creation
  Perineum
    Female ØW4NØ
    Male ØW4MØ
  Valve
    Aortic Ø24FØ
    Mitral Ø24GØ
    Tricuspid Ø24JØ
Cremaster muscle *use* Perineum Muscle
Cribriform plate
  use Ethmoid Bone, Left
  use Ethmoid Bone, Right
Cricoid cartilage *use* Trachea
Cricoidectomy *see* Excision, Larynx ØCBS
Cricothyroid artery
  use Thyroid Artery, Left
  use Thyroid Artery, Right
Cricothyroid muscle
  use Neck Muscle, Left
  use Neck Muscle, Right
Crisis Intervention GZ2ZZZZ
CRRT (Continuous renal replacement therapy) 5A1D90Z
Crural fascia
  use Subcutaneous Tissue and Fascia, Left Upper Leg

Crural fascia — *continued*
  use Subcutaneous Tissue and Fascia, Right Upper Leg
Crushing, nerve
  Cranial *see* Destruction, Central Nervous System and Cranial Nerves ØØ5
  Peripheral *see* Destruction, Peripheral Nervous System Ø15
Cryoablation *see* Destruction
Cryotherapy *see* Destruction
Cryptorchidectomy
  see Excision, Male Reproductive System ØVB
  see Resection, Male Reproductive System ØVT
Cryptorchiectomy
  see Excision, Male Reproductive System ØVB
  see Resection, Male Reproductive System ØVT
Cryptotomy
  see Division, Gastrointestinal System ØD8
  see Drainage, Gastrointestinal System ØD9
CT scan *see* Computerized Tomography (CT Scan)
CT sialogram *see* Computerized Tomography (CT Scan), Ear, Nose, Mouth and Throat B92
Cubital lymph node
  use Lymphatic, Left Upper Extremity
  use Lymphatic, Right Upper Extremity
Cubital nerve *use* Ulnar Nerve
Cuboid bone
  use Tarsal, Left
  use Tarsal, Right
Cuboideonavicular joint
  use Tarsal Joint, Left
  use Tarsal Joint, Right
Culdocentesis *see* Drainage, Cul-de-sac ØU9F
Culdoplasty
  see Repair, Cul-de-sac ØUQF
  see Supplement, Cul-de-sac ØUUF
Culdoscopy ØUJH8ZZ
Culdotomy *see* Drainage, Cul-de-sac ØU9F
Culmen *use* Cerebellum
Cultured epidermal cell autograft *use* Autologous Tissue Substitute
Cuneiform cartilage *use* Larynx
Cuneonavicular joint
  use Joint, Tarsal, Left
  use Joint, Tarsal, Right
Cuneonavicular ligament
  use Foot Bursa and Ligament, Left
  use Foot Bursa and Ligament, Right
Curettage
  see Excision
  see Extraction
Cutaneous (transverse) cervical nerve *use* Cervical Plexus
CVP (central venous pressure) *see* Measurement, Venous 4A04
Cyclodiathermy *see* Destruction, Eye Ø85
Cyclophotocoagulation *see* Destruction, Eye Ø85
CYPHER® Stent *use* Intraluminal Device, Drug-eluting in Heart and Great Vessels
Cystectomy
  see Excision, Bladder ØTBB
  see Resection, Bladder ØTTB
Cystocele repair *see* Repair, Subcutaneous Tissue and Fascia, Pelvic Region ØJQC
Cystography
  see Fluoroscopy, Urinary System BT1
  see Plain Radiography, Urinary System BT0
Cystolithotomy *see* Extirpation, Bladder ØTCB
Cystopexy
  see Repair, Bladder ØTQB
  see Reposition, Bladder ØTSB
Cystoplasty
  see Repair, Bladder ØTQB
  see Replacement, Bladder ØTRB
  see Supplement, Bladder ØTUB
Cystorrhaphy *see* Repair, Bladder ØTQB
Cystoscopy ØTJB8ZZ
Cystostomy *see* Bypass, Bladder ØT1B
Cystostomy tube *use* Drainage Device
Cystotomy *see* Drainage, Bladder ØT9B
Cystourethrography
  see Fluoroscopy, Urinary System BT1
  see Plain Radiography, Urinary System BT0
Cystourethroplasty
  see Repair, Urinary System ØTQ
  see Replacement, Urinary System ØTR

Cystourethroplasty — *continued*
  see Supplement, Urinary System ØTU
Cytarabine and Daunorubicin Liposome Antineoplastic XWØ

D

DBS lead *use* Neurostimulator Lead in Central Nervous System and Cranial Nerves
DeBakey Left Ventricular Assist Device *use* Implantable Heart Assist System in Heart and Great Vessels
Debridement
  Excisional *see* Excision
  Non-excisional *see* Extraction
Decompression, Circulatory 6A15
Decortication, lung
  see Extirpation, Respiratory System ØBC
  see Release, Respiratory System ØBN
Deep brain neurostimulator lead *use* Neurostimulator Lead in Central Nervous System and Cranial Nerves
Deep cervical fascia
  use Subcutaneous Tissue and Fascia, Left Neck
  use Subcutaneous Tissue and Fascia, Right Neck
Deep cervical vein
  use Vertebral Vein, Left
  use Vertebral Vein, Right
Deep circumflex iliac artery
  use External Iliac Artery, Left
  use External Iliac Artery, Right
Deep facial vein
  use Face Vein, Left
  use Face Vein, Right
Deep femoral artery
  use Femoral Artery, Left
  use Femoral Artery, Right
Deep femoral (profunda femoris) vein
  use Femoral Vein, Left
  use Femoral Vein, Right
Deep Inferior Epigastric Artery Perforator Flap
  Replacement
    Bilateral ØHRVØ77
    Left ØHRUØ77
    Right ØHRTØ77
  Transfer
    Left ØKXG
    Right ØKXF
Deep palmar arch
  use Hand Artery, Left
  use Hand Artery, Right
Deep transverse perineal muscle *use* Perineum Muscle
Deferential artery
  use Internal Iliac Artery, Left
  use Internal Iliac Artery, Right
Defibrillator Generator
  Abdomen ØJH8
  Chest ØJH6
Defibrotide Sodium Anticoagulant XWØ
Defitelio *use* Defibrotide Sodium Anticoagulant
Delivery
  Cesarean *see* Extraction, Products of Conception 1ØDØ
  Forceps *see* Extraction, Products of Conception 1ØDØ
  Manually assisted 1ØEØXZZ
  Products of Conception 1ØEØXZZ
  Vacuum assisted *see* Extraction, Products of Conception 1ØDØ
Delta frame external fixator
  use External Fixation Device, Hybrid in ØPH
  use External Fixation Device, Hybrid in ØPS
  use External Fixation Device, Hybrid in ØQH
  use External Fixation Device, Hybrid in ØQS
Delta III Reverse shoulder prosthesis *use* Synthetic Substitute, Reverse Ball and Socket in ØRR
Deltoid fascia
  use Subcutaneous Tissue and Fascia, Left Upper Arm
  use Subcutaneous Tissue and Fascia, Right Upper Arm
Deltoid ligament
  use Ankle Bursa and Ligament, Left
  use Ankle Bursa and Ligament, Right

Deltoid muscle
  use Shoulder Muscle, Left
  use Shoulder Muscle, Right
Deltopectoral (infraclavicular) lymph node
  use Lymphatic, Left Upper Extremity
  use Lymphatic, Right Upper Extremity
Denervation
  Cranial nerve *see* Destruction, Central Nervous System and Cranial Nerves ØØ5
  Peripheral nerve *see* Destruction, Peripheral Nervous System Ø15
Dens *use* Cervical Vertebra
Densitometry
  Plain Radiography
    Femur
      Left BQ04ZZ1
      Right BQ03ZZ1
    Hip
      Left BQ01ZZ1
      Right BQ00ZZ1
    Spine
      Cervical BR00ZZ1
      Lumbar BR09ZZ1
      Thoracic BR07ZZ1
      Whole BRØGZZ1
  Ultrasonography
    Elbow
      Left BP4HZZ1
      Right BP4GZZ1
    Hand
      Left BP4PZZ1
      Right BP4NZZ1
    Shoulder
      Left BP49ZZ1
      Right BP48ZZ1
    Wrist
      Left BP4MZZ1
      Right BP4LZZ1
Denticulate (dentate) ligament *use* Spinal Meninges
Depressor anguli oris muscle *use* Facial Muscle
Depressor labii inferioris muscle *use* Facial Muscle
Depressor septi nasi muscle *use* Facial Muscle
Depressor supercilii muscle *use* Facial Muscle
Dermabrasion *see* Extraction, Skin and Breast ØHD
Dermis *use* Skin
Descending genicular artery
  use Femoral Artery, Left
  use Femoral Artery, Right
Destruction
  Acetabulum
    Left ØQ55
    Right ØQ54
  Adenoids ØC5Q
  Ampulla of Vater ØF5C
  Anal Sphincter ØD5R
  Anterior Chamber
    Left Ø8533ZZ
    Right Ø8523ZZ
  Anus ØD5Q
  Aorta
    Abdominal
    Thoracic
      Ascending/Arch Ø25X
      Descending Ø25W
  Aortic Body ØG5D
  Appendix ØD5J
  Artery
    Anterior Tibial
      Left Ø45Q
      Right Ø45P
    Axillary
      Left Ø356
      Right Ø355
    Brachial
      Left Ø358
      Right Ø357
    Celiac Ø451
    Colic
      Left Ø457
      Middle Ø458
      Right Ø456
    Common Carotid
      Left Ø35J
      Right Ø35H
    Common Iliac
      Left Ø45D
      Right Ø45C

Destruction — *continued*
  Artery — *continued*
    External Carotid
      Left Ø35N
      Right Ø35M
    External Iliac
      Left Ø45J
      Right Ø45H
    Face Ø35R
    Femoral
      Left Ø45L
      Right Ø45K
    Foot
      Left Ø45W
      Right Ø45V
    Gastric Ø452
    Hand
      Left Ø35F
      Right Ø35D
    Hepatic Ø453
    Inferior Mesenteric Ø45B
    Innominate Ø352
    Internal Carotid
      Left Ø35L
      Right Ø35K
    Internal Iliac
      Left Ø45F
      Right Ø45E
    Internal Mammary
      Left Ø351
      Right Ø350
    Intracranial Ø35G
    Lower Ø45Y
    Peroneal
      Left Ø45U
      Right Ø45T
    Popliteal
      Left Ø45N
      Right Ø45M
    Posterior Tibial
      Left Ø45S
      Right Ø45R
    Pulmonary
      Left Ø25R
      Right Ø25Q
    Pulmonary Trunk Ø25P
    Radial
      Left Ø35C
      Right Ø35B
    Renal
      Left Ø45A
      Right Ø459
    Splenic Ø454
    Subclavian
      Left Ø354
      Right Ø353
    Superior Mesenteric Ø455
    Temporal
      Left Ø35T
      Right Ø35S
    Thyroid
      Left Ø35V
      Right Ø35U
    Ulnar
      Left Ø35A
      Right Ø359
    Upper Ø35Y
    Vertebral
      Left Ø35Q
      Right Ø35P
  Atrium
    Left Ø257
    Right Ø256
  Auditory Ossicle
    Left Ø95A
    Right Ø959
  Basal Ganglia ØØ58
  Bladder ØT5B
  Bladder Neck ØT5C
  Bone
    Ethmoid
      Left ØN5G
      Right ØN5F
    Frontal ØN51
    Hyoid ØN5X
    Lacrimal
      Left ØN5J
      Right ØN5H
    Nasal ØN5B

Destruction — *continued*

Bone — *continued*
- Occipital 0N57
- Palatine
  - Left 0N5L
  - Right 0N5K
- Parietal
  - Left 0N54
  - Right 0N53
- Pelvic
  - Left 0Q53
  - Right 0Q52
- Sphenoid 0N5C
- Temporal
  - Left 0N56
  - Right 0N55
- Zygomatic
  - Left 0N5N
  - Right 0N5M

Brain 0050

Breast
- Bilateral 0H5V
- Left 0H5U
- Right 0H5T

Bronchus
- Lingula 0B59
- Lower Lobe
  - Left 0B5B
  - Right 0B56
- Main
  - Left 0B57
  - Right 0B53
- Middle Lobe, Right 0B55
- Upper Lobe
  - Left 0B58
  - Right 0B54

Buccal Mucosa 0C54

Bursa and Ligament
- Abdomen
  - Left 0M5J
  - Right 0M5H
- Ankle
  - Left 0M5R
  - Right 0M5Q
- Elbow
  - Left 0M54
  - Right 0M53
- Foot
  - Left 0M5T
  - Right 0M5S
- Hand
  - Left 0M58
  - Right 0M57
- Head and Neck 0M50
- Hip
  - Left 0M5M
  - Right 0M5L
- Knee
  - Left 0M5P
  - Right 0M5N
- Lower Extremity
  - Left 0M5W
  - Right 0M5V
- Perineum 0M5K
- Rib(s) 0M5G
- Shoulder
  - Left 0M52
  - Right 0M51
- Spine
  - Lower 0M5D
  - Upper 0M5C
- Sternum 0M5F
- Upper Extremity
  - Left 0M5B
  - Right 0M59
- Wrist
  - Left 0M56
  - Right 0M55

Carina 0B52

Carotid Bodies, Bilateral 0G58

Carotid Body
- Left 0G56
- Right 0G57

Carpal
- Left 0P5N
- Right 0P5M

Cecum 0D5H

Cerebellum 005C

Cerebral Hemisphere 0057

Destruction — *continued*

Cerebral Meninges 0051

Cerebral Ventricle 0056

Cervix 0U5C

Chordae Tendineae 0259

Choroid
- Left 085B
- Right 085A

Cisterna Chyli 075L

Clavicle
- Left 0P5B
- Right 0P59

Clitoris 0U5J

Coccygeal Glomus 0G5B

Coccyx 0Q5S

Colon
- Ascending 0D5K
- Descending 0D5M
- Sigmoid 0D5N
- Transverse 0D5L

Conduction Mechanism 0258

Conjunctiva
- Left 085TXZZ
- Right 085SXZZ

Cord
- Bilateral 0V5H
- Left 0V5G
- Right 0V5F

Cornea
- Left 0859XZZ
- Right 0858XZZ

Cul-de-sac 0U5F

Diaphragm 0B5T

Disc
- Cervical Vertebral 0R53
- Cervicothoracic Vertebral 0R55
- Lumbar Vertebral 0S52
- Lumbosacral 0S54
- Thoracic Vertebral 0R59
- Thoracolumbar Vertebral 0R5B

Duct
- Common Bile 0F59
- Cystic 0F58
- Hepatic
  - Common 0F57
  - Left 0F56
  - Right 0F55
- Lacrimal
  - Left 085Y
  - Right 085X
- Pancreatic 0F5D
  - Accessory 0F5F
- Parotid
  - Left 0C5C
  - Right 0C5B

Duodenum 0D59

Dura Mater 0052

Ear
- External
  - Left 0951
  - Right 0950
- External Auditory Canal
  - Left 0954
  - Right 0953
- Inner
  - Left 095E
  - Right 095D
- Middle
  - Left 0956
  - Right 0955

Endometrium 0U5B

Epididymis
- Bilateral 0V5L
- Left 0V5K
- Right 0V5J

Epiglottis 0C5R

Esophagogastric Junction 0D54

Esophagus 0D55
- Lower 0D53
- Middle 0D52
- Upper 0D51

Eustachian Tube
- Left 095G
- Right 095F

Eye
- Left 0851XZZ
- Right 0850XZZ

Destruction — *continued*

Eyelid
- Lower
  - Left 085R
  - Right 085Q
- Upper
  - Left 085P
  - Right 085N

Fallopian Tube
- Left 0U56
- Right 0U55

Fallopian Tubes, Bilateral 0U57

Femoral Shaft
- Left 0Q59
- Right 0Q58

Femur
- Lower
  - Left 0Q5C
  - Right 0Q5B
- Upper
  - Left 0Q57
  - Right 0Q56

Fibula
- Left 0Q5K
- Right 0Q5J

Finger Nail 0H5QXZZ

Gallbladder 0F54

Gingiva
- Lower 0C56
- Upper 0C55

Gland
- Adrenal
  - Bilateral 0G54
  - Left 0G52
  - Right 0G53
- Lacrimal
  - Left 085W
  - Right 085V
- Minor Salivary 0C5J
- Parotid
  - Left 0C59
  - Right 0C58
- Pituitary 0G50
- Sublingual
  - Left 0C5F
  - Right 0C5D
- Submaxillary
  - Left 0C5H
  - Right 0C5G
- Vestibular 0U5L

Glenoid Cavity
- Left 0P58
- Right 0P57

Glomus Jugulare 0G5C

Humeral Head
- Left 0P5D
- Right 0P5C

Humeral Shaft
- Left 0P5G
- Right 0P5F

Hymen 0U5K

Hypothalamus 005A

Ileocecal Valve 0D5C

Ileum 0D5B

Intestine
- Large 0D5E
  - Left 0D5G
  - Right 0D5F
- Small 0D58

Iris
- Left 085D3ZZ
- Right 085C3ZZ

Jejunum 0D5A

Joint
- Acromioclavicular
  - Left 0R5H
  - Right 0R5G
- Ankle
  - Left 0S5G
  - Right 0S5F
- Carpal
  - Left 0R5R
  - Right 0R5Q
- Carpometacarpal
  - Left 0R5T
  - Right 0R5S
- Cervical Vertebral 0R51
- Cervicothoracic Vertebral 0R54
- Coccygeal 0S56

Destruction — *continued*
Joint — *continued*
Elbow
Left ØR5M
Right ØR5L
Finger Phalangeal
Left ØR5X
Right ØR5W
Hip
Left ØS5B
Right ØS59
Knee
Left ØS5D
Right ØS5C
Lumbar Vertebral ØS5Ø
Lumbosacral ØS53
Metacarpophalangeal
Left ØR5V
Right ØR5U
Metatarsal-Phalangeal
Left ØS5N
Right ØS5M
Occipital-cervical ØR5Ø
Sacrococcygeal ØS55
Sacroiliac
Left ØS58
Right ØS57
Shoulder
Left ØR5K
Right ØR5J
Sternoclavicular
Left ØR5F
Right ØR5E
Tarsal
Left ØS5J
Right ØS5H
Tarsometatarsal
Left ØS5L
Right ØS5K
Temporomandibular
Left ØR5D
Right ØR5C
Thoracic Vertebral ØR56
Thoracolumbar Vertebral ØR5A
Toe Phalangeal
Left ØS5Q
Right ØS5P
Wrist
Left ØR5P
Right ØR5N
Kidney
Left ØT51
Right ØT5Ø
Kidney Pelvis
Left ØT54
Right ØT53
Larynx ØC5S
Lens
Left Ø85K3ZZ
Right Ø85J3ZZ
Lip
Lower ØC51
Upper ØC5Ø
Liver ØF5Ø
Left Lobe ØF52
Right Lobe ØF51
Lung
Bilateral ØB5M
Left ØB5L
Lower Lobe
Left ØB5J
Right ØB5F
Middle Lobe, Right ØB5D
Right ØB5K
Upper Lobe
Left ØB5G
Right ØB5C
Lung Lingula ØB5H
Lymphatic
Aortic Ø75D
Axillary
Left Ø756
Right Ø755
Head Ø75Ø
Inguinal
Left Ø75J
Right Ø75H
Internal Mammary
Left Ø759

Destruction — *continued*
Lymphatic — *continued*
Internal Mammary — *continued*
Right Ø758
Lower Extremity
Left Ø75G
Right Ø75F
Mesenteric Ø75B
Neck
Left Ø752
Right Ø751
Pelvis Ø75C
Thoracic Duct Ø75K
Thorax Ø757
Upper Extremity
Left Ø754
Right Ø753
Mandible
Left ØN5V
Right ØN5T
Maxilla ØN5R
Medulla Oblongata ØØ5D
Mesentery ØD5V
Metacarpal
Left ØP5Q
Right ØP5P
Metatarsal
Left ØQ5P
Right ØQ5N
Muscle
Abdomen
Left ØK5L
Right ØK5K
Extraocular
Left Ø85M
Right Ø85L
Facial ØK51
Foot
Left ØK5W
Right ØK5V
Hand
Left ØK5D
Right ØK5C
Head ØK5Ø
Hip
Left ØK5P
Right ØK5N
Lower Arm and Wrist
Left ØK5B
Right ØK59
Lower Leg
Left ØK5T
Right ØK5S
Neck
Left ØK53
Right ØK52
Papillary Ø25D
Perineum ØK5M
Shoulder
Left ØK56
Right ØK55
Thorax
Left ØK5J
Right ØK5H
Tongue, Palate, Pharynx ØK54
Trunk
Left ØK5G
Right ØK5F
Upper Arm
Left ØK58
Right ØK57
Upper Leg
Left ØK5R
Right ØK5Q
Nasal Mucosa and Soft Tissue Ø95K
Nasopharynx Ø95N
Nerve
Abdominal Sympathetic Ø15M
Abducens ØØ5L
Accessory ØØ5R
Acoustic ØØ5N
Brachial Plexus Ø153
Cervical Ø151
Cervical Plexus Ø15Ø
Facial ØØ5M
Femoral Ø15D
Glossopharyngeal ØØ5P
Head and Neck Sympathetic Ø15K
Hypoglossal ØØ5S

Destruction — *continued*
Nerve — *continued*
Lumbar Ø15B
Lumbar Plexus Ø159
Lumbar Sympathetic Ø15N
Lumbosacral Plexus Ø15A
Median Ø155
Oculomotor ØØ5H
Olfactory ØØ5F
Optic ØØ5G
Peroneal Ø15H
Phrenic Ø152
Pudendal Ø15C
Radial Ø156
Sacral Ø15R
Sacral Plexus Ø15Q
Sacral Sympathetic Ø15P
Sciatic Ø15F
Thoracic Ø158
Thoracic Sympathetic Ø15L
Tibial Ø15G
Trigeminal ØØ5K
Trochlear ØØ5J
Ulnar Ø154
Vagus ØØ5Q
Nipple
Left ØH5X
Right ØH5W
Omentum ØD5U
Orbit
Left ØN5Q
Right ØN5P
Ovary
Bilateral ØU52
Left ØU51
Right ØU5Ø
Palate
Hard ØC52
Soft ØC53
Pancreas ØF5G
Para-aortic Body ØG59
Paraganglion Extremity ØG5F
Parathyroid Gland ØG5R
Inferior
Left ØG5P
Right ØG5N
Multiple ØG5Q
Superior
Left ØG5M
Right ØG5L
Patella
Left ØQ5F
Right ØQ5D
Penis ØV5S
Pericardium Ø25N
Peritoneum ØD5W
Phalanx
Finger
Left ØP5V
Right ØP5T
Thumb
Left ØP5S
Right ØP5R
Toe
Left ØQ5R
Right ØQ5Q
Pharynx ØC5M
Pineal Body ØG51
Pleura
Left ØB5P
Right ØB5N
Pons ØØ5B
Prepuce ØV5T
Prostate ØV5Ø
Robotic Waterjet Ablation XV5Ø8A4
Radius
Left ØP5J
Right ØP5H
Rectum ØD5P
Retina
Left Ø85F3ZZ
Right Ø85E3ZZ
Retinal Vessel
Left Ø85H3ZZ
Right Ø85G3ZZ
Ribs
1 to 2 ØP51
3 or More ØP52
Sacrum ØQ51

Destruction — *continued*

Scapula
  Left 0P56
  Right 0P55
Sclera
  Left 0857XZZ
  Right 0856XZZ
Scrotum 0V55
Septum
  Atrial 0255
  Nasal 095M
  Ventricular 025M
Sinus
  Accessory 095P
  Ethmoid
    Left 095V
    Right 095U
  Frontal
    Left 095T
    Right 095S
  Mastoid
    Left 095C
    Right 095B
  Maxillary
    Left 095R
    Right 095Q
  Sphenoid
    Left 095X
    Right 095W
Skin
  Abdomen 0H57XZ
  Back 0H56XZ
  Buttock 0H58XZ
  Chest 0H55XZ
  Ear
    Left 0H53XZ
    Right 0H52XZ
  Face 0H51XZ
  Foot
    Left 0H5NXZ
    Right 0H5MXZ
  Hand
    Left 0H5GXZ
    Right 0H5FXZ
  Inguinal 0H5AXZ
  Lower Arm
    Left 0H5EXZ
    Right 0H5DXZ
  Lower Leg
    Left 0H5LXZ
    Right 0H5KXZ
  Neck 0H54XZ
  Perineum 0H59XZ
  Scalp 0H50XZ
  Upper Arm
    Left 0H5CXZ
    Right 0H5BXZ
  Upper Leg
    Left 0H5JXZ
    Right 0H5HXZ
Skull 0N50
Spinal Cord
  Cervical 005W
  Lumbar 005Y
  Thoracic 005X
Spinal Meninges 005T
Spleen 075P
Sternum 0P50
Stomach 0D56
  Pylorus 0D57
Subcutaneous Tissue and Fascia
  Abdomen 0J58
  Back 0J57
  Buttock 0J59
  Chest 0J56
  Face 0J51
  Foot
    Left 0J5R
    Right 0J5Q
  Hand
    Left 0J5K
    Right 0J5J
  Lower Arm
    Left 0J5H
    Right 0J5G
  Lower Leg
    Left 0J5P
    Right 0J5N

Destruction — *continued*

Subcutaneous Tissue and Fascia — *continued*
  Neck
    Left 0J55
    Right 0J54
  Pelvic Region 0J5C
  Perineum 0J5B
  Scalp 0J50
  Upper Arm
    Left 0J5F
    Right 0J5D
  Upper Leg
    Left 0J5M
    Right 0J5L
Tarsal
  Left 0Q5M
  Right 0Q5L
Tendon
  Abdomen
    Left 0L5G
    Right 0L5F
  Ankle
    Left 0L5T
    Right 0L5S
  Foot
    Left 0L5W
    Right 0L5V
  Hand
    Left 0L58
    Right 0L57
  Head and Neck 0L50
  Hip
    Left 0L5K
    Right 0L5J
  Knee
    Left 0L5R
    Right 0L5Q
  Lower Arm and Wrist
    Left 0L56
    Right 0L55
  Lower Leg
    Left 0L5P
    Right 0L5N
  Perineum 0L5H
  Shoulder
    Left 0L52
    Right 0L51
  Thorax
    Left 0L5D
    Right 0L5C
  Trunk
    Left 0L5B
    Right 0L59
  Upper Arm
    Left 0L54
    Right 0L53
  Upper Leg
    Left 0L5M
    Right 0L5L
Testis
  Bilateral 0V5C
  Left 0V5B
  Right 0V59
Thalamus 0059
Thymus 075M
Thyroid Gland 0G5K
  Left Lobe 0G5G
  Right Lobe 0G5H
Tibia
  Left 0Q5H
  Right 0Q5G
Toe Nail 0H5RXZZ
Tongue 0C57
Tonsils 0C5P
Tooth
  Lower 0C5X
  Upper 0C5W
Trachea 0B51
Tunica Vaginalis
  Left 0V57
  Right 0V56
Turbinate, Nasal 095L
Tympanic Membrane
  Left 0958
  Right 0957
Ulna
  Left 0P5L
  Right 0P5K

Destruction — *continued*

Ureter
  Left 0T57
  Right 0T56
Urethra 0T5D
Uterine Supporting Structure 0U54
Uterus 0U59
Uvula 0C5N
Vagina 0U5G
Valve
  Aortic 025F
  Mitral 025G
  Pulmonary 025H
  Tricuspid 025J
Vas Deferens
  Bilateral 0V5Q
  Left 0V5P
  Right 0V5N
Vein
  Axillary
    Left 0558
    Right 0557
  Azygos 0550
  Basilic
    Left 055C
    Right 055B
  Brachial
    Left 055A
    Right 0559
  Cephalic
    Left 055F
    Right 055D
  Colic 0657
  Common Iliac
    Left 065D
    Right 065C
  Coronary 0254
  Esophageal 0653
  External Iliac
    Left 065G
    Right 065F
  External Jugular
    Left 055Q
    Right 055P
  Face
    Left 055V
    Right 055T
  Femoral
    Left 065N
    Right 065M
  Foot
    Left 065V
    Right 065T
  Gastric 0652
  Hand
    Left 055H
    Right 055G
  Hemiazygos 0551
  Hepatic 0654
  Hypogastric
    Left 065J
    Right 065H
  Inferior Mesenteric 0656
  Innominate
    Left 0554
    Right 0553
  Internal Jugular
    Left 055N
    Right 055M
  Intracranial 055L
  Lower 065Y
  Portal 0658
  Pulmonary
    Left 025T
    Right 025S
  Renal
    Left 065B
    Right 0659
  Saphenous
    Left 065Q
    Right 065P
  Splenic 0651
  Subclavian
    Left 0556
    Right 0555
  Superior Mesenteric 0655
  Upper 055Y
  Vertebral
    Left 055S

Destruction — *continued*
  Vein — *continued*
    Vertebral — *continued*
      Right Ø55R
  Vena Cava
    Inferior Ø65Ø
    Superior Ø25V
  Ventricle
    Left Ø25L
    Right Ø25K
  Vertebra
    Cervical ØP53
    Lumbar ØQ5Ø
    Thoracic ØP54
  Vesicle
    Bilateral ØV53
    Left ØV52
    Right ØV51
  Vitreous
    Left Ø8553ZZ
    Right Ø8543ZZ
  Vocal Cord
    Left ØC5V
    Right ØC5T
  Vulva ØU5M
Detachment
  Arm
    Lower
      Left ØX6FØZ
      Right ØX6DØZ
    Upper
      Left ØX69ØZ
      Right ØX68ØZ
  Elbow Region
    Left ØX6CØZZ
    Right ØX6BØZZ
  Femoral Region
    Left ØY68ØZZ
    Right ØY67ØZZ
  Finger
    Index
      Left ØX6PØZ
      Right ØX6NØZ
    Little
      Left ØX6WØZ
      Right ØX6VØZ
    Middle
      Left ØX6RØZ
      Right ØX6QØZ
    Ring
      Left ØX6TØZ
      Right ØX6SØZ
  Foot
    Left ØY6NØZ
    Right ØY6MØZ
  Forequarter
    Left ØX61ØZZ
    Right ØX6ØØZZ
  Hand
    Left ØX6KØZ
    Right ØX6JØZ
  Hindquarter
    Bilateral ØY64ØZZ
    Left ØY63ØZZ
    Right ØY62ØZZ
  Knee Region
    Left ØY6GØZZ
    Right ØY6FØZZ
  Leg
    Lower
      Left ØY6JØZ
      Right ØY6HØZ
    Upper
      Left ØY6DØZ
      Right ØY6CØZ
  Shoulder Region
    Left ØX63ØZZ
    Right ØX62ØZZ
  Thumb
    Left ØX6MØZ
    Right ØX6LØZ
  Toe
    1st
      Left ØY6QØZ
      Right ØY6PØZ
    2nd
      Left ØY6SØZ
      Right ØY6RØZ

Detachment — *continued*
  Toe — *continued*
    3rd
      Left ØY6UØZ
      Right ØY6TØZ
    4th
      Left ØY6WØZ
      Right ØY6VØZ
    5th
      Left ØY6YØZ
      Right ØY6XØZ
Determination, Mental status GZ14ZZZ
Detorsion
  see Release
  see Reposition
Detoxification Services, for substance abuse HZ2ZZZZ
Device Fitting FØDZ
Diagnostic Audiology *see* Audiology, Diagnostic
Diagnostic imaging *see* Imaging, Diagnostic
Diagnostic radiology *see* Imaging, Diagnostic
Dialysis
  Hemodialysis *see* Performance, Urinary 5A1D
  Peritoneal 3E1M39Z
Diaphragma sellae *use* Dura Mater
Diaphragmatic pacemaker generator *use* Stimulator Generator in Subcutaneous Tissue and Fascia
Diaphragmatic Pacemaker Lead
  Insertion of device in, Diaphragm ØBHT
  Removal of device from, Diaphragm ØBPT
  Revision of device in, Diaphragm ØBWT
Digital radiography, plain *see* Plain Radiography
Dilation
  Ampulla of Vater ØF7C
  Anus ØD7Q
  Aorta
    Abdominal
    Thoracic
      Ascending/Arch Ø27X
      Descending Ø27W
  Artery
    Anterior Tibial
      Left Ø47Q
        Sustained Release Drug-eluting
          Intraluminal Device
          X27Q385
          Four or More X27Q3C5
          Three X27Q3B5
          Two X27Q395
      Right Ø47P
        Sustained Release Drug-eluting
          Intraluminal Device
          X27P385
          Four or More X27P3C5
          Three X27P3B5
          Two X27P395
    Axillary
      Left Ø376
      Right Ø375
    Brachial
      Left Ø378
      Right Ø377
    Celiac Ø471
    Colic
      Left Ø477
      Middle Ø478
      Right Ø476
    Common Carotid
      Left Ø37J
      Right Ø37H
    Common Iliac
      Left Ø47D
      Right Ø47C
    Coronary
      Four or More Arteries Ø273
      One Artery Ø27Ø
      Three Arteries Ø272
      Two Arteries Ø271
    External Carotid
      Left Ø37N
      Right Ø37M
    External Iliac
      Left Ø47J
      Right Ø47H
    Face Ø37R
    Femoral
      Left Ø47L

Dilation — *continued*
  Artery — *continued*
    Femoral — *continued*
      Left — *continued*
        Sustained Release Drug-eluting
          Intraluminal Device
          X27J385
          Four or More X27J3C5
          Three X27J3B5
          Two X27J395
      Right Ø47K
        Sustained Release Drug-eluting
          Intraluminal Device
          X27H385
          Four or More X27H3C5
          Three X27H3B5
          Two X27H395
    Foot
      Left Ø47W
      Right Ø47V
    Gastric Ø472
    Hand
      Left Ø37F
      Right Ø37D
    Hepatic Ø473
    Inferior Mesenteric Ø47B
    Innominate Ø372
    Internal Carotid
      Left Ø37L
      Right Ø37K
    Internal Iliac
      Left Ø47F
      Right Ø47E
    Internal Mammary
      Left Ø371
      Right Ø37Ø
    Intracranial Ø37G
    Lower Ø47Y
    Peroneal
      Left Ø47U
        Sustained Release Drug-eluting
          Intraluminal Device
          X27U385
          Four or More X27U3C5
          Three X27U3B5
          Two X27U395
      Right Ø47T
        Sustained Release Drug-eluting
          Intraluminal Device
          X27T385
          Four or More X27T3C5
          Three X27T3B5
          Two X27T395
    Popliteal
      Left Ø47N
      Left Distal
        Sustained Release Drug-eluting
          Intraluminal Device
          X27N385
          Four or More X27N3C5
          Three X27N3B5
          Two X27N395
      Left Proximal
        Sustained Release Drug-eluting
          Intraluminal Device
          X27L385
          Four or More X27L3C5
          Three X27L3B5
          Two X27L395
      Right Ø47M
      Right Distal
        Sustained Release Drug-eluting
          Intraluminal Device
          X27M385
          Four or More X27M3C5
          Three X27M3B5
          Two X27M395
      Right Proximal
        Sustained Release Drug-eluting
          Intraluminal Device
          X27K385
          Four or More X27K3C5
          Three X27K3B5
          Two X27K395
    Posterior Tibial
      Left Ø47S
        Sustained Release Drug-eluting
          Intraluminal Device
          X27S385

Dilation — *continued*
  Artery — *continued*
    Posterior Tibial — *continued*
      Left — *continued*
        Sustained Release Drug-eluting Intraluminal Device — *continued*
          Four or More X27S3C5
          Three X27S3B5
          Two X27S395
        Right 047R
          Sustained Release Drug-eluting Intraluminal Device X27R385
            Four or More X27R3C5
            Three X27R3B5
            Two X27R395
    Pulmonary
      Left 027R
      Right 027Q
    Pulmonary Trunk 027P
    Radial
      Left 037C
      Right 037B
    Renal
      Left 047A
      Right 0479
    Splenic 0474
    Subclavian
      Left 0374
      Right 0373
    Superior Mesenteric 0475
    Temporal
      Left 037T
      Right 037S
    Thyroid
      Left 037V
      Right 037U
    Ulnar
      Left 037A
      Right 0379
    Upper 037Y
    Vertebral
      Left 037Q
      Right 037P
  Bladder 0T7B
  Bladder Neck 0T7C
  Bronchus
    Lingula 0B79
    Lower Lobe
      Left 0B7B
      Right 0B76
    Main
      Left 0B77
      Right 0B73
    Middle Lobe, Right 0B75
    Upper Lobe
      Left 0B78
      Right 0B74
  Carina 0B72
  Cecum 0D7H
  Cerebral Ventricle 0076
  Cervix 0U7C
  Colon
    Ascending 0D7K
    Descending 0D7M
    Sigmoid 0D7N
    Transverse 0D7L
  Duct
    Common Bile 0F79
    Cystic 0F78
    Hepatic
      Common 0F77
      Left 0F76
      Right 0F75
    Lacrimal
      Left 087Y
      Right 087X
    Pancreatic 0F7D
      Accessory 0F7F
    Parotid
      Left 0C7C
      Right 0C7B
  Duodenum 0D79
  Esophagogastric Junction 0D74
  Esophagus 0D75
    Lower 0D73
    Middle 0D72
    Upper 0D71

Dilation — *continued*
  Eustachian Tube
    Left 097G
    Right 097F
  Fallopian Tube
    Left 0U76
    Right 0U75
  Fallopian Tubes, Bilateral 0U77
  Hymen 0U7K
  Ileocecal Valve 0D7C
  Ileum 0D7B
  Intestine
    Large 0D7E
      Left 0D7G
      Right 0D7F
    Small 0D78
  Jejunum 0D7A
  Kidney Pelvis
    Left 0T74
    Right 0T73
  Larynx 0C7S
  Pharynx 0C7M
  Rectum 0D7P
  Stomach 0D76
    Pylorus 0D77
  Trachea 0B71
  Ureter
    Left 0T77
    Right 0T76
  Ureters, Bilateral 0T78
  Urethra 0T7D
  Uterus 0U79
  Vagina 0U7G
  Valve
    Aortic 027F
    Mitral 027G
    Pulmonary 027H
    Tricuspid 027J
  Vas Deferens
    Bilateral 0V7Q
    Left 0V7P
    Right 0V7N
  Vein
    Axillary
      Left 0578
      Right 0577
    Azygos 0570
    Basilic
      Left 057C
      Right 057B
    Brachial
      Left 057A
      Right 0579
    Cephalic
      Left 057F
      Right 057D
    Colic 0677
    Common Iliac
      Left 067D
      Right 067C
    Esophageal 0673
    External Iliac
      Left 067G
      Right 067F
    External Jugular
      Left 057Q
      Right 057P
    Face
      Left 057V
      Right 057T
    Femoral
      Left 067N
      Right 067M
    Foot
      Left 067V
      Right 067T
    Gastric 0672
    Hand
      Left 057H
      Right 057G
    Hemiazygos 0571
    Hepatic 0674
    Hypogastric
      Left 067J
      Right 067H
    Inferior Mesenteric 0676
    Innominate
      Left 0574
      Right 0573

Dilation — *continued*
  Vein — *continued*
    Internal Jugular
      Left 057N
      Right 057M
    Intracranial 057L
    Lower 067Y
    Portal 0678
    Pulmonary
      Left 027T
      Right 027S
    Renal
      Left 067B
      Right 0679
    Saphenous
      Left 067Q
      Right 067P
    Splenic 0671
    Subclavian
      Left 0576
      Right 0575
    Superior Mesenteric 0675
    Upper 057Y
    Vertebral
      Left 057S
      Right 057R
  Vena Cava
    Inferior 0670
    Superior 027V
  Ventricle
    Left 027L
    Right 027K
Direct Lateral Interbody Fusion (DLIF) device *use* Interbody Fusion Device in Lower Joints
Disarticulation *see* Detachment
Discectomy, diskectomy
  see Excision, Lower Joints 0SB
  see Excision, Upper Joints 0RB
  see Resection, Lower Joints 0ST
  see Resection, Upper Joints 0RT
Discography
  see Fluoroscopy, Axial Skeleton, Except Skull and Facial Bones BR1
  see Plain Radiography, Axial Skeleton, Except Skull and Facial Bones BR0
Dismembered pyeloplasty *see* Repair, Kidney Pelvis
Distal humerus
  use Humeral Shaft, Left
  use Humeral Shaft, Right
Distal humerus, involving joint
  use Elbow Joint, Left
  use Elbow Joint, Right
Distal radioulnar joint
  use Wrist Joint, Left
  use Wrist Joint, Right
Diversion *see* Bypass
Diverticulectomy *see* Excision, Gastrointestinal System 0DB
Division
  Acetabulum
    Left 0Q85
    Right 0Q84
  Anal Sphincter 0D8R
  Basal Ganglia 0088
  Bladder Neck 0T8C
  Bone
    Ethmoid
      Left 0N8G
      Right 0N8F
    Frontal 0N81
    Hyoid 0N8X
    Lacrimal
      Left 0N8J
      Right 0N8H
    Nasal 0N8B
    Occipital 0N87
    Palatine
      Left 0N8L
      Right 0N8K
    Parietal
      Left 0N84
      Right 0N83
    Pelvic
      Left 0Q83
      Right 0Q82
    Sphenoid 0N8C
    Temporal
      Left 0N86

Division — *continued*
Bone — *continued*
　　Temporal — *continued*
　　　Right 0N85
　　Zygomatic
　　　Left 0N8N
　　　Right 0N8M
Brain 0080
Bursa and Ligament
　　Abdomen
　　　Left 0M8J
　　　Right 0M8H
　　Ankle
　　　Left 0M8R
　　　Right 0M8Q
　　Elbow
　　　Left 0M84
　　　Right 0M83
　　Foot
　　　Left 0M8T
　　　Right 0M8S
　　Hand
　　　Left 0M88
　　　Right 0M87
　　Head and Neck 0M80
　　Hip
　　　Left 0M8M
　　　Right 0M8L
　　Knee
　　　Left 0M8P
　　　Right 0M8N
　　Lower Extremity
　　　Left 0M8W
　　　Right 0M8V
　　Perineum 0M8K
　　Rib(s) 0M8G
　　Shoulder
　　　Left 0M82
　　　Right 0M81
　　Spine
　　　Lower 0M8D
　　　Upper 0M8C
　　Sternum 0M8F
　　Upper Extremity
　　　Left 0M8B
　　　Right 0M89
　　Wrist
　　　Left 0M86
　　　Right 0M85
Carpal
　　Left 0P8N
　　Right 0P8M
Cerebral Hemisphere 0087
Chordae Tendineae 0289
Clavicle
　　Left 0P8B
　　Right 0P89
Coccyx 0Q8S
Conduction Mechanism 0288
Esophagogastric Junction 0D84
Femoral Shaft
　　Left 0Q89
　　Right 0Q88
Femur
　　Lower
　　　Left 0Q8C
　　　Right 0Q8B
　　Upper
　　　Left 0Q87
　　　Right 0Q86
Fibula
　　Left 0Q8K
　　Right 0Q8J
Gland, Pituitary 0G80
Glenoid Cavity
　　Left 0P88
　　Right 0P87
Humeral Head
　　Left 0P8D
　　Right 0P8C
Humeral Shaft
　　Left 0P8G
　　Right 0P8F
Hymen 0U8K
Kidneys, Bilateral 0T82
Mandible
　　Left 0N8V
　　Right 0N8T
Maxilla 0N8R

Metacarpal
　　Left 0P8Q
　　Right 0P8P
Metatarsal
　　Left 0Q8P
　　Right 0Q8N
Muscle
　　Abdomen
　　　Left 0K8L
　　　Right 0K8K
　　Facial 0K81
　　Foot
　　　Left 0K8W
　　　Right 0K8V
　　Hand
　　　Left 0K8D
　　　Right 0K8C
　　Head 0K80
　　Hip
　　　Left 0K8P
　　　Right 0K8N
　　Lower Arm and Wrist
　　　Left 0K8B
　　　Right 0K89
　　Lower Leg
　　　Left 0K8T
　　　Right 0K8S
　　Neck
　　　Left 0K83
　　　Right 0K82
　　Papillary 028D
　　Perineum 0K8M
　　Shoulder
　　　Left 0K86
　　　Right 0K85
　　Thorax
　　　Left 0K8J
　　　Right 0K8H
　　Tongue, Palate, Pharynx 0K84
　　Trunk
　　　Left 0K8G
　　　Right 0K8F
　　Upper Arm
　　　Left 0K88
　　　Right 0K87
　　Upper Leg
　　　Left 0K8R
　　　Right 0K8Q
Nerve
　　Abdominal Sympathetic 018M
　　Abducens 008L
　　Accessory 008R
　　Acoustic 008N
　　Brachial Plexus 0183
　　Cervical 0181
　　Cervical Plexus 0180
　　Facial 008M
　　Femoral 018D
　　Glossopharyngeal 008P
　　Head and Neck Sympathetic 018K
　　Hypoglossal 008S
　　Lumbar 018B
　　Lumbar Plexus 0189
　　Lumbar Sympathetic 018N
　　Lumbosacral Plexus 018A
　　Median 0185
　　Oculomotor 008H
　　Olfactory 008F
　　Optic 008G
　　Peroneal 018H
　　Phrenic 0182
　　Pudendal 018C
　　Radial 0186
　　Sacral 018R
　　Sacral Plexus 018Q
　　Sacral Sympathetic 018P
　　Sciatic 018F
　　Thoracic 0188
　　Thoracic Sympathetic 018L
　　Tibial 018G
　　Trigeminal 008K
　　Trochlear 008J
　　Ulnar 0184
　　Vagus 008Q
Orbit
　　Left 0N8Q
　　Right 0N8P

Ovary
　　Bilateral 0U82
　　Left 0U81
　　Right 0U80
Pancreas 0F8G
Patella
　　Left 0Q8F
　　Right 0Q8D
Perineum, Female 0W8NXZZ
Phalanx
　　Finger
　　　Left 0P8V
　　　Right 0P8T
　　Thumb
　　　Left 0P8S
　　　Right 0P8R
　　Toe
　　　Left 0Q8R
　　　Right 0Q8Q
Radius
　　Left 0P8J
　　Right 0P8H
Ribs
　　1 to 2 0P81
　　3 or More 0P82
Sacrum 0Q81
Scapula
　　Left 0P86
　　Right 0P85
Skin
　　Abdomen 0H87XZZ
　　Back 0H86XZZ
　　Buttock 0H88XZZ
　　Chest 0H85XZZ
　　Ear
　　　Left 0H83XZZ
　　　Right 0H82XZZ
　　Face 0H81XZZ
　　Foot
　　　Left 0H8NXZZ
　　　Right 0H8MXZZ
　　Hand
　　　Left 0H8GXZZ
　　　Right 0H8FXZZ
　　Inguinal 0H8AXZZ
　　Lower Arm
　　　Left 0H8EXZZ
　　　Right 0H8DXZZ
　　Lower Leg
　　　Left 0H8LXZZ
　　　Right 0H8KXZZ
　　Neck 0H84XZZ
　　Perineum 0H89XZZ
　　Scalp 0H80XZZ
　　Upper Arm
　　　Left 0H8CXZZ
　　　Right 0H8BXZZ
　　Upper Leg
　　　Left 0H8JXZZ
　　　Right 0H8HXZZ
Skull 0N80
Spinal Cord
　　Cervical 008W
　　Lumbar 008Y
　　Thoracic 008X
Sternum 0P80
Stomach, Pylorus 0D87
Subcutaneous Tissue and Fascia
　　Abdomen 0J88
　　Back 0J87
　　Buttock 0J89
　　Chest 0J86
　　Face 0J81
　　Foot
　　　Left 0J8R
　　　Right 0J8Q
　　Hand
　　　Left 0J8K
　　　Right 0J8J
　　Head and Neck 0J8S
　　Lower Arm
　　　Left 0J8H
　　　Right 0J8G
　　Lower Extremity 0J8W
　　Lower Leg
　　　Left 0J8P
　　　Right 0J8N

Division — *continued*
  Subcutaneous Tissue and Fascia — *continued*
    Neck
      Left 0J85
      Right 0J84
    Pelvic Region 0J8C
    Perineum 0J8B
    Scalp 0J80
    Trunk 0J8T
    Upper Arm
      Left 0J8F
      Right 0J8D
    Upper Extremity 0J8V
    Upper Leg
      Left 0J8M
      Right 0J8L
  Tarsal
    Left 0Q8M
    Right 0Q8L
  Tendon
    Abdomen
      Left 0L8G
      Right 0L8F
    Ankle
      Left 0L8T
      Right 0L8S
    Foot
      Left 0L8W
      Right 0L8V
    Hand
      Left 0L88
      Right 0L87
    Head and Neck 0L80
    Hip
      Left 0L8K
      Right 0L8J
    Knee
      Left 0L8R
      Right 0L8Q
    Lower Arm and Wrist
      Left 0L86
      Right 0L85
    Lower Leg
      Left 0L8P
      Right 0L8N
    Perineum 0L8H
    Shoulder
      Left 0L82
      Right 0L81
    Thorax
      Left 0L8D
      Right 0L8C
    Trunk
      Left 0L8B
      Right 0L89
    Upper Arm
      Left 0L84
      Right 0L83
    Upper Leg
      Left 0L8M
      Right 0L8L
  Thyroid Gland Isthmus 0G8J
  Tibia
    Left 0Q8H
    Right 0Q8G
  Turbinate, Nasal 098L
  Ulna
    Left 0P8L
    Right 0P8K
  Uterine Supporting Structure 0U84
  Vertebra
    Cervical 0P83
    Lumbar 0Q80
    Thoracic 0P84
Doppler study *see* Ultrasonography
Dorsal digital nerve *use* Radial Nerve
Dorsal metacarpal vein
  use Hand Vein, Left
  use Hand Vein, Right
Dorsal metatarsal artery
  use Foot Artery, Left
  use Foot Artery, Right
Dorsal metatarsal vein
  use Foot Vein, Left
  use Foot Vein, Right
Dorsal scapular artery
  use Subclavian Artery, Left
  use Subclavian Artery, Right

Dorsal scapular nerve *use* Brachial Plexus
Dorsal venous arch
  use Foot Vein, Left
  use Foot Vein, Right
Dorsalis pedis artery
  use Anterior Tibial Artery, Left
  use Anterior Tibial Artery, Right
DownStream® System 5A0512C, 5A0522C
Drainage
  Abdominal Wall 0W9F
  Acetabulum
    Left 0Q95
    Right 0Q94
  Adenoids 0C9Q
  Ampulla of Vater 0F9C
  Anal Sphincter 0D9R
  Ankle Region
    Left 0Y9L
    Right 0Y9K
  Anterior Chamber
    Left 0893
    Right 0892
  Anus 0D9Q
  Aorta, Abdominal 0490
  Aortic Body 0G9D
  Appendix 0D9J
  Arm
    Lower
      Left 0X9F
      Right 0X9D
    Upper
      Left 0X99
      Right 0X98
  Artery
    Anterior Tibial
      Left 049Q
      Right 049P
    Axillary
      Left 0396
      Right 0395
    Brachial
      Left 0398
      Right 0397
    Celiac 0491
    Colic
      Left 0497
      Middle 0498
      Right 0496
    Common Carotid
      Left 039J
      Right 039H
    Common Iliac
      Left 049D
      Right 049C
    External Carotid
      Left 039N
      Right 039M
    External Iliac
      Left 049J
      Right 049H
    Face 039R
    Femoral
      Left 049L
      Right 049K
    Foot
      Left 049W
      Right 049V
    Gastric 0492
    Hand
      Left 039F
      Right 039D
    Hepatic 0493
    Inferior Mesenteric 049B
    Innominate 0392
    Internal Carotid
      Left 039L
      Right 039K
    Internal Iliac
      Left 049F
      Right 049E
    Internal Mammary
      Left 0391
      Right 0390
    Intracranial 039G
    Lower 049Y
    Peroneal
      Left 049U
      Right 049T

Drainage — *continued*
  Artery — *continued*
    Popliteal
      Left 049N
      Right 049M
    Posterior Tibial
      Left 049S
      Right 049R
    Radial
      Left 039C
      Right 039B
    Renal
      Left 049A
      Right 0499
    Splenic 0494
    Subclavian
      Left 0394
      Right 0393
    Superior Mesenteric 0495
    Temporal
      Left 039T
      Right 039S
    Thyroid
      Left 039V
      Right 039U
    Ulnar
      Left 039A
      Right 0399
    Upper 039Y
    Vertebral
      Left 039Q
      Right 039P
  Auditory Ossicle
    Left 099A
    Right 0999
  Axilla
    Left 0X95
    Right 0X94
  Back
    Lower 0W9L
    Upper 0W9K
  Basal Ganglia 0098
  Bladder 0T9B
  Bladder Neck 0T9C
  Bone
    Ethmoid
      Left 0N9G
      Right 0N9F
    Frontal 0N91
    Hyoid 0N9X
    Lacrimal
      Left 0N9J
      Right 0N9H
    Nasal 0N9B
    Occipital 0N97
    Palatine
      Left 0N9L
      Right 0N9K
    Parietal
      Left 0N94
      Right 0N93
    Pelvic
      Left 0Q93
      Right 0Q92
    Sphenoid 0N9C
    Temporal
      Left 0N96
      Right 0N95
    Zygomatic
      Left 0N9N
      Right 0N9M
  Bone Marrow 079T
  Brain 0090
  Breast
    Bilateral 0H9V
    Left 0H9U
    Right 0H9T
  Bronchus
    Lingula 0B99
    Lower Lobe
      Left 0B9B
      Right 0B96
    Main
      Left 0B97
      Right 0B93
    Middle Lobe, Right 0B95
    Upper Lobe
      Left 0B98
      Right 0B94

Drainage — *continued*
Buccal Mucosa ØC94
Bursa and Ligament
  Abdomen
    Left ØM9J
    Right ØM9H
  Ankle
    Left ØM9R
    Right ØM9Q
  Elbow
    Left ØM94
    Right ØM93
  Foot
    Left ØM9T
    Right ØM9S
  Hand
    Left ØM98
    Right ØM97
  Head and Neck ØM90
  Hip
    Left ØM9M
    Right ØM9L
  Knee
    Left ØM9P
    Right ØM9N
  Lower Extremity
    Left ØM9W
    Right ØM9V
  Perineum ØM9K
  Rib(s) ØM9G
  Shoulder
    Left ØM92
    Right ØM91
  Spine
    Lower ØM9D
    Upper ØM9C
  Sternum ØM9F
  Upper Extremity
    Left ØM9B
    Right ØM99
  Wrist
    Left ØM96
    Right ØM95
Buttock
  Left ØY91
  Right ØY90
Carina ØB92
Carotid Bodies, Bilateral ØG98
Carotid Body
  Left ØG96
  Right ØG97
Carpal
  Left ØP9N
  Right ØP9M
Cavity, Cranial ØW91
Cecum ØD9H
Cerebellum ØØ9C
Cerebral Hemisphere ØØ97
Cerebral Meninges ØØ91
Cerebral Ventricle ØØ96
Cervix ØU9C
Chest Wall ØW98
Choroid
  Left Ø89B
  Right Ø89A
Cisterna Chyli Ø79L
Clavicle
  Left ØP9B
  Right ØP99
Clitoris ØU9J
Coccygeal Glomus ØG9B
Coccyx ØQ9S
Colon
  Ascending ØD9K
  Descending ØD9M
  Sigmoid ØD9N
  Transverse ØD9L
Conjunctiva
  Left Ø89T
  Right Ø89S
Cord
  Bilateral ØV9H
  Left ØV9G
  Right ØV9F
Cornea
  Left Ø899
  Right Ø898
Cul-de-sac ØU9F
Diaphragm ØB9T

Drainage — *continued*
Disc
  Cervical Vertebral ØR93
  Cervicothoracic Vertebral ØR95
  Lumbar Vertebral ØS92
  Lumbosacral ØS94
  Thoracic Vertebral ØR99
  Thoracolumbar Vertebral ØR9B
Duct
  Common Bile ØF99
  Cystic ØF98
  Hepatic
    Common ØF97
    Left ØF96
    Right ØF95
  Lacrimal
    Left Ø89Y
    Right Ø89X
  Pancreatic ØF9D
    Accessory ØF9F
  Parotid
    Left ØC9C
    Right ØC9B
Duodenum ØD99
Dura Mater ØØ92
Ear
  External
    Left Ø991
    Right Ø990
  External Auditory Canal
    Left Ø994
    Right Ø993
  Inner
    Left Ø99E
    Right Ø99D
  Middle
    Left Ø996
    Right Ø995
Elbow Region
  Left ØX9C
  Right ØX9B
Epididymis
  Bilateral ØV9L
  Left ØV9K
  Right ØV9J
Epidural Space, Intracranial ØØ93
Epiglottis ØC9R
Esophagogastric Junction ØD94
Esophagus ØD95
  Lower ØD93
  Middle ØD92
  Upper ØD91
Eustachian Tube
  Left Ø99G
  Right Ø99F
Extremity
  Lower
    Left ØY9B
    Right ØY99
  Upper
    Left ØX97
    Right ØX96
Eye
  Left Ø891
  Right Ø890
Eyelid
  Lower
    Left Ø89R
    Right Ø89Q
  Upper
    Left Ø89P
    Right Ø89N
Face ØW92
Fallopian Tube
  Left ØU96
  Right ØU95
Fallopian Tubes, Bilateral ØU97
Femoral Region
  Left ØY98
  Right ØY97
Femoral Shaft
  Left ØQ99
  Right ØQ98
Femur
  Lower
    Left ØQ9C
    Right ØQ9B
  Upper
    Left ØQ97

Drainage — *continued*
Femur — *continued*
  Upper — *continued*
    Right ØQ96
Fibula
  Left ØQ9K
  Right ØQ9J
Finger Nail ØH9Q
Foot
  Left ØY9N
  Right ØY9M
Gallbladder ØF94
Gingiva
  Lower ØC96
  Upper ØC95
Gland
  Adrenal
    Bilateral ØG94
    Left ØG92
    Right ØG93
  Lacrimal
    Left Ø89W
    Right Ø89V
  Minor Salivary ØC9J
  Parotid
    Left ØC99
    Right ØC98
  Pituitary ØG90
  Sublingual
    Left ØC9F
    Right ØC9D
  Submaxillary
    Left ØC9H
    Right ØC9G
  Vestibular ØU9L
Glenoid Cavity
  Left ØP98
  Right ØP97
Glomus Jugulare ØG9C
Hand
  Left ØX9K
  Right ØX9J
Head ØW90
Humeral Head
  Left ØP9D
  Right ØP9C
Humeral Shaft
  Left ØP9G
  Right ØP9F
Hymen ØU9K
Hypothalamus ØØ9A
Ileocecal Valve ØD9C
Ileum ØD9B
Inguinal Region
  Left ØY96
  Right ØY95
Intestine
  Large ØD9E
    Left ØD9G
    Right ØD9F
  Small ØD98
Iris
  Left Ø89D
  Right Ø89C
Jaw
  Lower ØW95
  Upper ØW94
Jejunum ØD9A
Joint
  Acromioclavicular
    Left ØR9H
    Right ØR9G
  Ankle
    Left ØS9G
    Right ØS9F
  Carpal
    Left ØR9R
    Right ØR9Q
  Carpometacarpal
    Left ØR9T
    Right ØR9S
  Cervical Vertebral ØR91
  Cervicothoracic Vertebral ØR94
  Coccygeal ØS96
  Elbow
    Left ØR9M
    Right ØR9L
  Finger Phalangeal
    Left ØR9X

⬤ **Subterms under main terms may continue to next column or page**

Drainage — *continued*
  Joint — *continued*
    Finger Phalangeal — *continued*
      Right ØR9W
    Hip
      Left ØS9B
      Right ØS99
    Knee
      Left ØS9D
      Right ØS9C
    Lumbar Vertebral ØS9Ø
    Lumbosacral ØS93
    Metacarpophalangeal
      Left ØR9V
      Right ØR9U
    Metatarsal-Phalangeal
      Left ØS9N
      Right ØS9M
    Occipital-cervical ØR9Ø
    Sacrococcygeal ØS95
    Sacroiliac
      Left ØS98
      Right ØS97
    Shoulder
      Left ØR9K
      Right ØR9J
    Sternoclavicular
      Left ØR9F
      Right ØR9E
    Tarsal
      Left ØS9J
      Right ØS9H
    Tarsometatarsal
      Left ØS9L
      Right ØS9K
    Temporomandibular
      Left ØR9D
      Right ØR9C
    Thoracic Vertebral ØR96
    Thoracolumbar Vertebral ØR9A
    Toe Phalangeal
      Left ØS9Q
      Right ØS9P
    Wrist
      Left ØR9P
      Right ØR9N
  Kidney
    Left ØT91
    Right ØT9Ø
  Kidney Pelvis
    Left ØT94
    Right ØT93
  Knee Region
    Left ØY9G
    Right ØY9F
  Larynx ØC9S
  Leg
    Lower
      Left ØY9J
      Right ØY9H
    Upper
      Left ØY9D
      Right ØY9C
  Lens
    Left Ø89K
    Right Ø89J
  Lip
    Lower ØC91
    Upper ØC9Ø
  Liver ØF9Ø
    Left Lobe ØF92
    Right Lobe ØF91
  Lung
    Bilateral ØB9M
    Left ØB9L
    Lower Lobe
      Left ØB9J
      Right ØB9F
    Middle Lobe, Right ØB9D
    Right ØB9K
    Upper Lobe
      Left ØB9G
      Right ØB9C
  Lung Lingula ØB9H
  Lymphatic
    Aortic Ø79D
    Axillary
      Left Ø796
      Right Ø795

Drainage — *continued*
  Lymphatic — *continued*
    Head Ø79Ø
    Inguinal
      Left Ø79J
      Right Ø79H
    Internal Mammary
      Left Ø799
      Right Ø798
    Lower Extremity
      Left Ø79G
      Right Ø79F
    Mesenteric Ø79B
    Neck
      Left Ø792
      Right Ø791
    Pelvis Ø79C
    Thoracic Duct Ø79K
    Thorax Ø797
    Upper Extremity
      Left Ø794
      Right Ø793
  Mandible
    Left ØN9V
    Right ØN9T
  Maxilla ØN9R
  Mediastinum ØW9C
  Medulla Oblongata ØØ9D
  Mesentery ØD9V
  Metacarpal
    Left ØP9Q
    Right ØP9P
  Metatarsal
    Left ØQ9P
    Right ØQ9N
  Muscle
    Abdomen
      Left ØK9L
      Right ØK9K
    Extraocular
      Left Ø89M
      Right Ø89L
    Facial ØK91
    Foot
      Left ØK9W
      Right ØK9V
    Hand
      Left ØK9D
      Right ØK9C
    Head ØK9Ø
    Hip
      Left ØK9P
      Right ØK9N
    Lower Arm and Wrist
      Left ØK9B
      Right ØK99
    Lower Leg
      Left ØK9T
      Right ØK9S
    Neck
      Left ØK93
      Right ØK92
    Perineum ØK9M
    Shoulder
      Left ØK96
      Right ØK95
    Thorax
      Left ØK9J
      Right ØK9H
    Tongue, Palate, Pharynx ØK94
    Trunk
      Left ØK9G
      Right ØK9F
    Upper Arm
      Left ØK98
      Right ØK97
    Upper Leg
      Left ØK9R
      Right ØK9Q
  Nasal Mucosa and Soft Tissue Ø99K
  Nasopharynx Ø99N
  Neck ØW96
  Nerve
    Abdominal Sympathetic Ø19M
    Abducens ØØ9L
    Accessory ØØ9R
    Acoustic ØØ9N
    Brachial Plexus Ø193
    Cervical Ø191

Drainage — *continued*
  Nerve — *continued*
    Cervical Plexus Ø19Ø
    Facial ØØ9M
    Femoral Ø19D
    Glossopharyngeal ØØ9P
    Head and Neck Sympathetic Ø19K
    Hypoglossal ØØ9S
    Lumbar Ø19B
    Lumbar Plexus Ø199
    Lumbar Sympathetic Ø19N
    Lumbosacral Plexus Ø19A
    Median Ø195
    Oculomotor ØØ9H
    Olfactory ØØ9F
    Optic ØØ9G
    Peroneal Ø19H
    Phrenic Ø192
    Pudendal Ø19C
    Radial Ø196
    Sacral Ø19R
    Sacral Plexus Ø19Q
    Sacral Sympathetic Ø19P
    Sciatic Ø19F
    Thoracic Ø198
    Thoracic Sympathetic Ø19L
    Tibial Ø19G
    Trigeminal ØØ9K
    Trochlear ØØ9J
    Ulnar Ø194
    Vagus ØØ9Q
  Nipple
    Left ØH9X
    Right ØH9W
  Omentum ØD9U
  Oral Cavity and Throat ØW93
  Orbit
    Left ØN9Q
    Right ØN9P
  Ovary
    Bilateral ØU92
    Left ØU91
    Right ØU9Ø
  Palate
    Hard ØC92
    Soft ØC93
  Pancreas ØF9G
  Para-aortic Body ØG99
  Paraganglion Extremity ØG9F
  Parathyroid Gland ØG9R
    Inferior
      Left ØG9P
      Right ØG9N
    Multiple ØG9Q
    Superior
      Left ØG9M
      Right ØG9L
  Patella
    Left ØQ9F
    Right ØQ9D
  Pelvic Cavity ØW9J
  Penis ØV9S
  Pericardial Cavity ØW9D
  Perineum
    Female ØW9N
    Male ØW9M
  Peritoneal Cavity ØW9G
  Peritoneum ØD9W
  Phalanx
    Finger
      Left ØP9V
      Right ØP9T
    Thumb
      Left ØP9S
      Right ØP9R
    Toe
      Left ØQ9R
      Right ØQ9Q
  Pharynx ØC9M
  Pineal Body ØG91
  Pleura
    Left ØB9P
    Right ØB9N
  Pleural Cavity
    Left ØW9B
    Right ØW99
  Pons ØØ9B
  Prepuce ØV9T

Drainage — *continued*
  Products of Conception
    Amniotic Fluid
      Diagnostic 1090
      Therapeutic 1090
    Fetal Blood 1090
    Fetal Cerebrospinal Fluid 1090
    Fetal Fluid, Other 1090
    Fluid, Other 1090
  Prostate 0V90
  Radius
    Left 0P9J
    Right 0P9H
  Rectum 0D9P
  Retina
    Left 089F
    Right 089E
  Retinal Vessel
    Left 089H
    Right 089G
  Retroperitoneum 0W9H
  Ribs
    1 to 2 0P91
    3 or More 0P92
  Sacrum 0Q91
  Scapula
    Left 0P96
    Right 0P95
  Sclera
    Left 0897
    Right 0896
  Scrotum 0V95
  Septum, Nasal 099M
  Shoulder Region
    Left 0X93
    Right 0X92
  Sinus
    Accessory 099P
    Ethmoid
      Left 099V
      Right 099U
    Frontal
      Left 099T
      Right 099S
    Mastoid
      Left 099C
      Right 099B
    Maxillary
      Left 099R
      Right 099Q
    Sphenoid
      Left 099X
      Right 099W
  Skin
    Abdomen 0H97
    Back 0H96
    Buttock 0H98
    Chest 0H95
    Ear
      Left 0H93
      Right 0H92
    Face 0H91
    Foot
      Left 0H9N
      Right 0H9M
    Hand
      Left 0H9G
      Right 0H9F
    Inguinal 0H9A
    Lower Arm
      Left 0H9E
      Right 0H9D
    Lower Leg
      Left 0H9L
      Right 0H9K
    Neck 0H94
    Perineum 0H99
    Scalp 0H90
    Upper Arm
      Left 0H9C
      Right 0H9B
    Upper Leg
      Left 0H9J
      Right 0H9H
  Skull 0N90
  Spinal Canal 009U
  Spinal Cord
    Cervical 009W
    Lumbar 009Y

Drainage — *continued*
  Spinal Cord — *continued*
    Thoracic 009X
  Spinal Meninges 009T
  Spleen 079P
  Sternum 0P90
  Stomach 0D96
    Pylorus 0D97
  Subarachnoid Space, Intracranial 0095
  Subcutaneous Tissue and Fascia
    Abdomen 0J98
    Back 0J97
    Buttock 0J99
    Chest 0J96
    Face 0J91
    Foot
      Left 0J9R
      Right 0J9Q
    Hand
      Left 0J9K
      Right 0J9J
    Lower Arm
      Left 0J9H
      Right 0J9G
    Lower Leg
      Left 0J9P
      Right 0J9N
    Neck
      Left 0J95
      Right 0J94
    Pelvic Region 0J9C
    Perineum 0J9B
    Scalp 0J90
    Upper Arm
      Left 0J9F
      Right 0J9D
    Upper Leg
      Left 0J9M
      Right 0J9L
  Subdural Space, Intracranial 0094
  Tarsal
    Left 0Q9M
    Right 0Q9L
  Tendon
    Abdomen
      Left 0L9G
      Right 0L9F
    Ankle
      Left 0L9T
      Right 0L9S
    Foot
      Left 0L9W
      Right 0L9V
    Hand
      Left 0L98
      Right 0L97
    Head and Neck 0L90
    Hip
      Left 0L9K
      Right 0L9J
    Knee
      Left 0L9R
      Right 0L9Q
    Lower Arm and Wrist
      Left 0L96
      Right 0L95
    Lower Leg
      Left 0L9P
      Right 0L9N
    Perineum 0L9H
    Shoulder
      Left 0L92
      Right 0L91
    Thorax
      Left 0L9D
      Right 0L9C
    Trunk
      Left 0L9B
      Right 0L99
    Upper Arm
      Left 0L94
      Right 0L93
    Upper Leg
      Left 0L9M
      Right 0L9L
  Testis
    Bilateral 0V9C
    Left 0V9B
    Right 0V99

Drainage — *continued*
  Thalamus 0099
  Thymus 079M
  Thyroid Gland 0G9K
    Left Lobe 0G9G
    Right Lobe 0G9H
  Tibia
    Left 0Q9H
    Right 0Q9G
  Toe Nail 0H9R
  Tongue 0C97
  Tonsils 0C9P
  Tooth
    Lower 0C9X
    Upper 0C9W
  Trachea 0B91
  Tunica Vaginalis
    Left 0V97
    Right 0V96
  Turbinate, Nasal 099L
  Tympanic Membrane
    Left 0998
    Right 0997
  Ulna
    Left 0P9L
    Right 0P9K
  Ureter
    Left 0T97
    Right 0T96
  Ureters, Bilateral 0T98
  Urethra 0T9D
  Uterine Supporting Structure 0U94
  Uterus 0U99
  Uvula 0C9N
  Vagina 0U9G
  Vas Deferens
    Bilateral 0V9Q
    Left 0V9P
    Right 0V9N
  Vein
    Axillary
      Left 0598
      Right 0597
    Azygos 0590
    Basilic
      Left 059C
      Right 059B
    Brachial
      Left 059A
      Right 0599
    Cephalic
      Left 059F
      Right 059D
    Colic 0697
    Common Iliac
      Left 069D
      Right 069C
    Esophageal 0693
    External Iliac
      Left 069G
      Right 069F
    External Jugular
      Left 059Q
      Right 059P
    Face
      Left 059V
      Right 059T
    Femoral
      Left 069N
      Right 069M
    Foot
      Left 069V
      Right 069T
    Gastric 0692
    Hand
      Left 059H
      Right 059G
    Hemiazygos 0591
    Hepatic 0694
    Hypogastric
      Left 069J
      Right 069H
    Inferior Mesenteric 0696
    Innominate
      Left 0594
      Right 0593
    Internal Jugular
      Left 059N
      Right 059M

▽ Subterms under main terms may continue to next column or page

Drainage — *continued*
  Vein — *continued*
    Intracranial Ø59L
    Lower Ø69Y
    Portal Ø698
    Renal
      Left Ø69B
      Right Ø699
    Saphenous
      Left Ø69Q
      Right Ø69P
    Splenic Ø691
    Subclavian
      Left Ø596
      Right Ø595
    Superior Mesenteric Ø695
    Upper Ø59Y
    Vertebral
      Left Ø59S
      Right Ø59R
    Vena Cava, Inferior Ø69Ø
  Vertebra
    Cervical ØP93
    Lumbar ØQ9Ø
    Thoracic ØP94
  Vesicle
    Bilateral ØV93
    Left ØV92
    Right ØV91
  Vitreous
    Left Ø895
    Right Ø894
  Vocal Cord
    Left ØC9V
    Right ØC9T
  Vulva ØU9M
  Wrist Region
    Left ØX9H
    Right ØX9G
Dressing
  Abdominal Wall 2W23X4Z
  Arm
    Lower
      Left 2W2DX4Z
      Right 2W2CX4Z
    Upper
      Left 2W2BX4Z
      Right 2W2AX4Z
  Back 2W25X4Z
  Chest Wall 2W24X4Z
  Extremity
    Lower
      Left 2W2MX4Z
      Right 2W2LX4Z
    Upper
      Left 2W29X4Z
      Right 2W28X4Z
  Face 2W21X4Z
  Finger
    Left 2W2KX4Z
    Right 2W2JX4Z
  Foot
    Left 2W2TX4Z
    Right 2W2SX4Z
  Hand
    Left 2W2FX4Z
    Right 2W2EX4Z
  Head 2W2ØX4Z
  Inguinal Region
    Left 2W27X4Z
    Right 2W26X4Z
  Leg
    Lower
      Left 2W2RX4Z
      Right 2W2QX4Z
    Upper
      Left 2W2PX4Z
      Right 2W2NX4Z
  Neck 2W22X4Z
  Thumb
    Left 2W2HX4Z
    Right 2W2GX4Z
  Toe
    Left 2W2VX4Z
    Right 2W2UX4Z
Driver stent (RX) (OTW) *use* Intraluminal Device
Drotrecogin alfa, infusion *see* Introduction of Recombinant Human-activated Protein C
Duct of Santorini *use* Pancreatic Duct, Accessory

Duct of Wirsung *use* Pancreatic Duct
Ductogram, mammary *see* Plain Radiography, Skin, Subcutaneous Tissue and Breast BHØ
Ductography, mammary *see* Plain Radiography, Skin, Subcutaneous Tissue and Breast BHØ
Ductus deferens
  use Vas Deferens
  use Vas Deferens, Bilateral
  use Vas Deferens, Left
  use Vas Deferens, Right
Duodenal ampulla *use* Ampulla of Vater
Duodenectomy
  see Excision, Duodenum ØDB9
  see Resection, Duodenum ØDT9
Duodenocholedochotomy *see* Drainage, Gallbladder ØF94
Duodenocystostomy
  see Bypass, Gallbladder ØF14
  see Drainage, Gallbladder ØF94
Duodenoenterostomy
  see Bypass, Gastrointestinal System ØD1
  see Drainage, Gastrointestinal System ØD9
Duodenojejunal flexure *use* Jejunum
Duodenolysis *see* Release, Duodenum ØDN9
Duodenorrhaphy *see* Repair, Duodenum ØDQ9
Duodenostomy
  see Bypass, Duodenum ØD19
  see Drainage, Duodenum ØD99
Duodenotomy *see* Drainage, Duodenum ØD99
Dura mater, intracranial *use* Dura Mater
Dura mater, spinal *use* Spinal Meninges
DuraGraft® Endothelial Damage Inhibitor *use* Endothelial Damage Inhibitor
DuraHeart Left Ventricular Assist System *use* Implantable Heart Assist System in Heart and Great Vessels
Dural venous sinus *use* Intracranial Vein
Durata® Defibrillation Lead *use* Cardiac Lead, Defibrillator in Ø2H
Dynesys® Dynamic Stabilization System
  use Spinal Stabilization Device, Pedicle-Based in ØRH
  use Spinal Stabilization Device, Pedicle-Based in ØSH

E

Earlobe
  use Ear, External, Bilateral
  use Ear, External, Left
  use Ear, External, Right
ECCO2R (Extracorporeal Carbon Dioxide Removal) 5AØ92ØZ
Echocardiogram *see* Ultrasonography, Heart B24
Echography *see* Ultrasonography
ECMO *see* Performance, Circulatory 5A15
ECMO, intraoperative *see* Performance, Circulatory 5A15A
EDWARDS INTUITY Elite valve system *use* Zooplastic Tissue, Rapid Deployment Technique in New Technology
EEG (electroencephalogram) *see* Measurement, Central Nervous 4AØØ
EGD (esophagogastroduodenoscopy) ØDJØ8ZZ
Eighth cranial nerve *use* Acoustic Nerve
Ejaculatory duct
  use Vas Deferens
  use Vas Deferens, Bilateral
  use Vas Deferens, Left
  use Vas Deferens, Right
EKG (electrocardiogram) *see* Measurement, Cardiac 4AØ2
Electrical bone growth stimulator (EBGS)
  use Bone Growth Stimulator in Head and Facial Bones
  use Bone Growth Stimulator in Lower Bones
  use Bone Growth Stimulator in Upper Bones
Electrical muscle stimulation (EMS) lead *use* Stimulator Lead in Muscles
Electrocautery
  Destruction *see* Destruction
  Repair *see* Repair
Electroconvulsive Therapy
  Bilateral-Multiple Seizure GZB3ZZZ
  Bilateral-Single Seizure GZB2ZZZ
  Electroconvulsive Therapy, Other GZB4ZZZ

Electroconvulsive Therapy — *continued*
  Unilateral-Multiple Seizure GZB1ZZZ
  Unilateral-Single Seizure GZBØZZZ
Electroencephalogram (EEG) *see* Measurement, Central Nervous 4AØØ
Electromagnetic Therapy
  Central Nervous 6A22
  Urinary 6A21
Electronic muscle stimulator lead *use* Stimulator Lead in Muscles
Electrophysiologic stimulation (EPS) *see* Measurement, Cardiac 4AØ2
Electroshock therapy *see* Electroconvulsive Therapy
Elevation, bone fragments, skull *see* Reposition, Head and Facial Bones ØNS
Eleventh cranial nerve *use* Accessory Nerve
Ellipsys® vascular access system
  Radial Artery, Left Ø31C3ZF
  Radial Artery, Right Ø31B3ZF
  Ulnar Artery, Left Ø31A3ZF
  Ulnar Artery, Right Ø3193ZF
E-Luminexx™ (Biliary) (Vascular) Stent *use* Intraluminal Device
Eluvia™ Drug-Eluting Vascular Stent System
  use Intraluminal Device, Sustained Release Drug-eluting in New Technology
  use Intraluminal Device, Sustained Release Drug-eluting, Two in New Technology
  use Intraluminal Device, Sustained Release Drug-eluting, Three in New Technology
  use Intraluminal Device, Sustained Release Drug-eluting, Four or More in New Technology
ELZONRIS™ *use* Tagraxofusp-erzs Antineoplastic
Embolectomy *see* Extirpation
Embolization
  see Occlusion
  see Restriction
Embolization coil(s) *use* Intraluminal Device
EMG (electromyogram) *see* Measurement, Musculoskeletal 4AØF
Encephalon *use* Brain
Endarterectomy
  see Extirpation, Lower Arteries Ø4C
  see Extirpation, Upper Arteries Ø3C
Endeavor® (III) (IV) (Sprint) Zotarolimus-eluting Coronary Stent System *use* Intraluminal Device, Drug-eluting in Heart and Great Vessels
EndoAVF procedure
  Radial Artery, Left Ø31C3ZF
  Radial Artery, Right Ø31B3ZF
  Ulnar Artery, Left Ø31A3ZF
  Ulnar Artery, Right Ø3193ZF
Endologix® AFX Endovascular AAA System *use* Intraluminal Device
EndoSure® sensor *use* Monitoring Device, Pressure Sensor in Ø2H
ENDOTAK RELIANCE® (G) Defibrillation Lead *use* Cardiac Lead, Defibrillator in Ø2H
Endothelial damage inhibitor, applied to vein graft XYØVX83
Endotracheal tube (cuffed) (double-lumen) *use* Intraluminal Device, Endotracheal Airway in Respiratory System
Endovascular fistula creation
  Radial Artery, Left Ø31C3ZF
  Radial Artery, Right Ø31B3ZF
  Ulnar Artery, Left Ø31A3ZF
  Ulnar Artery, Right Ø3193ZF
Endurant® Endovascular Stent Graft *use* Intraluminal Device
Endurant® II AAA stent graft system *use* Intraluminal Device
Engineered Autologous Chimeric Antigen Receptor T-cell Immunotherapy XWØ
Enlargement
  see Dilation
  see Repair
EnRhythm *use* Pacemaker, Dual Chamber in ØJH
Enterorrhaphy *see* Repair, Gastrointestinal System ØDQ
Enterra gastric neurostimulator *use* Stimulator Generator, Multiple Array in ØJH
Enucleation
  Eyeball *see* Resection, Eye Ø8T
  Eyeball with prosthetic implant *see* Replacement, Eye Ø8R
Ependyma *use* Cerebral Ventricle

Epicel® cultured epidermal autograft *use* Autologous Tissue Substitute
Epic™ Stented Tissue Valve (aortic) *use* Zooplastic Tissue in Heart and Great Vessels
Epidermis *use* Skin
Epididymectomy
see Excision, Male Reproductive System ØVB
see Resection, Male Reproductive System ØVT
Epididymoplasty
see Repair, Male Reproductive System ØVQ
see Supplement, Male Reproductive System ØVU
Epididymorrhaphy *see* Repair, Male Reproductive System ØVQ
Epididymotomy *see* Drainage, Male Reproductive System ØV9
Epidural space, spinal *use* Spinal Canal
Epiphysiodesis
see Insertion of device in, Lower Bones ØQH
see Insertion of device in, Upper Bones ØPH
see Repair, Lower Bones ØQQ
see Repair, Upper Bones ØPQ
Epiploic foramen *use* Peritoneum
Epiretinal Visual Prosthesis
Left Ø8H105Z
Right Ø8H0Ø5Z
Episiorrhaphy *see* Repair, Perineum, Female ØWQN
Episiotomy *see* Division, Perineum, Female ØW8N
Epithalamus *use* Thalamus
Epitrochlear lymph node
use Lymphatic, Left Upper Extremity
use Lymphatic, Right Upper Extremity
EPS (electrophysiologic stimulation) *see* Measurement, Cardiac 4AØ2
Eptifibatide, infusion *see* Introduction of Platelet Inhibitor
ERCP (endoscopic retrograde cholangiopancreatography) *see* Fluoroscopy, Hepatobiliary System and Pancreas BF1
Erdafitinib Antineoplastic XWØDXL5
Erector spinae muscle
use Trunk Muscle, Left
use Trunk Muscle, Right
ERLEADA™ *use* Apalutamide Antineoplastic
Esophageal artery *use* Upper Artery
Esophageal obturator airway (EOA) *use* Intraluminal Device, Airway in Gastrointestinal System
Esophageal plexus *use* Thoracic Sympathetic Nerve
Esophagectomy
see Excision, Gastrointestinal System ØDB
see Resection, Gastrointestinal System ØDT
Esophagocoloplasty
see Repair, Gastrointestinal System ØDQ
see Supplement, Gastrointestinal System ØDU
Esophagoenterostomy
see Bypass, Gastrointestinal System ØD1
see Drainage, Gastrointestinal System ØD9
Esophagoesophagostomy
see Bypass, Gastrointestinal System ØD1
see Drainage, Gastrointestinal System ØD9
Esophagogastrectomy
see Excision, Gastrointestinal System ØDB
see Resection, Gastrointestinal System ØDT
Esophagogastroduodenoscopy (EGD) ØDJØ8ZZ
Esophagogastroplasty
see Repair, Gastrointestinal System ØDQ
see Supplement, Gastrointestinal System ØDU
Esophagogastroscopy ØDJ68ZZ
Esophagogastrostomy
see Bypass, Gastrointestinal System ØD1
see Drainage, Gastrointestinal System ØD9
Esophagojejunoplasty *see* Supplement, Gastrointestinal System ØDU
Esophagojejunostomy
see Bypass, Gastrointestinal System ØD1
see Drainage, Gastrointestinal System ØD9
Esophagomyotomy *see* Division, Esophagogastric Junction ØD84
Esophagoplasty
see Repair, Gastrointestinal System ØDQ
see Replacement, Esophagus ØDR5
see Supplement, Gastrointestinal System ØDU
Esophagoplication *see* Restriction, Gastrointestinal System ØDV
Esophagorrhaphy *see* Repair, Gastrointestinal System ØDQ
Esophagoscopy ØDJØ8ZZ

Esophagotomy *see* Drainage, Gastrointestinal System ØD9
Esteem® implantable hearing system *use* Hearing Device in Ear, Nose, Sinus
ESWL (extracorporeal shock wave lithotripsy) *see* Fragmentation
Ethmoidal air cell
use Ethmoid Sinus, Left
use Ethmoid Sinus, Right
Ethmoidectomy
see Excision, Ear, Nose, Sinus Ø9B
see Excision, Head and Facial Bones ØNB
see Resection, Ear, Nose, Sinus Ø9T
see Resection, Head and Facial Bones ØNT
Ethmoidotomy *see* Drainage, Ear, Nose, Sinus Ø99
Evacuation
Hematoma *see* Extirpation
Other Fluid *see* Drainage
Evera (XT) (S) (DR/VR) *use* Defibrillator Generator in ØJH
Everolimus-eluting coronary stent *use* Intraluminal Device, Drug-eluting in Heart and Great Vessels
Evisceration
Eyeball *see* Resection, Eye Ø8T
Eyeball with prosthetic implant *see* Replacement, Eye Ø8R
Examination *see* Inspection
Exchange *see* Change device in
Excision
Abdominal Wall ØWBF
Acetabulum
Left ØQB5
Right ØQB4
Adenoids ØCBQ
Ampulla of Vater ØFBC
Anal Sphincter ØDBR
Ankle Region
Left ØYBL
Right ØYBK
Anus ØDBQ
Aorta
Abdominal
Thoracic
Ascending/Arch Ø2BX
Descending Ø2BW
Aortic Body ØGBD
Appendix ØDBJ
Arm
Lower
Left ØXBF
Right ØXBD
Upper
Left ØXB9
Right ØXB8
Artery
Anterior Tibial
Left Ø4BQ
Right Ø4BP
Axillary
Left Ø3B6
Right Ø3B5
Brachial
Left Ø3B8
Right Ø3B7
Celiac Ø4B1
Colic
Left Ø4B7
Middle Ø4B8
Right Ø4B6
Common Carotid
Left Ø3BJ
Right Ø3BH
Common Iliac
Left Ø4BD
Right Ø4BC
External Carotid
Left Ø3BN
Right Ø3BM
External Iliac
Left Ø4BJ
Right Ø4BH
Face Ø3BR
Femoral
Left Ø4BL
Right Ø4BK
Foot
Left Ø4BW
Right Ø4BV

Excision — *continued*
Artery — *continued*
Gastric Ø4B2
Hand
Left Ø3BF
Right Ø3BD
Hepatic Ø4B3
Inferior Mesenteric Ø4BB
Innominate Ø3B2
Internal Carotid
Left Ø3BL
Right Ø3BK
Internal Iliac
Left Ø4BF
Right Ø4BE
Internal Mammary
Left Ø3B1
Right Ø3BØ
Intracranial Ø3BG
Lower Ø4BY
Peroneal
Left Ø4BU
Right Ø4BT
Popliteal
Left Ø4BN
Right Ø4BM
Posterior Tibial
Left Ø4BS
Right Ø4BR
Pulmonary
Left Ø2BR
Right Ø2BQ
Pulmonary Trunk Ø2BP
Radial
Left Ø3BC
Right Ø3BB
Renal
Left Ø4BA
Right Ø4B9
Splenic Ø4B4
Subclavian
Left Ø3B4
Right Ø3B3
Superior Mesenteric Ø4B5
Temporal
Left Ø3BT
Right Ø3BS
Thyroid
Left Ø3BV
Right Ø3BU
Ulnar
Left Ø3BA
Right Ø3B9
Upper Ø3BY
Vertebral
Left Ø3BQ
Right Ø3BP
Atrium
Left Ø2B7
Right Ø2B6
Auditory Ossicle
Left Ø9BA
Right Ø9B9
Axilla
Left ØXB5
Right ØXB4
Back
Lower ØWBL
Upper ØWBK
Basal Ganglia ØØB8
Bladder ØTBB
Bladder Neck ØTBC
Bone
Ethmoid
Left ØNBG
Right ØNBF
Frontal ØNB1
Hyoid ØNBX
Lacrimal
Left ØNBJ
Right ØNBH
Nasal ØNBB
Occipital ØNB7
Palatine
Left ØNBL
Right ØNBK
Parietal
Left ØNB4
Right ØNB3

Excision — continued
  Bone — continued
    Pelvic
      Left ØQB3
      Right ØQB2
    Sphenoid ØNBC
    Temporal
      Left ØNB6
      Right ØNB5
    Zygomatic
      Left ØNBN
      Right ØNBM
  Brain ØØBØ
  Breast
    Bilateral ØHBV
    Left ØHBU
    Right ØHBT
    Supernumerary ØHBY
  Bronchus
    Lingula ØBB9
    Lower Lobe
      Left ØBBB
      Right ØBB6
    Main
      Left ØBB7
      Right ØBB3
    Middle Lobe, Right ØBB5
    Upper Lobe
      Left ØBB8
      Right ØBB4
  Buccal Mucosa ØCB4
  Bursa and Ligament
    Abdomen
      Left ØMBJ
      Right ØMBH
    Ankle
      Left ØMBR
      Right ØMBQ
    Elbow
      Left ØMB4
      Right ØMB3
    Foot
      Left ØMBT
      Right ØMBS
    Hand
      Left ØMB8
      Right ØMB7
    Head and Neck ØMBØ
    Hip
      Left ØMBM
      Right ØMBL
    Knee
      Left ØMBP
      Right ØMBN
    Lower Extremity
      Left ØMBW
      Right ØMBV
    Perineum ØMBK
    Rib(s) ØMBG
    Shoulder
      Left ØMB2
      Right ØMB1
    Spine
      Lower ØMBD
      Upper ØMBC
    Sternum ØMBF
    Upper Extremity
      Left ØMBB
      Right ØMB9
    Wrist
      Left ØMB6
      Right ØMB5
  Buttock
    Left ØYB1
    Right ØYBØ
  Carina ØBB2
  Carotid Bodies, Bilateral ØGB8
  Carotid Body
    Left ØGB6
    Right ØGB7
  Carpal
    Left ØPBN
    Right ØPBM
  Cecum ØDBH
  Cerebellum ØØBC
  Cerebral Hemisphere ØØB7
  Cerebral Meninges ØØB1
  Cerebral Ventricle ØØB6
  Cervix ØUBC

Excision — continued
  Chest Wall ØWB8
  Chordae Tendineae Ø2B9
  Choroid
    Left Ø8BB
    Right Ø8BA
  Cisterna Chyli Ø7BL
  Clavicle
    Left ØPBB
    Right ØPB9
  Clitoris ØUBJ
  Coccygeal Glomus ØGBB
  Coccyx ØQBS
  Colon
    Ascending ØDBK
    Descending ØDBM
    Sigmoid ØDBN
    Transverse ØDBL
  Conduction Mechanism Ø2B8
  Conjunctiva
    Left Ø8BTXZ
    Right Ø8BSXZ
  Cord
    Bilateral ØVBH
    Left ØVBG
    Right ØVBF
  Cornea
    Left Ø8B9XZ
    Right Ø8B8XZ
  Cul-de-sac ØUBF
  Diaphragm ØBBT
  Disc
    Cervical Vertebral ØRB3
    Cervicothoracic Vertebral ØRB5
    Lumbar Vertebral ØSB2
    Lumbosacral ØSB4
    Thoracic Vertebral ØRB9
    Thoracolumbar Vertebral ØRBB
  Duct
    Common Bile ØFB9
    Cystic ØFB8
    Hepatic
      Common ØFB7
      Left ØFB6
      Right ØFB5
    Lacrimal
      Left Ø8BY
      Right Ø8BX
    Pancreatic ØFBD
      Accessory ØFBF
    Parotid
      Left ØCBC
      Right ØCBB
  Duodenum ØDB9
  Dura Mater ØØB2
  Ear
    External
      Left Ø9B1
      Right Ø9BØ
    External Auditory Canal
      Left Ø9B4
      Right Ø9B3
    Inner
      Left Ø9BE
      Right Ø9BD
    Middle
      Left Ø9B6
      Right Ø9B5
  Elbow Region
    Left ØXBC
    Right ØXBB
  Epididymis
    Bilateral ØVBL
    Left ØVBK
    Right ØVBJ
  Epiglottis ØCBR
  Esophagogastric Junction ØDB4
  Esophagus ØDB5
    Lower ØDB3
    Middle ØDB2
    Upper ØDB1
  Eustachian Tube
    Left Ø9BG
    Right Ø9BF
  Extremity
    Lower
      Left ØYBB
      Right ØYB9

Excision — continued
  Extremity — continued
    Upper
      Left ØXB7
      Right ØXB6
  Eye
    Left Ø8B1
    Right Ø8BØ
  Eyelid
    Lower
      Left Ø8BR
      Right Ø8BQ
    Upper
      Left Ø8BP
      Right Ø8BN
  Face ØWB2
  Fallopian Tube
    Left ØUB6
    Right ØUB5
  Fallopian Tubes, Bilateral ØUB7
  Femoral Region
    Left ØYB8
    Right ØYB7
  Femoral Shaft
    Left ØQB9
    Right ØQB8
  Femur
    Lower
      Left ØQBC
      Right ØQBB
    Upper
      Left ØQB7
      Right ØQB6
  Fibula
    Left ØQBK
    Right ØQBJ
  Finger Nail ØHBQXZ
  Floor of mouth see Excision, Oral Cavity and Throat
    ØWB3
  Foot
    Left ØYBN
    Right ØYBM
  Gallbladder ØFB4
  Gingiva
    Lower ØCB6
    Upper ØCB5
  Gland
    Adrenal
      Bilateral ØGB4
      Left ØGB2
      Right ØGB3
    Lacrimal
      Left Ø8BW
      Right Ø8BV
    Minor Salivary ØCBJ
    Parotid
      Left ØCB9
      Right ØCB8
    Pituitary ØGBØ
    Sublingual
      Left ØCBF
      Right ØCBD
    Submaxillary
      Left ØCBH
      Right ØCBG
    Vestibular ØUBL
  Glenoid Cavity
    Left ØPB8
    Right ØPB7
  Glomus Jugulare ØGBC
  Hand
    Left ØXBK
    Right ØXBJ
  Head ØWBØ
  Humeral Head
    Left ØPBD
    Right ØPBC
  Humeral Shaft
    Left ØPBG
    Right ØPBF
  Hymen ØUBK
  Hypothalamus ØØBA
  Ileocecal Valve ØDBC
  Ileum ØDBB
  Inguinal Region
    Left ØYB6
    Right ØYB5
  Intestine
    Large ØDBE

Excision — *continued*
- Intestine — *continued*
  - Large — *continued*
    - Left ØDBG
    - Right ØDBF
  - Small ØDB8
- Iris
  - Left Ø8BD3Z
  - Right Ø8BC3Z
- Jaw
  - Lower ØWB5
  - Upper ØWB4
- Jejunum ØDBA
- Joint
  - Acromioclavicular
    - Left ØRBH
    - Right ØRBG
  - Ankle
    - Left ØSBG
    - Right ØSBF
  - Carpal
    - Left ØRBR
    - Right ØRBQ
  - Carpometacarpal
    - Left ØRBT
    - Right ØRBS
  - Cervical Vertebral ØRB1
  - Cervicothoracic Vertebral ØRB4
  - Coccygeal ØSB6
  - Elbow
    - Left ØRBM
    - Right ØRBL
  - Finger Phalangeal
    - Left ØRBX
    - Right ØRBW
  - Hip
    - Left ØSBB
    - Right ØSB9
  - Knee
    - Left ØSBD
    - Right ØSBC
  - Lumbar Vertebral ØSBØ
  - Lumbosacral ØSB3
  - Metacarpophalangeal
    - Left ØRBV
    - Right ØRBU
  - Metatarsal-Phalangeal
    - Left ØSBN
    - Right ØSBM
  - Occipital-cervical ØRBØ
  - Sacrococcygeal ØSB5
  - Sacroiliac
    - Left ØSB8
    - Right ØSB7
  - Shoulder
    - Left ØRBK
    - Right ØRBJ
  - Sternoclavicular
    - Left ØRBF
    - Right ØRBE
  - Tarsal
    - Left ØSBJ
    - Right ØSBH
  - Tarsometatarsal
    - Left ØSBL
    - Right ØSBK
  - Temporomandibular
    - Left ØRBD
    - Right ØRBC
  - Thoracic Vertebral ØRB6
  - Thoracolumbar Vertebral ØRBA
  - Toe Phalangeal
    - Left ØSBQ
    - Right ØSBP
  - Wrist
    - Left ØRBP
    - Right ØRBN
- Kidney
  - Left ØTB1
  - Right ØTBØ
- Kidney Pelvis
  - Left ØTB4
  - Right ØTB3
- Knee Region
  - Left ØYBG
  - Right ØYBF
- Larynx ØCBS

Excision — *continued*
- Leg
  - Lower
    - Left ØYBJ
    - Right ØYBH
  - Upper
    - Left ØYBD
    - Right ØYBC
- Lens
  - Left Ø8BK3Z
  - Right Ø8BJ3Z
- Lip
  - Lower ØCB1
  - Upper ØCBØ
- Liver ØFBØ
  - Left Lobe ØFB2
  - Right Lobe ØFB1
- Lung
  - Bilateral ØBBM
  - Left ØBBL
  - Lower Lobe
    - Left ØBBJ
    - Right ØBBF
  - Middle Lobe, Right ØBBD
  - Right ØBBK
  - Upper Lobe
    - Left ØBBG
    - Right ØBBC
- Lung Lingula ØBBH
- Lymphatic
  - Aortic Ø7BD
  - Axillary
    - Left Ø7B6
    - Right Ø7B5
  - Head Ø7BØ
  - Inguinal
    - Left Ø7BJ
    - Right Ø7BH
  - Internal Mammary
    - Left Ø7B9
    - Right Ø7B8
  - Lower Extremity
    - Left Ø7BG
    - Right Ø7BF
  - Mesenteric Ø7BB
  - Neck
    - Left Ø7B2
    - Right Ø7B1
  - Pelvis Ø7BC
  - Thoracic Duct Ø7BK
  - Thorax Ø7B7
  - Upper Extremity
    - Left Ø7B4
    - Right Ø7B3
- Mandible
  - Left ØNBV
  - Right ØNBT
- Maxilla ØNBR
- Mediastinum ØWBC
- Medulla Oblongata ØØBD
- Mesentery ØDBV
- Metacarpal
  - Left ØPBQ
  - Right ØPBP
- Metatarsal
  - Left ØQBP
  - Right ØQBN
- Muscle
  - Abdomen
    - Left ØKBL
    - Right ØKBK
  - Extraocular
    - Left Ø8BM
    - Right Ø8BL
  - Facial ØKB1
  - Foot
    - Left ØKBW
    - Right ØKBV
  - Hand
    - Left ØKBD
    - Right ØKBC
  - Head ØKBØ
  - Hip
    - Left ØKBP
    - Right ØKBN
  - Lower Arm and Wrist
    - Left ØKBB
    - Right ØKB9

Excision — *continued*
- Muscle — *continued*
  - Lower Leg
    - Left ØKBT
    - Right ØKBS
  - Neck
    - Left ØKB3
    - Right ØKB2
  - Papillary Ø2BD
  - Perineum ØKBM
  - Shoulder
    - Left ØKB6
    - Right ØKB5
  - Thorax
    - Left ØKBJ
    - Right ØKBH
  - Tongue, Palate, Pharynx ØKB4
  - Trunk
    - Left ØKBG
    - Right ØKBF
  - Upper Arm
    - Left ØKB8
    - Right ØKB7
  - Upper Leg
    - Left ØKBR
    - Right ØKBQ
- Nasal Mucosa and Soft Tissue Ø9BK
- Nasopharynx Ø9BN
- Neck ØWB6
- Nerve
  - Abdominal Sympathetic Ø1BM
  - Abducens ØØBL
  - Accessory ØØBR
  - Acoustic ØØBN
  - Brachial Plexus Ø1B3
  - Cervical Ø1B1
  - Cervical Plexus Ø1BØ
  - Facial ØØBM
  - Femoral Ø1BD
  - Glossopharyngeal ØØBP
  - Head and Neck Sympathetic Ø1BK
  - Hypoglossal ØØBS
  - Lumbar Ø1BB
  - Lumbar Plexus Ø1B9
  - Lumbar Sympathetic Ø1BN
  - Lumbosacral Plexus Ø1BA
  - Median Ø1B5
  - Oculomotor ØØBH
  - Olfactory ØØBF
  - Optic ØØBG
  - Peroneal Ø1BH
  - Phrenic Ø1B2
  - Pudendal Ø1BC
  - Radial Ø1B6
  - Sacral Ø1BR
  - Sacral Plexus Ø1BQ
  - Sacral Sympathetic Ø1BP
  - Sciatic Ø1BF
  - Thoracic Ø1B8
  - Thoracic Sympathetic Ø1BL
  - Tibial Ø1BG
  - Trigeminal ØØBK
  - Trochlear ØØBJ
  - Ulnar Ø1B4
  - Vagus ØØBQ
- Nipple
  - Left ØHBX
  - Right ØHBW
- Omentum ØDBU
- Oral Cavity and Throat ØWB3
- Orbit
  - Left ØNBQ
  - Right ØNBP
- Ovary
  - Bilateral ØUB2
  - Left ØUB1
  - Right ØUBØ
- Palate
  - Hard ØCB2
  - Soft ØCB3
- Pancreas ØFBG
- Para-aortic Body ØGB9
- Paraganglion Extremity ØGBF
- Parathyroid Gland ØGBR
  - Inferior
    - Left ØGBP
    - Right ØGBN
  - Multiple ØGBQ

Excision — continued
  Parathyroid Gland — continued
    Superior
      Left ØGBM
      Right ØGBL
  Patella
    Left ØQBF
    Right ØQBD
  Penis ØVBS
  Pericardium Ø2BN
  Perineum
    Female ØWBN
    Male ØWBM
  Peritoneum ØDBW
  Phalanx
    Finger
      Left ØPBV
      Right ØPBT
    Thumb
      Left ØPBS
      Right ØPBR
    Toe
      Left ØQBR
      Right ØQBQ
  Pharynx ØCBM
  Pineal Body ØGB1
  Pleura
    Left ØBBP
    Right ØBBN
  Pons ØØBB
  Prepuce ØVBT
  Prostate ØVBØ
  Radius
    Left ØPBJ
    Right ØPBH
  Rectum ØDBP
  Retina
    Left Ø8BF3Z
    Right Ø8BE3Z
  Retroperitoneum ØWBH
  Ribs
    1 to 2 ØPB1
    3 or More ØPB2
  Sacrum ØQB1
  Scapula
    Left ØPB6
    Right ØPB5
  Sclera
    Left Ø8B7XZ
    Right Ø8B6XZ
  Scrotum ØVB5
  Septum
    Atrial Ø2B5
    Nasal Ø9BM
    Ventricular Ø2BM
  Shoulder Region
    Left ØXB3
    Right ØXB2
  Sinus
    Accessory Ø9BP
    Ethmoid
      Left Ø9BV
      Right Ø9BU
    Frontal
      Left Ø9BT
      Right Ø9BS
    Mastoid
      Left Ø9BC
      Right Ø9BB
    Maxillary
      Left Ø9BR
      Right Ø9BQ
    Sphenoid
      Left Ø9BX
      Right Ø9BW
  Skin
    Abdomen ØHB7XZ
    Back ØHB6XZ
    Buttock ØHB8XZ
    Chest ØHB5XZ
    Ear
      Left ØHB3XZ
      Right ØHB2XZ
    Face ØHB1XZ
    Foot
      Left ØHBNXZ
      Right ØHBMXZ
    Hand
      Left ØHBGXZ

Excision — continued
  Skin — continued
    Hand — continued
      Right ØHBFXZ
    Inguinal ØHBAXZ
    Lower Arm
      Left ØHBEXZ
      Right ØHBDXZ
    Lower Leg
      Left ØHBLXZ
      Right ØHBKXZ
    Neck ØHB4XZ
    Perineum ØHB9XZ
    Scalp ØHBØXZ
    Upper Arm
      Left ØHBCXZ
      Right ØHBBXZ
    Upper Leg
      Left ØHBJXZ
      Right ØHBHXZ
  Skull ØNBØ
  Spinal Cord
    Cervical ØØBW
    Lumbar ØØBY
    Thoracic ØØBX
  Spinal Meninges ØØBT
  Spleen Ø7BP
  Sternum ØPBØ
  Stomach ØDB6
    Pylorus ØDB7
  Subcutaneous Tissue and Fascia
    Abdomen ØJB8
    Back ØJB7
    Buttock ØJB9
    Chest ØJB6
    Face ØJB1
    Foot
      Left ØJBR
      Right ØJBQ
    Hand
      Left ØJBK
      Right ØJBJ
    Lower Arm
      Left ØJBH
      Right ØJBG
    Lower Leg
      Left ØJBP
      Right ØJBN
    Neck
      Left ØJB5
      Right ØJB4
    Pelvic Region ØJBC
    Perineum ØJBB
    Scalp ØJBØ
    Upper Arm
      Left ØJBF
      Right ØJBD
    Upper Leg
      Left ØJBM
      Right ØJBL
  Tarsal
    Left ØQBM
    Right ØQBL
  Tendon
    Abdomen
      Left ØLBG
      Right ØLBF
    Ankle
      Left ØLBT
      Right ØLBS
    Foot
      Left ØLBW
      Right ØLBV
    Hand
      Left ØLB8
      Right ØLB7
    Head and Neck ØLBØ
    Hip
      Left ØLBK
      Right ØLBJ
    Knee
      Left ØLBR
      Right ØLBQ
    Lower Arm and Wrist
      Left ØLB6
      Right ØLB5
    Lower Leg
      Left ØLBP
      Right ØLBN

Excision — continued
  Tendon — continued
    Perineum ØLBH
    Shoulder
      Left ØLB2
      Right ØLB1
    Thorax
      Left ØLBD
      Right ØLBC
    Trunk
      Left ØLBB
      Right ØLB9
    Upper Arm
      Left ØLB4
      Right ØLB3
    Upper Leg
      Left ØLBM
      Right ØLBL
  Testis
    Bilateral ØVBC
    Left ØVBB
    Right ØVB9
  Thalamus ØØB9
  Thymus Ø7BM
  Thyroid Gland
    Left Lobe ØGBG
    Right Lobe ØGBH
  Thyroid Gland Isthmus ØGBJ
  Tibia
    Left ØQBH
    Right ØQBG
  Toe Nail ØHBRXZ
  Tongue ØCB7
  Tonsils ØCBP
  Tooth
    Lower ØCBX
    Upper ØCBW
  Trachea ØBB1
  Tunica Vaginalis
    Left ØVB7
    Right ØVB6
  Turbinate, Nasal Ø9BL
  Tympanic Membrane
    Left Ø9B8
    Right Ø9B7
  Ulna
    Left ØPBL
    Right ØPBK
  Ureter
    Left ØTB7
    Right ØTB6
  Urethra ØTBD
  Uterine Supporting Structure ØUB4
  Uterus ØUB9
  Uvula ØCBN
  Vagina ØUBG
  Valve
    Aortic Ø2BF
    Mitral Ø2BG
    Pulmonary Ø2BH
    Tricuspid Ø2BJ
  Vas Deferens
    Bilateral ØVBQ
    Left ØVBP
    Right ØVBN
  Vein
    Axillary
      Left Ø5B8
      Right Ø5B7
    Azygos Ø5BØ
    Basilic
      Left Ø5BC
      Right Ø5BB
    Brachial
      Left Ø5BA
      Right Ø5B9
    Cephalic
      Left Ø5BF
      Right Ø5BD
    Colic Ø6B7
    Common Iliac
      Left Ø6BD
      Right Ø6BC
    Coronary Ø2B4
    Esophageal Ø6B3
    External Iliac
      Left Ø6BG
      Right Ø6BF

Excision — *continued*
  Vein — *continued*
    External Jugular
      Left 05BQ
      Right 05BP
    Face
      Left 05BV
      Right 05BT
    Femoral
      Left 06BN
      Right 06BM
    Foot
      Left 06BV
      Right 06BT
    Gastric 06B2
    Hand
      Left 05BH
      Right 05BG
    Hemiazygos 05B1
    Hepatic 06B4
    Hypogastric
      Left 06BJ
      Right 06BH
    Inferior Mesenteric 06B6
    Innominate
      Left 05B4
      Right 05B3
    Internal Jugular
      Left 05BN
      Right 05BM
    Intracranial 05BL
    Lower 06BY
    Portal 06B8
    Pulmonary
      Left 02BT
      Right 02BS
    Renal
      Left 06BB
      Right 06B9
    Saphenous
      Left 06BQ
      Right 06BP
    Splenic 06B1
    Subclavian
      Left 05B6
      Right 05B5
    Superior Mesenteric 06B5
    Upper 05BY
    Vertebral
      Left 05BS
      Right 05BR
  Vena Cava
    Inferior 06B0
    Superior 02BV
  Ventricle
    Left 02BL
    Right 02BK
  Vertebra
    Cervical 0PB3
    Lumbar 0QB0
    Thoracic 0PB4
  Vesicle
    Bilateral 0VB3
    Left 0VB2
    Right 0VB1
  Vitreous
    Left 08B53Z
    Right 08B43Z
  Vocal Cord
    Left 0CBV
    Right 0CBT
  Vulva 0UBM
  Wrist Region
    Left 0XBH
    Right 0XBG
EXCLUDER® AAA Endoprosthesis
  use Intraluminal Device
  use Intraluminal Device, Branched or Fenestrated, One or Two Arteries in 04V
  use Intraluminal Device, Branched or Fenestrated, Three or More Arteries in 04V
EXCLUDER® IBE Endoprosthesis *use* Intraluminal Device, Branched or Fenestrated, One or Two Arteries in 04V
Exclusion, Left atrial appendage (LAA) *see* Occlusion, Atrium, Left 02L7
Exercise, rehabilitation *see* Motor Treatment, Rehabilitation F07

Exploration *see* Inspection
Express® Biliary SD Monorail® Premounted Stent System *use* Intraluminal Device
Express® (LD) Premounted Stent System *use* Intraluminal Device
Express® SD Renal Monorail® Premounted Stent System *use* Intraluminal Device
Ex-PRESS™ mini glaucoma shunt *use* Synthetic Substitute
Extensor carpi radialis muscle
  use Lower Arm and Wrist Muscle, Left
  use Lower Arm and Wrist Muscle, Right
Extensor carpi ulnaris muscle
  use Lower Arm and Wrist Muscle, Left
  use Lower Arm and Wrist Muscle, Right
Extensor digitorum brevis muscle
  use Foot Muscle, Left
  use Foot Muscle, Right
Extensor digitorum longus muscle
  use Lower Leg Muscle, Left
  use Lower Leg Muscle, Right
Extensor hallucis brevis muscle
  use Foot Muscle, Left
  use Foot Muscle, Right
Extensor hallucis longus muscle
  use Lower Leg Muscle, Left
  use Lower Leg Muscle, Right
External anal sphincter *use* Anal Sphincter
External auditory meatus
  use External Auditory Canal, Left
  use External Auditory Canal, Right
External fixator
  use External Fixation Device in Head and Facial Bones
  use External Fixation Device in Lower Bones
  use External Fixation Device in Lower Joints
  use External Fixation Device in Upper Bones
  use External Fixation Device in Upper Joints
External maxillary artery *use* Face Artery
External naris *use* Nasal Mucosa and Soft Tissue
External oblique aponeurosis *use* Subcutaneous Tissue and Fascia, Trunk
External oblique muscle
  use Abdomen Muscle, Left
  use Abdomen Muscle, Right
External popliteal nerve *use* Peroneal Nerve
External pudendal artery
  use Femoral Artery, Left
  use Femoral Artery, Right
External pudendal vein
  use Saphenous Vein, Left
  use Saphenous Vein, Right
External urethral sphincter *use* Urethra
Extirpation
  Acetabulum
    Left 0QC5
    Right 0QC4
  Adenoids 0CCQ
  Ampulla of Vater 0FCC
  Anal Sphincter 0DCR
  Anterior Chamber
    Left 08C3
    Right 08C2
  Anus 0DCQ
  Aorta
    Abdominal 04C0
    Thoracic
      Ascending/Arch 02CX
      Descending 02CW
  Aortic Body 0GCD
  Appendix 0DCJ
  Artery
    Anterior Tibial
      Left 04CQ
      Right 04CP
    Axillary
      Left 03C6
      Right 03C5
    Brachial
      Left 03C8
      Right 03C7
    Celiac 04C1
    Colic
      Left 04C7
      Middle 04C8
      Right 04C6

Extirpation — *continued*
  Artery — *continued*
    Common Carotid
      Left 03CJ
      Right 03CH
    Common Iliac
      Left 04CD
      Right 04CC
    Coronary
      Four or More Arteries 02C3
      One Artery 02C0
      Three Arteries 02C2
      Two Arteries 02C1
    External Carotid
      Left 03CN
      Right 03CM
    External Iliac
      Left 04CJ
      Right 04CH
    Face 03CR
    Femoral
      Left 04CL
      Right 04CK
    Foot
      Left 04CW
      Right 04CV
    Gastric 04C2
    Hand
      Left 03CF
      Right 03CD
    Hepatic 04C3
    Inferior Mesenteric 04CB
    Innominate 03C2
    Internal Carotid
      Left 03CL
      Right 03CK
    Internal Iliac
      Left 04CF
      Right 04CE
    Internal Mammary
      Left 03C1
      Right 03C0
    Intracranial 03CG
    Lower 04CY
    Peroneal
      Left 04CU
      Right 04CT
    Popliteal
      Left 04CN
      Right 04CM
    Posterior Tibial
      Left 04CS
      Right 04CR
    Pulmonary
      Left 02CR
      Right 02CQ
    Pulmonary Trunk 02CP
    Radial
      Left 03CC
      Right 03CB
    Renal
      Left 04CA
      Right 04C9
    Splenic 04C4
    Subclavian
      Left 03C4
      Right 03C3
    Superior Mesenteric 04C5
    Temporal
      Left 03CT
      Right 03CS
    Thyroid
      Left 03CV
      Right 03CU
    Ulnar
      Left 03CA
      Right 03C9
    Upper 03CY
    Vertebral
      Left 03CQ
      Right 03CP
  Atrium
    Left 02C7
    Right 02C6
  Auditory Ossicle
    Left 09CA
    Right 09C9
  Basal Ganglia 00C8
  Bladder 0TCB

Subterms under main terms may continue to next column or page

Extirpation — *continued*
Bladder Neck ØTCC
Bone
  Ethmoid
    Left ØNCG
    Right ØNCF
  Frontal ØNC1
  Hyoid ØNCX
  Lacrimal
    Left ØNCJ
    Right ØNCH
  Nasal ØNCB
  Occipital ØNC7
  Palatine
    Left ØNCL
    Right ØNCK
  Parietal
    Left ØNC4
    Right ØNC3
  Pelvic
    Left ØQC3
    Right ØQC2
  Sphenoid ØNCC
  Temporal
    Left ØNC6
    Right ØNC5
  Zygomatic
    Left ØNCN
    Right ØNCM
Brain ØØCØ
Breast
  Bilateral ØHCV
  Left ØHCU
  Right ØHCT
Bronchus
  Lingula ØBC9
  Lower Lobe
    Left ØBCB
    Right ØBC6
  Main
    Left ØBC7
    Right ØBC3
  Middle Lobe, Right ØBC5
  Upper Lobe
    Left ØBC8
    Right ØBC4
Buccal Mucosa ØCC4
Bursa and Ligament
  Abdomen
    Left ØMCJ
    Right ØMCH
  Ankle
    Left ØMCR
    Right ØMCQ
  Elbow
    Left ØMC4
    Right ØMC3
  Foot
    Left ØMCT
    Right ØMCS
  Hand
    Left ØMC8
    Right ØMC7
  Head and Neck ØMCØ
  Hip
    Left ØMCM
    Right ØMCL
  Knee
    Left ØMCP
    Right ØMCN
  Lower Extremity
    Left ØMCW
    Right ØMCV
  Perineum ØMCK
  Rib(s) ØMCG
  Shoulder
    Left ØMC2
    Right ØMC1
  Spine
    Lower ØMCD
    Upper ØMCC
  Sternum ØMCF
  Upper Extremity
    Left ØMCB
    Right ØMC9
  Wrist
    Left ØMC6
    Right ØMC5
Carina ØBC2

Extirpation — *continued*
Carotid Bodies, Bilateral ØGC8
Carotid Body
  Left ØGC6
  Right ØGC7
Carpal
  Left ØPCN
  Right ØPCM
Cavity, Cranial ØWC1
Cecum ØDCH
Cerebellum ØØCC
Cerebral Hemisphere ØØC7
Cerebral Meninges ØØC1
Cerebral Ventricle ØØC6
Cervix ØUCC
Chordae Tendineae Ø2C9
Choroid
  Left Ø8CB
  Right Ø8CA
Cisterna Chyli Ø7CL
Clavicle
  Left ØPCB
  Right ØPC9
Clitoris ØUCJ
Coccygeal Glomus ØGCB
Coccyx ØQCS
Colon
  Ascending ØDCK
  Descending ØDCM
  Sigmoid ØDCN
  Transverse ØDCL
Conduction Mechanism Ø2C8
Conjunctiva
  Left Ø8CTXZZ
  Right Ø8CSXZZ
Cord
  Bilateral ØVCH
  Left ØVCG
  Right ØVCF
Cornea
  Left Ø8C9XZZ
  Right Ø8C8XZZ
Cul-de-sac ØUCF
Diaphragm ØBCT
Disc
  Cervical Vertebral ØRC3
  Cervicothoracic Vertebral ØRC5
  Lumbar Vertebral ØSC2
  Lumbosacral ØSC4
  Thoracic Vertebral ØRC9
  Thoracolumbar Vertebral ØRCB
Duct
  Common Bile ØFC9
  Cystic ØFC8
  Hepatic
    Common ØFC7
    Left ØFC6
    Right ØFC5
  Lacrimal
    Left Ø8CY
    Right Ø8CX
  Pancreatic ØFCD
    Accessory ØFCF
  Parotid
    Left ØCCC
    Right ØCCB
Duodenum ØDC9
Dura Mater ØØC2
Ear
  External
    Left Ø9C1
    Right Ø9CØ
  External Auditory Canal
    Left Ø9C4
    Right Ø9C3
  Inner
    Left Ø9CE
    Right Ø9CD
  Middle
    Left Ø9C6
    Right Ø9C5
Endometrium ØUCB
Epididymis
  Bilateral ØVCL
  Left ØVCK
  Right ØVCJ
Epidural Space, Intracranial ØØC3
Epiglottis ØCCR
Esophagogastric Junction ØDC4

Extirpation — *continued*
Esophagus ØDC5
  Lower ØDC3
  Middle ØDC2
  Upper ØDC1
Eustachian Tube
  Left Ø9CG
  Right Ø9CF
Eye
  Left Ø8C1XZZ
  Right Ø8CØXZZ
Eyelid
  Lower
    Left Ø8CR
    Right Ø8CQ
  Upper
    Left Ø8CP
    Right Ø8CN
Fallopian Tube
  Left ØUC6
  Right ØUC5
Fallopian Tubes, Bilateral ØUC7
Femoral Shaft
  Left ØQC9
  Right ØQC8
Femur
  Lower
    Left ØQCC
    Right ØQCB
  Upper
    Left ØQC7
    Right ØQC6
Fibula
  Left ØQCK
  Right ØQCJ
Finger Nail ØHCQXZZ
Gallbladder ØFC4
Gastrointestinal Tract ØWCP
Genitourinary Tract ØWCR
Gingiva
  Lower ØCC6
  Upper ØCC5
Gland
  Adrenal
    Bilateral ØGC4
    Left ØGC2
    Right ØGC3
  Lacrimal
    Left Ø8CW
    Right Ø8CV
  Minor Salivary ØCCJ
  Parotid
    Left ØCC9
    Right ØCC8
  Pituitary ØGCØ
  Sublingual
    Left ØCCF
    Right ØCCD
  Submaxillary
    Left ØCCH
    Right ØCCG
  Vestibular ØUCL
Glenoid Cavity
  Left ØPC8
  Right ØPC7
Glomus Jugulare ØGCC
Humeral Head
  Left ØPCD
  Right ØPCC
Humeral Shaft
  Left ØPCG
  Right ØPCF
Hymen ØUCK
Hypothalamus ØØCA
Ileocecal Valve ØDCC
Ileum ØDCB
Intestine
  Large ØDCE
    Left ØDCG
    Right ØDCF
  Small ØDC8
Iris
  Left Ø8CD
  Right Ø8CC
Jaw
  Lower ØWC5
  Upper ØWC4
Jejunum ØDCA

Extirpation — *continued*
Joint
  Acromioclavicular
    Left ØRCH
    Right ØRCG
  Ankle
    Left ØSCG
    Right ØSCF
  Carpal
    Left ØRCR
    Right ØRCQ
  Carpometacarpal
    Left ØRCT
    Right ØRCS
  Cervical Vertebral ØRC1
  Cervicothoracic Vertebral ØRC4
  Coccygeal ØSC6
  Elbow
    Left ØRCM
    Right ØRCL
  Finger Phalangeal
    Left ØRCX
    Right ØRCW
  Hip
    Left ØSCB
    Right ØSC9
  Knee
    Left ØSCD
    Right ØSCC
  Lumbar Vertebral ØSCØ
  Lumbosacral ØSC3
  Metacarpophalangeal
    Left ØRCV
    Right ØRCU
  Metatarsal-Phalangeal
    Left ØSCN
    Right ØSCM
  Occipital-cervical ØRCØ
  Sacrococcygeal ØSC5
  Sacroiliac
    Left ØSC8
    Right ØSC7
  Shoulder
    Left ØRCK
    Right ØRCJ
  Sternoclavicular
    Left ØRCF
    Right ØRCE
  Tarsal
    Left ØSCJ
    Right ØSCH
  Tarsometatarsal
    Left ØSCL
    Right ØSCK
  Temporomandibular
    Left ØRCD
    Right ØRCC
  Thoracic Vertebral ØRC6
  Thoracolumbar Vertebral ØRCA
  Toe Phalangeal
    Left ØSCQ
    Right ØSCP
  Wrist
    Left ØRCP
    Right ØRCN
Kidney
  Left ØTC1
  Right ØTCØ
Kidney Pelvis
  Left ØTC4
  Right ØTC3
Larynx ØCCS
Lens
  Left Ø8CK
  Right Ø8CJ
Lip
  Lower ØCC1
  Upper ØCCØ
Liver ØFCØ
  Left Lobe ØFC2
  Right Lobe ØFC1
Lung
  Bilateral ØBCM
  Left ØBCL
  Lower Lobe
    Left ØBCJ
    Right ØBCF
  Middle Lobe, Right ØBCD
  Right ØBCK

Extirpation — *continued*
Lung — *continued*
  Upper Lobe
    Left ØBCG
    Right ØBCC
Lung Lingula ØBCH
Lymphatic
  Aortic Ø7CD
  Axillary
    Left Ø7C6
    Right Ø7C5
  Head Ø7CØ
  Inguinal
    Left Ø7CJ
    Right Ø7CH
  Internal Mammary
    Left Ø7C9
    Right Ø7C8
  Lower Extremity
    Left Ø7CG
    Right Ø7CF
  Mesenteric Ø7CB
  Neck
    Left Ø7C2
    Right Ø7C1
  Pelvis Ø7CC
  Thoracic Duct Ø7CK
  Thorax Ø7C7
  Upper Extremity
    Left Ø7C4
    Right Ø7C3
Mandible
  Left ØNCV
  Right ØNCT
Maxilla ØNCR
Mediastinum ØWCC
Medulla Oblongata ØØCD
Mesentery ØDCV
Metacarpal
  Left ØPCQ
  Right ØPCP
Metatarsal
  Left ØQCP
  Right ØQCN
Muscle
  Abdomen
    Left ØKCL
    Right ØKCK
  Extraocular
    Left Ø8CM
    Right Ø8CL
  Facial ØKC1
  Foot
    Left ØKCW
    Right ØKCV
  Hand
    Left ØKCD
    Right ØKCC
  Head ØKCØ
  Hip
    Left ØKCP
    Right ØKCN
  Lower Arm and Wrist
    Left ØKCB
    Right ØKC9
  Lower Leg
    Left ØKCT
    Right ØKCS
  Neck
    Left ØKC3
    Right ØKC2
  Papillary Ø2CD
  Perineum ØKCM
  Shoulder
    Left ØKC6
    Right ØKC5
  Thorax
    Left ØKCJ
    Right ØKCH
  Tongue, Palate, Pharynx ØKC4
  Trunk
    Left ØKCG
    Right ØKCF
  Upper Arm
    Left ØKC8
    Right ØKC7
  Upper Leg
    Left ØKCR
    Right ØKCQ

Extirpation — *continued*
Nasal Mucosa and Soft Tissue Ø9CK
Nasopharynx Ø9CN
Nerve
  Abdominal Sympathetic Ø1CM
  Abducens ØØCL
  Accessory ØØCR
  Acoustic ØØCN
  Brachial Plexus Ø1C3
  Cervical Ø1C1
  Cervical Plexus Ø1CØ
  Facial ØØCM
  Femoral Ø1CD
  Glossopharyngeal ØØCP
  Head and Neck Sympathetic Ø1CK
  Hypoglossal ØØCS
  Lumbar Ø1CB
  Lumbar Plexus Ø1C9
  Lumbar Sympathetic Ø1CN
  Lumbosacral Plexus Ø1CA
  Median Ø1C5
  Oculomotor ØØCH
  Olfactory ØØCF
  Optic ØØCG
  Peroneal Ø1CH
  Phrenic Ø1C2
  Pudendal Ø1CC
  Radial Ø1C6
  Sacral Ø1CR
  Sacral Plexus Ø1CQ
  Sacral Sympathetic Ø1CP
  Sciatic Ø1CF
  Thoracic Ø1C8
  Thoracic Sympathetic Ø1CL
  Tibial Ø1CG
  Trigeminal ØØCK
  Trochlear ØØCJ
  Ulnar Ø1C4
  Vagus ØØCQ
Nipple
  Left ØHCX
  Right ØHCW
Omentum ØDCU
Oral Cavity and Throat ØWC3
Orbit
  Left ØNCQ
  Right ØNCP
Orbital Atherectomy Technology X2C
Ovary
  Bilateral ØUC2
  Left ØUC1
  Right ØUCØ
Palate
  Hard ØCC2
  Soft ØCC3
Pancreas ØFCG
Para-aortic Body ØGC9
Paraganglion Extremity ØGCF
Parathyroid Gland ØGCR
  Inferior
    Left ØGCP
    Right ØGCN
  Multiple ØGCQ
  Superior
    Left ØGCM
    Right ØGCL
Patella
  Left ØQCF
  Right ØQCD
Pelvic Cavity ØWCJ
Penis ØVCS
Pericardial Cavity ØWCD
Pericardium Ø2CN
Peritoneal Cavity ØWCG
Peritoneum ØDCW
Phalanx
  Finger
    Left ØPCV
    Right ØPCT
  Thumb
    Left ØPCS
    Right ØPCR
  Toe
    Left ØQCR
    Right ØQCQ
Pharynx ØCCM
Pineal Body ØGC1
Pleura
  Left ØBCP

Extirpation — continued
- Pleura — continued
  - Right 0BCN
- Pleural Cavity
  - Left 0WCB
  - Right 0WC9
- Pons 00CB
- Prepuce 0VCT
- Prostate 0VC0
- Radius
  - Left 0PCJ
  - Right 0PCH
- Rectum 0DCP
- Respiratory Tract 0WCQ
- Retina
  - Left 08CF
  - Right 08CE
- Retinal Vessel
  - Left 08CH
  - Right 08CG
- Retroperitoneum 0WCH
- Ribs
  - 1 to 2 0PC1
  - 3 or More 0PC2
- Sacrum 0QC1
- Scapula
  - Left 0PC6
  - Right 0PC5
- Sclera
  - Left 08C7XZZ
  - Right 08C6XZZ
- Scrotum 0VC5
- Septum
  - Atrial 02C5
  - Nasal 09CM
  - Ventricular 02CM
- Sinus
  - Accessory 09CP
  - Ethmoid
    - Left 09CV
    - Right 09CU
  - Frontal
    - Left 09CT
    - Right 09CS
  - Mastoid
    - Left 09CC
    - Right 09CB
  - Maxillary
    - Left 09CR
    - Right 09CQ
  - Sphenoid
    - Left 09CX
    - Right 09CW
- Skin
  - Abdomen 0HC7XZZ
  - Back 0HC6XZZ
  - Buttock 0HC8XZZ
  - Chest 0HC5XZZ
  - Ear
    - Left 0HC3XZZ
    - Right 0HC2XZZ
  - Face 0HC1XZZ
  - Foot
    - Left 0HCNXZZ
    - Right 0HCMXZZ
  - Hand
    - Left 0HCGXZZ
    - Right 0HCFXZZ
  - Inguinal 0HCAXZZ
  - Lower Arm
    - Left 0HCEXZZ
    - Right 0HCDXZZ
  - Lower Leg
    - Left 0HCLXZZ
    - Right 0HCKXZZ
  - Neck 0HC4XZZ
  - Perineum 0HC9XZZ
  - Scalp 0HC0XZZ
  - Upper Arm
    - Left 0HCCXZZ
    - Right 0HCBXZZ
  - Upper Leg
    - Left 0HCJXZZ
    - Right 0HCHXZZ
- Spinal Canal 00CU
- Spinal Cord
  - Cervical 00CW
  - Lumbar 00CY
  - Thoracic 00CX

Extirpation — continued
- Spinal Meninges 00CT
- Spleen 07CP
- Sternum 0PC0
- Stomach 0DC6
  - Pylorus 0DC7
- Subarachnoid Space, Intracranial 00C5
- Subcutaneous Tissue and Fascia
  - Abdomen 0JC8
  - Back 0JC7
  - Buttock 0JC9
  - Chest 0JC6
  - Face 0JC1
  - Foot
    - Left 0JCR
    - Right 0JCQ
  - Hand
    - Left 0JCK
    - Right 0JCJ
  - Lower Arm
    - Left 0JCH
    - Right 0JCG
  - Lower Leg
    - Left 0JCP
    - Right 0JCN
  - Neck
    - Left 0JC5
    - Right 0JC4
  - Pelvic Region 0JCC
  - Perineum 0JCB
  - Scalp 0JC0
  - Upper Arm
    - Left 0JCF
    - Right 0JCD
  - Upper Leg
    - Left 0JCM
    - Right 0JCL
- Subdural Space, Intracranial 00C4
- Tarsal
  - Left 0QCM
  - Right 0QCL
- Tendon
  - Abdomen
    - Left 0LCG
    - Right 0LCF
  - Ankle
    - Left 0LCT
    - Right 0LCS
  - Foot
    - Left 0LCW
    - Right 0LCV
  - Hand
    - Left 0LC8
    - Right 0LC7
  - Head and Neck 0LC0
  - Hip
    - Left 0LCK
    - Right 0LCJ
  - Knee
    - Left 0LCR
    - Right 0LCQ
  - Lower Arm and Wrist
    - Left 0LC6
    - Right 0LC5
  - Lower Leg
    - Left 0LCP
    - Right 0LCN
  - Perineum 0LCH
  - Shoulder
    - Left 0LC2
    - Right 0LC1
  - Thorax
    - Left 0LCD
    - Right 0LCC
  - Trunk
    - Left 0LCB
    - Right 0LC9
  - Upper Arm
    - Left 0LC4
    - Right 0LC3
  - Upper Leg
    - Left 0LCM
    - Right 0LCL
- Testis
  - Bilateral 0VCC
  - Left 0VCB
  - Right 0VC9
- Thalamus 00C9
- Thymus 07CM

Extirpation — continued
- Thyroid Gland 0GCK
  - Left Lobe 0GCG
  - Right Lobe 0GCH
- Tibia
  - Left 0QCH
  - Right 0QCG
- Toe Nail 0HCRXZZ
- Tongue 0CC7
- Tonsils 0CCP
- Tooth
  - Lower 0CCX
  - Upper 0CCW
- Trachea 0BC1
- Tunica Vaginalis
  - Left 0VC7
  - Right 0VC6
- Turbinate, Nasal 09CL
- Tympanic Membrane
  - Left 09C8
  - Right 09C7
- Ulna
  - Left 0PCL
  - Right 0PCK
- Ureter
  - Left 0TC7
  - Right 0TC6
- Urethra 0TCD
- Uterine Supporting Structure 0UC4
- Uterus 0UC9
- Uvula 0CCN
- Vagina 0UCG
- Valve
  - Aortic 02CF
  - Mitral 02CG
  - Pulmonary 02CH
  - Tricuspid 02CJ
- Vas Deferens
  - Bilateral 0VCQ
  - Left 0VCP
  - Right 0VCN
- Vein
  - Axillary
    - Left 05C8
    - Right 05C7
  - Azygos 05C0
  - Basilic
    - Left 05CC
    - Right 05CB
  - Brachial
    - Left 05CA
    - Right 05C9
  - Cephalic
    - Left 05CF
    - Right 05CD
  - Colic 06C7
  - Common Iliac
    - Left 06CD
    - Right 06CC
  - Coronary 02C4
  - Esophageal 06C3
  - External Iliac
    - Left 06CG
    - Right 06CF
  - External Jugular
    - Left 05CQ
    - Right 05CP
  - Face
    - Left 05CV
    - Right 05CT
  - Femoral
    - Left 06CN
    - Right 06CM
  - Foot
    - Left 06CV
    - Right 06CT
  - Gastric 06C2
  - Hand
    - Left 05CH
    - Right 05CG
  - Hemiazygos 05C1
  - Hepatic 06C4
  - Hypogastric
    - Left 06CJ
    - Right 06CH
  - Inferior Mesenteric 06C6
  - Innominate
    - Left 05C4
    - Right 05C3

Extirpation — *continued*
Vein — *continued*
Internal Jugular
Left 05CN
Right 05CM
Intracranial 05CL
Lower 06CY
Portal 06C8
Pulmonary
Left 02CT
Right 02CS
Renal
Left 06CB
Right 06C9
Saphenous
Left 06CQ
Right 06CP
Splenic 06C1
Subclavian
Left 05C6
Right 05C5
Superior Mesenteric 06C5
Upper 05CY
Vertebral
Left 05CS
Right 05CR
Vena Cava
Inferior 06C0
Superior 02CV
Ventricle
Left 02CL
Right 02CK
Vertebra
Cervical 0PC3
Lumbar 0QC0
Thoracic 0PC4
Vesicle
Bilateral 0VC3
Left 0VC2
Right 0VC1
Vitreous
Left 08C5
Right 08C4
Vocal Cord
Left 0CCV
Right 0CCT
Vulva 0UCM
Extracorporeal Carbon Dioxide Removal (ECCO2R)
5A0920Z
Extracorporeal shock wave lithotripsy *see* Fragmentation
Extracranial-intracranial bypass (EC-IC) *see* Bypass, Upper Arteries 031
Extraction
Acetabulum
Left 0QD50ZZ
Right 0QD40ZZ
Ampulla of Vater 0FDC
Anus 0DDQ
Appendix 0DDJ
Auditory Ossicle
Left 09DA0ZZ
Right 09D90ZZ
Bone
Ethmoid
Left 0NDG0ZZ
Right 0NDF0ZZ
Frontal 0ND10ZZ
Hyoid 0NDX0ZZ
Lacrimal
Left 0NDJ0ZZ
Right 0NDH0ZZ
Nasal 0NDB0ZZ
Occipital 0ND70ZZ
Palatine
Left 0NDL0ZZ
Right 0NDK0ZZ
Parietal
Left 0ND40ZZ
Right 0ND30ZZ
Pelvic
Left 0QD30ZZ
Right 0QD20ZZ
Sphenoid 0NDC0ZZ
Temporal
Left 0ND60ZZ
Right 0ND50ZZ
Zygomatic
Left 0NDN0ZZ

Extraction — *continued*
Bone — *continued*
Zygomatic — *continued*
Right 0NDM0ZZ
Bone Marrow
Iliac 07DR
Sternum 07DQ
Vertebral 07DS
Breast
Bilateral 0HDV0ZZ
Left 0HDU0ZZ
Right 0HDT0ZZ
Supernumerary 0HDY0ZZ
Bronchus
Lingula 0BD9
Lower Lobe
Left 0BDB
Right 0BD6
Main
Left 0BD7
Right 0BD3
Middle Lobe, Right 0BD5
Upper Lobe
Left 0BD8
Right 0BD4
Bursa and Ligament
Abdomen
Left 0MDJ
Right 0MDH
Ankle
Left 0MDR
Right 0MDQ
Elbow
Left 0MD4
Right 0MD3
Foot
Left 0MDT
Right 0MDS
Hand
Left 0MD8
Right 0MD7
Head and Neck 0MD0
Hip
Left 0MDM
Right 0MDL
Knee
Left 0MDP
Right 0MDN
Lower Extremity
Left 0MDW
Right 0MDV
Perineum 0MDK
Rib(s) 0MDG
Shoulder
Left 0MD2
Right 0MD1
Spine
Lower 0MDD
Upper 0MDC
Sternum 0MDF
Upper Extremity
Left 0MDB
Right 0MD9
Wrist
Left 0MD6
Right 0MD5
Carina 0BD2
Carpal
Left 0PDN0ZZ
Right 0PDM0ZZ
Cecum 0DDH
Cerebral Meninges 00D1
Cisterna Chyli 07DL
Clavicle
Left 0PDB0ZZ
Right 0PD90ZZ
Coccyx 0QDS0ZZ
Colon
Ascending 0DDK
Descending 0DDM
Sigmoid 0DDN
Transverse 0DDL
Cornea
Left 08D9XZ
Right 08D8XZ
Duct
Common Bile 0FD9
Cystic 0FD8

Extraction — *continued*
Duct — *continued*
Hepatic
Common 0FD7
Left 0FD6
Right 0FD5
Pancreatic 0FDD
Accessory 0FDF
Duodenum 0DD9
Dura Mater 00D2
Endometrium 0UDB
Esophagogastric Junction 0DD4
Esophagus 0DD5
Lower 0DD3
Middle 0DD2
Upper 0DD1
Femoral Shaft
Left 0QD90ZZ
Right 0QD80ZZ
Femur
Lower
Left 0QDC0ZZ
Right 0QDB0ZZ
Upper
Left 0QD70ZZ
Right 0QD60ZZ
Fibula
Left 0QDK0ZZ
Right 0QDJ0ZZ
Finger Nail 0HDQXZZ
Gallbladder 0FD4
Glenoid Cavity
Left 0PD80ZZ
Right 0PD70ZZ
Hair 0HDSXZZ
Humeral Head
Left 0PDD0ZZ
Right 0PDC0ZZ
Humeral Shaft
Left 0PDG0ZZ
Right 0PDF0ZZ
Ileocecal Valve 0DDC
Ileum 0DDB
Intestine
Large 0DDE
Left 0DDG
Right 0DDF
Small 0DD8
Jejunum 0DDA
Kidney
Left 0TD1
Right 0TD0
Lens
Left 08DK3ZZ
Right 08DJ3ZZ
Liver 0FD0
Left Lobe 0FD2
Right Lobe 0FD1
Lung
Bilateral 0BDM
Left 0BDL
Lower Lobe
Left 0BDJ
Right 0BDF
Middle Lobe, Right 0BDD
Right 0BDK
Upper Lobe
Left 0BDG
Right 0BDC
Lung Lingula 0BDH
Lymphatic
Aortic 07DD
Axillary
Left 07D6
Right 07D5
Head 07D0
Inguinal
Left 07DJ
Right 07DH
Internal Mammary
Left 07D9
Right 07D8
Lower Extremity
Left 07DG
Right 07DF
Mesenteric 07DB
Neck
Left 07D2
Right 07D1

Extraction — *continued*
  Lymphatic — *continued*
    Pelvis 07DC
    Thoracic Duct 07DK
    Thorax 07D7
    Upper Extremity
      Left 07D4
      Right 07D3
  Mandible
    Left 0NDV0ZZ
    Right 0NDT0ZZ
  Maxilla 0NDR0ZZ
  Metacarpal
    Left 0PDQ0ZZ
    Right 0PDP0ZZ
  Metatarsal
    Left 0QDP0ZZ
    Right 0QDN0ZZ
  Muscle
    Abdomen
      Left 0KDL0ZZ
      Right 0KDK0ZZ
    Facial 0KD10ZZ
    Foot
      Left 0KDW0ZZ
      Right 0KDV0ZZ
    Hand
      Left 0KDD0ZZ
      Right 0KDC0ZZ
    Head 0KD00ZZ
    Hip
      Left 0KDP0ZZ
      Right 0KDN0ZZ
    Lower Arm and Wrist
      Left 0KDB0ZZ
      Right 0KD90ZZ
    Lower Leg
      Left 0KDT0ZZ
      Right 0KDS0ZZ
    Neck
      Left 0KD30ZZ
      Right 0KD20ZZ
    Perineum 0KDM0ZZ
    Shoulder
      Left 0KD60ZZ
      Right 0KD50ZZ
    Thorax
      Left 0KDJ0ZZ
      Right 0KDH0ZZ
    Tongue, Palate, Pharynx 0KD40ZZ
    Trunk
      Left 0KDG0ZZ
      Right 0KDF0ZZ
    Upper Arm
      Left 0KD80ZZ
      Right 0KD70ZZ
    Upper Leg
      Left 0KDR0ZZ
      Right 0KDQ0ZZ
  Nerve
    Abdominal Sympathetic 01DM
    Abducens 00DL
    Accessory 00DR
    Acoustic 00DN
    Brachial Plexus 01D3
    Cervical 01D1
    Cervical Plexus 01D0
    Facial 00DM
    Femoral 01DD
    Glossopharyngeal 00DP
    Head and Neck Sympathetic 01DK
    Hypoglossal 00DS
    Lumbar 01DB
    Lumbar Plexus 01D9
    Lumbar Sympathetic 01DN
    Lumbosacral Plexus 01DA
    Median 01D5
    Oculomotor 00DH
    Olfactory 00DF
    Optic 00DG
    Peroneal 01DH
    Phrenic 01D2
    Pudendal 01DC
    Radial 01D6
    Sacral 01DR
    Sacral Plexus 01DQ
    Sacral Sympathetic 01DP
    Sciatic 01DF
    Thoracic 01D8

Extraction — *continued*
  Nerve — *continued*
    Thoracic Sympathetic 01DL
    Tibial 01DG
    Trigeminal 00DK
    Trochlear 00DJ
    Ulnar 01D4
    Vagus 00DQ
  Orbit
    Left 0NDQ0ZZ
    Right 0NDP0ZZ
  Ova 0UDN
  Pancreas 0FDG
  Patella
    Left 0QDF0ZZ
    Right 0QDD0ZZ
  Phalanx
    Finger
      Left 0PDV0ZZ
      Right 0PDT0ZZ
    Thumb
      Left 0PDS0ZZ
      Right 0PDR0ZZ
    Toe
      Left 0QDR0ZZ
      Right 0QDQ0ZZ
  Pleura
    Left 0BDP
    Right 0BDN
  Products of Conception
    Ectopic 10D2
    Extraperitoneal 10D00Z2
    High 10D00Z0
    High Forceps 10D07Z5
    Internal Version 10D07Z7
    Low 10D00Z1
    Low Forceps 10D07Z3
    Mid Forceps 10D07Z4
    Other 10D07Z8
    Retained 10D1
    Vacuum 10D07Z6
  Radius
    Left 0PDJ0ZZ
    Right 0PDH0ZZ
  Rectum 0DDP
  Ribs
    1 to 2 0PD10ZZ
    3 or More 0PD20ZZ
  Sacrum 0QD10ZZ
  Scapula
    Left 0PD60ZZ
    Right 0PD50ZZ
  Septum, Nasal 09DM
  Sinus
    Accessory 09DP
    Ethmoid
      Left 09DV
      Right 09DU
    Frontal
      Left 09DT
      Right 09DS
    Mastoid
      Left 09DC
      Right 09DB
    Maxillary
      Left 09DR
      Right 09DQ
    Sphenoid
      Left 09DX
      Right 09DW
  Skin
    Abdomen 0HD7XZZ
    Back 0HD6XZZ
    Buttock 0HD8XZZ
    Chest 0HD5XZZ
    Ear
      Left 0HD3XZZ
      Right 0HD2XZZ
    Face 0HD1XZZ
    Foot
      Left 0HDNXZZ
      Right 0HDMXZZ
    Hand
      Left 0HDGXZZ
      Right 0HDFXZZ
    Inguinal 0HDAXZZ
    Lower Arm
      Left 0HDEXZZ
      Right 0HDDXZZ

Extraction — *continued*
  Skin — *continued*
    Lower Leg
      Left 0HDLXZZ
      Right 0HDKXZZ
    Neck 0HD4XZZ
    Perineum 0HD9XZZ
    Scalp 0HD0XZZ
    Upper Arm
      Left 0HDCXZZ
      Right 0HDBXZZ
    Upper Leg
      Left 0HDJXZZ
      Right 0HDHXZZ
  Skull 0ND00ZZ
  Spinal Meninges 00DT
  Spleen 07DP
  Sternum 0PD00ZZ
  Stomach 0DD6
    Pylorus 0DD7
  Subcutaneous Tissue and Fascia
    Abdomen 0JD8
    Back 0JD7
    Buttock 0JD9
    Chest 0JD6
    Face 0JD1
    Foot
      Left 0JDR
      Right 0JDQ
    Hand
      Left 0JDK
      Right 0JDJ
    Lower Arm
      Left 0JDH
      Right 0JDG
    Lower Leg
      Left 0JDP
      Right 0JDN
    Neck
      Left 0JD5
      Right 0JD4
    Pelvic Region 0JDC
    Perineum 0JDB
    Scalp 0JD0
    Upper Arm
      Left 0JDF
      Right 0JDD
    Upper Leg
      Left 0JDM
      Right 0JDL
  Tarsal
    Left 0QDM0ZZ
    Right 0QDL0ZZ
  Tendon
    Abdomen
      Left 0LDG0ZZ
      Right 0LDF0ZZ
    Ankle
      Left 0LDT0ZZ
      Right 0LDS0ZZ
    Foot
      Left 0LDW0ZZ
      Right 0LDV0ZZ
    Hand
      Left 0LD80ZZ
      Right 0LD70ZZ
    Head and Neck 0LD00ZZ
    Hip
      Left 0LDK0ZZ
      Right 0LDJ0ZZ
    Knee
      Left 0LDR0ZZ
      Right 0LDQ0ZZ
    Lower Arm and Wrist
      Left 0LD60ZZ
      Right 0LD50ZZ
    Lower Leg
      Left 0LDP0ZZ
      Right 0LDN0ZZ
    Perineum 0LDH0ZZ
    Shoulder
      Left 0LD20ZZ
      Right 0LD10ZZ
    Thorax
      Left 0LDD0ZZ
      Right 0LDC0ZZ
    Trunk
      Left 0LDB0ZZ
      Right 0LD90ZZ

Extraction — *continued*
　Tendon — *continued*
　　Upper Arm
　　　Left 0LD40ZZ
　　　Right 0LD30ZZ
　　Upper Leg
　　　Left 0LDM0ZZ
　　　Right 0DLL0ZZ
　Thymus 07DM
　Tibia
　　Left 0QDH0ZZ
　　Right 0QDG0ZZ
　Toe Nail 0HDRXZZ
　Tooth
　　Lower 0CDXXZ
　　Upper 0CDWXZ
　Trachea 0BD1
　Turbinate, Nasal 09DL
　Tympanic Membrane
　　Left 09D8
　　Right 09D7
　Ulna
　　Left 0PDL0ZZ
　　Right 0PDK0ZZ
　Vein
　　Basilic
　　　Left 05DC
　　　Right 05DB
　　Brachial
　　　Left 05DA
　　　Right 05D9
　　Cephalic
　　　Left 05DF
　　　Right 05DD
　　Femoral
　　　Left 06DN
　　　Right 06DM
　　Foot
　　　Left 06DV
　　　Right 06DT
　　Hand
　　　Left 05DH
　　　Right 05DG
　　Lower 06DY
　　Saphenous
　　　Left 06DQ
　　　Right 06DP
　　Upper 05DY
　Vertebra
　　Cervical 0PD30ZZ
　　Lumbar 0QD00ZZ
　　Thoracic 0PD40ZZ
　Vocal Cord
　　Left 0CDV
　　Right 0CDT
Extradural space, intracranial *use* Epidural Space, Intracranial
Extradural space, spinal *use* Spinal Canal
EXtreme Lateral Interbody Fusion (XLIF) device *use* Interbody Fusion Device in Lower Joints

F

Face lift *see* Alteration, Face 0W02
Facet replacement spinal stabilization device
　use Spinal Stabilization Device, Facet Replacement in 0RH
　use Spinal Stabilization Device, Facet Replacement in 0SH
Facial artery *use* Face Artery
Factor Xa Inhibitor Reversal Agent, Andexanet Alfa *use* Coagulation Factor Xa, Inactivated
False vocal cord *use* Larynx
Falx cerebri *use* Dura Mater
Fascia lata
　use Subcutaneous Tissue and Fascia, Left Upper Leg
　use Subcutaneous Tissue and Fascia, Right Upper Leg
Fasciaplasty, fascioplasty
　see Repair, Subcutaneous Tissue and Fascia 0JQ
　see Replacement, Subcutaneous Tissue and Fascia 0JR
Fasciectomy *see* Excision, Subcutaneous Tissue and Fascia 0JB
Fasciorrhaphy *see* Repair, Subcutaneous Tissue and Fascia 0JQ

Fasciotomy
　see Division, Subcutaneous Tissue and Fascia 0J8
　see Drainage, Subcutaneous Tissue and Fascia 0J9
　see Release
Feeding Device
　Change device in
　　Lower 0D2DXUZ
　　Upper 0D20XUZ
　Insertion of device in
　　Duodenum 0DH9
　　Esophagus 0DH5
　　Ileum 0DHB
　　Intestine, Small 0DH8
　　Jejunum 0DHA
　　Stomach 0DH6
　Removal of device from
　　Esophagus 0DP5
　　Intestinal Tract
　　　Lower 0DPD
　　　Upper 0DP0
　　Stomach 0DP6
　Revision of device in
　　Intestinal Tract
　　　Lower 0DWD
　　　Upper 0DW0
　　Stomach 0DW6
Femoral head
　use Upper Femur, Left
　use Upper Femur, Right
Femoral lymph node
　use Lymphatic, Left Lower Extremity
　use Lymphatic, Right Lower Extremity
Femoropatellar joint
　use Knee Joint, Left
　use Knee Joint, Left, Tibial Surface
　use Knee Joint, Right
　use Knee Joint, Right, Femoral Surface
Femorotibial joint
　use Knee Joint, Left
　use Knee Joint, Left, Tibial Surface
　use Knee Joint, Right
　use Knee Joint, Right, Tibial Surface
FGS (fluorescence-guided surgery) *see* Fluorescence Guided Procedure
Fibular artery
　use Peroneal Artery, Left
　use Peroneal Artery, Right
Fibularis brevis muscle
　use Lower Leg Muscle, Left
　use Lower Leg Muscle, Right
Fibularis longus muscle
　use Lower Leg Muscle, Left
　use Lower Leg Muscle, Right
Fifth cranial nerve *use* Trigeminal Nerve
Filum terminale *use* Spinal Meninges
Fimbriectomy
　see Excision, Female Reproductive System 0UB
　see Resection, Female Reproductive System 0UT
Fine needle aspiration
　Fluid or gas *see* Drainage
　Tissue biopsy
　　see Excision
　　see Extraction
First cranial nerve *use* Olfactory Nerve
First intercostal nerve *use* Brachial Plexus
Fistulization
　see Bypass
　see Drainage
　see Repair
Fitting
　Arch bars, for fracture reduction *see* Reposition, Mouth and Throat 0CS
　Arch bars, for immobilization *see* Immobilization, Face 2W31
　Artificial limb *see* Device Fitting, Rehabilitation F0D
　Hearing aid *see* Device Fitting, Rehabilitation F0D
　Ocular prosthesis F0DZ8UZ
　Prosthesis, limb *see* Device Fitting, Rehabilitation F0D
　Prosthesis, ocular F0DZ8UZ
Fixation, bone
　External, with fracture reduction *see* Reposition
　External, without fracture reduction *see* Insertion
　Internal, with fracture reduction *see* Reposition
　Internal, without fracture reduction *see* Insertion

FLAIR® Endovascular Stent Graft *use* Intraluminal Device
Flexible Composite Mesh *use* Synthetic Substitute
Flexor carpi radialis muscle
　use Lower Arm and Wrist Muscle, Left
　use Lower Arm and Wrist Muscle, Right
Flexor carpi ulnaris muscle
　use Lower Arm and Wrist Muscle, Left
　use Lower Arm and Wrist Muscle, Right
Flexor digitorum brevis muscle
　use Foot Muscle, Left
　use Foot Muscle, Right
Flexor digitorum longus muscle
　use Lower Leg Muscle, Left
　use Lower Leg Muscle, Right
Flexor hallucis brevis muscle
　use Foot Muscle, Left
　use Foot Muscle, Right
Flexor hallucis longus muscle
　use Lower Leg Muscle, Left
　use Lower Leg Muscle, Right
Flexor pollicis longus muscle
　use Lower Arm and Wrist Muscle, Left
　use Lower Arm and Wrist Muscle, Right
Flow Diverter embolization device *use* Intraluminal Device, Flow Diverter in 03V
Fluorescence Guided Procedure
　Extremity
　　Lower 8E0Y
　　Upper 8E0X
　Head and Neck Region 8E09
　　Aminolevulinic Acid 8E090EM
　　No Qualifier 8E090EZ
　Trunk Region 8E0W
Fluorescent Pyrazine, Kidney XT25XE5
Fluoroscopy
　Abdomen and Pelvis BW11
　Airway, Upper BB1DZZZ
　Ankle
　　Left BQ1H
　　Right BQ1G
　Aorta
　　Abdominal B410
　　　Laser, Intraoperative B410
　　Thoracic B310
　　　Laser, Intraoperative B310
　　Thoraco-Abdominal B31P
　　　Laser, Intraoperative B31P
　Aorta and Bilateral Lower Extremity Arteries B41D
　　Laser, Intraoperative B41D
　Arm
　　Left BP1FZZZ
　　Right BP1EZZZ
　Artery
　　Brachiocephalic-Subclavian
　　　Laser, Intraoperative B311
　　　Right B311
　　Bronchial B31L
　　　Laser, Intraoperative B31L
　　Bypass Graft, Other B21F
　　Cervico-Cerebral Arch B31Q
　　　Laser, Intraoperative B31Q
　　Common Carotid
　　　Bilateral B315
　　　　Laser, Intraoperative B315
　　　Left B314
　　　　Laser, Intraoperative B314
　　　Right B313
　　　　Laser, Intraoperative B313
　　Coronary
　　　Bypass Graft
　　　　Multiple B213
　　　　　Laser, Intraoperative B213
　　　　Single B212
　　　　　Laser, Intraoperative B212
　　　Multiple B211
　　　　Laser, Intraoperative B211
　　　Single B210
　　　　Laser, Intraoperative B210
　　External Carotid
　　　Bilateral B31C
　　　　Laser, Intraoperative B31C
　　　Left B31B
　　　　Laser, Intraoperative B31B
　　　Right B319
　　　　Laser, Intraoperative B319
　　Hepatic B412
　　　Laser, Intraoperative B412

Fluoroscopy — *continued*
  Artery — *continued*
    Inferior Mesenteric B415
      Laser, Intraoperative B415
    Intercostal B31L
      Laser, Intraoperative B31L
    Internal Carotid
      Bilateral B318
        Laser, Intraoperative B318
      Left B317
        Laser, Intraoperative B317
      Right B316
        Laser, Intraoperative B316
    Internal Mammary Bypass Graft
      Left B218
      Right B217
    Intra-Abdominal
      Laser, Intraoperative B41B
      Other B41B
    Intracranial B31R
      Laser, Intraoperative B31R
    Lower
      Laser, Intraoperative B41J
      Other B41J
    Lower Extremity
      Bilateral and Aorta B41D
        Laser, Intraoperative B41D
      Left B41G
        Laser, Intraoperative B41G
      Right B41F
        Laser, Intraoperative B41F
    Lumbar B419
      Laser, Intraoperative B419
    Pelvic B41C
      Laser, Intraoperative B41C
    Pulmonary
      Left B31T
        Laser, Intraoperative B31T
      Right B31S
        Laser, Intraoperative B31S
    Pulmonary Trunk B31U
      Laser, Intraoperative B31U
    Renal
      Bilateral B418
        Laser, Intraoperative B418
      Left B417
        Laser, Intraoperative B417
      Right B416
        Laser, Intraoperative B416
    Spinal B31M
      Laser, Intraoperative B31M
    Splenic B413
      Laser, Intraoperative B413
    Subclavian
      Laser, Intraoperative B312
      Left B312
    Superior Mesenteric B414
      Laser, Intraoperative B414
    Upper
      Laser, Intraoperative B31N
      Other B31N
    Upper Extremity
      Bilateral B31K
        Laser, Intraoperative B31K
      Left B31J
        Laser, Intraoperative B31J
      Right B31H
        Laser, Intraoperative B31H
    Vertebral
      Bilateral B31G
        Laser, Intraoperative B31G
      Left B31F
        Laser, Intraoperative B31F
      Right B31D
        Laser, Intraoperative B31D
  Bile Duct BF10
    Pancreatic Duct and Gallbladder BF14
  Bile Duct and Gallbladder BF13
  Biliary Duct BF11
  Bladder BT10
    Kidney and Ureter BT14
    Left BT1F
    Right BT1D
  Bladder and Urethra BT1B
  Bowel, Small BD1
  Calcaneus
    Left BQ1KZZZ
    Right BQ1JZZZ

Fluoroscopy — *continued*
  Clavicle
    Left BP15ZZZ
    Right BP14ZZZ
  Coccyx BR1F
  Colon BD14
  Corpora Cavernosa BV10
  Dialysis Fistula B51W
  Dialysis Shunt B51W
  Diaphragm BB16ZZZ
  Disc
    Cervical BR11
    Lumbar BR13
    Thoracic BR12
  Duodenum BD19
  Elbow
    Left BP1H
    Right BP1G
  Epiglottis B91G
  Esophagus BD11
  Extremity
    Lower BW1C
    Upper BW1J
  Facet Joint
    Cervical BR14
    Lumbar BR16
    Thoracic BR15
  Fallopian Tube
    Bilateral BU12
    Left BU11
    Right BU10
  Fallopian Tube and Uterus BU18
  Femur
    Left BQ14ZZZ
    Right BQ13ZZZ
  Finger
    Left BP1SZZZ
    Right BP1RZZZ
  Foot
    Left BQ1MZZZ
    Right BQ1LZZZ
  Forearm
    Left BP1KZZZ
    Right BP1JZZZ
  Gallbladder BF12
    Bile Duct and Pancreatic Duct BF14
  Gallbladder and Bile Duct BF13
  Gastrointestinal, Upper BD1
  Hand
    Left BP1PZZZ
    Right BP1NZZZ
  Head and Neck BW19
  Heart
    Left B215
    Right B214
    Right and Left B216
  Hip
    Left BQ11
    Right BQ10
  Humerus
    Left BP1BZZZ
    Right BP1AZZZ
  Ileal Diversion Loop BT1C
  Ileal Loop, Ureters and Kidney BT1G
  Intracranial Sinus B512
  Joint
    Acromioclavicular, Bilateral BP13ZZZ
    Finger
      Left BP1D
      Right BP1C
    Foot
      Left BQ1Y
      Right BQ1X
    Hand
      Left BP1D
      Right BP1C
    Lumbosacral BR1B
    Sacroiliac BR1D
    Sternoclavicular
      Bilateral BP12ZZZ
      Left BP11ZZZ
      Right BP10ZZZ
    Temporomandibular
      Bilateral BN19
      Left BN18
      Right BN17
    Thoracolumbar BR18
    Toe
      Left BQ1Y

Fluoroscopy — *continued*
  Joint — *continued*
    Toe — *continued*
      Right BQ1X
  Kidney
    Bilateral BT13
    Ileal Loop and Ureter BT1G
    Left BT12
    Right BT11
    Ureter and Bladder BT14
      Left BT1F
      Right BT1D
  Knee
    Left BQ18
    Right BQ17
  Larynx B91J
  Leg
    Left BQ1FZZZ
    Right BQ1DZZZ
  Lung
    Bilateral BB14ZZZ
    Left BB13ZZZ
    Right BB12ZZZ
  Mediastinum BB1CZZZ
  Mouth BD1B
  Neck and Head BW19
  Oropharynx BD1B
  Pancreatic Duct BF1
    Gallbladder and Bile Buct BF14
  Patella
    Left BQ1WZZZ
    Right BQ1VZZZ
  Pelvis BR1C
  Pelvis and Abdomen BW11
  Pharynix B91G
  Ribs
    Left BP1YZZZ
    Right BP1XZZZ
  Sacrum BR1F
  Scapula
    Left BP17ZZZ
    Right BP16ZZZ
  Shoulder
    Left BP19
    Right BP18
  Sinus, Intracranial B512
  Spinal Cord B01B
  Spine
    Cervical BR10
    Lumbar BR19
    Thoracic BR17
    Whole BR1G
  Sternum BR1H
  Stomach BD12
  Toe
    Left BQ1QZZZ
    Right BQ1PZZZ
  Tracheobronchial Tree
    Bilateral BB19YZZ
    Left BB18YZZ
    Right BB17YZZ
  Ureter
    Ileal Loop and Kidney BT1G
    Kidney and Bladder BT14
      Left BT1F
      Right BT1D
    Left BT17
    Right BT16
  Urethra BT15
  Urethra and Bladder BT1B
  Uterus BU16
  Uterus and Fallopian Tube BU18
  Vagina BU19
  Vasa Vasorum BV18
  Vein
    Cerebellar B511
    Cerebral B511
    Epidural B510
    Jugular
      Bilateral B515
      Left B514
      Right B513
    Lower Extremity
      Bilateral B51D
      Left B51C
      Right B51B
    Other B51V
    Pelvic (Iliac)
      Left B51G

Fluoroscopy — *continued*
  Vein — *continued*
    Pelvic — *continued*
      Right B51F
    Pelvic (Iliac) Bilateral B51H
    Portal B51T
    Pulmonary
      Bilateral B51S
      Left B51R
      Right B51Q
    Renal
      Bilateral B51L
      Left B51K
      Right B51J
    Spanchnic B51T
    Subclavian
      Left B517
      Right B516
    Upper Extremity
      Bilateral B51P
      Left B51N
      Right B51M
  Vena Cava
    Inferior B519
    Superior B518
  Wrist
    Left BP1M
    Right BP1L

Fluoroscopy, laser intraoperative
  see Fluoroscopy, Heart B21
  see Fluoroscopy, Lower Arteries B41
  see Fluoroscopy, Upper Arteries B31
Flushing *see* Irrigation
Foley catheter *use* Drainage Device
Fontan completion procedure Stage II *see* Bypass, Vena Cava, Inferior 0610
Foramen magnum *use* Occipital Bone
Foramen of Monro (intraventricular) *use* Cerebral Ventricle
Foreskin *use* Prepuce
Formula™ Balloon-Expandable Renal Stent System *use* Intraluminal Device
Fosfomycin Anti-infective XW0
Fosfomycin injection *use* Fosfomycin Anti-infective
Fossa of Rosenmuller *use* Nasopharynx
Fourth cranial nerve *use* Trochlear Nerve
Fourth ventricle *use* Cerebral Ventricle
Fovea
  use Retina, Left
  use Retina, Right
Fragmentation
  Ampulla of Vater 0FFC
  Anus 0DFQ
  Appendix 0DFJ
  Bladder 0TFB
  Bladder Neck 0TFC
  Bronchus
    Lingula 0BF9
    Lower Lobe
      Left 0BFB
      Right 0BF6
    Main
      Left 0BF7
      Right 0BF3
    Middle Lobe, Right 0BF5
    Upper Lobe
      Left 0BF8
      Right 0BF4
  Carina 0BF2
  Cavity, Cranial 0WF1
  Cecum 0DFH
  Cerebral Ventricle 00F6
  Colon
    Ascending 0DFK
    Descending 0DFM
    Sigmoid 0DFN
    Transverse 0DFL
  Duct
    Common Bile 0FF9
    Cystic 0FF8
    Hepatic
      Common 0FF7
      Left 0FF6
      Right 0FF5
    Pancreatic 0FFD
      Accessory 0FFF
    Parotid
      Left 0CFC

Fragmentation — *continued*
  Duct — *continued*
    Parotid — *continued*
      Right 0CFB
  Duodenum 0DF9
  Epidural Space, Intracranial 00F3
  Esophagus 0DF5
  Fallopian Tube
    Left 0UF6
    Right 0UF5
  Fallopian Tubes, Bilateral 0UF7
  Gallbladder 0FF4
  Gastrointestinal Tract 0WFP
  Genitourinary Tract 0WFR
  Ileum 0DFB
  Intestine
    Large 0DFE
      Left 0DFG
      Right 0DFF
    Small 0DF8
  Jejunum 0DFA
  Kidney Pelvis
    Left 0TF4
    Right 0TF3
  Mediastinum 0WFC
  Oral Cavity and Throat 0WF3
  Pelvic Cavity 0WFJ
  Pericardial Cavity 0WFD
  Pericardium 02FN
  Peritoneal Cavity 0WFG
  Pleural Cavity
    Left 0WFB
    Right 0WF9
  Rectum 0DFP
  Respiratory Tract 0WFQ
  Spinal Canal 00FU
  Stomach 0DF6
  Subarachnoid Space, Intracranial 00F5
  Subdural Space, Intracranial 00F4
  Trachea 0BF1
  Ureter
    Left 0TF7
    Right 0TF6
  Urethra 0TFD
  Uterus 0UF9
  Vitreous
    Left 08F5
    Right 08F4
Freestyle (Stentless) Aortic Root Bioprosthesis *use* Zooplastic Tissue in Heart and Great Vessels
Frenectomy
  see Excision, Mouth and Throat 0CB
  see Resection, Mouth and Throat 0CT
Frenoplasty, frenuloplasty
  see Repair, Mouth and Throat 0CQ
  see Replacement, Mouth and Throat 0CR
  see Supplement, Mouth and Throat 0CU
Frenotomy
  see Drainage, Mouth and Throat 0C9
  see Release, Mouth and Throat 0CN
Frenulotomy
  see Drainage, Mouth and Throat 0C9
  see Release, Mouth and Throat 0CN
Frenulum labii inferioris *use* Lower Lip
Frenulum labii superioris *use* Upper Lip
Frenulum linguae *use* Tongue
Frenulumectomy
  see Excision, Mouth and Throat 0CB
  see Resection, Mouth and Throat 0CT
Frontal lobe *use* Cerebral Hemisphere
Frontal vein
  use Face Vein, Left
  use Face Vein, Right
Fulguration *see* Destruction
Fundoplication, gastroesophageal *see* Restriction, Esophagogastric Junction 0DV4
Fundus uteri *use* Uterus
Fusion
  Acromioclavicular
    Left 0RGH
    Right 0RGG
  Ankle
    Left 0SGG
    Right 0SGF
  Carpal
    Left 0RGR
    Right 0RGQ

Fusion — *continued*
  Carpometacarpal
    Left 0RGT
    Right 0RGS
  Cervical Vertebral 0RG1
    2 or more 0RG2
      Interbody Fusion Device
        Nanotextured Surface XRG2092
        Radiolucent Porous XRG20F3
    Interbody Fusion Device
      Nanotextured Surface XRG1092
      Radiolucent Porous XRG10F3
  Cervicothoracic Vertebral 0RG4
    Interbody Fusion Device
      Nanotextured Surface XRG4092
      Radiolucent Porous XRG40F3
  Coccygeal 0SG6
  Elbow
    Left 0RGM
    Right 0RGL
  Finger Phalangeal
    Left 0RGX
    Right 0RGW
  Hip
    Left 0SGB
    Right 0SG9
  Knee
    Left 0SGD
    Right 0SGC
  Lumbar Vertebral 0SG0
    2 or more 0SG1
      Interbody Fusion Device
        Nanotextured Surface XRGC092
        Radiolucent Porous XRGC0F3
    Interbody Fusion Device
      Nanotextured Surface XRGB092
      Radiolucent Porous XRGB0F3
  Lumbosacral 0SG3
    Interbody Fusion Device
      Nanotextured Surface XRGD092
      Radiolucent Porous XRGD0F3
  Metacarpophalangeal
    Left 0RGV
    Right 0RGU
  Metatarsal-Phalangeal
    Left 0SGN
    Right 0SGM
  Occipital-cervical 0RG0
    Interbody Fusion Device
      Nanotextured Surface XRG0092
      Radiolucent Porous XRG00F3
  Sacrococcygeal 0SG5
  Sacroiliac
    Left 0SG8
    Right 0SG7
  Shoulder
    Left 0RGK
    Right 0RGJ
  Sternoclavicular
    Left 0RGF
    Right 0RGE
  Tarsal
    Left 0SGJ
    Right 0SGH
  Tarsometatarsal
    Left 0SGL
    Right 0SGK
  Temporomandibular
    Left 0RGD
    Right 0RGC
  Thoracic Vertebral 0RG6
    2 to 7 0RG7
      Interbody Fusion Device
        Nanotextured Surface XRG7092
        Radiolucent Porous XRG70F3
    8 or more 0RG8
      Interbody Fusion Device
        Nanotextured Surface XRG8092
        Radiolucent Porous XRG80F3
    Interbody Fusion Device
      Nanotextured Surface XRG6092
      Radiolucent Porous XRG60F3
  Thoracolumbar Vertebral 0RGA
    Interbody Fusion Device
      Nanotextured Surface XRGA092
      Radiolucent Porous XRGA0F3
  Toe Phalangeal
    Left 0SGQ
    Right 0SGP

Fusion — *continued*
Wrist
Left ØRGP
Right ØRGN
Fusion screw (compression) (lag) (locking)
use Internal Fixation Device in Lower Joints
use Internal Fixation Device in Upper Joints

G

Gait training *see* Motor Treatment, Rehabilitation F07
Galea aponeurotica *use* Subcutaneous Tissue and Fascia, Scalp
GammaTile™ *use* Radioactive Element, Cesium-131 Collagen Implant in 00H
Ganglion impar (ganglion of Walther) *use* Sacral Sympathetic Nerve
Ganglionectomy
Destruction of lesion *see* Destruction
Excision of lesion *see* Excision
Gasserian ganglion *use* Trigeminal Nerve
Gastrectomy
Partial *see* Excision, Stomach ØDB6
Total *see* Resection, Stomach ØDT6
Vertical (sleeve) *see* Excision, Stomach ØDB6
Gastric electrical stimulation (GES) lead *use* Stimulator Lead in Gastrointestinal System
Gastric lymph node *use* Lymphatic, Aortic
Gastric pacemaker lead *use* Stimulator Lead in Gastrointestinal System
Gastric plexus *use* Abdominal Sympathetic Nerve
Gastrocnemius muscle
use Lower Leg Muscle, Left
use Lower Leg Muscle, Right
Gastrocolic ligament *use* Omentum
Gastrocolic omentum *use* Omentum
Gastrocolostomy
see Bypass, Gastrointestinal System ØD1
see Drainage, Gastrointestinal System ØD9
Gastroduodenal artery *use* Hepatic Artery
Gastroduodenectomy
see Excision, Gastrointestinal System ØDB
see Resection, Gastrointestinal System ØDT
Gastroduodenoscopy ØDJ08ZZ
Gastroenteroplasty
see Repair, Gastrointestinal System ØDQ
see Supplement, Gastrointestinal System ØDU
Gastroenterostomy
see Bypass, Gastrointestinal System ØD1
see Drainage, Gastrointestinal System ØD9
Gastroesophageal (GE) junction *use* Esophagogastric Junction
Gastrogastrostomy
see Bypass, Stomach ØD16
see Drainage, Stomach ØD96
Gastrohepatic omentum *use* Omentum
Gastrojejunostomy
see Bypass, Stomach ØD16
see Drainage, Stomach ØD96
Gastrolysis *see* Release, Stomach ØDN6
Gastropexy
see Repair, Stomach ØDQ6
see Reposition, Stomach ØDS6
Gastrophrenic ligament *use* Omentum
Gastroplasty
see Repair, Stomach ØDQ6
see Supplement, Stomach ØDU6
Gastroplication *see* Restriction, Stomach ØDV6
Gastropylorectomy *see* Excision, Gastrointestinal System ØDB
Gastrorrhaphy *see* Repair, Stomach ØDQ6
Gastroscopy ØDJ68ZZ
Gastrosplenic ligament *use* Omentum
Gastrostomy
see Bypass, Stomach ØD16
see Drainage, Stomach ØD96
Gastrotomy *see* Drainage, Stomach ØD96
Gemellus muscle
use Hip Muscle, Left
use Hip Muscle, Right
Geniculate ganglion *use* Facial Nerve
Geniculate nucleus *use* Thalamus
Genioglossus muscle *use* Tongue, Palate, Pharynx Muscle
Genioplasty *see* Alteration, Jaw, Lower ØW05
Genitofemoral nerve *use* Lumbar Plexus

GIAPREZA™ *use* Synthetic Human Angiotensin II
Gilteritinib Antineoplastic XW0DXV5
Gingivectomy *see* Excision, Mouth and Throat ØCB
Gingivoplasty
see Repair, Mouth and Throat ØCQ
see Replacement, Mouth and Throat ØCR
see Supplement, Mouth and Throat ØCU
Glans penis *use* Prepuce
Glenohumeral joint
use Shoulder Joint, Left
use Shoulder Joint, Right
Glenohumeral ligament
use Shoulder Bursa and Ligament, Left
use Shoulder Bursa and Ligament, Right
Glenoid fossa (of scapula)
use Glenoid Cavity, Left
use Glenoid Cavity, Right
Glenoid ligament (labrum)
use Shoulder Joint, Left
use Shoulder Joint, Right
Globus pallidus *use* Basal Ganglia
Glomectomy
see Excision, Endocrine System ØGB
see Resection, Endocrine System ØGT
Glossectomy
see Excision, Tongue ØCB7
see Resection, Tongue ØCT7
Glossoepiglottic fold *use* Epiglottis
Glossopexy
see Repair, Tongue ØCQ7
see Reposition, Tongue ØCS7
Glossoplasty
see Repair, Tongue ØCQ7
see Replacement, Tongue ØCR7
see Supplement, Tongue ØCU7
Glossorrhaphy *see* Repair, Tongue ØCQ7
Glossotomy *see* Drainage, Tongue ØC97
Glottis *use* Larynx
Gluteal Artery Perforator Flap
Replacement
Bilateral ØHRVØ79
Left ØHRUØ79
Right ØHRTØ79
Transfer
Left ØKXG
Right ØKXF
Gluteal lymph node *use* Lymphatic, Pelvis
Gluteal vein
use Hypogastric Vein, Left
use Hypogastric Vein, Right
Gluteus maximus muscle
use Hip Muscle, Left
use Hip Muscle, Right
Gluteus medius muscle
use Hip Muscle, Left
use Hip Muscle, Right
Gluteus minimus muscle
use Hip Muscle, Left
use Hip Muscle, Right
GORE EXCLUDER® AAA Endoprosthesis
use Intraluminal Device
use Intraluminal Device, Branched or Fenestrated, One or Two Arteries in 04V
use Intraluminal Device, Branched or Fenestrated, Three or More Arteries in 04V
GORE EXCLUDER® IBE Endoprosthesis *use* Intraluminal Device, Branched or Fenestrated, One or Two Arteries in 04V
GORE TAG® Thoracic Endoprosthesis *use* Intraluminal Device
GORE® DUALMESH® *use* Synthetic Substitute
Gracilis muscle
use Upper Leg Muscle, Left
use Upper Leg Muscle, Right
Graft
see Replacement
see Supplement
Great auricular nerve *use* Cervical Plexus
Great cerebral vein *use* Intracranial Vein
Great(er) saphenous vein
use Saphenous Vein, Left
use Saphenous Vein, Right
Greater alar cartilage *use* Nasal Mucosa and Soft Tissue
Greater occipital nerve *use* Cervical Nerve
Greater Omentum *use* Omentum

Greater splanchnic nerve *use* Thoracic Sympathetic Nerve
Greater superficial petrosal nerve *use* Facial Nerve
Greater trochanter
use Upper Femur, Left
use Upper Femur, Right
Greater tuberosity
use Humeral Head, Left
use Humeral Head, Right
Greater vestibular (Bartholin's) gland *use* Vestibular Gland
Greater wing *use* Sphenoid Bone
Guedel airway *use* Intraluminal Device, Airway in Mouth and Throat
Guidance, catheter placement
EKG *see* Measurement, Physiological Systems 4A0
Fluoroscopy *see* Fluoroscopy, Veins B51
Ultrasound *see* Ultrasonography, Veins B54

H

Hallux
use 1st Toe, Left
use 1st Toe, Right
Hamate bone
use Carpal, Left
use Carpal, Right
Hancock Bioprosthesis (aortic) (mitral) valve *use* Zooplastic Tissue in Heart and Great Vessels
Hancock Bioprosthetic Valved Conduit *use* Zooplastic Tissue in Heart and Great Vessels
Harvesting, stem cells *see* Pheresis, Circulatory 6A55
Head of fibula
use Fibula, Left
use Fibula, Right
Hearing Aid Assessment F14Z
Hearing Assessment F13Z
Hearing Device
Bone Conduction
Left 09HE
Right 09HD
Insertion of device in
Left 0NH6
Right 0NH5
Multiple Channel Cochlear Prosthesis
Left 09HE
Right 09HD
Removal of device from, Skull 0NP0
Revision of device in, Skull 0NW0
Single Channel Cochlear Prosthesis
Left 09HE
Right 09HD
Hearing Treatment F09Z
Heart Assist System
Implantable
Insertion of device in, Heart 02HA
Removal of device from, Heart 02PA
Revision of device in, Heart 02WA
Short-term External
Insertion of device in, Heart 02HA
Removal of device from, Heart 02PA
Revision of device in, Heart 02WA
HeartMate 3™ LVAS *use* Implantable Heart Assist System in Heart and Great Vessels
HeartMate II® Left Ventricular Assist Device (LVAD) *use* Implantable Heart Assist System in Heart and Great Vessels
HeartMate XVE® Left Ventricular Assist Device (LVAD) *use* Implantable Heart Assist System in Heart and Great Vessels
HeartMate® implantable heart assist system *see* Insertion of device in, Heart 02HA
Helix
use Ear, External, Bilateral
use Ear, External, Left
use Ear, External, Right
Hematopoietic cell transplant (HCT) *see* Transfusion, Circulatory 302
Hemicolectomy *see* Resection, Gastrointestinal System 0DT
Hemicystectomy *see* Excision, Urinary System 0TB
Hemigastrectomy *see* Excision, Gastrointestinal System 0DB
Hemiglossectomy *see* Excision, Mouth and Throat 0CB
Hemilaminectomy
see Excision, Lower Bones 0QB

Hemilaminectomy — *continued*
  see Excision, Upper Bones ØPB
Hemilaminotomy
  see Drainage, Lower Bones ØQ9
  see Drainage, Upper Bones ØP9
  see Excision, Lower Bones ØQB
  see Excision, Upper Bones ØPB
  see Release, Central Nervous System and Cranial
    Nerves ØØN
  see Release, Lower Bones ØQN
  see Release, Peripheral Nervous System Ø1N
  see Release, Upper Bones ØPN
Hemilaryngectomy *see* Excision, Larynx ØCBS
Hemimandibulectomy *see* Excision, Head and Facial
  Bones ØNB
Hemimaxillectomy *see* Excision, Head and Facial Bones
  ØNB
Hemipylorectomy *see* Excision, Gastrointestinal System ØDB
Hemispherectomy
  see Excision, Central Nervous System and Cranial
    Nerves ØØB
  see Resection, Central Nervous System and Cranial
    Nerves ØØT
Hemithyroidectomy
  see Excision, Endocrine System ØGB
  see Resection, Endocrine System ØGT
Hemodialysis *see* Performance, Urinary 5A1D
Hemolung® Respiratory Assist System (RAS)
  5AØ92ØZ
Hepatectomy
  see Excision, Hepatobiliary System and Pancreas
    ØFB
  see Resection, Hepatobiliary System and Pancreas
    ØFT
Hepatic artery proper *use* Hepatic Artery
Hepatic flexure *use* Transverse Colon
Hepatic lymph node *use* Lymphatic, Aortic
Hepatic plexus *use* Abdominal Sympathetic Nerve
Hepatic portal vein *use* Portal Vein
Hepaticoduodenostomy
  see Bypass, Hepatobiliary System and Pancreas
    ØF1
  see Drainage, Hepatobiliary System and Pancreas
    ØF9
Hepaticotomy *see* Drainage, Hepatobiliary System and
  Pancreas ØF9
Hepatocholedochostomy *see* Drainage, Duct, Common Bile ØF99
Hepatogastric ligament *use* Omentum
Hepatopancreatic ampulla *use* Ampulla of Vater
Hepatopexy
  see Repair, Hepatobiliary System and Pancreas ØFQ
  see Reposition, Hepatobiliary System and Pancreas
    ØFS
Hepatorrhaphy *see* Repair, Hepatobiliary System and
  Pancreas ØFQ
Hepatotomy *see* Drainage, Hepatobiliary System and
  Pancreas ØF9
Herculink (RX) Elite Renal Stent System *use* Intraluminal Device
Herniorrhaphy
  see Repair, Anatomical Regions, General ØWQ
  see Repair, Anatomical Regions, Lower Extremities
    ØYQ
  With synthetic substitute
    see Supplement, Anatomical Regions, General ØWU
    see Supplement, Anatomical Regions, Lower
      Extremities ØYU
Hip (joint) liner *use* Liner in Lower Joints
HIPEC (hyperthermic intraperitoneal chemotherapy) 3EØM3ØY
Holter monitoring 4A12X45
Holter valve ventricular shunt *use* Synthetic Substitute
Human angiotensin II, synthetic *use* Synthetic Human Angiotensin II
Humeroradial joint
  use Elbow Joint, Left
  use Elbow Joint, Right
Humeroulnar joint
  use Elbow Joint, Left
  use Elbow Joint, Right
Humerus, distal
  use Humeral Shaft, Left
  use Humeral Shaft, Right

Hydrocelectomy *see* Excision, Male Reproductive System ØVB
Hydrotherapy
  Assisted exercise in pool *see* Motor Treatment,
    Rehabilitation FØ7
  Whirlpool *see* Activities of Daily Living Treatment,
    Rehabilitation FØ8
Hymenectomy
  see Excision, Hymen ØUBK
  see Resection, Hymen ØUTK
Hymenoplasty
  see Repair, Hymen ØUQK
  see Supplement, Hymen ØUUK
Hymenorrhaphy *see* Repair, Hymen ØUQK
Hymenotomy
  see Division, Hymen ØU8K
  see Drainage, Hymen ØU9K
Hyoglossus muscle *use* Tongue, Palate, Pharynx
  Muscle
Hyoid artery
  use Thyroid Artery, Left
  use Thyroid Artery, Right
Hyperalimentation *see* Introduction of substance in
  or on
Hyperbaric oxygenation
  Decompression sickness treatment *see* Decompression, Circulatory 6A15
  Wound treatment *see* Assistance, Circulatory 5AØ5
Hyperthermia
  Radiation Therapy
    Abdomen DWY38ZZ
    Adrenal Gland DGY28ZZ
    Bile Ducts DFY28ZZ
    Bladder DTY28ZZ
    Bone Marrow D7YØ8ZZ
    Bone, Other DPYC8ZZ
    Brain DØYØ8ZZ
    Brain Stem DØY18ZZ
    Breast
      Left DMYØ8ZZ
      Right DMY18ZZ
    Bronchus DBY18ZZ
    Cervix DUY18ZZ
    Chest DWY28ZZ
    Chest Wall DBY78ZZ
    Colon DDY58ZZ
    Diaphragm DBY88ZZ
    Duodenum DDY28ZZ
    Ear D9YØ8ZZ
    Esophagus DDYØ8ZZ
    Eye D8YØ8ZZ
    Femur DPY98ZZ
    Fibula DPYB8ZZ
    Gallbladder DFY18ZZ
    Gland
      Adrenal DGY28ZZ
      Parathyroid DGY48ZZ
      Pituitary DGYØ8ZZ
      Thyroid DGY58ZZ
    Glands, Salivary D9Y68ZZ
    Head and Neck DWY18ZZ
    Hemibody DWY48ZZ
    Humerus DPY68ZZ
    Hypopharynx D9Y38ZZ
    Ileum DDY48ZZ
    Jejunum DDY38ZZ
    Kidney DTYØ8ZZ
    Larynx D9YB8ZZ
    Liver DFYØ8ZZ
    Lung DBY28ZZ
    Lymphatics
      Abdomen D7Y68ZZ
      Axillary D7Y48ZZ
      Inguinal D7Y88ZZ
      Neck D7Y38ZZ
      Pelvis D7Y78ZZ
      Thorax D7Y58ZZ
    Mandible DPY38ZZ
    Maxilla DPY28ZZ
    Mediastinum DBY68ZZ
    Mouth D9Y48ZZ
    Nasopharynx D9YD8ZZ
    Neck and Head DWY18ZZ
    Nerve, Peripheral DØY78ZZ
    Nose D9Y18ZZ
    Oropharynx D9YF8ZZ
    Ovary DUYØ8ZZ

Hyperthermia — *continued*
  Radiation Therapy — *continued*
    Palate
      Hard D9Y88ZZ
      Soft D9Y98ZZ
    Pancreas DFY38ZZ
    Parathyroid Gland DGY48ZZ
    Pelvic Bones DPY88ZZ
    Pelvic Region DWY68ZZ
    Pineal Body DGY18ZZ
    Pituitary Gland DGYØ8ZZ
    Pleura DBY58ZZ
    Prostate DVYØ8ZZ
    Radius DPY78ZZ
    Rectum DDY78ZZ
    Rib DPY58ZZ
    Sinuses D9Y78ZZ
    Skin
      Abdomen DHY88ZZ
      Arm DHY48ZZ
      Back DHY78ZZ
      Buttock DHY98ZZ
      Chest DHY68ZZ
      Face DHY28ZZ
      Leg DHYB8ZZ
      Neck DHY38ZZ
    Skull DPYØ8ZZ
    Spinal Cord DØY68ZZ
    Spleen D7Y28ZZ
    Sternum DPY48ZZ
    Stomach DDY18ZZ
    Testis DVY18ZZ
    Thymus D7Y18ZZ
    Thyroid Gland DGY58ZZ
    Tibia DPYB8ZZ
    Tongue D9Y58ZZ
    Trachea DBYØ8ZZ
    Ulna DPY78ZZ
    Ureter DTY18ZZ
    Urethra DTY38ZZ
    Uterus DUY28ZZ
    Whole Body DWY58ZZ
  Whole Body 6A3Z
**Hyperthermic intraperitoneal chemotherapy
  (HIPEC)** 3EØM3ØY
Hypnosis GZFZZZZ
Hypogastric artery
  use Internal Iliac Artery, Left
  use Internal Iliac Artery, Right
Hypopharynx *use* Pharynx
Hypophysectomy
  see Excision, Gland, Pituitary ØGBØ
  see Resection, Gland, Pituitary ØGTØ
Hypophysis *use* Pituitary Gland
Hypothalamotomy *see* Destruction, Thalamus ØØ59
Hypothenar muscle
  use Hand Muscle, Left
  use Hand Muscle, Right
Hypothermia, Whole Body 6A4Z
Hysterectomy
  Supracervical *see* Resection, Uterus ØUT9
  Total *see* Resection, Uterus ØUT9
Hysterolysis *see* Release, Uterus ØUN9
Hysteropexy
  see Repair, Uterus ØUQ9
  see Reposition, Uterus ØUS9
Hysteroplasty *see* Repair, Uterus ØUQ9
Hysterorrhaphy *see* Repair, Uterus ØUQ9
Hysteroscopy ØUJD8ZZ
Hysterotomy *see* Drainage, Uterus ØU99
Hysterotrachelectomy
  see Resection, Cervix ØUTC
  see Resection, Uterus ØUT9
Hysterotracheloplasty *see* Repair, Uterus ØUQ9
Hysterotrachelorrhaphy *see* Repair, Uterus ØUQ9

I

IABP (Intra-aortic balloon pump) *see* Assistance,
  Cardiac 5AØ2
IAEMT (Intraoperative anesthetic effect monitoring and titration) *see* Monitoring, Central Nervous 4A1Ø
Idarucizumab, Dabigatran Reversal Agent XWØ
IHD (Intermittent hemodialysis) 5A1D7ØZ
Ileal artery *use* Superior Mesenteric Artery

Ileectomy
  see Excision, Ileum ØDBB
  see Resection, Ileum ØDTB
Ileocolic artery *use* Superior Mesenteric Artery
Ileocolic vein *use* Colic Vein
Ileopexy
  see Repair, Ileum ØDQB
  see Reposition, Ileum ØDSB
Ileorrhaphy *see* Repair, Ileum ØDQB
Ileoscopy ØDJD8ZZ
Ileostomy
  see Bypass, Ileum ØD1B
  see Drainage, Ileum ØD9B
Ileotomy *see* Drainage, Ileum ØD9B
Ileoureterostomy *see* Bypass, Urinary System ØT1
Iliac crest
  use Pelvic Bone, Left
  use Pelvic Bone, Right
Iliac fascia
  use Subcutaneous Tissue and Fascia, Left Upper
    Leg
  use Subcutaneous Tissue and Fascia, Right Upper
    Leg
Iliac lymph node *use* Lymphatic, Pelvis
Iliacus muscle
  use Hip Muscle, Left
  use Hip Muscle, Right
Iliofemoral ligament
  use Hip Bursa and Ligament, Left
  use Hip Bursa and Ligament, Right
Iliohypogastric nerve *use* Lumbar Plexus
Ilioinguinal nerve *use* Lumbar Plexus
Iliolumbar artery
  use Internal Iliac Artery, Left
  use Internal Iliac Artery, Right
Iliolumbar ligament *use* Lower Spine Bursa and Ligament
Iliotibial tract (band)
  use Subcutaneous Tissue and Fascia, Left Upper
    Leg
  use Subcutaneous Tissue and Fascia, Right Upper
    Leg
Ilium
  use Pelvic Bone, Left
  use Pelvic Bone, Right
Ilizarov external fixator
  use External Fixation Device, Ring in ØPH
  use External Fixation Device, Ring in ØPS
  use External Fixation Device, Ring in ØQH
  use External Fixation Device, Ring in ØQS
Ilizarov-Vecklich device
  use External Fixation Device, Limb Lengthening in
    ØPH
  use External Fixation Device, Limb Lengthening in
    ØQH
Imaging, diagnostic
  see Computerized Tomography (CT Scan)
  see Fluoroscopy
  see Magnetic Resonance Imaging (MRI)
  see Plain Radiography
  see Ultrasonography
Imipenem-cilastatin-relebactam Anti-infective
  XW0
IMI/REL *use* Imipenem-cilastatin-relebactam Anti-infec-
  tive
Immobilization
  Abdominal Wall 2W33X
  Arm
    Lower
      Left 2W3DX
      Right 2W3CX
    Upper
      Left 2W3BX
      Right 2W3AX
  Back 2W35X
  Chest Wall 2W34X
  Extremity
    Lower
      Left 2W3MX
      Right 2W3LX
    Upper
      Left 2W39X
      Right 2W38X
  Face 2W31X
  Finger
    Left 2W3KX
    Right 2W3JX

Immobilization — *continued*
  Foot
    Left 2W3TX
    Right 2W3SX
  Hand
    Left 2W3FX
    Right 2W3EX
  Head 2W30X
  Inguinal Region
    Left 2W37X
    Right 2W36X
  Leg
    Lower
      Left 2W3RX
      Right 2W3QX
    Upper
      Left 2W3PX
      Right 2W3NX
  Neck 2W32X
  Thumb
    Left 2W3HX
    Right 2W3GX
  Toe
    Left 2W3VX
    Right 2W3UX
Immunization *see* Introduction of Serum, Toxoid, and
  Vaccine
Immunotherapy *see* Introduction of Immunotherapeu-
  tic Substance
Immunotherapy, antineoplastic
  Interferon *see* Introduction of Low-dose Inter-
    leukin-2
  Interleukin-2, high-dose *see* Introduction of High-
    dose Interleukin-2
  Interleukin-2, low-dose *see* Introduction of Low-
    dose Interleukin-2
  Monoclonal antibody *see* Introduction of Mono-
    clonal Antibody
  Proleukin, high-dose *see* Introduction of High-dose
    Interleukin-2
  Proleukin, low-dose *see* Introduction of Low-dose
    Interleukin-2
Impella® heart pump *use* Short-term External Heart
  Assist System in Heart and Great Vessels
Impeller Pump
  Continuous, Output 5A0221D
  Intermittent, Output 5A0211D
Implantable cardioverter-defibrillator (ICD) *use*
  Defibrillator Generator in ØJH
Implantable drug infusion pump (anti-spasmodic)
  (chemotherapy) (pain) *use* Infusion Device,
  Pump in Subcutaneous Tissue and Fascia
Implantable glucose monitoring device *use* Moni-
  toring Device
Implantable hemodynamic monitor (IHM) *use*
  Monitoring Device, Hemodynamic in ØJH
Implantable hemodynamic monitoring system
  (IHMS) *use* Monitoring Device, Hemodynamic in
  ØJH
Implantable Miniature Telescope™ (IMT) *use* Syn-
  thetic Substitute, Intraocular Telescope in Ø8R
Implantation
  see Insertion
  see Replacement
Implanted (venous)(access) port *use* Vascular Access
  Device, Totally Implantable in Subcutaneous Tis-
  sue and Fascia
IMV (intermittent mandatory ventilation) *see* Assis-
  tance, Respiratory 5A09
In Vitro Fertilization 8E0ZXY1
Incision, abscess *see* Drainage
Incudectomy
  see Excision, Ear, Nose, Sinus Ø9B
  see Resection, Ear, Nose, Sinus Ø9T
Incudopexy
  see Repair, Ear, Nose, Sinus Ø9Q
  see Reposition, Ear, Nose, Sinus Ø9S
Incus
  use Auditory Ossicle, Left
  use Auditory Ossicle, Right
Induction of labor
  Artificial rupture of membranes *see* Drainage,
    Pregnancy 1Ø9
  Oxytocin *see* Introduction of Hormone
InDura, intrathecal catheter (1P) (spinal) *use* Infu-
  sion Device

Infection, Whole Blood Nucleic Acid-base Microbial
  Detection, Measurement XXE5XM5
Inferior cardiac nerve *use* Thoracic Sympathetic Nerve
Inferior cerebellar vein *use* Intracranial Vein
Inferior cerebral vein *use* Intracranial Vein
Inferior epigastric artery
  use External Iliac Artery, Left
  use External Iliac Artery, Right
Inferior epigastric lymph node *use* Lymphatic, Pelvis
Inferior genicular artery
  use Popliteal Artery, Left
  use Popliteal Artery, Right
Inferior gluteal artery
  use Internal Iliac Artery, Left
  use Internal Iliac Artery, Right
Inferior gluteal nerve *use* Sacral Plexus
Inferior hypogastric plexus *use* Abdominal Sympa-
  thetic Nerve
Inferior labial artery *use* Face Artery
Inferior longitudinal muscle *use* Tongue, Palate,
  Pharynx Muscle
Inferior mesenteric ganglion *use* Abdominal Sympa-
  thetic Nerve
Inferior mesenteric lymph node *use* Lymphatic,
  Mesenteric
Inferior mesenteric plexus *use* Abdominal Sympathet-
  ic Nerve
Inferior oblique muscle
  use Extraocular Muscle, Left
  use Extraocular Muscle, Right
Inferior pancreaticoduodenal artery *use* Superior
  Mesenteric Artery
Inferior phrenic artery *use* Abdominal Aorta
Inferior rectus muscle
  use Extraocular Muscle, Left
  use Extraocular Muscle, Right
Inferior suprarenal artery
  use Renal Artery, Left
  use Renal Artery, Right
Inferior tarsal plate
  use Lower Eyelid, Left
  use Lower Eyelid, Right
Inferior thyroid vein
  use Innominate Vein, Left
  use Innominate Vein, Right
Inferior tibiofibular joint
  use Ankle Joint, Left
  use Ankle Joint, Right
Inferior turbinate *use* Nasal Turbinate
Inferior ulnar collateral artery
  use Brachial Artery, Left
  use Brachial Artery, Right
Inferior vesical artery
  use Internal Iliac Artery, Left
  use Internal Iliac Artery, Right
Infraauricular lymph node *use* Lymphatic, Head
Infraclavicular (deltopectoral) lymph node
  use Lymphatic, Left Upper Extremity
  use Lymphatic, Right Upper Extremity
Infrahyoid muscle
  use Neck Muscle, Left
  use Neck Muscle, Right
Infraparotid lymph node *use* Lymphatic, Head
Infraspinatus fascia
  use Subcutaneous Tissue and Fascia, Left Upper
    Arm
  use Subcutaneous Tissue and Fascia, Right Upper
    Arm
Infraspinatus muscle
  use Shoulder Muscle, Left
  use Shoulder Muscle, Right
Infundibulopelvic ligament *use* Uterine Supporting
  Structure
Infusion *see* Introduction of substance in or on
Infusion Device, Pump
  Insertion of device in
    Abdomen ØJH8
    Back ØJH7
    Chest ØJH6
    Lower Arm
      Left ØJHH
      Right ØJHG
    Lower Leg
      Left ØJHP
      Right ØJHN
    Trunk ØJHT

Infusion Device, Pump — *continued*
  Insertion of device in — *continued*
    Upper Arm
      Left 0JHF
      Right 0JHD
    Upper Leg
      Left 0JHM
      Right 0JHL
  Removal of device from
    Lower Extremity 0JPW
    Trunk 0JPT
    Upper Extremity 0JPV
  Revision of device in
    Lower Extremity 0JWW
    Trunk 0JWT
    Upper Extremity 0JWV
Infusion, glucarpidase
  Central Vein 3E043GQ
  Peripheral Vein 3E033GQ
Inguinal canal
  use Inguinal Region, Bilateral
  use Inguinal Region, Left
  use Inguinal Region, Right
Inguinal triangle
  use Inguinal Region, Bilateral
  use Inguinal Region, Left
  use Inguinal Region, Right
Injection *see* Introduction of substance in or on
Injection, Concentrated Bone Marrow Aspirate (CBMA), intramuscular XK02303
Injection reservoir, port *use* Vascular Access Device, Totally Implantable in Subcutaneous Tissue and Fascia
Injection reservoir, pump *use* Infusion Device, Pump in Subcutaneous Tissue and Fascia
Insemination, artificial 3E0P7LZ
Insertion
  Antimicrobial envelope *see* Introduction of Anti-infective
  Aqueous drainage shunt
    see Bypass, Eye 081
    see Drainage, Eye 089
  Products of Conception 10H0
  Spinal Stabilization Device
    see Insertion of device in, Lower Joints 0SH
    see Insertion of device in, Upper Joints 0RH
Insertion of device in
  Abdominal Wall 0WHF
  Acetabulum
    Left 0QH5
    Right 0QH4
  Anal Sphincter 0DHR
  Ankle Region
    Left 0YHL
    Right 0YHK
  Anus 0DHQ
  Aorta
    Abdominal 04H0
    Thoracic
      Ascending/Arch 02HX
      Descending 02HW
  Arm
    Lower
      Left 0XHF
      Right 0XHD
    Upper
      Left 0XH9
      Right 0XH8
  Artery
    Anterior Tibial
      Left 04HQ
      Right 04HP
    Axillary
      Left 03H6
      Right 03H5
    Brachial
      Left 03H8
      Right 03H7
    Celiac 04H1
    Colic
      Left 04H7
      Middle 04H8
      Right 04H6
    Common Carotid
      Left 03HJ
      Right 03HH
    Common Iliac
      Left 04HD

Insertion of device in — *continued*
  Artery — *continued*
    Common Iliac — *continued*
      Right 04HC
    Coronary
      Four or More Arteries 02H3
      One Artery 02H0
      Three Arteries 02H2
      Two Arteries 02H1
    External Carotid
      Left 03HN
      Right 03HM
    External Iliac
      Left 04HJ
      Right 04HH
    Face 03HR
    Femoral
      Left 04HL
      Right 04HK
    Foot
      Left 04HW
      Right 04HV
    Gastric 04H2
    Hand
      Left 03HF
      Right 03HD
    Hepatic 04H3
    Inferior Mesenteric 04HB
    Innominate 03H2
    Internal Carotid
      Left 03HL
      Right 03HK
    Internal Iliac
      Left 04HF
      Right 04HE
    Internal Mammary
      Left 03H1
      Right 03H0
    Intracranial 03HG
    Lower 04HY
    Peroneal
      Left 04HU
      Right 04HT
    Popliteal
      Left 04HN
      Right 04HM
    Posterior Tibial
      Left 04HS
      Right 04HR
    Pulmonary
      Left 02HR
      Right 02HQ
    Pulmonary Trunk 02HP
    Radial
      Left 03HC
      Right 03HB
    Renal
      Left 04HA
      Right 04H9
    Splenic 04H4
    Subclavian
      Left 03H4
      Right 03H3
    Superior Mesenteric 04H5
    Temporal
      Left 03HT
      Right 03HS
    Thyroid
      Left 03HV
      Right 03HU
    Ulnar
      Left 03HA
      Right 03H9
    Upper 03HY
    Vertebral
      Left 03HQ
      Right 03HP
  Atrium
    Left 02H7
    Right 02H6
  Axilla
    Left 0XH5
    Right 0XH4
  Back
    Lower 0WHL
    Upper 0WHK
  Bladder 0THB
  Bladder Neck 0THC

Insertion of device in — *continued*
  Bone
    Ethmoid
      Left 0NHG
      Right 0NHF
    Facial 0NHW
    Frontal 0NH1
    Hyoid 0NHX
    Lacrimal
      Left 0NHJ
      Right 0NHH
    Lower 0QHY
    Nasal 0NHB
    Occipital 0NH7
    Palatine
      Left 0NHL
      Right 0NHK
    Parietal
      Left 0NH4
      Right 0NH3
    Pelvic
      Left 0QH3
      Right 0QH2
    Sphenoid 0NHC
    Temporal
      Left 0NH6
      Right 0NH5
    Upper 0PHY
    Zygomatic
      Left 0NHN
      Right 0NHM
  Brain 00H0
  Breast
    Bilateral 0HHV
    Left 0HHU
    Right 0HHT
  Bronchus
    Lingula 0BH9
    Lower Lobe
      Left 0BHB
      Right 0BH6
    Main
      Left 0BH7
      Right 0BH3
    Middle Lobe, Right 0BH5
    Upper Lobe
      Left 0BH8
      Right 0BH4
  Bursa and Ligament
    Lower 0MHY
    Upper 0MHX
  Buttock
    Left 0YH1
    Right 0YH0
  Carpal
    Left 0PHN
    Right 0PHM
  Cavity, Cranial 0WH1
  Cerebral Ventricle 00H6
  Cervix 0UHC
  Chest Wall 0WH8
  Cisterna Chyli 07HL
  Clavicle
    Left 0PHB
    Right 0PH9
  Coccyx 0QHS
  Cul-de-sac 0UHF
  Diaphragm 0BHT
  Disc
    Cervical Vertebral 0RH3
    Cervicothoracic Vertebral 0RH5
    Lumbar Vertebral 0SH2
    Lumbosacral 0SH4
    Thoracic Vertebral 0RH9
    Thoracolumbar Vertebral 0RHB
  Duct
    Hepatobiliary 0FHB
    Pancreatic 0FHD
  Duodenum 0DH9
  Ear
    Inner
      Left 09HE
      Right 09HD
    Left 09HJ
    Right 09HH
  Elbow Region
    Left 0XHC
    Right 0XHB
  Epididymis and Spermatic Cord 0VHM

Insertion of device in — *continued*
- Esophagus ØDH5
- Extremity
  - Lower
    - Left ØYHB
    - Right ØYH9
  - Upper
    - Left ØXH7
    - Right ØXH6
- Eye
  - Left Ø8H1
  - Right Ø8HØ
- Face ØWH2
- Fallopian Tube ØUH8
- Femoral Region
  - Left ØYH8
  - Right ØYH7
- Femoral Shaft
  - Left ØQH9
  - Right ØQH8
- Femur
  - Lower
    - Left ØQHC
    - Right ØQHB
  - Upper
    - Left ØQH7
    - Right ØQH6
- Fibula
  - Left ØQHK
  - Right ØQHJ
- Foot
  - Left ØYHN
  - Right ØYHM
- Gallbladder ØFH4
- Gastrointestinal Tract ØWHP
- Genitourinary Tract ØWHR
- Gland
  - Endocrine ØGHS
  - Salivary ØCHA
- Glenoid Cavity
  - Left ØPH8
  - Right ØPH7
- Hand
  - Left ØXHK
  - Right ØXHJ
- Head ØWHØ
- Heart Ø2HA
- Humeral Head
  - Left ØPHD
  - Right ØPHC
- Humeral Shaft
  - Left ØPHG
  - Right ØPHF
- Ileum ØDHB
- Inguinal Region
  - Left ØYH6
  - Right ØYH5
- Intestinal Tract
  - Lower ØDHD
  - Upper ØDHØ
- Intestine
  - Large ØDHE
  - Small ØDH8
- Jaw
  - Lower ØWH5
  - Upper ØWH4
- Jejunum ØDHA
- Joint
  - Acromioclavicular
    - Left ØRHH
    - Right ØRHG
  - Ankle
    - Left ØSHG
    - Right ØSHF
  - Carpal
    - Left ØRHR
    - Right ØRHQ
  - Carpometacarpal
    - Left ØRHT
    - Right ØRHS
  - Cervical Vertebral ØRH1
  - Cervicothoracic Vertebral ØRH4
  - Coccygeal ØSH6
  - Elbow
    - Left ØRHM
    - Right ØRHL
  - Finger Phalangeal
    - Left ØRHX
    - Right ØRHW

Insertion of device in — *continued*
- Joint — *continued*
  - Hip
    - Left ØSHB
    - Right ØSH9
  - Knee
    - Left ØSHD
    - Right ØSHC
  - Lumbar Vertebral ØSHØ
  - Lumbosacral ØSH3
  - Metacarpophalangeal
    - Left ØRHV
    - Right ØRHU
  - Metatarsal-Phalangeal
    - Left ØSHN
    - Right ØSHM
  - Occipital-cervical ØRHØ
  - Sacrococcygeal ØSH5
  - Sacroiliac
    - Left ØSH8
    - Right ØSH7
  - Shoulder
    - Left ØRHK
    - Right ØRHJ
  - Sternoclavicular
    - Left ØRHF
    - Right ØRHE
  - Tarsal
    - Left ØSHJ
    - Right ØSHH
  - Tarsometatarsal
    - Left ØSHL
    - Right ØSHK
  - Temporomandibular
    - Left ØRHD
    - Right ØRHC
  - Thoracic Vertebral ØRH6
  - Thoracolumbar Vertebral ØRHA
  - Toe Phalangeal
    - Left ØSHQ
    - Right ØSHP
  - Wrist
    - Left ØRHP
    - Right ØRHN
- Kidney ØTH5
- Knee Region
  - Left ØYHG
  - Right ØYHF
- Larynx ØCHS
- Leg
  - Lower
    - Left ØYHJ
    - Right ØYHH
  - Upper
    - Left ØYHD
    - Right ØYHC
- Liver ØFHØ
  - Left Lobe ØFH2
  - Right Lobe ØFH1
- Lung
  - Left ØBHL
  - Right ØBHK
- Lymphatic Ø7HN
  - Thoracic Duct Ø7HK
- Mandible
  - Left ØNHV
  - Right ØNHT
- Maxilla ØNHR
- Mediastinum ØWHC
- Metacarpal
  - Left ØPHQ
  - Right ØPHP
- Metatarsal
  - Left ØQHP
  - Right ØQHN
- Mouth and Throat ØCHY
- Muscle
  - Lower ØKHY
  - Upper ØKHX
- Nasal Mucosa and Soft Tissue Ø9HK
- Nasopharynx Ø9HN
- Neck ØWH6
- Nerve
  - Cranial ØØHE
  - Peripheral Ø1HY
- Nipple
  - Left ØHHX
  - Right ØHHW
- Oral Cavity and Throat ØWH3

Insertion of device in — *continued*
- Orbit
  - Left ØNHQ
  - Right ØNHP
- Ovary ØUH3
- Pancreas ØFHG
- Patella
  - Left ØQHF
  - Right ØQHD
- Pelvic Cavity ØWHJ
- Penis ØVHS
- Pericardial Cavity ØWHD
- Pericardium Ø2HN
- Perineum
  - Female ØWHN
  - Male ØWHM
- Peritoneal Cavity ØWHG
- Phalanx
  - Finger
    - Left ØPHV
    - Right ØPHT
  - Thumb
    - Left ØPHS
    - Right ØPHR
  - Toe
    - Left ØQHR
    - Right ØQHQ
- Pleura ØBHQ
- Pleural Cavity
  - Left ØWHB
  - Right ØWH9
- Prostate ØVHØ
- Prostate and Seminal Vesicles ØVH4
- Radius
  - Left ØPHJ
  - Right ØPHH
- Rectum ØDHP
- Respiratory Tract ØWHQ
- Retroperitoneum ØWHH
- Ribs
  - 1 to 2 ØPH1
  - 3 or More ØPH2
- Sacrum ØQH1
- Scapula
  - Left ØPH6
  - Right ØPH5
- Scrotum and Tunica Vaginalis ØVH8
- Shoulder Region
  - Left ØXH3
  - Right ØXH2
- Sinus Ø9HY
- Skin ØHHPXYZ
- Skull ØNHØ
- Spinal Canal ØØHU
- Spinal Cord ØØHV
- Spleen Ø7HP
- Sternum ØPHØ
- Stomach ØDH6
- Subcutaneous Tissue and Fascia
  - Abdomen ØJH8
  - Back ØJH7
  - Buttock ØJH9
  - Chest ØJH6
  - Face ØJH1
  - Foot
    - Left ØJHR
    - Right ØJHQ
  - Hand
    - Left ØJHK
    - Right ØJHJ
  - Head and Neck ØJHS
  - Lower Arm
    - Left ØJHH
    - Right ØJHG
  - Lower Extremity ØJHW
  - Lower Leg
    - Left ØJHP
    - Right ØJHN
  - Neck
    - Left ØJH5
    - Right ØJH4
  - Pelvic Region ØJHC
  - Perineum ØJHB
  - Scalp ØJHØ
  - Trunk ØJHT
  - Upper Arm
    - Left ØJHF
    - Right ØJHD
  - Upper Extremity ØJHV

Insertion of device in — *continued*

Subcutaneous Tissue and Fascia — *continued*
- Upper Leg
  - Left ØJHM
  - Right ØJHL
- Tarsal
  - Left ØQHM
  - Right ØQHL
- Tendon
  - Lower ØLHY
  - Upper ØLHX
- Testis ØVHD
- Thymus Ø7HM
- Tibia
  - Left ØQHH
  - Right ØQHG
- Tongue ØCH7
- Trachea ØBH1
- Tracheobronchial Tree ØBHØ
- Ulna
  - Left ØPHL
  - Right ØPHK
- Ureter ØTH9
- Urethra ØTHD
- Uterus ØUH9
- Uterus and Cervix ØUHD
- Vagina ØUHG
- Vagina and Cul-de-sac ØUHH
- Vas Deferens ØVHR
- Vein
  - Axillary
    - Left Ø5H8
    - Right Ø5H7
  - Azygos Ø5HØ
  - Basilic
    - Left Ø5HC
    - Right Ø5HB
  - Brachial
    - Left Ø5HA
    - Right Ø5H9
  - Cephalic
    - Left Ø5HF
    - Right Ø5HD
  - Colic Ø6H7
  - Common Iliac
    - Left Ø6HD
    - Right Ø6HC
  - Coronary Ø2H4
  - Esophageal Ø6H3
  - External Iliac
    - Left Ø6HG
    - Right Ø6HF
  - External Jugular
    - Left Ø5HQ
    - Right Ø5HP
  - Face
    - Left Ø5HV
    - Right Ø5HT
  - Femoral
    - Left Ø6HN
    - Right Ø6HM
  - Foot
    - Left Ø6HV
    - Right Ø6HT
  - Gastric Ø6H2
  - Hand
    - Left Ø5HH
    - Right Ø5HG
  - Hemiazygos Ø5H1
  - Hepatic Ø6H4
  - Hypogastric
    - Left Ø6HJ
    - Right Ø6HH
  - Inferior Mesenteric Ø6H6
  - Innominate
    - Left Ø5H4
    - Right Ø5H3
  - Internal Jugular
    - Left Ø5HN
    - Right Ø5HM
  - Intracranial Ø5HL
  - Lower Ø6HY
  - Portal Ø6H8
  - Pulmonary
    - Left Ø2HT
    - Right Ø2HS
  - Renal
    - Left Ø6HB
    - Right Ø6H9

Insertion of device in — *continued*

Vein — *continued*
- Saphenous
  - Left Ø6HQ
  - Right Ø6HP
- Splenic Ø6H1
- Subclavian
  - Left Ø5H6
  - Right Ø5H5
- Superior Mesenteric Ø6H5
- Upper Ø5HY
- Vertebral
  - Left Ø5HS
  - Right Ø5HR
- Vena Cava
  - Inferior Ø6HØ
  - Superior Ø2HV
- Ventricle
  - Left Ø2HL
  - Right Ø2HK
- Vertebra
  - Cervical ØPH3
  - Lumbar ØQHØ
  - Thoracic ØPH4
- Wrist Region
  - Left ØXHH
  - Right ØXHG

Inspection
- Abdominal Wall ØWJF
- Ankle Region
  - Left ØYJL
  - Right ØYJK
- Arm
  - Lower
    - Left ØXJF
    - Right ØXJD
  - Upper
    - Left ØXJ9
    - Right ØXJ8
- Artery
  - Lower Ø4JY
  - Upper Ø3JY
- Axilla
  - Left ØXJ5
  - Right ØXJ4
- Back
  - Lower ØWJL
  - Upper ØWJK
- Bladder ØTJB
- Bone
  - Facial ØNJW
  - Lower ØQJY
  - Nasal ØNJB
  - Upper ØPJY
- Bone Marrow Ø7JT
- Brain ØØJØ
- Breast
  - Left ØHJU
  - Right ØHJT
- Bursa and Ligament
  - Lower ØMJY
  - Upper ØMJX
- Buttock
  - Left ØYJ1
  - Right ØYJØ
- Cavity, Cranial ØWJ1
- Chest Wall ØWJ8
- Cisterna Chyli Ø7JL
- Diaphragm ØBJT
- Disc
  - Cervical Vertebral ØRJ3
  - Cervicothoracic Vertebral ØRJ5
  - Lumbar Vertebral ØSJ2
  - Lumbosacral ØSJ4
  - Thoracic Vertebral ØRJ9
  - Thoracolumbar Vertebral ØRJB
- Duct
  - Hepatobiliary ØFJB
  - Pancreatic ØFJD
- Ear
  - Inner
    - Left Ø9JE
    - Right Ø9JD
  - Left Ø9JJ
  - Right Ø9JH
- Elbow Region
  - Left ØXJC
  - Right ØXJB
- Epididymis and Spermatic Cord ØVJM

Inspection — *continued*
- Extremity
  - Lower
    - Left ØYJB
    - Right ØYJ9
  - Upper
    - Left ØXJ7
    - Right ØXJ6
- Eye
  - Left Ø8J1XZZ
  - Right Ø8JØXZZ
- Face ØWJ2
- Fallopian Tube ØUJ8
- Femoral Region
  - Bilateral ØYJE
  - Left ØYJ8
  - Right ØYJ7
- Finger Nail ØHJQXZZ
- Foot
  - Left ØYJN
  - Right ØYJM
- Gallbladder ØFJ4
- Gastrointestinal Tract ØWJP
- Genitourinary Tract ØWJR
- Gland
  - Adrenal ØGJ5
  - Endocrine ØGJS
  - Pituitary ØGJØ
  - Salivary ØCJA
- Great Vessel Ø2JY
- Hand
  - Left ØXJK
  - Right ØXJJ
- Head ØWJØ
- Heart Ø2JA
- Inguinal Region
  - Bilateral ØYJA
  - Left ØYJ6
  - Right ØYJ5
- Intestinal Tract
  - Lower ØDJD
  - Upper ØDJØ
- Jaw
  - Lower ØWJ5
  - Upper ØWJ4
- Joint
  - Acromioclavicular
    - Left ØRJH
    - Right ØRJG
  - Ankle
    - Left ØSJG
    - Right ØSJF
  - Carpal
    - Left ØRJR
    - Right ØRJQ
  - Carpometacarpal
    - Left ØRJT
    - Right ØRJS
  - Cervical Vertebral ØRJ1
  - Cervicothoracic Vertebral ØRJ4
  - Coccygeal ØSJ6
  - Elbow
    - Left ØRJM
    - Right ØRJL
  - Finger Phalangeal
    - Left ØRJX
    - Right ØRJW
  - Hip
    - Left ØSJB
    - Right ØSJ9
  - Knee
    - Left ØSJD
    - Right ØSJC
  - Lumbar Vertebral ØSJØ
  - Lumbosacral ØSJ3
  - Metacarpophalangeal
    - Left ØRJV
    - Right ØRJU
  - Metatarsal-Phalangeal
    - Left ØSJN
    - Right ØSJM
  - Occipital-cervical ØRJØ
  - Sacrococcygeal ØSJ5
  - Sacroiliac
    - Left ØSJ8
    - Right ØSJ7
  - Shoulder
    - Left ØRJK
    - Right ØRJJ

Inspection — *continued*
  Joint — *continued*
    Sternoclavicular
      Left ØRJF
      Right ØRJE
    Tarsal
      Left ØSJJ
      Right ØSJH
    Tarsometatarsal
      Left ØSJL
      Right ØSJK
    Temporomandibular
      Left ØRJD
      Right ØRJC
    Thoracic Vertebral ØRJ6
    Thoracolumbar Vertebral ØRJA
    Toe Phalangeal
      Left ØSJQ
      Right ØSJP
    Wrist
      Left ØRJP
      Right ØRJN
  Kidney ØTJ5
  Knee Region
    Left ØYJG
    Right ØYJF
  Larynx ØCJS
  Leg
    Lower
      Left ØYJJ
      Right ØYJH
    Upper
      Left ØYJD
      Right ØYJC
  Lens
    Left Ø8JKXZZ
    Right Ø8JJXZZ
  Liver ØFJØ
  Lung
    Left ØBJL
    Right ØBJK
  Lymphatic Ø7JN
    Thoracic Duct Ø7JK
  Mediastinum ØWJC
  Mesentery ØDJV
  Mouth and Throat ØCJY
  Muscle
    Extraocular
      Left Ø8JM
      Right Ø8JL
    Lower ØKJY
    Upper ØKJX
  Nasal Mucosa and Soft Tissue Ø9JK
  Neck ØWJ6
  Nerve
    Cranial ØØJE
    Peripheral Ø1JY
  Omentum ØDJU
  Oral Cavity and Throat ØWJ3
  Ovary ØUJ3
  Pancreas ØFJG
  Parathyroid Gland ØGJR
  Pelvic Cavity ØWJJ
  Penis ØVJS
  Pericardial Cavity ØWJD
  Perineum
    Female ØWJN
    Male ØWJM
  Peritoneal Cavity ØWJG
  Peritoneum ØDJW
  Pineal Body ØGJ1
  Pleura ØBJQ
  Pleural Cavity
    Left ØWJB
    Right ØWJ9
  Products of Conception 1ØJØ
    Ectopic 1ØJ2
    Retained 1ØJ1
  Prostate and Seminal Vesicles ØVJ4
  Respiratory Tract ØWJQ
  Retroperitoneum ØWJH
  Scrotum and Tunica Vaginalis ØVJ8
  Shoulder Region
    Left ØXJ3
    Right ØXJ2
  Sinus Ø9JY
  Skin ØHJPXZZ
  Skull ØNJØ
  Spinal Canal ØØJU

Inspection — *continued*
  Spinal Cord ØØJV
  Spleen Ø7JP
  Stomach ØDJ6
  Subcutaneous Tissue and Fascia
    Head and Neck ØJJS
    Lower Extremity ØJJW
    Trunk ØJJT
    Upper Extremity ØJJV
  Tendon
    Lower ØLJY
    Upper ØLJX
  Testis ØVJD
  Thymus Ø7JM
  Thyroid Gland ØGJK
  Toe Nail ØHJRXZZ
  Trachea ØBJ1
  Tracheobronchial Tree ØBJØ
  Tympanic Membrane
    Left Ø9J8
    Right Ø9J7
  Ureter ØTJ9
  Urethra ØTJD
  Uterus and Cervix ØUJD
  Vagina and Cul-de-sac ØUJH
  Vas Deferens ØVJR
  Vein
    Lower Ø6JY
    Upper Ø5JY
  Vulva ØUJM
  Wrist Region
    Left ØXJH
    Right ØXJG
Instillation *see* Introduction of substance in or on
Insufflation *see* Introduction of substance in or on
Interatrial septum *use* Atrial Septum
Interbody fusion (spine) cage
  use Interbody Fusion Device in Lower Joints
  use Interbody Fusion Device in Upper Joints
Interbody Fusion Device
  Nanotextured Surface
    Cervical Vertebral XRG1Ø92
      2 or more XRG2Ø92
    Cervicothoracic Vertebral XRG4Ø92
    Lumbar Vertebral XRGBØ92
      2 or more XRGCØ92
    Lumbosacral XRGDØ92
    Occipital-cervical XRGØØ92
    Thoracic Vertebral XRG6Ø92
      2 to 7 XRG7Ø92
      8 or more XRG8Ø92
    Thoracolumbar Vertebral XRGAØ92
  Radiolucent Porous
    Cervical Vertebral XRG1ØF3
      2 or more XRG2ØF3
    Cervicothoracic Vertebral XRG4ØF3
    Lumbar Vertebral XRGBØF3
      2 or more XRGCØF3
    Lumbosacral XRGDØF3
    Occipital-cervical XRGØØF3
    Thoracic Vertebral XRG6ØF3
      2 to 7 XRG7ØF3
      8 or more XRG8ØF3
    Thoracolumbar Vertebral XRGAØF3
Intercarpal joint
  use Carpal Joint, Left
  use Carpal Joint, Right
Intercarpal ligament
  use Hand Bursa and Ligament, Left
  use Hand Bursa and Ligament, Right
Interclavicular ligament
  use Shoulder Bursa and Ligament, Left
  use Shoulder Bursa and Ligament, Right
Intercostal lymph node *use* Lymphatic, Thorax
Intercostal muscle
  use Thorax Muscle, Left
  use Thorax Muscle, Right
Intercostal nerve *use* Thoracic Nerve
Intercostobrachial nerve *use* Thoracic Nerve
Intercuneiform joint
  use Tarsal Joint, Left
  use Tarsal Joint, Right
Intercuneiform ligament
  use Foot Bursa and Ligament, Left
  use Foot Bursa and Ligament, Right
Intermediate bronchus *use* Main Bronchus, Right
Intermediate cuneiform bone
  use Tarsal, Left

Intermediate cuneiform bone — *continued*
  use Tarsal, Right
Intermittent hemodialysis (IHD) 5A1D7ØZ
Intermittent mandatory ventilation *see* Assistance, Respiratory 5AØ9
Intermittent Negative Airway Pressure
  24-96 Consecutive Hours, Ventilation 5AØ945B
  Greater than 96 Consecutive Hours, Ventilation 5AØ955B
  Less than 24 Consecutive Hours, Ventilation 5AØ935B
Intermittent Positive Airway Pressure
  24-96 Consecutive Hours, Ventilation 5AØ9458
  Greater than 96 Consecutive Hours, Ventilation 5AØ9558
  Less than 24 Consecutive Hours, Ventilation 5AØ9358
Intermittent positive pressure breathing *see* Assistance, Respiratory 5AØ9
Internal anal sphincter *use* Anal Sphincter
Internal carotid artery, intracranial portion *use* Intracranial Artery
Internal carotid plexus *use* Head and Neck Sympathetic Nerve
Internal (basal) cerebral vein *use* Intracranial Vein
Internal iliac vein
  use Hypogastric Vein, Left
  use Hypogastric Vein, Right
Internal maxillary artery
  use External Carotid Artery, Left
  use External Carotid Artery, Right
Internal naris *use* Nasal Mucosa and Soft Tissue
Internal oblique muscle
  use Abdomen Muscle, Left
  use Abdomen Muscle, Right
Internal pudendal artery
  use Internal Iliac Artery, Left
  use Internal Iliac Artery, Right
Internal pudendal vein
  use Hypogastric Vein, Left
  use Hypogastric Vein, Right
Internal thoracic artery
  use Internal Mammary Artery, Left
  use Internal Mammary Artery, Right
  use Subclavian Artery, Left
  use Subclavian Artery, Right
Internal urethral sphincter *use* Urethra
Interphalangeal (IP) joint
  use Finger Phalangeal Joint, Left
  use Finger Phalangeal Joint, Right
  use Toe Phalangeal Joint, Left
  use Toe Phalangeal Joint, Right
Interphalangeal ligament
  use Foot Bursa and Ligament, Left
  use Foot Bursa and Ligament, Right
  use Hand Bursa and Ligament, Left
  use Hand Bursa and Ligament, Right
Interrogation, cardiac rhythm related device
  Interrogation only *see* Measurement, Cardiac 4BØ2
  With cardiac function testing *see* Measurement, Cardiac 4AØ2
Interruption *see* Occlusion
Interspinalis muscle
  use Trunk Muscle, Left
  use Trunk Muscle, Right
Interspinous ligament, cervical *use* Head and Neck Bursa and Ligament
Interspinous ligament, lumbar *use* Lower Spine Bursa and Ligament
Interspinous ligament, thoracic *use* Upper Spine Bursa and Ligament
Interspinous process spinal stabilization device
  use Spinal Stabilization Device, Interspinous Process in ØRH
  use Spinal Stabilization Device, Interspinous Process in ØSH
InterStim® Therapy lead *use* Neurostimulator Lead in Peripheral Nervous System
InterStim® Therapy neurostimulator *use* Stimulator Generator, Single Array in ØJH
Intertransversarius muscle
  use Trunk Muscle, Left
  use Trunk Muscle, Right
Intertransverse ligament, cervical *use* Head and Neck Bursa and Ligament
Intertransverse ligament, lumbar *use* Lower Spine Bursa and Ligament

Intertransverse ligament, thoracic *use* Upper Spine Bursa and Ligament
Interventricular foramen (Monro) *use* Cerebral Ventricle
Interventricular septum *use* Ventricular Septum
Intestinal lymphatic trunk *use* Cisterna Chyli
Intraluminal Device
  Airway
    Esophagus 0DH5
    Mouth and Throat 0CHY
    Nasopharynx 09HN
  Bioactive
    Occlusion
      Common Carotid
        Left 03LJ
        Right 03LH
      External Carotid
        Left 03LN
        Right 03LM
      Internal Carotid
        Left 03LL
        Right 03LK
      Intracranial 03LG
      Vertebral
        Left 03LQ
        Right 03LP
    Restriction
      Common Carotid
        Left 03VJ
        Right 03VH
      External Carotid
        Left 03VN
        Right 03VM
      Internal Carotid
        Left 03VL
        Right 03VK
      Intracranial 03VG
      Vertebral
        Left 03VQ
        Right 03VP
  Endobronchial Valve
    Lingula 0BH9
    Lower Lobe
      Left 0BHB
      Right 0BH6
    Main
      Left 0BH7
      Right 0BH3
    Middle Lobe, Right 0BH5
    Upper Lobe
      Left 0BH8
      Right 0BH4
  Endotracheal Airway
    Change device in, Trachea 0B21XEZ
    Insertion of device in, Trachea 0BH1
  Pessary
    Change device in, Vagina and Cul-de-sac 0U2HXGZ
    Insertion of device in
      Cul-de-sac 0UHF
      Vagina 0UHG
Intramedullary (IM) rod (nail)
  use Internal Fixation Device, Intramedullary in Lower Bones
  use Internal Fixation Device, Intramedullary in Upper Bones
Intramedullary skeletal kinetic distractor (ISKD)
  use Internal Fixation Device, Intramedullary in Lower Bones
  use Internal Fixation Device, Intramedullary in Upper Bones
Intraocular Telescope
  Left 08RK30Z
  Right 08RJ30Z
Intraoperative Knee Replacement Sensor XR2
Intraoperative Radiation Therapy (IORT)
  Anus DDY8CZZ
  Bile Ducts DFY2CZZ
  Bladder DTY2CZZ
  Cervix DUY1CZZ
  Colon DDY5CZZ
  Duodenum DDY2CZZ
  Gallbladder DFY1CZZ
  Ileum DDY4CZZ
  Jejunum DDY3CZZ
  Kidney DTY0CZZ
  Larynx D9YBCZZ
  Liver DFY0CZZ

Intraoperative Radiation Therapy (IORT) — *continued*
  Mouth D9Y4CZZ
  Nasopharynx D9YDCZZ
  Ovary DUY0CZZ
  Pancreas DFY3CZZ
  Pharynx D9YCCZZ
  Prostate DVY0CZZ
  Rectum DDY7CZZ
  Stomach DDY1CZZ
  Ureter DTY1CZZ
  Urethra DTY3CZZ
  Uterus DUY2CZZ
Intrauterine Device (IUD) *use* Contraceptive Device in Female Reproductive System
Intravascular fluorescence angiography (IFA) *see* Monitoring, Physiological Systems 4A1
Introduction of substance in or on
  Artery
    Central 3E06
      Analgesics 3E06
      Anesthetic, Intracirculatory 3E06
      Antiarrhythmic 3E06
      Anti-infective 3E06
      Anti-inflammatory 3E06
      Antineoplastic 3E06
      Destructive Agent 3E06
      Diagnostic Substance, Other 3E06
      Electrolytic Substance 3E06
      Hormone 3E06
      Hypnotics 3E06
      Immunotherapeutic 3E06
      Nutritional Substance 3E06
      Platelet Inhibitor 3E06
      Radioactive Substance 3E06
      Sedatives 3E06
      Serum 3E06
      Thrombolytic 3E06
      Toxoid 3E06
      Vaccine 3E06
      Vasopressor 3E06
      Water Balance Substance 3E06
    Coronary 3E07
      Diagnostic Substance, Other 3E07
      Platelet Inhibitor 3E07
      Thrombolytic 3E07
    Peripheral 3E05
      Analgesics 3E05
      Anesthetic, Intracirculatory 3E05
      Antiarrhythmic 3E05
      Anti-infective 3E05
      Anti-inflammatory 3E05
      Antineoplastic 3E05
      Destructive Agent 3E05
      Diagnostic Substance, Other 3E05
      Electrolytic Substance 3E05
      Hormone 3E05
      Hypnotics 3E05
      Immunotherapeutic 3E05
      Nutritional Substance 3E05
      Platelet Inhibitor 3E05
      Radioactive Substance 3E05
      Sedatives 3E05
      Serum 3E05
      Thrombolytic 3E05
      Toxoid 3E05
      Vaccine 3E05
      Vasopressor 3E05
      Water Balance Substance 3E05
  Biliary Tract 3E0J
    Analgesics 3E0J
    Anesthetic Agent 3E0J
    Anti-infective 3E0J
    Anti-inflammatory 3E0J
    Antineoplastic 3E0J
    Destructive Agent 3E0J
    Diagnostic Substance, Other 3E0J
    Electrolytic Substance 3E0J
    Gas 3E0J
    Hypnotics 3E0J
    Islet Cells, Pancreatic 3E0J
    Nutritional Substance 3E0J
    Radioactive Substance 3E0J
    Sedatives 3E0J
    Water Balance Substance 3E0J
  Bone 3E0V
    Analgesics 3E0V3NZ
    Anesthetic Agent 3E0V3BZ
    Anti-infective 3E0V32

Introduction of substance in or on — *continued*
  Bone — *continued*
    Anti-inflammatory 3E0V33Z
    Antineoplastic 3E0V30
    Destructive Agent 3E0V3TZ
    Diagnostic Substance, Other 3E0V3KZ
    Electrolytic Substance 3E0V37Z
    Hypnotics 3E0V3NZ
    Nutritional Substance 3E0V36Z
    Radioactive Substance 3E0V3HZ
    Sedatives 3E0V3NZ
    Water Balance Substance 3E0V37Z
  Bone Marrow 3E0A3GC
    Antineoplastic 3E0A30
  Brain 3E0Q
    Analgesics 3E0Q
    Anesthetic Agent 3E0Q
    Anti-infective 3E0Q
    Anti-inflammatory 3E0Q
    Antineoplastic 3E0Q
    Destructive Agent 3E0Q
    Diagnostic Substance, Other 3E0Q
    Electrolytic Substance 3E0Q
    Gas 3E0Q
    Hypnotics 3E0Q
    Nutritional Substance 3E0Q
    Radioactive Substance 3E0Q
    Sedatives 3E0Q
    Stem Cells
      Embryonic 3E0Q
      Somatic 3E0Q
    Water Balance Substance 3E0Q
  Cranial Cavity 3E0Q
    Analgesics 3E0Q
    Anesthetic Agent 3E0Q
    Anti-infective 3E0Q
    Anti-inflammatory 3E0Q
    Antineoplastic 3E0Q
    Destructive Agent 3E0Q
    Diagnostic Substance, Other 3E0Q
    Electrolytic Substance 3E0Q
    Gas 3E0Q
    Hypnotics 3E0Q
    Nutritional Substance 3E0Q
    Radioactive Substance 3E0Q
    Sedatives 3E0Q
    Stem Cells
      Embryonic 3E0Q
      Somatic 3E0Q
    Water Balance Substance 3E0Q
  Ear 3E0B
    Analgesics 3E0B
    Anesthetic Agent 3E0B
    Anti-infective 3E0B
    Anti-inflammatory 3E0B
    Antineoplastic 3E0B
    Destructive Agent 3E0B
    Diagnostic Substance, Other 3E0B
    Hypnotics 3E0B
    Radioactive Substance 3E0B
    Sedatives 3E0B
  Epidural Space 3E0S3GC
    Analgesics 3E0S3NZ
    Anesthetic Agent 3E0S3BZ
    Anti-infective 3E0S32
    Anti-inflammatory 3E0S33Z
    Antineoplastic 3E0S30
    Destructive Agent 3E0S3TZ
    Diagnostic Substance, Other 3E0S3KZ
    Electrolytic Substance 3E0S37Z
    Gas 3E0S
    Hypnotics 3E0S3NZ
    Nutritional Substance 3E0S36Z
    Radioactive Substance 3E0S3HZ
    Sedatives 3E0S3NZ
    Water Balance Substance 3E0S37Z
  Eye 3E0C
    Analgesics 3E0C
    Anesthetic Agent 3E0C
    Anti-infective 3E0C
    Anti-inflammatory 3E0C
    Antineoplastic 3E0C
    Destructive Agent 3E0C
    Diagnostic Substance, Other 3E0C
    Gas 3E0C
    Hypnotics 3E0C
    Pigment 3E0C
    Radioactive Substance 3E0C
    Sedatives 3E0C

⬩ Subterms under main terms may continue to next column or page

Introduction of substance in or on — *continued*
  Reproductive — *continued*
    Female — *continued*
      Gas 3E0P
      Hormone 3E0P
      Hypnotics 3E0P
      Nutritional Substance 3E0P
      Ovum, Fertilized 3E0P
      Radioactive Substance 3E0P
      Sedatives 3E0P
      Sperm 3E0P
      Water Balance Substance 3E0P
    Male 3E0N
      Analgesics 3E0N
      Anesthetic Agent 3E0N
      Anti-infective 3E0N
      Anti-inflammatory 3E0N
      Antineoplastic 3E0N
      Destructive Agent 3E0N
      Diagnostic Substance, Other 3E0N
      Electrolytic Substance 3E0N
      Gas 3E0N
      Hypnotics 3E0N
      Nutritional Substance 3E0N
      Radioactive Substance 3E0N
      Sedatives 3E0N
      Water Balance Substance 3E0N
  Respiratory Tract 3E0F
    Analgesics 3E0F
    Anesthetic Agent 3E0F
    Anti-infective 3E0F
    Anti-inflammatory 3E0F
    Antineoplastic 3E0F
    Destructive Agent 3E0F
    Diagnostic Substance, Other 3E0F
    Electrolytic Substance 3E0F
    Gas 3E0F
    Hypnotics 3E0F
    Nutritional Substance 3E0F
    Radioactive Substance 3E0F
    Sedatives 3E0F
    Water Balance Substance 3E0F
  Skin 3E00XGC
    Analgesics 3E00XNZ
    Anesthetic Agent 3E00XBZ
    Anti-infective 3E00X2
    Anti-inflammatory 3E00X3Z
    Antineoplastic 3E00X0
    Destructive Agent 3E00XTZ
    Diagnostic Substance, Other 3E00XKZ
    Hypnotics 3E00XNZ
    Pigment 3E00XMZ
    Sedatives 3E00XNZ
    Serum 3E00X4Z
    Toxoid 3E00X4Z
    Vaccine 3E00X4Z
  Spinal Canal 3E0R3GC
    Analgesics 3E0R3NZ
    Anesthetic Agent 3E0R3BZ
    Anti-infective 3E0R32
    Anti-inflammatory 3E0R33Z
    Antineoplastic 3E0R30
    Destructive Agent 3E0R3TZ
    Diagnostic Substance, Other 3E0R3KZ
    Electrolytic Substance 3E0R37Z
    Gas 3E0R
    Hypnotics 3E0R3NZ
    Nutritional Substance 3E0R36Z
    Radioactive Substance 3E0R3HZ
    Sedatives 3E0R3NZ
    Stem Cells
      Embryonic 3E0R
      Somatic 3E0R
    Water Balance Substance 3E0R37Z
  Subcutaneous Tissue 3E013GC
    Analgesics 3E013NZ
    Anesthetic Agent 3E013BZ
    Anti-infective 3E01
    Anti-inflammatory 3E0133Z
    Antineoplastic 3E0130
    Destructive Agent 3E013TZ
    Diagnostic Substance, Other 3E013KZ
    Electrolytic Substance 3E0137Z
    Hormone 3E013V
    Hypnotics 3E013NZ
    Nutritional Substance 3E0136Z
    Radioactive Substance 3E013HZ
    Sedatives 3E013NZ
    Serum 3E0134Z

Introduction of substance in or on — *continued*
  Subcutaneous Tissue — *continued*
    Toxoid 3E0134Z
    Vaccine 3E0134Z
    Water Balance Substance 3E0137Z
  Vein
    Central 3E04
      Analgesics 3E04
      Anesthetic, Intracirculatory 3E04
      Antiarrhythmic 3E04
      Anti-infective 3E04
      Anti-inflammatory 3E04
      Antineoplastic 3E04
      Destructive Agent 3E04
      Diagnostic Substance, Other 3E04
      Electrolytic Substance 3E04
      Hormone 3E04
      Hypnotics 3E04
      Immunotherapeutic 3E04
      Nutritional Substance 3E04
      Platelet Inhibitor 3E04
      Radioactive Substance 3E04
      Sedatives 3E04
      Serum 3E04
      Thrombolytic 3E04
      Toxoid 3E04
      Vaccine 3E04
      Vasopressor 3E04
      Water Balance Substance 3E04
    Peripheral 3E03
      Analgesics 3E03
      Anesthetic, Intracirculatory 3E03
      Antiarrhythmic 3E03
      Anti-infective 3E03
      Anti-inflammatory 3E03
      Antineoplastic 3E03
      Destructive Agent 3E03
      Diagnostic Substance, Other 3E03
      Electrolytic Substance 3E03
      Hormone 3E03
      Hypnotics 3E03
      Immunotherapeutic 3E03
      Islet Cells, Pancreatic 3E03
      Nutritional Substance 3E03
      Platelet Inhibitor 3E03
      Radioactive Substance 3E03
      Sedatives 3E03
      Serum 3E03
      Thrombolytic 3E03
      Toxoid 3E03
      Vaccine 3E03
      Vasopressor 3E03
      Water Balance Substance 3E03

Intubation
  Airway
    see Insertion of device in, Esophagus 0DH5
    see Insertion of device in, Mouth and Throat 0CHY
    see Insertion of device in, Trachea 0BH1
  Drainage device *see* Drainage
  Feeding Device *see* Insertion of device in, Gastrointestinal System 0DH
INTUITY Elite valve system, EDWARDS *use* Zooplastic Tissue, Rapid Deployment Technique in New Technology
Iobenguane I-131 Antineoplastic XW0
Iobenguane I-131, High Specific Activity (HSA) *use* Iobenguane I-131 Antineoplastic
IPPB (intermittent positive pressure breathing) *see* Assistance, Respiratory 5A09
IRE (Irreversible Electroporation) *see* Destruction, Hepatobiliary System and Pancreas 0F5
Iridectomy
  see Excision, Eye 08B
  see Resection, Eye 08T
Iridoplasty
  see Repair, Eye 08Q
  see Replacement, Eye 08R
  see Supplement, Eye 08U
Iridotomy *see* Drainage, Eye 089
Irreversible Electroporation (IRE) *see* Destruction, Hepatobiliary System and Pancreas 0F5
Irrigation
  Biliary Tract, Irrigating Substance 3E1J
  Brain, Irrigating Substance 3E1Q38Z
  Cranial Cavity, Irrigating Substance 3E1Q38Z
  Ear, Irrigating Substance 3E1B
  Epidural Space, Irrigating Substance 3E1S38Z

Irrigation — *continued*
  Eye, Irrigating Substance 3E1C
  Gastrointestinal Tract
    Lower, Irrigating Substance 3E1H
    Upper, Irrigating Substance 3E1G
  Genitourinary Tract, Irrigating Substance 3E1K
  Irrigating Substance 3C1ZX8Z
  Joint, Irrigating Substance 3E1U
  Mucous Membrane, Irrigating Substance 3E10
  Nose, Irrigating Substance 3E19
  Pancreatic Tract, Irrigating Substance 3E1J
  Pericardial Cavity, Irrigating Substance 3E1Y38Z
  Peritoneal Cavity
    Dialysate 3E1M39Z
    Irrigating Substance 3E1M38Z
  Pleural Cavity, Irrigating Substance 3E1L38Z
  Reproductive
    Female, Irrigating Substance 3E1P
    Male, Irrigating Substance 3E1N
  Respiratory Tract, Irrigating Substance 3E1F
  Skin, Irrigating Substance 3E10
  Spinal Canal, Irrigating Substance 3E1R38Z
Isavuconazole Anti-infective XW0
Ischiatic nerve *use* Sciatic Nerve
Ischiocavernosus muscle *use* Perineum Muscle
Ischiofemoral ligament
  use Hip Bursa and Ligament, Left
  use Hip Bursa and Ligament, Right
Ischium
  use Pelvic Bone, Left
  use Pelvic Bone, Right
Isolation 8E0ZXY6
Isotope Administration, Whole Body DWY5G
Itrel (3) (4) neurostimulator *use* Stimulator Generator, Single Array in 0JH

J

Jakafi® *use* Ruxolitinib
Jejunal artery *use* Superior Mesenteric Artery
Jejunectomy
  see Excision, Jejunum 0DBA
  see Resection, Jejunum 0DTA
Jejunocolostomy
  see Bypass, Gastrointestinal System 0D1
  see Drainage, Gastrointestinal System 0D9
Jejunopexy
  see Repair, Jejunum 0DQA
  see Reposition, Jejunum 0DSA
Jejunostomy
  see Bypass, Jejunum 0D1A
  see Drainage, Jejunum 0D9A
Jejunotomy *see* Drainage, Jejunum 0D9A
Joint fixation plate
  use Internal Fixation Device in Lower Joints
  use Internal Fixation Device in Upper Joints
Joint liner (insert) *use* Liner in Lower Joints
Joint spacer (antibiotic)
  use Spacer in Lower Joints
  use Spacer in Upper Joints
Jugular body *use* Glomus Jugulare
Jugular lymph node
  use Lymphatic, Left Neck
  use Lymphatic, Right Neck

K

Kappa *use* Pacemaker, Dual Chamber in 0JH
Kcentra *use* 4-Factor Prothrombin Complex Concentrate
Keratectomy, kerectomy
  see Excision, Eye 08B
  see Resection, Eye 08T
Keratocentesis *see* Drainage, Eye 089
Keratoplasty
  see Repair, Eye 08Q
  see Replacement, Eye 08R
  see Supplement, Eye 08U
Keratotomy
  see Drainage, Eye 089
  see Repair, Eye 08Q
Keystone Heart TriGuard 3™ CEPD (cerebral embolic protection device) X2A6325

Kirschner wire (K-wire)
 use Internal Fixation Device in Head and Facial
  Bones
 use Internal Fixation Device in Lower Bones
 use Internal Fixation Device in Lower Joints
 use Internal Fixation Device in Upper Bones
 use Internal Fixation Device in Upper Joints
Knee (implant) insert *use* Liner in Lower Joints
KUB x-ray *see* Plain Radiography, Kidney, Ureter and
 Bladder BT04
Kuntscher nail
 use Internal Fixation Device, Intramedullary in
  Lower Bones
 use Internal Fixation Device, Intramedullary in
  Upper Bones
KYMRIAH *use* Engineered Autologous Chimeric Antigen
 Receptor T-cell Immunotherapy

L

Labia majora *use* Vulva
Labia minora *use* Vulva
Labial gland
 use Lower Lip
 use Upper Lip
Labiectomy
 see Excision, Female Reproductive System 0UB
 see Resection, Female Reproductive System 0UT
Lacrimal canaliculus
 use Lacrimal Duct, Left
 use Lacrimal Duct, Right
Lacrimal punctum
 use Lacrimal Duct, Left
 use Lacrimal Duct, Right
Lacrimal sac
 use Lacrimal Duct, Left
 use Lacrimal Duct, Right
LAGB (laparoscopic adjustable gastric banding)
 Initial procedure 0DV64CZ
 Surgical correction *see* Revision of device in,
  Stomach 0DW6
Laminectomy
 see Excision, Lower Bones 0QB
 see Excision, Upper Bones 0PB
 see Release, Central Nervous System and Cranial
  Nerves 00N
 see Release, Peripheral Nervous System 01N
Laminotomy
 see Drainage, Lower Bones 0Q9
 see Drainage, Upper Bones 0P9
 see Excision, Lower Bones 0QB
 see Excision, Upper Bones 0PB
 see Release, Central Nervous System and Cranial
  Nerves 00N
 see Release, Lower Bones 0QN
 see Release, Peripheral Nervous System 01N
 see Release, Upper Bones 0PN
Laparoscopic-assisted transanal pull-through
 see Excision, Gastrointestinal System 0DB
 see Resection, Gastrointestinal System 0DT
Laparoscopy *see* Inspection
Laparotomy
 Drainage *see* Drainage, Peritoneal Cavity 0W9G
 Exploratory *see* Inspection, Peritoneal Cavity 0WJG
LAP-BAND® Adjustable Gastric Banding System
 use Extraluminal Device
Laryngectomy
 see Excision, Larynx 0CBS
 see Resection, Larynx 0CTS
Laryngocentesis *see* Drainage, Larynx 0C9S
Laryngogram *see* Fluoroscopy, Larynx B91J
Laryngopexy *see* Repair, Larynx 0CQS
Laryngopharynx *use* Pharynx
Laryngoplasty
 see Repair, Larynx 0CQS
 see Replacement, Larynx 0CRS
 see Supplement, Larynx 0CUS
Laryngorrhaphy *see* Repair, Larynx 0CQS
Laryngoscopy 0CJS8ZZ
Laryngotomy *see* Drainage, Larynx 0C9S
Laser Interstitial Thermal Therapy
 Adrenal Gland DGY2KZZ
 Anus DDY8KZZ
 Bile Ducts DFY2KZZ
 Brain D0Y0KZZ
 Brain Stem D0Y1KZZ

Laser Interstitial Thermal Therapy — *continued*
 Breast
  Left DMY0KZZ
  Right DMY1KZZ
 Bronchus DBY1KZZ
 Chest Wall DBY7KZZ
 Colon DDY5KZZ
 Diaphragm DBY8KZZ
 Duodenum DDY2KZZ
 Esophagus DDY0KZZ
 Gallbladder DFY1KZZ
 Gland
  Adrenal DGY2KZZ
  Parathyroid DGY4KZZ
  Pituitary DGY0KZZ
  Thyroid DGY5KZZ
 Ileum DDY4KZZ
 Jejunum DDY3KZZ
 Liver DFY0KZZ
 Lung DBY2KZZ
 Mediastinum DBY6KZZ
 Nerve, Peripheral D0Y7KZZ
 Pancreas DFY3KZZ
 Parathyroid Gland DGY4KZZ
 Pineal Body DGY1KZZ
 Pituitary Gland DGY0KZZ
 Pleura DBY5KZZ
 Prostate DVY0KZZ
 Rectum DDY7KZZ
 Spinal Cord D0Y6KZZ
 Stomach DDY1KZZ
 Thyroid Gland DGY5KZZ
 Trachea DBY0KZZ
Lateral canthus
 use Upper Eyelid, Left
 use Upper Eyelid, Right
Lateral collateral ligament (LCL)
 use Knee Bursa and Ligament, Left
 use Knee Bursa and Ligament, Right
Lateral condyle of femur
 use Lower Femur, Left
 use Lower Femur, Right
Lateral condyle of tibia
 use Tibia, Left
 use Tibia, Right
Lateral cuneiform bone
 use Tarsal, Left
 use Tarsal, Right
Lateral epicondyle of femur
 use Lower Femur, Left
 use Lower Femur, Right
Lateral epicondyle of humerus
 use Humeral Shaft, Left
 use Humeral Shaft, Right
Lateral femoral cutaneous nerve *use* Lumbar Plexus
Lateral (brachial) lymph node
 use Lymphatic, Left Axillary
 use Lymphatic, Right Axillary
Lateral malleolus
 use Fibula, Left
 use Fibula, Right
Lateral meniscus
 use Knee Joint, Left
 use Knee Joint, Right
Lateral nasal cartilage *use* Nasal Mucosa and Soft
 Tissue
Lateral plantar artery
 use Foot Artery, Left
 use Foot Artery, Right
Lateral plantar nerve *use* Tibial Nerve
Lateral rectus muscle
 use Extraocular Muscle, Left
 use Extraocular Muscle, Right
Lateral sacral artery
 use Internal Iliac Artery, Left
 use Internal Iliac Artery, Right
Lateral sacral vein
 use Hypogastric Vein, Left
 use Hypogastric Vein, Right
Lateral sural cutaneous nerve *use* Peroneal Nerve
Lateral tarsal artery
 use Foot Artery, Left
 use Foot Artery, Right
Lateral temporomandibular ligament *use* Head and
 Neck Bursa and Ligament
Lateral thoracic artery
 use Axillary Artery, Left

Lateral thoracic artery — *continued*
 use Axillary Artery, Right
Latissimus dorsi muscle
 use Trunk Muscle, Left
 use Trunk Muscle, Right
Latissimus Dorsi Myocutaneous Flap
 Replacement
  Bilateral 0HRV075
  Left 0HRU075
  Right 0HRT075
 Transfer
  Left 0KXG
  Right 0KXF
Lavage
 see Irrigation
 Bronchial alveolar, diagnostic *see* Drainage, Respi-
  ratory System 0B9
Least splanchnic nerve *use* Thoracic Sympathetic
 Nerve
Left ascending lumbar vein *use* Hemiazygos Vein
Left atrioventricular valve *use* Mitral Valve
Left auricular appendix *use* Atrium, Left
Left colic vein *use* Colic Vein
Left coronary sulcus *use* Heart, Left
Left gastric artery *use* Gastric Artery
Left gastroepiploic artery *use* Splenic Artery
Left gastroepiploic vein *use* Splenic Vein
Left inferior phrenic vein *use* Renal Vein, Left
Left inferior pulmonary vein *use* Pulmonary Vein,
 Left
Left jugular trunk *use* Thoracic Duct
Left lateral ventricle *use* Cerebral Ventricle
Left ovarian vein *use* Renal Vein, Left
Left second lumbar vein *use* Renal Vein, Left
Left subclavian trunk *use* Thoracic Duct
Left subcostal vein *use* Hemiazygos Vein
Left superior pulmonary vein *use* Pulmonary Vein,
 Left
Left suprarenal vein *use* Renal Vein, Left
Left testicular vein *use* Renal Vein, Left
Lengthening
 Bone, with device *see* Insertion of Limb Lengthen-
  ing Device
 Muscle, by incision *see* Division, Muscles 0K8
 Tendon, by incision *see* Division, Tendons 0L8
Leptomeninges, intracranial *use* Cerebral Meninges
Leptomeninges, spinal *use* Spinal Meninges
Lesser alar cartilage *use* Nasal Mucosa and Soft Tissue
Lesser occipital nerve *use* Cervical Plexus
Lesser Omentum *use* Omentum
Lesser saphenous vein
 use Saphenous Vein, Left
 use Saphenous Vein, Right
Lesser splanchnic nerve *use* Thoracic Sympathetic
 Nerve
Lesser trochanter
 use Upper Femur, Left
 use Upper Femur, Right
Lesser tuberosity
 use Humeral Head, Left
 use Humeral Head, Right
Lesser wing *use* Sphenoid Bone
Leukopheresis, therapeutic *see* Pheresis, Circulatory
 6A55
Levator anguli oris muscle *use* Facial Muscle
Levator ani muscle *use* Perineum Muscle
Levator labii superioris alaeque nasi muscle *use*
 Facial Muscle
Levator labii superioris muscle *use* Facial Muscle
Levator palpebrae superioris muscle
 use Upper Eyelid, Left
 use Upper Eyelid, Right
Levator scapulae muscle
 use Neck Muscle, Left
 use Neck Muscle, Right
Levator veli palatini muscle *use* Tongue, Palate,
 Pharynx Muscle
Levatores costarum muscle
 use Thorax Muscle, Left
 use Thorax Muscle, Right
LifeStent® (Flexstar) (XL) Vascular Stent System
 use Intraluminal Device
Ligament of head of fibula
 use Knee Bursa and Ligament, Left
 use Knee Bursa and Ligament, Right
Ligament of the lateral malleolus
 use Ankle Bursa and Ligament, Left

Ligament of the lateral malleolus — *continued*
  use Ankle Bursa and Ligament, Right
Ligamentum flavum, cervical *use* Head and Neck
  Bursa and Ligament
Ligamentum flavum, lumbar *use* Lower Spine Bursa
  and Ligament
Ligamentum flavum, thoracic *use* Upper Spine Bursa
  and Ligament
Ligation *see* Occlusion
Ligation, hemorrhoid *see* Occlusion, Lower Veins,
  Hemorrhoidal Plexus
Light Therapy GZJZZZZ
Liner
  Removal of device from
    Hip
      Left ØSPBØ9Z
      Right ØSP9Ø9Z
    Knee
      Left ØSPDØ9Z
      Right ØSPCØ9Z
  Revision of device in
    Hip
      Left ØSWBØ9Z
      Right ØSW9Ø9Z
    Knee
      Left ØSWDØ9Z
      Right ØSWCØ9Z
  Supplement
    Hip
      Left ØSUBØ9Z
        Acetabular Surface ØSUEØ9Z
        Femoral Surface ØSUSØ9Z
      Right ØSU9Ø9Z
        Acetabular Surface ØSUAØ9Z
        Femoral Surface ØSURØ9Z
    Knee
      Left ØSUDØ9
        Femoral Surface ØSUUØ9Z
        Tibial Surface ØSUWØ9Z
      Right ØSUCØ9
        Femoral Surface ØSUTØ9Z
        Tibial Surface ØSUVØ9Z
Lingual artery
  use External Carotid Artery, Left
  use External Carotid Artery, Right
Lingual tonsil *use* Pharynx
Lingulectomy, lung
  see Excision, Lung Lingula ØBBH
  see Resection, Lung Lingula ØBTH
Lithotripsy
  see Fragmentation
  With removal of fragments *see* Extirpation
LITT (laser interstitial thermal therapy) *see* Laser
  Interstitial Thermal Therapy
LIVIAN™ CRT-D *use* Cardiac Resynchronization Defibrillator Pulse Generator in ØJH
Lobectomy
  see Excision, Central Nervous System and Cranial
    Nerves ØØB
  see Excision, Endocrine System ØGB
  see Excision, Hepatobiliary System and Pancreas
    ØFB
  see Excision, Respiratory System ØBB
  see Resection, Endocrine System ØGT
  see Resection, Hepatobiliary System and Pancreas
    ØFT
  see Resection, Respiratory System ØBT
Lobotomy *see* Division, Brain ØØ8Ø
Localization
  see Imaging
  see Map
Locus ceruleus *use* Pons
Long thoracic nerve *use* Brachial Plexus
Loop ileostomy *see* Bypass, Ileum ØD1B
Loop recorder, implantable *use* Monitoring Device
Lower GI series *see* Fluoroscopy, Colon BD14
Lumbar artery *use* Abdominal Aorta
Lumbar facet joint *use* Lumbar Vertebral Joint
Lumbar ganglion *use* Lumbar Sympathetic Nerve
Lumbar lymph node *use* Lymphatic, Aortic
Lumbar lymphatic trunk *use* Cisterna Chyli
Lumbar splanchnic nerve *use* Lumbar Sympathetic
  Nerve
Lumbosacral facet joint *use* Lumbosacral Joint
Lumbosacral trunk *use* Lumbar Nerve
Lumpectomy *see* Excision

Lunate bone
  use Carpal, Left
  use Carpal, Right
Lunotriquetral ligament
  use Hand Bursa and Ligament, Left
  use Hand Bursa and Ligament, Right
Lymphadenectomy
  see Excision, Lymphatic and Hemic Systems Ø7B
  see Resection, Lymphatic and Hemic Systems Ø7T
Lymphadenotomy *see* Drainage, Lymphatic and Hemic
  Systems Ø79
Lymphangiectomy
  see Excision, Lymphatic and Hemic Systems Ø7B
  see Resection, Lymphatic and Hemic Systems Ø7T
Lymphangiogram *see* Plain Radiography, Lymphatic
  System B7Ø
Lymphangioplasty
  see Repair, Lymphatic and Hemic Systems Ø7Q
  see Supplement, Lymphatic and Hemic Systems
    Ø7U
Lymphangiorrhaphy *see* Repair, Lymphatic and Hemic
  Systems Ø7Q
Lymphangiotomy *see* Drainage, Lymphatic and Hemic
  Systems Ø79
Lysis *see* Release

M

Macula
  use Retina, Left
  use Retina, Right
MAGEC® Spinal Bracing and Distraction System
  use Magnetically Controlled Growth Rod(s) in New
    Technology
Magnet extraction, ocular foreign body *see* Extirpa-
  tion, Eye Ø8C
Magnetic Resonance Imaging (MRI)
  Abdomen BW3Ø
  Ankle
    Left BQ3H
    Right BQ3G
  Aorta
    Abdominal B43Ø
    Thoracic B33Ø
  Arm
    Left BP3F
    Right BP3E
  Artery
    Celiac B431
    Cervico-Cerebral Arch B33Q
    Common Carotid, Bilateral B335
    Coronary
      Bypass Graft, Multiple B233
      Multiple B231
    Internal Carotid, Bilateral B338
    Intracranial B33R
    Lower Extremity
      Bilateral B43H
      Left B43G
      Right B43F
    Pelvic B43C
    Renal, Bilateral B438
    Spinal B33M
    Superior Mesenteric B434
    Upper Extremity
      Bilateral B33K
      Left B33J
      Right B33H
    Vertebral, Bilateral B33G
  Bladder BT3Ø
  Brachial Plexus BW3P
  Brain BØ3Ø
  Breast
    Bilateral BH32
    Left BH31
    Right BH3Ø
  Calcaneus
    Left BQ3K
    Right BQ3J
  Chest BW33Y
  Coccyx BR3F
  Connective Tissue
    Lower Extremity BL31
    Upper Extremity BL3Ø
  Corpora Cavernosa BV3Ø
  Disc
    Cervical BR31

Magnetic Resonance Imaging (MRI) — *continued*
  Disc — *continued*
    Lumbar BR33
    Thoracic BR32
  Ear B93Ø
  Elbow
    Left BP3H
    Right BP3G
  Eye
    Bilateral B837
    Left B836
    Right B835
  Femur
    Left BQ34
    Right BQ33
  Fetal Abdomen BY33
  Fetal Extremity BY35
  Fetal Head BY3Ø
  Fetal Heart BY31
  Fetal Spine BY34
  Fetal Thorax BY32
  Fetus, Whole BY36
  Foot
    Left BQ3M
    Right BQ3L
  Forearm
    Left BP3K
    Right BP3J
  Gland
    Adrenal, Bilateral BG32
    Parathyroid BG33
    Parotid, Bilateral B936
    Salivary, Bilateral B93D
    Submandibular, Bilateral B939
    Thyroid BG34
  Head BW38
  Heart, Right and Left B236
  Hip
    Left BQ31
    Right BQ3Ø
  Intracranial Sinus B532
  Joint
    Finger
      Left BP3D
      Right BP3C
    Hand
      Left BP3D
      Right BP3C
    Temporomandibular, Bilateral BN39
  Kidney
    Bilateral BT33
    Left BT32
    Right BT31
    Transplant BT39
  Knee
    Left BQ38
    Right BQ37
  Larynx B93J
  Leg
    Left BQ3F
    Right BQ3D
  Liver BF35
  Liver and Spleen BF36
  Lung Apices BB3G
  Nasopharynx B93F
  Neck BW3F
  Nerve
    Acoustic BØ3C
    Brachial Plexus BW3P
  Oropharynx B93F
  Ovary
    Bilateral BU35
    Left BU34
    Right BU33
  Ovary and Uterus BU3C
  Pancreas BF37
  Patella
    Left BQ3W
    Right BQ3V
  Pelvic Region BW3G
  Pelvis BR3C
  Pituitary Gland BØ39
  Plexus, Brachial BW3P
  Prostate BV33
  Retroperitoneum BW3H
  Sacrum BR3F
  Scrotum BV34
  Sella Turcica BØ39

Magnetic Resonance Imaging (MRI) — *continued*
  Shoulder
    Left BP39
    Right BP38
  Sinus
    Intracranial B532
    Paranasal B932
  Spinal Cord B03B
  Spine
    Cervical BR30
    Lumbar BR39
    Thoracic BR37
  Spleen and Liver BF36
  Subcutaneous Tissue
    Abdomen BH3H
    Extremity
      Lower BH3J
      Upper BH3F
    Head BH3D
    Neck BH3D
    Pelvis BH3H
    Thorax BH3G
  Tendon
    Lower Extremity BL33
    Upper Extremity BL32
  Testicle
    Bilateral BV37
    Left BV36
    Right BV35
  Toe
    Left BQ3Q
    Right BQ3P
  Uterus BU36
    Pregnant BU3B
  Uterus and Ovary BU3C
  Vagina BU39
  Vein
    Cerebellar B531
    Cerebral B531
    Jugular, Bilateral B535
    Lower Extremity
      Bilateral B53D
      Left B53C
      Right B53B
    Other B53V
    Pelvic (Iliac) Bilateral B53H
    Portal B53T
    Pulmonary, Bilateral B53S
    Renal, Bilateral B53L
    Spanchnic B53T
    Upper Extremity
      Bilateral B53P
      Left B53N
      Right B53M
  Vena Cava
    Inferior B539
    Superior B538
  Wrist
    Left BP3M
    Right BP3L
Magnetically Controlled Growth Rod(s)
  Cervical XNS3
  Lumbar XNS0
  Thoracic XNS4
Magnetic-guided radiofrequency endovascular fistula
  Radial Artery, Left 031C3ZF
  Radial Artery, Right 031B3ZF
  Ulnar Artery, Left 031A3ZF
  Ulnar Artery, Right 03193ZF
Malleotomy *see* Drainage, Ear, Nose, Sinus 099
Malleus
  use Auditory Ossicle, Left
  use Auditory Ossicle, Right
Mammaplasty, mammoplasty
  see Alteration, Skin and Breast 0H0
  see Repair, Skin and Breast 0HQ
  see Replacement, Skin and Breast 0HR
  see Supplement, Skin and Breast 0HU
Mammary duct
  use Breast, Bilateral
  use Breast, Left
  use Breast, Right
Mammary gland
  use Breast, Bilateral
  use Breast, Left
  use Breast, Right

Mammectomy
  see Excision, Skin and Breast 0HB
  see Resection, Skin and Breast 0HT
Mammillary body *use* Hypothalamus
Mammography *see* Plain Radiography, Skin, Subcutaneous Tissue and Breast BH0
Mammotomy *see* Drainage, Skin and Breast 0H9
Mandibular nerve *use* Trigeminal Nerve
Mandibular notch
  use Mandible, Left
  use Mandible, Right
Mandibulectomy
  see Excision, Head and Facial Bones 0NB
  see Resection, Head and Facial Bones 0NT
Manipulation
  Adhesions *see* Release
  Chiropractic *see* Chiropractic Manipulation
Manual removal, retained placenta *see* Extraction, Products of Conception, Retained 10D1
Manubrium *use* Sternum
Map
  Basal Ganglia 00K8
  Brain 00K0
  Cerebellum 00KC
  Cerebral Hemisphere 00K7
  Conduction Mechanism 02K8
  Hypothalamus 00KA
  Medulla Oblongata 00KD
  Pons 00KB
  Thalamus 00K9
Mapping
  Doppler ultrasound *see* Ultrasonography
  Electrocardiogram only *see* Measurement, Cardiac 4A02
Mark IV Breathing Pacemaker System *use* Stimulator Generator in Subcutaneous Tissue and Fascia
Marsupialization
  see Drainage
  see Excision
Massage, cardiac
  External 5A12012
  Open 02QA0ZZ
Masseter muscle *use* Head Muscle
Masseteric fascia *use* Subcutaneous Tissue and Fascia, Face
Mastectomy
  see Excision, Skin and Breast 0HB
  see Resection, Skin and Breast 0HT
Mastoid air cells
  use Mastoid Sinus, Left
  use Mastoid Sinus, Right
Mastoid (postauricular) lymph node
  use Lymphatic, Left Neck
  use Lymphatic, Right Neck
Mastoid process
  use Temporal Bone, Left
  use Temporal Bone, Right
Mastoidectomy
  see Excision, Ear, Nose, Sinus 09B
  see Resection, Ear, Nose, Sinus 09T
Mastoidotomy *see* Drainage, Ear, Nose, Sinus 099
Mastopexy
  see Repair, Skin and Breast 0HQ
  see Reposition, Skin and Breast 0HS
Mastorrhaphy *see* Repair, Skin and Breast 0HQ
Mastotomy *see* Drainage, Skin and Breast 0H9
Maxillary artery
  use External Carotid Artery, Left
  use External Carotid Artery, Right
Maxillary nerve *use* Trigeminal Nerve
Maximo II DR (VR) *use* Defibrillator Generator in 0JH
Maximo II DR CRT-D *use* Cardiac Resynchronization Defibrillator Pulse Generator in 0JH
Measurement
  Arterial
    Flow
      Coronary 4A03
      Peripheral 4A03
      Pulmonary 4A03
    Pressure
      Coronary 4A03
      Peripheral 4A03
      Pulmonary 4A03
      Thoracic, Other 4A03
    Pulse
      Coronary 4A03
      Peripheral 4A03

Measurement — *continued*
  Arterial — *continued*
    Pulse — *continued*
      Pulmonary 4A03
    Saturation, Peripheral 4A03
    Sound, Peripheral 4A03
  Biliary
    Flow 4A0C
    Pressure 4A0C
  Cardiac
    Action Currents 4A02
    Defibrillator 4B02XTZ
    Electrical Activity 4A02
      Guidance 4A02X4A
      No Qualifier 4A02X4Z
    Output 4A02
    Pacemaker 4B02XSZ
    Rate 4A02
    Rhythm 4A02
    Sampling and Pressure
      Bilateral 4A02
      Left Heart 4A02
      Right Heart 4A02
    Sound 4A02
    Total Activity, Stress 4A02XM4
  Central Nervous
    Conductivity 4A00
    Electrical Activity 4A00
    Pressure 4A000BZ
      Intracranial 4A00
    Saturation, Intracranial 4A00
    Stimulator 4B00XVZ
    Temperature, Intracranial 4A00
  Circulatory, Volume 4A05XLZ
  Gastrointestinal
    Motility 4A0B
    Pressure 4A0B
    Secretion 4A0B
  Infection, Whole Blood Nucleic Acid-base Microbial Detection XXE5XM5
  Lymphatic
    Flow 4A06
    Pressure 4A06
  Metabolism 4A0Z
  Musculoskeletal
    Contractility 4A0F
    Stimulator 4B0FXVZ
  Olfactory, Acuity 4A08X0Z
  Peripheral Nervous
    Conductivity
      Motor 4A01
      Sensory 4A01
    Electrical Activity 4A01
    Stimulator 4B01XVZ
  Products of Conception
    Cardiac
      Electrical Activity 4A0H
      Rate 4A0H
      Rhythm 4A0H
      Sound 4A0H
    Nervous
      Conductivity 4A0J
      Electrical Activity 4A0J
      Pressure 4A0J
  Respiratory
    Capacity 4A09
    Flow 4A09
    Pacemaker 4B09XSZ
    Rate 4A09
    Resistance 4A09
    Total Activity 4A09
    Volume 4A09
  Sleep 4A0ZXQZ
  Temperature 4A0Z
  Urinary
    Contractility 4A0D
    Flow 4A0D
    Pressure 4A0D
    Resistance 4A0D
    Volume 4A0D
  Venous
    Flow
      Central 4A04
      Peripheral 4A04
      Portal 4A04
      Pulmonary 4A04
    Pressure
      Central 4A04
      Peripheral 4A04

Subterms under main terms may continue to next column or page

New Technology — *continued*
  Dilation — *continued*
    Anterior Tibial — *continued*
      Right — *continued*
        Two X27P395
      Femoral
        Left
          Sustained Release Drug-eluting
            Intraluminal Device
              X27J385
          Four or More X27J3C5
          Three X27J3B5
          Two X27J395
        Right
          Sustained Release Drug-eluting
            Intraluminal Device
              X27H385
          Four or More X27H3C5
          Three X27H3B5
          Two X27H395
      Peroneal
        Left
          Sustained Release Drug-eluting
            Intraluminal Device
              X27U385
          Four or More X27U3C5
          Three X27U3B5
          Two X27U395
        Right
          Sustained Release Drug-eluting
            Intraluminal Device
              X27T385
          Four or More X27T3C5
          Three X27T3B5
          Two X27T395
      Popliteal
        Left Distal
          Sustained Release Drug-eluting
            Intraluminal Device
              X27N385
          Four or More X27N3C5
          Three X27N3B5
          Two X27N395
        Left Proximal
          Sustained Release Drug-eluting
            Intraluminal Device
              X27L385
          Four or More X27L3C5
          Three X27L3B5
          Two X27L395
        Right Distal
          Sustained Release Drug-eluting
            Intraluminal Device
              X27M385
          Four or More X27M3C5
          Three X27M3B5
          Two X27M395
        Right Proximal
          Sustained Release Drug-eluting
            Intraluminal Device
              X27K385
          Four or More X27K3C5
          Three X27K3B5
          Two X27K395
      Posterior Tibial
        Left
          Sustained Release Drug-eluting
            Intraluminal Device
              X27S385
          Four or More X27S3C5
          Three X27S3B5
          Two X27S395
        Right
          Sustained Release Drug-eluting
            Intraluminal Device
              X27R385
          Four or More X27R3C5
          Three X27R3B5
          Two X27R395
  Endothelial Damage Inhibitor XY0VX83
  Engineered Autologous Chimeric Antigen Receptor
    T-cell Immunotherapy XW0
  Erdafitinib Antineoplastic XW0DXL5
  Fosfomycin Anti-infective XW0
  Fusion
    Cervical Vertebral
      2 or more
        Nanotextured Surface XRG2092
        Radiolucent Porous XRG20F3

New Technology — *continued*
  Fusion
    Cervical Vertebral — *continued*
      Interbody Fusion Device
        Nanotextured Surface XRG1092
        Radiolucent Porous XRG10F3
    Cervicothoracic Vertebral
      Nanotextured Surface XRG4092
      Radiolucent Porous XRG40F3
    Lumbar Vertebral
      2 or more
        Nanotextured Surface XRGC092
        Radiolucent Porous XRGC0F3
      Interbody Fusion Device
        Nanotextured Surface XRGB092
        Radiolucent Porous XRGB0F3
    Lumbosacral
      Nanotextured Surface XRGD092
      Radiolucent Porous XRGD0F3
    Occipital-cervical
      Nanotextured Surface XRG0092
      Radiolucent Porous XRG00F3
    Thoracic Vertebral
      2 to 7
        Nanotextured Surface XRG7092
        Radiolucent Porous XRG70F3
      8 or more
        Nanotextured Surface XRG8092
        Radiolucent Porous XRG80F3
      Interbody Fusion Device
        Nanotextured Surface XRG6092
        Radiolucent Porous XRG60F3
    Thoracolumbar Vertebral
      Nanotextured Surface XRGA092
      Radiolucent Porous XRGA0F3
  Gilteritinib Antineoplastic XW0DXV5
  Idarucizumab, Dabigatran Reversal Agent XW0
  Imipenem-cilastatin-relebactam Anti-infective
    XW0
  Intraoperative Knee Replacement Sensor XR2
  Iobenguane I-131 Antineoplastic XW0
  Isavuconazole Anti-infective XW0
  Kidney, Fluorescent Pyrazine XT25XE5
  Measurement, Infection, Whole Blood Nucleic
    Acid-base Microbial Detection XXE5XM5
  Meropenem-vaborbactam Anti-infective XW0
  Orbital Atherectomy Technology X2C
  Other New Technology Therapeutic Substance
    XW0
  Plazomicin Anti-infective XW0
  Replacement
    Skin Substitute, Porcine Liver Derived
      XHRPXL2
    Zooplastic Tissue, Rapid Deployment Tech-
      nique X2RF
  Reposition
    Cervical, Magnetically Controlled Growth
      Rod(s) XNS3
    Lumbar, Magnetically Controlled Growth
      Rod(s) XNS0
    Thoracic, Magnetically Controlled Growth
      Rod(s) XNS4
  Ruxolitinib XW0DXT5
  Synthetic Human Angiotensin II XW0
  Tagraxofusp-erzs Antineoplastic XW0
  Uridine Triacetate XW0DX82
  Venetoclax Antineoplastic XW0DXR5
Ninth cranial nerve *use* Glossopharyngeal Nerve
Nitinol framed polymer mesh *use* Synthetic Substi-
  tute
Nonimaging Nuclear Medicine Assay
  Bladder, Kidneys and Ureters CT63
  Blood C763
  Kidneys, Ureters and Bladder CT63
  Lymphatics and Hematologic System C76YYZZ
  Ureters, Kidneys and Bladder CT63
  Urinary System CT6YYZZ
Nonimaging Nuclear Medicine Probe
  Abdomen CW50
  Abdomen and Chest CW54
  Abdomen and Pelvis CW51
  Brain C050
  Central Nervous System C05YYZZ
  Chest CW53
  Chest and Abdomen CW54
  Chest and Neck CW56
  Extremity
    Lower CP5PZZZ
    Upper CP5NZZZ

Nonimaging Nuclear Medicine Probe — *continued*
  Head and Neck CW5B
  Heart C25YYZZ
    Right and Left C256
  Lymphatics
    Head C75J
    Head and Neck C755
    Lower Extremity C75P
    Neck C75K
    Pelvic C75D
    Trunk C75M
    Upper Chest C75L
    Upper Extremity C75N
  Lymphatics and Hematologic System C75YYZZ
  Musculoskeletal System, Other CP5YYZZ
  Neck and Chest CW56
  Neck and Head CW5B
  Pelvic Region CW5J
  Pelvis and Abdomen CW51
  Spine CP55ZZZ
Nonimaging Nuclear Medicine Uptake
  Endocrine System CG4YYZZ
  Gland, Thyroid CG42
Non-tunneled central venous catheter *use* Infusion
  Device
Nostril *use* Nasal Mucosa and Soft Tissue
Novacor Left Ventricular Assist Device *use* Im-
  plantable Heart Assist System in Heart and Great
  Vessels
Novation® Ceramic AHS® (Articulation Hip System)
  use Synthetic Substitute, Ceramic in 0SR
Nuclear medicine
  see Nonimaging Nuclear Medicine Assay
  see Nonimaging Nuclear Medicine Probe
  see Nonimaging Nuclear Medicine Uptake
  see Planar Nuclear Medicine Imaging
  see Positron Emission Tomographic (PET) Imaging
  see Systemic Nuclear Medicine Therapy
  see Tomographic (Tomo) Nuclear Medicine Imag-
    ing
Nuclear scintigraphy *see* Nuclear Medicine
Nutrition, concentrated substances
  Enteral infusion 3E0G36Z
  Parenteral (peripheral) infusion *see* Introduction
    of Nutritional Substance

O

Obliteration *see* Destruction
Obturator artery
  use Internal Iliac Artery, Left
  use Internal Iliac Artery, Right
Obturator lymph node *use* Lymphatic, Pelvis
Obturator muscle
  use Hip Muscle, Left
  use Hip Muscle, Right
Obturator nerve *use* Lumbar Plexus
Obturator vein
  use Hypogastric Vein, Left
  use Hypogastric Vein, Right
Obtuse margin *use* Heart, Left
Occipital artery
  use External Carotid Artery, Left
  use External Carotid Artery, Right
Occipital lobe *use* Cerebral Hemisphere
Occipital lymph node
  use Lymphatic, Left Neck
  use Lymphatic, Right Neck
Occipitofrontalis muscle *use* Facial Muscle
Occlusion
  Ampulla of Vater 0FLC
  Anus 0DLQ
  Aorta
    Abdominal 04L0
    Thoracic, Descending 02LW3DJ
  Artery
    Anterior Tibial
      Left 04LQ
      Right 04LP
    Axillary
      Left 03L6
      Right 03L5
    Brachial
      Left 03L8
      Right 03L7
    Celiac 04L1

▽ **Subterms under main terms may continue to next column or page**

Occlusion — *continued*
  Artery — *continued*
    Colic
      Left 04L7
      Middle 04L8
      Right 04L6
    Common Carotid
      Left 03LJ
      Right 03LH
    Common Iliac
      Left 04LD
      Right 04LC
    External Carotid
      Left 03LN
      Right 03LM
    External Iliac
      Left 04LJ
      Right 04LH
    Face 03LR
    Femoral
      Left 04LL
      Right 04LK
    Foot
      Left 04LW
      Right 04LV
    Gastric 04L2
    Hand
      Left 03LF
      Right 03LD
    Hepatic 04L3
    Inferior Mesenteric 04LB
    Innominate 03L2
    Internal Carotid
      Left 03LL
      Right 03LK
    Internal Iliac
      Left 04LF
      Right 04LE
    Internal Mammary
      Left 03L1
      Right 03L0
    Intracranial 03LG
    Lower 04LY
    Peroneal
      Left 04LU
      Right 04LT
    Popliteal
      Left 04LN
      Right 04LM
    Posterior Tibial
      Left 04LS
      Right 04LR
    Pulmonary
      Left 02LR
      Right 02LQ
    Pulmonary Trunk 02LP
    Radial
      Left 03LC
      Right 03LB
    Renal
      Left 04LA
      Right 04L9
    Splenic 04L4
    Subclavian
      Left 03L4
      Right 03L3
    Superior Mesenteric 04L5
    Temporal
      Left 03LT
      Right 03LS
    Thyroid
      Left 03LV
      Right 03LU
    Ulnar
      Left 03LA
      Right 03L9
    Upper 03LY
    Vertebral
      Left 03LQ
      Right 03LP
  Atrium, Left 02L7
  Bladder 0TLB
  Bladder Neck 0TLC
  Bronchus
    Lingula 0BL9
    Lower Lobe
      Left 0BLB
      Right 0BL6

Occlusion — *continued*
  Bronchus — *continued*
    Main
      Left 0BL7
      Right 0BL3
    Middle Lobe, Right 0BL5
    Upper Lobe
      Left 0BL8
      Right 0BL4
  Carina 0BL2
  Cecum 0DLH
  Cisterna Chyli 07LL
  Colon
    Ascending 0DLK
    Descending 0DLM
    Sigmoid 0DLN
    Transverse 0DLL
  Cord
    Bilateral 0VLH
    Left 0VLG
    Right 0VLF
  Cul-de-sac 0ULF
  Duct
    Common Bile 0FL9
    Cystic 0FL8
    Hepatic
      Common 0FL7
      Left 0FL6
      Right 0FL5
    Lacrimal
      Left 08LY
      Right 08LX
    Pancreatic 0FLD
      Accessory 0FLF
    Parotid
      Left 0CLC
      Right 0CLB
  Duodenum 0DL9
  Esophagogastric Junction 0DL4
  Esophagus 0DL5
    Lower 0DL3
    Middle 0DL2
    Upper 0DL1
  Fallopian Tube
    Left 0UL6
    Right 0UL5
  Fallopian Tubes, Bilateral 0UL7
  Ileocecal Valve 0DLC
  Ileum 0DLB
  Intestine
    Large 0DLE
      Left 0DLG
      Right 0DLF
    Small 0DL8
  Jejunum 0DLA
  Kidney Pelvis
    Left 0TL4
    Right 0TL3
  Left atrial appendage (LAA) *see* Occlusion, Atrium, Left 02L7
  Lymphatic
    Aortic 07LD
    Axillary
      Left 07L6
      Right 07L5
    Head 07L0
    Inguinal
      Left 07LJ
      Right 07LH
    Internal Mammary
      Left 07L9
      Right 07L8
    Lower Extremity
      Left 07LG
      Right 07LF
    Mesenteric 07LB
    Neck
      Left 07L2
      Right 07L1
    Pelvis 07LC
    Thoracic Duct 07LK
    Thorax 07L7
    Upper Extremity
      Left 07L4
      Right 07L3
  Rectum 0DLP
  Stomach 0DL6
    Pylorus 0DL7
  Trachea 0BL1

Occlusion — *continued*
  Ureter
    Left 0TL7
    Right 0TL6
  Urethra 0TLD
  Vagina 0ULG
  Valve, Pulmonary 02LH
  Vas Deferens
    Bilateral 0VLQ
    Left 0VLP
    Right 0VLN
  Vein
    Axillary
      Left 05L8
      Right 05L7
    Azygos 05L0
    Basilic
      Left 05LC
      Right 05LB
    Brachial
      Left 05LA
      Right 05L9
    Cephalic
      Left 05LF
      Right 05LD
    Colic 06L7
    Common Iliac
      Left 06LD
      Right 06LC
    Esophageal 06L3
    External Iliac
      Left 06LG
      Right 06LF
    External Jugular
      Left 05LQ
      Right 05LP
    Face
      Left 05LV
      Right 05LT
    Femoral
      Left 06LN
      Right 06LM
    Foot
      Left 06LV
      Right 06LT
    Gastric 06L2
    Hand
      Left 05LH
      Right 05LG
    Hemiazygos 05L1
    Hepatic 06L4
    Hypogastric
      Left 06LJ
      Right 06LH
    Inferior Mesenteric 06L6
    Innominate
      Left 05L4
      Right 05L3
    Internal Jugular
      Left 05LN
      Right 05LM
    Intracranial 05LL
    Lower 06LY
    Portal 06L8
    Pulmonary
      Left 02LT
      Right 02LS
    Renal
      Left 06LB
      Right 06L9
    Saphenous
      Left 06LQ
      Right 06LP
    Splenic 06L1
    Subclavian
      Left 05L6
      Right 05L5
    Superior Mesenteric 06L5
    Upper 05LY
    Vertebral
      Left 05LS
      Right 05LR
  Vena Cava
    Inferior 06L0
    Superior 02LV

Occlusion, REBOA (resuscitative endovascular balloon occlusion of the aorta)
02LW3DJ
04L03DJ
Occupational therapy *see* Activities of Daily Living Treatment, Rehabilitation F08
Odentectomy
see Excision, Mouth and Throat 0CB
see Resection, Mouth and Throat 0CT
Odontoid process *use* Cervical Vertebra
Olecranon bursa
use Elbow Bursa and Ligament, Left
use Elbow Bursa and Ligament, Right
Olecranon process
use Ulna, Left
use Ulna, Right
Olfactory bulb *use* Olfactory Nerve
Omentectomy, omentumectomy
see Excision, Gastrointestinal System 0DB
see Resection, Gastrointestinal System 0DT
Omentofixation *see* Repair, Gastrointestinal System 0DQ
Omentoplasty
see Repair, Gastrointestinal System 0DQ
see Replacement, Gastrointestinal System 0DR
see Supplement, Gastrointestinal System 0DU
Omentorrhaphy *see* Repair, Gastrointestinal System 0DQ
Omentotomy *see* Drainage, Gastrointestinal System 0D9
Omnilink Elite Vascular Balloon Expandable Stent System *use* Intraluminal Device
Onychectomy
see Excision, Skin and Breast 0HB
see Resection, Skin and Breast 0HT
Onychoplasty
see Repair, Skin and Breast 0HQ
see Replacement, Skin and Breast 0HR
Onychotomy *see* Drainage, Skin and Breast 0H9
Oophorectomy
see Excision, Female Reproductive System 0UB
see Resection, Female Reproductive System 0UT
Oophoropexy
see Repair, Female Reproductive System 0UQ
see Reposition, Female Reproductive System 0US
Oophoroplasty
see Repair, Female Reproductive System 0UQ
see Supplement, Female Reproductive System 0UU
Oophorrhaphy *see* Repair, Female Reproductive System 0UQ
Oophorostomy *see* Drainage, Female Reproductive System 0U9
Oophorotomy
see Division, Female Reproductive System 0U8
see Drainage, Female Reproductive System 0U9
Oophorrhaphy *see* Repair, Female Reproductive System 0UQ
Open Pivot Aortic Valve Graft (AVG) *use* Synthetic Substitute
Open Pivot (mechanical) Valve *use* Synthetic Substitute
Ophthalmic artery *use* Intracranial Artery
Ophthalmic nerve *use* Trigeminal Nerve
Ophthalmic vein *use* Intracranial Vein
Opponensplasty
Tendon replacement *see* Replacement, Tendons 0LR
Tendon transfer *see* Transfer, Tendons 0LX
Optic chiasma *use* Optic Nerve
Optic disc
use Retina, Left
use Retina, Right
Optic foramen *use* Sphenoid Bone
Optical coherence tomography, intravascular *see* Computerized Tomography (CT Scan)
Optimizer™ III implantable pulse generator *use* Contractility Modulation Device in 0JH
Orbicularis oculi muscle
use Upper Eyelid, Left
use Upper Eyelid, Right
Orbicularis oris muscle *use* Facial Muscle
Orbital Atherectomy Technology X2C
Orbital fascia *use* Subcutaneous Tissue and Fascia, Face
Orbital portion of ethmoid bone
use Orbit, Left

Orbital portion of ethmoid bone — *continued*
use Orbit, Right
Orbital portion of frontal bone
use Orbit, Left
use Orbit, Right
Orbital portion of lacrimal bone
use Orbit, Left
use Orbit, Right
Orbital portion of maxilla
use Orbit, Left
use Orbit, Right
Orbital portion of palatine bone
use Orbit, Left
use Orbit, Right
Orbital portion of sphenoid bone
use Orbit, Left
use Orbit, Right
Orbital portion of zygomatic bone
use Orbit, Left
use Orbit, Right
Orchectomy, orchidectomy, orchiectomy
see Excision, Male Reproductive System 0VB
see Resection, Male Reproductive System 0VT
Orchidoplasty, orchioplasty
see Repair, Male Reproductive System 0VQ
see Replacement, Male Reproductive System 0VR
see Supplement, Male Reproductive System 0VU
Orchidorrhaphy, orchiorrhaphy *see* Repair, Male Reproductive System 0VQ
Orchidotomy, orchiotomy, orchotomy *see* Drainage, Male Reproductive System 0V9
Orchiopexy
see Repair, Male Reproductive System 0VQ
see Reposition, Male Reproductive System 0VS
Oropharyngeal airway (OPA) *use* Intraluminal Device, Airway in Mouth and Throat
Oropharynx *use* Pharynx
Ossiculectomy
see Excision, Ear, Nose, Sinus 09B
see Resection, Ear, Nose, Sinus 09T
Ossiculotomy *see* Drainage, Ear, Nose, Sinus 099
Ostectomy
see Excision, Head and Facial Bones 0NB
see Excision, Lower Bones 0QB
see Excision, Upper Bones 0PB
see Resection, Head and Facial Bones 0NT
see Resection, Lower Bones 0QT
see Resection, Upper Bones 0PT
Osteoclasis
see Division, Head and Facial Bones 0N8
see Division, Lower Bones 0Q8
see Division, Upper Bones 0P8
Osteolysis
see Release, Head and Facial Bones 0NN
see Release, Lower Bones 0QN
see Release, Upper Bones 0PN
Osteopathic Treatment
Abdomen 7W09X
Cervical 7W01X
Extremity
Lower 7W06X
Upper 7W07X
Head 7W00X
Lumbar 7W03X
Pelvis 7W05X
Rib Cage 7W08X
Sacrum 7W04X
Thoracic 7W02X
Osteopexy
see Repair, Head and Facial Bones 0NQ
see Repair, Lower Bones 0QQ
see Repair, Upper Bones 0PQ
see Reposition, Head and Facial Bones 0NS
see Reposition, Lower Bones 0QS
see Reposition, Upper Bones 0PS
Osteoplasty
see Repair, Head and Facial Bones 0NQ
see Repair, Lower Bones 0QQ
see Repair, Upper Bones 0PQ
see Replacement, Head and Facial Bones 0NR
see Replacement, Lower Bones 0QR
see Replacement, Upper Bones 0PR
see Supplement, Head and Facial Bones 0NU
see Supplement, Lower Bones 0QU
see Supplement, Upper Bones 0PU

Osteorrhaphy
see Repair, Head and Facial Bones 0NQ
see Repair, Lower Bones 0QQ
see Repair, Upper Bones 0PQ
Osteotomy, ostotomy
see Division, Head and Facial Bones 0N8
see Division, Lower Bones 0Q8
see Division, Upper Bones 0P8
see Drainage, Head and Facial Bones 0N9
see Drainage, Lower Bones 0Q9
see Drainage, Upper Bones 0P9
Otic ganglion *use* Head and Neck Sympathetic Nerve
Otoplasty
see Repair, Ear, Nose, Sinus 09Q
see Replacement, Ear, Nose, Sinus 09R
see Supplement, Ear, Nose, Sinus 09U
Otoscopy *see* Inspection, Ear, Nose, Sinus 09J
Oval window
use Middle Ear, Left
use Middle Ear, Right
Ovarian artery *use* Abdominal Aorta
Ovarian ligament *use* Uterine Supporting Structure
Ovariectomy
see Excision, Female Reproductive System 0UB
see Resection, Female Reproductive System 0UT
Ovariocentesis *see* Drainage, Female Reproductive System 0U9
Ovariopexy
see Repair, Female Reproductive System 0UQ
see Reposition, Female Reproductive System 0US
Ovariotomy
see Division, Female Reproductive System 0U8
see Drainage, Female Reproductive System 0U9
Ovatio™ CRT-D *use* Cardiac Resynchronization Defibrillator Pulse Generator in 0JH
Oversewing
Gastrointestinal ulcer *see* Repair, Gastrointestinal System 0DQ
Pleural bleb *see* Repair, Respiratory System 0BQ
Oviduct
use Fallopian Tube, Left
use Fallopian Tube, Right
Oximetry, Fetal pulse 10H073Z
OXINIUM *use* Synthetic Substitute, Oxidized Zirconium on Polyethylene in 0SR
Oxygenation
Extracorporeal membrane (ECMO) *see* Performance, Circulatory 5A15
Hyperbaric *see* Assistance, Circulatory 5A05
Supersaturated *see* Assistance, Circulatory 5A05

P

Pacemaker
Dual Chamber
Abdomen 0JH8
Chest 0JH6
Intracardiac
Insertion of device in
Atrium
Left 02H7
Right 02H6
Vein, Coronary 02H4
Ventricle
Left 02HL
Right 02HK
Removal of device from, Heart 02PA
Revision of device in, Heart 02WA
Single Chamber
Abdomen 0JH8
Chest 0JH6
Single Chamber Rate Responsive
Abdomen 0JH8
Chest 0JH6
Packing
Abdominal Wall 2W43X5Z
Anorectal 2Y43X5Z
Arm
Lower
Left 2W4DX5Z
Right 2W4CX5Z
Upper
Left 2W4BX5Z
Right 2W4AX5Z
Back 2W45X5Z
Chest Wall 2W44X5Z

Subterms under main terms may continue to next column or page

Packing — *continued*
  Ear 2Y42X5Z
  Extremity
    Lower
      Left 2W4MX5Z
      Right 2W4LX5Z
    Upper
      Left 2W49X5Z
      Right 2W48X5Z
  Face 2W41X5Z
  Finger
    Left 2W4KX5Z
    Right 2W4JX5Z
  Foot
    Left 2W4TX5Z
    Right 2W4SX5Z
  Genital Tract, Female 2Y44X5Z
  Hand
    Left 2W4FX5Z
    Right 2W4EX5Z
  Head 2W40X5Z
  Inguinal Region
    Left 2W47X5Z
    Right 2W46X5Z
  Leg
    Lower
      Left 2W4RX5Z
      Right 2W4QX5Z
    Upper
      Left 2W4PX5Z
      Right 2W4NX5Z
  Mouth and Pharynx 2Y40X5Z
  Nasal 2Y41X5Z
  Neck 2W42X5Z
  Thumb
    Left 2W4HX5Z
    Right 2W4GX5Z
  Toe
    Left 2W4VX5Z
    Right 2W4UX5Z
  Urethra 2Y45X5Z
Paclitaxel-eluting coronary stent *use* Intraluminal Device, Drug-eluting in Heart and Great Vessels
Paclitaxel-eluting peripheral stent
  use Intraluminal Device, Drug-eluting in Lower Arteries
  use Intraluminal Device, Drug-eluting in Upper Arteries
Palatine gland *use* Buccal Mucosa
Palatine tonsil *use* Tonsils
Palatine uvula *use* Uvula
Palatoglossal muscle *use* Tongue, Palate, Pharynx Muscle
Palatopharyngeal muscle *use* Tongue, Palate, Pharynx Muscle
Palatoplasty
  see Repair, Mouth and Throat 0CQ
  see Replacement, Mouth and Throat 0CR
  see Supplement, Mouth and Throat 0CU
Palatorrhaphy *see* Repair, Mouth and Throat 0CQ
Palmar cutaneous nerve
  use Median Nerve
  use Radial Nerve
Palmar (volar) digital vein
  use Hand Vein, Left
  use Hand Vein, Right
Palmar fascia (aponeurosis)
  use Subcutaneous Tissue and Fascia, Left Hand
  use Subcutaneous Tissue and Fascia, Right Hand
Palmar interosseous muscle
  use Hand Muscle, Left
  use Hand Muscle, Right
Palmar (volar) metacarpal vein
  use Hand Vein, Left
  use Hand Vein, Right
Palmar ulnocarpal ligament
  use Wrist Bursa and Ligament, Left
  use Wrist Bursa and Ligament, Right
Palmaris longus muscle
  use Lower Arm and Wrist Muscle, Left
  use Lower Arm and Wrist Muscle, Right
Pancreatectomy
  see Excision, Pancreas 0FBG
  see Resection, Pancreas 0FTG
Pancreatic artery *use* Splenic Artery
Pancreatic plexus *use* Abdominal Sympathetic Nerve
Pancreatic vein *use* Splenic Vein

Pancreaticoduodenostomy *see* Bypass, Hepatobiliary System and Pancreas 0F1
Pancreaticosplenic lymph node *use* Lymphatic, Aortic
Pancreatogram, endoscopic retrograde *see* Fluoroscopy, Pancreatic Duct BF18
Pancreatolithotomy *see* Extirpation, Pancreas 0FCG
Pancreatotomy
  see Division, Pancreas 0F8G
  see Drainage, Pancreas 0F9G
Panniculectomy
  see Excision, Skin, Abdomen 0HB7
  see Excision, Subcutaneous Tissue and Fascia, Abdomen 0JB8
Paraaortic lymph node *use* Lymphatic, Aortic
Paracentesis
  Eye *see* Drainage, Eye 089
  Peritoneal Cavity *see* Drainage, Peritoneal Cavity 0W9G
  Tympanum *see* Drainage, Ear, Nose, Sinus 099
Pararectal lymph node *use* Lymphatic, Mesenteric
Parasternal lymph node *use* Lymphatic, Thorax
Parathyroidectomy
  see Excision, Endocrine System 0GB
  see Resection, Endocrine System 0GT
Paratracheal lymph node *use* Lymphatic, Thorax
Paraurethral (Skene's) gland *use* Vestibular Gland
Parenteral nutrition, total *see* Introduction of Nutritional Substance
Parietal lobe *use* Cerebral Hemisphere
Parotid lymph node *use* Lymphatic, Head
Parotid plexus *use* Facial Nerve
Parotidectomy
  see Excision, Mouth and Throat 0CB
  see Resection, Mouth and Throat 0CT
Pars flaccida
  use Tympanic Membrane, Left
  use Tympanic Membrane, Right
Partial joint replacement
  Hip *see* Replacement, Lower Joints 0SR
  Knee *see* Replacement, Lower Joints 0SR
  Shoulder *see* Replacement, Upper Joints 0RR
Partially absorbable mesh *use* Synthetic Substitute
Patch, blood, spinal 3E0R3GC
Patellapexy
  see Repair, Lower Bones 0QQ
  see Reposition, Lower Bones 0QS
Patellaplasty
  see Repair, Lower Bones 0QQ
  see Replacement, Lower Bones 0QR
  see Supplement, Lower Bones 0QU
Patellar ligament
  use Knee Bursa and Ligament, Left
  use Knee Bursa and Ligament, Right
Patellar tendon
  use Knee Tendon, Left
  use Knee Tendon, Right
Patellectomy
  see Excision, Lower Bones 0QB
  see Resection, Lower Bones 0QT
Patellofemoral joint
  use Knee Joint, Left
  use Knee Joint, Left, Femoral Surface
  use Knee Joint, Right
  use Knee Joint, Right, Femoral Surface
Pectineus muscle
  use Upper Leg Muscle, Left
  use Upper Leg Muscle, Right
Pectoral fascia *use* Subcutaneous Tissue and Fascia, Chest
Pectoral (anterior) lymph node
  use Lymphatic Left, Axillary
  use Lymphatic Right, Axillary
Pectoralis major muscle
  use Thorax Muscle, Left
  use Thorax Muscle, Right
Pectoralis minor muscle
  use Thorax Muscle, Left
  use Thorax Muscle, Right
Pedicle-based dynamic stabilization device
  use Spinal Stabilization Device, Pedicle-Based in 0SH
  use Spinal Stabilization Device, Pedicle-Based in 0RH
PEEP (positive end expiratory pressure) *see* Assistance, Respiratory 5A09

PEG (percutaneous endoscopic gastrostomy) 0DH63UZ
PEJ (percutaneous endoscopic jejunostomy) 0DHA3UZ
Pelvic splanchnic nerve
  use Abdominal Sympathetic Nerve
  use Sacral Sympathetic Nerve
Penectomy
  see Excision, Male Reproductive System 0VB
  see Resection, Male Reproductive System 0VT
Penile urethra *use* Urethra
Perceval sutureless valve *use* Zooplastic Tissue, Rapid Deployment Technique in New Technology
Percutaneous endoscopic gastrojejunostomy (PEG/J) tube *use* Feeding Device in Gastrointestinal System
Percutaneous endoscopic gastrostomy (PEG) tube *use* Feeding Device in Gastrointestinal System
Percutaneous nephrostomy catheter *use* Drainage Device
Percutaneous transluminal coronary angioplasty (PTCA) *see* Dilation, Heart and Great Vessels 027
Performance
  Biliary
    Multiple, Filtration 5A1C60Z
    Single, Filtration 5A1C00Z
  Cardiac
    Continuous
      Output 5A1221Z
      Pacing 5A1223Z
    Intermittent, Pacing 5A1213Z
    Single, Output, Manual 5A12012
  Circulatory
    Continuous
      Central Membrane 5A1522F
      Peripheral Veno-arterial Membrane 5A1522G
      Peripheral Veno-venous Membrane 5A1522H
    Intraoperative
      Central Membrane 5A15A2F
      Peripheral Veno-arterial Membrane 5A15A2G
      Peripheral Veno-venous Membrane 5A15A2H
  Respiratory
    24-96 Consecutive Hours, Ventilation 5A1945Z
    Greater than 96 Consecutive Hours, Ventilation 5A1955Z
    Less than 24 Consecutive Hours, Ventilation 5A1935Z
    Single, Ventilation, Nonmechanical 5A19054
  Urinary
    Continuous, Greater than 18 hours per day, Filtration 5A1D90Z
    Intermittent, Less than 6 Hours Per Day, Filtration 5A1D70Z
    Prolonged Intermittent, 6-18 hours per day, Filtration 5A1D80Z
Perfusion *see* Introduction of substance in or on
Perfusion, donor organ
  Heart 6AB50BZ
  Kidney(s) 6ABT0BZ
  Liver 6ABF0BZ
  Lung(s) 6ABB0BZ
Pericardiectomy
  see Excision, Pericardium 02BN
  see Resection, Pericardium 02TN
Pericardiocentesis *see* Drainage, Pericardial Cavity 0W9D
Pericardiolysis *see* Release, Pericardium 02NN
Pericardiophrenic artery
  use Internal Mammary Artery, Left
  use Internal Mammary Artery, Right
Pericardioplasty
  see Repair, Pericardium 02QN
  see Replacement, Pericardium 02RN
  see Supplement, Pericardium 02UN
Pericardiorrhaphy *see* Repair, Pericardium 02QN
Pericardiostomy *see* Drainage, Pericardial Cavity 0W9D
Pericardiotomy *see* Drainage, Pericardial Cavity 0W9D
Perimetrium *use* Uterus
Peripheral parenteral nutrition *see* Introduction of Nutritional Substance
Peripherally inserted central catheter (PICC) *use* Infusion Device
Peritoneal dialysis 3E1M39Z

Peritoneocentesis
 see Drainage, Peritoneal Cavity ØW9G
 see Drainage, Peritoneum ØD9W
Peritoneoplasty
 see Repair, Peritoneum ØDQW
 see Replacement, Peritoneum ØDRW
 see Supplement, Peritoneum ØDUW
Peritoneoscopy ØDJW4ZZ
Peritoneotomy *see* Drainage, Peritoneum ØD9W
Peritoneumectomy *see* Excision, Peritoneum ØDBW
Peroneus brevis muscle
 use Lower Leg Muscle, Left
 use Lower Leg Muscle, Right
Peroneus longus muscle
 use Lower Leg Muscle, Left
 use Lower Leg Muscle, Right
Pessary ring *use* Intraluminal Device, Pessary in Female
 Reproductive System
PET scan *see* Positron Emission Tomographic (PET)
 Imaging
Petrous part of temoporal bone
 use Temporal Bone, Left
 use Temporal Bone, Right
Phacoemulsification, lens
 With IOL implant *see* Replacement, Eye Ø8R
 Without IOL implant *see* Extraction, Eye Ø8D
Phalangectomy
 see Excision, Lower Bones ØQB
 see Excision, Upper Bones ØPB
 see Resection, Lower Bones ØQT
 see Resection, Upper Bones ØPT
Phallectomy
 see Excision, Penis ØVBS
 see Resection, Penis ØVTS
Phalloplasty
 see Repair, Penis ØVQS
 see Supplement, Penis ØVUS
Phallotomy *see* Drainage, Penis ØV9S
Pharmacotherapy, for substance abuse
 Antabuse HZ93ZZZ
 Bupropion HZ97ZZZ
 Clonidine HZ96ZZZ
 Levo-alpha-acetyl-methadol (LAAM) HZ92ZZZ
 Methadone Maintenance HZ91ZZZ
 Naloxone HZ95ZZZ
 Naltrexone HZ94ZZZ
 Nicotine Replacement HZ90ZZZ
 Psychiatric Medication HZ98ZZZ
 Replacement Medication, Other HZ99ZZZ
Pharyngeal constrictor muscle *use* Tongue, Palate,
 Pharynx Muscle
Pharyngeal plexus *use* Vagus Nerve
Pharyngeal recess *use* Nasopharynx
Pharyngeal tonsil *use* Adenoids
Pharyngogram *see* Fluoroscopy, Pharynix B91G
Pharyngoplasty
 see Repair, Mouth and Throat ØCQ
 see Replacement, Mouth and Throat ØCR
 see Supplement, Mouth and Throat ØCU
Pharyngorrhaphy *see* Repair, Mouth and Throat ØCQ
Pharyngotomy *see* Drainage, Mouth and Throat ØC9
Pharyngotympanic tube
 use Eustachian Tube, Left
 use Eustachian Tube, Right
Pheresis
 Erythrocytes 6A55
 Leukocytes 6A55
 Plasma 6A55
 Platelets 6A55
 Stem Cells
  Cord Blood 6A55
  Hematopoietic 6A55
Phlebectomy
 see Excision, Lower Veins Ø6B
 see Excision, Upper Veins Ø5B
 see Extraction, Lower Veins Ø6D
 see Extraction, Upper Veins Ø5D
Phlebography
 see Plain Radiography, Veins B5Ø
 Impedance 4AØ4X51
Phleborrhaphy
 see Repair, Lower Veins Ø6Q
 see Repair, Upper Veins Ø5Q
Phlebotomy
 see Drainage, Lower Veins Ø69
 see Drainage, Upper Veins Ø59

Photocoagulation
 For Destruction *see* Destruction
 For Repair *see* Repair
Photopheresis, therapeutic *see* Phototherapy, Circu-
 latory 6A65
Phototherapy
 Circulatory 6A65
 Skin 6A6Ø
 Ultraviolet light *see* Ultraviolet Light Therapy,
  Physiological Systems 6A8
Phrenectomy, phrenoneurectomy *see* Excision,
 Nerve, Phrenic Ø1B2
Phrenemphraxis *see* Destruction, Nerve, Phrenic Ø152
Phrenic nerve stimulator generator *use* Stimulator
 Generator in Subcutaneous Tissue and Fascia
Phrenic nerve stimulator lead *use* Diaphragmatic
 Pacemaker Lead in Respiratory System
Phreniclasis *see* Destruction, Nerve, Phrenic Ø152
Phrenicoexeresis *see* Extraction, Nerve, Phrenic Ø1D2
Phrenicotomy *see* Division, Nerve, Phrenic Ø182
Phrenicotripsy *see* Destruction, Nerve, Phrenic Ø152
Phrenoplasty
 see Repair, Respiratory System ØBQ
 see Supplement, Respiratory System ØBU
Phrenotomy *see* Drainage, Respiratory System ØB9
Physiatry *see* Motor Treatment, Rehabilitation FØ7
Physical medicine *see* Motor Treatment, Rehabilitation
 FØ7
Physical therapy *see* Motor Treatment, Rehabilitation
 FØ7
PHYSIOMESH™ Flexible Composite Mesh *use* Syn-
 thetic Substitute
Pia mater, intracranial *use* Cerebral Meninges
Pia mater, spinal *use* Spinal Meninges
Pinealectomy
 see Excision, Pineal Body ØGB1
 see Resection, Pineal Body ØGT1
Pinealoscopy ØGJ14ZZ
Pinealotomy *see* Drainage, Pineal Body ØG91
Pinna
 use External Ear, Bilateral
 use External Ear, Left
 use External Ear, Right
Pipeline™ (Flex) embolization device *use* Intraluminal Device, Flow Diverter in Ø3V
Piriform recess (sinus) *use* Pharynx
Piriformis muscle
 use Hip Muscle, Left
 use Hip Muscle, Right
**PIRRT (Prolonged intermittent renal replacement
 therapy)** 5A1D8ØZ
Pisiform bone
 use Carpal, Left
 use Carpal, Right
Pisohamate ligament
 use Hand Bursa and Ligament, Left
 use Hand Bursa and Ligament, Right
Pisometacarpal ligament
 use Hand Bursa and Ligament, Left
 use Hand Bursa and Ligament, Right
Pituitectomy
 see Excision, Gland, Pituitary ØGBØ
 see Resection, Gland, Pituitary ØGTØ
Plain film radiology *see* Plain Radiography
Plain Radiography
 Abdomen BWØØZZZ
 Abdomen and Pelvis BWØ1ZZZ
 Abdominal Lymphatic
  Bilateral B7Ø1
  Unilateral B7ØØ
 Airway, Upper BBØDZZZ
 Ankle
  Left BQØH
  Right BQØG
 Aorta
  Abdominal B4ØØ
  Thoracic B3ØØ
  Thoraco-Abdominal B3ØP
 Aorta and Bilateral Lower Extremity Arteries B4ØD
 Arch
  Bilateral BNØDZZZ
  Left BNØCZZZ
  Right BNØBZZZ
 Arm
  Left BPØFZZZ
  Right BPØEZZZ

Plain Radiography — *continued*
 Artery
  Brachiocephalic-Subclavian, Right B3Ø1
  Bronchial B3ØL
  Bypass Graft, Other B2ØF
  Cervico-Cerebral Arch B3ØQ
  Common Carotid
   Bilateral B3Ø5
   Left B3Ø4
   Right B3Ø3
  Coronary
   Bypass Graft
    Multiple B2Ø3
    Single B2Ø2
   Multiple B2Ø1
   Single B2ØØ
  External Carotid
   Bilateral B3ØC
   Left B3ØB
   Right B3Ø9
  Hepatic B4Ø2
  Inferior Mesenteric B4Ø5
  Intercostal B3ØL
  Internal Carotid
   Bilateral B3Ø8
   Left B3Ø7
   Right B3Ø6
  Internal Mammary Bypass Graft
   Left B2Ø8
   Right B2Ø7
  Intra-Abdominal, Other B4ØB
  Intracranial B3ØR
  Lower Extremity
   Bilateral and Aorta B4ØD
   Left B4ØG
   Right B4ØF
  Lower, Other B4ØJ
  Lumbar B4Ø9
  Pelvic B4ØC
  Pulmonary
   Left B3ØT
   Right B3ØS
  Renal
   Bilateral B4Ø8
   Left B4Ø7
   Right B4Ø6
   Transplant B4ØM
  Spinal B3ØM
  Splenic B4Ø3
  Subclavian, Left B3Ø2
  Superior Mesenteric B4Ø4
  Upper Extremity
   Bilateral B3ØK
   Left B3ØJ
   Right B3ØH
  Upper, Other B3ØN
  Vertebral
   Bilateral B3ØG
   Left B3ØF
   Right B3ØD
 Bile Duct BFØØ
 Bile Duct and Gallbladder BFØ3
 Bladder BTØØ
  Kidney and Ureter BTØ4
 Bladder and Urethra BTØB
 Bone
  Facial BNØ5ZZZ
  Nasal BNØ4ZZZ
 Bones, Long, All BWØBZZZ
 Breast
  Bilateral BHØ2ZZZ
  Left BHØ1ZZZ
  Right BHØØZZZ
 Calcaneus
  Left BQØKZZZ
  Right BQØJZZZ
 Chest BWØ3ZZZ
 Clavicle
  Left BPØ5ZZZ
  Right BPØ4ZZZ
 Coccyx BRØFZZZ
 Corpora Cavernosa BVØØ
 Dialysis Fistula B5ØW
 Dialysis Shunt B5ØW
 Disc
  Cervical BRØ1
  Lumbar BRØ3
  Thoracic BRØ2

⚕ **Subterms under main terms may continue to next column or page**

Plain Radiography — *continued*
Duct
  Lacrimal
    Bilateral B802
    Left B801
    Right B800
  Mammary
    Multiple
      Left BH06
      Right BH05
    Single
      Left BH04
      Right BH03
Elbow
  Left BP0H
  Right BP0G
Epididymis
  Left BV02
  Right BV01
Extremity
  Lower BW0CZZZ
  Upper BW0JZZZ
Eye
  Bilateral B807ZZZ
  Left B806ZZZ
  Right B805ZZZ
Facet Joint
  Cervical BR04
  Lumbar BR06
  Thoracic BR05
Fallopian Tube
  Bilateral BU02
  Left BU01
  Right BU00
Fallopian Tube and Uterus BU08
Femur
  Left, Densitometry BQ04ZZ1
  Right, Densitometry BQ03ZZ1
Finger
  Left BP0SZZZ
  Right BP0RZZZ
Foot
  Left BQ0MZZZ
  Right BQ0LZZZ
Forearm
  Left BP0KZZZ
  Right BP0JZZZ
Gallbladder and Bile Duct BF03
Gland
  Parotid
    Bilateral B906
    Left B905
    Right B904
  Salivary
    Bilateral B90D
    Left B90C
    Right B90B
  Submandibular
    Bilateral B909
    Left B908
    Right B907
Hand
  Left BP0PZZZ
  Right BP0NZZZ
Heart
  Left B205
  Right B204
  Right and Left B206
Hepatobiliary System, All BF0C
Hip
  Left BQ01
    Densitometry BQ01ZZ1
  Right BQ00
    Densitometry BQ00ZZ1
Humerus
  Left BP0BZZZ
  Right BP0AZZZ
Ileal Diversion Loop BT0C
Intracranial Sinus B502
Joint
  Acromioclavicular, Bilateral BP03ZZZ
  Finger
    Left BP0D
    Right BP0C
  Foot
    Left BQ0Y
    Right BQ0X
  Hand
    Left BP0D

Plain Radiography — *continued*
Joint — *continued*
  Hand — *continued*
    Right BP0C
  Lumbosacral BR0BZZZ
  Sacroiliac BR0D
  Sternoclavicular
    Bilateral BP02ZZZ
    Left BP01ZZZ
    Right BP00ZZZ
  Temporomandibular
    Bilateral BN09
    Left BN08
    Right BN07
  Thoracolumbar BR08ZZZ
  Toe
    Left BQ0Y
    Right BQ0X
Kidney
  Bilateral BT03
  Left BT02
  Right BT01
  Ureter and Bladder BT04
Knee
  Left BQ08
  Right BQ07
Leg
  Left BQ0FZZZ
  Right BQ0DZZZ
Lymphatic
  Head B704
  Lower Extremity
    Bilateral B70B
    Left B709
    Right B708
  Neck B704
  Pelvic B70C
  Upper Extremity
    Bilateral B707
    Left B706
    Right B705
Mandible BN06ZZZ
Mastoid B90HZZZ
Nasopharynx B90FZZZ
Optic Foramina
  Left B804ZZZ
  Right B803ZZZ
Orbit
  Bilateral BN03ZZZ
  Left BN02ZZZ
  Right BN01ZZZ
Oropharynx B90FZZZ
Patella
  Left BQ0WZZZ
  Right BQ0VZZZ
Pelvis BR0CZZZ
Pelvis and Abdomen BW01ZZZ
Prostate BV03
Retroperitoneal Lymphatic
  Bilateral B701
  Unilateral B700
Ribs
  Left BP0YZZZ
  Right BP0XZZZ
Sacrum BR0FZZZ
Scapula
  Left BP07ZZZ
  Right BP06ZZZ
Shoulder
  Left BP09
  Right BP08
Sinus
  Intracranial B502
  Paranasal B902ZZZ
Skull BN00ZZZ
Spinal Cord B00B
Spine
  Cervical, Densitometry BR00ZZ1
  Lumbar, Densitometry BR09ZZ1
  Thoracic, Densitometry BR07ZZ1
  Whole, Densitometry BR0GZZ1
Sternum BR0HZZZ
Teeth
  All BN0JZZZ
  Multiple BN0HZZZ
Testicle
  Left BV06
  Right BV05

Plain Radiography — *continued*
Toe
  Left BQ0QZZZ
  Right BQ0PZZZ
Tooth, Single BN0GZZZ
Tracheobronchial Tree
  Bilateral BB09YZZ
  Left BB08YZZ
  Right BB07YZZ
Ureter
  Bilateral BT08
  Kidney and Bladder BT04
  Left BT07
  Right BT06
Urethra BT05
Urethra and Bladder BT0B
Uterus BU06
Uterus and Fallopian Tube BU08
Vagina BU09
Vasa Vasorum BV08
Vein
  Cerebellar B501
  Cerebral B501
  Epidural B500
  Jugular
    Bilateral B505
    Left B504
    Right B503
  Lower Extremity
    Bilateral B50D
    Left B50C
    Right B50B
  Other B50V
  Pelvic (Iliac)
    Left B50G
    Right B50F
  Pelvic (Iliac) Bilateral B50H
  Portal B50T
  Pulmonary
    Bilateral B50S
    Left B50R
    Right B50Q
  Renal
    Bilateral B50L
    Left B50K
    Right B50J
  Spanchnic B50T
  Subclavian
    Left B507
    Right B506
  Upper Extremity
    Bilateral B50P
    Left B50N
    Right B50M
Vena Cava
  Inferior B509
  Superior B508
Whole Body BW0KZZZ
  Infant BW0MZZZ
Whole Skeleton BW0LZZZ
Wrist
  Left BP0M
  Right BP0L
Planar Nuclear Medicine Imaging
Abdomen CW10
Abdomen and Chest CW14
Abdomen and Pelvis CW11
Anatomical Region, Other CW1ZZZZ
Anatomical Regions, Multiple CW1YYZZ
Bladder and Ureters CT1H
Bladder, Kidneys and Ureters CT13
Blood C713
Bone Marrow C710
Brain C010
Breast CH1YYZZ
  Bilateral CH12
  Left CH11
  Right CH10
Bronchi and Lungs CB12
Central Nervous System C01YYZZ
Cerebrospinal Fluid C015
Chest CW13
Chest and Abdomen CW14
Chest and Neck CW16
Digestive System CD1YYZZ
Ducts, Lacrimal, Bilateral C819
Ear, Nose, Mouth and Throat C91YYZZ
Endocrine System CG1YYZZ

Subterms under main terms may continue to next column or page

Positron Emission Tomographic (PET) Imaging —
continued
Respiratory System CB3YYZZ
Whole Body CW3NYZZ
Positron emission tomography *see* Positron Emission Tomographic (PET) Imaging
Postauricular (mastoid) lymph node
use Lymphatic, Left Neck
use Lymphatic, Right Neck
Postcava *use* Inferior Vena Cava
Posterior auricular artery
use External Carotid Artery, Left
use External Carotid Artery, Right
Posterior auricular nerve *use* Facial Nerve
Posterior auricular vein
use External Jugular Vein, Left
use External Jugular Vein, Right
Posterior cerebral artery *use* Intracranial Artery
Posterior chamber
use Eye, Left
use Eye, Right
Posterior circumflex humeral artery
use Axillary Artery, Left
use Axillary Artery, Right
Posterior communicating artery *use* Intracranial Artery
Posterior cruciate ligament (PCL)
use Knee Bursa and Ligament, Left
use Knee Bursa and Ligament, Right
Posterior facial (retromandibular) vein
use Face Vein, Left
use Face Vein, Right
Posterior femoral cutaneous nerve *use* Sacral Plexus
Posterior inferior cerebellar artery (PICA) *use* Intracranial Artery
Posterior interosseous nerve *use* Radial Nerve
Posterior labial nerve *use* Pudendal Nerve
Posterior (subscapular) lymph node
use Lymphatic, Left Axillary
use Lymphatic, Right Axillary
Posterior scrotal nerve *use* Pudendal Nerve
Posterior spinal artery
use Vertebral Artery, Left
use Vertebral Artery, Right
Posterior tibial recurrent artery
use Anterior Tibial Artery, Left
use Anterior Tibial Artery, Right
Posterior ulnar recurrent artery
use Ulnar Artery, Left
use Ulnar Artery, Right
Posterior vagal trunk *use* Vagus Nerve
PPN (peripheral parenteral nutrition) *see* Introduction of Nutritional Substance
Preauricular lymph node *use* Lymphatic, Head
Precava *use* Superior Vena Cava
PRECICE intramedullary limb lengthening system
use Internal Fixation Device, Intramedullary Limb Lengthening in ØPH
use Internal Fixation Device, Intramedullary Limb Lengthening in ØQH
Prepatellar bursa
use Knee Bursa and Ligament, Left
use Knee Bursa and Ligament, Right
Preputiotomy *see* Drainage, Male Reproductive System ØV9
Pressure support ventilation *see* Performance, Respiratory 5A19
PRESTIGE® Cervical Disc *use* Synthetic Substitute
Pretracheal fascia
use Subcutaneous Tissue and Fascia, Left Neck
use Subcutaneous Tissue and Fascia, Right Neck
Prevertebral fascia
use Subcutaneous Tissue and Fascia, Left Neck
use Subcutaneous Tissue and Fascia, Right Neck
PrimeAdvanced neurostimulator (SureScan) (MRI Safe) *use* Stimulator Generator, Multiple Array in ØJH
Princeps pollicis artery
use Hand Artery, Left
use Hand Artery, Right
Probing, duct
Diagnostic *see* Inspection
Dilation *see* Dilation
PROCEED™ Ventral Patch *use* Synthetic Substitute
Procerus muscle *use* Facial Muscle

Proctectomy
see Excision, Rectum ØDBP
see Resection, Rectum ØDTP
Proctoclysis *see* Introduction of substance in or on, Gastrointestinal Tract, Lower 3EØH
Proctocolectomy
see Excision, Gastrointestinal System ØDB
see Resection, Gastrointestinal System ØDT
Proctocolpoplasty
see Repair, Gastrointestinal System ØDQ
see Supplement, Gastrointestinal System ØDU
Proctoperineoplasty
see Repair, Gastrointestinal System ØDQ
see Supplement, Gastrointestinal System ØDU
Proctoperineorrhaphy *see* Repair, Gastrointestinal System ØDQ
Proctopexy
see Repair, Rectum ØDQP
see Reposition, Rectum ØDSP
Proctoplasty
see Repair, Rectum ØDQP
see Supplement, Rectum ØDUP
Proctorrhaphy *see* Repair, Rectum ØDQP
Proctoscopy ØDJD8ZZ
Proctosigmoidectomy
see Excision, Gastrointestinal System ØDB
see Resection, Gastrointestinal System ØDT
Proctosigmoidoscopy ØDJD8ZZ
Proctostomy *see* Drainage, Rectum ØD9P
Proctotomy *see* Drainage, Rectum ØD9P
Prodisc-C *use* Synthetic Substitute
Prodisc-L *use* Synthetic Substitute
Production, atrial septal defect *see* Excision, Septum, Atrial Ø2B5
Profunda brachii
use Brachial Artery, Left
use Brachial Artery, Right
Profunda femoris (deep femoral) vein
use Femoral Vein, Left
use Femoral Vein, Right
PROLENE Polypropylene Hernia System (PHS) *use* Synthetic Substitute
Prolonged intermittent renal replacement therapy (PIRRT) 5A1D8ØZ
Pronator quadratus muscle
use Lower Arm and Wrist Muscle, Left
use Lower Arm and Wrist Muscle, Right
Pronator teres muscle
use Lower Arm and Wrist Muscle, Left
use Lower Arm and Wrist Muscle, Right
Prostatectomy
see Excision, Prostate ØVBØ
see Resection, Prostate ØVTØ
Prostatic urethra *use* Urethra
Prostatomy, prostatotomy *see* Drainage, Prostate ØV9Ø
Protecta XT CRT-D *use* Cardiac Resynchronization Defibrillator Pulse Generator in ØJH
Protecta XT DR (XT VR) *use* Defibrillator Generator in ØJH
Protégé® RX Carotid Stent System *use* Intraluminal Device
Proximal radioulnar joint
use Elbow Joint, Left
use Elbow Joint, Right
Psoas muscle
use Hip Muscle, Left
use Hip Muscle, Right
PSV (pressure support ventilation) *see* Performance, Respiratory 5A19
Psychoanalysis GZ54ZZZ
Psychological Tests
Cognitive Status GZ14ZZZ
Developmental GZ1ØZZZ
Intellectual and Psychoeducational GZ12ZZZ
Neurobehavioral Status GZ14ZZZ
Neuropsychological GZ13ZZZ
Personality and Behavioral GZ11ZZZ
Psychotherapy
Family, Mental Health Services GZ72ZZZ
Group GZHZZZZ
Mental Health Services GZHZZZZ
Individual
see Psychotherapy, Individual, Mental Health Services
for substance abuse
12-Step HZ53ZZZ

Psychotherapy — *continued*
Individual — *continued*
for substance abuse — *continued*
Behavioral HZ51ZZZ
Cognitive HZ5ØZZZ
Cognitive-Behavioral HZ52ZZZ
Confrontational HZ58ZZZ
Interactive HZ55ZZZ
Interpersonal HZ54ZZZ
Motivational Enhancement HZ57ZZZ
Psychoanalysis HZ5BZZZ
Psychodynamic HZ5CZZZ
Psychoeducation HZ56ZZZ
Psychophysiological HZ5DZZZ
Supportive HZ59ZZZ
Mental Health Services
Behavioral GZ51ZZZ
Cognitive GZ52ZZZ
Cognitive-Behavioral GZ58ZZZ
Interactive GZ5ØZZZ
Interpersonal GZ53ZZZ
Psychoanalysis GZ54ZZZ
Psychodynamic GZ55ZZZ
Psychophysiological GZ59ZZZ
Supportive GZ56ZZZ
PTCA (percutaneous transluminal coronary angioplasty) *see* Dilation, Heart and Great Vessels Ø27
Pterygoid muscle *use* Head Muscle
Pterygoid process *use* Sphenoid Bone
Pterygopalatine (sphenopalatine) ganglion *use* Head and Neck Sympathetic Nerve
Pubis
use Pelvic Bone, Left
use Pelvic Bone, Right
Pubofemoral ligament
use Hip Bursa and Ligament, Left
use Hip Bursa and Ligament, Right
Pudendal nerve *use* Sacral Plexus
Pull-through, laparoscopic-assisted transanal
see Excision, Gastrointestinal System ØDB
see Resection, Gastrointestinal System ØDT
Pull-through, rectal *see* Resection, Rectum ØDTP
Pulmoaortic canal *use* Pulmonary Artery, Left
Pulmonary annulus *use* Pulmonary Valve
Pulmonary artery wedge monitoring *see* Monitoring, Arterial 4A13
Pulmonary plexus
use Thoracic Sympathetic Nerve
use Vagus Nerve
Pulmonic valve *use* Pulmonary Valve
Pulpectomy *see* Excision, Mouth and Throat ØCB
Pulverization *see* Fragmentation
Pulvinar *use* Thalamus
Pump reservoir *use* Infusion Device, Pump in Subcutaneous Tissue and Fascia
Punch biopsy *see* Excision with qualifier Diagnostic
Puncture *see* Drainage
Puncture, lumbar *see* Drainage, Spinal Canal ØØ9U
Pyelography
see Fluoroscopy, Urinary System BT1
see Plain Radiography, Urinary System BTØ
Pyeloileostomy, urinary diversion *see* Bypass, Urinary System ØT1
Pyeloplasty
see Repair, Urinary System ØTQ
see Replacement, Urinary System ØTR
see Supplement, Urinary System ØTU
Pyeloplasty, dismembered *see* Repair, Kidney Pelvis
Pyelorrhaphy *see* Repair, Urinary System ØTQ
Pyeloscopy ØTJ58ZZ
Pyelostomy
see Bypass, Urinary System ØT1
see Drainage, Urinary System ØT9
Pyelotomy *see* Drainage, Urinary System ØT9
Pylorectomy
see Excision, Stomach, Pylorus ØDB7
see Resection, Stomach, Pylorus ØDT7
Pyloric antrum *use* Stomach, Pylorus
Pyloric canal *use* Stomach, Pylorus
Pyloric sphincter *use* Stomach, Pylorus
Pylorodiosis *see* Dilation, Stomach, Pylorus ØD77
Pylorogastrectomy
see Excision, Gastrointestinal System ØDB
see Resection, Gastrointestinal System ØDT
Pyloroplasty
see Repair, Stomach, Pylorus ØDQ7
see Supplement, Stomach, Pylorus ØDU7

Pyloroscopy ØDJ68ZZ
Pylorotomy *see* Drainage, Stomach, Pylorus ØD97
Pyramidalis muscle
  use Abdomen Muscle, Left
  use Abdomen Muscle, Right

Q

Quadrangular cartilage *use* Nasal Septum
Quadrant resection of breast *see* Excision, Skin and
    Breast ØHB
Quadrate lobe *use* Liver
Quadratus femoris muscle
  use Hip Muscle, Left
  use Hip Muscle, Right
Quadratus lumborum muscle
  use Trunk Muscle, Left
  use Trunk Muscle, Right
Quadratus plantae muscle
  use Foot Muscle, Left
  use Foot Muscle, Right
Quadriceps (femoris)
  use Upper Leg Muscle, Left
  use Upper Leg Muscle, Right
Quarantine 8EØZXY6

R

Radial collateral carpal ligament
  use Wrist Bursa and Ligament, Left
  use Wrist Bursa and Ligament, Right
Radial collateral ligament
  use Elbow Bursa and Ligament, Left
  use Elbow Bursa and Ligament, Right
Radial notch
  use Ulna, Left
  use Ulna, Right
Radial recurrent artery
  use Radial Artery, Left
  use Radial Artery, Right
Radial vein
  use Brachial Vein, Left
  use Brachial Vein, Right
Radialis indicis
  use Hand Artery, Left
  use Hand Artery, Right
Radiation Therapy
  see Beam Radiation
  see Brachytherapy
  see Stereotactic Radiosurgery
Radiation treatment *see* Radiation Therapy
Radiocarpal joint
  use Wrist Joint, Left
  use Wrist Joint, Right
Radiocarpal ligament
  use Wrist Bursa and Ligament, Left
  use Wrist Bursa and Ligament, Right
Radiography *see* Plain Radiography
Radiology, analog *see* Plain Radiography
Radiology, diagnostic *see* Imaging, Diagnostic
Radioulnar ligament
  use Wrist Bursa and Ligament, Left
  use Wrist Bursa and Ligament, Right
Range of motion testing *see* Motor Function Assess-
    ment, Rehabilitation FØ1
REALIZE® Adjustable Gastric Band *use* Extraluminal
    Device
Reattachment
  Abdominal Wall ØWMFØZZ
  Ampulla of Vater ØFMC
  Ankle Region
    Left ØYMLØZZ
    Right ØYMKØZZ
  Arm
    Lower
      Left ØXMFØZZ
      Right ØXMDØZZ
    Upper
      Left ØXM9ØZZ
      Right ØXM8ØZZ
  Axilla
    Left ØXM5ØZZ
    Right ØXM4ØZZ
  Back
    Lower ØWMLØZZ

Reattachment — *continued*
  Back — *continued*
    Upper ØWMKØZZ
  Bladder ØTMB
  Bladder Neck ØTMC
  Breast
    Bilateral ØHMVXZZ
    Left ØHMUXZZ
    Right ØHMTXZZ
  Bronchus
    Lingula ØBM9ØZZ
    Lower Lobe
      Left ØBMBØZZ
      Right ØBM6ØZZ
    Main
      Left ØBM7ØZZ
      Right ØBM3ØZZ
    Middle Lobe, Right ØBM5ØZZ
    Upper Lobe
      Left ØBM8ØZZ
      Right ØBM4ØZZ
  Bursa and Ligament
    Abdomen
      Left ØMMJ
      Right ØMMH
    Ankle
      Left ØMMR
      Right ØMMQ
    Elbow
      Left ØMM4
      Right ØMM3
    Foot
      Left ØMMT
      Right ØMMS
    Hand
      Left ØMM8
      Right ØMM7
    Head and Neck ØMMØ
    Hip
      Left ØMMM
      Right ØMML
    Knee
      Left ØMMP
      Right ØMMN
    Lower Extremity
      Left ØMMW
      Right ØMMV
    Perineum ØMMK
    Rib(s) ØMMG
    Shoulder
      Left ØMM2
      Right ØMM1
    Spine
      Lower ØMMD
      Upper ØMMC
    Sternum ØMMF
    Upper Extremity
      Left ØMMB
      Right ØMM9
    Wrist
      Left ØMM6
      Right ØMM5
  Buttock
    Left ØYM1ØZZ
    Right ØYMØØZZ
  Carina ØBM2ØZZ
  Cecum ØDMH
  Cervix ØUMC
  Chest Wall ØWM8ØZZ
  Clitoris ØUMJXZZ
  Colon
    Ascending ØDMK
    Descending ØDMM
    Sigmoid ØDMN
    Transverse ØDML
  Cord
    Bilateral ØVMH
    Left ØVMG
    Right ØVMF
  Cul-de-sac ØUMF
  Diaphragm ØBMTØZZ
  Duct
    Common Bile ØFM9
    Cystic ØFM8
    Hepatic
      Common ØFM7
      Left ØFM6
      Right ØFM5
    Pancreatic ØFMD

Reattachment — *continued*
  Duct — *continued*
    Pancreatic — *continued*
      Accessory ØFMF
  Duodenum ØDM9
  Ear
    Left Ø9M1XZZ
    Right Ø9MØXZZ
  Elbow Region
    Left ØXMCØZZ
    Right ØXMBØZZ
  Esophagus ØDM5
  Extremity
    Lower
      Left ØYMBØZZ
      Right ØYM9ØZZ
    Upper
      Left ØXM7ØZZ
      Right ØXM6ØZZ
  Eyelid
    Lower
      Left Ø8MRXZZ
      Right Ø8MQXZZ
    Upper
      Left Ø8MPXZZ
      Right Ø8MNXZZ
  Face ØWM2ØZZ
  Fallopian Tube
    Left ØUM6
    Right ØUM5
  Fallopian Tubes, Bilateral ØUM7
  Femoral Region
    Left ØYM8ØZZ
    Right ØYM7ØZZ
  Finger
    Index
      Left ØXMPØZZ
      Right ØXMNØZZ
    Little
      Left ØXMWØZZ
      Right ØXMVØZZ
    Middle
      Left ØXMRØZZ
      Right ØXMQØZZ
    Ring
      Left ØXMTØZZ
      Right ØXMSØZZ
  Foot
    Left ØYMNØZZ
    Right ØYMMØZZ
  Forequarter
    Left ØXM1ØZZ
    Right ØXMØØZZ
  Gallbladder ØFM4
  Gland
    Left ØGM2
    Right ØGM3
  Hand
    Left ØXMKØZZ
    Right ØXMJØZZ
  Hindquarter
    Bilateral ØYM4ØZZ
    Left ØYM3ØZZ
    Right ØYM2ØZZ
  Hymen ØUMK
  Ileum ØDMB
  Inguinal Region
    Left ØYM6ØZZ
    Right ØYM5ØZZ
  Intestine
    Large ØDME
      Left ØDMG
      Right ØDMF
    Small ØDM8
  Jaw
    Lower ØWM5ØZZ
    Upper ØWM4ØZZ
  Jejunum ØDMA
  Kidney
    Left ØTM1
    Right ØTMØ
  Kidney Pelvis
    Left ØTM4
    Right ØTM3
  Kidneys, Bilateral ØTM2
  Knee Region
    Left ØYMGØZZ
    Right ØYMFØZZ

Reattachment — *continued*
- Leg
  - Lower
    - Left ØYMJØZZ
    - Right ØYMHØZZ
  - Upper
    - Left ØYMDØZZ
    - Right ØYMCØZZ
- Lip
  - Lower ØCM1ØZZ
  - Upper ØCMØØZZ
- Liver ØFMØ
  - Left Lobe ØFM2
  - Right Lobe ØFM1
- Lung
  - Left ØBMLØZZ
  - Lower Lobe
    - Left ØBMJØZZ
    - Right ØBMFØZZ
  - Middle Lobe, Right ØBMDØZZ
  - Right ØBMKØZZ
  - Upper Lobe
    - Left ØBMGØZZ
    - Right ØBMCØZZ
- Lung Lingula ØBMHØZZ
- Muscle
  - Abdomen
    - Left ØKML
    - Right ØKMK
  - Facial ØKM1
  - Foot
    - Left ØKMW
    - Right ØKMV
  - Hand
    - Left ØKMD
    - Right ØKMC
  - Head ØKMØ
  - Hip
    - Left ØKMP
    - Right ØKMN
  - Lower Arm and Wrist
    - Left ØKMB
    - Right ØKM9
  - Lower Leg
    - Left ØKMT
    - Right ØKMS
  - Neck
    - Left ØKM3
    - Right ØKM2
  - Perineum ØKMM
  - Shoulder
    - Left ØKM6
    - Right ØKM5
  - Thorax
    - Left ØKMJ
    - Right ØKMH
  - Tongue, Palate, Pharynx ØKM4
  - Trunk
    - Left ØKMG
    - Right ØKMF
  - Upper Arm
    - Left ØKM8
    - Right ØKM7
  - Upper Leg
    - Left ØKMR
    - Right ØKMQ
- Nasal Mucosa and Soft Tissue Ø9MKXZZ
- Neck ØWM6ØZZ
- Nipple
  - Left ØHMXXZZ
  - Right ØHMWXZZ
- Ovary
  - Bilateral ØUM2
  - Left ØUM1
  - Right ØUMØ
- Palate, Soft ØCM3ØZZ
- Pancreas ØFMG
- Parathyroid Gland ØGMR
  - Inferior
    - Left ØGMP
    - Right ØGMN
  - Multiple ØGMQ
  - Superior
    - Left ØGMM
    - Right ØGML
- Penis ØVMSXZZ
- Perineum
  - Female ØWMNØZZ
  - Male ØWMMØZZ

Reattachment — *continued*
- Rectum ØDMP
- Scrotum ØVM5XZZ
- Shoulder Region
  - Left ØXM3ØZZ
  - Right ØXM2ØZZ
- Skin
  - Abdomen ØHM7XZZ
  - Back ØHM6XZZ
  - Buttock ØHM8XZZ
  - Chest ØHM5XZZ
  - Ear
    - Left ØHM3XZZ
    - Right ØHM2XZZ
  - Face ØHM1XZZ
  - Foot
    - Left ØHMNXZZ
    - Right ØHMMXZZ
  - Hand
    - Left ØHMGXZZ
    - Right ØHMFXZZ
  - Inguinal ØHMAXZZ
  - Lower Arm
    - Left ØHMEXZZ
    - Right ØHMDXZZ
  - Lower Leg
    - Left ØHMLXZZ
    - Right ØHMKXZZ
  - Neck ØHM4XZZ
  - Perineum ØHM9XZZ
  - Scalp ØHMØXZZ
  - Upper Arm
    - Left ØHMCXZZ
    - Right ØHMBXZZ
  - Upper Leg
    - Left ØHMJXZZ
    - Right ØHMHXZZ
- Stomach ØDM6
- Tendon
  - Abdomen
    - Left ØLMG
    - Right ØLMF
  - Ankle
    - Left ØLMT
    - Right ØLMS
  - Foot
    - Left ØLMW
    - Right ØLMV
  - Hand
    - Left ØLM8
    - Right ØLM7
  - Head and Neck ØLMØ
  - Hip
    - Left ØLMK
    - Right ØLMJ
  - Knee
    - Left ØLMR
    - Right ØLMQ
  - Lower Arm and Wrist
    - Left ØLM6
    - Right ØLM5
  - Lower Leg
    - Left ØLMP
    - Right ØLMN
  - Perineum ØLMH
  - Shoulder
    - Left ØLM2
    - Right ØLM1
  - Thorax
    - Left ØLMD
    - Right ØLMC
  - Trunk
    - Left ØLMB
    - Right ØLM9
  - Upper Arm
    - Left ØLM4
    - Right ØLM3
  - Upper Leg
    - Left ØLMM
    - Right ØLML
- Testis
  - Bilateral ØVMC
  - Left ØVMB
  - Right ØVM9
- Thumb
  - Left ØXMMØZZ
  - Right ØXMLØZZ
- Thyroid Gland
  - Left Lobe ØGMG

Reattachment — *continued*
- Thyroid Gland — *continued*
  - Right Lobe ØGMH
- Toe
  - 1st
    - Left ØYMQØZZ
    - Right ØYMPØZZ
  - 2nd
    - Left ØYMSØZZ
    - Right ØYMRØZZ
  - 3rd
    - Left ØYMUØZZ
    - Right ØYMTØZZ
  - 4th
    - Left ØYMWØZZ
    - Right ØYMVØZZ
  - 5th
    - Left ØYMYØZZ
    - Right ØYMXØZZ
- Tongue ØCM7ØZZ
- Tooth
  - Lower ØCMX
  - Upper ØCMW
- Trachea ØBM1ØZZ
- Tunica Vaginalis
  - Left ØVM7
  - Right ØVM6
- Ureter
  - Left ØTM7
  - Right ØTM6
- Ureters, Bilateral ØTM8
- Urethra ØTMD
- Uterine Supporting Structure ØUM4
- Uterus ØUM9
- Uvula ØCMNØZZ
- Vagina ØUMG
- Vulva ØUMMXZZ
- Wrist Region
  - Left ØXMHØZZ
  - Right ØXMGØZZ

REBOA (resuscitative endovascular balloon occlusion of the aorta)
- Ø2LW3DJ
- Ø4LØ3DJ

Rebound HRD® (Hernia Repair Device) *use* Synthetic Substitute

RECELL® cell suspension autograft *see* Replacement, Skin and Breast ØHR

Recession
- *see* Repair
- *see* Reposition

Reclosure, disrupted abdominal wall ØWQFXZZ

Reconstruction
- *see* Repair
- *see* Replacement
- *see* Supplement

Rectectomy
- *see* Excision, Rectum ØDBP
- *see* Resection, Rectum ØDTP

Rectocele repair *see* Repair, Subcutaneous Tissue and Fascia, Pelvic Region ØJQC

Rectopexy
- *see* Repair, Gastrointestinal System ØDQ
- *see* Reposition, Gastrointestinal System ØDS

Rectoplasty
- *see* Repair, Gastrointestinal System ØDQ
- *see* Supplement, Gastrointestinal System ØDU

Rectorrhaphy *see* Repair, Gastrointestinal System ØDQ

Rectoscopy ØDJD8ZZ

Rectosigmoid junction *use* Sigmoid Colon

Rectosigmoidectomy
- *see* Excision, Gastrointestinal System ØDB
- *see* Resection, Gastrointestinal System ØDT

Rectostomy *see* Drainage, Rectum ØD9P

Rectotomy *see* Drainage, Rectum ØD9P

Rectus abdominis muscle
- *use* Abdomen Muscle, Left
- *use* Abdomen Muscle, Right

Rectus femoris muscle
- *use* Upper Leg Muscle, Left
- *use* Upper Leg Muscle, Right

Recurrent laryngeal nerve *use* Vagus Nerve

Reduction
- Dislocation *see* Reposition
- Fracture *see* Reposition
- Intussusception, intestinal *see* Reposition, Gastrointestinal System ØDS

Reduction — *continued*
Mammoplasty *see* Excision, Skin and Breast ØHB
Prolapse *see* Reposition
Torsion *see* Reposition
Volvulus, gastrointestinal *see* Reposition, Gastrointestinal System ØDS

Refusion *see* Fusion

Rehabilitation
see Activities of Daily Living Assessment, Rehabilitation FØ2
see Activities of Daily Living Treatment, Rehabilitation FØ8
see Caregiver Training, Rehabilitation FØF
see Cochlear Implant Treatment, Rehabilitation FØB
see Device Fitting, Rehabilitation FØD
see Hearing Treatment, Rehabilitation FØ9
see Motor Function Assessment, Rehabilitation FØ1
see Motor Treatment, Rehabilitation FØ7
see Speech Assessment, Rehabilitation FØØ
see Speech Treatment, Rehabilitation FØ6
see Vestibular Treatment, Rehabilitation FØC

Reimplantation
see Reattachment
see Reposition
see Transfer

Reinforcement
see Repair
see Supplement

Relaxation, scar tissue *see* Release

Release
Acetabulum
Left ØQN5
Right ØQN4
Adenoids ØCNQ
Ampulla of Vater ØFNC
Anal Sphincter ØDNR
Anterior Chamber
Left Ø8N33ZZ
Right Ø8N23ZZ
Anus ØDNQ
Aorta
Abdominal Ø4NØ
Thoracic
Ascending/Arch Ø2NX
Descending Ø2NW
Aortic Body ØGND
Appendix ØDNJ
Artery
Anterior Tibial
Left Ø4NQ
Right Ø4NP
Axillary
Left Ø3N6
Right Ø3N5
Brachial
Left Ø3N8
Right Ø3N7
Celiac Ø4N1
Colic
Left Ø4N7
Middle Ø4N8
Right Ø4N6
Common Carotid
Left Ø3NJ
Right Ø3NH
Common Iliac
Left Ø4ND
Right Ø4NC
Coronary
Four or More Arteries Ø2N3
One Artery Ø2NØ
Three Arteries Ø2N2
Two Arteries Ø2N1
External Carotid
Left Ø3NN
Right Ø3NM
External Iliac
Left Ø4NJ
Right Ø4NH
Face Ø3NR
Femoral
Left Ø4NL
Right Ø4NK
Foot
Left Ø4NW
Right Ø4NV

Release — *continued*
Artery — *continued*
Gastric Ø4N2
Hand
Left Ø3NF
Right Ø3ND
Hepatic Ø4N3
Inferior Mesenteric Ø4NB
Innominate Ø3N2
Internal Carotid
Left Ø3NL
Right Ø3NK
Internal Iliac
Left Ø4NF
Right Ø4NE
Internal Mammary
Left Ø3N1
Right Ø3NØ
Intracranial Ø3NG
Lower Ø4NY
Peroneal
Left Ø4NU
Right Ø4NT
Popliteal
Left Ø4NN
Right Ø4NM
Posterior Tibial
Left Ø4NS
Right Ø4NR
Pulmonary
Left Ø2NR
Right Ø2NQ
Pulmonary Trunk Ø2NP
Radial
Left Ø3NC
Right Ø3NB
Renal
Left Ø4NA
Right Ø4N9
Splenic Ø4N4
Subclavian
Left Ø3N4
Right Ø3N3
Superior Mesenteric Ø4N5
Temporal
Left Ø3NT
Right Ø3NS
Thyroid
Left Ø3NV
Right Ø3NU
Ulnar
Left Ø3NA
Right Ø3N9
Upper Ø3NY
Vertebral
Left Ø3NQ
Right Ø3NP
Atrium
Left Ø2N7
Right Ø2N6
Auditory Ossicle
Left Ø9NA
Right Ø9N9
Basal Ganglia ØØN8
Bladder ØTNB
Bladder Neck ØTNC
Bone
Ethmoid
Left ØNNG
Right ØNNF
Frontal ØNN1
Hyoid ØNNX
Lacrimal
Left ØNNJ
Right ØNNH
Nasal ØNNB
Occipital ØNN7
Palatine
Left ØNNL
Right ØNNK
Parietal
Left ØNN4
Right ØNN3
Pelvic
Left ØQN3
Right ØQN2
Sphenoid ØNNC
Temporal
Left ØNN6

Release — *continued*
Bone — *continued*
Temporal — *continued*
Right ØNN5
Zygomatic
Left ØNNN
Right ØNNM
Brain ØØNØ
Breast
Bilateral ØHNV
Left ØHNU
Right ØHNT
Bronchus
Lingula ØBN9
Lower Lobe
Left ØBNB
Right ØBN6
Main
Left ØBN7
Right ØBN3
Middle Lobe, Right ØBN5
Upper Lobe
Left ØBN8
Right ØBN4
Buccal Mucosa ØCN4
Bursa and Ligament
Abdomen
Left ØMNJ
Right ØMNH
Ankle
Left ØMNR
Right ØMNQ
Elbow
Left ØMN4
Right ØMN3
Foot
Left ØMNT
Right ØMNS
Hand
Left ØMN8
Right ØMN7
Head and Neck ØMNØ
Hip
Left ØMNM
Right ØMNL
Knee
Left ØMNP
Right ØMNN
Lower Extremity
Left ØMNW
Right ØMNV
Perineum ØMNK
Rib(s) ØMNG
Shoulder
Left ØMN2
Right ØMN1
Spine
Lower ØMND
Upper ØMNC
Sternum ØMNF
Upper Extremity
Left ØMNB
Right ØMN9
Wrist
Left ØMN6
Right ØMN5
Carina ØBN2
Carotid Bodies, Bilateral ØGN8
Carotid Body
Left ØGN6
Right ØGN7
Carpal
Left ØPNN
Right ØPNM
Cecum ØDNH
Cerebellum ØØNC
Cerebral Hemisphere ØØN7
Cerebral Meninges ØØN1
Cerebral Ventricle ØØN6
Cervix ØUNC
Chordae Tendineae Ø2N9
Choroid
Left Ø8NB
Right Ø8NA
Cisterna Chyli Ø7NL
Clavicle
Left ØPNB
Right ØPN9
Clitoris ØUNJ

▽ **Subterms under main terms may continue to next column or page**

Release — continued
Coccygeal Glomus ØGNB
Coccyx ØQNS
Colon
  Ascending ØDNK
  Descending ØDNM
  Sigmoid ØDNN
  Transverse ØDNL
Conduction Mechanism Ø2N8
Conjunctiva
  Left Ø8NTXZZ
  Right Ø8NSXZZ
Cord
  Bilateral ØVNH
  Left ØVNG
  Right ØVNF
Cornea
  Left Ø8N9XZZ
  Right Ø8N8XZZ
Cul-de-sac ØUNF
Diaphragm ØBNT
Disc
  Cervical Vertebral ØRN3
  Cervicothoracic Vertebral ØRN5
  Lumbar Vertebral ØSN2
  Lumbosacral ØSN4
  Thoracic Vertebral ØRN9
  Thoracolumbar Vertebral ØRNB
Duct
  Common Bile ØFN9
  Cystic ØFN8
  Hepatic
    Common ØFN7
    Left ØFN6
    Right ØFN5
  Lacrimal
    Left Ø8NY
    Right Ø8NX
  Pancreatic ØFND
    Accessory ØFNF
  Parotid
    Left ØCNC
    Right ØCNB
Duodenum ØDN9
Dura Mater ØØN2
Ear
  External
    Left Ø9N1
    Right Ø9NØ
  External Auditory Canal
    Left Ø9N4
    Right Ø9N3
  Inner
    Left Ø9NE
    Right Ø9ND
  Middle
    Left Ø9N6
    Right Ø9N5
Epididymis
  Bilateral ØVNL
  Left ØVNK
  Right ØVNJ
Epiglottis ØCNR
Esophagogastric Junction ØDN4
Esophagus ØDN5
  Lower ØDN3
  Middle ØDN2
  Upper ØDN1
Eustachian Tube
  Left Ø9NG
  Right Ø9NF
Eye
  Left Ø8N1XZZ
  Right Ø8NØXZZ
Eyelid
  Lower
    Left Ø8NR
    Right Ø8NQ
  Upper
    Left Ø8NP
    Right Ø8NN
Fallopian Tube
  Left ØUN6
  Right ØUN5
Fallopian Tubes, Bilateral ØUN7
Femoral Shaft
  Left ØQN9
  Right ØQN8

Release — continued
Femur
  Lower
    Left ØQNC
    Right ØQNB
  Upper
    Left ØQN7
    Right ØQN6
Fibula
  Left ØQNK
  Right ØQNJ
Finger Nail ØHNQXZZ
Gallbladder ØFN4
Gingiva
  Lower ØCN6
  Upper ØCN5
Gland
  Adrenal
    Bilateral ØGN4
    Left ØGN2
    Right ØGN3
  Lacrimal
    Left Ø8NW
    Right Ø8NV
  Minor Salivary ØCNJ
  Parotid
    Left ØCN9
    Right ØCN8
  Pituitary ØGNØ
  Sublingual
    Left ØCNF
    Right ØCND
  Submaxillary
    Left ØCNH
    Right ØCNG
  Vestibular ØUNL
Glenoid Cavity
  Left ØPN8
  Right ØPN7
Glomus Jugulare ØGNC
Humeral Head
  Left ØPND
  Right ØPNC
Humeral Shaft
  Left ØPNG
  Right ØPNF
Hymen ØUNK
Hypothalamus ØØNA
Ileocecal Valve ØDNC
Ileum ØDNB
Intestine
  Large ØDNE
    Left ØDNG
    Right ØDNF
  Small ØDN8
Iris
  Left Ø8ND3ZZ
  Right Ø8NC3ZZ
Jejunum ØDNA
Joint
  Acromioclavicular
    Left ØRNH
    Right ØRNG
  Ankle
    Left ØSNG
    Right ØSNF
  Carpal
    Left ØRNR
    Right ØRNQ
  Carpometacarpal
    Left ØRNT
    Right ØRNS
  Cervical Vertebral ØRN1
  Cervicothoracic Vertebral ØRN4
  Coccygeal ØSN6
  Elbow
    Left ØRNM
    Right ØRNL
  Finger Phalangeal
    Left ØRNX
    Right ØRNW
  Hip
    Left ØSNB
    Right ØSN9
  Knee
    Left ØSND
    Right ØSNC
  Lumbar Vertebral ØSNØ
  Lumbosacral ØSN3

Release — continued
Joint — continued
  Metacarpophalangeal
    Left ØRNV
    Right ØRNU
  Metatarsal-Phalangeal
    Left ØSNN
    Right ØSNM
  Occipital-cervical ØRNØ
  Sacrococcygeal ØSN5
  Sacroiliac
    Left ØSN8
    Right ØSN7
  Shoulder
    Left ØRNK
    Right ØRNJ
  Sternoclavicular
    Left ØRNF
    Right ØRNE
  Tarsal
    Left ØSNJ
    Right ØSNH
  Tarsometatarsal
    Left ØSNL
    Right ØSNK
  Temporomandibular
    Left ØRND
    Right ØRNC
  Thoracic Vertebral ØRN6
  Thoracolumbar Vertebral ØRNA
  Toe Phalangeal
    Left ØSNQ
    Right ØSNP
  Wrist
    Left ØRNP
    Right ØRNN
Kidney
  Left ØTN1
  Right ØTNØ
Kidney Pelvis
  Left ØTN4
  Right ØTN3
Larynx ØCNS
Lens
  Left Ø8NK3ZZ
  Right Ø8NJ3ZZ
Lip
  Lower ØCN1
  Upper ØCNØ
Liver ØFNØ
  Left Lobe ØFN2
  Right Lobe ØFN1
Lung
  Bilateral ØBNM
  Left ØBNL
  Lower Lobe
    Left ØBNJ
    Right ØBNF
  Middle Lobe, Right ØBND
  Right ØBNK
  Upper Lobe
    Left ØBNG
    Right ØBNC
Lung Lingula ØBNH
Lymphatic
  Aortic Ø7ND
  Axillary
    Left Ø7N6
    Right Ø7N5
  Head Ø7NØ
  Inguinal
    Left Ø7NJ
    Right Ø7NH
  Internal Mammary
    Left Ø7N9
    Right Ø7N8
  Lower Extremity
    Left Ø7NG
    Right Ø7NF
  Mesenteric Ø7NB
  Neck
    Left Ø7N2
    Right Ø7N1
  Pelvis Ø7NC
  Thoracic Duct Ø7NK
  Thorax Ø7N7
  Upper Extremity
    Left Ø7N4
    Right Ø7N3

Release — continued
- Mandible
  - Left ØNNV
  - Right ØNNT
- Maxilla ØNNR
- Medulla Oblongata ØØND
- Mesentery ØDNV
- Metacarpal
  - Left ØPNQ
  - Right ØPNP
- Metatarsal
  - Left ØQNP
  - Right ØQNN
- Muscle
  - Abdomen
    - Left ØKNL
    - Right ØKNK
  - Extraocular
    - Left Ø8NM
    - Right Ø8NL
  - Facial ØKN1
  - Foot
    - Left ØKNW
    - Right ØKNV
  - Hand
    - Left ØKND
    - Right ØKNC
  - Head ØKNØ
  - Hip
    - Left ØKNP
    - Right ØKNN
  - Lower Arm and Wrist
    - Left ØKNB
    - Right ØKN9
  - Lower Leg
    - Left ØKNT
    - Right ØKNS
  - Neck
    - Left ØKN3
    - Right ØKN2
  - Papillary Ø2ND
  - Perineum ØKNM
  - Shoulder
    - Left ØKN6
    - Right ØKN5
  - Thorax
    - Left ØKNJ
    - Right ØKNH
  - Tongue, Palate, Pharynx ØKN4
  - Trunk
    - Left ØKNG
    - Right ØKNF
  - Upper Arm
    - Left ØKN8
    - Right ØKN7
  - Upper Leg
    - Left ØKNR
    - Right ØKNQ
- Myocardial Bridge *see* Release, Artery, Coronary
- Nasal Mucosa and Soft Tissue Ø9NK
- Nasopharynx Ø9NN
- Nerve
  - Abdominal Sympathetic Ø1NM
  - Abducens ØØNL
  - Accessory ØØNR
  - Acoustic ØØNN
  - Brachial Plexus Ø1N3
  - Cervical Ø1N1
  - Cervical Plexus Ø1NØ
  - Facial ØØNM
  - Femoral Ø1ND
  - Glossopharyngeal ØØNP
  - Head and Neck Sympathetic Ø1NK
  - Hypoglossal ØØNS
  - Lumbar Ø1NB
  - Lumbar Plexus Ø1N9
  - Lumbar Sympathetic Ø1NN
  - Lumbosacral Plexus Ø1NA
  - Median Ø1N5
  - Oculomotor ØØNH
  - Olfactory ØØNF
  - Optic ØØNG
  - Peroneal Ø1NH
  - Phrenic Ø1N2
  - Pudendal Ø1NC
  - Radial Ø1N6
  - Sacral Ø1NR
  - Sacral Plexus Ø1NQ
  - Sacral Sympathetic Ø1NP

Release — continued
- Nerve — continued
  - Sciatic Ø1NF
  - Thoracic Ø1N8
  - Thoracic Sympathetic Ø1NL
  - Tibial Ø1NG
  - Trigeminal ØØNK
  - Trochlear ØØNJ
  - Ulnar Ø1N4
  - Vagus ØØNQ
- Nipple
  - Left ØHNX
  - Right ØHNW
- Omentum ØDNU
- Orbit
  - Left ØNNQ
  - Right ØNNP
- Ovary
  - Bilateral ØUN2
  - Left ØUN1
  - Right ØUNØ
- Palate
  - Hard ØCN2
  - Soft ØCN3
- Pancreas ØFNG
- Para-aortic Body ØGN9
- Paraganglion Extremity ØGNF
- Parathyroid Gland ØGNR
  - Inferior
    - Left ØGNP
    - Right ØGNN
  - Multiple ØGNQ
  - Superior
    - Left ØGNM
    - Right ØGNL
- Patella
  - Left ØQNF
  - Right ØQND
- Penis ØVNS
- Pericardium Ø2NN
- Peritoneum ØDNW
- Phalanx
  - Finger
    - Left ØPNV
    - Right ØPNT
  - Thumb
    - Left ØPNS
    - Right ØPNR
  - Toe
    - Left ØQNR
    - Right ØQNQ
- Pharynx ØCNM
- Pineal Body ØGN1
- Pleura
  - Left ØBNP
  - Right ØBNN
- Pons ØØNB
- Prepuce ØVNT
- Prostate ØVNØ
- Radius
  - Left ØPNJ
  - Right ØPNH
- Rectum ØDNP
- Retina
  - Left Ø8NF3ZZ
  - Right Ø8NE3ZZ
- Retinal Vessel
  - Left Ø8NH3ZZ
  - Right Ø8NG3ZZ
- Ribs
  - 1 to 2 ØPN1
  - 3 or More ØPN2
- Sacrum ØQN1
- Scapula
  - Left ØPN6
  - Right ØPN5
- Sclera
  - Left Ø8N7XZZ
  - Right Ø8N6XZZ
- Scrotum ØVN5
- Septum
  - Atrial Ø2N5
  - Nasal Ø9NM
  - Ventricular Ø2NM
- Sinus
  - Accessory Ø9NP
  - Ethmoid
    - Left Ø9NV
    - Right Ø9NU

Release — continued
- Sinus — continued
  - Frontal
    - Left Ø9NT
    - Right Ø9NS
  - Mastoid
    - Left Ø9NC
    - Right Ø9NB
  - Maxillary
    - Left Ø9NR
    - Right Ø9NQ
  - Sphenoid
    - Left Ø9NX
    - Right Ø9NW
- Skin
  - Abdomen ØHN7XZZ
  - Back ØHN6XZZ
  - Buttock ØHN8XZZ
  - Chest ØHN5XZZ
  - Ear
    - Left ØHN3XZZ
    - Right ØHN2XZZ
  - Face ØHN1XZZ
  - Foot
    - Left ØHNNXZZ
    - Right ØHNMXZZ
  - Hand
    - Left ØHNGXZZ
    - Right ØHNFXZZ
  - Inguinal ØHNAXZZ
  - Lower Arm
    - Left ØHNEXZZ
    - Right ØHNDXZZ
  - Lower Leg
    - Left ØHNLXZZ
    - Right ØHNKXZZ
  - Neck ØHN4XZZ
  - Perineum ØHN9XZZ
  - Scalp ØHNØXZZ
  - Upper Arm
    - Left ØHNCXZZ
    - Right ØHNBXZZ
  - Upper Leg
    - Left ØHNJXZZ
    - Right ØHNHXZZ
- Spinal Cord
  - Cervical ØØNW
  - Lumbar ØØNY
  - Thoracic ØØNX
- Spinal Meninges ØØNT
- Spleen Ø7NP
- Sternum ØPNØ
- Stomach ØDN6
  - Pylorus ØDN7
- Subcutaneous Tissue and Fascia
  - Abdomen ØJN8
  - Back ØJN7
  - Buttock ØJN9
  - Chest ØJN6
  - Face ØJN1
  - Foot
    - Left ØJNR
    - Right ØJNQ
  - Hand
    - Left ØJNK
    - Right ØJNJ
  - Lower Arm
    - Left ØJNH
    - Right ØJNG
  - Lower Leg
    - Left ØJNP
    - Right ØJNN
  - Neck
    - Left ØJN5
    - Right ØJN4
  - Pelvic Region ØJNC
  - Perineum ØJNB
  - Scalp ØJNØ
  - Upper Arm
    - Left ØJNF
    - Right ØJND
  - Upper Leg
    - Left ØJNM
    - Right ØJNL
- Tarsal
  - Left ØQNM
  - Right ØQNL

Release — *continued*
Tendon
  Abdomen
    Left ØLNG
    Right ØLNF
  Ankle
    Left ØLNT
    Right ØLNS
  Foot
    Left ØLNW
    Right ØLNV
  Hand
    Left ØLN8
    Right ØLN7
  Head and Neck ØLNØ
  Hip
    Left ØLNK
    Right ØLNJ
  Knee
    Left ØLNR
    Right ØLNQ
  Lower Arm and Wrist
    Left ØLN6
    Right ØLN5
  Lower Leg
    Left ØLNP
    Right ØLNN
  Perineum ØLNH
  Shoulder
    Left ØLN2
    Right ØLN1
  Thorax
    Left ØLND
    Right ØLNC
  Trunk
    Left ØLNB
    Right ØLN9
  Upper Arm
    Left ØLN4
    Right ØLN3
  Upper Leg
    Left ØLNM
    Right ØLNL
Testis
  Bilateral ØVNC
  Left ØVNB
  Right ØVN9
Thalamus ØØN9
Thymus Ø7NM
Thyroid Gland ØGNK
  Left Lobe ØGNG
  Right Lobe ØGNH
Tibia
  Left ØQNH
  Right ØQNG
Toe Nail ØHNRXZZ
Tongue ØCN7
Tonsils ØCNP
Tooth
  Lower ØCNX
  Upper ØCNW
Trachea ØBN1
Tunica Vaginalis
  Left ØVN7
  Right ØVN6
Turbinate, Nasal Ø9NL
Tympanic Membrane
  Left Ø9N8
  Right Ø9N7
Ulna
  Left ØPNL
  Right ØPNK
Ureter
  Left ØTN7
  Right ØTN6
Urethra ØTND
Uterine Supporting Structure ØUN4
Uterus ØUN9
Uvula ØCNN
Vagina ØUNG
Valve
  Aortic Ø2NF
  Mitral Ø2NG
  Pulmonary Ø2NH
  Tricuspid Ø2NJ
Vas Deferens
  Bilateral ØVNQ
  Left ØVNP
  Right ØVNN

Release — *continued*
Vein
  Axillary
    Left Ø5N8
    Right Ø5N7
  Azygos Ø5NØ
  Basilic
    Left Ø5NC
    Right Ø5NB
  Brachial
    Left Ø5NA
    Right Ø5N9
  Cephalic
    Left Ø5NF
    Right Ø5ND
  Colic Ø6N7
  Common Iliac
    Left Ø6ND
    Right Ø6NC
  Coronary Ø2N4
  Esophageal Ø6N3
  External Iliac
    Left Ø6NG
    Right Ø6NF
  External Jugular
    Left Ø5NQ
    Right Ø5NP
  Face
    Left Ø5NV
    Right Ø5NT
  Femoral
    Left Ø6NN
    Right Ø6NM
  Foot
    Left Ø6NV
    Right Ø6NT
  Gastric Ø6N2
  Hand
    Left Ø5NH
    Right Ø5NG
  Hemiazygos Ø5N1
  Hepatic Ø6N4
  Hypogastric
    Left Ø6NJ
    Right Ø6NH
  Inferior Mesenteric Ø6N6
  Innominate
    Left Ø5N4
    Right Ø5N3
  Internal Jugular
    Left Ø5NN
    Right Ø5NM
  Intracranial Ø5NL
  Lower Ø6NY
  Portal Ø6N8
  Pulmonary
    Left Ø2NT
    Right Ø2NS
  Renal
    Left Ø6NB
    Right Ø6N9
  Saphenous
    Left Ø6NQ
    Right Ø6NP
  Splenic Ø6N1
  Subclavian
    Left Ø5N6
    Right Ø5N5
  Superior Mesenteric Ø6N5
  Upper Ø5NY
  Vertebral
    Left Ø5NS
    Right Ø5NR
  Vena Cava
    Inferior Ø6NØ
    Superior Ø2NV
  Ventricle
    Left Ø2NL
    Right Ø2NK
  Vertebra
    Cervical ØPN3
    Lumbar ØQNØ
    Thoracic ØPN4
  Vesicle
    Bilateral ØVN3
    Left ØVN2
    Right ØVN1
  Vitreous
    Left Ø8N53ZZ

Release — *continued*
Vitreous — *continued*
    Right Ø8N43ZZ
Vocal Cord
  Left ØCNV
  Right ØCNT
Vulva ØUNM
Relocation *see* Reposition
Removal
Abdominal Wall 2W53X
Anorectal 2Y53X5Z
Arm
  Lower
    Left 2W5DX
    Right 2W5CX
  Upper
    Left 2W5BX
    Right 2W5AX
Back 2W55X
Chest Wall 2W54X
Ear 2Y52X5Z
Extremity
  Lower
    Left 2W5MX
    Right 2W5LX
  Upper
    Left 2W59X
    Right 2W58X
Face 2W51X
Finger
  Left 2W5KX
  Right 2W5JX
Foot
  Left 2W5TX
  Right 2W5SX
Genital Tract, Female 2Y54X5Z
Hand
  Left 2W5FX
  Right 2W5EX
Head 2W5ØX
Inguinal Region
  Left 2W57X
  Right 2W56X
Leg
  Lower
    Left 2W5RX
    Right 2W5QX
  Upper
    Left 2W5PX
    Right 2W5NX
Mouth and Pharynx 2Y5ØX5Z
Nasal 2Y51X5Z
Neck 2W52X
Thumb
  Left 2W5HX
  Right 2W5GX
Toe
  Left 2W5VX
  Right 2W5UX
Urethra 2Y55X5Z
Removal of device from
Abdominal Wall ØWPF
Acetabulum
  Left ØQP5
  Right ØQP4
Anal Sphincter ØDPR
Anus ØDPQ
Artery
  Lower Ø4PY
  Upper Ø3PY
Back
  Lower ØWPL
  Upper ØWPK
Bladder ØTPB
Bone
  Facial ØNPW
  Lower ØQPY
  Nasal ØNPB
  Pelvic
    Left ØQP3
    Right ØQP2
  Upper ØPPY
Bone Marrow Ø7PT
Brain ØØPØ
Breast
  Left ØHPU
  Right ØHPT
Bursa and Ligament
  Lower ØMPY

Removal of device from — *continued*
  Bursa and Ligament — *continued*
    Upper ØMPX
  Carpal
    Left ØPPN
    Right ØPPM
  Cavity, Cranial ØWP1
  Cerebral Ventricle ØØP6
  Chest Wall ØWP8
  Cisterna Chyli Ø7PL
  Clavicle
    Left ØPPB
    Right ØPP9
  Coccyx ØQPS
  Diaphragm ØBPT
  Disc
    Cervical Vertebral ØRP3
    Cervicothoracic Vertebral ØRP5
    Lumbar Vertebral ØSP2
    Lumbosacral ØSP4
    Thoracic Vertebral ØRP9
    Thoracolumbar Vertebral ØRPB
  Duct
    Hepatobiliary ØFPB
    Pancreatic ØFPD
  Ear
    Inner
      Left Ø9PJ
      Right Ø9PD
    Left Ø9PJ
    Right Ø9PH
  Epididymis and Spermatic Cord ØVPM
  Esophagus ØDP5
  Extremity
    Lower
      Left ØYPB
      Right ØYP9
    Upper
      Left ØXP7
      Right ØXP6
  Eye
    Left Ø8P1
    Right Ø8PØ
  Face ØWP2
  Fallopian Tube ØUP8
  Femoral Shaft
    Left ØQP9
    Right ØQP8
  Femur
    Lower
      Left ØQPC
      Right ØQPB
    Upper
      Left ØQP7
      Right ØQP6
  Fibula
    Left ØQPK
    Right ØQPJ
  Finger Nail ØHPQX
  Gallbladder ØFP4
  Gastrointestinal Tract ØWPP
  Genitourinary Tract ØWPR
  Gland
    Adrenal ØGP5
    Endocrine ØGPS
    Pituitary ØGPØ
    Salivary ØCPA
  Glenoid Cavity
    Left ØPP8
    Right ØPP7
  Great Vessel Ø2PY
  Hair ØHPSX
  Head ØWPØ
  Heart Ø2PA
  Humeral Head
    Left ØPPD
    Right ØPPC
  Humeral Shaft
    Left ØPPG
    Right ØPPF
  Intestinal Tract
    Lower ØDPD
    Upper ØDPØ
  Jaw
    Lower ØWP5
    Upper ØWP4
  Joint
    Acromioclavicular
      Left ØRPH

Removal of device from — *continued*
  Joint — *continued*
    Acromioclavicular — *continued*
      Right ØRPG
    Ankle
      Left ØSPG
      Right ØSPF
    Carpal
      Left ØRPR
      Right ØRPQ
    Carpometacarpal
      Left ØRPT
      Right ØRPS
    Cervical Vertebral ØRP1
    Cervicothoracic Vertebral ØRP4
    Coccygeal ØSP6
    Elbow
      Left ØRPM
      Right ØRPL
    Finger Phalangeal
      Left ØRPX
      Right ØRPW
    Hip
      Left ØSPB
        Acetabular Surface ØSPE
        Femoral Surface ØSPS
      Right ØSP9
        Acetabular Surface ØSPA
        Femoral Surface ØSPR
    Knee
      Left ØSPD
        Femoral Surface ØSPU
        Tibial Surface ØSPW
      Right ØSPC
        Femoral Surface ØSPT
        Tibial Surface ØSPV
    Lumbar Vertebral ØSPØ
    Lumbosacral ØSP3
    Metacarpophalangeal
      Left ØRPV
      Right ØRPU
    Metatarsal-Phalangeal
      Left ØSPN
      Right ØSPM
    Occipital-cervical ØRPØ
    Sacrococcygeal ØSP5
    Sacroiliac
      Left ØSP8
      Right ØSP7
    Shoulder
      Left ØRPK
      Right ØRPJ
    Sternoclavicular
      Left ØRPF
      Right ØRPE
    Tarsal
      Left ØSPJ
      Right ØSPH
    Tarsometatarsal
      Left ØSPL
      Right ØSPK
    Temporomandibular
      Left ØRPD
      Right ØRPC
    Thoracic Vertebral ØRP6
    Thoracolumbar Vertebral ØRPA
    Toe Phalangeal
      Left ØSPQ
      Right ØSPP
    Wrist
      Left ØRPP
      Right ØRPN
  Kidney ØTP5
  Larynx ØCPS
  Lens
    Left Ø8PK3
    Right Ø8PJ3
  Liver ØFPØ
  Lung
    Left ØBPL
    Right ØBPK
  Lymphatic Ø7PN
    Thoracic Duct Ø7PK
  Mediastinum ØWPC
  Mesentery ØDPV
  Metacarpal
    Left ØPPQ
    Right ØPPP

Removal of device from — *continued*
  Metatarsal
    Left ØQPP
    Right ØQPN
  Mouth and Throat ØCPY
  Muscle
    Extraocular
      Left Ø8PM
      Right Ø8PL
    Lower ØKPY
    Upper ØKPX
  Nasal Mucosa and Soft Tissue Ø9PK
  Neck ØWP6
  Nerve
    Cranial ØØPE
    Peripheral Ø1PY
  Omentum ØDPU
  Ovary ØUP3
  Pancreas ØFPG
  Parathyroid Gland ØGPR
  Patella
    Left ØQPF
    Right ØQPD
  Pelvic Cavity ØWPJ
  Penis ØVPS
  Pericardial Cavity ØWPD
  Perineum
    Female ØWPN
    Male ØWPM
  Peritoneal Cavity ØWPG
  Peritoneum ØDPW
  Phalanx
    Finger
      Left ØPPV
      Right ØPPT
    Thumb
      Left ØPPS
      Right ØPPR
    Toe
      Left ØQPR
      Right ØQPQ
  Pineal Body ØGP1
  Pleura ØBPQ
  Pleural Cavity
    Left ØWPB
    Right ØWP9
  Products of Conception 10PØ
  Prostate and Seminal Vesicles ØVP4
  Radius
    Left ØPPJ
    Right ØPPH
  Rectum ØDPP
  Respiratory Tract ØWPQ
  Retroperitoneum ØWPH
  Ribs
    1 to 2 ØPP1
    3 or More ØPP2
  Sacrum ØQP1
  Scapula
    Left ØPP6
    Right ØPP5
  Scrotum and Tunica Vaginalis ØVP8
  Sinus Ø9PY
  Skin ØHPPX
  Skull ØNPØ
  Spinal Canal ØØPU
  Spinal Cord ØØPV
  Spleen Ø7PP
  Sternum ØPPØ
  Stomach ØDP6
  Subcutaneous Tissue and Fascia
    Head and Neck ØJPS
    Lower Extremity ØJPW
    Trunk ØJPT
    Upper Extremity ØJPV
  Tarsal
    Left ØQPM
    Right ØQPL
  Tendon
    Lower ØLPY
    Upper ØLPX
  Testis ØVPD
  Thymus Ø7PM
  Thyroid Gland ØGPK
  Tibia
    Left ØQPH
    Right ØQPG
  Toe Nail ØHPRX
  Trachea ØBP1

Subterms under main terms may continue to next column or page

Removal of device from — *continued*
Tracheobronchial Tree 0BP0
Tympanic Membrane
　Left 09P8
　Right 09P7
Ulna
　Left 0PPL
　Right 0PPK
Ureter 0TP9
Urethra 0TPD
Uterus and Cervix 0UPD
Vagina and Cul-de-sac 0UPH
Vas Deferens 0VPR
Vein
　Azygos 05P0
　Innominate
　　Left 05P4
　　Right 05P3
　Lower 06PY
　Upper 05PY
Vertebra
　Cervical 0PP3
　Lumbar 0QP0
　Thoracic 0PP4
Vulva 0UPM
Renal calyx
use Kidney
use Kidney, Left
use Kidney, Right
use Kidneys, Bilateral
Renal capsule
use Kidney
use Kidney, Left
use Kidney, Right
use Kidneys, Bilateral
Renal cortex
use Kidney
use Kidney, Left
use Kidney, Right
use Kidneys, Bilateral
Renal dialysis *see* Performance, Urinary 5A1D
Renal plexus *use* Abdominal Sympathetic Nerve
Renal segment
use Kidney
use Kidney, Left
use Kidney, Right
use Kidneys, Bilateral
Renal segmental artery
use Renal Artery, Left
use Renal Artery, Right
Reopening, operative site
Control of bleeding *see* Control bleeding in
Inspection only *see* Inspection
Repair
Abdominal Wall 0WQF
Acetabulum
　Left 0QQ5
　Right 0QQ4
Adenoids 0CQQ
Ampulla of Vater 0FQC
Anal Sphincter 0DQR
Ankle Region
　Left 0YQL
　Right 0YQK
Anterior Chamber
　Left 08Q33ZZ
　Right 08Q23ZZ
Anus 0DQQ
Aorta
　Abdominal 04Q0
　Thoracic
　　Ascending/Arch 02QX
　　Descending 02QW
Aortic Body 0GQD
Appendix 0DQJ
Arm
　Lower
　　Left 0XQF
　　Right 0XQD
　Upper
　　Left 0XQ9
　　Right 0XQ8
Artery
　Anterior Tibial
　　Left 04QQ
　　Right 04QP
　Axillary
　　Left 03Q6

Repair — *continued*
Artery — *continued*
　Axillary — *continued*
　　Right 03Q5
　Brachial
　　Left 03Q8
　　Right 03Q7
　Celiac 04Q1
　Colic
　　Left 04Q7
　　Middle 04Q8
　　Right 04Q6
　Common Carotid
　　Left 03QJ
　　Right 03QH
　Common Iliac
　　Left 04QD
　　Right 04QC
　Coronary
　　Four or More Arteries 02Q3
　　One Artery 02Q0
　　Three Arteries 02Q2
　　Two Arteries 02Q1
　External Carotid
　　Left 03QN
　　Right 03QM
　External Iliac
　　Left 04QJ
　　Right 04QH
　Face 03QR
　Femoral
　　Left 04QL
　　Right 04QK
　Foot
　　Left 04QW
　　Right 04QV
　Gastric 04Q2
　Hand
　　Left 03QF
　　Right 03QD
　Hepatic 04Q3
　Inferior Mesenteric 04QB
　Innominate 03Q2
　Internal Carotid
　　Left 03QL
　　Right 03QK
　Internal Iliac
　　Left 04QF
　　Right 04QE
　Internal Mammary
　　Left 03Q1
　　Right 03Q0
　Intracranial 03QG
　Lower 04QY
　Peroneal
　　Left 04QU
　　Right 04QT
　Popliteal
　　Left 04QN
　　Right 04QM
　Posterior Tibial
　　Left 04QS
　　Right 04QR
　Pulmonary
　　Left 02QR
　　Right 02QQ
　Pulmonary Trunk 02QP
　Radial
　　Left 03QC
　　Right 03QB
　Renal
　　Left 04QA
　　Right 04Q9
　Splenic 04Q4
　Subclavian
　　Left 03Q4
　　Right 03Q3
　Superior Mesenteric 04Q5
　Temporal
　　Left 03QT
　　Right 03QS
　Thyroid
　　Left 03QV
　　Right 03QU
　Ulnar
　　Left 03QA
　　Right 03Q9
　Upper 03QY

Repair — *continued*
Artery — *continued*
　Vertebral
　　Left 03QQ
　　Right 03QP
Atrium
　Left 02Q7
　Right 02Q6
Auditory Ossicle
　Left 09QA
　Right 09Q9
Axilla
　Left 0XQ5
　Right 0XQ4
Back
　Lower 0WQL
　Upper 0WQK
Basal Ganglia 00Q8
Bladder 0TQB
Bladder Neck 0TQC
Bone
　Ethmoid
　　Left 0NQG
　　Right 0NQF
　Frontal 0NQ1
　Hyoid 0NQX
　Lacrimal
　　Left 0NQJ
　　Right 0NQH
　Nasal 0NQB
　Occipital 0NQ7
　Palatine
　　Left 0NQL
　　Right 0NQK
　Parietal
　　Left 0NQ4
　　Right 0NQ3
　Pelvic
　　Left 0QQ3
　　Right 0QQ2
　Sphenoid 0NQC
　Temporal
　　Left 0NQ6
　　Right 0NQ5
　Zygomatic
　　Left 0NQN
　　Right 0NQM
Brain 00Q0
Breast
　Bilateral 0HQV
　Left 0HQU
　Right 0HQT
　Supernumerary 0HQY
Bronchus
　Lingula 0BQ9
　Lower Lobe
　　Left 0BQB
　　Right 0BQ6
　Main
　　Left 0BQ7
　　Right 0BQ3
　Middle Lobe, Right 0BQ5
　Upper Lobe
　　Left 0BQ8
　　Right 0BQ4
Buccal Mucosa 0CQ4
Bursa and Ligament
　Abdomen
　　Left 0MQJ
　　Right 0MQH
　Ankle
　　Left 0MQR
　　Right 0MQQ
　Elbow
　　Left 0MQ4
　　Right 0MQ3
　Foot
　　Left 0MQT
　　Right 0MQS
　Hand
　　Left 0MQ8
　　Right 0MQ7
　Head and Neck 0MQ0
　Hip
　　Left 0MQM
　　Right 0MQL
　Knee
　　Left 0MQP
　　Right 0MQN

Repair — *continued*
  Bursa and Ligament — *continued*
    Lower Extremity
      Left ØMQW
      Right ØMQV
    Perineum ØMQK
    Rib(s) ØMQG
    Shoulder
      Left ØMQ2
      Right ØMQ1
    Spine
      Lower ØMQD
      Upper ØMQC
    Sternum ØMQF
    Upper Extremity
      Left ØMQB
      Right ØMQ9
    Wrist
      Left ØMQ6
      Right ØMQ5
  Buttock
    Left ØYQ1
    Right ØYQØ
  Carina ØBQ2
  Carotid Bodies, Bilateral ØGQ8
  Carotid Body
    Left ØGQ6
    Right ØGQ7
  Carpal
    Left ØPQN
    Right ØPQM
  Cecum ØDQH
  Cerebellum ØØQC
  Cerebral Hemisphere ØØQ7
  Cerebral Meninges ØØQ1
  Cerebral Ventricle ØØQ6
  Cervix ØUQC
  Chest Wall ØWQ8
  Chordae Tendineae Ø2Q9
  Choroid
    Left Ø8QB
    Right Ø8QA
  Cisterna Chyli Ø7QL
  Clavicle
    Left ØPQB
    Right ØPQ9
  Clitoris ØUQJ
  Coccygeal Glomus ØGQB
  Coccyx ØQQS
  Colon
    Ascending ØDQK
    Descending ØDQM
    Sigmoid ØDQN
    Transverse ØDQL
  Conduction Mechanism Ø2Q8
  Conjunctiva
    Left Ø8QTXZZ
    Right Ø8QSXZZ
  Cord
    Bilateral ØVQH
    Left ØVQG
    Right ØVQF
  Cornea
    Left Ø8Q9XZZ
    Right Ø8Q8XZZ
  Cul-de-sac ØUQF
  Diaphragm ØBQT
  Disc
    Cervical Vertebral ØRQ3
    Cervicothoracic Vertebral ØRQ5
    Lumbar Vertebral ØSQ2
    Lumbosacral ØSQ4
    Thoracic Vertebral ØRQ9
    Thoracolumbar Vertebral ØRQB
  Duct
    Common Bile ØFQ9
    Cystic ØFQ8
    Hepatic
      Common ØFQ7
      Left ØFQ6
      Right ØFQ5
    Lacrimal
      Left Ø8QY
      Right Ø8QX
    Pancreatic ØFQD
      Accessory ØFQF
  Parotid
    Left ØCQC
    Right ØCQB

Repair — *continued*
  Duodenum ØDQ9
  Dura Mater ØØQ2
  Ear
    External
      Bilateral Ø9Q2
      Left Ø9Q1
      Right Ø9QØ
    External Auditory Canal
      Left Ø9Q4
      Right Ø9Q3
    Inner
      Left Ø9QE
      Right Ø9QD
    Middle
      Left Ø9Q6
      Right Ø9Q5
  Elbow Region
    Left ØXQC
    Right ØXQB
  Epididymis
    Bilateral ØVQL
    Left ØVQK
    Right ØVQJ
  Epiglottis ØCQR
  Esophagogastric Junction ØDQ4
  Esophagus ØDQ5
    Lower ØDQ3
    Middle ØDQ2
    Upper ØDQ1
  Eustachian Tube
    Left Ø9QG
    Right Ø9QF
  Extremity
    Lower
      Left ØYQB
      Right ØYQ9
    Upper
      Left ØXQ7
      Right ØXQ6
  Eye
    Left Ø8Q1XZZ
    Right Ø8QØXZZ
  Eyelid
    Lower
      Left Ø8QR
      Right Ø8QQ
    Upper
      Left Ø8QP
      Right Ø8QN
  Face ØWQ2
  Fallopian Tube
    Left ØUQ6
    Right ØUQ5
  Fallopian Tubes, Bilateral ØUQ7
  Femoral Region
    Bilateral ØYQE
    Left ØYQ8
    Right ØYQ7
  Femoral Shaft
    Left ØQQ9
    Right ØQQ8
  Femur
    Lower
      Left ØQQC
      Right ØQQB
    Upper
      Left ØQQ7
      Right ØQQ6
  Fibula
    Left ØQQK
    Right ØQQJ
  Finger
    Index
      Left ØXQP
      Right ØXQN
    Little
      Left ØXQW
      Right ØXQV
    Middle
      Left ØXQR
      Right ØXQQ
    Ring
      Left ØXQT
      Right ØXQS
  Finger Nail ØHQQXZZ
  Floor of mouth *see* Repair, Oral Cavity and Throat ØWQ3

Repair — *continued*
  Foot
    Left ØYQN
    Right ØYQM
  Gallbladder ØFQ4
  Gingiva
    Lower ØCQ6
    Upper ØCQ5
  Gland
    Adrenal
      Bilateral ØGQ4
      Left ØGQ2
      Right ØGQ3
    Lacrimal
      Left Ø8QW
      Right Ø8QV
    Minor Salivary ØCQJ
    Parotid
      Left ØCQ9
      Right ØCQ8
    Pituitary ØGQØ
    Sublingual
      Left ØCQF
      Right ØCQD
    Submaxillary
      Left ØCQH
      Right ØCQG
    Vestibular ØUQL
  Glenoid Cavity
    Left ØPQ8
    Right ØPQ7
  Glomus Jugulare ØGQC
  Hand
    Left ØXQK
    Right ØXQJ
  Head ØWQØ
  Heart Ø2QA
    Left Ø2QC
    Right Ø2QB
  Humeral Head
    Left ØPQD
    Right ØPQC
  Humeral Shaft
    Left ØPQG
    Right ØPQF
  Hymen ØUQK
  Hypothalamus ØØQA
  Ileocecal Valve ØDQC
  Ileum ØDQB
  Inguinal Region
    Bilateral ØYQA
    Left ØYQ6
    Right ØYQ5
  Intestine
    Large ØDQE
      Left ØDQG
      Right ØDQF
    Small ØDQ8
  Iris
    Left Ø8QD3ZZ
    Right Ø8QC3ZZ
  Jaw
    Lower ØWQ5
    Upper ØWQ4
  Jejunum ØDQA
  Joint
    Acromioclavicular
      Left ØRQH
      Right ØRQG
    Ankle
      Left ØSQG
      Right ØSQF
    Carpal
      Left ØRQR
      Right ØRQQ
    Carpometacarpal
      Left ØRQT
      Right ØRQS
    Cervical Vertebral ØRQ1
    Cervicothoracic Vertebral ØRQ4
    Coccygeal ØSQ6
    Elbow
      Left ØRQM
      Right ØRQL
    Finger Phalangeal
      Left ØRQX
      Right ØRQW
    Hip
      Left ØSQB

△ Subterms under main terms may continue to next column or page

Repair — continued
  Joint — continued
    Hip — continued
      Right 0SQ9
    Knee
      Left 0SQD
      Right 0SQC
    Lumbar Vertebral 0SQ0
    Lumbosacral 0SQ3
    Metacarpophalangeal
      Left 0RQV
      Right 0RQU
    Metatarsal-Phalangeal
      Left 0SQN
      Right 0SQM
    Occipital-cervical 0RQ0
    Sacrococcygeal 0SQ5
    Sacroiliac
      Left 0SQ8
      Right 0SQ7
    Shoulder
      Left 0RQK
      Right 0RQJ
    Sternoclavicular
      Left 0RQF
      Right 0RQE
    Tarsal
      Left 0SQJ
      Right 0SQH
    Tarsometatarsal
      Left 0SQL
      Right 0SQK
    Temporomandibular
      Left 0RQD
      Right 0RQC
    Thoracic Vertebral 0RQ6
    Thoracolumbar Vertebral 0RQA
    Toe Phalangeal
      Left 0SQQ
      Right 0SQP
    Wrist
      Left 0RQP
      Right 0RQN
  Kidney
    Left 0TQ1
    Right 0TQ0
  Kidney Pelvis
    Left 0TQ4
    Right 0TQ3
  Knee Region
    Left 0YQG
    Right 0YQF
  Larynx 0CQS
  Leg
    Lower
      Left 0YQJ
      Right 0YQH
    Upper
      Left 0YQD
      Right 0YQC
  Lens
    Left 08QK3ZZ
    Right 08QJ3ZZ
  Lip
    Lower 0CQ1
    Upper 0CQ0
  Liver 0FQ0
    Left Lobe 0FQ2
    Right Lobe 0FQ1
  Lung
    Bilateral 0BQM
    Left 0BQL
    Lower Lobe
      Left 0BQJ
      Right 0BQF
    Middle Lobe, Right 0BQD
    Right 0BQK
    Upper Lobe
      Left 0BQG
      Right 0BQC
  Lung Lingula 0BQH
  Lymphatic
    Aortic 07QD
    Axillary
      Left 07Q6
      Right 07Q5
    Head 07Q0
    Inguinal
      Left 07QJ

Repair — continued
  Lymphatic — continued
    Inguinal — continued
      Right 07QH
    Internal Mammary
      Left 07Q9
      Right 07Q8
    Lower Extremity
      Left 07QG
      Right 07QF
    Mesenteric 07QB
    Neck
      Left 07Q2
      Right 07Q1
    Pelvis 07QC
    Thoracic Duct 07QK
    Thorax 07Q7
    Upper Extremity
      Left 07Q4
      Right 07Q3
  Mandible
    Left 0NQV
    Right 0NQT
  Maxilla 0NQR
  Mediastinum 0WQC
  Medulla Oblongata 00QD
  Mesentery 0DQV
  Metacarpal
    Left 0PQQ
    Right 0PQP
  Metatarsal
    Left 0QQP
    Right 0QQN
  Muscle
    Abdomen
      Left 0KQL
      Right 0KQK
    Extraocular
      Left 08QM
      Right 08QL
    Facial 0KQ1
    Foot
      Left 0KQW
      Right 0KQV
    Hand
      Left 0KQD
      Right 0KQC
    Head 0KQ0
    Hip
      Left 0KQP
      Right 0KQN
    Lower Arm and Wrist
      Left 0KQB
      Right 0KQ9
    Lower Leg
      Left 0KQT
      Right 0KQS
    Neck
      Left 0KQ3
      Right 0KQ2
    Papillary 02QD
    Perineum 0KQM
    Shoulder
      Left 0KQ6
      Right 0KQ5
    Thorax
      Left 0KQJ
      Right 0KQH
    Tongue, Palate, Pharynx 0KQ4
    Trunk
      Left 0KQG
      Right 0KQF
    Upper Arm
      Left 0KQ8
      Right 0KQ7
    Upper Leg
      Left 0KQR
      Right 0KQQ
  Nasal Mucosa and Soft Tissue 09QK
  Nasopharynx 09QN
  Neck 0WQ6
  Nerve
    Abdominal Sympathetic 01QM
    Abducens 00QL
    Accessory 00QR
    Acoustic 00QN
    Brachial Plexus 01Q3
    Cervical 01Q1
    Cervical Plexus 01Q0

Repair — continued
  Nerve — continued
    Facial 00QM
    Femoral 01QD
    Glossopharyngeal 00QP
    Head and Neck Sympathetic 01QK
    Hypoglossal 00QS
    Lumbar 01QB
    Lumbar Plexus 01Q9
    Lumbar Sympathetic 01QN
    Lumbosacral Plexus 01QA
    Median 01Q5
    Oculomotor 00QH
    Olfactory 00QF
    Optic 00QG
    Peroneal 01QH
    Phrenic 01Q2
    Pudendal 01QC
    Radial 01Q6
    Sacral 01QR
    Sacral Plexus 01QQ
    Sacral Sympathetic 01QP
    Sciatic 01QF
    Thoracic 01Q8
    Thoracic Sympathetic 01QL
    Tibial 01QG
    Trigeminal 00QK
    Trochlear 00QJ
    Ulnar 01Q4
    Vagus 00QQ
  Nipple
    Left 0HQX
    Right 0HQW
  Omentum 0DQU
  Oral Cavity and Throat 0WQ3
  Orbit
    Left 0NQQ
    Right 0NQP
  Ovary
    Bilateral 0UQ2
    Left 0UQ1
    Right 0UQ0
  Palate
    Hard 0CQ2
    Soft 0CQ3
  Pancreas 0FQG
  Para-aortic Body 0GQ9
  Paraganglion Extremity 0GQF
  Parathyroid Gland 0GQR
    Inferior
      Left 0GQP
      Right 0GQN
    Multiple 0GQQ
    Superior
      Left 0GQM
      Right 0GQL
  Patella
    Left 0QQF
    Right 0QQD
  Penis 0VQS
  Pericardium 02QN
  Perineum
    Female 0WQN
    Male 0WQM
  Peritoneum 0DQW
  Phalanx
    Finger
      Left 0PQV
      Right 0PQT
    Thumb
      Left 0PQS
      Right 0PQR
    Toe
      Left 0QQR
      Right 0QQQ
  Pharynx 0CQM
  Pineal Body 0GQ1
  Pleura
    Left 0BQP
    Right 0BQN
  Pons 00QB
  Prepuce 0VQT
  Products of Conception 10Q0
  Prostate 0VQ0
  Radius
    Left 0PQJ
    Right 0PQH
  Rectum 0DQP

Repair — *continued*
    Vein — *continued*
        Hand — *continued*
            Right 05QG
        Hemiazygos 05Q1
        Hepatic 06Q4
        Hypogastric
            Left 06QJ
            Right 06QH
        Inferior Mesenteric 06Q6
        Innominate
            Left 05Q4
            Right 05Q3
        Internal Jugular
            Left 05QN
            Right 05QM
        Intracranial 05QL
        Lower 06QY
        Portal 06Q8
        Pulmonary
            Left 02QT
            Right 02QS
        Renal
            Left 06QB
            Right 06Q9
        Saphenous
            Left 06QQ
            Right 06QP
        Splenic 06Q1
        Subclavian
            Left 05Q6
            Right 05Q5
        Superior Mesenteric 06Q5
        Upper 05QY
        Vertebral
            Left 05QS
            Right 05QR
    Vena Cava
        Inferior 06Q0
        Superior 02QV
    Ventricle
        Left 02QL
        Right 02QK
    Vertebra
        Cervical 0PQ3
        Lumbar 0QQ0
        Thoracic 0PQ4
    Vesicle
        Bilateral 0VQ3
        Left 0VQ2
        Right 0VQ1
    Vitreous
        Left 08Q53ZZ
        Right 08Q43ZZ
    Vocal Cord
        Left 0CQV
        Right 0CQT
    Vulva 0UQM
    Wrist Region
        Left 0XQH
        Right 0XQG
Repair, obstetric laceration, periurethral 0UQMXZZ
Replacement
    Acetabulum
        Left 0QR5
        Right 0QR4
    Ampulla of Vater 0FRC
    Anal Sphincter 0DRR
    Aorta
        Abdominal 04R0
        Thoracic
            Ascending/Arch 02RX
            Descending 02RW
    Artery
        Anterior Tibial
            Left 04RQ
            Right 04RP
        Axillary
            Left 03R6
            Right 03R5
        Brachial
            Left 03R8
            Right 03R7
        Celiac 04R1
        Colic
            Left 04R7
            Middle 04R8
            Right 04R6

Replacement — *continued*
    Artery — *continued*
        Common Carotid
            Left 03RJ
            Right 03RH
        Common Iliac
            Left 04RD
            Right 04RC
        External Carotid
            Left 03RN
            Right 03RM
        External Iliac
            Left 04RJ
            Right 04RH
        Face 03RR
        Femoral
            Left 04RL
            Right 04RK
        Foot
            Left 04RW
            Right 04RV
        Gastric 04R2
        Hand
            Left 03RF
            Right 03RD
        Hepatic 04R3
        Inferior Mesenteric 04RB
        Innominate 03R2
        Internal Carotid
            Left 03RL
            Right 03RK
        Internal Iliac
            Left 04RF
            Right 04RE
        Internal Mammary
            Left 03R1
            Right 03R0
        Intracranial 03RG
        Lower 04RY
        Peroneal
            Left 04RU
            Right 04RT
        Popliteal
            Left 04RN
            Right 04RM
        Posterior Tibial
            Left 04RS
            Right 04RR
        Pulmonary
            Left 02RR
            Right 02RQ
        Pulmonary Trunk 02RP
        Radial
            Left 03RC
            Right 03RB
        Renal
            Left 04RA
            Right 04R9
        Splenic 04R4
        Subclavian
            Left 03R4
            Right 03R3
        Superior Mesenteric 04R5
        Temporal
            Left 03RT
            Right 03RS
        Thyroid
            Left 03RV
            Right 03RU
        Ulnar
            Left 03RA
            Right 03R9
        Upper 03RY
        Vertebral
            Left 03RQ
            Right 03RP
    Atrium
        Left 02R7
        Right 02R6
    Auditory Ossicle
        Left 09RA0
        Right 09R90
    Bladder 0TRB
    Bladder Neck 0TRC
    Bone
        Ethmoid
            Left 0NRG
            Right 0NRF
        Frontal 0NR1

Replacement — *continued*
    Bone — *continued*
        Hyoid 0NRX
        Lacrimal
            Left 0NRJ
            Right 0NRH
        Nasal 0NRB
        Occipital 0NR7
        Palatine
            Left 0NRL
            Right 0NRK
        Parietal
            Left 0NR4
            Right 0NR3
        Pelvic
            Left 0QR3
            Right 0QR2
        Sphenoid 0NRC
        Temporal
            Left 0NR6
            Right 0NR5
        Zygomatic
            Left 0NRN
            Right 0NRM
    Breast
        Bilateral 0HRV
        Left 0HRU
        Right 0HRT
    Bronchus
        Lingula 0BR9
        Lower Lobe
            Left 0BRB
            Right 0BR6
        Main
            Left 0BR7
            Right 0BR3
        Middle Lobe, Right 0BR5
        Upper Lobe
            Left 0BR8
            Right 0BR4
    Buccal Mucosa 0CR4
    Bursa and Ligament
        Abdomen
            Left 0MRJ
            Right 0MRH
        Ankle
            Left 0MRR
            Right 0MRQ
        Elbow
            Left 0MR4
            Right 0MR3
        Foot
            Left 0MRT
            Right 0MRS
        Hand
            Left 0MR8
            Right 0MR7
        Head and Neck 0MR0
        Hip
            Left 0MRM
            Right 0MRL
        Knee
            Left 0MRP
            Right 0MRN
        Lower Extremity
            Left 0MRW
            Right 0MRV
        Perineum 0MRK
        Rib(s) 0MRG
        Shoulder
            Left 0MR2
            Right 0MR1
        Spine
            Lower 0MRD
            Upper 0MRC
        Sternum 0MRF
        Upper Extremity
            Left 0MRB
            Right 0MR9
        Wrist
            Left 0MR6
            Right 0MR5
    Carina 0BR2
    Carpal
        Left 0PRN
        Right 0PRM
    Cerebral Meninges 00R1
    Cerebral Ventricle 00R6
    Chordae Tendineae 02R9

Replacement — *continued*
Choroid
  Left Ø8RB
  Right Ø8RA
Clavicle
  Left ØPRB
  Right ØPR9
Coccyx ØQRS
Conjunctiva
  Left Ø8RTX
  Right Ø8RSX
Cornea
  Left Ø8R9
  Right Ø8R8
Diaphragm ØBRT
Disc
  Cervical Vertebral ØRR3Ø
  Cervicothoracic Vertebral ØRR5Ø
  Lumbar Vertebral ØSR2Ø
  Lumbosacral ØSR4Ø
  Thoracic Vertebral ØRR9Ø
  Thoracolumbar Vertebral ØRRBØ
Duct
  Common Bile ØFR9
  Cystic ØFR8
  Hepatic
    Common ØFR7
    Left ØFR6
    Right ØFR5
  Lacrimal
    Left Ø8RY
    Right Ø8RX
  Pancreatic ØFRD
    Accessory ØFRF
  Parotid
    Left ØCRC
    Right ØCRB
Dura Mater ØØR2
Ear
  External
    Bilateral Ø9R2
    Left Ø9R1
    Right Ø9RØ
  Inner
    Left Ø9REØ
    Right Ø9RDØ
  Middle
    Left Ø9R6Ø
    Right Ø9R5Ø
Epiglottis ØCRR
Esophagus ØDR5
Eye
  Left Ø8R1
  Right Ø8RØ
Eyelid
  Lower
    Left Ø8RR
    Right Ø8RQ
  Upper
    Left Ø8RP
    Right Ø8RN
Femoral Shaft
  Left ØQR9
  Right ØQR8
Femur
  Lower
    Left ØQRC
    Right ØQRB
  Upper
    Left ØQR7
    Right ØQR6
Fibula
  Left ØQRK
  Right ØQRJ
Finger Nail ØHRQX
Gingiva
  Lower ØCR6
  Upper ØCR5
Glenoid Cavity
  Left ØPR8
  Right ØPR7
Hair ØHRSX
Humeral Head
  Left ØPRD
  Right ØPRC
Humeral Shaft
  Left ØPRG
  Right ØPRF

Replacement — *continued*
Iris
  Left Ø8RD3
  Right Ø8RC3
Joint
  Acromioclavicular
    Left ØRRHØ
    Right ØRRGØ
  Ankle
    Left ØSRG
    Right ØSRF
  Carpal
    Left ØRRRØ
    Right ØRRQØ
  Carpometacarpal
    Left ØRRTØ
    Right ØRRSØ
  Cervical Vertebral ØRR1Ø
  Cervicothoracic Vertebral ØRR4Ø
  Coccygeal ØSR6Ø
  Elbow
    Left ØRRMØ
    Right ØRRLØ
  Finger Phalangeal
    Left ØRRXØ
    Right ØRRWØ
  Hip
    Left ØSRB
      Acetabular Surface ØSRE
      Femoral Surface ØSRS
    Right ØSR9
      Acetabular Surface ØSRA
      Femoral Surface ØSRR
  Knee
    Left ØSRD
      Femoral Surface ØSRU
      Tibial Surface ØSRW
    Right ØSRC
      Femoral Surface ØSRT
      Tibial Surface ØSRV
  Lumbar Vertebral ØSRØØ
  Lumbosacral ØSR3Ø
  Metacarpophalangeal
    Left ØRRVØ
    Right ØRRUØ
  Metatarsal-Phalangeal
    Left ØSRNØ
    Right ØSRMØ
  Occipital-cervical ØRRØØ
  Sacrococcygeal ØSR5Ø
  Sacroiliac
    Left ØSR8Ø
    Right ØSR7Ø
  Shoulder
    Left ØRRK
    Right ØRRJ
  Sternoclavicular
    Left ØRRFØ
    Right ØRREØ
  Tarsal
    Left ØSRJØ
    Right ØSRHØ
  Tarsometatarsal
    Left ØSRLØ
    Right ØSRKØ
  Temporomandibular
    Left ØRRDØ
    Right ØRRCØ
  Thoracic Vertebral ØRR6Ø
  Thoracolumbar Vertebral ØRRAØ
  Toe Phalangeal
    Left ØSRQØ
    Right ØSRPØ
  Wrist
    Left ØRRPØ
    Right ØRRNØ
Kidney Pelvis
  Left ØTR4
  Right ØTR3
Larynx ØCRS
Lens
  Left Ø8RK3ØZ
  Right Ø8RJ3ØZ
Lip
  Lower ØCR1
  Upper ØCRØ
Mandible
  Left ØNRV
  Right ØNRT

Replacement — *continued*
Maxilla ØNRR
Mesentery ØDRV
Metacarpal
  Left ØPRQ
  Right ØPRP
Metatarsal
  Left ØQRP
  Right ØQRN
Muscle
  Abdomen
    Left ØKRL
    Right ØKRK
  Facial ØKR1
  Foot
    Left ØKRW
    Right ØKRV
  Hand
    Left ØKRD
    Right ØKRC
  Head ØKRØ
  Hip
    Left ØKRP
    Right ØKRN
  Lower Arm and Wrist
    Left ØKRB
    Right ØKR9
  Lower Leg
    Left ØKRT
    Right ØKRS
  Neck
    Left ØKR3
    Right ØKR2
  Papillary Ø2RD
  Perineum ØKRM
  Shoulder
    Left ØKR6
    Right ØKR5
  Thorax
    Left ØKRJ
    Right ØKRH
  Tongue, Palate, Pharynx ØKR4
  Trunk
    Left ØKRG
    Right ØKRF
  Upper Arm
    Left ØKR8
    Right ØKR7
  Upper Leg
    Left ØKRR
    Right ØKRQ
Nasal Mucosa and Soft Tissue Ø9RK
Nasopharynx Ø9RN
Nerve
  Abducens ØØRL
  Accessory ØØRR
  Acoustic ØØRN
  Cervical Ø1R1
  Facial ØØRM
  Femoral Ø1RD
  Glossopharyngeal ØØRP
  Hypoglossal ØØRS
  Lumbar Ø1RB
  Median Ø1R5
  Oculomotor ØØRH
  Olfactory ØØRF
  Optic ØØRG
  Peroneal Ø1RH
  Phrenic Ø1R2
  Pudendal Ø1RC
  Radial Ø1R6
  Sacral Ø1RR
  Sciatic Ø1RF
  Thoracic Ø1R8
  Tibial Ø1RG
  Trigeminal ØØRK
  Trochlear ØØRJ
  Ulnar Ø1R4
  Vagus ØØRQ
Nipple
  Left ØHRX
  Right ØHRW
Omentum ØDRU
Orbit
  Left ØNRQ
  Right ØNRP
Palate
  Hard ØCR2
  Soft ØCR3

Subterms under main terms may continue to next column or page

Replacement — *continued*
- Patella
  - Left ØQRF
  - Right ØQRD
- Pericardium Ø2RN
- Peritoneum ØDRW
- Phalanx
  - Finger
    - Left ØPRV
    - Right ØPRT
  - Thumb
    - Left ØPRS
    - Right ØPRR
  - Toe
    - Left ØQRR
    - Right ØQRQ
- Pharynx ØCRM
- Radius
  - Left ØPRJ
  - Right ØPRH
- Retinal Vessel
  - Left Ø8RH3
  - Right Ø8RG3
- Ribs
  - 1 to 2 ØPR1
  - 3 or More ØPR2
- Sacrum ØQR1
- Scapula
  - Left ØPR6
  - Right ØPR5
- Sclera
  - Left Ø8R7X
  - Right Ø8R6X
- Septum
  - Atrial Ø2R5
  - Nasal Ø9RM
  - Ventricular Ø2RM
- Skin
  - Abdomen ØHR7
  - Back ØHR6
  - Buttock ØHR8
  - Chest ØHR5
  - Ear
    - Left ØHR3
    - Right ØHR2
  - Face ØHR1
  - Foot
    - Left ØHRN
    - Right ØHRM
  - Hand
    - Left ØHRG
    - Right ØHRF
  - Inguinal ØHRA
  - Lower Arm
    - Left ØHRE
    - Right ØHRD
  - Lower Leg
    - Left ØHRL
    - Right ØHRK
  - Neck ØHR4
  - Perineum ØHR9
  - Scalp ØHRØ
  - Upper Arm
    - Left ØHRC
    - Right ØHRB
  - Upper Leg
    - Left ØHRJ
    - Right ØHRH
- Skin Substitute, Porcine Liver Derived XHRPXL2
- Skull ØNRØ
- Spinal Meninges ØØRT
- Sternum ØPRØ
- Subcutaneous Tissue and Fascia
  - Abdomen ØJR8
  - Back ØJR7
  - Buttock ØJR9
  - Chest ØJR6
  - Face ØJR1
  - Foot
    - Left ØJRR
    - Right ØJRQ
  - Hand
    - Left ØJRK
    - Right ØJRJ
  - Lower Arm
    - Left ØJRH
    - Right ØJRG
  - Lower Leg
    - Left ØJRP

Replacement — *continued*
- Subcutaneous Tissue and Fascia — *continued*
  - Lower Leg — *continued*
    - Right ØJRN
  - Neck
    - Left ØJR5
    - Right ØJR4
  - Pelvic Region ØJRC
  - Perineum ØJRB
  - Scalp ØJRØ
  - Upper Arm
    - Left ØJRF
    - Right ØJRD
  - Upper Leg
    - Left ØJRM
    - Right ØJRL
- Tarsal
  - Left ØQRM
  - Right ØQRL
- Tendon
  - Abdomen
    - Left ØLRG
    - Right ØLRF
  - Ankle
    - Left ØLRT
    - Right ØLRS
  - Foot
    - Left ØLRW
    - Right ØLRV
  - Hand
    - Left ØLR8
    - Right ØLR7
  - Head and Neck ØLRØ
  - Hip
    - Left ØLRK
    - Right ØLRJ
  - Knee
    - Left ØLRR
    - Right ØLRQ
  - Lower Arm and Wrist
    - Left ØLR6
    - Right ØLR5
  - Lower Leg
    - Left ØLRP
    - Right ØLRN
  - Perineum ØLRH
  - Shoulder
    - Left ØLR2
    - Right ØLR1
  - Thorax
    - Left ØLRD
    - Right ØLRC
  - Trunk
    - Left ØLRB
    - Right ØLR9
  - Upper Arm
    - Left ØLR4
    - Right ØLR3
  - Upper Leg
    - Left ØLRM
    - Right ØLRL
- Testis
  - Bilateral ØVRCØJZ
  - Left ØVRBØJZ
  - Right ØVR9ØJZ
- Thumb
  - Left ØXRM
  - Right ØXRL
- Tibia
  - Left ØQRH
  - Right ØQRG
- Toe Nail ØHRRX
- Tongue ØCR7
- Tooth
  - Lower ØCRX
  - Upper ØCRW
- Trachea ØBR1
- Turbinate, Nasal Ø9RL
- Tympanic Membrane
  - Left Ø9R8
  - Right Ø9R7
- Ulna
  - Left ØPRL
  - Right ØPRK
- Ureter
  - Left ØTR7
  - Right ØTR6
- Urethra ØTRD
- Uvula ØCRN

Replacement — *continued*
- Valve
  - Aortic Ø2RF
  - Mitral Ø2RG
  - Pulmonary Ø2RH
  - Tricuspid Ø2RJ
- Vein
  - Axillary
    - Left Ø5R8
    - Right Ø5R7
  - Azygos Ø5RØ
  - Basilic
    - Left Ø5RC
    - Right Ø5RB
  - Brachial
    - Left Ø5RA
    - Right Ø5R9
  - Cephalic
    - Left Ø5RF
    - Right Ø5RD
  - Colic Ø6R7
  - Common Iliac
    - Left Ø6RD
    - Right Ø6RC
  - Esophageal Ø6R3
  - External Iliac
    - Left Ø6RG
    - Right Ø6RF
  - External Jugular
    - Left Ø5RQ
    - Right Ø5RP
  - Face
    - Left Ø5RV
    - Right Ø5RT
  - Femoral
    - Left Ø6RN
    - Right Ø6RM
  - Foot
    - Left Ø6RV
    - Right Ø6RT
  - Gastric Ø6R2
  - Hand
    - Left Ø5RH
    - Right Ø5RG
  - Hemiazygos Ø5R1
  - Hepatic Ø6R4
  - Hypogastric
    - Left Ø6RJ
    - Right Ø6RH
  - Inferior Mesenteric Ø6R6
  - Innominate
    - Left Ø5R4
    - Right Ø5R3
  - Internal Jugular
    - Left Ø5RN
    - Right Ø5RM
  - Intracranial Ø5RL
  - Lower Ø6RY
  - Portal Ø6R8
  - Pulmonary
    - Left Ø2RT
    - Right Ø2RS
  - Renal
    - Left Ø6RB
    - Right Ø6R9
  - Saphenous
    - Left Ø6RQ
    - Right Ø6RP
  - Splenic Ø6R1
  - Subclavian
    - Left Ø5R6
    - Right Ø5R5
  - Superior Mesenteric Ø6R5
  - Upper Ø5RY
  - Vertebral
    - Left Ø5RS
    - Right Ø5RR
- Vena Cava
  - Inferior Ø6RØ
  - Superior Ø2RV
- Ventricle
  - Left Ø2RL
  - Right Ø2RK
- Vertebra
  - Cervical ØPR3
  - Lumbar ØQRØ
  - Thoracic ØPR4
- Vitreous
  - Left Ø8R53

Replacement — *continued*
  Vitreous — *continued*
    Right Ø8R43
  Vocal Cord
    Left ØCRV
    Right ØCRT
  Zooplastic Tissue, Rapid Deployment Technique
    X2RF
Replacement, hip
  Partial or total *see* Replacement, Lower Joints ØSR
  Resurfacing only *see* Supplement, Lower Joints
    ØSU
Replantation *see* Reposition
Replantation, scalp *see* Reattachment, Skin, Scalp
  ØHMØ
Reposition
  Acetabulum
    Left ØQS5
    Right ØQS4
  Ampulla of Vater ØFSC
  Anus ØDSQ
  Aorta
    Abdominal Ø4SØ
    Thoracic
      Ascending/Arch Ø2SXØZZ
      Descending Ø2SWØZZ
  Artery
    Anterior Tibial
      Left Ø4SQ
      Right Ø4SP
    Axillary
      Left Ø3S6
      Right Ø3S5
    Brachial
      Left Ø3S8
      Right Ø3S7
    Celiac Ø4S1
    Colic
      Left Ø4S7
      Middle Ø4S8
      Right Ø4S6
    Common Carotid
      Left Ø3SJ
      Right Ø3SH
    Common Iliac
      Left Ø4SD
      Right Ø4SC
    Coronary
      One Artery Ø2SØØZZ
      Two Arteries Ø2S1ØZZ
    External Carotid
      Left Ø3SN
      Right Ø3SM
    External Iliac
      Left Ø4SJ
      Right Ø4SH
    Face Ø3SR
    Femoral
      Left Ø4SL
      Right Ø4SK
    Foot
      Left Ø4SW
      Right Ø4SV
    Gastric Ø4S2
    Hand
      Left Ø3SF
      Right Ø3SD
    Hepatic Ø4S3
    Inferior Mesenteric Ø4SB
    Innominate Ø3S2
    Internal Carotid
      Left Ø3SL
      Right Ø3SK
    Internal Iliac
      Left Ø4SF
      Right Ø4SE
    Internal Mammary
      Left Ø3S1
      Right Ø3SØ
    Intracranial Ø3SG
    Lower Ø4SY
    Peroneal
      Left Ø4SU
      Right Ø4ST
    Popliteal
      Left Ø4SN
      Right Ø4SM
    Posterior Tibial
      Left Ø4SS

Reposition — *continued*
  Artery — *continued*
    Posterior Tibial — *continued*
      Right Ø4SR
    Pulmonary
      Left Ø2SRØZZ
      Right Ø2SQØZZ
    Pulmonary Trunk Ø2SPØZZ
    Radial
      Left Ø3SC
      Right Ø3SB
    Renal
      Left Ø4SA
      Right Ø4S9
    Splenic Ø4S4
    Subclavian
      Left Ø3S4
      Right Ø3S3
    Superior Mesenteric Ø4S5
    Temporal
      Left Ø3ST
      Right Ø3SS
    Thyroid
      Left Ø3SV
      Right Ø3SU
    Ulnar
      Left Ø3SA
      Right Ø3S9
    Upper Ø3SY
    Vertebral
      Left Ø3SQ
      Right Ø3SP
  Auditory Ossicle
    Left Ø9SA
    Right Ø9S9
  Bladder ØTSB
  Bladder Neck ØTSC
  Bone
    Ethmoid
      Left ØNSG
      Right ØNSF
    Frontal ØNS1
    Hyoid ØNSX
    Lacrimal
      Left ØNSJ
      Right ØNSH
    Nasal ØNSB
    Occipital ØNS7
    Palatine
      Left ØNSL
      Right ØNSK
    Parietal
      Left ØNS4
      Right ØNS3
    Pelvic
      Left ØQS3
      Right ØQS2
    Sphenoid ØNSC
    Temporal
      Left ØNS6
      Right ØNS5
    Zygomatic
      Left ØNSN
      Right ØNSM
  Breast
    Bilateral ØHSVØZZ
    Left ØHSUØZZ
    Right ØHSTØZZ
  Bronchus
    Lingula ØBS9ØZZ
    Lower Lobe
      Left ØBSBØZZ
      Right ØBS6ØZZ
    Main
      Left ØBS7ØZZ
      Right ØBS3ØZZ
    Middle Lobe, Right ØBS5ØZZ
    Upper Lobe
      Left ØBS8ØZZ
      Right ØBS4ØZZ
  Bursa and Ligament
    Abdomen
      Left ØMSJ
      Right ØMSH
    Ankle
      Left ØMSR
      Right ØMSQ
    Elbow
      Left ØMS4

Reposition — *continued*
  Bursa and Ligament — *continued*
    Elbow — *continued*
      Right ØMS3
    Foot
      Left ØMST
      Right ØMSS
    Hand
      Left ØMS8
      Right ØMS7
    Head and Neck ØMSØ
    Hip
      Left ØMSM
      Right ØMSL
    Knee
      Left ØMSP
      Right ØMSN
    Lower Extremity
      Left ØMSW
      Right ØMSV
    Perineum ØMSK
    Rib(s) ØMSG
    Shoulder
      Left ØMS2
      Right ØMS1
    Spine
      Lower ØMSD
      Upper ØMSC
    Sternum ØMSF
    Upper Extremity
      Left ØMSB
      Right ØMS9
    Wrist
      Left ØMS6
      Right ØMS5
  Carina ØBS2ØZZ
  Carpal
    Left ØPSN
    Right ØPSM
  Cecum ØDSH
  Cervix ØUSC
  Clavicle
    Left ØPSB
    Right ØPS9
  Coccyx ØQSS
  Colon
    Ascending ØDSK
    Descending ØDSM
    Sigmoid ØDSN
    Transverse ØDSL
  Cord
    Bilateral ØVSH
    Left ØVSG
    Right ØVSF
  Cul-de-sac ØUSF
  Diaphragm ØBSTØZZ
  Duct
    Common Bile ØFS9
    Cystic ØFS8
    Hepatic
      Common ØFS7
      Left ØFS6
      Right ØFS5
    Lacrimal
      Left Ø8SY
      Right Ø8SX
    Pancreatic ØFSD
      Accessory ØFSF
    Parotid
      Left ØCSC
      Right ØCSB
  Duodenum ØDS9
  Ear
    Bilateral Ø9S2
    Left Ø9S1
    Right Ø9SØ
  Epiglottis ØCSR
  Esophagus ØDS5
  Eustachian Tube
    Left Ø9SG
    Right Ø9SF
  Eyelid
    Lower
      Left Ø8SR
      Right Ø8SQ
    Upper
      Left Ø8SP
      Right Ø8SN

Subterms under main terms may continue to next column or page

Reposition — continued

Fallopian Tube
Left 0US6
Right 0US5
Fallopian Tubes, Bilateral 0US7
Femoral Shaft
Left 0QS9
Right 0QS8
Femur
Lower
Left 0QSC
Right 0QSB
Upper
Left 0QS7
Right 0QS6
Fibula
Left 0QSK
Right 0QSJ
Gallbladder 0FS4
Gland
Adrenal
Left 0GS2
Right 0GS3
Lacrimal
Left 08SW
Right 08SV
Glenoid Cavity
Left 0PS8
Right 0PS7
Hair 0HSSXZZ
Humeral Head
Left 0PSD
Right 0PSC
Humeral Shaft
Left 0PSG
Right 0PSF
Ileum 0DSB
Intestine
Large 0DSE
Small 0DS8
Iris
Left 08SD3ZZ
Right 08SC3ZZ
Jejunum 0DSA
Joint
Acromioclavicular
Left 0RSH
Right 0RSG
Ankle
Left 0SSG
Right 0SSF
Carpal
Left 0RSR
Right 0RSQ
Carpometacarpal
Left 0RST
Right 0RSS
Cervical Vertebral 0RS1
Cervicothoracic Vertebral 0RS4
Coccygeal 0SS6
Elbow
Left 0RSM
Right 0RSL
Finger Phalangeal
Left 0RSX
Right 0RSW
Hip
Left 0SSB
Right 0SS9
Knee
Left 0SSD
Right 0SSC
Lumbar Vertebral 0SS0
Lumbosacral 0SS3
Metacarpophalangeal
Left 0RSV
Right 0RSU
Metatarsal-Phalangeal
Left 0SSN
Right 0SSM
Occipital-cervical 0RS0
Sacrococcygeal 0SS5
Sacroiliac
Left 0SS8
Right 0SS7
Shoulder
Left 0RSK
Right 0RSJ

Reposition — continued

Joint — continued
Sternoclavicular
Left 0RSF
Right 0RSE
Tarsal
Left 0SSJ
Right 0SSH
Tarsometatarsal
Left 0SSL
Right 0SSK
Temporomandibular
Left 0RSD
Right 0RSC
Thoracic Vertebral 0RS6
Thoracolumbar Vertebral 0RSA
Toe Phalangeal
Left 0SSQ
Right 0SSP
Wrist
Left 0RSP
Right 0RSN
Kidney
Left 0TS1
Right 0TS0
Kidney Pelvis
Left 0TS4
Right 0TS3
Kidneys, Bilateral 0TS2
Lens
Left 08SK3ZZ
Right 08SJ3ZZ
Lip
Lower 0CS1
Upper 0CS0
Liver 0FS0
Lung
Left 0BSL0ZZ
Lower Lobe
Left 0BSJ0ZZ
Right 0BSF0ZZ
Middle Lobe, Right 0BSD0ZZ
Right 0BSK0ZZ
Upper Lobe
Left 0BSG0ZZ
Right 0BSC0ZZ
Lung Lingula 0BSH0ZZ
Mandible
Left 0NSV
Right 0NST
Maxilla 0NSR
Metacarpal
Left 0PSQ
Right 0PSP
Metatarsal
Left 0QSP
Right 0QSN
Muscle
Abdomen
Left 0KSL
Right 0KSK
Extraocular
Left 08SM
Right 08SL
Facial 0KS1
Foot
Left 0KSW
Right 0KSV
Hand
Left 0KSD
Right 0KSC
Head 0KS0
Hip
Left 0KSP
Right 0KSN
Lower Arm and Wrist
Left 0KSB
Right 0KS9
Lower Leg
Left 0KST
Right 0KSS
Neck
Left 0KS3
Right 0KS2
Perineum 0KSM
Shoulder
Left 0KS6
Right 0KS5

Reposition — continued

Muscle — continued
Thorax
Left 0KSJ
Right 0KSH
Tongue, Palate, Pharynx 0KS4
Trunk
Left 0KSG
Right 0KSF
Upper Arm
Left 0KS8
Right 0KS7
Upper Leg
Left 0KSR
Right 0KSQ
Nasal Mucosa and Soft Tissue 09SK
Nerve
Abducens 00SL
Accessory 00SR
Acoustic 00SN
Brachial Plexus 01S3
Cervical 01S1
Cervical Plexus 01S0
Facial 00SM
Femoral 01SD
Glossopharyngeal 00SP
Hypoglossal 00SS
Lumbar 01SB
Lumbar Plexus 01S9
Lumbosacral Plexus 01SA
Median 01S5
Oculomotor 00SH
Olfactory 00SF
Optic 00SG
Peroneal 01SH
Phrenic 01S2
Pudendal 01SC
Radial 01S6
Sacral 01SR
Sacral Plexus 01SQ
Sciatic 01SF
Thoracic 01S8
Tibial 01SG
Trigeminal 00SK
Trochlear 00SJ
Ulnar 01S4
Vagus 00SQ
Nipple
Left 0HSXXZZ
Right 0HSWXZZ
Orbit
Left 0NSQ
Right 0NSP
Ovary
Bilateral 0US2
Left 0US1
Right 0US0
Palate
Hard 0CS2
Soft 0CS3
Pancreas 0FSG
Parathyroid Gland 0GSR
Inferior
Left 0GSP
Right 0GSN
Multiple 0GSQ
Superior
Left 0GSM
Right 0GSL
Patella
Left 0QSF
Right 0QSD
Phalanx
Finger
Left 0PSV
Right 0PST
Thumb
Left 0PSS
Right 0PSR
Toe
Left 0QSR
Right 0QSQ
Products of Conception 10S0
Ectopic 10S2
Radius
Left 0PSJ
Right 0PSH
Rectum 0DSP

Reposition — *continued*

Retinal Vessel
  Left 08SH3ZZ
  Right 08SG3ZZ
Ribs
  1 to 2 0PS1
  3 or More 0PS2
Sacrum 0QS1
Scapula
  Left 0PS6
  Right 0PS5
Septum, Nasal 09SM
Sesamoid Bone(s) 1st Toe
  see Reposition, Metatarsal, Left 0QSP
  see Reposition, Metatarsal, Right 0QSN
Skull 0NS0
Spinal Cord
  Cervical 00SW
  Lumbar 00SY
  Thoracic 00SX
Spleen 07SP0ZZ
Sternum 0PS0
Stomach 0DS6
Tarsal
  Left 0QSM
  Right 0QSL
Tendon
  Abdomen
    Left 0LSG
    Right 0LSF
  Ankle
    Left 0LST
    Right 0LSS
  Foot
    Left 0LSW
    Right 0LSV
  Hand
    Left 0LS8
    Right 0LS7
  Head and Neck 0LS0
  Hip
    Left 0LSK
    Right 0LSJ
  Knee
    Left 0LSR
    Right 0LSQ
  Lower Arm and Wrist
    Left 0LS6
    Right 0LS5
  Lower Leg
    Left 0LSP
    Right 0LSN
  Perineum 0LSH
  Shoulder
    Left 0LS2
    Right 0LS1
  Thorax
    Left 0LSD
    Right 0LSC
  Trunk
    Left 0LSB
    Right 0LS9
  Upper Arm
    Left 0LS4
    Right 0LS3
  Upper Leg
    Left 0LSM
    Right 0LSL
Testis
  Bilateral 0VSC
  Left 0VSB
  Right 0VS9
Thymus 07SM0ZZ
Thyroid Gland
  Left Lobe 0GSG
  Right Lobe 0GSH
Tibia
  Left 0QSH
  Right 0QSG
Tongue 0CS7
Tooth
  Lower 0CSX
  Upper 0CSW
Trachea 0BS10ZZ
Turbinate, Nasal 09SL
Tympanic Membrane
  Left 09S8
  Right 09S7

Reposition — *continued*

Ulna
  Left 0PSL
  Right 0PSK
Ureter
  Left 0TS7
  Right 0TS6
Ureters, Bilateral 0TS8
Urethra 0TSD
Uterine Supporting Structure 0US4
Uterus 0US9
Uvula 0CSN
Vagina 0USG
Vein
  Axillary
    Left 05S8
    Right 05S7
  Azygos 05S0
  Basilic
    Left 05SC
    Right 05SB
  Brachial
    Left 05SA
    Right 05S9
  Cephalic
    Left 05SF
    Right 05SD
  Colic 06S7
  Common Iliac
    Left 06SD
    Right 06SC
  Esophageal 06S3
  External Iliac
    Left 06SG
    Right 06SF
  External Jugular
    Left 05SQ
    Right 05SP
  Face
    Left 05SV
    Right 05ST
  Femoral
    Left 06SN
    Right 06SM
  Foot
    Left 06SV
    Right 06ST
  Gastric 06S2
  Hand
    Left 05SH
    Right 05SG
  Hemiazygos 05S1
  Hepatic 06S4
  Hypogastric
    Left 06SJ
    Right 06SH
  Inferior Mesenteric 06S6
  Innominate
    Left 05S4
    Right 05S3
  Internal Jugular
    Left 05SN
    Right 05SM
  Intracranial 05SL
  Lower 06SY
  Portal 06S8
  Pulmonary
    Left 02ST0ZZ
    Right 02SS0ZZ
  Renal
    Left 06SB
    Right 06S9
  Saphenous
    Left 06SQ
    Right 06SP
  Splenic 06S1
  Subclavian
    Left 05S6
    Right 05S5
  Superior Mesenteric 06S5
  Upper 05SY
  Vertebral
    Left 05SS
    Right 05SR
Vena Cava
  Inferior 06S0
  Superior 02SV0ZZ
Vertebra
  Cervical 0PS3

Reposition — *continued*

Vertebra — *continued*
  Cervical — *continued*
    Magnetically Controlled Growth Rod(s)
      XNS3
    Lumbar 0QS0
    Magnetically Controlled Growth Rod(s)
      XNS0
    Thoracic 0PS4
    Magnetically Controlled Growth Rod(s)
      XNS4
Vocal Cord
  Left 0CSV
  Right 0CST

Resection
Acetabulum
  Left 0QT50ZZ
  Right 0QT40ZZ
Adenoids 0CTQ
Ampulla of Vater 0FTC
Anal Sphincter 0DTR
Anus 0DTQ
Aortic Body 0GTD
Appendix 0DTJ
Auditory Ossicle
  Left 09TA
  Right 09T9
Bladder 0TTB
Bladder Neck 0TTC
Bone
  Ethmoid
    Left 0NTG0ZZ
    Right 0NTF0ZZ
  Frontal 0NT10ZZ
  Hyoid 0NTX0ZZ
  Lacrimal
    Left 0NTJ0ZZ
    Right 0NTH0ZZ
  Nasal 0NTB0ZZ
  Occipital 0NT70ZZ
  Palatine
    Left 0NTL0ZZ
    Right 0NTK0ZZ
  Parietal
    Left 0NT40ZZ
    Right 0NT30ZZ
  Pelvic
    Left 0QT30ZZ
    Right 0QT20ZZ
  Sphenoid 0NTC0ZZ
  Temporal
    Left 0NT60ZZ
    Right 0NT50ZZ
  Zygomatic
    Left 0NTN0ZZ
    Right 0NTM0ZZ
Breast
  Bilateral 0HTV0ZZ
  Left 0HTU0ZZ
  Right 0HTT0ZZ
  Supernumerary 0HTY0ZZ
Bronchus
  Lingula 0BT9
  Lower Lobe
    Left 0BTB
    Right 0BT6
  Main
    Left 0BT7
    Right 0BT3
  Middle Lobe, Right 0BT5
  Upper Lobe
    Left 0BT8
    Right 0BT4
Bursa and Ligament
  Abdomen
    Left 0MTJ
    Right 0MTH
  Ankle
    Left 0MTR
    Right 0MTQ
  Elbow
    Left 0MT4
    Right 0MT3
  Foot
    Left 0MTT
    Right 0MTS
  Hand
    Left 0MT8
    Right 0MT7

Subterms under main terms may continue to next column or page

Resection — continued
  Bursa and Ligament — continued
    Head and Neck ØMTØ
    Hip
      Left ØMTM
      Right ØMTL
    Knee
      Left ØMTP
      Right ØMTN
    Lower Extremity
      Left ØMTW
      Right ØMTV
    Perineum ØMTK
    Rib(s) ØMTG
    Shoulder
      Left ØMT2
      Right ØMT1
    Spine
      Lower ØMTD
      Upper ØMTC
    Sternum ØMTF
    Upper Extremity
      Left ØMTB
      Right ØMT9
    Wrist
      Left ØMT6
      Right ØMT5
  Carina ØBT2
  Carotid Bodies, Bilateral ØGT8
  Carotid Body
    Left ØGT6
    Right ØGT7
  Carpal
    Left ØPTNØZZ
    Right ØPTMØZZ
  Cecum ØDTH
  Cerebral Hemisphere ØØT7
  Cervix ØUTC
  Chordae Tendineae Ø2T9
  Cisterna Chyli Ø7TL
  Clavicle
    Left ØPTBØZZ
    Right ØPT9ØZZ
  Clitoris ØUTJ
  Coccygeal Glomus ØGTB
  Coccyx ØQTSØZZ
  Colon
    Ascending ØDTK
    Descending ØDTM
    Sigmoid ØDTN
    Transverse ØDTL
  Conduction Mechanism Ø2T8
  Cord
    Bilateral ØVTH
    Left ØVTG
    Right ØVTF
  Cornea
    Left Ø8T9XZZ
    Right Ø8T8XZZ
  Cul-de-sac ØUTF
  Diaphragm ØBTT
  Disc
    Cervical Vertebral ØRT3ØZZ
    Cervicothoracic Vertebral ØRT5ØZZ
    Lumbar Vertebral ØST2ØZZ
    Lumbosacral ØST4ØZZ
    Thoracic Vertebral ØRT9ØZZ
    Thoracolumbar Vertebral ØRTBØZZ
  Duct
    Common Bile ØFT9
    Cystic ØFT8
    Hepatic
      Common ØFT7
      Left ØFT6
      Right ØFT5
    Lacrimal
      Left Ø8TY
      Right Ø8TX
    Pancreatic ØFTD
      Accessory ØFTF
    Parotid
      Left ØCTCØZZ
      Right ØCTBØZZ
  Duodenum ØDT9
  Ear
    External
      Left Ø9T1
      Right Ø9TØ

Resection — continued
  Ear — continued
    Inner
      Left Ø9TE
      Right Ø9TD
    Middle
      Left Ø9T6
      Right Ø9T5
  Epididymis
    Bilateral ØVTL
    Left ØVTK
    Right ØVTJ
  Epiglottis ØCTR
  Esophagogastric Junction ØDT4
  Esophagus ØDT5
    Lower ØDT3
    Middle ØDT2
    Upper ØDT1
  Eustachian Tube
    Left Ø9TG
    Right Ø9TF
  Eye
    Left Ø8T1XZZ
    Right Ø8TØXZZ
  Eyelid
    Lower
      Left Ø8TR
      Right Ø8TQ
    Upper
      Left Ø8TP
      Right Ø8TN
  Fallopian Tube
    Left ØUT6
    Right ØUT5
  Fallopian Tubes, Bilateral ØUT7
  Femoral Shaft
    Left ØQT9ØZZ
    Right ØQT8ØZZ
  Femur
    Lower
      Left ØQTCØZZ
      Right ØQTBØZZ
    Upper
      Left ØQT7ØZZ
      Right ØQT6ØZZ
  Fibula
    Left ØQTKØZZ
    Right ØQTJØZZ
  Finger Nail ØHTQXZZ
  Gallbladder ØFT4
  Gland
    Adrenal
      Bilateral ØGT4
      Left ØGT2
      Right ØGT3
    Lacrimal
      Left Ø8TW
      Right Ø8TV
    Minor Salivary ØCTJØZZ
    Parotid
      Left ØCT9ØZZ
      Right ØCT8ØZZ
    Pituitary ØGTØ
    Sublingual
      Left ØCTFØZZ
      Right ØCTDØZZ
    Submaxillary
      Left ØCTHØZZ
      Right ØCTGØZZ
    Vestibular ØUTL
  Glenoid Cavity
    Left ØPT8ØZZ
    Right ØPT7ØZZ
  Glomus Jugulare ØGTC
  Humeral Head
    Left ØPTDØZZ
    Right ØPTCØZZ
  Humeral Shaft
    Left ØPTGØZZ
    Right ØPTFØZZ
  Hymen ØUTK
  Ileocecal Valve ØDTC
  Ileum ØDTB
  Intestine
    Large ØDTE
      Left ØDTG
      Right ØDTF
    Small ØDT8

Resection — continued
  Iris
    Left Ø8TD3ZZ
    Right Ø8TC3ZZ
  Jejunum ØDTA
  Joint
    Acromioclavicular
      Left ØRTHØZZ
      Right ØRTGØZZ
    Ankle
      Left ØSTGØZZ
      Right ØSTFØZZ
    Carpal
      Left ØRTRØZZ
      Right ØRTQØZZ
    Carpometacarpal
      Left ØRTTØZZ
      Right ØRTSØZZ
    Cervicothoracic Vertebral ØRT4ØZZ
    Coccygeal ØST6ØZZ
    Elbow
      Left ØRTMØZZ
      Right ØRTLØZZ
    Finger Phalangeal
      Left ØRTXØZZ
      Right ØRTWØZZ
    Hip
      Left ØSTBØZZ
      Right ØST9ØZZ
    Knee
      Left ØSTDØZZ
      Right ØSTCØZZ
    Metacarpophalangeal
      Left ØRTVØZZ
      Right ØRTUØZZ
    Metatarsal-Phalangeal
      Left ØSTNØZZ
      Right ØSTMØZZ
    Sacrococcygeal ØST5ØZZ
    Sacroiliac
      Left ØST8ØZZ
      Right ØST7ØZZ
    Shoulder
      Left ØRTKØZZ
      Right ØRTJØZZ
    Sternoclavicular
      Left ØRTFØZZ
      Right ØRTEØZZ
    Tarsal
      Left ØSTJØZZ
      Right ØSTHØZZ
    Tarsometatarsal
      Left ØSTLØZZ
      Right ØSTKØZZ
    Temporomandibular
      Left ØRTDØZZ
      Right ØRTCØZZ
    Toe Phalangeal
      Left ØSTQØZZ
      Right ØSTPØZZ
    Wrist
      Left ØRTPØZZ
      Right ØRTNØZZ
  Kidney
    Left ØTT1
    Right ØTTØ
  Kidney Pelvis
    Left ØTT4
    Right ØTT3
  Kidneys, Bilateral ØTT2
  Larynx ØCTS
  Lens
    Left Ø8TK3ZZ
    Right Ø8TJ3ZZ
  Lip
    Lower ØCT1
    Upper ØCTØ
  Liver ØFTØ
    Left Lobe ØFT2
    Right Lobe ØFT1
  Lung
    Bilateral ØBTM
    Left ØBTL
    Lower Lobe
      Left ØBTJ
      Right ØBTF
    Middle Lobe, Right ØBTD
    Right ØBTK

Resection — *continued*
Lung — *continued*
Upper Lobe
Left ØBTG
Right ØBTC
Lung Lingula ØBTH
Lymphatic
Aortic 07TD
Axillary
Left 07T6
Right 07T5
Head 07TØ
Inguinal
Left 07TJ
Right 07TH
Internal Mammary
Left 07T9
Right 07T8
Lower Extremity
Left 07TG
Right 07TF
Mesenteric 07TB
Neck
Left 07T2
Right 07T1
Pelvis 07TC
Thoracic Duct 07TK
Thorax 07T7
Upper Extremity
Left 07T4
Right 07T3
Mandible
Left ØNTVØZZ
Right ØNTTØZZ
Maxilla ØNTRØZZ
Metacarpal
Left ØPTQØZZ
Right ØPTPØZZ
Metatarsal
Left ØQTPØZZ
Right ØQTNØZZ
Muscle
Abdomen
Left ØKTL
Right ØKTK
Extraocular
Left Ø8TM
Right Ø8TL
Facial ØKT1
Foot
Left ØKTW
Right ØKTV
Hand
Left ØKTD
Right ØKTC
Head ØKTØ
Hip
Left ØKTP
Right ØKTN
Lower Arm and Wrist
Left ØKTB
Right ØKT9
Lower Leg
Left ØKTT
Right ØKTS
Neck
Left ØKT3
Right ØKT2
Papillary Ø2TD
Perineum ØKTM
Shoulder
Left ØKT6
Right ØKT5
Thorax
Left ØKTJ
Right ØKTH
Tongue, Palate, Pharynx ØKT4
Trunk
Left ØKTG
Right ØKTF
Upper Arm
Left ØKT8
Right ØKT7
Upper Leg
Left ØKTR
Right ØKTQ
Nasal Mucosa and Soft Tissue Ø9TK
Nasopharynx Ø9TN

Resection — *continued*
Nipple
Left ØHTXXZZ
Right ØHTWXZZ
Omentum ØDTU
Orbit
Left ØNTQØZZ
Right ØNTPØZZ
Ovary
Bilateral ØUT2
Left ØUT1
Right ØUTØ
Palate
Hard ØCT2
Soft ØCT3
Pancreas ØFTG
Para-aortic Body ØGT9
Paraganglion Extremity ØGTF
Parathyroid Gland ØGTR
Inferior
Left ØGTP
Right ØGTN
Multiple ØGTQ
Superior
Left ØGTM
Right ØGTL
Patella
Left ØQTFØZZ
Right ØQTDØZZ
Penis ØVTS
Pericardium Ø2TN
Phalanx
Finger
Left ØPTVØZZ
Right ØPTTØZZ
Thumb
Left ØPTSØZZ
Right ØPTRØZZ
Toe
Left ØQTRØZZ
Right ØQTQØZZ
Pharynx ØCTM
Pineal Body ØGT1
Prepuce ØVTT
Products of Conception, Ectopic 1ØT2
Prostate ØVTØ
Radius
Left ØPTJØZZ
Right ØPTHØZZ
Rectum ØDTP
Ribs
1 to 2 ØPT1ØZZ
3 or More ØPT2ØZZ
Scapula
Left ØPT6ØZZ
Right ØPT5ØZZ
Scrotum ØVT5
Septum
Atrial Ø2T5
Nasal Ø9TM
Ventricular Ø2TM
Sinus
Accessory Ø9TP
Ethmoid
Left Ø9TV
Right Ø9TU
Frontal
Left Ø9TT
Right Ø9TS
Mastoid
Left Ø9TC
Right Ø9TB
Maxillary
Left Ø9TR
Right Ø9TQ
Sphenoid
Left Ø9TX
Right Ø9TW
Spleen Ø7TP
Sternum ØPTØØZZ
Stomach ØDT6
Pylorus ØDT7
Tarsal
Left ØQTMØZZ
Right ØQTLØZZ
Tendon
Abdomen
Left ØLTG
Right ØLTF

Resection — *continued*
Tendon — *continued*
Ankle
Left ØLTT
Right ØLTS
Foot
Left ØLTW
Right ØLTV
Hand
Left ØLT8
Right ØLT7
Head and Neck ØLTØ
Hip
Left ØLTK
Right ØLTJ
Knee
Left ØLTR
Right ØLTQ
Lower Arm and Wrist
Left ØLT6
Right ØLT5
Lower Leg
Left ØLTP
Right ØLTN
Perineum ØLTH
Shoulder
Left ØLT2
Right ØLT1
Thorax
Left ØLTD
Right ØLTC
Trunk
Left ØLTB
Right ØLT9
Upper Arm
Left ØLT4
Right ØLT3
Upper Leg
Left ØLTM
Right ØLTL
Testis
Bilateral ØVTC
Left ØVTB
Right ØVT9
Thymus Ø7TM
Thyroid Gland ØGTK
Left Lobe ØGTG
Right Lobe ØGTH
Thyroid Gland Isthmus ØGTJ
Tibia
Left ØQTHØZZ
Right ØQTGØZZ
Toe Nail ØHTRXZZ
Tongue ØCT7
Tonsils ØCTP
Tooth
Lower ØCTXØZ
Upper ØCTWØZ
Trachea ØBT1
Tunica Vaginalis
Left ØVT7
Right ØVT6
Turbinate, Nasal Ø9TL
Tympanic Membrane
Left Ø9T8
Right Ø9T7
Ulna
Left ØPTLØZZ
Right ØPTKØZZ
Ureter
Left ØTT7
Right ØTT6
Urethra ØTTD
Uterine Supporting Structure ØUT4
Uterus ØUT9
Uvula ØCTN
Vagina ØUTG
Valve, Pulmonary Ø2TH
Vas Deferens
Bilateral ØVTQ
Left ØVTP
Right ØVTN
Vesicle
Bilateral ØVT3
Left ØVT2
Right ØVT1
Vitreous
Left Ø8T53ZZ
Right Ø8T43ZZ

Subterms under main terms may continue to next column or page

Resection — *continued*
- Vocal Cord
  - Left 0CTV
  - Right 0CTT
- Vulva 0UTM

Resection, Left ventricular outflow tract obstruction (LVOT) *see* Dilation, Ventricle, Left 027L

Resection, Subaortic membrane (Left ventricular outflow tract obstruction) *see* Dilation, Ventricle, Left 027L

Restoration, Cardiac, Single, Rhythm 5A2204Z

RestoreAdvanced neurostimulator (SureScan) (MRI Safe) *use* Stimulator Generator, Multiple Array Rechargeable in 0JH

RestoreSensor neurostimulator (SureScan) (MRI Safe) *use* Stimulator Generator, Multiple Array Rechargeable in 0JH

RestoreUltra neurostimulator (SureScan) (MRI Safe) *use* Stimulator Generator, Multiple Array Rechargeable in 0JH

Restriction
- Ampulla of Vater 0FVC
- Anus 0DVQ
- Aorta
  - Abdominal 04V0
    - Intraluminal Device, Branched or Fenestrated 04V0
  - Thoracic
    - Ascending/Arch, Intraluminal Device, Branched or Fenestrated 02VX
    - Descending, Intraluminal Device, Branched or Fenestrated 02VW
- Artery
  - Anterior Tibial
    - Left 04VQ
    - Right 04VP
  - Axillary
    - Left 03V6
    - Right 03V5
  - Brachial
    - Left 03V8
    - Right 03V7
  - Celiac 04V1
  - Colic
    - Left 04V7
    - Middle 04V8
    - Right 04V6
  - Common Carotid
    - Left 03VJ
    - Right 03VH
  - Common Iliac
    - Left 04VD
    - Right 04VC
  - External Carotid
    - Left 03VN
    - Right 03VM
  - External Iliac
    - Left 04VJ
    - Right 04VH
  - Face 03VR
  - Femoral
    - Left 04VL
    - Right 04VK
  - Foot
    - Left 04VW
    - Right 04VV
  - Gastric 04V2
  - Hand
    - Left 03VF
    - Right 03VD
  - Hepatic 04V3
  - Inferior Mesenteric 04VB
  - Innominate 03V2
  - Internal Carotid
    - Left 03VL
    - Right 03VK
  - Internal Iliac
    - Left 04VF
    - Right 04VE
  - Internal Mammary
    - Left 03V1
    - Right 03V0
  - Intracranial 03VG
  - Lower 04VY
  - Peroneal
    - Left 04VU
    - Right 04VT

Restriction — *continued*
- Artery — *continued*
  - Popliteal
    - Left 04VN
    - Right 04VM
  - Posterior Tibial
    - Left 04VS
    - Right 04VR
  - Pulmonary
    - Left 02VR
    - Right 02VQ
  - Pulmonary Trunk 02VP
  - Radial
    - Left 03VC
    - Right 03VB
  - Renal
    - Left 04VA
    - Right 04V9
  - Splenic 04V4
  - Subclavian
    - Left 03V4
    - Right 03V3
  - Superior Mesenteric 04V5
  - Temporal
    - Left 03VT
    - Right 03VS
  - Thyroid
    - Left 03VV
    - Right 03VU
  - Ulnar
    - Left 03VA
    - Right 03V9
  - Upper 03VY
  - Vertebral
    - Left 03VQ
    - Right 03VP
- Bladder 0TVB
- Bladder Neck 0TVC
- Bronchus
  - Lingula 0BV9
  - Lower Lobe
    - Left 0BVB
    - Right 0BV6
  - Main
    - Left 0BV7
    - Right 0BV3
  - Middle Lobe, Right 0BV5
  - Upper Lobe
    - Left 0BV8
    - Right 0BV4
- Carina 0BV2
- Cecum 0DVH
- Cervix 0UVC
- Cisterna Chyli 07VL
- Colon
  - Ascending 0DVK
  - Descending 0DVM
  - Sigmoid 0DVN
  - Transverse 0DVL
- Duct
  - Common Bile 0FV9
  - Cystic 0FV8
  - Hepatic
    - Common 0FV7
    - Left 0FV6
    - Right 0FV5
  - Lacrimal
    - Left 08VY
    - Right 08VX
  - Pancreatic 0FVD
    - Accessory 0FVF
  - Parotid
    - Left 0CVC
    - Right 0CVB
- Duodenum 0DV9
- Esophagogastric Junction 0DV4
- Esophagus 0DV5
  - Lower 0DV3
  - Middle 0DV2
  - Upper 0DV1
- Heart 02VA
- Ileocecal Valve 0DVC
- Ileum 0DVB
- Intestine
  - Large 0DVE
    - Left 0DVG
    - Right 0DVF
  - Small 0DV8
- Jejunum 0DVA

Restriction — *continued*
- Kidney Pelvis
  - Left 0TV4
  - Right 0TV3
- Lymphatic
  - Aortic 07VD
  - Axillary
    - Left 07V6
    - Right 07V5
  - Head 07V0
  - Inguinal
    - Left 07VJ
    - Right 07VH
  - Internal Mammary
    - Left 07V9
    - Right 07V8
  - Lower Extremity
    - Left 07V7
    - Right 07VF
  - Mesenteric 07VB
  - Neck
    - Left 07V2
    - Right 07V1
  - Pelvis 07VC
  - Thoracic Duct 07VK
  - Thorax 07V7
  - Upper Extremity
    - Left 07V4
    - Right 07V3
- Rectum 0DVP
- Stomach 0DV6
  - Pylorus 0DV7
- Trachea 0BV1
- Ureter
  - Left 0TV7
  - Right 0TV6
- Urethra 0TVD
- Valve, Mitral 02VG
- Vein
  - Axillary
    - Left 05V8
    - Right 05V7
  - Azygos 05V0
  - Basilic
    - Left 05VC
    - Right 05VB
  - Brachial
    - Left 05VA
    - Right 05V9
  - Cephalic
    - Left 05VF
    - Right 05VD
  - Colic 06V7
  - Common Iliac
    - Left 06VD
    - Right 06VC
  - Esophageal 06V3
  - External Iliac
    - Left 06VG
    - Right 06VF
  - External Jugular
    - Left 05VQ
    - Right 05VP
  - Face
    - Left 05VV
    - Right 05VT
  - Femoral
    - Left 06VN
    - Right 06VM
  - Foot
    - Left 06VV
    - Right 06VT
  - Gastric 06V2
  - Hand
    - Left 05VH
    - Right 05VG
  - Hemiazygos 05V1
  - Hepatic 06V4
  - Hypogastric
    - Left 06VJ
    - Right 06VH
  - Inferior Mesenteric 06V6
  - Innominate
    - Left 05V4
    - Right 05V3
  - Internal Jugular
    - Left 05VN
    - Right 05VM
  - Intracranial 05VL

Restriction — *continued*
Vein — *continued*
Lower 06VY
Portal 06V8
Pulmonary
Left 02VT
Right 02VS
Renal
Left 06VB
Right 06V9
Saphenous
Left 06VQ
Right 06VP
Splenic 06V1
Subclavian
Left 05V6
Right 05V5
Superior Mesenteric 06V5
Upper 05VY
Vertebral
Left 05VS
Right 05VR
Vena Cava
Inferior 06V0
Superior 02VV
Resurfacing Device
Removal of device from
Left 0SPB0BZ
Right 0SP90BZ
Revision of device in
Left 0SWB0BZ
Right 0SW90BZ
Supplement
Left 0SUB0BZ
Acetabular Surface 0SUE0BZ
Femoral Surface 0SUS0BZ
Right 0SU90BZ
Acetabular Surface 0SUA0BZ
Femoral Surface 0SUR0BZ
Resuscitation
Cardiopulmonary *see* Assistance, Cardiac 5A02
Cardioversion 5A2204Z
Defibrillation 5A2204Z
Endotracheal intubation *see* Insertion of device in, Trachea 0BH1
External chest compression 5A12012
Pulmonary 5A19054
Resuscitative endovascular balloon occlusion of the aorta (REBOA)
02LW3DJ
04L03DJ
Resuture, Heart valve prosthesis *see* Revision of device in, Heart and Great Vessels 02W
Retained placenta, manual removal *see* Extraction, Products of Conception, Retained 10D1
Retraining
Cardiac *see* Motor Treatment, Rehabilitation F07
Vocational *see* Activities of Daily Living Treatment, Rehabilitation F08
Retrogasserian rhizotomy *see* Division, Nerve, Trigeminal 008K
Retroperitoneal cavity *use* Retroperitoneum
Retroperitoneal lymph node *use* Lymphatic, Aortic
Retroperitoneal space *use* Retroperitoneum
Retropharyngeal lymph node
use Lymphatic, Left Neck
use Lymphatic, Right Neck
Retropubic space *use* Pelvic Cavity
Reveal (LINQ) (DX) (XT) *use* Monitoring Device
Reverse total shoulder replacement *see* Replacement, Upper Joints 0RR
Reverse® Shoulder Prosthesis *use* Synthetic Substitute, Reverse Ball and Socket in 0RR
Revision
Correcting a portion of existing device *see* Revision of device in
Removal of device without replacement *see* Removal of device from
Replacement of existing device
see Removal of device from
see Root operation to place new device, e.g., Insertion, Replacement, Supplement
Revision of device in
Abdominal Wall 0WWF
Acetabulum
Left 0QW5
Right 0QW4
Anal Sphincter 0DWR

Revision of device in — *continued*
Anus 0DWQ
Artery
Lower 04WY
Upper 03WY
Auditory Ossicle
Left 09WA
Right 09W9
Back
Lower 0WWL
Upper 0WWK
Bladder 0TWB
Bone
Facial 0NWW
Lower 0QWY
Nasal 0NWB
Pelvic
Left 0QW3
Right 0QW2
Upper 0PWY
Bone Marrow 07WT
Brain 00W0
Breast
Left 0HWU
Right 0HWT
Bursa and Ligament
Lower 0MWY
Upper 0MWX
Carpal
Left 0PWN
Right 0PWM
Cavity, Cranial 0WW1
Cerebral Ventricle 00W6
Chest Wall 0WW8
Cisterna Chyli 07WL
Clavicle
Left 0PWB
Right 0PW9
Coccyx 0QWS
Diaphragm 0BWT
Disc
Cervical Vertebral 0RW3
Cervicothoracic Vertebral 0RW5
Lumbar Vertebral 0SW2
Lumbosacral 0SW4
Thoracic Vertebral 0RW9
Thoracolumbar Vertebral 0RWB
Duct
Hepatobiliary 0FWB
Pancreatic 0FWD
Ear
Inner
Left 09WE
Right 09WD
Left 09WJ
Right 09WH
Epididymis and Spermatic Cord 0VWM
Esophagus 0DW5
Extremity
Lower
Left 0YWB
Right 0YW9
Upper
Left 0XW7
Right 0XW6
Eye
Left 08W1
Right 08W0
Face 0WW2
Fallopian Tube 0UW8
Femoral Shaft
Left 0QW9
Right 0QW8
Femur
Lower
Left 0QWC
Right 0QWB
Upper
Left 0QW7
Right 0QW6
Fibula
Left 0QWK
Right 0QWJ
Finger Nail 0HWQX
Gallbladder 0FW4
Gastrointestinal Tract 0WWP
Genitourinary Tract 0WWR
Gland
Adrenal 0GW5

Revision of device in — *continued*
Gland — *continued*
Endocrine 0GWS
Pituitary 0GW0
Salivary 0CWA
Glenoid Cavity
Left 0PW8
Right 0PW7
Great Vessel 02WY
Hair 0HWSX
Head 0WW0
Heart 02WA
Humeral Head
Left 0PWD
Right 0PWC
Humeral Shaft
Left 0PWG
Right 0PWF
Intestinal Tract
Lower 0DWD
Upper 0DW0
Intestine
Large 0DWE
Small 0DW8
Jaw
Lower 0WW5
Upper 0WW4
Joint
Acromioclavicular
Left 0RWH
Right 0RWG
Ankle
Left 0SWG
Right 0SWF
Carpal
Left 0RWR
Right 0RWQ
Carpometacarpal
Left 0RWT
Right 0RWS
Cervical Vertebral 0RW1
Cervicothoracic Vertebral 0RW4
Coccygeal 0SW6
Elbow
Left 0RWM
Right 0RWL
Finger Phalangeal
Left 0RWX
Right 0RWW
Hip
Left 0SWB
Acetabular Surface 0SWE
Femoral Surface 0SWS
Right 0SW9
Acetabular Surface 0SWA
Femoral Surface 0SWR
Knee
Left 0SWD
Femoral Surface 0SWU
Tibial Surface 0SWW
Right 0SWC
Femoral Surface 0SWT
Tibial Surface 0SWV
Lumbar Vertebral 0SW0
Lumbosacral 0SW3
Metacarpophalangeal
Left 0RWV
Right 0RWU
Metatarsal-Phalangeal
Left 0SWN
Right 0SWM
Occipital-cervical 0RW0
Sacrococcygeal 0SW5
Sacroiliac
Left 0SW8
Right 0SW7
Shoulder
Left 0RWK
Right 0RWJ
Sternoclavicular
Left 0RWF
Right 0RWE
Tarsal
Left 0SWJ
Right 0SWH
Tarsometatarsal
Left 0SWL
Right 0SWK

Revision of device in — *continued*

Joint — *continued*
  Temporomandibular
    Left ØRWD
    Right ØRWC
  Thoracic Vertebral ØRW6
  Thoracolumbar Vertebral ØRWA
  Toe Phalangeal
    Left ØSWQ
    Right ØSWP
  Wrist
    Left ØRWP
    Right ØRWN
Kidney ØTW5
Larynx ØCWS
Lens
  Left Ø8WK
  Right Ø8WJ
Liver ØFWØ
Lung
  Left ØBWL
  Right ØBWK
Lymphatic Ø7WN
  Thoracic Duct Ø7WK
Mediastinum ØWWC
Mesentery ØDWV
Metacarpal
  Left ØPWQ
  Right ØPWP
Metatarsal
  Left ØQWP
  Right ØQWN
Mouth and Throat ØCWY
Muscle
  Extraocular
    Left Ø8WM
    Right Ø8WL
  Lower ØKWY
  Upper ØKWX
Nasal Mucosa and Soft Tissue Ø9WK
Neck ØWW6
Nerve
  Cranial ØØWE
  Peripheral Ø1WY
Omentum ØDWU
Ovary ØUW3
Pancreas ØFWG
Parathyroid Gland ØGWR
Patella
  Left ØQWF
  Right ØQWD
Pelvic Cavity ØWWJ
Penis ØVWS
Pericardial Cavity ØWWD
Perineum
  Female ØWWN
  Male ØWWM
Peritoneal Cavity ØWWG
Peritoneum ØDWW
Phalanx
  Finger
    Left ØPWV
    Right ØPWT
  Thumb
    Left ØPWS
    Right ØPWR
  Toe
    Left ØQWR
    Right ØQWQ
Pineal Body ØGW1
Pleura ØBWQ
Pleural Cavity
  Left ØWWB
  Right ØWW9
Prostate and Seminal Vesicles ØVW4
Radius
  Left ØPWJ
  Right ØPWH
Respiratory Tract ØWWQ
Retroperitoneum ØWWH
Ribs
  1 to 2 ØPW1
  3 or More ØPW2
Sacrum ØQW1
Scapula
  Left ØPW6
  Right ØPW5
Scrotum and Tunica Vaginalis ØVW8

Revision of device in — *continued*

Septum
  Atrial Ø2W5
  Ventricular Ø2WM
Sinus Ø9WY
Skin ØHWPX
Skull ØNWØ
Spinal Canal ØØWU
Spinal Cord ØØWV
Spleen Ø7WP
Sternum ØPWØ
Stomach ØDW6
Subcutaneous Tissue and Fascia
  Head and Neck ØJWS
  Lower Extremity ØJWW
  Trunk ØJWT
  Upper Extremity ØJWV
Tarsal
  Left ØQWM
  Right ØQWL
Tendon
  Lower ØLWY
  Upper ØLWX
Testis ØVWD
Thymus Ø7WM
Thyroid Gland ØGWK
Tibia
  Left ØQWH
  Right ØQWG
Toe Nail ØHWRX
Trachea ØBW1
Tracheobronchial Tree ØBWØ
Tympanic Membrane
  Left Ø9W8
  Right Ø9W7
Ulna
  Left ØPWL
  Right ØPWK
Ureter ØTW9
Urethra ØTWD
Uterus and Cervix ØUWD
Vagina and Cul-de-sac ØUWH
Valve
  Aortic Ø2WF
  Mitral Ø2WG
  Pulmonary Ø2WH
  Tricuspid Ø2WJ
Vas Deferens ØVWR
Vein
  Azygos Ø5WØ
  Innominate
    Left Ø5W4
    Right Ø5W3
  Lower Ø6WY
  Upper Ø5WY
Vertebra
  Cervical ØPW3
  Lumbar ØQWØ
  Thoracic ØPW4
Vulva ØUWM
Revo MRI™ SureScan® pacemaker *use* Pacemaker, Dual Chamber in ØJH
rhBMP-2 *use* Recombinant Bone Morphogenetic Protein
Rheos® System device *use* Stimulator Generator in Subcutaneous Tissue and Fascia
Rheos® System lead *use* Stimulator Lead in Upper Arteries
Rhinopharynx *use* Nasopharynx
Rhinoplasty
  see Alteration, Nasal Mucosa and Soft Tissue Ø9ØK
  see Repair, Nasal Mucosa and Soft Tissue Ø9QK
  see Replacement, Nasal Mucosa and Soft Tissue Ø9RK
  see Supplement, Nasal Mucosa and Soft Tissue Ø9UK
Rhinorrhaphy *see* Repair, Nasal Mucosa and Soft Tissue Ø9QK
Rhinoscopy Ø9JKXZZ
Rhizotomy
  see Division, Central Nervous System and Cranial Nerves ØØ8
  see Division, Peripheral Nervous System Ø18
Rhomboid major muscle
  use Trunk Muscle, Left
  use Trunk Muscle, Right
Rhomboid minor muscle
  use Trunk Muscle, Left

Rhomboid minor muscle — *continued*
  use Trunk Muscle, Right
Rhythm electrocardiogram *see* Measurement, Cardiac 4AØ2
Rhytidectomy *see* Alteration, Face ØWØ2
Right ascending lumbar vein *use* Azygos Vein
Right atrioventricular valve *use* Tricuspid Valve
Right auricular appendix *use* Atrium, Right
Right colic vein *use* Colic Vein
Right coronary sulcus *use* Heart, Right
Right gastric artery *use* Gastric Artery
Right gastroepiploic vein *use* Superior Mesenteric Vein
Right inferior phrenic vein *use* Inferior Vena Cava
Right inferior pulmonary vein *use* Pulmonary Vein, Right
Right jugular trunk *use* Lymphatic, Right Neck
Right lateral ventricle *use* Cerebral Ventricle
Right lymphatic duct *use* Lymphatic, Right Neck
Right ovarian vein *use* Inferior Vena Cava
Right second lumbar vein *use* Inferior Vena Cava
Right subclavian trunk *use* Lymphatic, Right Neck
Right subcostal vein *use* Azygos Vein
Right superior pulmonary vein *use* Pulmonary Vein, Right
Right suprarenal vein *use* Inferior Vena Cava
Right testicular vein *use* Inferior Vena Cava
Rima glottidis *use* Larynx
Risorius muscle *use* Facial Muscle
RNS System lead *use* Neurostimulator Lead in Central Nervous System and Cranial Nerves
RNS system neurostimulator generator *use* Neurostimulator Generator in Head and Facial Bones
Robotic Assisted Procedure
  Extremity
    Lower 8EØY
    Upper 8EØX
  Head and Neck Region 8EØ9
  Trunk Region 8EØW
Robotic Waterjet Ablation, Destruction, Prostate XV5Ø8A4
Rotation of fetal head
  Forceps 1ØSØ7ZZ
  Manual 1ØSØXZZ
Round ligament of uterus *use* Uterine Supporting Structure
Round window
  use Inner Ear, Left
  use Inner Ear, Right
Roux-en-Y operation
  see Bypass, Gastrointestinal System ØD1
  see Bypass, Hepatobiliary System and Pancreas ØF1
Rupture
  Adhesions *see* Release
  Fluid collection *see* Drainage
Ruxolitinib XWØDXT5

S

Sacral ganglion *use* Sacral Sympathetic Nerve
Sacral lymph node *use* Lymphatic, Pelvis
Sacral nerve modulation (SNM) lead *use* Stimulator Lead in Urinary System
Sacral neuromodulation lead *use* Stimulator Lead in Urinary System
Sacral splanchnic nerve *use* Sacral Sympathetic Nerve
Sacrectomy *see* Excision, Lower Bones ØQB
Sacrococcygeal ligament *use* Lower Spine Bursa and Ligament
Sacrococcygeal symphysis *use* Sacrococcygeal Joint
Sacroiliac ligament *use* Lower Spine Bursa and Ligament
Sacrospinous ligament *use* Lower Spine Bursa and Ligament
Sacrotuberous ligament *use* Lower Spine Bursa and Ligament
Salpingectomy
  see Excision, Female Reproductive System ØUB
  see Resection, Female Reproductive System ØUT
Salpingolysis *see* Release, Female Reproductive System ØUN
Salpingopexy
  see Repair, Female Reproductive System ØUQ
  see Reposition, Female Reproductive System ØUS

Salpingopharyngeus muscle use Tongue, Palate, Pharynx Muscle

Salpingoplasty
see Repair, Female Reproductive System ØUQ
see Supplement, Female Reproductive System ØUU

Salpingorrhaphy see Repair, Female Reproductive System ØUQ

Salpingoscopy ØUJ88ZZ

Salpingostomy see Drainage, Female Reproductive System ØU9

Salpingotomy see Drainage, Female Reproductive System ØU9

Salpinx
use Fallopian Tube, Left
use Fallopian Tube, Right

Saphenous nerve use Femoral Nerve

SAPIEN transcatheter aortic valve use Zooplastic Tissue in Heart and Great Vessels

Sartorius muscle
use Upper Leg Muscle, Left
use Upper Leg Muscle, Right

SAVAL below-the-knee (BTK) drug-eluting stent system
use Intraluminal Device, Sustained Release Drug-eluting in New Technology
use Intraluminal Device, Sustained Release Drug-eluting, Two in New Technology
use Intraluminal Device, Sustained Release Drug-eluting, Three in New Technology
use Intraluminal Device, Sustained Release Drug-eluting, Four or More in New Technology

Scalene muscle
use Neck Muscle, Left
use Neck Muscle, Right

Scan
Computerized Tomography (CT) see Computerized Tomography (CT Scan)
Radioisotope see Planar Nuclear Medicine Imaging

Scaphoid bone
use Carpal, Left
use Carpal, Right

Scapholunate ligament
use Hand Bursa and Ligament, Left
use Hand Bursa and Ligament, Right

Scaphotrapezium ligament
use Hand Bursa and Ligament, Left
use Hand Bursa and Ligament, Right

Scapulectomy
see Excision, Upper Bones ØPB
see Resection, Upper Bones ØPT

Scapulopexy
see Repair, Upper Bones ØPQ
see Reposition, Upper Bones ØPS

Scarpa's (vestibular) ganglion use Acoustic Nerve

Sclerectomy see Excision, Eye Ø8B

Sclerotherapy, mechanical see Destruction

Sclerotherapy, via injection of sclerosing agent
see Introduction, Destructive Agent

Sclerotomy see Drainage, Eye Ø89

Scrotectomy
see Excision, Male Reproductive System ØVB
see Resection, Male Reproductive System ØVT

Scrotoplasty
see Repair, Male Reproductive System ØVQ
see Supplement, Male Reproductive System ØVU

Scrotorrhaphy see Repair, Male Reproductive System ØVQ

Scrototomy see Drainage, Male Reproductive System ØV9

Sebaceous gland use Skin

Second cranial nerve use Optic Nerve

Section, cesarean see Extraction, Pregnancy 1ØD

Secura (DR) (VR) use Defibrillator Generator in ØJH

Sella turcica use Sphenoid Bone

Semicircular canal
use Inner Ear, Left
use Inner Ear, Right

Semimembranosus muscle
use Upper Leg Muscle, Left
use Upper Leg Muscle, Right

Semitendinosus muscle
use Upper Leg Muscle, Left
use Upper Leg Muscle, Right

Seprafilm use Adhesion Barrier

Septal cartilage use Nasal Septum

Septectomy
see Excision, Ear, Nose, Sinus Ø9B
see Excision, Heart and Great Vessels Ø2B
see Resection, Ear, Nose, Sinus Ø9T
see Resection, Heart and Great Vessels Ø2T

Septoplasty
see Repair, Ear, Nose, Sinus Ø9Q
see Repair, Heart and Great Vessels Ø2Q
see Replacement, Ear, Nose, Sinus Ø9R
see Replacement, Heart and Great Vessels Ø2R
see Reposition, Ear, Nose, Sinus Ø9S
see Supplement, Ear, Nose, Sinus Ø9U
see Supplement, Heart and Great Vessels Ø2U

Septostomy, balloon atrial Ø2163Z7

Septotomy see Drainage, Ear, Nose, Sinus Ø99

Sequestrectomy, bone see Extirpation

Serratus anterior muscle
use Thorax Muscle, Left
use Thorax Muscle, Right

Serratus posterior muscle
use Trunk Muscle, Left
use Trunk Muscle, Right

Seventh cranial nerve use Facial Nerve

Sheffield hybrid external fixator
use External Fixation Device, Hybrid in ØPH
use External Fixation Device, Hybrid in ØPS
use External Fixation Device, Hybrid in ØQH
use External Fixation Device, Hybrid in ØQS

Sheffield ring external fixator
use External Fixation Device, Ring in ØPH
use External Fixation Device, Ring in ØPS
use External Fixation Device, Ring in ØQH
use External Fixation Device, Ring in ØQS

Shirodkar cervical cerclage ØUVC7ZZ

Shock Wave Therapy, Musculoskeletal 6A93

Short gastric artery use Splenic Artery

Shortening
see Excision
see Repair
see Reposition

Shunt creation see Bypass

Sialoadenectomy
Complete see Resection, Mouth and Throat ØCT
Partial see Excision, Mouth and Throat ØCB

Sialodochoplasty
see Repair, Mouth and Throat ØCQ
see Replacement, Mouth and Throat ØCR
see Supplement, Mouth and Throat ØCU

Sialoectomy
see Excision, Mouth and Throat ØCB
see Resection, Mouth and Throat ØCT

Sialography see Plain Radiography, Ear, Nose, Mouth and Throat B9Ø

Sialolithotomy see Extirpation, Mouth and Throat ØCC

S-ICD™ lead use Subcutaneous Defibrillator Lead in Subcutaneous Tissue and Fascia

Sigmoid artery use Inferior Mesenteric Artery

Sigmoid flexure use Sigmoid Colon

Sigmoid vein use Inferior Mesenteric Vein

Sigmoidectomy
see Excision, Gastrointestinal System ØDB
see Resection, Gastrointestinal System ØDT

Sigmoidorrhaphy see Repair, Gastrointestinal System ØDQ

Sigmoidoscopy ØDJD8ZZ

Sigmoidotomy see Drainage, Gastrointestinal System ØD9

Single lead pacemaker (atrium) (ventricle) use Pacemaker, Single Chamber in ØJH

Single lead rate responsive pacemaker (atrium) (ventricle) use Pacemaker, Single Chamber Rate Responsive in ØJH

Sinoatrial node use Conduction Mechanism

Sinogram
Abdominal Wall see Fluoroscopy, Abdomen and Pelvis BW11
Chest Wall see Plain Radiography, Chest BWØ3
Retroperitoneum see Fluoroscopy, Abdomen and Pelvis BW11

Sinus venosus use Atrium, Right

Sinusectomy
see Excision, Ear, Nose, Sinus Ø9B
see Resection, Ear, Nose, Sinus Ø9T

Sinusoscopy Ø9JY4ZZ

Sinusotomy see Drainage, Ear, Nose, Sinus Ø99

Sirolimus-eluting coronary stent use Intraluminal Device, Drug-eluting in Heart and Great Vessels

Sixth cranial nerve use Abducens Nerve

Size reduction, breast see Excision, Skin and Breast ØHB

SJM Biocor® Stented Valve System use Zooplastic Tissue in Heart and Great Vessels

Skene's (paraurethral) gland use Vestibular Gland

Skin Substitute, Porcine Liver Derived, Replacement XHRPXL2

Sling
Fascial, orbicularis muscle (mouth) see Supplement, Muscle, Facial ØKU1
Levator muscle, for urethral suspension see Reposition, Bladder Neck ØTSC
Pubococcygeal, for urethral suspension see Reposition, Bladder Neck ØTSC
Rectum see Reposition, Rectum ØDSP

Small bowel series see Fluoroscopy, Bowel, Small BD13

Small saphenous vein
use Saphenous Vein, Left
use Saphenous Vein, Right

Snaring, polyp, colon see Excision, Gastrointestinal System ØDB

Solar (celiac) plexus use Abdominal Sympathetic Nerve

Soleus muscle
use Lower Leg Muscle, Left
use Lower Leg Muscle, Right

Spacer
Insertion of device in
Disc
Lumbar Vertebral ØSH2
Lumbosacral ØSH4
Joint
Acromioclavicular
Left ØRHH
Right ØRHG
Ankle
Left ØSHG
Right ØSHF
Carpal
Left ØRHR
Right ØRHQ
Carpometacarpal
Left ØRHT
Right ØRHS
Cervical Vertebral ØRH1
Cervicothoracic Vertebral ØRH4
Coccygeal ØSH6
Elbow
Left ØRHM
Right ØRHL
Finger Phalangeal
Left ØRHX
Right ØRHW
Hip
Left ØSHB
Right ØSH9
Knee
Left ØSHD
Right ØSHC
Lumbar Vertebral ØSHØ
Lumbosacral ØSH3
Metacarpophalangeal
Left ØRHV
Right ØRHU
Metatarsal-Phalangeal
Left ØSHN
Right ØSHM
Occipital-cervical ØRHØ
Sacrococcygeal ØSH5
Sacroiliac
Left ØSH8
Right ØSH7
Shoulder
Left ØRHK
Right ØRHJ
Sternoclavicular
Left ØRHF
Right ØRHE
Tarsal
Left ØSHJ
Right ØSHH
Tarsometatarsal
Left ØSHL
Right ØSHK

Spacer — *continued*
Insertion of device in — *continued*
Joint — *continued*
Temporomandibular
Left ØRHD
Right ØRHC
Thoracic Vertebral ØRH6
Thoracolumbar Vertebral ØRHA
Toe Phalangeal
Left ØSHQ
Right ØSHP
Wrist
Left ØRHP
Right ØRHN
Removal of device from
Acromioclavicular
Left ØRPH
Right ØRPG
Ankle
Left ØSPG
Right ØSPF
Carpal
Left ØRPR
Right ØRPQ
Carpometacarpal
Left ØRPT
Right ØRPS
Cervical Vertebral ØRP1
Cervicothoracic Vertebral ØRP4
Coccygeal ØSP6
Elbow
Left ØRPM
Right ØRPL
Finger Phalangeal
Left ØRPX
Right ØRPW
Hip
Left ØSPB
Right ØSP9
Knee
Left ØSPD
Right ØSPC
Lumbar Vertebral ØSPØ
Lumbosacral ØSP3
Metacarpophalangeal
Left ØRPV
Right ØRPU
Metatarsal-Phalangeal
Left ØSPN
Right ØSPM
Occipital-cervical ØRPØ
Sacrococcygeal ØSP5
Sacroiliac
Left ØSP8
Right ØSP7
Shoulder
Left ØRPK
Right ØRPJ
Sternoclavicular
Left ØRPF
Right ØRPE
Tarsal
Left ØSPJ
Right ØSPH
Tarsometatarsal
Left ØSPL
Right ØSPK
Temporomandibular
Left ØRPD
Right ØRPC
Thoracic Vertebral ØRP6
Thoracolumbar Vertebral ØRPA
Toe Phalangeal
Left ØSPQ
Right ØSPP
Wrist
Left ØRPP
Right ØRPN
Revision of device in
Acromioclavicular
Left ØRWH
Right ØRWG
Ankle
Left ØSWG
Right ØSWF
Carpal
Left ØRWR
Right ØRWQ

Spacer — *continued*
Revision of device in — *continued*
Carpometacarpal
Left ØRWT
Right ØRWS
Cervical Vertebral ØRW1
Cervicothoracic Vertebral ØRW4
Coccygeal ØSW6
Elbow
Left ØRWM
Right ØRWL
Finger Phalangeal
Left ØRWX
Right ØRWW
Hip
Left ØSWB
Right ØSW9
Knee
Left ØSWD
Right ØSWC
Lumbar Vertebral ØSWØ
Lumbosacral ØSW3
Metacarpophalangeal
Left ØRWV
Right ØRWU
Metatarsal-Phalangeal
Left ØSWN
Right ØSWM
Occipital-cervical ØRWØ
Sacrococcygeal ØSW5
Sacroiliac
Left ØSW8
Right ØSW7
Shoulder
Left ØRWK
Right ØRWJ
Sternoclavicular
Left ØRWF
Right ØRWE
Tarsal
Left ØSWJ
Right ØSWH
Tarsometatarsal
Left ØSWL
Right ØSWK
Temporomandibular
Left ØRWD
Right ØRWC
Thoracic Vertebral ØRW6
Thoracolumbar Vertebral ØRWA
Toe Phalangeal
Left ØSWQ
Right ØSWP
Wrist
Left ØRWP
Right ØRWN
Spacer, Articulating (Antibiotic) *use* Articulating Spacer in Lower Joints
Spacer, Static (Antibiotic) *use* Spacer in Lower Joints
Spectroscopy
Intravascular 8E023DZ
Near infrared 8E023DZ
Speech Assessment FØØ
Speech therapy *see* Speech Treatment, Rehabilitation FØ6
Speech Treatment FØ6
Sphenoidectomy
see Excision, Ear, Nose, Sinus Ø9B
see Excision, Head and Facial Bones ØNB
see Resection, Ear, Nose, Sinus Ø9T
see Resection, Head and Facial Bones ØNT
Sphenoidotomy *see* Drainage, Ear, Nose, Sinus Ø99
Sphenomandibular ligament *use* Head and Neck Bursa and Ligament
Sphenopalatine (pterygopalatine) ganglion *use* Head and Neck Sympathetic Nerve
Sphincterorrhaphy, anal *see* Repair, Anal Sphincter ØDQR
Sphincterotomy, anal
see Division, Anal Sphincter ØD8R
see Drainage, Anal Sphincter ØD9R
Spinal cord neurostimulator lead *use* Neurostimulator Lead in Central Nervous System and Cranial Nerves
Spinal growth rods, magnetically controlled *use* Magnetically Controlled Growth Rod(s) in New Technology
Spinal nerve, cervical *use* Cervical Nerve

Spinal nerve, lumbar *use* Lumbar Nerve
Spinal nerve, sacral *use* Sacral Nerve
Spinal nerve, thoracic *use* Thoracic Nerve
Spinal Stabilization Device
Facet Replacement
Cervical Vertebral ØRH1
Cervicothoracic Vertebral ØRH4
Lumbar Vertebral ØSHØ
Lumbosacral ØSH3
Occipital-cervical ØRHØ
Thoracic Vertebral ØRH6
Thoracolumbar Vertebral ØRHA
Interspinous Process
Cervical Vertebral ØRH1
Cervicothoracic Vertebral ØRH4
Lumbar Vertebral ØSHØ
Lumbosacral ØSH3
Occipital-cervical ØRHØ
Thoracic Vertebral ØRH6
Thoracolumbar Vertebral ØRHA
Pedicle-Based
Cervical Vertebral ØRH1
Cervicothoracic Vertebral ØRH4
Lumbar Vertebral ØSHØ
Lumbosacral ØSH3
Occipital-cervical ØRHØ
Thoracic Vertebral ØRH6
Thoracolumbar Vertebral ØRHA
Spinous process
use Cervical Vertebra
use Lumbar Vertebra
use Thoracic Vertebra
Spiral ganglion *use* Acoustic Nerve
Spiration IBV™ Valve System *use* Intraluminal Device, Endobronchial Valve in Respiratory System
Splenectomy
see Excision, Lymphatic and Hemic Systems Ø7B
see Resection, Lymphatic and Hemic Systems Ø7T
Splenic flexure *use* Transverse Colon
Splenic plexus *use* Abdominal Sympathetic Nerve
Splenius capitis muscle *use* Head Muscle
Splenius cervicis muscle
use Neck Muscle, Left
use Neck Muscle, Right
Splenolysis *see* Release, Lymphatic and Hemic Systems Ø7N
Splenopexy
see Repair, Lymphatic and Hemic Systems Ø7Q
see Reposition, Lymphatic and Hemic Systems Ø7S
Splenoplasty *see* Repair, Lymphatic and Hemic Systems Ø7Q
Splenorrhaphy *see* Repair, Lymphatic and Hemic Systems Ø7Q
Splenotomy *see* Drainage, Lymphatic and Hemic Systems Ø79
Splinting, musculoskeletal *see* Immobilization, Anatomical Regions 2W3
SPY PINPOINT fluorescence imaging system *see* Monitoring, Physiological Systems 4A1
SPY system intravascular fluorescence angiography *see* Monitoring, Physiological Systems 4A1
Stapedectomy
see Excision, Ear, Nose, Sinus Ø9B
see Resection, Ear, Nose, Sinus Ø9T
Stapediolysis *see* Release, Ear, Nose, Sinus Ø9N
Stapedioplasty
see Repair, Ear, Nose, Sinus Ø9Q
see Replacement, Ear, Nose, Sinus Ø9R
see Supplement, Ear, Nose, Sinus Ø9U
Stapedotomy *see* Drainage, Ear, Nose, Sinus Ø99
Stapes
use Auditory Ossicle, Left
use Auditory Ossicle, Right
Static Spacer (Antibiotic) *use* Spacer in Lower Joints
STELARA® *use* Other New Technology Therapeutic Substance
Stellate ganglion *use* Head and Neck Sympathetic Nerve
Stem cell transplant *see* Transfusion, Circulatory 3Ø2
Stensen's duct
use Parotid Duct, Left
use Parotid Duct, Right
Stent, intraluminal (cardiovascular) (gastrointestinal) (hepatobiliary) (urinary) *use* Intraluminal Device
Stent retriever thrombectomy *see* Extirpation, Upper Arteries Ø3C

Stented tissue valve use Zooplastic Tissue in Heart and Great Vessels

Stereotactic Radiosurgery
Abdomen DW23
Adrenal Gland DG22
Bile Ducts DF22
Bladder DT22
Bone Marrow D720
Brain D020
Brain Stem D021
Breast
   Left DM20
   Right DM21
Bronchus DB21
Cervix DU21
Chest DW22
Chest Wall DB27
Colon DD25
Diaphragm DB28
Duodenum DD22
Ear D920
Esophagus DD20
Eye D820
Gallbladder DF21
Gamma Beam
   Abdomen DW23JZZ
   Adrenal Gland DG22JZZ
   Bile Ducts DF22JZZ
   Bladder DT22JZZ
   Bone Marrow D720JZZ
   Brain D020JZZ
   Brain Stem D021JZZ
   Breast
      Left DM20JZZ
      Right DM21JZZ
   Bronchus DB21JZZ
   Cervix DU21JZZ
   Chest DW22JZZ
   Chest Wall DB27JZZ
   Colon DD25JZZ
   Diaphragm DB28JZZ
   Duodenum DD22JZZ
   Ear D920JZZ
   Esophagus DD20JZZ
   Eye D820JZZ
   Gallbladder DF21JZZ
   Gland
      Adrenal DG22JZZ
      Parathyroid DG24JZZ
      Pituitary DG20JZZ
      Thyroid DG25JZZ
   Glands, Salivary D926JZZ
   Head and Neck DW21JZZ
   Ileum DD24JZZ
   Jejunum DD23JZZ
   Kidney DT20JZZ
   Larynx D92BJZZ
   Liver DF20JZZ
   Lung DB22JZZ
   Lymphatics
      Abdomen D726JZZ
      Axillary D724JZZ
      Inguinal D728JZZ
      Neck D723JZZ
      Pelvis D727JZZ
      Thorax D725JZZ
   Mediastinum DB26JZZ
   Mouth D924JZZ
   Nasopharynx D92DJZZ
   Neck and Head DW21JZZ
   Nerve, Peripheral D027JZZ
   Nose D921JZZ
   Ovary DU20JZZ
   Palate
      Hard D928JZZ
      Soft D929JZZ
   Pancreas DF23JZZ
   Parathyroid Gland DG24JZZ
   Pelvic Region DW26JZZ
   Pharynx D92CJZZ
   Pineal Body DG21JZZ
   Pituitary Gland DG20JZZ
   Pleura DB25JZZ
   Prostate DV20JZZ
   Rectum DD27JZZ
   Sinuses D927JZZ
   Spinal Cord D026JZZ
   Spleen D722JZZ
   Stomach DD21JZZ

Stereotactic Radiosurgery — continued
Gamma Beam — continued
   Testis DV21JZZ
   Thymus D721JZZ
   Thyroid Gland DG25JZZ
   Tongue D925JZZ
   Trachea DB20JZZ
   Ureter DT21JZZ
   Urethra DT23JZZ
   Uterus DU22JZZ
Gland
   Adrenal DG22
   Parathyroid DG24
   Pituitary DG20
   Thyroid DG25
Glands, Salivary D926
Head and Neck DW21
Ileum DD24
Jejunum DD23
Kidney DT20
Larynx D92B
Liver DF20
Lung DB22
Lymphatics
   Abdomen D726
   Axillary D724
   Inguinal D728
   Neck D723
   Pelvis D727
   Thorax D725
Mediastinum DB26
Mouth D924
Nasopharynx D92D
Neck and Head DW21
Nerve, Peripheral D027
Nose D921
Other Photon
   Abdomen DW23DZZ
   Adrenal Gland DG22DZZ
   Bile Ducts DF22DZZ
   Bladder DT22DZZ
   Bone Marrow D720DZZ
   Brain D020DZZ
   Brain Stem D021DZZ
   Breast
      Left DM20DZZ
      Right DM21DZZ
   Bronchus DB21DZZ
   Cervix DU21DZZ
   Chest DW22DZZ
   Chest Wall DB27DZZ
   Colon DD25DZZ
   Diaphragm DB28DZZ
   Duodenum DD22DZZ
   Ear D920DZZ
   Esophagus DD20DZZ
   Eye D820DZZ
   Gallbladder DF21DZZ
   Gland
      Adrenal DG22DZZ
      Parathyroid DG24DZZ
      Pituitary DG20DZZ
      Thyroid DG25DZZ
   Glands, Salivary D926DZZ
   Head and Neck DW21DZZ
   Ileum DD24DZZ
   Jejunum DD23DZZ
   Kidney DT20DZZ
   Larynx D92BDZZ
   Liver DF20DZZ
   Lung DB22DZZ
   Lymphatics
      Abdomen D726DZZ
      Axillary D724DZZ
      Inguinal D728DZZ
      Neck D723DZZ
      Pelvis D727DZZ
      Thorax D725DZZ
   Mediastinum DB26DZZ
   Mouth D924DZZ
   Nasopharynx D92DDZZ
   Neck and Head DW21DZZ
   Nerve, Peripheral D027DZZ
   Nose D921DZZ
   Ovary DU20DZZ
   Palate
      Hard D928DZZ
      Soft D929DZZ
   Pancreas DF23DZZ

Stereotactic Radiosurgery — continued
Other Photon — continued
   Parathyroid Gland DG24DZZ
   Pelvic Region DW26DZZ
   Pharynx D92CDZZ
   Pineal Body DG21DZZ
   Pituitary Gland DG20DZZ
   Pleura DB25DZZ
   Prostate DV20DZZ
   Rectum DD27DZZ
   Sinuses D927DZZ
   Spinal Cord D026DZZ
   Spleen D722DZZ
   Stomach DD21DZZ
   Testis DV21DZZ
   Thymus D721DZZ
   Thyroid Gland DG25DZZ
   Tongue D925DZZ
   Trachea DB20DZZ
   Ureter DT21DZZ
   Urethra DT23DZZ
   Uterus DU22DZZ
Ovary DU20
Palate
   Hard D928
   Soft D929
Pancreas DF23
Parathyroid Gland DG24
Particulate
   Abdomen DW23HZZ
   Adrenal Gland DG22HZZ
   Bile Ducts DF22HZZ
   Bladder DT22HZZ
   Bone Marrow D720HZZ
   Brain D020HZZ
   Brain Stem D021HZZ
   Breast
      Left DM20HZZ
      Right DM21HZZ
   Bronchus DB21HZZ
   Cervix DU21HZZ
   Chest DW22HZZ
   Chest Wall DB27HZZ
   Colon DD25HZZ
   Diaphragm DB28HZZ
   Duodenum DD22HZZ
   Ear D920HZZ
   Esophagus DD20HZZ
   Eye D820HZZ
   Gallbladder DF21HZZ
   Gland
      Adrenal DG22HZZ
      Parathyroid DG24HZZ
      Pituitary DG20HZZ
      Thyroid DG25HZZ
   Glands, Salivary D926HZZ
   Head and Neck DW21HZZ
   Ileum DD24HZZ
   Jejunum DD23HZZ
   Kidney DT20HZZ
   Larynx D92BHZZ
   Liver DF20HZZ
   Lung DB22HZZ
   Lymphatics
      Abdomen D726HZZ
      Axillary D724HZZ
      Inguinal D728HZZ
      Neck D723HZZ
      Pelvis D727HZZ
      Thorax D725HZZ
   Mediastinum DB26HZZ
   Mouth D924HZZ
   Nasopharynx D92DHZZ
   Neck and Head DW21HZZ
   Nerve, Peripheral D027HZZ
   Nose D921HZZ
   Ovary DU20HZZ
   Palate
      Hard D928HZZ
      Soft D929HZZ
   Pancreas DF23HZZ
   Parathyroid Gland DG24HZZ
   Pelvic Region DW26HZZ
   Pharynx D92CHZZ
   Pineal Body DG21HZZ
   Pituitary Gland DG20HZZ
   Pleura DB25HZZ
   Prostate DV20HZZ
   Rectum DD27HZZ

Subterms under main terms may continue to next column or page

Stereotactic Radiosurgery — *continued*
Particulate — *continued*
Sinuses D927HZZ
Spinal Cord D026HZZ
Spleen D722HZZ
Stomach DD21HZZ
Testis DV21HZZ
Thymus D721HZZ
Thyroid Gland DG25HZZ
Tongue D925HZZ
Trachea DB20HZZ
Ureter DT21HZZ
Urethra DT23HZZ
Uterus DU22HZZ
Pelvic Region DW26
Pharynx D92C
Pineal Body DG21
Pituitary Gland DG20
Pleura DB25
Prostate DV20
Rectum DD27
Sinuses D927
Spinal Cord D026
Spleen D722
Stomach DD21
Testis DV21
Thymus D721
Thyroid Gland DG25
Tongue D925
Trachea DB20
Ureter DT21
Urethra DT23
Uterus DU22
Sternoclavicular ligament
use Shoulder Bursa and Ligament, Left
use Shoulder Bursa and Ligament, Right
Sternocleidomastoid artery
use Thyroid Artery, Left
use Thyroid Artery, Right
Sternocleidomastoid muscle
use Neck Muscle, Left
use Neck Muscle, Right
Sternocostal ligament *use* Sternum Bursa and Ligament
Sternotomy
see Division, Sternum 0P80
see Drainage, Sternum 0P90
Stimulation, cardiac
Cardioversion 5A2204Z
Electrophysiologic testing *see* Measurement, Cardiac 4A02
Stimulator Generator
Insertion of device in
Abdomen 0JH8
Back 0JH7
Chest 0JH6
Multiple Array
Abdomen 0JH8
Back 0JH7
Chest 0JH6
Multiple Array Rechargeable
Abdomen 0JH8
Back 0JH7
Chest 0JH6
Removal of device from, Subcutaneous Tissue and Fascia, Trunk 0JPT
Revision of device in, Subcutaneous Tissue and Fascia, Trunk 0JWT
Single Array
Abdomen 0JH8
Back 0JH7
Chest 0JH6
Single Array Rechargeable
Abdomen 0JH8
Back 0JH7
Chest 0JH6
Stimulator Lead
Insertion of device in
Anal Sphincter 0DHR
Artery
Left 03HL
Right 03HK
Bladder 0THB
Muscle
Lower 0KHY
Upper 0KHX
Stomach 0DH6
Ureter 0TH9

Stimulator Lead — *continued*
Removal of device from
Anal Sphincter 0DPR
Artery, Upper 03PY
Bladder 0TPB
Muscle
Lower 0KPY
Upper 0KPX
Stomach 0DP6
Ureter 0TP9
Revision of device in
Anal Sphincter 0DWR
Artery, Upper 03WY
Bladder 0TWB
Muscle
Lower 0KWY
Upper 0KWX
Stomach 0DW6
Ureter 0TW9
Stoma
Excision
Abdominal Wall 0WBFXZ2
Neck 0WB6XZ2
Repair
Abdominal Wall 0WQFXZ2
Neck 0WQ6XZ2
Stomatoplasty
see Repair, Mouth and Throat 0CQ
see Replacement, Mouth and Throat 0CR
see Supplement, Mouth and Throat 0CU
Stomatorrhaphy *see* Repair, Mouth and Throat 0CQ
Stratos LV *use* Cardiac Resynchronization Pacemaker Pulse Generator in 0JH
Stress test 4A02XM4, 4A12XM4
Stripping *see* Extraction
Study
Electrophysiologic stimulation, cardiac *see* Measurement, Cardiac 4A02
Ocular motility 4A07X7Z
Pulmonary airway flow measurement *see* Measurement, Respiratory 4A09
Visual acuity 4A07X0Z
Styloglossus muscle *use* Tongue, Palate, Pharynx Muscle
Stylomandibular ligament *use* Head and Neck Bursa and Ligament
Stylopharyngeus muscle *use* Tongue, Palate, Pharynx Muscle
Subacromial bursa
use Shoulder Bursa and Ligament, Left
use Shoulder Bursa and Ligament, Right
Subaortic (common iliac) lymph node *use* Lymphatic, Pelvis
Subarachnoid space, spinal *use* Spinal Canal
Subclavicular (apical) lymph node
use Lymphatic, Left Axillary
use Lymphatic, Right Axillary
Subclavius muscle
use Thorax Muscle, Left
use Thorax Muscle, Right
Subclavius nerve *use* Brachial Plexus
Subcostal artery *use* Upper Artery
Subcostal muscle
use Thorax Muscle, Left
use Thorax Muscle, Right
Subcostal nerve *use* Thoracic Nerve
Subcutaneous Defibrillator Lead
Insertion of device in, Subcutaneous Tissue and Fascia, Chest 0JH6
Removal of device from, Subcutaneous Tissue and Fascia, Trunk 0JPT
Revision of device in, Subcutaneous Tissue and Fascia, Trunk 0JWT
Subcutaneous injection reservoir, port *use* Vascular Access Device, Totally Implantable in Subcutaneous Tissue and Fascia
Subcutaneous injection reservoir, pump *use* Infusion Device, Pump in Subcutaneous Tissue and Fascia
Subdermal progesterone implant *use* Contraceptive Device in Subcutaneous Tissue and Fascia
Subdural space, spinal *use* Spinal Canal
Submandibular ganglion
use Facial Nerve
use Head and Neck Sympathetic Nerve
Submandibular gland
use Submaxillary Gland, Left

Submandibular gland — *continued*
use Submaxillary Gland, Right
Submandibular lymph node *use* Lymphatic, Head
Submandibular space *use* Subcutaneous Tissue and Fascia, Face
Submaxillary ganglion *use* Head and Neck Sympathetic Nerve
Submaxillary lymph node *use* Lymphatic, Head
Submental artery *use* Face Artery
Submental lymph node *use* Lymphatic, Head
Submucous (Meissner's) plexus *use* Abdominal Sympathetic Nerve
Suboccipital nerve *use* Cervical Nerve
Suboccipital venous plexus
use Vertebral Vein, Left
use Vertebral Vein, Right
Subparotid lymph node *use* Lymphatic, Head
Subscapular aponeurosis
use Subcutaneous Tissue and Fascia, Left Upper Arm
use Subcutaneous Tissue and Fascia, Right Upper Arm
Subscapular artery
use Axillary Artery, Left
use Axillary Artery, Right
Subscapular (posterior) lymph node
use Lymphatic, Axillary, Left
use Lymphatic, Axillary, Right
Subscapularis muscle
use Shoulder Muscle, Left
use Shoulder Muscle, Right
Substance Abuse Treatment
Counseling
Family, for substance abuse, Other Family Counseling HZ63ZZZ
Group
12-Step HZ43ZZZ
Behavioral HZ41ZZZ
Cognitive HZ40ZZZ
Cognitive-Behavioral HZ42ZZZ
Confrontational HZ48ZZZ
Continuing Care HZ49ZZZ
Infectious Disease
Post-Test HZ4CZZZ
Pre-Test HZ4CZZZ
Interpersonal HZ44ZZZ
Motivational Enhancement HZ47ZZZ
Psychoeducation HZ46ZZZ
Spiritual HZ4BZZZ
Vocational HZ45ZZZ
Individual
12-Step HZ33ZZZ
Behavioral HZ31ZZZ
Cognitive HZ30ZZZ
Cognitive-Behavioral HZ32ZZZ
Confrontational HZ38ZZZ
Continuing Care HZ39ZZZ
Infectious Disease
Post-Test HZ3CZZZ
Pre-Test HZ3CZZZ
Interpersonal HZ34ZZZ
Motivational Enhancement HZ37ZZZ
Psychoeducation HZ36ZZZ
Spiritual HZ3BZZZ
Vocational HZ35ZZZ
Detoxification Services, for substance abuse HZ2ZZZZ
Medication Management
Antabuse HZ83ZZZ
Bupropion HZ87ZZZ
Clonidine HZ86ZZZ
Levo-alpha-acetyl-methadol (LAAM) HZ82ZZZ
Methadone Maintenance HZ81ZZZ
Naloxone HZ85ZZZ
Naltrexone HZ84ZZZ
Nicotine Replacement HZ80ZZZ
Other Replacement Medication HZ89ZZZ
Psychiatric Medication HZ88ZZZ
Pharmacotherapy
Antabuse HZ93ZZZ
Bupropion HZ97ZZZ
Clonidine HZ96ZZZ
Levo-alpha-acetyl-methadol (LAAM) HZ92ZZZ
Methadone Maintenance HZ91ZZZ
Naloxone HZ95ZZZ
Naltrexone HZ94ZZZ

Substance Abuse Treatment — *continued*
  Pharmacotherapy — *continued*
    Nicotine Replacement HZ90ZZZ
    Psychiatric Medication HZ98ZZZ
    Replacement Medication, Other HZ99ZZZ
  Psychotherapy
    12-Step HZ53ZZZ
    Behavioral HZ51ZZZ
    Cognitive HZ50ZZZ
    Cognitive-Behavioral HZ52ZZZ
    Confrontational HZ58ZZZ
    Interactive HZ55ZZZ
    Interpersonal HZ54ZZZ
    Motivational Enhancement HZ57ZZZ
    Psychoanalysis HZ5BZZZ
    Psychodynamic HZ5CZZZ
    Psychoeducation HZ56ZZZ
    Psychophysiological HZ5DZZZ
    Supportive HZ59ZZZ
Substantia nigra *use* Basal Ganglia
Subtalar (talocalcaneal) joint
  use Tarsal Joint, Left
  use Tarsal Joint, Right
Subtalar ligament
  use Foot Bursa and Ligament, Left
  use Foot Bursa and Ligament, Right
Subthalamic nucleus *use* Basal Ganglia
Suction curettage (D&C), nonobstetric *see* Extraction, Endometrium 0UDB
Suction curettage, obstetric post-delivery *see* Extraction, Products of Conception, Retained 10D1
Superficial circumflex iliac vein
  use Saphenous Vein, Left
  use Saphenous Vein, Right
Superficial epigastric artery
  use Femoral Artery, Left
  use Femoral Artery, Right
Superficial epigastric vein
  use Saphenous Vein, Left
  use Saphenous Vein, Right
Superficial Inferior Epigastric Artery Flap
  Replacement
    Bilateral 0HRV078
    Left 0HRU078
    Right 0HRT078
  Transfer
    Left 0KXG
    Right 0KXF
Superficial palmar arch
  use Hand Artery, Left
  use Hand Artery, Right
Superficial palmar venous arch
  use Hand Vein, Left
  use Hand Vein, Right
Superficial temporal artery
  use Temporal Artery, Left
  use Temporal Artery, Right
Superficial transverse perineal muscle *use* Perineum Muscle
Superior cardiac nerve *use* Thoracic Sympathetic Nerve
Superior cerebellar vein *use* Intracranial Vein
Superior cerebral vein *use* Intracranial Vein
Superior clunic (cluneal) nerve *use* Lumbar Nerve
Superior epigastric artery
  use Internal Mammary Artery, Left
  use Internal Mammary Artery, Right
Superior genicular artery
  use Popliteal Artery, Left
  use Popliteal Artery, Right
Superior gluteal artery
  use Internal Iliac Artery, Left
  use Internal Iliac Artery, Right
Superior gluteal nerve *use* Lumbar Plexus
Superior hypogastric plexus *use* Abdominal Sympathetic Nerve
Superior labial artery *use* Face Artery
Superior laryngeal artery
  use Thyroid Artery, Left
  use Thyroid Artery, Right
Superior laryngeal nerve *use* Vagus Nerve
Superior longitudinal muscle *use* Tongue, Palate, Pharynx Muscle
Superior mesenteric ganglion *use* Abdominal Sympathetic Nerve
Superior mesenteric lymph node *use* Lymphatic, Mesenteric

Superior mesenteric plexus *use* Abdominal Sympathetic Nerve
Superior oblique muscle
  use Extraocular Muscle, Left
  use Extraocular Muscle, Right
Superior olivary nucleus *use* Pons
Superior rectal artery *use* Inferior Mesenteric Artery
Superior rectal vein *use* Inferior Mesenteric Vein
Superior rectus muscle
  use Extraocular Muscle, Left
  use Extraocular Muscle, Right
Superior tarsal plate
  use Upper Eyelid, Left
  use Upper Eyelid, Right
Superior thoracic artery
  use Axillary Artery, Left
  use Axillary Artery, Right
Superior thyroid artery
  use External Carotid Artery, Left
  use External Carotid Artery, Right
  use Thyroid Artery, Left
  use Thyroid Artery, Right
Superior turbinate *use* Nasal Turbinate
Superior ulnar collateral artery
  use Brachial Artery, Left
  use Brachial Artery, Right
Supersaturated Oxygen therapy 5A0512C, 5A0522C
Supplement
  Abdominal Wall 0WUF
  Acetabulum
    Left 0QU5
    Right 0QU4
  Ampulla of Vater 0FUC
  Anal Sphincter 0DUR
  Ankle Region
    Left 0YUL
    Right 0YUK
  Anus 0DUQ
  Aorta
    Abdominal 04U0
    Thoracic
      Ascending/Arch 02UX
      Descending 02UW
  Arm
    Lower
      Left 0XUF
      Right 0XUD
    Upper
      Left 0XU9
      Right 0XU8
  Artery
    Anterior Tibial
      Left 04UQ
      Right 04UP
    Axillary
      Left 03U6
      Right 03U5
    Brachial
      Left 03U8
      Right 03U7
    Celiac 04U1
    Colic
      Left 04U7
      Middle 04U8
      Right 04U6
    Common Carotid
      Left 03UJ
      Right 03UH
    Common Iliac
      Left 04UD
      Right 04UC
    Coronary
      Four or More Arteries 02U3
      One Artery 02U0
      Three Arteries 02U2
      Two Arteries 02U1
    External Carotid
      Left 03UN
      Right 03UM
    External Iliac
      Left 04UJ
      Right 04UH
    Face 03UR
    Femoral
      Left 04UL
      Right 04UK
    Foot
      Left 04UW

Supplement — *continued*
  Artery — *continued*
    Foot — *continued*
      Right 04UV
    Gastric 04U2
    Hand
      Left 03UF
      Right 03UD
    Hepatic 04U3
    Inferior Mesenteric 04UB
    Innominate 03U2
    Internal Carotid
      Left 03UL
      Right 03UK
    Internal Iliac
      Left 04UF
      Right 04UE
    Internal Mammary
      Left 03U1
      Right 03U0
    Intracranial 03UG
    Lower 04UY
    Peroneal
      Left 04UU
      Right 04UT
    Popliteal
      Left 04UN
      Right 04UM
    Posterior Tibial
      Left 04US
      Right 04UR
    Pulmonary
      Left 02UR
      Right 02UQ
    Pulmonary Trunk 02UP
    Radial
      Left 03UC
      Right 03UB
    Renal
      Left 04UA
      Right 04U9
    Splenic 04U4
    Subclavian
      Left 03U4
      Right 03U3
    Superior Mesenteric 04U5
    Temporal
      Left 03UT
      Right 03US
    Thyroid
      Left 03UV
      Right 03UU
    Ulnar
      Left 03UA
      Right 03U9
    Upper 03UY
    Vertebral
      Left 03UQ
      Right 03UP
  Atrium
    Left 02U7
    Right 02U6
  Auditory Ossicle
    Left 09UA
    Right 09U9
  Axilla
    Left 0XU5
    Right 0XU4
  Back
    Lower 0WUL
    Upper 0WUK
  Bladder 0TUB
  Bladder Neck 0TUC
  Bone
    Ethmoid
      Left 0NUG
      Right 0NUF
    Frontal 0NU1
    Hyoid 0NUX
    Lacrimal
      Left 0NUJ
      Right 0NUH
    Nasal 0NUB
    Occipital 0NU7
    Palatine
      Left 0NUL
      Right 0NUK
    Parietal
      Left 0NU4

Supplement — *continued*
 Bone — *continued*
  Parietal — *continued*
   Right ØNU3
  Pelvic
   Left ØQU3
   Right ØQU2
  Sphenoid ØNUC
  Temporal
   Left ØNU6
   Right ØNU5
  Zygomatic
   Left ØNUN
   Right ØNUM
 Breast
  Bilateral ØHUV
  Left ØHUU
  Right ØHUT
 Bronchus
  Lingula ØBU9
  Lower Lobe
   Left ØBUB
   Right ØBU6
  Main
   Left ØBU7
   Right ØBU3
  Middle Lobe, Right ØBU5
  Upper Lobe
   Left ØBU8
   Right ØBU4
 Buccal Mucosa ØCU4
 Bursa and Ligament
  Abdomen
   Left ØMUJ
   Right ØMUH
  Ankle
   Left ØMUR
   Right ØMUQ
  Elbow
   Left ØMU4
   Right ØMU3
  Foot
   Left ØMUT
   Right ØMUS
  Hand
   Left ØMU8
   Right ØMU7
  Head and Neck ØMUØ
  Hip
   Left ØMUM
   Right ØMUL
  Knee
   Left ØMUP
   Right ØMUN
  Lower Extremity
   Left ØMUW
   Right ØMUV
  Perineum ØMUK
  Rib(s) ØMUG
  Shoulder
   Left ØMU2
   Right ØMU1
  Spine
   Lower ØMUD
   Upper ØMUC
  Sternum ØMUF
  Upper Extremity
   Left ØMUB
   Right ØMU9
  Wrist
   Left ØMU6
   Right ØMU5
 Buttock
  Left ØYU1
  Right ØYUØ
 Carina ØBU2
 Carpal
  Left ØPUN
  Right ØPUM
 Cecum ØDUH
 Cerebral Meninges ØØU1
 Cerebral Ventricle ØØU6
 Chest Wall ØWU8
 Chordae Tendineae Ø2U9
 Cisterna Chyli Ø7UL
 Clavicle
  Left ØPUB
  Right ØPU9
 Clitoris ØUUJ

Supplement — *continued*
 Coccyx ØQUS
 Colon
  Ascending ØDUK
  Descending ØDUM
  Sigmoid ØDUN
  Transverse ØDUL
 Cord
  Bilateral ØVUH
  Left ØVUG
  Right ØVUF
 Cornea
  Left Ø8U9
  Right Ø8U8
 Cul-de-sac ØUUF
 Diaphragm ØBUT
 Disc
  Cervical Vertebral ØRU3
  Cervicothoracic Vertebral ØRU5
  Lumbar Vertebral ØSU2
  Lumbosacral ØSU4
  Thoracic Vertebral ØRU9
  Thoracolumbar Vertebral ØRUB
 Duct
  Common Bile ØFU9
  Cystic ØFU8
  Hepatic
   Common ØFU7
   Left ØFU6
   Right ØFU5
  Lacrimal
   Left Ø8UY
   Right Ø8UX
  Pancreatic ØFUD
   Accessory ØFUF
 Duodenum ØDU9
 Dura Mater ØØU2
 Ear
  External
   Bilateral Ø9U2
   Left Ø9U1
   Right Ø9UØ
  Inner
   Left Ø9UE
   Right Ø9UD
  Middle
   Left Ø9U6
   Right Ø9U5
 Elbow Region
  Left ØXUC
  Right ØXUB
 Epididymis
  Bilateral ØVUL
  Left ØVUK
  Right ØVUJ
 Epiglottis ØCUR
 Esophagogastric Junction ØDU4
 Esophagus ØDU5
  Lower ØDU3
  Middle ØDU2
  Upper ØDU1
 Extremity
  Lower
   Left ØYUB
   Right ØYU9
  Upper
   Left ØXU7
   Right ØXU6
 Eye
  Left Ø8U1
  Right Ø8UØ
 Eyelid
  Lower
   Left Ø8UR
   Right Ø8UQ
  Upper
   Left Ø8UP
   Right Ø8UN
 Face ØWU2
 Fallopian Tube
  Left ØUU6
  Right ØUU5
 Fallopian Tubes, Bilateral ØUU7
 Femoral Region
  Bilateral ØYUE
  Left ØYU8
  Right ØYU7
 Femoral Shaft
  Left ØQU9

Supplement — *continued*
 Femoral Shaft — *continued*
  Right ØQU8
 Femur
  Lower
   Left ØQUC
   Right ØQUB
  Upper
   Left ØQU7
   Right ØQU6
 Fibula
  Left ØQUK
  Right ØQUJ
 Finger
  Index
   Left ØXUP
   Right ØXUN
  Little
   Left ØXUW
   Right ØXUV
  Middle
   Left ØXUR
   Right ØXUQ
  Ring
   Left ØXUT
   Right ØXUS
 Foot
  Left ØYUN
  Right ØYUM
 Gingiva
  Lower ØCU6
  Upper ØCU5
 Glenoid Cavity
  Left ØPU8
  Right ØPU7
 Hand
  Left ØXUK
  Right ØXUJ
 Head ØWUØ
 Heart Ø2UA
 Humeral Head
  Left ØPUD
  Right ØPUC
 Humeral Shaft
  Left ØPUG
  Right ØPUF
 Hymen ØUUK
 Ileocecal Valve ØDUC
 Ileum ØDUB
 Inguinal Region
  Bilateral ØYUA
  Left ØYU6
  Right ØYU5
 Intestine
  Large ØDUE
   Left ØDUG
   Right ØDUF
  Small ØDU8
 Iris
  Left Ø8UD
  Right Ø8UC
 Jaw
  Lower ØWU5
  Upper ØWU4
 Jejunum ØDUA
 Joint
  Acromioclavicular
   Left ØRUH
   Right ØRUG
  Ankle
   Left ØSUG
   Right ØSUF
  Carpal
   Left ØRUR
   Right ØRUQ
  Carpometacarpal
   Left ØRUT
   Right ØRUS
  Cervical Vertebral ØRU1
  Cervicothoracic Vertebral ØRU4
  Coccygeal ØSU6
  Elbow
   Left ØRUM
   Right ØRUL
  Finger Phalangeal
   Left ØRUX
   Right ØRUW
  Hip
   Left ØSUB

Subterms under main terms may continue to next column or page

Index

Supplement — *continued*
  Subcutaneous Tissue and Fascia — *continued*
    Face ØJU1
    Foot
      Left ØJUR
      Right ØJUQ
    Hand
      Left ØJUK
      Right ØJUJ
    Lower Arm
      Left ØJUH
      Right ØJUG
    Lower Leg
      Left ØJUP
      Right ØJUN
    Neck
      Left ØJU5
      Right ØJU4
    Pelvic Region ØJUC
    Perineum ØJUB
    Scalp ØJUØ
    Upper Arm
      Left ØJUF
      Right ØJUD
    Upper Leg
      Left ØJUM
      Right ØJUL
  Tarsal
    Left ØQUM
    Right ØQUL
  Tendon
    Abdomen
      Left ØLUG
      Right ØLUF
    Ankle
      Left ØLUT
      Right ØLUS
    Foot
      Left ØLUW
      Right ØLUV
    Hand
      Left ØLU8
      Right ØLU7
    Head and Neck ØLUØ
    Hip
      Left ØLUK
      Right ØLUJ
    Knee
      Left ØLUR
      Right ØLUQ
    Lower Arm and Wrist
      Left ØLU6
      Right ØLU5
    Lower Leg
      Left ØLUP
      Right ØLUN
    Perineum ØLUH
    Shoulder
      Left ØLU2
      Right ØLU1
    Thorax
      Left ØLUD
      Right ØLUC
    Trunk
      Left ØLUB
      Right ØLU9
    Upper Arm
      Left ØLU4
      Right ØLU3
    Upper Leg
      Left ØLUM
      Right ØLUL
  Testis
    Bilateral ØVUCØ
    Left ØVUBØ
    Right ØVU9Ø
  Thumb
    Left ØXUM
    Right ØXUL
  Tibia
    Left ØQUH
    Right ØQUG
  Toe
    1st
      Left ØYUQ
      Right ØYUP
    2nd
      Left ØYUS
      Right ØYUR

Supplement — *continued*
  Toe — *continued*
    3rd
      Left ØYUU
      Right ØYUT
    4th
      Left ØYUW
      Right ØYUV
    5th
      Left ØYUY
      Right ØYUX
  Tongue ØCU7
  Trachea ØBU1
  Tunica Vaginalis
    Left ØVU7
    Right ØVU6
  Turbinate, Nasal Ø9UL
  Tympanic Membrane
    Left Ø9U8
    Right Ø9U7
  Ulna
    Left ØPUL
    Right ØPUK
  Ureter
    Left ØTU7
    Right ØTU6
  Urethra ØTUD
  Uterine Supporting Structure ØUU4
  Uvula ØCUN
  Vagina ØUUG
  Valve
    Aortic Ø2UF
    Mitral Ø2UG
    Pulmonary Ø2UH
    Tricuspid Ø2UJ
  Vas Deferens
    Bilateral ØVUQ
    Left ØVUP
    Right ØVUN
  Vein
    Axillary
      Left Ø5U8
      Right Ø5U7
    Azygos Ø5UØ
    Basilic
      Left Ø5UC
      Right Ø5UB
    Brachial
      Left Ø5UA
      Right Ø5U9
    Cephalic
      Left Ø5UF
      Right Ø5UD
    Colic Ø6U7
    Common Iliac
      Left Ø6UD
      Right Ø6UC
    Esophageal Ø6U3
    External Iliac
      Left Ø6UG
      Right Ø6UF
    External Jugular
      Left Ø5UQ
      Right Ø5UP
    Face
      Left Ø5UV
      Right Ø5UT
    Femoral
      Left Ø6UN
      Right Ø6UM
    Foot
      Left Ø6UV
      Right Ø6UT
    Gastric Ø6U2
    Hand
      Left Ø5UH
      Right Ø5UG
    Hemiazygos Ø5U1
    Hepatic Ø6U4
    Hypogastric
      Left Ø6UJ
      Right Ø6UH
    Inferior Mesenteric Ø6U6
    Innominate
      Left Ø5U4
      Right Ø5U3
    Internal Jugular
      Left Ø5UN
      Right Ø5UM

Supplement — *continued*
  Vein — *continued*
    Intracranial Ø5UL
    Lower Ø6UY
    Portal Ø6U8
    Pulmonary
      Left Ø2UT
      Right Ø2US
    Renal
      Left Ø6UB
      Right Ø6U9
    Saphenous
      Left Ø6UQ
      Right Ø6UP
    Splenic Ø6U1
    Subclavian
      Left Ø5U6
      Right Ø5U5
    Superior Mesenteric Ø6U5
    Upper Ø5UY
    Vertebral
      Left Ø5US
      Right Ø5UR
  Vena Cava
    Inferior Ø6UØ
    Superior Ø2UV
  Ventricle
    Left Ø2UL
    Right Ø2UK
  Vertebra
    Cervical ØPU3
    Lumbar ØQUØ
    Thoracic ØPU4
  Vesicle
    Bilateral ØVU3
    Left ØVU2
    Right ØVU1
  Vocal Cord
    Left ØCUV
    Right ØCUT
  Vulva ØUUM
  Wrist Region
    Left ØXUH
    Right ØXUG

Supraclavicular (Virchow's) lymph node
  use Lymphatic, Left Neck
  use Lymphatic, Right Neck
Supraclavicular nerve *use* Cervical Plexus
Suprahyoid lymph node *use* Lymphatic, Head
Suprahyoid muscle
  use Neck Muscle, Left
  use Neck Muscle, Right
Suprainguinal lymph node *use* Lymphatic, Pelvis
Supraorbital vein
  use Face Vein, Left
  use Face Vein, Right
Suprarenal gland
  use Adrenal Gland
  use Adrenal Gland, Bilateral
  use Adrenal Gland, Left
  use Adrenal Gland, Right
Suprarenal plexus *use* Abdominal Sympathetic Nerve
Suprascapular nerve *use* Brachial Plexus
Supraspinatus fascia
  use Subcutaneous Tissue and Fascia, Left Upper Arm
  use Subcutaneous Tissue and Fascia, Right Upper Arm
Supraspinatus muscle
  use Shoulder Muscle, Left
  use Shoulder Muscle, Right
Supraspinous ligament
  use Lower Spine Bursa and Ligament
  use Upper Spine Bursa and Ligament
Suprasternal notch *use* Sternum
Supratrochlear lymph node
  use Lymphatic, Left Upper Extremity
  use Lymphatic, Right Upper Extremity
Sural artery
  use Popliteal Artery, Left
  use Popliteal Artery, Right
Surpass Streamline™ Flow Diverter *use* Intraluminal Device, Flow Diverter in Ø3V
Suspension
  Bladder Neck *see* Reposition, Bladder Neck ØTSC
  Kidney *see* Reposition, Urinary System ØTS
  Urethra *see* Reposition, Urinary System ØTS

Supplement — Suspension

Suspension — *continued*
　Urethrovesical *see* Reposition, Bladder Neck ØTSC
　Uterus *see* Reposition, Uterus ØUS9
　Vagina *see* Reposition, Vagina ØUSG
Sustained Release Drug-eluting Intraluminal Device
　Dilation
　　Anterior Tibial
　　　Left X27Q385
　　　Right X27P385
　　Femoral
　　　Left X27J385
　　　Right X27H385
　　Peroneal
　　　Left X27U385
　　　Right X27T385
　　Popliteal
　　　Left Distal X27N385
　　　Left Proximal X27L385
　　　Right Distal X27M385
　　　Right Proximal X27K385
　　Posterior Tibial
　　　Left X27S385
　　　Right X27R385
　　Four or More
　　　Anterior Tibial
　　　　Left X27Q3C5
　　　　Right X27P3C5
　　　Femoral
　　　　Left X27J3C5
　　　　Right X27H3C5
　　　Peroneal
　　　　Left X27U3C5
　　　　Right X27T3C5
　　　Popliteal
　　　　Left Distal X27N3C5
　　　　Left Proximal X27L3C5
　　　　Right Distal X27M3C5
　　　　Right Proximal X27K3C5
　　　Posterior Tibial
　　　　Left X27S3C5
　　　　Right X27R3C5
　　Three
　　　Anterior Tibial
　　　　Left X27Q3B5
　　　　Right X27P3B5
　　　Femoral
　　　　Left X27J3B5
　　　　Right X27H3B5
　　　Peroneal
　　　　Left X27U3B5
　　　　Right X27T3B5
　　　Popliteal
　　　　Left Distal X27N3B5
　　　　Left Proximal X27L3B5
　　　　Right Distal X27M3B5
　　　　Right Proximal X27K3B5
　　　Posterior Tibial
　　　　Left X27S3B5
　　　　Right X27R3B5
　　Two
　　　Anterior Tibial
　　　　Left X27Q395
　　　　Right X27P395
　　　Femoral
　　　　Left X27J395
　　　　Right X27H395
　　　Peroneal
　　　　Left X27U395
　　　　Right X27T395
　　　Popliteal
　　　　Left Distal X27N395
　　　　Left Proximal X27L395
　　　　Right Distal X27M395
　　　　Right Proximal X27K395
　　　Posterior Tibial
　　　　Left X27S395
　　　　Right X27R395
Suture
　Laceration repair *see* Repair
　Ligation *see* Occlusion
Suture Removal
　Extremity
　　Lower 8EØYXY8
　　Upper 8EØXXY8
　Head and Neck Region 8EØ9XY8
　Trunk Region 8EØWXY8

Sutureless valve, Perceval *use* Zooplastic Tissue, Rapid Deployment Technique in New Technology
Sweat gland *use* Skin
Sympathectomy *see* Excision, Peripheral Nervous System Ø1B
SynCardia Total Artificial Heart *use* Synthetic Substitute
Synchra CRT-P *use* Cardiac Resynchronization Pacemaker Pulse Generator in ØJH
SynchroMed pump *use* Infusion Device, Pump in Subcutaneous Tissue and Fascia
Synechiotomy, iris *see* Release, Eye Ø8N
Synovectomy
　Lower joint *see* Excision, Lower Joints ØSB
　Upper joint *see* Excision, Upper Joints ØRB
Synthetic Human Angiotensin II XWØ
Systemic Nuclear Medicine Therapy
　Abdomen CW7Ø
　Anatomical Regions, Multiple CW7YYZZ
　Chest CW73
　Thyroid CW7G
　Whole Body CW7N

T

Tagraxofusp-erzs Antineoplastic XWØ
Takedown
　Arteriovenous shunt *see* Removal of device from, Upper Arteries Ø3P
　Arteriovenous shunt, with creation of new shunt *see* Bypass, Upper Arteries Ø31
　Stoma
　　see Excision
　　see Reposition
Talent® Converter *use* Intraluminal Device
Talent® Occluder *use* Intraluminal Device
Talent® Stent Graft (abdominal) (thoracic) *use* Intraluminal Device
Talocalcaneal (subtalar) joint
　use Tarsal Joint, Left
　use Tarsal Joint, Right
Talocalcaneal ligament
　use Foot Bursa and Ligament, Left
　use Foot Bursa and Ligament, Right
Talocalcaneonavicular joint
　use Tarsal Joint, Left
　use Tarsal Joint, Right
Talocalcaneonavicular ligament
　use Foot Bursa and Ligament, Left
　use Foot Bursa and Ligament, Right
Talocrural joint
　use Ankle Joint, Left
　use Joint, Ankle, Right
Talofibular ligament
　use Ankle Bursa and Ligament, Left
　use Ankle Bursa and Ligament, Right
Talus bone
　use Tarsal, Left
　use Tarsal, Right
TandemHeart® System *use* Short-term External Heart Assist System in Heart and Great Vessels
Tarsectomy
　see Excision, Lower Bones ØQB
　see Resection, Lower Bones ØQT
Tarsometatarsal ligament
　use Foot Bursa and Ligament, Left
　use Foot Bursa and Ligament, Right
Tarsorrhaphy *see* Repair, Eye Ø8Q
Tattooing
　Cornea 3EØCXMZ
　Skin *see* Introduction of substance in or on, Skin 3EØØ
TAXUS® Liberté® Paclitaxel-eluting Coronary Stent System *use* Intraluminal Device, Drug-eluting in Heart and Great Vessels
TBNA (transbronchial needle aspiration)
　Fluid or gas *see* Drainage, Respiratory System ØB9
　Tissue biopsy *see* Extraction, Respiratory System ØBD
Telemetry 4A12X4Z
　Ambulatory 4A12X45
Temperature gradient study 4AØZXKZ
Temporal lobe *use* Cerebral Hemisphere
Temporalis muscle *use* Head Muscle
Temporoparietalis muscle *use* Head Muscle
Tendolysis *see* Release, Tendons ØLN

Tendonectomy
　see Excision, Tendons ØLB
　see Resection, Tendons ØLT
Tendonoplasty, tenoplasty
　see Repair, Tendons ØLQ
　see Replacement, Tendons ØLR
　see Supplement, Tendons ØLU
Tendorrhaphy *see* Repair, Tendons ØLQ
Tendototomy
　see Division, Tendons ØL8
　see Drainage, Tendons ØL9
Tenectomy, tenonectomy
　see Excision, Tendons ØLB
　see Resection, Tendons ØLT
Tenolysis *see* Release, Tendons ØLN
Tenontorrhaphy *see* Repair, Tendons ØLQ
Tenontotomy
　see Division, Tendons ØL8
　see Drainage, Tendons ØL9
Tenorrhaphy *see* Repair, Tendons ØLQ
Tenosynovectomy
　see Excision, Tendons ØLB
　see Resection, Tendons ØLT
Tenotomy
　see Division, Tendons ØL8
　see Drainage, Tendons ØL9
Tensor fasciae latae muscle
　use Hip Muscle, Left
　use Hip Muscle, Right
Tensor veli palatini muscle *use* Tongue, Palate, Pharynx Muscle
Tenth cranial nerve *use* Vagus Nerve
Tentorium cerebelli *use* Dura Mater
Teres major muscle
　use Shoulder Muscle, Left
　use Shoulder Muscle, Right
Teres minor muscle
　use Shoulder Muscle, Left
　use Shoulder Muscle, Right
Termination of pregnancy
　Aspiration curettage 1ØAØ7ZZ
　Dilation and curettage 1ØAØ7ZZ
　Hysterotomy 1ØAØØZZ
　Intra-amniotic injection 1ØAØ3ZZ
　Laminaria 1ØAØ7ZW
　Vacuum 1ØAØ7Z6
Testectomy
　see Excision, Male Reproductive System ØVB
　see Resection, Male Reproductive System ØVT
Testicular artery *use* Abdominal Aorta
Testing
　Glaucoma 4AØ7XBZ
　Hearing *see* Hearing Assessment, Diagnostic Audiology F13
　Mental health *see* Psychological Tests
　Muscle function, electromyography (EMG) *see* Measurement, Musculoskeletal 4AØF
　Muscle function, manual *see* Motor Function Assessment, Rehabilitation FØ1
　Neurophysiologic monitoring, intra-operative *see* Monitoring, Physiological Systems 4A1
　Range of motion *see* Motor Function Assessment, Rehabilitation FØ1
　Vestibular function *see* Vestibular Assessment, Diagnostic Audiology F15
Thalamectomy *see* Excision, Thalamus ØØB9
Thalamotomy *see* Drainage, Thalamus ØØ99
Thenar muscle
　use Hand Muscle, Left
　use Hand Muscle, Right
Therapeutic Massage
　Musculoskeletal System 8EØKX1Z
　Reproductive System
　　Prostate 8EØVX1C
　　Rectum 8EØVX1D
Therapeutic occlusion coil(s) *use* Intraluminal Device
Thermography 4AØZXKZ
Thermotherapy, prostate *see* Destruction, Prostate ØV5Ø
Third cranial nerve *use* Oculomotor Nerve
Third occipital nerve *use* Cervical Nerve
Third ventricle *use* Cerebral Ventricle
Thoracectomy *see* Excision, Anatomical Regions, General ØWB
Thoracentesis *see* Drainage, Anatomical Regions, General ØW9
Thoracic aortic plexus *use* Thoracic Sympathetic Nerve

Subterms under main terms may continue to next column or page

Thoracic esophagus *use* Esophagus, Middle
Thoracic facet joint *use* Thoracic Vertebral Joint
Thoracic ganglion *use* Thoracic Sympathetic Nerve
Thoracoacromial artery
   use Axillary Artery, Left
   use Axillary Artery, Right
Thoracentesis *see* Drainage, Anatomical Regions, General 0W9
Thoracolumbar facet joint *use* Thoracolumbar Vertebral Joint
Thoracoplasty
   see Repair, Anatomical Regions, General 0WQ
   see Supplement, Anatomical Regions, General 0WU
Thoracostomy, for lung collapse *see* Drainage, Respiratory System 0B9
Thoracostomy tube *use* Drainage Device
Thoracotomy *see* Drainage, Anatomical Regions, General 0W9
Thoratec IVAD (Implantable Ventricular Assist Device) *use* Implantable Heart Assist System in Heart and Great Vessels
Thoratec Paracorporeal Ventricular Assist Device *use* Short-term External Heart Assist System in Heart and Great Vessels
Thrombectomy *see* Extirpation
Thymectomy
   see Excision, Lymphatic and Hemic Systems 07B
   see Resection, Lymphatic and Hemic Systems 07T
Thymopexy
   see Repair, Lymphatic and Hemic Systems 07Q
   see Reposition, Lymphatic and Hemic Systems 07S
Thymus gland *use* Thymus
Thyroarytenoid muscle
   use Neck Muscle, Left
   use Neck Muscle, Right
Thyrocervical trunk
   use Thyroid Artery, Left
   use Thyroid Artery, Right
Thyroid cartilage *use* Larynx
Thyroidectomy
   see Excision, Endocrine System 0GB
   see Resection, Endocrine System 0GT
Thyroidorrhaphy *see* Repair, Endocrine System 0GQ
Thyroidoscopy 0GJK4ZZ
Thyroidotomy *see* Drainage, Endocrine System 0G9
Tibial insert *use* Liner in Lower Joints
Tibialis anterior muscle
   use Lower Leg Muscle, Left
   use Lower Leg Muscle, Right
Tibialis posterior muscle
   use Lower Leg Muscle, Left
   use Lower Leg Muscle, Right
Tibiofemoral joint
   use Knee Joint, Left
   use Knee Joint, Right
   use Knee Joint, Tibial Surface, Left
   use Knee Joint, Tibial Surface, Right
Tibioperoneal trunk
   use Popliteal Artery, Left
   use Popliteal Artery, Right
Tisagenlecleucel *use* Engineered Autologous Chimeric Antigen Receptor T-cell Immunotherapy
Tissue bank graft *use* Nonautologous Tissue Substitute
Tissue expander (inflatable) (injectable)
   use Tissue Expander in Skin and Breast
   use Tissue Expander in Subcutaneous Tissue and Fascia
Tissue Expander
   Insertion of device in
     Breast
       Bilateral 0HHV
       Left 0HHU
       Right 0HHT
     Nipple
       Left 0HHX
       Right 0HHW
     Subcutaneous Tissue and Fascia
       Abdomen 0JH8
       Back 0JH7
       Buttock 0JH9
       Chest 0JH6
       Face 0JH1
       Foot
         Left 0JHR
         Right 0JHQ
       Hand
         Left 0JHK

Tissue Expander — *continued*
   Insertion of device in — *continued*
     Subcutaneous Tissue and Fascia — *continued*
       Hand — *continued*
         Right 0JHJ
       Lower Arm
         Left 0JHH
         Right 0JHG
       Lower Leg
         Left 0JHP
         Right 0JHN
       Neck
         Left 0JH5
         Right 0JH4
       Pelvic Region 0JHC
       Perineum 0JHB
       Scalp 0JH0
       Upper Arm
         Left 0JHF
         Right 0JHD
       Upper Leg
         Left 0JHM
         Right 0JHL
   Removal of device from
     Breast
       Left 0HPU
       Right 0HPT
     Subcutaneous Tissue and Fascia
       Head and Neck 0JPS
       Lower Extremity 0JPW
       Trunk 0JPT
       Upper Extremity 0JPV
   Revision of device in
     Breast
       Left 0HWU
       Right 0HWT
     Subcutaneous Tissue and Fascia
       Head and Neck 0JWS
       Lower Extremity 0JWW
       Trunk 0JWT
       Upper Extremity 0JWV
Tissue Plasminogen Activator (tPA) (r-tPA) *use* Other Thrombolytic
Titanium Sternal Fixation System (TSFS)
   use Internal Fixation Device, Rigid Plate in 0PS
   use Internal Fixation Device, Rigid Plate in 0PH
Tomographic (Tomo) Nuclear Medicine Imaging
   Abdomen CW20
   Abdomen and Chest CW24
   Abdomen and Pelvis CW21
   Anatomical Regions, Multiple CW2YYZZ
   Bladder, Kidneys and Ureters CT23
   Brain C020
   Breast CH2YYZZ
     Bilateral CH22
     Left CH21
     Right CH20
   Bronchi and Lungs CB22
   Central Nervous System C02YYZZ
   Cerebrospinal Fluid C025
   Chest CW23
   Chest and Abdomen CW24
   Chest and Neck CW26
   Digestive System CD2YYZZ
   Endocrine System CG2YYZZ
   Extremity
     Lower CW2D
       Bilateral CP2F
       Left CP2D
       Right CP2C
     Upper CW2M
       Bilateral CP2B
       Left CP29
       Right CP28
   Gallbladder CF24
   Gastrointestinal Tract CD27
   Gland, Parathyroid CG21
   Head and Neck CW2B
   Heart C22YYZZ
     Right and Left C226
   Hepatobiliary System and Pancreas CF2YYZZ
   Kidneys, Ureters and Bladder CT23
   Liver CF25
   Liver and Spleen CF26
   Lungs and Bronchi CB22
   Lymphatics and Hematologic System C72YYZZ
   Musculoskeletal System, Other CP2YYZZ
   Myocardium C22G

Tomographic (Tomo) Nuclear Medicine Imaging — *continued*
   Neck and Chest CW26
   Neck and Head CW2B
   Pancreas and Hepatobiliary System CF2YYZZ
   Pelvic Region CW2J
   Pelvis CP26
   Pelvis and Abdomen CW21
   Pelvis and Spine CP27
   Respiratory System CB2YYZZ
   Skin CH2YYZZ
   Skull CP21
   Skull and Cervical Spine CP23
   Spine
     Cervical CP22
     Cervical and Skull CP23
     Lumbar CP2H
     Thoracic CP2G
     Thoracolumbar CP2J
   Spine and Pelvis CP27
   Spleen C722
   Spleen and Liver CF26
   Subcutaneous Tissue CH2YYZZ
   Thorax CP24
   Ureters, Kidneys and Bladder CT23
   Urinary System CT2YYZZ
Tomography, computerized *see* Computerized Tomography (CT Scan)
Tongue, base of *use* Pharynx
Tonometry 4A07XBZ
Tonsillectomy
   see Excision, Mouth and Throat 0CB
   see Resection, Mouth and Throat 0CT
Tonsillotomy *see* Drainage, Mouth and Throat 0C9
Total Anomalous Pulmonary Venous Return (TAPVR) repair
   see Bypass, Atrium, Left 0217
   see Bypass, Vena Cava, Superior 021V
Total artificial (replacement) heart *use* Synthetic Substitute
Total parenteral nutrition (TPN) *see* Introduction of Nutritional Substance
Trachectomy
   see Excision, Trachea 0BB1
   see Resection, Trachea 0BT1
Trachelectomy
   see Excision, Cervix 0UBC
   see Resection, Cervix 0UTC
Trachelopexy
   see Repair, Cervix 0UQC
   see Reposition, Cervix 0USC
Tracheloplasty *see* Repair, Cervix 0UQC
Trachelorrhaphy *see* Repair, Cervix 0UQC
Trachelotomy *see* Drainage, Cervix 0U9C
Tracheobronchial lymph node *use* Lymphatic, Thorax
Tracheoesophageal fistulization 0B110D6
Tracheolysis *see* Release, Respiratory System 0BN
Tracheoplasty
   see Repair, Respiratory System 0BQ
   see Supplement, Respiratory System 0BU
Tracheorrhaphy *see* Repair, Respiratory System 0BQ
Tracheoscopy 0BJ18ZZ
Tracheostomy *see* Bypass, Respiratory System 0B1
Tracheostomy Device
   Bypass, Trachea 0B11
   Change device in, Trachea 0B21XFZ
   Removal of device from, Trachea 0BP1
   Revision of device in, Trachea 0BW1
Tracheostomy tube *use* Tracheostomy Device in Respiratory System
Tracheotomy *see* Drainage, Respiratory System 0B9
Traction
   Abdominal Wall 2W63X
   Arm
     Lower
       Left 2W6DX
       Right 2W6CX
     Upper
       Left 2W6BX
       Right 2W6AX
   Back 2W65X
   Chest Wall 2W64X
   Extremity
     Lower
       Left 2W6MX
       Right 2W6LX
     Upper
       Left 2W69X

Traction — *continued*
Extremity — *continued*
Upper — *continued*
Right 2W68X
Face 2W61X
Finger
Left 2W6KX
Right 2W6JX
Foot
Left 2W6TX
Right 2W6SX
Hand
Left 2W6FX
Right 2W6EX
Head 2W60X
Inguinal Region
Left 2W67X
Right 2W66X
Leg
Lower
Left 2W6RX
Right 2W6QX
Upper
Left 2W6PX
Right 2W6NX
Neck 2W62X
Thumb
Left 2W6HX
Right 2W6GX
Toe
Left 2W6VX
Right 2W6UX
Tractotomy *see* Division, Central Nervous System and Cranial Nerves 008
Tragus
use External Ear, Bilateral
use External Ear, Left
use External Ear, Right
Training, caregiver *see* Caregiver Training
TRAM (transverse rectus abdominis myocutaneous) flap reconstruction
Free *see* Replacement, Skin and Breast 0HR
Pedicled *see* Transfer, Muscles 0KX
Transdermal Glomerular Filtration Rate (GFR) Measurement System XT25XE5
Transection *see* Division
Transfer
Buccal Mucosa 0CX4
Bursa and Ligament
Abdomen
Left 0MXJ
Right 0MXH
Ankle
Left 0MXR
Right 0MXQ
Elbow
Left 0MX4
Right 0MX3
Foot
Left 0MXT
Right 0MXS
Hand
Left 0MX8
Right 0MX7
Head and Neck 0MX0
Hip
Left 0MXM
Right 0MXL
Knee
Left 0MXP
Right 0MXN
Lower Extremity
Left 0MXW
Right 0MXV
Perineum 0MXK
Rib(s) 0MXG
Shoulder
Left 0MX2
Right 0MX1
Spine
Lower 0MXD
Upper 0MXC
Sternum 0MXF
Upper Extremity
Left 0MXB
Right 0MX9
Wrist
Left 0MX6

Transfer — *continued*
Bursa and Ligament — *continued*
Wrist — *continued*
Right 0MX5
Finger
Left 0XXP0ZM
Right 0XXN0ZL
Gingiva
Lower 0CX6
Upper 0CX5
Intestine
Large 0DXE
Small 0DX8
Lip
Lower 0CX1
Upper 0CX0
Muscle
Abdomen
Left 0KXL
Right 0KXK
Extraocular
Left 08XM
Right 08XL
Facial 0KX1
Foot
Left 0KXW
Right 0KXV
Hand
Left 0KXD
Right 0KXC
Head 0KX0
Hip
Left 0KXP
Right 0KXN
Lower Arm and Wrist
Left 0KXB
Right 0KX9
Lower Leg
Left 0KXT
Right 0KXS
Neck
Left 0KX3
Right 0KX2
Perineum 0KXM
Shoulder
Left 0KX6
Right 0KX5
Thorax
Left 0KXJ
Right 0KXH
Tongue, Palate, Pharynx 0KX4
Trunk
Left 0KXG
Right 0KXF
Upper Arm
Left 0KX8
Right 0KX7
Upper Leg
Left 0KXR
Right 0KXQ
Nerve
Abducens 00XL
Accessory 00XR
Acoustic 00XN
Cervical 01X1
Facial 00XM
Femoral 01XD
Glossopharyngeal 00XP
Hypoglossal 00XS
Lumbar 01XB
Median 01X5
Oculomotor 00XH
Olfactory 00XF
Optic 00XG
Peroneal 01XH
Phrenic 01X2
Pudendal 01XC
Radial 01X6
Sciatic 01XF
Thoracic 01X8
Tibial 01XG
Trigeminal 00XK
Trochlear 00XJ
Ulnar 01X4
Vagus 00XQ
Palate, Soft 0CX3
Prepuce 0VXT
Skin
Abdomen 0HX7XZZ

Transfer — *continued*
Skin — *continued*
Back 0HX6XZZ
Buttock 0HX8XZZ
Chest 0HX5XZZ
Ear
Left 0HX3XZZ
Right 0HX2XZZ
Face 0HX1XZZ
Foot
Left 0HXNXZZ
Right 0HXMXZZ
Hand
Left 0HXGXZZ
Right 0HXFXZZ
Inguinal 0HXAXZZ
Lower Arm
Left 0HXEXZZ
Right 0HXDXZZ
Lower Leg
Left 0HXLXZZ
Right 0HXKXZZ
Neck 0HX4XZZ
Perineum 0HX9XZZ
Scalp 0HX0XZZ
Upper Arm
Left 0HXCXZZ
Right 0HXBXZZ
Upper Leg
Left 0HXJXZZ
Right 0HXHXZZ
Stomach 0DX6
Subcutaneous Tissue and Fascia
Abdomen 0JX8
Back 0JX7
Buttock 0JX9
Chest 0JX6
Face 0JX1
Foot
Left 0JXR
Right 0JXQ
Hand
Left 0JXK
Right 0JXJ
Lower Arm
Left 0JXH
Right 0JXG
Lower Leg
Left 0JXP
Right 0JXN
Neck
Left 0JX5
Right 0JX4
Pelvic Region 0JXC
Perineum 0JXB
Scalp 0JX0
Upper Arm
Left 0JXF
Right 0JXD
Upper Leg
Left 0JXM
Right 0JXL
Tendon
Abdomen
Left 0LXG
Right 0LXF
Ankle
Left 0LXT
Right 0LXS
Foot
Left 0LXW
Right 0LXV
Hand
Left 0LX8
Right 0LX7
Head and Neck 0LX0
Hip
Left 0LXK
Right 0LXJ
Knee
Left 0LXR
Right 0LXQ
Lower Arm and Wrist
Left 0LX6
Right 0LX5
Lower Leg
Left 0LXP
Right 0LXN
Perineum 0LXH

▽ **Subterms under main terms may continue to next column or page**

Transfer — *continued*
  Tendon — *continued*
    Shoulder
      Left 0LX2
      Right 0LX1
    Thorax
      Left 0LXD
      Right 0LXC
    Trunk
      Left 0LXB
      Right 0LX9
    Upper Arm
      Left 0LX4
      Right 0LX3
    Upper Leg
      Left 0LXM
      Right 0LXL
  Tongue 0CX7
Transfusion
  Products of Conception
    Antihemophilic Factors 3027
    Blood
      Platelets 3027
      Red Cells 3027
        Frozen 3027
      White Cells 3027
      Whole 3027
    Factor IX 3027
    Fibrinogen 3027
    Globulin 3027
    Plasma
      Fresh 3027
      Frozen 3027
    Plasma Cryoprecipitate 3027
    Serum Albumin 3027
  Vein
    4-Factor Prothrombin Complex Concentrate
      30280B1
    Central
      Antihemophilic Factors 3024
      Blood
        Platelets 3024
        Red Cells 3024
          Frozen 3024
        White Cells 3024
        Whole 3024
      Bone Marrow 3024
      Factor IX 3024
      Fibrinogen 3024
      Globulin 3024
      Plasma
        Fresh 3024
        Frozen 3024
      Plasma Cryoprecipitate 3024
      Serum Albumin 3024
      Stem Cells
        Cord Blood 3024
        Embryonic 3024
        Hematopoietic 3024
        T-cell Depleted Hematopoietic
          3024
    Peripheral
      Antihemophilic Factors 3023
      Blood
        Platelets 3023
        Red Cells 3023
          Frozen 3023
        White Cells 3023
        Whole 3023
      Bone Marrow 3023
      Factor IX 3023
      Fibrinogen 3023
      Globulin 3023
      Plasma
        Fresh 3023
        Frozen 3023
      Plasma Cryoprecipitate 3023
      Serum Albumin 3023
      Stem Cells
        Cord Blood 3023
        Embryonic 3023
        Hematopoietic 3023
        T-cell Depleted Hematopoietic
          3023
Transplant *see* Transplantation
Transplantation
  Bone marrow *see* Transfusion, Circulatory 302
  Esophagus 0DY50Z
  Face 0WY20Z

Transplantation — *continued*
  Hand
    Left 0XYK0Z
    Right 0XYJ0Z
  Heart 02YA0Z
  Hematopoietic cell *see* Transfusion, Circulatory
    302
  Intestine
    Large 0DYE0Z
    Small 0DY80Z
  Kidney
    Left 0TY10Z
    Right 0TY00Z
  Liver 0FY00Z
  Lung
    Bilateral 0BYM0Z
    Left 0BYL0Z
    Lower Lobe
      Left 0BYJ0Z
      Right 0BYF0Z
    Middle Lobe, Right 0BYD0Z
    Right 0BYK0Z
    Upper Lobe
      Left 0BYG0Z
      Right 0BYC0Z
  Lung Lingula 0BYH0Z
  Ovary
    Left 0UY10Z
    Right 0UY00Z
  Pancreas 0FYG0Z
  Products of Conception 10Y0
  Spleen 07YP0Z
  Stem cell *see* Transfusion, Circulatory 302
  Stomach 0DY60Z
  Thymus 07YM0Z
  Uterus 0UY90Z
Transposition
  see Bypass
  see Reposition
  see Transfer
Transversalis fascia *use* Subcutaneous Tissue and
  Fascia, Trunk
Transverse acetabular ligament
  use Hip Bursa and Ligament, Left
  use Hip Bursa and Ligament, Right
Transverse (cutaneous) cervical nerve *use* Cervical
  Plexus
Transverse facial artery
  use Temporal Artery, Left
  use Temporal Artery, Right
Transverse foramen *use* Cervical Vertebra
Transverse humeral ligament
  use Shoulder Bursa and Ligament, Left
  use Shoulder Bursa and Ligament, Right
Transverse ligament of atlas *use* Head and Neck
  Bursa and Ligament
Transverse process
  use Cervical Vertebra
  use Lumbar Vertebra
  use Thoracic Vertebra
Transverse Rectus Abdominis Myocutaneous Flap
  Replacement
    Bilateral 0HRV076
    Left 0HRU076
    Right 0HRT076
  Transfer
    Left 0KXL
    Right 0KXK
Transverse scapular ligament
  use Shoulder Bursa and Ligament, Left
  use Shoulder Bursa and Ligament, Right
Transverse thoracis muscle
  use Thorax Muscle, Left
  use Thorax Muscle, Right
Transversospinalis muscle
  use Trunk Muscle, Left
  use Trunk Muscle, Right
Transversus abdominis muscle
  use Abdomen Muscle, Left
  use Abdomen Muscle, Right
Trapezium bone
  use Carpal, Left
  use Carpal, Right
Trapezius muscle
  use Trunk Muscle, Left
  use Trunk Muscle, Right

Trapezoid bone
  use Carpal, Left
  use Carpal, Right
Triceps brachii muscle
  use Upper Arm Muscle, Left
  use Upper Arm Muscle, Right
Tricuspid annulus *use* Tricuspid Valve
Trifacial nerve *use* Trigeminal Nerve
Trifecta™ Valve (aortic) *use* Zooplastic Tissue in Heart
  and Great Vessels
Trigone of bladder *use* Bladder
**TriGuard 3™ CEPD (cerebral embolic protection
  device)** X2A6325
Trimming, excisional *see* Excision
Triquetral bone
  use Carpal, Left
  use Carpal, Right
Trochanteric bursa
  use Hip Bursa and Ligament, Left
  use Hip Bursa and Ligament, Right
**TUMT (transurethral microwave thermotherapy
  of prostate)** 0V507ZZ
TUNA (transurethral needle ablation of prostate)
  0V507ZZ
Tunneled central venous catheter *use* Vascular Access Device, Tunneled in Subcutaneous Tissue
  and Fascia
Tunneled spinal (intrathecal) catheter *use* Infusion
  Device
Turbinectomy
  see Excision, Ear, Nose, Sinus 09B
  see Resection, Ear, Nose, Sinus 09T
Turbinoplasty
  see Repair, Ear, Nose, Sinus 09Q
  see Replacement, Ear, Nose, Sinus 09R
  see Supplement, Ear, Nose, Sinus 09U
Turbinotomy
  see Division, Ear, Nose, Sinus 098
  see Drainage, Ear, Nose, Sinus 099
TURP (transurethral resection of prostate) 0VB07ZZ
  see Excision, Prostate 0VB0
  see Resection, Prostate 0VT0
Twelfth cranial nerve *use* Hypoglossal Nerve
Two lead pacemaker *use* Pacemaker, Dual Chamber
  in 0JH
Tympanic cavity
  use Middle Ear, Left
  use Middle Ear, Right
Tympanic nerve *use* Glossopharyngeal Nerve
Tympanic part of temporal bone
  use Temporal Bone, Left
  use Temporal Bone, Right
Tympanogram *see* Hearing Assessment, Diagnostic
  Audiology F13
Tympanoplasty
  see Repair, Ear, Nose, Sinus 09Q
  see Replacement, Ear, Nose, Sinus 09R
  see Supplement, Ear, Nose, Sinus 09U
Tympanosympathectomy *see* Excision, Nerve, Head
  and Neck Sympathetic 01BK
Tympanotomy *see* Drainage, Ear, Nose, Sinus 099
TYRX Antibacterial Envelope *use* Anti-Infective Envelope

U

Ulnar collateral carpal ligament
  use Wrist Bursa and Ligament, Left
  use Wrist Bursa and Ligament, Right
Ulnar collateral ligament
  use Elbow Bursa and Ligament, Left
  use Elbow Bursa and Ligament, Right
Ulnar notch
  use Radius, Left
  use Radius, Right
Ulnar vein
  use Brachial Vein, Left
  use Brachial Vein, Right
Ultrafiltration
  Hemodialysis *see* Performance, Urinary 5A1D
  Therapeutic plasmapheresis *see* Pheresis, Circula-
    tory 6A55
Ultraflex™ Precision Colonic Stent System *use* Intraluminal Device
ULTRAPRO Hernia System (UHS) *use* Synthetic Substitute

ULTRAPRO Partially Absorbable Lightweight Mesh
   use Synthetic Substitute
ULTRAPRO Plug *use* Synthetic Substitute
Ultrasonic osteogenic stimulator
   use Bone Growth Stimulator in Head and Facial
     Bones
   use Bone Growth Stimulator in Lower Bones
   use Bone Growth Stimulator in Upper Bones
Ultrasonography
   Abdomen BW40ZZZ
   Abdomen and Pelvis BW41ZZZ
   Abdominal Wall BH49ZZZ
   Aorta
     Abdominal, Intravascular B440ZZ3
     Thoracic, Intravascular B340ZZ3
   Appendix BD48ZZZ
   Artery
     Brachiocephalic-Subclavian, Right, Intravas-
      cular B341ZZ3
     Celiac and Mesenteric, Intravascular B44KZZ3
     Common Carotid
      Bilateral, Intravascular B345ZZ3
      Left, Intravascular B344ZZ3
      Right, Intravascular B343ZZ3
     Coronary
      Multiple B241YZZ
       Intravascular B241ZZ3
       Transesophageal B241ZZ4
      Single B240YZZ
       Intravascular B240ZZ3
       Transesophageal B240ZZ4
     Femoral, Intravascular B44LZZ3
     Inferior Mesenteric, Intravascular B445ZZ3
     Internal Carotid
      Bilateral, Intravascular B348ZZ3
      Left, Intravascular B347ZZ3
      Right, Intravascular B346ZZ3
     Intra-Abdominal, Other, Intravascular
      B44BZZ3
     Intracranial, Intravascular B34RZZ3
     Lower Extremity
      Bilateral, Intravascular B44HZZ3
      Left, Intravascular B44GZZ3
      Right, Intravascular B44FZZ3
     Mesenteric and Celiac, Intravascular B44KZZ3
     Ophthalmic, Intravascular B34VZZ3
     Penile, Intravascular B44NZZ3
     Pulmonary
      Left, Intravascular B34TZZ3
      Right, Intravascular B34SZZ3
     Renal
      Bilateral, Intravascular B448ZZ3
      Left, Intravascular B447ZZ3
      Right, Intravascular B446ZZ3
     Subclavian, Left, Intravascular B342ZZ3
     Superior Mesenteric, Intravascular B444ZZ3
     Upper Extremity
      Bilateral, Intravascular B34KZZ3
      Left, Intravascular B34JZZ3
      Right, Intravascular B34HZZ3
   Bile Duct BF40ZZZ
   Bile Duct and Gallbladder BF43ZZZ
   Bladder BT40ZZZ
     and Kidney BT4JZZZ
   Brain B040ZZZ
   Breast
     Bilateral BH42ZZZ
     Left BH41ZZZ
     Right BH40ZZZ
   Chest Wall BH4BZZZ
   Coccyx BR4FZZZ
   Connective Tissue
     Lower Extremity BL41ZZZ
     Upper Extremity BL40ZZZ
   Duodenum BD49ZZZ
   Elbow
     Left, Densitometry BP4HZZ1
     Right, Densitometry BP4GZZ1
   Esophagus BD41ZZZ
   Extremity
     Lower BH48ZZZ
     Upper BH47ZZZ
   Eye
     Bilateral B847ZZZ
     Left B846ZZZ
     Right B845ZZZ
   Fallopian Tube
     Bilateral BU42

Ultrasonography — *continued*
   Fallopian Tube — *continued*
     Left BU41
     Right BU40
   Fetal Umbilical Cord BY47ZZZ
   Fetus
     First Trimester, Multiple Gestation BY4BZZZ
     Second Trimester, Multiple Gestation
      BY4DZZZ
     Single
      First Trimester BY49ZZZ
      Second Trimester BY4CZZZ
      Third Trimester BY4FZZZ
     Third Trimester, Multiple Gestation BY4GZZZ
   Gallbladder BF42ZZZ
   Gallbladder and Bile Duct BF43ZZZ
   Gastrointestinal Tract BD47ZZZ
   Gland
     Adrenal
      Bilateral BG42ZZZ
      Left BG41ZZZ
      Right BG40ZZZ
     Parathyroid BG43ZZZ
     Thyroid BG44ZZZ
   Hand
     Left, Densitometry BP4PZZ1
     Right, Densitometry BP4NZZ1
   Head and Neck BH4CZZZ
   Heart
     Left B245YZZ
      Intravascular B245ZZ3
      Transesophageal B245ZZ4
     Pediatric B24DYZZ
      Intravascular B24DZZ3
      Transesophageal B24DZZ4
     Right B244YZZ
      Intravascular B244ZZ3
      Transesophageal B244ZZ4
     Right and Left B246YZZ
      Intravascular B246ZZ3
      Transesophageal B246ZZ4
   Heart with Aorta B24BYZZ
     Intravascular B24BZZ3
     Transesophageal B24BZZ4
   Hepatobiliary System, All BF4CZZZ
   Hip
     Bilateral BQ42ZZZ
     Left BQ41ZZZ
     Right BQ40ZZZ
   Kidney
     and Bladder BT4JZZZ
     Bilateral BT43ZZZ
     Left BT42ZZZ
     Right BT41ZZZ
     Transplant BT49ZZZ
   Knee
     Bilateral BQ49ZZZ
     Left BQ48ZZZ
     Right BQ47ZZZ
   Liver BF45ZZZ
   Liver and Spleen BF46ZZZ
   Mediastinum BB4CZZZ
   Neck BW4FZZZ
   Ovary
     Bilateral BU45
     Left BU44
     Right BU43
   Ovary and Uterus BU4C
   Pancreas BF47ZZZ
   Pelvic Region BW4GZZZ
   Pelvis and Abdomen BW41ZZZ
   Penis BV4BZZZ
   Pericardium B24CYZZ
     Intravascular B24CZZ3
     Transesophageal B24CZZ4
   Placenta BY48ZZZ
   Pleura BB4BZZZ
   Prostate and Seminal Vesicle BV49ZZZ
   Rectum BD4CZZZ
   Sacrum BR4FZZZ
   Scrotum BV44ZZZ
   Seminal Vesicle and Prostate BV49ZZZ
   Shoulder
     Left, Densitometry BP49ZZ1
     Right, Densitometry BP48ZZ1
   Spinal Cord B04BZZZ
   Spine
     Cervical BR40ZZZ
     Lumbar BR49ZZZ

Ultrasonography — *continued*
   Spine — *continued*
     Thoracic BR47ZZZ
   Spleen and Liver BF46ZZZ
   Stomach BD42ZZZ
   Tendon
     Lower Extremity BL43ZZZ
     Upper Extremity BL42ZZZ
   Ureter
     Bilateral BT48ZZZ
     Left BT47ZZZ
     Right BT46ZZZ
   Urethra BT45ZZZ
   Uterus BU46
   Uterus and Ovary BU4C
   Vein
     Jugular
      Left, Intravascular B544ZZ3
      Right, Intravascular B543ZZ3
     Lower Extremity
      Bilateral, Intravascular B54DZZ3
      Left, Intravascular B54CZZ3
      Right, Intravascular B54BZZ3
     Portal, Intravascular B54TZZ3
     Renal
      Bilateral, Intravascular B54LZZ3
      Left, Intravascular B54KZZ3
      Right, Intravascular B54JZZ3
     Spanchnic, Intravascular B54TZZ3
     Subclavian
      Left, Intravascular B547ZZ3
      Right, Intravascular B546ZZ3
     Upper Extremity
      Bilateral, Intravascular B54PZZ3
      Left, Intravascular B54NZZ3
      Right, Intravascular B54MZZ3
   Vena Cava
     Inferior, Intravascular B549ZZ3
     Superior, Intravascular B548ZZ3
   Wrist
     Left, Densitometry BP4MZZ1
     Right, Densitometry BP4LZZ1
Ultrasound bone healing system
   use Bone Growth Stimulator in Head and Facial
     Bones
   use Bone Growth Stimulator in Lower Bones
   use Bone Growth Stimulator in Upper Bones
Ultrasound Therapy
   Heart 6A75
   No Qualifier 6A75
   Vessels
     Head and Neck 6A75
     Other 6A75
     Peripheral 6A75
Ultraviolet Light Therapy, Skin 6A80
Umbilical artery
   use Internal Iliac Artery, Left
   use Internal Iliac Artery, Right
   use Lower Artery
Uniplanar external fixator
   use External Fixation Device, Monoplanar in 0PH
   use External Fixation Device, Monoplanar in 0PS
   use External Fixation Device, Monoplanar in 0QH
   use External Fixation Device, Monoplanar in 0QS
Upper GI series *see* Fluoroscopy, Gastrointestinal, Upper BD15
Ureteral orifice
   use Ureter
   use Ureter, Left
   use Ureter, Right
   use Ureters, Bilateral
Ureterectomy
   see Excision, Urinary System 0TB
   see Resection, Urinary System 0TT
Ureterocolostomy *see* Bypass, Urinary System 0T1
Ureterocystostomy *see* Bypass, Urinary System 0T1
Ureteroenterostomy *see* Bypass, Urinary System 0T1
Ureteroileostomy *see* Bypass, Urinary System 0T1
Ureterolithotomy *see* Extirpation, Urinary System 0TC
Ureterolysis *see* Release, Urinary System 0TN
Ureteroneocystostomy
   see Bypass, Urinary System 0T1
   see Reposition, Urinary System 0TS
Ureteropelvic junction (UPJ)
   use Kidney Pelvis, Left
   use Kidney Pelvis, Right
Ureteropexy
   see Repair, Urinary System 0TQ

Subterms under main terms may continue to next column or page

Ureteropexy — continued
see Reposition, Urinary System ØTS
Ureteroplasty
see Repair, Urinary System ØTQ
see Replacement, Urinary System ØTR
see Supplement, Urinary System ØTU
Ureteroplication see Restriction, Urinary System ØTV
Ureteropyelography see Fluoroscopy, Urinary System BT1
Ureterorrhaphy see Repair, Urinary System ØTQ
Ureteroscopy ØTJ98ZZ
Ureterostomy
see Bypass, Urinary System ØT1
see Drainage, Urinary System ØT9
Ureterotomy see Drainage, Urinary System ØT9
Ureteroureterostomy see Bypass, Urinary System ØT1
Ureterovesical orifice
use Ureter
use Ureter, Left
use Ureter, Right
use Ureters, Bilateral
Urethral catheterization, indwelling ØT9B70Z
Urethrectomy
see Excision, Urethra ØTBD
see Resection, Urethra ØTTD
Urethrolithotomy see Extirpation, Urethra ØTCD
Urethrolysis see Release, Urethra ØTND
Urethropexy
see Repair, Urethra ØTQD
see Reposition, Urethra ØTSD
Urethroplasty
see Repair, Urethra ØTQD
see Replacement, Urethra ØTRD
see Supplement, Urethra ØTUD
Urethrorrhaphy see Repair, Urethra ØTQD
Urethroscopy ØTJD8ZZ
Urethrotomy see Drainage, Urethra ØT9D
Uridine Triacetate XWØDX82
Urinary incontinence stimulator lead use Stimulator Lead in Urinary System
Urography see Fluoroscopy, Urinary System BT1
Ustekinumab use Other New Technology Therapeutic Substance
Uterine Artery
use Internal Iliac Artery, Left
use Internal Iliac Artery, Right
Uterine artery embolization (UAE) see Occlusion, Lower Arteries Ø4L
Uterine cornu use Uterus
Uterine tube
use Fallopian Tube, Left
use Fallopian Tube, Right
Uterine vein
use Hypogastric Vein, Left
use Hypogastric Vein, Right
Uvulectomy
see Excision, Uvula ØCBN
see Resection, Uvula ØCTN
Uvulorrhaphy see Repair, Uvula ØCQN
Uvulotomy see Drainage, Uvula ØC9N

V

Vabomere™ use Meropenem-vaborbactam Anti-infective
Vaccination see Introduction of Serum, Toxoid, and Vaccine
Vacuum extraction, obstetric 10DØ7Z6
Vaginal artery
use Internal Iliac Artery, Left
use Internal Iliac Artery, Right
Vaginal pessary use Intraluminal Device, Pessary in Female Reproductive System
Vaginal vein
use Hypogastric Vein, Left
use Hypogastric Vein, Right
Vaginectomy
see Excision, Vagina ØUBG
see Resection, Vagina ØUTG
Vaginofixation
see Repair, Vagina ØUQG
see Reposition, Vagina ØUSG
Vaginoplasty
see Repair, Vagina ØUQG
see Supplement, Vagina ØUUG
Vaginorrhaphy see Repair, Vagina ØUQG

Vaginoscopy ØUJH8ZZ
Vaginotomy see Drainage, Female Reproductive System ØU9
Vagotomy see Division, Nerve, Vagus ØØ8Q
Valiant Thoracic Stent Graft use Intraluminal Device
Valvotomy, valvulotomy
see Division, Heart and Great Vessels Ø28
see Release, Heart and Great Vessels Ø2N
Valvuloplasty
see Repair, Heart and Great Vessels Ø2Q
see Replacement, Heart and Great Vessels Ø2R
see Supplement, Heart and Great Vessels Ø2U
Valvuloplasty, Alfieri Stitch see Restriction, Valve, Mitral Ø2VG
Vascular Access Device
Totally Implantable
Insertion of device in
Abdomen ØJH8
Chest ØJH6
Lower Arm
Left ØJHH
Right ØJHG
Lower Leg
Left ØJHP
Right ØJHN
Upper Arm
Left ØJHF
Right ØJHD
Upper Leg
Left ØJHM
Right ØJHL
Removal of device from
Lower Extremity ØJPW
Trunk ØJPT
Upper Extremity ØJPV
Revision of device in
Lower Extremity ØJWW
Trunk ØJWT
Upper Extremity ØJWV
Tunneled
Insertion of device in
Abdomen ØJH8
Chest ØJH6
Lower Arm
Left ØJHH
Right ØJHG
Lower Leg
Left ØJHP
Right ØJHN
Upper Arm
Left ØJHF
Right ØJHD
Upper Leg
Left ØJHM
Right ØJHL
Removal of device from
Lower Extremity ØJPW
Trunk ØJPT
Upper Extremity ØJPV
Revision of device in
Lower Extremity ØJWW
Trunk ØJWT
Upper Extremity ØJWV
Vasectomy see Excision, Male Reproductive System ØVB
Vasography
see Fluoroscopy, Male Reproductive System BV1
see Plain Radiography, Male Reproductive System BVØ
Vasoligation see Occlusion, Male Reproductive System ØVL
Vasorrhaphy see Repair, Male Reproductive System ØVQ
Vasostomy see Bypass, Male Reproductive System ØV1
Vasotomy
Drainage see Drainage, Male Reproductive System ØV9
With ligation see Occlusion, Male Reproductive System ØVL
Vasovasostomy see Repair, Male Reproductive System ØVQ
Vastus intermedius muscle
use Upper Leg Muscle, Left
use Upper Leg Muscle, Right
Vastus lateralis muscle
use Upper Leg Muscle, Left
use Upper Leg Muscle, Right

Vastus medialis muscle
use Upper Leg Muscle, Left
use Upper Leg Muscle, Right
VCG (vectorcardiogram) see Measurement, Cardiac 4AØ2
Vectra® Vascular Access Graft use Vascular Access Device, Tunneled in Subcutaneous Tissue and Fascia
Venclexta® use Venetoclax Antineoplastic
Venectomy
see Excision, Lower Veins Ø6B
see Excision, Upper Veins Ø5B
Venetoclax Antineoplastic XWØDXR5
Venography
see Fluoroscopy, Veins B51
see Plain Radiography, Veins B5Ø
Venorrhaphy
see Repair, Lower Veins Ø6Q
see Repair, Upper Veins Ø5Q
Venotripsy
see Occlusion, Lower Veins Ø6L
see Occlusion, Upper Veins Ø5L
Ventricular fold use Larynx
Ventriculoatriostomy see Bypass, Central Nervous System and Cranial Nerves ØØ1
Ventriculocisternostomy see Bypass, Central Nervous System and Cranial Nerves ØØ1
Ventriculogram, cardiac
Combined left and right heart see Fluoroscopy, Heart, Right and Left B216
Left ventricle see Fluoroscopy, Heart, Left B215
Right ventricle see Fluoroscopy, Heart, Right B214
Ventriculopuncture, through previously implanted catheter 8CØ1X6J
Ventriculoscopy ØØJØ4ZZ
Ventriculostomy
External drainage see Drainage, Cerebral Ventricle ØØ96
Internal shunt see Bypass, Cerebral Ventricle ØØ16
Ventriculovenostomy see Bypass, Cerebral Ventricle ØØ16
Ventrio™ Hernia Patch use Synthetic Substitute
VEP (visual evoked potential) 4AØ7X0Z
Vermiform appendix use Appendix
Vermilion border
use Lower Lip
use Upper Lip
Versa use Pacemaker, Dual Chamber in ØJH
Version, obstetric
External 10SØXZZ
Internal 10SØ7ZZ
Vertebral arch
use Cervical Vertebra
use Lumbar Vertebra
use Thoracic Vertebra
Vertebral body
use Cervical Vertebra
use Lumbar Vertebra
use Thoracic Vertebra
Vertebral canal use Spinal Canal
Vertebral foramen
use Cervical Vertebra
use Lumbar Vertebra
use Thoracic Vertebra
Vertebral lamina
use Cervical Vertebra
use Lumbar Vertebra
use Thoracic Vertebra
Vertebral pedicle
use Cervical Vertebra
use Lumbar Vertebra
use Thoracic Vertebra
Vesical vein
use Hypogastric Vein, Left
use Hypogastric Vein, Right
Vesicotomy see Drainage, Urinary System ØT9
Vesiculectomy
see Excision, Male Reproductive System ØVB
see Resection, Male Reproductive System ØVT
Vesiculogram, seminal see Plain Radiography, Male Reproductive System BVØ
Vesiculotomy see Drainage, Male Reproductive System ØV9
Vestibular Assessment F15Z
Vestibular (Scarpa's) ganglion use Acoustic Nerve
Vestibular nerve use Acoustic Nerve

Vestibular Treatment F0C
Vestibulocochlear nerve *use* Acoustic Nerve
VH-IVUS (virtual histology intravascular ultrasound) *see* Ultrasonography, Heart B24
Virchow's (supraclavicular) lymph node
   use Lymphatic, Left Neck
   use Lymphatic, Right Neck
Virtuoso (II) (DR) (VR) *use* Defibrillator Generator in 0JH
Vistogard(R) *use* Uridine Triacetate
Vitrectomy
   see Excision, Eye 08B
   see Resection, Eye 08T
Vitreous body
   use Vitreous, Left
   use Vitreous, Right
Viva (XT) (S) *use* Cardiac Resynchronization Defibrillator Pulse Generator in 0JH
Vocal fold
   use Vocal Cord, Left
   use Vocal Cord, Right
Vocational
   Assessment *see* Activities of Daily Living Assessment, Rehabilitation F02
   Retraining *see* Activities of Daily Living Treatment, Rehabilitation F08
Volar (palmar) digital vein
   use Hand Vein, Left
   use Hand Vein, Right
Volar (palmar) metacarpal vein
   use Hand Vein, Left
   use Hand Vein, Right
Vomer bone *use* Nasal Septum
Vomer of nasal septum *use* Nasal Bone
Voraxaze *use* Glucarpidase
Vulvectomy
   see Excision, Female Reproductive System 0UB
   see Resection, Female Reproductive System 0UT
VYXEOS™ *use* Cytarabine and Daunorubicin Liposome Antineoplastic

W

WALLSTENT® Endoprosthesis *use* Intraluminal Device
Washing *see* Irrigation
WavelinQ EndoAVF system
   Radial Artery, Left 031C3ZF
   Radial Artery, Right 031B3ZF
   Ulnar Artery, Left 031A3ZF
   Ulnar Artery, Right 03193ZF
Wedge resection, pulmonary *see* Excision, Respiratory System 0BB
Window *see* Drainage
Wiring, dental 2W31X9Z

X

Xact Carotid Stent System *use* Intraluminal Device
Xenograft *use* Zooplastic Tissue in Heart and Great Vessels
XIENCE Everolimus Eluting Coronary Stent System *use* Intraluminal Device, Drug-eluting in Heart and Great Vessels
Xiphoid process *use* Sternum
XLIF® System *use* Interbody Fusion Device in Lower Joints
XOSPATA® *use* Gilteritinib Antineoplastic
X-ray *see* Plain Radiography
X-STOP® Spacer
   use Spinal Stabilization Device, Interspinous Process in 0RH
   use Spinal Stabilization Device, Interspinous Process in 0SH

Y

Yoga Therapy 8E0ZXY4

Z

Zenith AAA Endovascular Graft
   use Intraluminal Device
   use Intraluminal Device, Branched or Fenestrated, One or Two Arteries in 04V
   use Intraluminal Device, Branched or Fenestrated, Three or More Arteries in 04V
Zenith Flex® AAA Endovascular Graft *use* Intraluminal Device
Zenith TX2® TAA Endovascular Graft *use* Intraluminal Device
Zenith® Renu™ AAA Ancillary Graft *use* Intraluminal Device
Zilver® PTX® (paclitaxel) Drug-Eluting Peripheral Stent
   use Intraluminal Device, Drug-eluting in Lower Arteries
   use Intraluminal Device, Drug-eluting in Upper Arteries
Zimmer® NexGen® LPS Mobile Bearing Knee *use* Synthetic Substitute
Zimmer® NexGen® LPS-Flex Mobile Knee *use* Synthetic Substitute
ZINPLAVA™ *use* Bezlotoxumab Monoclonal Antibody
Zonule of Zinn
   use Lens, Left
   use Lens, Right
Zooplastic Tissue, Rapid Deployment Technique, Replacement X2RF
Zotarolimus-eluting Coronary Stent *use* Intraluminal Device, Drug-eluting in Heart and Great Vessels
Z-plasty, skin for scar contracture *see* Release, Skin and Breast 0HN
Zygomatic process of frontal bone *use* Frontal Bone
Zygomatic process of temporal bone
   use Temporal Bone, Left
   use Temporal Bone, Right
Zygomaticus muscle *use* Facial Muscle
Zyvox *use* Oxazolidinones

ICD-10-PCS Tables

Central Nervous System and Cranial Nerves ØØ1–ØØX

Character Meanings

This Character Meaning table is provided as a guide to assist the user in the identification of character members that may be found in this section of code tables. It **SHOULD NOT** be used to build a PCS code.

Operation–Character 3		Body Part–Character 4		Approach–Character 5		Device–Character 6		Qualifier–Character 7	
1	Bypass	Ø	Brain	Ø	Open	Ø	Drainage Device	Ø	Nasopharynx
2	Change	1	Cerebral Meninges	3	Percutaneous	2	Monitoring Device	1	Mastoid Sinus
5	Destruction	2	Dura Mater	4	Percutaneous Endoscopic	3	Infusion Device	2	Atrium
7	Dilation	3	Epidural Space, Intracranial	X	External	4	Radioactive Element, Cesium-131 Collagen Implant	3	Blood Vessel
8	Division	4	Subdural Space, Intracranial			7	Autologous Tissue Substitute	4	Pleural Cavity
9	Drainage	5	Subarachnoid Space, Intracranial			J	Synthetic Substitute	5	Intestine
B	Excision	6	Cerebral Ventricle			K	Nonautologous Tissue Substitute	6	Peritoneal Cavity
C	Extirpation	7	Cerebral Hemisphere			M	Neurostimulator Lead	7	Urinary Tract
D	Extraction	8	Basal Ganglia			Y	Other Device	8	Bone Marrow
F	Fragmentation	9	Thalamus			Z	No Device	9	Fallopian Tube
H	Insertion	A	Hypothalamus					A	Subgaleal Space
J	Inspection	B	Pons					B	Cerebral Cisterns
K	Map	C	Cerebellum					F	Olfactory Nerve
N	Release	D	Medulla Oblongata					G	Optic Nerve
P	Removal	E	Cranial Nerve					H	Oculomotor Nerve
Q	Repair	F	Olfactory Nerve					J	Trochlear Nerve
R	Replacement	G	Optic Nerve					K	Trigeminal Nerve
S	Reposition	H	Oculomotor Nerve					L	Abducens Nerve
T	Resection	J	Trochlear Nerve					M	Facial Nerve
U	Supplement	K	Trigeminal Nerve					N	Acoustic Nerve
W	Revision	L	Abducens Nerve					P	Glossopharyngeal Nerve
X	Transfer	M	Facial Nerve					Q	Vagus Nerve
		N	Acoustic Nerve					R	Accessory Nerve
		P	Glossopharyngeal Nerve					S	Hypoglossal Nerve
		Q	Vagus Nerve					X	Diagnostic
		R	Accessory Nerve					Z	No Qualifier
		S	Hypoglossal Nerve						
		T	Spinal Meninges						
		U	Spinal Canal						
		V	Spinal Cord						
		W	Cervical Spinal Cord						
		X	Thoracic Spinal Cord						
		Y	Lumbar Spinal Cord						

AHA Coding Clinic for table 001

2018, 4Q, 86	Placement of lumboatrial shunt
2017, 4Q, 39-41	Dilation and bypass of cerebral ventricle
2015, 2Q, 9	Revision of ventriculoperitoneal (VP) shunt
2013, 2Q, 36	Insertion of ventriculoperitoneal shunt with laparoscopic assistance

AHA Coding Clinic for table 007

2017, 4Q, 39-41	Dilation and bypass of cerebral ventricle

AHA Coding Clinic for table 009

2018, 4Q, 85	Externalization of lumboatrial shunt
2017, 1Q, 50	Failed lumbar puncture
2015, 3Q, 10	Open evacuation of subdural hematoma
2015, 3Q, 11	Percutaneous drainage of subdural hematoma
2015, 3Q, 12	Subdural evacuation portal system (SEPS) placement
2015, 3Q, 12	Placement of ventriculostomy catheter via burr hole
2015, 2Q, 30	Drainage of syrinx
2015, 1Q, 31	Intrathecal chemotherapy
2014, 1Q, 8	Diagnostic lumbar tap
2014, 1Q, 8	Lumbar drainage port aspiration

AHA Coding Clinic for table 00B

2017, 3Q, 17	Resection of schwannoma and placement of DuraGen and Lorenz cranial plating system
2016, 2Q, 12	Resection of malignant neoplasm of infratemporal fossa
2016, 2Q, 18	Amygdalohippocampectomy
2014, 4Q, 34	Resection of brain malignancy with implantation of chemotherapeutic wafer
2014, 3Q, 24	Repair of lipomyelomeningocele and tethered cord

AHA Coding Clinic for table 00C

2017, 4Q, 48	New and revised body part values - Extirpation spinal canal
2016, 2Q, 29	Decompressive craniectomy with cryopreservation and storage of bone flap
2015, 3Q, 10	Open evacuation of subdural hematoma
2015, 3Q, 11	Percutaneous drainage of subdural hematoma
2015, 3Q, 13	Evacuation of intracerebral hematoma

AHA Coding Clinic for table 00D

2015, 3Q, 13	Nonexcisional debridement of cranial wound with removal and replacement of hardware

AHA Coding Clinic for table 00H

2017, 4Q, 30-31	Radiotherapeutic brain implant
2017, 3Q, 13	Implantation of bilateral neurostimulator electrodes
2014, 3Q, 19	End of life replacement of Baclofen pump

AHA Coding Clinic for table 00J

2017, 1Q, 50	Failed lumbar puncture

AHA Coding Clinic for table 00N

2019, 1Q, 28	Decompressive laminectomy of both spinal cord and nerve roots
2018, 3Q, 30	Decompressive laminectomy (release of spinal cord versus release of spinal meninges)
2017, 3Q, 10	Repair of Chiari malformation
2017, 2Q, 23	Decompression of spinal cord and placement of instrumentation
2016, 2Q, 29	Decompressive craniectomy with cryopreservation and storage of bone flap
2015, 2Q, 20	Cervical laminoplasty
2015, 2Q, 21	Multiple decompressive cervical laminectomies
2015, 2Q, 34	Decompressive laminectomy
2014, 3Q, 24	Repair of lipomyelomeningocele and tethered cord

AHA Coding Clinic for table 00P

2014, 3Q, 19	End of life replacement of Baclofen pump

AHA Coding Clinic for table 00Q

2014, 3Q, 7	Hemi-cranioplasty for repair of cranial defect
2013, 3Q, 25	Fracture of frontal bone with repair and coagulation for hemostasis

AHA Coding Clinic for table 00S

2014, 4Q, 35	Reimplantation of buccal nerve

AHA Coding Clinic for table 00U

2018, 1Q, 9	Craniectomy with DuraGaurd placement
2017, 4Q, 62	Added and revised device values - Nerve substitutes
2017, 3Q, 10	Repair of Chiari malformation
2017, 3Q, 17	Resection of schwannoma and placement of DuraGen and Lorenz cranial plating system
2015, 4Q, 39	Dural patch graft
2014, 3Q, 24	Repair of lipomyelomeningocele and tethered cord

AHA Coding Clinic for table 00W

2018, 4Q, 86	Placement of lumboatrial shunt

Brain

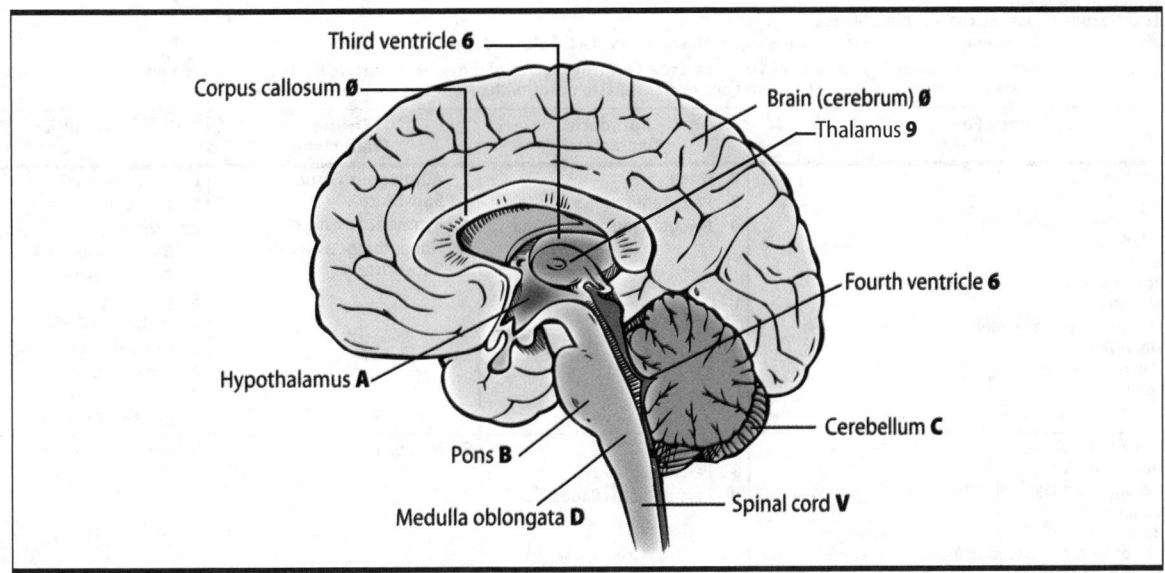

Third ventricle **6**
Corpus callosum **Ø**
Brain (cerebrum) **Ø**
Thalamus **9**
Fourth ventricle **6**
Hypothalamus **A**
Cerebellum **C**
Pons **B**
Medulla oblongata **D**
Spinal cord **V**

Cranial Nerves

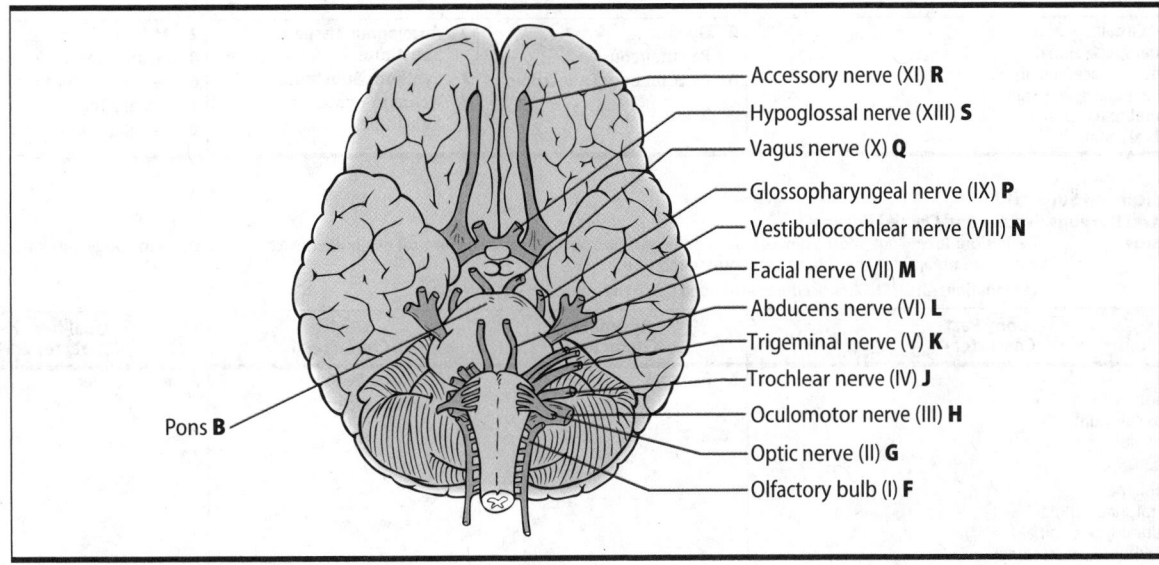

Accessory nerve (XI) **R**
Hypoglossal nerve (XIII) **S**
Vagus nerve (X) **Q**
Glossopharyngeal nerve (IX) **P**
Vestibulocochlear nerve (VIII) **N**
Facial nerve (VII) **M**
Abducens nerve (VI) **L**
Trigeminal nerve (V) **K**
Trochlear nerve (IV) **J**
Oculomotor nerve (III) **H**
Optic nerve (II) **G**
Olfactory bulb (I) **F**
Pons **B**

Ø   Medical and Surgical
Ø   Central Nervous System and Cranial Nerves
1   Bypass   Definition: Altering the route of passage of the contents of a tubular body part

                     Explanation: Rerouting contents of a body part to a downstream area of the normal route, to a similar route and body part, or to an abnormal route and dissimilar body part. Includes one or more anastomoses, with or without the use of a device.

Body Part Character 4	Approach Character 5	Device Character 6	Qualifier Character 7

6 Cerebral Ventricle
Aqueduct of Sylvius
Cerebral aqueduct (Sylvius)
Choroid plexus
Ependyma
Foramen of Monro (intraventricular)
Fourth ventricle
Interventricular foramen (Monro)
Left lateral ventricle
Right lateral ventricle
Third ventricle
	Ø Open
	3 Percutaneous
	4 Percutaneous Endoscopic
		7 Autologous Tissue
		   Substitute
		J Synthetic Substitute
		K Nonautologous Tissue
		   Substitute
			Ø Nasopharynx
			1 Mastoid Sinus
			2 Atrium
			3 Blood Vessel
			4 Pleural Cavity
			5 Intestine
			6 Peritoneal Cavity
			7 Urinary Tract
			8 Bone Marrow
			A Subgaleal Space
			B Cerebral Cisterns

6 Cerebral Ventricle Aqueduct of Sylvius Cerebral aqueduct (Sylvius) Choroid plexus Ependyma Foramen of Monro (intraventricular) Fourth ventricle Interventricular foramen (Monro) Left lateral ventricle Right lateral ventricle Third ventricle	**Ø** Open **3** Percutaneous **4** Percutaneous Endoscopic	**Z** No Device	**B** Cerebral Cisterns

U Spinal Canal
Epidural space, spinal
Extradural space, spinal
Subarachnoid space, spinal
Subdural space, spinal
Vertebral canal
	Ø Open
	3 Percutaneous
	4 Percutaneous Endoscopic
		7 Autologous Tissue
		   Substitute
		J Synthetic Substitute
		K Nonautologous Tissue
		   Substitute
			2 Atrium
			4 Pleural Cavity
			6 Peritoneal Cavity
			7 Urinary Tract
			9 Fallopian Tube

Ø   Medical and Surgical
Ø   Central Nervous System and Cranial Nerves
2   Change   Definition: Taking out or off a device from a body part and putting back an identical or similar device in or on the same body part without cutting or puncturing the skin or a mucous membrane

                     Explanation: All CHANGE procedures are coded using the approach EXTERNAL

Body Part Character 4	Approach Character 5	Device Character 6	Qualifier Character 7
Ø Brain Cerebrum Corpus callosum Encephalon **E Cranial Nerve** **U Spinal Canal** Epidural space, spinal Extradural space, spinal Subarachnoid space, spinal Subdural space, spinal Vertebral canal	**X** External	**Ø** Drainage Device **Y** Other Device	**Z** No Qualifier

Non-OR   All body part, approach, device, and qualifier values

Ø   **Medical and Surgical**
Ø   **Central Nervous System and Cranial Nerves**
5   **Destruction**   Definition: Physical eradication of all or a portion of a body part by the direct use of energy, force, or a destructive agent

                   Explanation: None of the body part is physically taken out

Body Part Character 4		Approach Character 5	Device Character 6	Qualifier Character 7

Ø Brain
Cerebrum
Corpus callosum
Encephalon
1 Cerebral Meninges
Arachnoid mater,
  intracranial
Leptomeninges,
  intracranial
Pia mater, intracranial
2 Dura Mater
Diaphragma sellae
Dura mater, intracranial
Falx cerebri
Tentorium cerebelli
6 Cerebral Ventricle
Aqueduct of Sylvius
Cerebral aqueduct (Sylvius)
Choroid plexus
Ependyma
Foramen of Monro
  (intraventricular)
Fourth ventricle
Interventricular foramen
  (Monro)
Left lateral ventricle
Right lateral ventricle
Third ventricle
7 Cerebral Hemisphere
Frontal lobe
Occipital lobe
Parietal lobe
Temporal lobe
8 Basal Ganglia
Basal nuclei
Claustrum
Corpus striatum
Globus pallidus
Substantia nigra
Subthalamic nucleus
9 Thalamus
Epithalamus
Geniculate nucleus
Metathalamus
Pulvinar
A Hypothalamus
Mammillary body
B Pons
Apneustic center
Basis pontis
Locus ceruleus
Pneumotaxic center
Pontine tegmentum
Superior olivary nucleus
C Cerebellum
Culmen
D Medulla Oblongata
Myelencephalon
F Olfactory Nerve
First cranial nerve
Olfactory bulb
G Optic Nerve
Optic chiasma
Second cranial nerve
	H Oculomotor Nerve
	Third cranial nerve
	J Trochlear Nerve
	Fourth cranial nerve
	K Trigeminal Nerve
	Fifth cranial nerve
	Gasserian ganglion
	Mandibular nerve
	Maxillary nerve
	Ophthalmic nerve
	Trifacial nerve
	L Abducens Nerve
	Sixth cranial nerve
	M Facial Nerve
	Chorda tympani
	Geniculate ganglion
	Greater superficial petrosal
	  nerve
	Nerve to the stapedius
	Parotid plexus
	Posterior auricular nerve
	Seventh cranial nerve
	Submandibular ganglion
	N Acoustic Nerve
	Cochlear nerve
	Eighth cranial nerve
	Scarpa's (vestibular)
	  ganglion
	Spiral ganglion
	Vestibular (Scarpa's)
	  ganglion
	Vestibular nerve
	Vestibulocochlear nerve
	P Glossopharyngeal Nerve
	Carotid sinus nerve
	Ninth cranial nerve
	Tympanic nerve
	Q Vagus Nerve
	Anterior vagal trunk
	Pharyngeal plexus
	Pneumogastric nerve
	Posterior vagal trunk
	Pulmonary plexus
	Recurrent laryngeal nerve
	Superior laryngeal nerve
	Tenth cranial nerve
	R Accessory Nerve
	Eleventh cranial nerve
	S Hypoglossal Nerve
	Twelfth cranial nerve
	T Spinal Meninges
	Arachnoid mater, spinal
	Denticulate (dentate)
	  ligament
	Dura mater, spinal
	Filum terminale
	Leptomeninges, spinal
	Pia mater, spinal
	W Cervical Spinal Cord
	X Thoracic Spinal Cord
	Y Lumbar Spinal Cord
	Cauda equina
	Conus medullaris
		Ø Open
		3 Percutaneous
		4 Percutaneous Endoscopic
			Z No Device	**Z No Qualifier**

Non-OR   Ø05[F,G,H,J,K,L,M,N,P,Q,R,S][Ø,3,4]ZZ

LG Limited Coverage   **NC** Noncovered   ⊞ Combination Member   HAC associated procedure   Combination Only   DRG Non-OR   Non-OR   New/Revised in GREEN

ICD-10-PCS 2020   133

Ø Medical and Surgical
Ø Central Nervous System and Cranial Nerves
7 Dilation   Definition: Expanding an orifice or the lumen of a tubular body part

Explanation: The orifice can be a natural orifice or an artificially created orifice. Accomplished by stretching a tubular body part using intraluminal pressure or by cutting part of the orifice or wall of the tubular body part.

Body Part Character 4	Approach Character 5	Device Character 6	Qualifier Character 7
6 Cerebral Ventricle Aqueduct of Sylvius Cerebral aqueduct (Sylvius) Choroid plexus Ependyma Foramen of Monro (intraventricular) Fourth ventricle Interventricular foramen (Monro) Left lateral ventricle Right lateral ventricle Third ventricle	Ø Open 3 Percutaneous 4 Percutaneous Endoscopic	Z No Device	Z No Qualifier

Ø Medical and Surgical
Ø Central Nervous System and Cranial Nerves
8 Division   Definition: Cutting into a body part, without draining fluids and/or gases from the body part, in order to separate or transect a body part

Explanation: All or a portion of the body part is separated into two or more portions

Body Part Character 4	Approach Character 5	Device Character 6	Qualifier Character 7

Ø Brain
Cerebrum
Corpus callosum
Encephalon
7 Cerebral Hemisphere
Frontal lobe
Occipital lobe
Parietal lobe
Temporal lobe
8 Basal Ganglia
Basal nuclei
Claustrum
Corpus striatum
Globus pallidus
Substantia nigra
Subthalamic nucleus
F Olfactory Nerve
First cranial nerve
Olfactory bulb
G Optic Nerve
Optic chiasma
Second cranial nerve
H Oculomotor Nerve
Third cranial nerve
J Trochlear Nerve
Fourth cranial nerve
K Trigeminal Nerve
Fifth cranial nerve
Gasserian ganglion
Mandibular nerve
Maxillary nerve
Ophthalmic nerve
Trifacial nerve
L Abducens Nerve
Sixth cranial nerve
M Facial Nerve
Chorda tympani
Geniculate ganglion
Greater superficial petrosal
  nerve
Nerve to the stapedius
Parotid plexus
Posterior auricular nerve
Seventh cranial nerve
Submandibular ganglion
 	
N Acoustic Nerve
Cochlear nerve
Eighth cranial nerve
Scarpa's (vestibular)
  ganglion
Spiral ganglion
Vestibular (Scarpa's)
  ganglion
Vestibular nerve
Vestibulocochlear nerve
P Glossopharyngeal Nerve
Carotid sinus nerve
Ninth cranial nerve
Tympanic nerve
Q Vagus Nerve
Anterior vagal trunk
Pharyngeal plexus
Pneumogastric nerve
Posterior vagal trunk
Pulmonary plexus
Recurrent laryngeal nerve
Superior laryngeal nerve
Tenth cranial nerve
R Accessory Nerve
Eleventh cranial nerve
S Hypoglossal Nerve
Twelfth cranial nerve
W Cervical Spinal Cord
X Thoracic Spinal Cord
Y Lumbar Spinal Cord
Cauda equina
Conus medullaris
	Ø Open
	3 Percutaneous
	4 Percutaneous Endoscopic
		Z No Device	Z No Qualifier

Ø   Medical and Surgical
Ø   Central Nervous System and Cranial Nerves
9   Drainage   Definition: Taking or letting out fluids and/or gases from a body part
                         Explanation: The qualifier DIAGNOSTIC is used to identify drainage procedures that are biopsies

Body Part Character 4		Approach Character 5	Device Character 6	Qualifier Character 7

Ø Brain
Cerebrum
Corpus callosum
Encephalon
1 Cerebral Meninges
Arachnoid mater,
  intracranial
Leptomeninges,
  intracranial
Pia mater, intracranial
2 Dura Mater
Diaphragma sellae
Dura mater, intracranial
Falx cerebri
Tentorium cerebelli
3 Epidural Space,
Intracranial
Extradural space,
  intracranial
4 Subdural Space,
Intracranial
5 Subarachnoid Space,
Intracranial
6 Cerebral Ventricle
Aqueduct of Sylvius
Cerebral aqueduct (Sylvius)
Choroid plexus
Ependyma
Foramen of Monro
  (intraventricular)
Fourth ventricle
Interventricular foramen
  (Monro)
Left lateral ventricle
Right lateral ventricle
Third ventricle
7 Cerebral Hemisphere
Frontal lobe
Occipital lobe
Parietal lobe
Temporal lobe
8 Basal Ganglia
Basal nuclei
Claustrum
Corpus striatum
Globus pallidus
Substantia nigra
Subthalamic nucleus
9 Thalamus
Epithalamus
Geniculate nucleus
Metathalamus
Pulvinar
A Hypothalamus
Mammillary body
B Pons
Apneustic center
Basis pontis
Locus ceruleus
Pneumotaxic center
Pontine tegmentum
Superior olivary nucleus
C Cerebellum
Culmen
D Medulla Oblongata
Myelencephalon
F Olfactory Nerve
First cranial nerve
Olfactory bulb
	G Optic Nerve
	Optic chiasma
	Second cranial nerve
	H Oculomotor Nerve
	Third cranial nerve
	J Trochlear Nerve
	Fourth cranial nerve
	K Trigeminal Nerve
	Fifth cranial nerve
	Gasserian ganglion
	Mandibular nerve
	Maxillary nerve
	Ophthalmic nerve
	Trifacial nerve
	L Abducens Nerve
	Sixth cranial nerve
	M Facial Nerve
	Chorda tympani
	Geniculate ganglion
	Greater superficial petrosal
	  nerve
	Nerve to the stapedius
	Parotid plexus
	Posterior auricular nerve
	Seventh cranial nerve
	Submandibular ganglion
	N Acoustic Nerve
	Cochlear nerve
	Eighth cranial nerve
	Scarpa's (vestibular) ganglion
	Spiral ganglion
	Vestibular (Scarpa's) ganglion
	Vestibular nerve
	Vestibulocochlear nerve
	P Glossopharyngeal Nerve
	Carotid sinus nerve
	Ninth cranial nerve
	Tympanic nerve
	Q Vagus Nerve
	Anterior vagal trunk
	Pharyngeal plexus
	Pneumogastric nerve
	Posterior vagal trunk
	Pulmonary plexus
	Recurrent laryngeal nerve
	Superior laryngeal nerve
	Tenth cranial nerve
	R Accessory Nerve
	Eleventh cranial nerve
	S Hypoglossal Nerve
	Twelfth cranial nerve
	T Spinal Meninges
	Arachnoid mater, spinal
	Denticulate (dentate)
	  ligament
	Dura mater, spinal
	Filum terminale
	Leptomeninges, spinal
	Pia mater, spinal
	U Spinal Canal
	Epidural space, spinal
	Extradural space, spinal
	Subarachnoid space, spinal
	Subdural space, spinal
	Vertebral canal
	W Cervical Spinal Cord
	X Thoracic Spinal Cord
	Y Lumbar Spinal Cord
	Cauda equina
	Conus medullaris
		Ø Open
		3 Percutaneous
		4 Percutaneous Endoscopic
			Ø Drainage Device	**Z No Qualifier**

009 Continued on next page

Non-OR	009[T,W,X,Y]30Z
Non-OR	009U[3,4]0Z

LC Limited Coverage   **NC** Noncovered   ⊞ Combination Member   HAC associated procedure   Combination Only   DRG Non-OR   Non-OR   New/Revised in GREEN

ICD-10-PCS 2020   135

0   **Medical and Surgical**   *009 Continued*
0   **Central Nervous System and Cranial Nerves**
9   **Drainage**   Definition: Taking or letting out fluids and/or gases from a body part

                      Explanation: The qualifier DIAGNOSTIC is used to identify drainage procedures that are biopsies

Body Part Character 4		Approach Character 5	Device Character 6	Qualifier Character 7
0 Brain Cerebrum Corpus callosum Encephalon **1 Cerebral Meninges** Arachnoid mater, intracranial Leptomeninges, intracranial Pia mater, intracranial **2 Dura Mater** Diaphragma sellae Dura mater, intracranial Falx cerebri Tentorium cerebelli **3 Epidural Space, Intracranial** Extradural space, intracranial **4 Subdural Space, Intracranial** **5 Subarachnoid Space, Intracranial** **6 Cerebral Ventricle** Aqueduct of Sylvius Cerebral aqueduct (Sylvius) Choroid plexus Ependyma Foramen of Monro (intraventricular) Fourth ventricle Interventricular foramen (Monro) Left lateral ventricle Right lateral ventricle Third ventricle **7 Cerebral Hemisphere** Frontal lobe Occipital lobe Parietal lobe Temporal lobe **8 Basal Ganglia** Basal nuclei Claustrum Corpus striatum Globus pallidus Substantia nigra Subthalamic nucleus **9 Thalamus** Epithalamus Geniculate nucleus Metathalamus Pulvinar **A Hypothalamus** Mammillary body **B Pons** Apneustic center Basis pontis Locus ceruleus Pneumotaxic center Pontine tegmentum Superior olivary nucleus **C Cerebellum** Culmen **D Medulla Oblongata** Myelencephalon **F Olfactory Nerve** First cranial nerve Olfactory bulb	**G Optic Nerve** Optic chiasma Second cranial nerve **H Oculomotor Nerve** Third cranial nerve **J Trochlear Nerve** Fourth cranial nerve **K Trigeminal Nerve** Fifth cranial nerve Gasserian ganglion Mandibular nerve Maxillary nerve Ophthalmic nerve Trifacial nerve **L Abducens Nerve** Sixth cranial nerve **M Facial Nerve** Chorda tympani Geniculate ganglion Greater superficial petrosal nerve Nerve to the stapedius Parotid plexus Posterior auricular nerve Seventh cranial nerve Submandibular ganglion **N Acoustic Nerve** Cochlear nerve Eighth cranial nerve Scarpa's (vestibular) ganglion Spiral ganglion Vestibular (Scarpa's) ganglion Vestibular nerve Vestibulocochlear nerve **P Glossopharyngeal Nerve** Carotid sinus nerve Ninth cranial nerve Tympanic nerve **Q Vagus Nerve** Anterior vagal trunk Pharyngeal plexus Pneumogastric nerve Posterior vagal trunk Pulmonary plexus Recurrent laryngeal nerve Superior laryngeal nerve Tenth cranial nerve **R Accessory Nerve** Eleventh cranial nerve **S Hypoglossal Nerve** Twelfth cranial nerve **T Spinal Meninges** Arachnoid mater, spinal Denticulate (dentate) ligament Dura mater, spinal Filum terminale Leptomeninges, spinal Pia mater, spinal **U Spinal Canal** Epidural space, spinal Extradural space, spinal Subarachnoid space, spinal Subdural space, spinal Vertebral canal **W Cervical Spinal Cord** **X Thoracic Spinal Cord** **Y Lumbar Spinal Cord** Cauda equina Conus medullaris	**0 Open** **3 Percutaneous** **4 Percutaneous Endoscopic**	**Z No Device**	**X Diagnostic** **Z No Qualifier**

Non-OR   009[0,1,2,3,4,5,6,7,8,9,A,B,C,D,F,G,H,J,K,L,M,N,P,Q,R,S][3,4]ZX
Non-OR   009[T,W,X,Y]3Z[X,Z]
Non-OR   009U[3,4]Z[X,Z]

LC Limited Coverage   NC Noncovered   ⊞ Combination Member   HAC associated procedure   Combination Only   DRG Non-OR   Non-OR   New/Revised in GREEN

136   ICD-10-PCS 2020

Ø   **Medical and Surgical**
Ø   **Central Nervous System and Cranial Nerves**
B   **Excision**   Definition: Cutting out or off, without replacement, a portion of a body part
                Explanation: The qualifier DIAGNOSTIC is used to identify excision procedures that are biopsies

Body Part Character 4		Approach Character 5	Device Character 6	Qualifier Character 7

Ø **Brain**
  Cerebrum
  Corpus callosum
  Encephalon
1 **Cerebral Meninges**
  Arachnoid mater,
    intracranial
  Leptomeninges,
    intracranial
  Pia mater, intracranial
2 **Dura Mater**
  Diaphragma sellae
  Dura mater, intracranial
  Falx cerebri
  Tentorium cerebelli
6 **Cerebral Ventricle**
  Aqueduct of Sylvius
  Cerebral aqueduct (Sylvius)
  Choroid plexus
  Ependyma
  Foramen of Monro
    (intraventricular)
  Fourth ventricle
  Interventricular foramen
    (Monro)
  Left lateral ventricle
  Right lateral ventricle
  Third ventricle
7 **Cerebral Hemisphere**
  Frontal lobe
  Occipital lobe
  Parietal lobe
  Temporal lobe
8 **Basal Ganglia**
  Basal nuclei
  Claustrum
  Corpus striatum
  Globus pallidus
  Substantia nigra
  Subthalamic nucleus
9 **Thalamus**
  Epithalamus
  Geniculate nucleus
  Metathalamus
  Pulvinar
A **Hypothalamus**
  Mammillary body
B **Pons**
  Apneustic center
  Basis pontis
  Locus ceruleus
  Pneumotaxic center
  Pontine tegmentum
  Superior olivary nucleus
C **Cerebellum**
  Culmen
D **Medulla Oblongata**
  Myelencephalon
F **Olfactory Nerve**
  First cranial nerve
  Olfactory bulb
G **Optic Nerve**
  Optic chiasma
  Second cranial nerve
	H **Oculomotor Nerve**
	  Third cranial nerve
	J **Trochlear Nerve**
	  Fourth cranial nerve
	K **Trigeminal Nerve**
	  Fifth cranial nerve
	  Gasserian ganglion
	  Mandibular nerve
	  Maxillary nerve
	  Ophthalmic nerve
	  Trifacial nerve
	L **Abducens Nerve**
	  Sixth cranial nerve
	M **Facial Nerve**
	  Chorda tympani
	  Geniculate ganglion
	  Greater superficial petrosal
	    nerve
	  Nerve to the stapedius
	  Parotid plexus
	  Posterior auricular nerve
	  Seventh cranial nerve
	  Submandibular ganglion
	N **Acoustic Nerve**
	  Cochlear nerve
	  Eighth cranial nerve
	  Scarpa's (vestibular)
	    ganglion
	  Spiral ganglion
	  Vestibular (Scarpa's)
	    ganglion
	  Vestibular nerve
	  Vestibulocochlear nerve
	P **Glossopharyngeal Nerve**
	  Carotid sinus nerve
	  Ninth cranial nerve
	  Tympanic nerve
	Q **Vagus Nerve**
	  Anterior vagal trunk
	  Pharyngeal plexus
	  Pneumogastric nerve
	  Posterior vagal trunk
	  Pulmonary plexus
	  Recurrent laryngeal nerve
	  Superior laryngeal nerve
	  Tenth cranial nerve
	R **Accessory Nerve**
	  Eleventh cranial nerve
	S **Hypoglossal Nerve**
	  Twelfth cranial nerve
	T **Spinal Meninges**
	  Arachnoid mater, spinal
	  Denticulate (dentate)
	    ligament
	  Dura mater, spinal
	  Filum terminale
	  Leptomeninges, spinal
	  Pia mater, spinal
	W **Cervical Spinal Cord**
	X **Thoracic Spinal Cord**
	Y **Lumbar Spinal Cord**
	  Cauda equina
	  Conus medullaris
		Ø Open
		3 Percutaneous
		4 Percutaneous Endoscopic
			Z No Device	X Diagnostic
				Z No Qualifier

Non-OR   ØØB[F,G,H,J,K,L,M,N,P,Q,R,S][3,4]ZX

LC Limited Coverage   NC Noncovered   ⊞ Combination Member   HAC associated procedure   Combination Only   DRG Non-OR   Non-OR   New/Revised in GREEN

ICD-10-PCS 2020   **137**

ØØB–ØØB

0 Medical and Surgical
0 Central Nervous System and Cranial Nerves
C Extirpation   Definition: Taking or cutting out solid matter from a body part

Explanation: The solid matter may be an abnormal byproduct of a biological function or a foreign body; it may be imbedded in a body part or in the lumen of a tubular body part. The solid matter may or may not have been previously broken into pieces.

Body Part Character 4		Approach Character 5	Device Character 6	Qualifier Character 7

0 Brain
Cerebrum
Corpus callosum
Encephalon
1 Cerebral Meninges
Arachnoid mater,
   intracranial
Leptomeninges,
   intracranial
Pia mater, intracranial
2 Dura Mater
Diaphragma sellae
Dura mater, intracranial
Falx cerebri
Tentorium cerebelli
3 Epidural Space,
Intracranial
Extradural space,
   intracranial
4 Subdural Space,
Intracranial
5 Subarachnoid Space,
Intracranial
6 Cerebral Ventricle
Aqueduct of Sylvius
Cerebral aqueduct (Sylvius)
Choroid plexus
Ependyma
Foramen of Monro
   (intraventricular)
Fourth ventricle
Interventricular foramen
   (Monro)
Left lateral ventricle
Right lateral ventricle
Third ventricle
7 Cerebral Hemisphere
Frontal lobe
Occipital lobe
Parietal lobe
Temporal lobe
8 Basal Ganglia
Basal nuclei
Claustrum
Corpus striatum
Globus pallidus
Substantia nigra
Subthalamic nucleus
9 Thalamus
Epithalamus
Geniculate nucleus
Metathalamus
Pulvinar
A Hypothalamus
Mammillary body
B Pons
Apneustic center
Basis pontis
Locus ceruleus
Pneumotaxic center
Pontine tegmentum
Superior olivary nucleus
C Cerebellum
Culmen
D Medulla Oblongata
Myelencephalon
F Olfactory Nerve
First cranial nerve
Olfactory bulb
	G Optic Nerve
	Optic chiasma
	Second cranial nerve
	H Oculomotor Nerve
	Third cranial nerve
	J Trochlear Nerve
	Fourth cranial nerve
	K Trigeminal Nerve
	Fifth cranial nerve
	Gasserian ganglion
	Mandibular nerve
	Maxillary nerve
	Ophthalmic nerve
	Trifacial nerve
	L Abducens Nerve
	Sixth cranial nerve
	M Facial Nerve
	Chorda tympani
	Geniculate ganglion
	Greater superficial petrosal
	   nerve
	Nerve to the stapedius
	Parotid plexus
	Posterior auricular nerve
	Seventh cranial nerve
	Submandibular ganglion
	N Acoustic Nerve
	Cochlear nerve
	Eighth cranial nerve
	Scarpa's (vestibular)
	   ganglion
	Spiral ganglion
	Vestibular (Scarpa's)
	   ganglion
	Vestibular nerve
	Vestibulocochlear nerve
	P Glossopharyngeal Nerve
	Carotid sinus nerve
	Ninth cranial nerve
	Tympanic nerve
	Q Vagus Nerve
	Anterior vagal trunk
	Pharyngeal plexus
	Pneumogastric nerve
	Posterior vagal trunk
	Pulmonary plexus
	Recurrent laryngeal nerve
	Superior laryngeal nerve
	Tenth cranial nerve
	R Accessory Nerve
	Eleventh cranial nerve
	S Hypoglossal Nerve
	Twelfth cranial nerve
	T Spinal Meninges
	Arachnoid mater, spinal
	Denticulate (dentate)
	   ligament
	Dura mater, spinal
	Filum terminale
	Leptomeninges, spinal
	Pia mater, spinal
	U Spinal Canal
	W Cervical Spinal Cord
	X Thoracic Spinal Cord
	Y Lumbar Spinal Cord
	Cauda equina
	Conus medullaris
		0 Open
		3 Percutaneous
		4 Percutaneous Endoscopic
			Z No Device	**Z No Qualifier**

LC Limited Coverage   NC Noncovered   ⊞ Combination Member   HAC associated procedure   Combination Only   DRG Non-OR   Non-OR   New/Revised in GREEN

138   ICD-10-PCS 2020

Ø   **Medical and Surgical**
Ø   **Central Nervous System and Cranial Nerves**
D   **Extraction**   Definition: Pulling or stripping out or off all or a portion of a body part by the use of force
                Explanation: The qualifier DIAGNOSTIC is used to identify extraction procedures that are biopsies

Body Part Character 4		Approach Character 5	Device Character 6	Qualifier Character 7

1 **Cerebral Meninges**
  Arachnoid mater, intracranial
  Leptomeninges, intracranial
  Pia mater, intracranial
2 **Dura Mater**
  Diaphragma sellae
  Dura mater, intracranial
  Falx cerebri
  Tentorium cerebelli
F **Olfactory Nerve**
  First cranial nerve
  Olfactory bulb
G **Optic Nerve**
  Optic chiasma
  Second cranial nerve
H **Oculomotor Nerve**
  Third cranial nerve
J **Trochlear Nerve**
  Fourth cranial nerve
K **Trigeminal Nerve**
  Fifth cranial nerve
  Gasserian ganglion
  Mandibular nerve
  Maxillary nerve
  Ophthalmic nerve
  Trifacial nerve
L **Abducens Nerve**
  Sixth cranial nerve
M **Facial Nerve**
  Chorda tympani
  Geniculate ganglion
  Greater superficial petrosal nerve
  Nerve to the stapedius
  Parotid plexus
  Posterior auricular nerve
  Seventh cranial nerve
  Submandibular ganglion
	N **Acoustic Nerve**
	  Cochlear nerve
	  Eighth cranial nerve
	  Scarpa's (vestibular) ganglion
	  Spiral ganglion
	  Vestibular (Scarpa's) ganglion
	  Vestibular nerve
	  Vestibulocochlear nerve
	P **Glossopharyngeal Nerve**
	  Carotid sinus nerve
	  Ninth cranial nerve
	  Tympanic nerve
	Q **Vagus Nerve**
	  Anterior vagal trunk
	  Pharyngeal plexus
	  Pneumogastric nerve
	  Posterior vagal trunk
	  Pulmonary plexus
	  Recurrent laryngeal nerve
	  Superior laryngeal nerve
	  Tenth cranial nerve
	R **Accessory Nerve**
	  Eleventh cranial nerve
	S **Hypoglossal Nerve**
	  Twelfth cranial nerve
	T **Spinal Meninges**
	  Arachnoid mater, spinal
	  Denticulate (dentate) ligament
	  Dura mater, spinal
	  Filum terminale
	  Leptomeninges, spinal
	  Pia mater, spinal
		Ø Open
		3 Percutaneous
		4 Percutaneous Endoscopic
			Z No Device	Z No Qualifier

Ø   **Medical and Surgical**
Ø   **Central Nervous System and Cranial Nerves**
F   **Fragmentation**   Definition: Breaking solid matter in a body part into pieces
                Explanation: Physical force (e.g., manual, ultrasonic) applied directly or indirectly is used to break the solid matter into pieces. The solid matter may be an abnormal byproduct of a biological function or a foreign body. The pieces of solid matter are not taken out.

Body Part Character 4	Approach Character 5	Device Character 6	Qualifier Character 7

3 **Epidural Space, Intracranial** `NC`
  Extradural space, intracranial
4 **Subdural Space, Intracranial** `NC`
5 **Subarachnoid Space, Intracranial** `NC`
6 **Cerebral Ventricle** `NC`
  Aqueduct of Sylvius
  Cerebral aqueduct (Sylvius)
  Choroid plexus
  Ependyma
  Foramen of Monro (intraventricular)
  Fourth ventricle
  Interventricular foramen (Monro)
  Left lateral ventricle
  Right lateral ventricle
  Third ventricle
U **Spinal Canal**
  Epidural space, spinal
  Extradural space, spinal
  Subarachnoid space, spinal
  Subdural space, spinal
  Vertebral canal
	Ø Open
	3 Percutaneous
	4 Percutaneous Endoscopic
	X External
		Z No Device	Z No Qualifier

Non-OR   00F[3,4,5,6]XZZ
`NC`   00F[3,4,5,6]XZZ

Central Nervous System and Cranial Nerves

Ø Medical and Surgical
Ø Central Nervous System and Cranial Nerves
H Insertion   Definition: Putting in a nonbiological appliance that monitors, assists, performs, or prevents a physiological function but does not physically take the place of a body part

Explanation: None

Body Part Character 4		Approach Character 5	Device Character 6	Qualifier Character 7

Ø Brain ⊞
Cerebrum
Corpus callosum
Encephalon
		Ø Open	**2 Monitoring Device**
			3 Infusion Device
			4 Radioactive Element,
			    Cesium-131 Collagen
			    Implant
			M Neurostimulator Lead
			Y Other Device
				Z No Qualifier

Ø Brain ⊞ Cerebrum Corpus callosum Encephalon		**3 Percutaneous** **4 Percutaneous Endoscopic**	**2 Monitoring Device** **3 Infusion Device** **M Neurostimulator Lead** **Y Other Device**	**Z No Qualifier**

6 Cerebral Ventricle ⊞
Aqueduct of Sylvius
Cerebral aqueduct (Sylvius)
Choroid plexus
Ependyma
Foramen of Monro
  (intraventricular)
Fourth ventricle Interventricular
  foramen (Monro)
Left lateral ventricle
Right lateral ventricle
Third ventricle
	E Cranial Nerve ⊞
	U Spinal Canal ⊞
	  Epidural space, spinal
	  Extradural space, spinal
	  Subarachnoid space,
	    spinal
	  Subdural space, spinal
	  Vertebral canal
	V Spinal Cord ⊞
		Ø Open
		3 Percutaneous
		4 Percutaneous Endoscopic
			2 Monitoring Device
			3 Infusion Device
			M Neurostimulator Lead
			Y Other Device
				Z No Qualifier

DRG Non-OR	00H004Z		
Non-OR	00H[E,U,V]32Z	**See Appendix L for Procedure Combinations**	
Non-OR	00H[E,U][3,4]YZ	⊞ 00H00MZ	
Non-OR	00H[U,V][0,3,4]3Z	⊞ 00H0[3,4]MZ	
		⊞ 00H[6,E,U,V][0,3,4]MZ	

Ø Medical and Surgical
Ø Central Nervous System and Cranial Nerves
J Inspection   Definition: Visually and/or manually exploring a body part

Explanation: Visual exploration may be performed with or without optical instrumentation. Manual exploration may be performed directly or through intervening body layers.

Body Part Character 4		Approach Character 5	Device Character 6	Qualifier Character 7

Ø Brain
Cerebrum
Corpus callosum
Encephalon
E Cranial Nerve
	U Spinal Canal
	  Epidural space, spinal
	  Extradural space, spinal
	  Subarachnoid space, spinal
	  Subdural space, spinal
	  Vertebral canal
	V Spinal Cord
		Ø Open
		3 Percutaneous
		4 Percutaneous Endoscopic
			Z No Device	**Z No Qualifier**

Non-OR	00J[0,E,U,V]3ZZ

Ø Medical and Surgical
Ø Central Nervous System and Cranial Nerves
K Map   Definition: Locating the route of passage of electrical impulses and/or locating functional areas in a body part

Explanation: Applicable only to the cardiac conduction mechanism and the central nervous system

Body Part Character 4		Approach Character 5	Device Character 6	Qualifier Character 7
Ø Brain Cerebrum Corpus callosum Encephalon **7 Cerebral Hemisphere** Frontal lobe Occipital lobe Parietal lobe Temporal lobe **8 Basal Ganglia** Basal nuclei Claustrum Corpus striatum Globus pallidus Substantia nigra Subthalamic nucleus	**9 Thalamus** Epithalamus Geniculate nucleus Metathalamus Pulvinar **A Hypothalamus** Mammillary body **B Pons** Apneustic center Basis pontis Locus ceruleus Pneumotaxic center Pontine tegmentum Superior olivary nucleus **C Cerebellum** Culmen **D Medulla Oblongata** Myelencephalon	**Ø Open** **3 Percutaneous** **4 Percutaneous Endoscopic**	**Z No Device**	**Z No Qualifier**

⬛ Limited Coverage   ⬛ Noncovered   ⊞ Combination Member   HAC associated procedure   Combination Only   DRG Non-OR   Non-OR   New/Revised in GREEN

Ø **Medical and Surgical**
Ø **Central Nervous System and Cranial Nerves**
N **Release**   Definition: Freeing a body part from an abnormal physical constraint by cutting or by the use of force
               Explanation: Some of the restraining tissue may be taken out but none of the body part is taken out

Body Part Character 4		Approach Character 5	Device Character 6	Qualifier Character 7
Ø **Brain**	**H** **Oculomotor Nerve**	**Ø** Open	**Z** No Device	**Z** No Qualifier
Cerebrum	Third cranial nerve	**3** Percutaneous		
Corpus callosum	**J** **Trochlear Nerve**	**4** Percutaneous Endoscopic		
Encephalon	Fourth cranial nerve			
1 **Cerebral Meninges**	**K** **Trigeminal Nerve**			
Arachnoid mater,	Fifth cranial nerve			
intracranial	Gasserian ganglion			
Leptomeninges,	Mandibular nerve			
intracranial	Maxillary nerve			
Pia mater, intracranial	Ophthalmic nerve			
2 **Dura Mater**	Trifacial nerve			
Diaphragma sellae	**L** **Abducens Nerve**			
Dura mater, intracranial	Sixth cranial nerve			
Falx cerebri	**M** **Facial Nerve**			
Tentorium cerebelli	Chorda tympani			
6 **Cerebral Ventricle**	Geniculate ganglion			
Aqueduct of Sylvius	Greater superficial petrosal			
Cerebral aqueduct (Sylvius)	nerve			
Choroid plexus	Nerve to the stapedius			
Ependyma	Parotid plexus			
Foramen of Monro	Posterior auricular nerve			
(intraventricular)	Seventh cranial nerve			
Fourth ventricle	Submandibular ganglion			
Interventricular foramen	**N** **Acoustic Nerve**			
(Monro)	Cochlear nerve			
Left lateral ventricle	Eighth cranial nerve			
Right lateral ventricle	Scarpa's (vestibular)			
Third ventricle	ganglion			
7 **Cerebral Hemisphere**	Spiral ganglion			
Frontal lobe	Vestibular (Scarpa's)			
Occipital lobe	ganglion			
Parietal lobe	Vestibular nerve			
Temporal lobe	Vestibulocochlear nerve			
8 **Basal Ganglia**	**P** **Glossopharyngeal Nerve**			
Basal nuclei	Carotid sinus nerve			
Claustrum	Ninth cranial nerve			
Corpus striatum	Tympanic nerve			
Globus pallidus	**Q** **Vagus Nerve**			
Substantia nigra	Anterior vagal trunk			
Subthalamic nucleus	Pharyngeal plexus			
9 **Thalamus**	Pneumogastric nerve			
Epithalamus	Posterior vagal trunk			
Geniculate nucleus	Pulmonary plexus			
Metathalamus	Recurrent laryngeal nerve			
Pulvinar	Superior laryngeal nerve			
A **Hypothalamus**	Tenth cranial nerve			
Mammillary body	**R** **Accessory Nerve**			
B **Pons**	Eleventh cranial nerve			
Apneustic center	**S** **Hypoglossal Nerve**			
Basis pontis	Twelfth cranial nerve			
Locus ceruleus	**T** **Spinal Meninges**			
Pneumotaxic center	Arachnoid mater, spinal			
Pontine tegmentum	Denticulate (dentate)			
Superior olivary nucleus	ligament			
C **Cerebellum**	Dura mater, spinal			
Culmen	Filum terminale			
D **Medulla Oblongata**	Leptomeninges, spinal			
Myelencephalon	Pia mater, spinal			
F **Olfactory Nerve**	**W** **Cervical Spinal Cord**			
First cranial nerve	**X** **Thoracic Spinal Cord**			
Olfactory bulb	**Y** **Lumbar Spinal Cord**			
G **Optic Nerve**	Cauda equina			
Optic chiasma	Conus medullaris			
Second cranial nerve				

0   Medical and Surgical
0   Central Nervous System and Cranial Nerves
P   Removal   Definition: Taking out or off a device from a body part
                          Explanation: If a device is taken out and a similar device put in without cutting or puncturing the skin or mucous membrane, the procedure is
                          coded to the root operation CHANGE. Otherwise, the procedure for taking out a device is coded to the root operation REMOVAL.

Body Part Character 4	Approach Character 5	Device Character 6	Qualifier Character 7
0 Brain Cerebrum Corpus callosum Encephalon **V Spinal Cord**	**0 Open** **3 Percutaneous** **4 Percutaneous Endoscopic**	**0 Drainage Device** **2 Monitoring Device** **3 Infusion Device** **7 Autologous Tissue Substitute** **J Synthetic Substitute** **K Nonautologous Tissue Substitute** **M Neurostimulator Lead** **Y Other Device**	**Z No Qualifier**
0 Brain Cerebrum Corpus callosum Encephalon **V Spinal Cord**	**X External**	**0 Drainage Device** **2 Monitoring Device** **3 Infusion Device** **M Neurostimulator Lead**	**Z No Qualifier**
6 Cerebral Ventricle Aqueduct of Sylvius Cerebral aqueduct (Sylvius) Choroid plexus Ependyma Foramen of Monro (intraventricular) Fourth ventricle Interventricular foramen (Monro) Left lateral ventricle Right lateral ventricle Third ventricle **U Spinal Canal** Epidural space, spinal Extradural space, spinal Subarachnoid space, spinal Subdural space, spinal Vertebral canal	**0 Open** **3 Percutaneous** **4 Percutaneous Endoscopic**	**0 Drainage Device** **2 Monitoring Device** **3 Infusion Device** **J Synthetic Substitute** **M Neurostimulator Lead** **Y Other Device**	**Z No Qualifier**
6 Cerebral Ventricle Aqueduct of Sylvius Cerebral aqueduct (Sylvius) Choroid plexus Ependyma Foramen of Monro (intraventricular) Fourth ventricle Interventricular foramen (Monro) Left lateral ventricle Right lateral ventricle Third ventricle **U Spinal Canal** Epidural space, spinal Extradural space, spinal Subarachnoid space, spinal Subdural space, spinal Vertebral canal	**X External**	**0 Drainage Device** **2 Monitoring Device** **3 Infusion Device** **M Neurostimulator Lead**	**Z No Qualifier**
E Cranial Nerve	**0 Open** **3 Percutaneous** **4 Percutaneous Endoscopic**	**0 Drainage Device** **2 Monitoring Device** **3 Infusion Device** **7 Autologous Tissue Substitute** **M Neurostimulator Lead** **Y Other Device**	**Z No Qualifier**
E Cranial Nerve	**X External**	**0 Drainage Device** **2 Monitoring Device** **3 Infusion Device** **M Neurostimulator Lead**	**Z No Qualifier**

Non-OR   00P[0,V]3[0,2,3]Z
Non-OR   00P[0,V][3,4]YZ
Non-OR   00P[0,V]X[0,2,3,M]Z
Non-OR   00P[6,U]3[0,2,3]Z
Non-OR   00P[6,U][3,4]YZ
Non-OR   00P[6,U]X[0,2,3,M]Z
Non-OR   00PE3[0,2,3]Z
Non-OR   00PE[3,4]YZ
Non-OR   00PEX[0,2,3,M]Z

Ø **Medical and Surgical**
Ø **Central Nervous System and Cranial Nerves**
Q **Repair** Definition: Restoring, to the extent possible, a body part to its normal anatomic structure and function
Explanation: Used only when the method to accomplish the repair is not one of the other root operations

Body Part Character 4		Approach Character 5	Device Character 6	Qualifier Character 7

Ø **Brain**
 Cerebrum
 Corpus callosum
 Encephalon
1 **Cerebral Meninges**
 Arachnoid mater,
  intracranial
 Leptomeninges,
  intracranial
 Pia mater, intracranial
2 **Dura Mater**
 Diaphragma sellae
 Dura mater, intracranial
 Falx cerebri
 Tentorium cerebelli
6 **Cerebral Ventricle**
 Aqueduct of Sylvius
 Cerebral aqueduct (Sylvius)
 Choroid plexus
 Ependyma
 Foramen of Monro
  (intraventricular)
 Fourth ventricle
 Interventricular foramen
  (Monro)
 Left lateral ventricle
 Right lateral ventricle
 Third ventricle
7 **Cerebral Hemisphere**
 Frontal lobe
 Occipital lobe
 Parietal lobe
 Temporal lobe
8 **Basal Ganglia**
 Basal nuclei
 Claustrum
 Corpus striatum
 Globus pallidus
 Substantia nigra
 Subthalamic nucleus
9 **Thalamus**
 Epithalamus
 Geniculate nucleus
 Metathalamus
 Pulvinar
A **Hypothalamus**
 Mammillary body
B **Pons**
 Apneustic center
 Basis pontis
 Locus ceruleus
 Pneumotaxic center
 Pontine tegmentum
 Superior olivary nucleus
C **Cerebellum**
 Culmen
D **Medulla Oblongata**
 Myelencephalon
F **Olfactory Nerve**
 First cranial nerve
 Olfactory bulb
G **Optic Nerve**
 Optic chiasma
 Second cranial nerve
	H **Oculomotor Nerve**
	 Third cranial nerve
	J **Trochlear Nerve**
	 Fourth cranial nerve
	K **Trigeminal Nerve**
	 Fifth cranial nerve
	 Gasserian ganglion
	 Mandibular nerve
	 Maxillary nerve
	 Ophthalmic nerve
	 Trifacial nerve
	L **Abducens Nerve**
	 Sixth cranial nerve
	M **Facial Nerve**
	 Chorda tympani
	 Geniculate ganglion
	 Greater superficial petrosal
	  nerve
	 Nerve to the stapedius
	 Parotid plexus
	 Posterior auricular nerve
	 Seventh cranial nerve
	 Submandibular ganglion
	N **Acoustic Nerve**
	 Cochlear nerve
	 Eighth cranial nerve
	 Scarpa's (vestibular)
	  ganglion
	 Spiral ganglion
	 Vestibular (Scarpa's)
	  ganglion
	 Vestibular nerve
	 Vestibulocochlear nerve
	P **Glossopharyngeal Nerve**
	 Carotid sinus nerve
	 Ninth cranial nerve
	 Tympanic nerve
	Q **Vagus Nerve**
	 Anterior vagal trunk
	 Pharyngeal plexus
	 Pneumogastric nerve
	 Posterior vagal trunk
	 Pulmonary plexus
	 Recurrent laryngeal nerve
	 Superior laryngeal nerve
	 Tenth cranial nerve
	R **Accessory Nerve**
	 Eleventh cranial nerve
	S **Hypoglossal Nerve**
	 Twelfth cranial nerve
	T **Spinal Meninges**
	 Arachnoid mater, spinal
	 Denticulate (dentate)
	  ligament
	 Dura mater, spinal
	 Filum terminale
	 Leptomeninges, spinal
	 Pia mater, spinal
	W **Cervical Spinal Cord**
	X **Thoracic Spinal Cord**
	Y **Lumbar Spinal Cord**
	 Cauda equina
	 Conus medullaris
		Ø **Open**
		3 **Percutaneous**
		4 **Percutaneous Endoscopic**
			Z **No Device**	Z **No Qualifier**

Central Nervous System and Cranial Nerves

Ø   **Medical and Surgical**
Ø   **Central Nervous System and Cranial Nerves**
R   **Replacement**   Definition: Putting in or on biological or synthetic material that physically takes the place and/or function of all or a portion of a body part

Explanation: The body part may have been taken out or replaced, or may be taken out, physically eradicated, or rendered nonfunctional during the REPLACEMENT procedure. A REMOVAL procedure is coded for taking out the device used in a previous replacement procedure.

Body Part Character 4		Approach Character 5	Device Character 6	Qualifier Character 7

1 **Cerebral Meninges**
  Arachnoid mater,
    intracranial
  Leptomeninges,
    intracranial
  Pia mater, intracranial
2 **Dura Mater**
  Diaphragma sellae
  Dura mater, intracranial
  Falx cerebri
  Tentorium cerebelli
6 **Cerebral Ventricle**
  Aqueduct of Sylvius
  Cerebral aqueduct (Sylvius)
  Choroid plexus
  Ependyma
  Foramen of Monro
    (intraventricular)
  Fourth ventricle
  Interventricular foramen
    (Monro)
  Left lateral ventricle
  Right lateral ventricle
  Third ventricle
F **Olfactory Nerve**
  First cranial nerve
  Olfactory bulb
G **Optic Nerve**
  Optic chiasma
  Second cranial nerve
H **Oculomotor Nerve**
  Third cranial nerve
J **Trochlear Nerve**
  Fourth cranial nerve
K **Trigeminal Nerve**
  Fifth cranial nerve
  Gasserian ganglion
  Mandibular nerve
  Maxillary nerve
  Ophthalmic nerve
  Trifacial nerve
L **Abducens Nerve**
  Sixth cranial nerve
	M **Facial Nerve**
	  Chorda tympani
	  Geniculate ganglion
	  Greater superficial petrosal
	    nerve
	  Nerve to the stapedius
	  Parotid plexus
	  Posterior auricular nerve
	  Seventh cranial nerve
	  Submandibular ganglion
	N **Acoustic Nerve**
	  Cochlear nerve
	  Eighth cranial nerve
	  Scarpa's (vestibular)
	    ganglion
	  Spiral ganglion
	  Vestibular (Scarpa's)
	    ganglion
	  Vestibular nerve
	  Vestibulocochlear nerve
	P **Glossopharyngeal Nerve**
	  Carotid sinus nerve
	  Ninth cranial nerve
	  Tympanic nerve
	Q **Vagus Nerve**
	  Anterior vagal trunk
	  Pharyngeal plexus
	  Pneumogastric nerve
	  Posterior vagal trunk
	  Pulmonary plexus
	  Recurrent laryngeal nerve
	  Superior laryngeal nerve
	  Tenth cranial nerve
	R **Accessory Nerve**
	  Eleventh cranial nerve
	S **Hypoglossal Nerve**
	  Twelfth cranial nerve
	T **Spinal Meninges**
	  Arachnoid mater, spinal
	  Denticulate (dentate)
	    ligament
	  Dura mater, spinal
	  Filum terminale
	  Leptomeninges, spinal
	  Pia mater, spinal
		Ø **Open**
		4 **Percutaneous Endoscopic**
			7 **Autologous Tissue**
			  Substitute
			J **Synthetic Substitute**
			K **Nonautologous Tissue**
			  Substitute
				Z **No Qualifier**

0   **Medical and Surgical**
0   **Central Nervous System and Cranial Nerves**
S   **Reposition**   Definition: Moving to its normal location, or other suitable location, all or a portion of a body part

Explanation: The body part is moved to a new location from an abnormal location, or from a normal location where it is not functioning correctly. The body part may or may not be cut out or off to be moved to the new location.

Body Part Character 4		Approach Character 5	Device Character 6	Qualifier Character 7

F **Olfactory Nerve**
   First cranial nerve
   Olfactory bulb
G **Optic Nerve**
   Optic chiasma
   Second cranial nerve
H **Oculomotor Nerve**
   Third cranial nerve
J **Trochlear Nerve**
   Fourth cranial nerve
K **Trigeminal Nerve**
   Fifth cranial nerve
   Gasserian ganglion
   Mandibular nerve
   Maxillary nerve
   Ophthalmic nerve
   Trifacial nerve
L **Abducens Nerve**
   Sixth cranial nerve
M **Facial Nerve**
   Chorda tympani
   Geniculate ganglion
   Greater superficial petrosal
     nerve
   Nerve to the stapedius
   Parotid plexus
   Posterior auricular nerve
   Seventh cranial nerve
   Submandibular ganglion
	N **Acoustic Nerve**
	   Cochlear nerve
	   Eighth cranial nerve
	   Scarpa's (vestibular)
	     ganglion
	   Spiral ganglion
	   Vestibular (Scarpa's)
	     ganglion
	   Vestibular nerve
	   Vestibulocochlear nerve
	P **Glossopharyngeal Nerve**
	   Carotid sinus nerve
	   Ninth cranial nerve
	   Tympanic nerve
	Q **Vagus Nerve**
	   Anterior vagal trunk
	   Pharyngeal plexus
	   Pneumogastric nerve
	   Posterior vagal trunk
	   Pulmonary plexus
	   Recurrent laryngeal nerve
	   Superior laryngeal nerve
	   Tenth cranial nerve
	R **Accessory Nerve**
	   Eleventh cranial nerve
	S **Hypoglossal Nerve**
	   Twelfth cranial nerve
	W **Cervical Spinal Cord**
	X **Thoracic Spinal Cord**
	Y **Lumbar Spinal Cord**
	   Cauda equina
	   Conus medullaris
		0 Open
		3 Percutaneous
		4 Percutaneous Endoscopic
			Z No Device	**Z** No Qualifier

0   **Medical and Surgical**
0   **Central Nervous System and Cranial Nerves**
T   **Resection**   Definition: Cutting out or off, without replacement, all of a body part

Explanation: None

Body Part Character 4	Approach Character 5	Device Character 6	Qualifier Character 7

7 **Cerebral Hemisphere**
   Frontal lobe
   Occipital lobe
   Parietal lobe
   Temporal lobe
	0 Open
	3 Percutaneous
	4 Percutaneous Endoscopic
		Z No Device	**Z** No Qualifier

Central Nervous System and Cranial Nerves *(side tab)*

Ø   **Medical and Surgical**
Ø   **Central Nervous System and Cranial Nerves**
U   **Supplement**   Definition: Putting in or on biological or synthetic material that physically reinforces and/or augments the function of a portion of a body part
                  Explanation: The biological material is non-living, or is living and from the same individual. The body part may have been previously replaced, and the SUPPLEMENT procedure is performed to physically reinforce and/or augment the function of the replaced body part.

Body Part Character 4		Approach Character 5	Device Character 6	Qualifier Character 7

1 Cerebral Meninges
Arachnoid mater,
  intracranial
Leptomeninges,
  intracranial
Pia mater, intracranial
2 Dura Mater
Diaphragma sellae
Dura mater, intracranial
Falx cerebri
Tentorium cerebelli
6 Cerebral Ventricle
Aqueduct of Sylvius
Cerebral aqueduct (Sylvius)
Choroid plexus
Ependyma
Foramen of Monro
  (intraventricular)
Fourth ventricle
Interventricular foramen
  (Monro)
Left lateral ventricle
Right lateral ventricle
Third ventricle
F Olfactory Nerve
First cranial nerve
Olfactory bulb
G Optic Nerve
Optic chiasma
Second cranial nerve
H Oculomotor Nerve
Third cranial nerve
J Trochlear Nerve
Fourth cranial nerve
K Trigeminal Nerve
Fifth cranial nerve
Gasserian ganglion
Mandibular nerve
Maxillary nerve
Ophthalmic nerve
Trifacial nerve
L Abducens Nerve
Sixth cranial nerve
	M Facial Nerve
	Chorda tympani
	Geniculate ganglion
	Greater superficial petrosal
	  nerve
	Nerve to the stapedius
	Parotid plexus
	Posterior auricular nerve
	Seventh cranial nerve
	Submandibular ganglion
	N Acoustic Nerve
	Cochlear nerve
	Eighth cranial nerve
	Scarpa's (vestibular)
	  ganglion
	Spiral ganglion
	Vestibular (Scarpa's)
	  ganglion
	Vestibular nerve
	Vestibulocochlear nerve
	P Glossopharyngeal Nerve
	Carotid sinus nerve
	Ninth cranial nerve
	Tympanic nerve
	Q Vagus Nerve
	Anterior vagal trunk
	Pharyngeal plexus
	Pneumogastric nerve
	Posterior vagal trunk
	Pulmonary plexus
	Recurrent laryngeal nerve
	Superior laryngeal nerve
	Tenth cranial nerve
	R Accessory Nerve
	Eleventh cranial nerve
	S Hypoglossal Nerve
	Twelfth cranial nerve
	T Spinal Meninges
	Arachnoid mater, spinal
	Denticulate (dentate)
	  ligament
	Dura mater, spinal
	Filum terminale
	Leptomeninges, spinal
	Pia mater, spinal
		Ø Open
		3 Percutaneous
		4 Percutaneous Endoscopic
			7 Autologous Tissue
			  Substitute
			J Synthetic Substitute
			K Nonautologous Tissue
			  Substitute
				Z No Qualifier

LC Limited Coverage   NC Noncovered   ⊞ Combination Member   HAC associated procedure   Combination Only   DRG Non-OR   Non-OR   New/Revised in GREEN

146   ICD-10-PCS 2020

0   **Medical and Surgical**
0   **Central Nervous System and Cranial Nerves**
W   **Revision**   Definition: Correcting, to the extent possible, a portion of a malfunctioning device or the position of a displaced device

Explanation: Revision can include correcting a malfunctioning or displaced device by taking out or putting in components of the device such as a screw or pin

Body Part Character 4	Approach Character 5	Device Character 6	Qualifier Character 7
0 **Brain** Cerebrum Corpus callosum Encephalon **V** **Spinal Cord**	**0** Open **3** Percutaneous **4** Percutaneous Endoscopic	**0** Drainage Device **2** Monitoring Device **3** Infusion Device **7** Autologous Tissue Substitute **J** Synthetic Substitute **K** Nonautologous Tissue Substitute **M** Neurostimulator Lead **Y** Other Device	**Z** No Qualifier
0 **Brain** Cerebrum Corpus callosum Encephalon **V** **Spinal Cord**	**X** External	**0** Drainage Device **2** Monitoring Device **3** Infusion Device **7** Autologous Tissue Substitute **J** Synthetic Substitute **K** Nonautologous Tissue Substitute **M** Neurostimulator Lead	**Z** No Qualifier
6 **Cerebral Ventricle** Aqueduct of Sylvius Cerebral aqueduct (Sylvius) Choroid plexus Ependyma Foramen of Monro (intraventricular) Fourth ventricle Interventricular foramen (Monro) Left lateral ventricle Right lateral ventricle Third ventricle **U** **Spinal Canal** Epidural space, spinal Extradural space, spinal Subarachnoid space, spinal Subdural space, spinal Vertebral canal	**0** Open **3** Percutaneous **4** Percutaneous Endoscopic	**0** Drainage Device **2** Monitoring Device **3** Infusion Device **J** Synthetic Substitute **M** Neurostimulator Lead **Y** Other Device	**Z** No Qualifier
6 **Cerebral Ventricle** Aqueduct of Sylvius Cerebral aqueduct (Sylvius) Choroid plexus Ependyma Foramen of Monro (intraventricular) Fourth ventricle Interventricular foramen (Monro) Left lateral ventricle Right lateral ventricle Third ventricle **U** **Spinal Canal** Epidural space, spinal Extradural space, spinal Subarachnoid space, spinal Subdural space, spinal Vertebral canal	**X** External	**0** Drainage Device **2** Monitoring Device **3** Infusion Device **J** Synthetic Substitute **M** Neurostimulator Lead	**Z** No Qualifier
E **Cranial Nerve**	**0** Open **3** Percutaneous **4** Percutaneous Endoscopic	**0** Drainage Device **2** Monitoring Device **3** Infusion Device **7** Autologous Tissue Substitute **M** Neurostimulator Lead **Y** Other Device	**Z** No Qualifier
E **Cranial Nerve**	**X** External	**0** Drainage Device **2** Monitoring Device **3** Infusion Device **7** Autologous Tissue Substitute **M** Neurostimulator Lead	**Z** No Qualifier

Non-OR	00W[0,V][3,4]YZ
Non-OR	00W[0,V]X[0,2,3,7,J,K,M]Z
Non-OR	00W[6,U][3,4]YZ
Non-OR	00W[6,U]X[0,2,3,J,M]Z
Non-OR	00WE[3,4]YZ
Non-OR	00WEX[0,2,3,7,M]Z

LC Limited Coverage   NC Noncovered   ⊞ Combination Member   HAC associated procedure   Combination Only   DRG Non-OR   Non-OR   New/Revised in GREEN

ICD-10-PCS 2020   147

00W–00W

0   **Medical and Surgical**
0   **Central Nervous System and Cranial Nerves**
X   **Transfer**   Definition: Moving, without taking out, all or a portion of a body part to another location to take over the function of all or a portion of a body part
                    Explanation: The body part transferred remains connected to its vascular and nervous supply

Body Part Character 4	Approach Character 5	Device Character 6	Qualifier Character 7

F **Olfactory Nerve**
  First cranial nerve
  Olfactory bulb
	0 Open
	4 Percutaneous Endoscopic
		Z No Device	**F** Olfactory Nerve
			G Optic Nerve
			H Oculomotor Nerve

G **Optic Nerve**
  Optic chiasma
  Second cranial nerve
			J Trochlear Nerve
			K Trigeminal Nerve
			L Abducens Nerve

H **Oculomotor Nerve** Third cranial nerve			**M** Facial Nerve **N** Acoustic Nerve
J **Trochlear Nerve** Fourth cranial nerve			**P** Glossopharyngeal Nerve **Q** Vagus Nerve

K **Trigeminal Nerve**
  Fifth cranial nerve
  Gasserian ganglion
  Mandibular nerve
  Maxillary nerve
  Ophthalmic nerve
  Trifacial nerve
			R Accessory Nerve
			S Hypoglossal Nerve

L **Abducens Nerve** Sixth cranial nerve			

M **Facial Nerve**
  Chorda tympani
  Geniculate ganglion
  Greater superficial petrosal nerve
  Nerve to the stapedius
  Parotid plexus
  Posterior auricular nerve
  Seventh cranial nerve
  Submandibular ganglion			

N **Acoustic Nerve**
  Cochlear nerve
  Eighth cranial nerve
  Scarpa's (vestibular) ganglion
  Spiral ganglion
  Vestibular (Scarpa's) ganglion
  Vestibular nerve
  Vestibulocochlear nerve			

P **Glossopharyngeal Nerve**
  Carotid sinus nerve
  Ninth cranial nerve
  Tympanic nerve			

Q **Vagus Nerve**
  Anterior vagal trunk
  Pharyngeal plexus
  Pneumogastric nerve
  Posterior vagal trunk
  Pulmonary plexus
  Recurrent laryngeal nerve
  Superior laryngeal nerve
  Tenth cranial nerve			

R **Accessory Nerve** Eleventh cranial nerve			
S **Hypoglossal Nerve** Twelfth cranial nerve			

Peripheral Nervous System Ø12–Ø1X

Character Meanings

This Character Meaning table is provided as a guide to assist the user in the identification of character members that may be found in this section of code tables. It **SHOULD NOT** be used to build a PCS code.

Operation–Character 3	Body Part–Character 4	Approach–Character 5	Device–Character 6	Qualifier–Character 7
2 Change	Ø Cervical Plexus	Ø Open	Ø Drainage Device	1 Cervical Nerve
5 Destruction	1 Cervical Nerve	3 Percutaneous	2 Monitoring Device	2 Phrenic Nerve
8 Division	2 Phrenic Nerve	4 Percutaneous Endoscopic	7 Autologous Tissue Substitute	4 Ulnar Nerve
9 Drainage	3 Brachial Plexus	X External	M Neurostimulator Lead	5 Median Nerve
B Excision	4 Ulnar Nerve		Y Other Device	6 Radial Nerve
C Extirpation	5 Median Nerve		Z No Device	8 Thoracic Nerve
D Extraction	6 Radial Nerve			B Lumbar Nerve
H Insertion	8 Thoracic Nerve			C Perineal Nerve
J Inspection	9 Lumbar Plexus			D Femoral Nerve
N Release	A Lumbosacral Plexus			F Sciatic Nerve
P Removal	B Lumbar Nerve			G Tibial Nerve
Q Repair	C Pudendal Nerve			H Peroneal Nerve
R Replacement	D Femoral Nerve			X Diagnostic
S Reposition	F Sciatic Nerve			Z No Qualifier
U Supplement	G Tibial Nerve			
W Revision	H Peroneal Nerve			
X Transfer	K Head and Neck Sympathetic Nerve			
	L Thoracic Sympathetic Nerve			
	M Abdominal Sympathetic Nerve			
	N Lumbar Sympathetic Nerve			
	P Sacral Sympathetic Nerve			
	Q Sacral Plexus			
	R Sacral Nerve			
	Y Peripheral Nerve			

AHA Coding Clinic for table Ø1B
2018, 2Q, 22   Excision of synovial cyst
2017, 2Q, 19   Thoracic outlet decompression with sympathectomy

AHA Coding Clinic for table Ø1N
2019, 1Q, 28   Decompressive laminectomy of both spinal cord and nerve roots
2018, 2Q, 22   Excision of synovial cyst
2017, 2Q, 19   Thoracic outlet decompression with sympathectomy
2016, 2Q, 16   Decompressive laminectomy/foraminotomy and lumbar discectomy
2016, 2Q, 17   Removal of longitudinal ligament to decompress cervical nerve root
2016, 2Q, 23   Thoracic outlet syndrome and release of brachial plexus
2015, 2Q, 34   Decompressive laminectomy
2014, 3Q, 33   Radial fracture treatment with open reduction internal fixation, and release of carpal ligament

AHA Coding Clinic for table Ø1U
2017, 4Q, 62   Added and revised device values - Nerve substitutes

Median and Ulnar Nerves

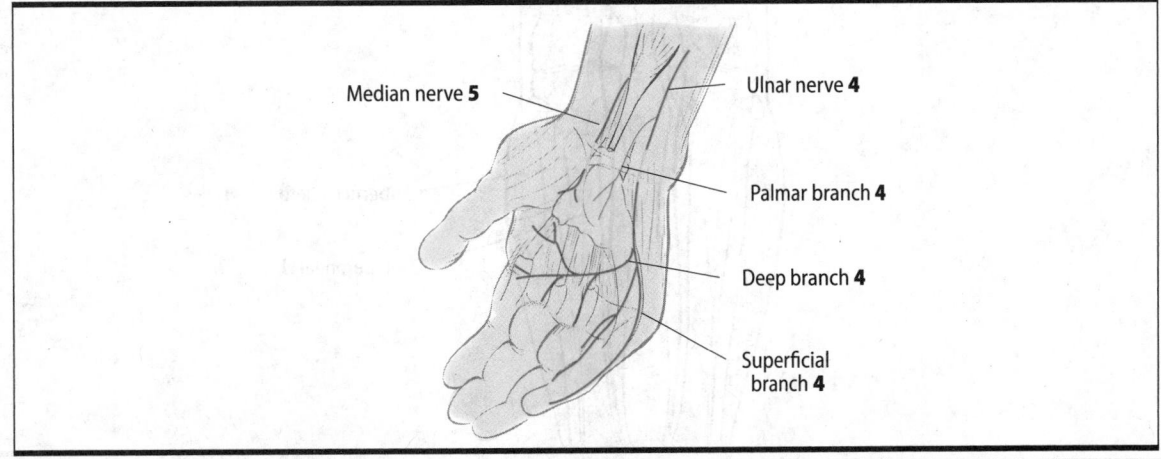

Median nerve **5**

Ulnar nerve **4**

Palmar branch **4**

Deep branch **4**

Superficial branch **4**

Peripheral Nervous System

Great auricular ⎤ Cervical plexus Ø
Lesser occiptial ⎦

Greater occipital ⎤
Suboccipital ⎬ Cervical nerve 1
3rd occiptial ⎦

Ansa cervicalis
Transverse cervical
Cervical plexus Ø

L. phrenic 2
Supraclavicular Ø

Dorsal scapular
First intercostal
Subclavian
Long thoracic
Axillary
Musculocutaneous
Brachial plexus 3

Median 5

Ulnar 4
Radial 6
Thoracic splanchnic L

Intercostal nerves 8

Lumbar splanchnic N
Genitofemoral
Iliohypogastric
Ilioinguinal
Obturator
Lateral femoral cutaneous
Accessory obturator
Superior gluteal
Lumbar plexus 9

Subcostal 8

Sacral R

Inferior gluteal Q
Sacral splanchnic P
Pelvic splanchnic P
Pudendal Q
Posterior femoral cutaneous Q
Sacral plexus and sacral sympathetic nerves

Posterior scrotal/labial C
Femoral D

Sciatic F

Saphenous D

Common peroneal H

Tibial G

Superficial peroneal H

Deep peroneal H

Ø   Medical and Surgical
1   Peripheral Nervous System
2   Change   Definition: Taking out or off a device from a body part and putting back an identical or similar device in or on the same body part without cutting or puncturing the skin or a mucous membrane
                 Explanation: All CHANGE procedures are coded using the approach EXTERNAL

Body Part Character 4	Approach Character 5	Device Character 6	Qualifier Character 7
Y Peripheral Nerve	X External	Ø Drainage Device Y Other Device	Z No Qualifier

Non-OR   All body part, approach, device, and qualifier values

Ø   Medical and Surgical
1   Peripheral Nervous System
5   Destruction   Definition: Physical eradication of all or a portion of a body part by the direct use of energy, force, or a destructive agent
                 Explanation: None of the body part is physically taken out

Body Part Character 4		Approach Character 5	Device Character 6	Qualifier Character 7

Ø   **Cervical Plexus**
    Ansa cervicalis
    Cutaneous (transverse) cervical nerve
    Great auricular nerve
    Lesser occipital nerve
    Supraclavicular nerve
    Transverse (cutaneous) cervical nerve
1   **Cervical Nerve**
    Greater occipital nerve
    Spinal nerve, cervical
    Suboccipital nerve
    Third occipital nerve
2   **Phrenic Nerve**
    Accessory phrenic nerve
3   **Brachial Plexus**
    Axillary nerve
    Dorsal scapular nerve
    First intercostal nerve
    Long thoracic nerve
    Musculocutaneous nerve
    Subclavius nerve
    Suprascapular nerve
4   **Ulnar Nerve**
    Cubital nerve
5   **Median Nerve**
    Anterior interosseous nerve
    Palmar cutaneous nerve
6   **Radial Nerve**
    Dorsal digital nerve
    Musculospiral nerve
    Palmar cutaneous nerve
    Posterior interosseous nerve
8   **Thoracic Nerve**
    Intercostal nerve
    Intercostobrachial nerve
    Spinal nerve, thoracic
    Subcostal nerve
9   **Lumbar Plexus**
    Accessory obturator nerve
    Genitofemoral nerve
    Iliohypogastric nerve
    Ilioinguinal nerve
    Lateral femoral cutaneous nerve
    Obturator nerve
    Superior gluteal nerve
A   **Lumbosacral Plexus**
B   **Lumbar Nerve**
    Lumbosacral trunk
    Spinal nerve, lumbar
    Superior clunic (cluneal) nerve
C   **Pudendal Nerve**
    Posterior labial nerve
    Posterior scrotal nerve
D   **Femoral Nerve**
    Anterior crural nerve
    Saphenous nerve
F   **Sciatic Nerve**
    Ischiatic nerve
G   **Tibial Nerve**
    Lateral plantar nerve
    Medial plantar nerve
    Medial popliteal nerve
    Medial sural cutaneous nerve
	H **Peroneal Nerve**
	    Common fibular nerve
	    Common peroneal nerve
	    External popliteal nerve
	    Lateral sural cutaneous nerve
	K **Head and Neck Sympathetic Nerve**
	    Cavernous plexus
	    Cervical ganglion
	    Ciliary ganglion
	    Internal carotid plexus
	    Otic ganglion
	    Pterygopalatine (sphenopalatine)
	      ganglion
	    Sphenopalatine (pterygopalatine)
	      ganglion
	    Stellate ganglion
	    Submandibular ganglion
	    Submaxillary ganglion
	L **Thoracic Sympathetic Nerve**
	    Cardiac plexus
	    Esophageal plexus
	    Greater splanchnic nerve
	    Inferior cardiac nerve
	    Least splanchnic nerve
	    Lesser splanchnic nerve
	    Middle cardiac nerve
	    Pulmonary plexus
	    Superior cardiac nerve
	    Thoracic aortic plexus
	    Thoracic ganglion
	M **Abdominal Sympathetic Nerve**
	    Abdominal aortic plexus
	    Auerbach's (myenteric) plexus
	    Celiac (solar) plexus
	    Celiac ganglion
	    Gastric plexus
	    Hepatic plexus
	    Inferior hypogastric plexus
	    Inferior mesenteric ganglion
	    Inferior mesenteric plexus
	    Meissner's (submucous) plexus
	    Myenteric (Auerbach's) plexus
	    Pancreatic plexus
	    Pelvic splanchnic nerve
	    Renal plexus
	    Solar (celiac) plexus
	    Splenic plexus
	    Submucous (Meissner's) plexus
	    Superior hypogastric plexus
	    Superior mesenteric ganglion
	    Superior mesenteric plexus
	    Suprarenal plexus
	N **Lumbar Sympathetic Nerve**
	    Lumbar ganglion
	    Lumbar splanchnic nerve
	P **Sacral Sympathetic Nerve**
	    Ganglion impar (ganglion of
	      Walther)
	    Pelvic splanchnic nerve
	    Sacral ganglion
	    Sacral splanchnic nerve
	Q **Sacral Plexus**
	    Inferior gluteal nerve
	    Posterior femoral cutaneous nerve
	    Pudendal nerve
	R **Sacral Nerve**
	    Spinal nerve, sacral
		Ø Open
		3 Percutaneous
		4 Percutaneous
		    Endoscopic
			Z No Device	Z No Qualifier

Non-OR   Ø15[Ø,2,3,4,5,6,9,A,C,D,F,G,H,Q][Ø,3,4]ZZ   Non-OR   Ø15[1,8,B,R]3ZZ

Peripheral Nervous System

Ø　Medical and Surgical
1　Peripheral Nervous System
8　Division　　　Definition: Cutting into a body part, without draining fluids and/or gases from the body part, in order to separate or transect a body part
　　　　　　　　　　Explanation: All or a portion of the body part is separated into two or more portions

Body Part Character 4		Approach Character 5	Device Character 6	Qualifier Character 7
Ø Cervical Plexus Ansa cervicalis Cutaneous (transverse) cervical 　nerve Great auricular nerve Lesser occipital nerve Supraclavicular nerve Transverse (cutaneous) cervical 　nerve **1 Cervical Nerve** Greater occipital nerve Spinal nerve, cervical Suboccipital nerve Third occipital nerve **2 Phrenic Nerve** Accessory phrenic nerve **3 Brachial Plexus** Axillary nerve Dorsal scapular nerve First intercostal nerve Long thoracic nerve Musculocutaneous nerve Subclavius nerve Suprascapular nerve **4 Ulnar Nerve** Cubital nerve **5 Median Nerve** Anterior interosseous nerve Palmar cutaneous nerve **6 Radial Nerve** Dorsal digital nerve Musculospiral nerve Palmar cutaneous nerve Posterior interosseous nerve **8 Thoracic Nerve** Intercostal nerve Intercostobrachial nerve Spinal nerve, thoracic Subcostal nerve **9 Lumbar Plexus** Accessory obturator nerve Genitofemoral nerve Iliohypogastric nerve Ilioinguinal nerve Lateral femoral cutaneous 　nerve Obturator nerve Superior gluteal nerve **A Lumbosacral Plexus** **B Lumbar Nerve** Lumbosacral trunk Spinal nerve, lumbar Superior clunic (cluneal) nerve **C Pudendal Nerve** Posterior labial nerve Posterior scrotal nerve **D Femoral Nerve** Anterior crural nerve Saphenous nerve **F Sciatic Nerve** Ischiatic nerve	**G Tibial Nerve** Lateral plantar nerve Medial plantar nerve Medial popliteal nerve Medial sural cutaneous nerve **H Peroneal Nerve** Common fibular nerve Common peroneal nerve External popliteal nerve Lateral sural cutaneous nerve **K Head and Neck Sympathetic 　Nerve** Cavernous plexus Cervical ganglion Ciliary ganglion Internal carotid plexus Otic ganglion Pterygopalatine 　(sphenopalatine) ganglion Sphenopalatine 　(pterygopalatine) ganglion Stellate ganglion Submandibular ganglion Submaxillary ganglion **L Thoracic Sympathetic Nerve** Cardiac plexus Esophageal plexus Greater splanchnic nerve Inferior cardiac nerve Least splanchnic nerve Lesser splanchnic nerve Middle cardiac nerve Pulmonary plexus Superior cardiac nerve Thoracic aortic plexus Thoracic ganglion **M Abdominal Sympathetic 　Nerve** Abdominal aortic plexus Auerbach's (myenteric) plexus Celiac (solar) plexus Celiac ganglion Gastric plexus Hepatic plexus Inferior hypogastric plexus Inferior mesenteric ganglion Inferior mesenteric plexus Meissner's (submucous) plexus Myenteric (Auerbach's) plexus Pancreatic plexus Pelvic splanchnic nerve Renal plexus Solar (celiac) plexus Splenic plexus Submucous (Meissner's) plexus Superior hypogastric plexus Superior mesenteric ganglion Superior mesenteric plexus Suprarenal plexus **N Lumbar Sympathetic Nerve** Lumbar ganglion Lumbar splanchnic nerve **P Sacral Sympathetic Nerve** Ganglion impar (ganglion of 　Walther) Pelvic splanchnic nerve Sacral ganglion Sacral splanchnic nerve **Q Sacral Plexus** Inferior gluteal nerve Posterior femoral cutaneous 　nerve Pudendal nerve **R Sacral Nerve** Spinal nerve, sacral	**Ø** Open **3** Percutaneous **4** Percutaneous Endoscopic	**Z** No Device	**Z** No Qualifier

Ø   **Medical and Surgical**
1   **Peripheral Nervous System**
9   **Drainage**   Definition: Taking or letting out fluids and/or gases from a body part
                        Explanation: The qualifier DIAGNOSTIC is used to identify drainage procedures that are biopsies

Body Part Character 4		Approach Character 5	Device Character 6	Qualifier Character 7

Ø Cervical Plexus
Ansa cervicalis
Cutaneous (transverse) cervical
   nerve
Great auricular nerve
Lesser occipital nerve
Supraclavicular nerve
Transverse (cutaneous) cervical
   nerve
1 Cervical Nerve
Greater occipital nerve
Spinal nerve, cervical
Suboccipital nerve
Third occipital nerve
2 Phrenic Nerve
Accessory phrenic nerve
3 Brachial Plexus
Axillary nerve
Dorsal scapular nerve
First intercostal nerve
Long thoracic nerve
Musculocutaneous nerve
Subclavius nerve
Suprascapular nerve
4 Ulnar Nerve
Cubital nerve
5 Median Nerve
Anterior interosseous nerve
Palmar cutaneous nerve
6 Radial Nerve
Dorsal digital nerve
Musculospiral nerve
Palmar cutaneous nerve
Posterior interosseous nerve
8 Thoracic Nerve
Intercostal nerve
Intercostobrachial nerve
Spinal nerve, thoracic
Subcostal nerve
9 Lumbar Plexus
Accessory obturator nerve
Genitofemoral nerve
Iliohypogastric nerve
Ilioinguinal nerve
Lateral femoral cutaneous
   nerve
Obturator nerve
Superior gluteal nerve
A Lumbosacral Plexus
B Lumbar Nerve
Lumbosacral trunk
Spinal nerve, lumbar
Superior clunic (cluneal) nerve
C Pudendal Nerve
Posterior labial nerve
Posterior scrotal nerve
D Femoral Nerve
Anterior crural nerve
Saphenous nerve
F Sciatic Nerve
Ischiatic nerve
G Tibial Nerve
Lateral plantar nerve
Medial plantar nerve
Medial popliteal nerve
Medial sural cutaneous nerve
	H Peroneal Nerve
	Common fibular nerve
	Common peroneal nerve
	External popliteal nerve
	Lateral sural cutaneous nerve
	K Head and Neck Sympathetic
	Nerve
	Cavernous plexus
	Cervical ganglion
	Ciliary ganglion
	Internal carotid plexus
	Otic ganglion
	Pterygopalatine
	   (sphenopalatine) ganglion
	Sphenopalatine
	   (pterygopalatine) ganglion
	Stellate ganglion
	Submandibular ganglion
	Submaxillary ganglion
	L Thoracic Sympathetic Nerve
	Cardiac plexus
	Esophageal plexus
	Greater splanchnic nerve
	Inferior cardiac nerve
	Least splanchnic nerve
	Lesser splanchnic nerve
	Middle cardiac nerve
	Pulmonary plexus
	Superior cardiac nerve
	Thoracic aortic plexus
	Thoracic ganglion
	M Abdominal Sympathetic
	Nerve
	Abdominal aortic plexus
	Auerbach's (myenteric) plexus
	Celiac (solar) plexus
	Celiac ganglion
	Gastric plexus
	Hepatic plexus
	Inferior hypogastric plexus
	Inferior mesenteric ganglion
	Inferior mesenteric plexus
	Meissner's (submucous) plexus
	Myenteric (Auerbach's) plexus
	Pancreatic plexus
	Pelvic splanchnic nerve
	Renal plexus
	Solar (celiac) plexus
	Splenic plexus
	Submucous (Meissner's) plexus
	Superior hypogastric plexus
	Superior mesenteric ganglion
	Superior mesenteric plexus
	Suprarenal plexus
	N Lumbar Sympathetic Nerve
	Lumbar ganglion
	Lumbar splanchnic nerve
	P Sacral Sympathetic Nerve
	Ganglion impar (ganglion of
	   Walther)
	Pelvic splanchnic nerve
	Sacral ganglion
	Sacral splanchnic nerve
	Q Sacral Plexus
	Inferior gluteal nerve
	Posterior femoral cutaneous
	   nerve
	Pudendal nerve
	R Sacral Nerve
	Spinal nerve, sacral
		Ø Open
		3 Percutaneous
		4 Percutaneous Endoscopic
			Ø Drainage Device	**Z No Qualifier**

Ø19 Continued on next page

Non-OR   Ø19[Ø,1,2,3,4,5,6,8,9,A,B,C,D,F,G,H,K,L,M,N,P,Q,R]3ØZ

Peripheral Nervous System

Ø   **Medical and Surgical**
1   **Peripheral Nervous System**
9   **Drainage**   Definition: Taking or letting out fluids and/or gases from a body part

Ø19 Continued

                 Explanation: The qualifier DIAGNOSTIC is used to identify drainage procedures that are biopsies

Body Part Character 4		Approach Character 5	Device Character 6	Qualifier Character 7

Ø Cervical Plexus
Ansa cervicalis
Cutaneous (transverse) cervical
   nerve
Great auricular nerve
Lesser occipital nerve
Supraclavicular nerve
Transverse (cutaneous) cervical
   nerve
1 Cervical Nerve
Greater occipital nerve
Spinal nerve, cervical
Suboccipital nerve
Third occipital nerve
2 Phrenic Nerve
Accessory phrenic nerve
3 Brachial Plexus
Axillary nerve
Dorsal scapular nerve
First intercostal nerve
Long thoracic nerve
Musculocutaneous nerve
Subclavius nerve
Suprascapular nerve
4 Ulnar Nerve
Cubital nerve
5 Median Nerve
Anterior interosseous nerve
Palmar cutaneous nerve
6 Radial Nerve
Dorsal digital nerve
Musculospiral nerve
Palmar cutaneous nerve
Posterior interosseous nerve
8 Thoracic Nerve
Intercostal nerve
Intercostobrachial nerve
Spinal nerve, thoracic
Subcostal nerve
9 Lumbar Plexus
Accessory obturator nerve
Genitofemoral nerve
Iliohypogastric nerve
Ilioinguinal nerve
Lateral femoral cutaneous
   nerve
Obturator nerve
Superior gluteal nerve
A Lumbosacral Plexus
B Lumbar Nerve
Lumbosacral trunk
Spinal nerve, lumbar
Superior clunic (cluneal) nerve
C Pudendal Nerve
Posterior labial nerve
Posterior scrotal nerve
D Femoral Nerve
Anterior crural nerve
Saphenous nerve
F Sciatic Nerve
Ischiatic nerve
G Tibial Nerve
Lateral plantar nerve
Medial plantar nerve
Medial popliteal nerve
Medial sural cutaneous nerve
	H Peroneal Nerve
	Common fibular nerve
	Common peroneal nerve
	External popliteal nerve
	Lateral sural cutaneous nerve
	K Head and Neck Sympathetic Nerve
	Cavernous plexus
	Cervical ganglion
	Ciliary ganglion
	Internal carotid plexus
	Otic ganglion
	Pterygopalatine
	   (sphenopalatine) ganglion
	Sphenopalatine
	   (pterygopalatine) ganglion
	Stellate ganglion
	Submandibular ganglion
	Submaxillary ganglion
	L Thoracic Sympathetic Nerve
	Cardiac plexus
	Esophageal plexus
	Greater splanchnic nerve
	Inferior cardiac nerve
	Least splanchnic nerve
	Lesser splanchnic nerve
	Middle cardiac nerve
	Pulmonary plexus
	Superior cardiac nerve
	Thoracic aortic plexus
	Thoracic ganglion
	M Abdominal Sympathetic Nerve
	Abdominal aortic plexus
	Auerbach's (myenteric) plexus
	Celiac (solar) plexus
	Celiac ganglion
	Gastric plexus
	Hepatic plexus
	Inferior hypogastric plexus
	Inferior mesenteric ganglion
	Inferior mesenteric plexus
	Meissner's (submucous) plexus
	Myenteric (Auerbach's) plexus
	Pancreatic plexus
	Pelvic splanchnic nerve
	Renal plexus
	Solar (celiac) plexus
	Splenic plexus
	Submucous (Meissner's) plexus
	Superior hypogastric plexus
	Superior mesenteric ganglion
	Superior mesenteric plexus
	Suprarenal plexus
	N Lumbar Sympathetic Nerve
	Lumbar ganglion
	Lumbar splanchnic nerve
	P Sacral Sympathetic Nerve
	Ganglion impar (ganglion of
	   Walther)
	Pelvic splanchnic nerve
	Sacral ganglion
	Sacral splanchnic nerve
	Q Sacral Plexus
	Inferior gluteal nerve
	Posterior femoral cutaneous
	   nerve
	Pudendal nerve
	R Sacral Nerve
	Spinal nerve, sacral
		Ø Open
		3 Percutaneous
		4 Percutaneous Endoscopic
			Z No Device	**X Diagnostic**
				Z No Qualifier

Non-OR	Ø19[Ø,1,2,3,4,5,6,8,9,A,B,C,D,F,G,H,Q,R][3,4]ZX
Non-OR	Ø19[Ø,1,2,3,4,5,6,8,9,A,B,C,D,F,G,H,K,L,M,N,P,Q,R]3ZZ

LC Limited Coverage   **NC** Noncovered   ⊞ Combination Member   HAC associated procedure   Combination Only   DRG Non-OR   Non-OR   New/Revised in GREEN

154   ICD-10-PCS 2020

Ø   Medical and Surgical
1   Peripheral Nervous System
B   Excision   Definition: Cutting out or off, without replacement, a portion of a body part
               Explanation: The qualifier DIAGNOSTIC is used to identify excision procedures that are biopsies

Body Part Character 4		Approach Character 5	Device Character 6	Qualifier Character 7

Ø Cervical Plexus
Ansa cervicalis
Cutaneous (transverse) cervical
   nerve
Great auricular nerve
Lesser occipital nerve
Supraclavicular nerve
Transverse (cutaneous) cervical
   nerve
1 Cervical Nerve
Greater occipital nerve
Spinal nerve, cervical
Suboccipital nerve
Third occipital nerve
2 Phrenic Nerve
Accessory phrenic nerve
3 Brachial Plexus
Axillary nerve
Dorsal scapular nerve
First intercostal nerve
Long thoracic nerve
Musculocutaneous nerve
Subclavius nerve
Suprascapular nerve
4 Ulnar Nerve
Cubital nerve
5 Median Nerve
Anterior interosseous nerve
Palmar cutaneous nerve
6 Radial Nerve
Dorsal digital nerve
Musculospiral nerve
Palmar cutaneous nerve
Posterior interosseous nerve
8 Thoracic Nerve
Intercostal nerve
Intercostobrachial nerve
Spinal nerve, thoracic
Subcostal nerve
9 Lumbar Plexus
Accessory obturator nerve
Genitofemoral nerve
Iliohypogastric nerve
Ilioinguinal nerve
Lateral femoral cutaneous
   nerve
Obturator nerve
Superior gluteal nerve
A Lumbosacral Plexus
B Lumbar Nerve
Lumbosacral trunk
Spinal nerve, lumbar
Superior clunic (cluneal) nerve
C Pudendal Nerve
Posterior labial nerve
Posterior scrotal nerve
D Femoral Nerve
Anterior crural nerve
Saphenous nerve
F Sciatic Nerve
Ischiatic nerve
G Tibial Nerve
Lateral plantar nerve
Medial plantar nerve
Medial popliteal nerve
Medial sural cutaneous nerve
	H Peroneal Nerve
	Common fibular nerve
	Common peroneal nerve
	External popliteal nerve
	Lateral sural cutaneous nerve
	K Head and Neck Sympathetic
	Nerve
	Cavernous plexus
	Cervical ganglion
	Ciliary ganglion
	Internal carotid plexus
	Otic ganglion
	Pterygopalatine
	   (sphenopalatine) ganglion
	Sphenopalatine
	   (pterygopalatine) ganglion
	Stellate ganglion
	Submandibular ganglion
	Submaxillary ganglion
	L Thoracic Sympathetic
	Nerve
	Cardiac plexus
	Esophageal plexus
	Greater splanchnic nerve
	Inferior cardiac nerve
	Least splanchnic nerve
	Lesser splanchnic nerve
	Middle cardiac nerve
	Pulmonary plexus
	Superior cardiac nerve
	Thoracic aortic plexus
	Thoracic ganglion
	M Abdominal Sympathetic
	Nerve
	Abdominal aortic plexus
	Auerbach's (myenteric) plexus
	Celiac (solar) plexus
	Celiac ganglion
	Gastric plexus
	Hepatic plexus
	Inferior hypogastric plexus
	Inferior mesenteric ganglion
	Inferior mesenteric plexus
	Meissner's (submucous) plexus
	Myenteric (Auerbach's) plexus
	Pancreatic plexus
	Pelvic splanchnic nerve
	Renal plexus
	Solar (celiac) plexus
	Splenic plexus
	Submucous (Meissner's) plexus
	Superior hypogastric plexus
	Superior mesenteric ganglion
	Superior mesenteric plexus
	Suprarenal plexus
	N Lumbar Sympathetic Nerve
	Lumbar ganglion
	Lumbar splanchnic nerve
	P Sacral Sympathetic Nerve
	Ganglion impar (ganglion of
	   Walther)
	Pelvic splanchnic nerve
	Sacral ganglion
	Sacral splanchnic nerve
	Q Sacral Plexus
	Inferior gluteal nerve
	Posterior femoral cutaneous
	   nerve
	Pudendal nerve
	R Sacral Nerve
	Spinal nerve, sacral
		Ø Open
		3 Percutaneous
		4 Percutaneous Endoscopic
			Z No Device	**X Diagnostic**
				Z No Qualifier

Non-OR   Ø1B[Ø,1,2,3,4,5,6,8,9,A,B,C,D,F,G,H,Q,R][3,4]ZX

LC Limited Coverage   NC Noncovered   ⊞ Combination Member   HAC associated procedure   Combination Only   DRG Non-OR   Non-OR   New/Revised in GREEN

ICD-10-PCS 2020   155

Ø   Medical and Surgical
1   Peripheral Nervous System
C   Extirpation   Definition: Taking or cutting out solid matter from a body part

Explanation: The solid matter may be an abnormal byproduct of a biological function or a foreign body; it may be imbedded in a body part or in the lumen of a tubular body part. The solid matter may or may not have been previously broken into pieces.

Body Part Character 4		Approach Character 5	Device Character 6	Qualifier Character 7

Ø Cervical Plexus
  Ansa cervicalis
  Cutaneous (transverse) cervical
    nerve
  Great auricular nerve
  Lesser occipital nerve
  Supraclavicular nerve
  Transverse (cutaneous) cervical
    nerve
1 Cervical Nerve
  Greater occipital nerve
  Spinal nerve, cervical
  Suboccipital nerve
  Third occipital nerve
2 Phrenic Nerve
  Accessory phrenic nerve
3 Brachial Plexus
  Axillary nerve
  Dorsal scapular nerve
  First intercostal nerve
  Long thoracic nerve
  Musculocutaneous nerve
  Subclavius nerve
  Suprascapular nerve
4 Ulnar Nerve
  Cubital nerve
5 Median Nerve
  Anterior interosseous nerve
  Palmar cutaneous nerve
6 Radial Nerve
  Dorsal digital nerve
  Musculospiral nerve
  Palmar cutaneous nerve
  Posterior interosseous nerve
8 Thoracic Nerve
  Intercostal nerve
  Intercostobrachial nerve
  Spinal nerve, thoracic
  Subcostal nerve
9 Lumbar Plexus
  Accessory obturator nerve
  Genitofemoral nerve
  Iliohypogastric nerve
  Ilioinguinal nerve
  Lateral femoral cutaneous
    nerve
  Obturator nerve
  Superior gluteal nerve
A Lumbosacral Plexus
B Lumbar Nerve
  Lumbosacral trunk
  Spinal nerve, lumbar
  Superior clunic (cluneal) nerve
C Pudendal Nerve
  Posterior labial nerve
  Posterior scrotal nerve
D Femoral Nerve
  Anterior crural nerve
  Saphenous nerve
F Sciatic Nerve
  Ischiatic nerve
G Tibial Nerve
  Lateral plantar nerve
  Medial plantar nerve
  Medial popliteal nerve
  Medial sural cutaneous nerve
	H Peroneal Nerve
	  Common fibular nerve
	  Common peroneal nerve
	  External popliteal nerve
	  Lateral sural cutaneous nerve
	K Head and Neck Sympathetic
	  Nerve
	  Cavernous plexus
	  Cervical ganglion
	  Ciliary ganglion
	  Internal carotid plexus
	  Otic ganglion
	  Pterygopalatine
	    (sphenopalatine) ganglion
	  Sphenopalatine
	    (pterygopalatine) ganglion
	  Stellate ganglion
	  Submandibular ganglion
	  Submaxillary ganglion
	L Thoracic Sympathetic Nerve
	  Cardiac plexus
	  Esophageal plexus
	  Greater splanchnic nerve
	  Inferior cardiac nerve
	  Least splanchnic nerve
	  Lesser splanchnic nerve
	  Middle cardiac nerve
	  Pulmonary plexus
	  Superior cardiac nerve
	  Thoracic aortic plexus
	  Thoracic ganglion
	M Abdominal Sympathetic
	  Nerve
	  Abdominal aortic plexus
	  Auerbach's (myenteric) plexus
	  Celiac (solar) plexus
	  Celiac ganglion
	  Gastric plexus
	  Hepatic plexus
	  Inferior hypogastric plexus
	  Inferior mesenteric ganglion
	  Inferior mesenteric plexus
	  Meissner's (submucous) plexus
	  Myenteric (Auerbach's) plexus
	  Pancreatic plexus
	  Pelvic splanchnic nerve
	  Renal plexus
	  Solar (celiac) plexus
	  Splenic plexus
	  Submucous (Meissner's) plexus
	  Superior hypogastric plexus
	  Superior mesenteric ganglion
	  Superior mesenteric plexus
	  Suprarenal plexus
	N Lumbar Sympathetic Nerve
	  Lumbar ganglion
	  Lumbar splanchnic nerve
	P Sacral Sympathetic Nerve
	  Ganglion impar (ganglion of
	    Walther)
	  Pelvic splanchnic nerve
	  Sacral ganglion
	  Sacral splanchnic nerve
	Q Sacral Plexus
	  Inferior gluteal nerve
	  Posterior femoral cutaneous
	    nerve
	  Pudendal nerve
	R Sacral Nerve
	  Spinal nerve, sacral
		Ø Open
		3 Percutaneous
		4 Percutaneous Endoscopic
			Z No Device	**Z No Qualifier**

Ø   **Medical and Surgical**
1   **Peripheral Nervous System**
D   **Extraction**   Definition: Pulling or stripping out or off all or a portion of a body part by the use of force
                  Explanation: The qualifier DIAGNOSTIC is used to identify extraction procedures that are biopsies

Body Part Character 4	Approach Character 5	Device Character 6	Qualifier Character 7

Ø Cervical Plexus
  Ansa cervicalis
  Cutaneous (transverse) cervical
    nerve
  Great auricular nerve
  Lesser occipital nerve
  Supraclavicular nerve
  Transverse (cutaneous) cervical
    nerve
1 Cervical Nerve
  Greater occipital nerve
  Spinal nerve, cervical
  Suboccipital nerve
  Third occipital nerve
2 Phrenic Nerve
  Accessory phrenic nerve
3 Brachial Plexus
  Axillary nerve
  Dorsal scapular nerve
  First intercostal nerve
  Long thoracic nerve
  Musculocutaneous nerve
  Subclavius nerve
  Suprascapular nerve
4 Ulnar Nerve
  Cubital nerve
5 Median Nerve
  Anterior interosseous nerve
  Palmar cutaneous nerve
6 Radial Nerve
  Dorsal digital nerve
  Musculospiral nerve
  Palmar cutaneous nerve
  Posterior interosseous nerve
8 Thoracic Nerve
  Intercostal nerve
  Intercostobrachial nerve
  Spinal nerve, thoracic
  Subcostal nerve
9 Lumbar Plexus
  Accessory obturator nerve
  Genitofemoral nerve
  Iliohypogastric nerve
  Ilioinguinal nerve
  Lateral femoral cutaneous nerve
  Obturator nerve
  Superior gluteal nerve
A Lumbosacral Plexus
B Lumbar Nerve
  Lumbosacral trunk
  Spinal nerve, lumbar
  Superior clunic (cluneal) nerve
C Pudendal Nerve]
  Posterior labial nerve
  Posterior scrotal nerve
D Femoral Nerve
  Anterior crural nerve
  Saphenous nerve
F Sciatic Nerve
  Ischiatic nerve
G Tibial Nerve
  Lateral plantar nerve
  Medial plantar nerve
  Medial popliteal nerve
  Medial sural cutaneous nerve
	H Peroneal Nerve
	  Common fibular nerve
	  Common peroneal nerve
	  External popliteal nerve
	  Lateral sural cutaneous nerve
	K Head and Neck Sympathetic
	  Nerve
	  Cavernous plexus
	  Cervical ganglion
	  Ciliary ganglion
	  Internal carotid plexus
	  Otic ganglion
	  Pterygopalatine
	    (sphenopalatine) ganglion
	  Sphenopalatine
	    (pterygopalatine) ganglion
	  Stellate ganglion
	  Submandibular ganglion
	  Submaxillary ganglion
	L Thoracic Sympathetic Nerve
	  Cardiac plexus
	  Esophageal plexus
	  Greater splanchnic nerve
	  Inferior cardiac nerve
	  Least splanchnic nerve
	  Lesser splanchnic nerve
	  Middle cardiac nerve
	  Pulmonary plexus
	  Superior cardiac nerve
	  Thoracic aortic plexus
	  Thoracic ganglion
	M Abdominal Sympathetic Nerve
	  Abdominal aortic plexus
	  Auerbach's (myenteric) plexus
	  Celiac (solar) plexus
	  Celiac ganglion
	  Gastric plexus
	  Hepatic plexus
	  Inferior hypogastric plexus
	  Inferior mesenteric ganglion
	  Inferior mesenteric plexus
	  Meissner's (submucous) plexus
	  Myenteric (Auerbach's) plexus
	  Pancreatic plexus
	  Pelvic splanchnic nerve
	  Renal plexus
	  Solar (celiac) plexus
	  Splenic plexus
	  Submucous (Meissner's) plexus
	  Superior hypogastric plexus
	  Superior mesenteric ganglion
	  Superior mesenteric plexus
	  Suprarenal plexus
	N Lumbar Sympathetic Nerve
	  Lumbar ganglion
	  Lumbar splanchnic nerve
	P Sacral Sympathetic Nerve
	  Ganglion impar (ganglion of
	    Walther)
	  Pelvic splanchnic nerve
	  Sacral ganglion
	  Sacral splanchnic nerve
	Q Sacral Plexus
	  Inferior gluteal nerve
	  Posterior femoral cutaneous
	    nerve
	  Pudendal nerve
	R Sacral Nerve
	  Spinal nerve, sacral
		Ø Open
		3 Percutaneous
		4 Percutaneous Endoscopic
			Z No Device	**Z No Qualifier**

LC Limited Coverage **NC** Noncovered ⊞ Combination Member HAC associated procedure Combination Only DRG Non-OR Non-OR New/Revised in GREEN

ICD-10-PCS 2020   157

Ø **Medical and Surgical**
1 **Peripheral Nervous System**
H **Insertion**   Definition: Putting in a nonbiological appliance that monitors, assists, performs, or prevents a physiological function but does not physically take the place of a body part
Explanation: None

Body Part Character 4	Approach Character 5	Device Character 6	Qualifier Character 7
Y Peripheral Nerve ⊞	Ø Open 3 Percutaneous 4 Percutaneous Endoscopic	2 Monitoring Device M Neurostimulator Lead Y Other Device	Z No Qualifier

Non-OR Ø1HY[3,4]YZ

See Appendix L for Procedure Combinations
⊞ Ø1HY[Ø,3,4]MZ

Ø **Medical and Surgical**
1 **Peripheral Nervous System**
J **Inspection**   Definition: Visually and/or manually exploring a body part
Explanation: Visual exploration may be performed with or without optical instrumentation. Manual exploration may be performed directly or through intervening body layers.

Body Part Character 4	Approach Character 5	Device Character 6	Qualifier Character 7
Y Peripheral Nerve	Ø Open 3 Percutaneous 4 Percutaneous Endoscopic	Z No Device	Z No Qualifier

Non-OR Ø1JY3ZZ

LC Limited Coverage NC Noncovered ⊞ Combination Member HAC associated procedure Combination Only DRG Non-OR Non-OR New/Revised in GREEN
158 ICD-10-PCS 2020

Peripheral Nervous System

01H–01J

Ø   Medical and Surgical
1   Peripheral Nervous System
N   Release   Definition: Freeing a body part from an abnormal physical constraint by cutting or by the use of force
                      Explanation: Some of the restraining tissue may be taken out but none of the body part is taken out

Body Part Character 4		Approach Character 5	Device Character 6	Qualifier Character 7

Ø Cervical Plexus
Ansa cervicalis
Cutaneous (transverse) cervical
   nerve
Great auricular nerve
Lesser occipital nerve
Supraclavicular nerve
Transverse (cutaneous) cervical
   nerve
1 Cervical Nerve
Greater occipital nerve
Spinal nerve, cervical
Suboccipital nerve
Third occipital nerve
2 Phrenic Nerve
Accessory phrenic nerve
3 Brachial Plexus
Axillary nerve
Dorsal scapular nerve
First intercostal nerve
Long thoracic nerve
Musculocutaneous nerve
Subclavius nerve
Suprascapular nerve
4 Ulnar Nerve
Cubital nerve
5 Median Nerve
Anterior interosseous nerve
Palmar cutaneous nerve
6 Radial Nerve
Dorsal digital nerve
Musculospiral nerve
Palmar cutaneous nerve
Posterior interosseous nerve
8 Thoracic Nerve
Intercostal nerve
Intercostobrachial nerve
Spinal nerve, thoracic
Subcostal nerve
9 Lumbar Plexus
Accessory obturator nerve
Genitofemoral nerve
Iliohypogastric nerve
Ilioinguinal nerve
Lateral femoral cutaneous nerve
Obturator nerve
Superior gluteal nerve
A Lumbosacral Plexus
B Lumbar Nerve
Lumbosacral trunk
Spinal nerve, lumbar
Superior clunic (cluneal) nerve
C Pudendal Nerve
Posterior labial nerve
Posterior scrotal nerve
D Femoral Nerve
Anterior crural nerve
Saphenous nerve
F Sciatic Nerve
Ischiatic nerve
G Tibial Nerve
Lateral plantar nerve
Medial plantar nerve
Medial popliteal nerve
Medial sural cutaneous nerve
	H Peroneal Nerve
	Common fibular nerve
	Common peroneal nerve
	External popliteal nerve
	Lateral sural cutaneous nerve
	**K Head and Neck Sympathetic
	Nerve**
	Cavernous plexus
	Cervical ganglion
	Ciliary ganglion
	Internal carotid plexus
	Otic ganglion
	Pterygopalatine
	   (sphenopalatine) ganglion
	Sphenopalatine
	   (pterygopalatine) ganglion
	Stellate ganglion
	Submandibular ganglion
	Submaxillary ganglion
	L Thoracic Sympathetic Nerve
	Cardiac plexus
	Esophageal plexus
	Greater splanchnic nerve
	Inferior cardiac nerve
	Least splanchnic nerve
	Lesser splanchnic nerve
	Middle cardiac nerve
	Pulmonary plexus
	Superior cardiac nerve
	Thoracic aortic plexus
	Thoracic ganglion
	**M Abdominal Sympathetic
	Nerve**
	Abdominal aortic plexus
	Auerbach's (myenteric) plexus
	Celiac (solar) plexus
	Celiac ganglion
	Gastric plexus
	Hepatic plexus
	Inferior hypogastric plexus
	Inferior mesenteric ganglion
	Inferior mesenteric plexus
	Meissner's (submucous) plexus
	Myenteric (Auerbach's) plexus
	Pancreatic plexus
	Pelvic splanchnic nerve
	Renal plexus
	Solar (celiac) plexus
	Splenic plexus
	Submucous (Meissner's) plexus
	Superior hypogastric plexus
	Superior mesenteric ganglion
	Superior mesenteric plexus
	Suprarenal plexus
	N Lumbar Sympathetic Nerve
	Lumbar ganglion
	Lumbar splanchnic nerve
	P Sacral Sympathetic Nerve
	Ganglion impar (ganglion of
	   Walther)
	Pelvic splanchnic nerve
	Sacral ganglion
	Sacral splanchnic nerve
	Q Sacral Plexus
	Inferior gluteal nerve
	Posterior femoral cutaneous
	   nerve
	Pudendal nerve
	R Sacral Nerve
	Spinal nerve, sacral
		Ø Open
		3 Percutaneous
		4 Percutaneous Endoscopic
			Z No Device	**Z No Qualifier**

LC Limited Coverage   **NC** Noncovered   ⊞ Combination Member   HAC associated procedure   Combination Only   DRG Non-OR   Non-OR   New/Revised in GREEN

ICD-10-PCS 2020   **159**

Ø1N–Ø1N

Peripheral Nervous System

Ø   **Medical and Surgical**
1   **Peripheral Nervous System**
P   **Removal**   Definition: Taking out or off a device from a body part

Explanation: If a device is taken out and a similar device put in without cutting or puncturing the skin or mucous membrane, the procedure is coded to the root operation CHANGE. Otherwise, the procedure for taking out a device is coded to the root operation REMOVAL.

Body Part Character 4	Approach Character 5	Device Character 6	Qualifier Character 7
Y Peripheral Nerve	Ø Open 3 Percutaneous 4 Percutaneous Endoscopic	Ø Drainage Device 2 Monitoring Device 7 Autologous Tissue Substitute M Neurostimulator Lead Y Other Device	Z No Qualifier
Y Peripheral Nerve	X External	Ø Drainage Device 2 Monitoring Device M Neurostimulator Lead	Z No Qualifier

Non-OR   Ø1PY3[Ø,2]Z
Non-OR   Ø1PY[3,4]YZ
Non-OR   Ø1PYX[Ø,2,M]Z

Ø   Medical and Surgical
1   Peripheral Nervous System
Q   Repair   Definition: Restoring, to the extent possible, a body part to its normal anatomic structure and function
                 Explanation: Used only when the method to accomplish the repair is not one of the other root operations

Body Part Character 4		Approach Character 5	Device Character 6	Qualifier Character 7

Ø Cervical Plexus
Ansa cervicalis
Cutaneous (transverse) cervical
   nerve
Great auricular nerve
Lesser occipital nerve
Supraclavicular nerve
Transverse (cutaneous) cervical
   nerve
1 Cervical Nerve
Greater occipital nerve
Spinal nerve, cervical
Suboccipital nerve
Third occipital nerve
2 Phrenic Nerve
Accessory phrenic nerve
3 Brachial Plexus
Axillary nerve
Dorsal scapular nerve
First intercostal nerve
Long thoracic nerve
Musculocutaneous nerve
Subclavius nerve
Suprascapular nerve
4 Ulnar Nerve
Cubital nerve
5 Median Nerve
Anterior interosseous nerve
Palmar cutaneous nerve
6 Radial Nerve
Dorsal digital nerve
Musculospiral nerve
Palmar cutaneous nerve
Posterior interosseous nerve
8 Thoracic Nerve
Intercostal nerve
Intercostobrachial nerve
Spinal nerve, thoracic
Subcostal nerve
9 Lumbar Plexus
Accessory obturator nerve
Genitofemoral nerve
Iliohypogastric nerve
Ilioinguinal nerve
Lateral femoral cutaneous
   nerve
Obturator nerve
Superior gluteal nerve
A Lumbosacral Plexus
B Lumbar Nerve
Lumbosacral trunk
Spinal nerve, lumbar
Superior clunic (cluneal) nerve
C Pudendal Nerve
Posterior labial nerve
Posterior scrotal nerve
D Femoral Nerve
Anterior crural nerve
Saphenous nerve
F Sciatic Nerve
Ischiatic nerve
G Tibial Nerve
Lateral plantar nerve
Medial plantar nerve
Medial popliteal nerve
Medial sural cutaneous nerve
	H Peroneal Nerve
	Common fibular nerve
	Common peroneal nerve
	External popliteal nerve
	Lateral sural cutaneous nerve
	**K Head and Neck Sympathetic
	   Nerve**
	Cavernous plexus
	Cervical ganglion
	Ciliary ganglion
	Internal carotid plexus
	Otic ganglion
	Pterygopalatine
	   (sphenopalatine) ganglion
	Sphenopalatine
	   (pterygopalatine) ganglion
	Stellate ganglion
	Submandibular ganglion
	Submaxillary ganglion
	L Thoracic Sympathetic Nerve
	Cardiac plexus
	Esophageal plexus
	Greater splanchnic nerve
	Inferior cardiac nerve
	Least splanchnic nerve
	Lesser splanchnic nerve
	Middle cardiac nerve
	Pulmonary plexus
	Superior cardiac nerve
	Thoracic aortic plexus
	Thoracic ganglion
	**M Abdominal Sympathetic
	   Nerve**
	Abdominal aortic plexus
	Auerbach's (myenteric) plexus
	Celiac (solar) plexus
	Celiac ganglion
	Gastric plexus
	Hepatic plexus
	Inferior hypogastric plexus
	Inferior mesenteric ganglion
	Inferior mesenteric plexus
	Meissner's (submucous) plexus
	Myenteric (Auerbach's) plexus
	Pancreatic plexus
	Pelvic splanchnic nerve
	Renal plexus
	Solar (celiac) plexus
	Splenic plexus
	Submucous (Meissner's) plexus
	Superior hypogastric plexus
	Superior mesenteric ganglion
	Superior mesenteric plexus
	Suprarenal plexus
	N Lumbar Sympathetic Nerve
	Lumbar ganglion
	Lumbar splanchnic nerve
	P Sacral Sympathetic Nerve
	Ganglion impar (ganglion of
	   Walther)
	Pelvic splanchnic nerve
	Sacral ganglion
	Sacral splanchnic nerve
	Q Sacral Plexus
	Inferior gluteal nerve
	Posterior femoral cutaneous
	   nerve
	Pudendal nerve
	R Sacral Nerve
	Spinal nerve, sacral
		Ø Open
		3 Percutaneous
		4 Percutaneous Endoscopic
			Z No Device	**Z No Qualifier**

Peripheral Nervous System

Ø   Medical and Surgical
1   Peripheral Nervous System
R   Replacement   Definition: Putting in or on biological or synthetic material that physically takes the place and/or function of all or a portion of a body part

Explanation: The body part may have been taken out or replaced, or may be taken out, physically eradicated, or rendered nonfunctional during the REPLACEMENT procedure. A REMOVAL procedure is coded for taking out the device used in a previous replacement procedure.

Body Part Character 4	Approach Character 5	Device Character 6	Qualifier Character 7

1 Cervical Nerve
  Greater occipital nerve
  Spinal nerve, cervical
  Suboccipital nerve
  Third occipital nerve
2 Phrenic Nerve
  Accessory phrenic nerve
4 Ulnar Nerve
  Cubital nerve
5 Median Nerve
  Anterior interosseous nerve
  Palmar cutaneous nerve
6 Radial Nerve
  Dorsal digital nerve
  Musculospiral nerve
  Palmar cutaneous nerve
  Posterior interosseous nerve
8 Thoracic Nerve
  Intercostal nerve
  Intercostobrachial nerve
  Spinal nerve, thoracic
  Subcostal nerve
B Lumbar Nerve
  Lumbosacral trunk
  Spinal nerve, lumbar
  Superior clunic (cluneal) nerve
C Pudendal Nerve
  Posterior labial nerve
  Posterior scrotal nerve
D Femoral Nerve
  Anterior crural nerve
  Saphenous nerve
F Sciatic Nerve
  Ischiatic nerve
G Tibial Nerve
  Lateral plantar nerve
  Medial plantar nerve
  Medial popliteal nerve
  Medial sural cutaneous nerve
H Peroneal Nerve
  Common fibular nerve
  Common peroneal nerve
  External popliteal nerve
  Lateral sural cutaneous nerve
R Sacral Nerve
  Spinal nerve, sacral
	Ø Open
	4 Percutaneous Endoscopic
		7 Autologous Tissue Substitute
		J Synthetic Substitute
		K Nonautologous Tissue Substitute
			Z No Qualifier

[LC] Limited Coverage   [NC] Noncovered   ⊞ Combination Member   HAC associated procedure   Combination Only   DRG Non-OR   Non-OR   New/Revised in GREEN

162   ICD-10-PCS 2020

Ø **Medical and Surgical**
1 **Peripheral Nervous System**
S **Reposition**   Definition: Moving to its normal location, or other suitable location, all or a portion of a body part

         Explanation: The body part is moved to a new location from an abnormal location, or from a normal location where it is not functioning
         correctly. The body part may or may not be cut out or off to be moved to the new location.

Body Part Character 4	Approach Character 5	Device Character 6	Qualifier Character 7
Ø Cervical Plexus Ansa cervicalis Cutaneous (transverse) cervical nerve Great auricular nerve Lesser occipital nerve Supraclavicular nerve Transverse (cutaneous) cervical nerve **1 Cervical Nerve** Greater occipital nerve Spinal nerve, cervical Suboccipital nerve Third occipital nerve **2 Phrenic Nerve** Accessory phrenic nerve **3 Brachial Plexus** Axillary nerve Dorsal scapular nerve First intercostal nerve Long thoracic nerve Musculocutaneous nerve Subclavius nerve Suprascapular nerve **4 Ulnar Nerve** Cubital nerve **5 Median Nerve** Anterior interosseous nerve Palmar cutaneous nerve **6 Radial Nerve** Dorsal digital nerve Musculospiral nerve Palmar cutaneous nerve Posterior interosseous nerve **8 Thoracic Nerve** Intercostal nerve Intercostobrachial nerve Spinal nerve, thoracic Subcostal nerve **9 Lumbar Plexus** Accessory obturator nerve Genitofemoral nerve Iliohypogastric nerve Ilioinguinal nerve Lateral femoral cutaneous nerve Obturator nerve Superior gluteal nerve **A Lumbosacral Plexus** **B Lumbar Nerve** Lumbosacral trunk Spinal nerve, lumbar Superior clunic (cluneal) nerve **C Pudendal Nerve** Posterior labial nerve Posterior scrotal nerve **D Femoral Nerve** Anterior crural nerve Saphenous nerve **F Sciatic Nerve** Ischiatic nerve **G Tibial Nerve** Lateral plantar nerve Medial plantar nerve Medial popliteal nerve Medial sural cutaneous nerve **H Peroneal Nerve** Common fibular nerve Common peroneal nerve External popliteal nerve Lateral sural cutaneous nerve **Q Sacral Plexus** Inferior gluteal nerve Posterior femoral cutaneous nerve Pudendal nerve **R Sacral Nerve** Spinal nerve, sacral	**Ø Open** **3 Percutaneous** **4 Percutaneous Endoscopic**	**Z No Device**	**Z No Qualifier**

Peripheral Nervous System *(side margin)*

Ø **Medical and Surgical**
1 **Peripheral Nervous System**
U **Supplement**   Definition: Putting in or on biological or synthetic material that physically reinforces and/or augments the function of a portion of a body part
  Explanation: The biological material is non-living, or is living and from the same individual. The body part may have been previously replaced, and the SUPPLEMENT procedure is performed to physically reinforce and/or augment the function of the replaced body part.

Body Part Character 4	Approach Character 5	Device Character 6	Qualifier Character 7

1 **Cervical Nerve**
  Greater occipital nerve
  Spinal nerve, cervical
  Suboccipital nerve
  Third occipital nerve
2 **Phrenic Nerve**
  Accessory phrenic nerve
4 **Ulnar Nerve**
  Cubital nerve
5 **Median Nerve**
  Anterior interosseous nerve
  Palmar cutaneous nerve
6 **Radial Nerve**
  Dorsal digital nerve
  Musculospiral nerve
  Palmar cutaneous nerve
  Posterior interosseous nerve
8 **Thoracic Nerve**
  Intercostal nerve
  Intercostobrachial nerve
  Spinal nerve, thoracic
  Subcostal nerve
B **Lumbar Nerve**
  Lumbosacral trunk
  Spinal nerve, lumbar
  Superior clunic (cluneal) nerve
C **Pudendal Nerve**
  Posterior labial nerve
  Posterior scrotal nerve
D **Femoral Nerve**
  Anterior crural nerve
  Saphenous nerve
F **Sciatic Nerve**
  Ischiatic nerve
G **Tibial Nerve**
  Lateral plantar nerve
  Medial plantar nerve
  Medial popliteal nerve
  Medial sural cutaneous nerve
H **Peroneal Nerve**
  Common fibular nerve
  Common peroneal nerve
  External popliteal nerve
  Lateral sural cutaneous nerve
R **Sacral Nerve**
  Spinal nerve, sacral
	Ø Open
	3 Percutaneous
	4 Percutaneous Endoscopic
		7 Autologous Tissue Substitute
		J Synthetic Substitute
		K Nonautologous Tissue Substitute
			Z No Qualifier

Ø **Medical and Surgical**
1 **Peripheral Nervous System**
W **Revision**   Definition: Correcting, to the extent possible, a portion of a malfunctioning device or the position of a displaced device
  Explanation: Revision can include correcting a malfunctioning or displaced device by taking out or putting in components of the device such as a screw or pin

Body Part Character 4	Approach Character 5	Device Character 6	Qualifier Character 7
Y Peripheral Nerve	**Ø** Open **3** Percutaneous **4** Percutaneous Endoscopic	**Ø** Drainage Device **2** Monitoring Device **7** Autologous Tissue Substitute **M** Neurostimulator Lead **Y** Other Device	**Z** No Qualifier
Y Peripheral Nerve	**X** External	**Ø** Drainage Device **2** Monitoring Device **7** Autologous Tissue Substitute **M** Neurostimulator Lead	**Z** No Qualifier

Non-OR Ø1WY[3,4]YZ
Non-OR Ø1WYX[Ø,2,7,M]Z

Ø   Medical and Surgical
1   Peripheral Nervous System
X   Transfer   Definition: Moving, without taking out, all or a portion of a body part to another location to take over the function of all or a portion of a body part
                              Explanation: The body part transferred remains connected to its vascular and nervous supply

Body Part Character 4	Approach Character 5	Device Character 6	Qualifier Character 7

1 Cervical Nerve
    Greater occipital nerve
    Spinal nerve, cervical
    Suboccipital nerve
    Third occipital nerve
2 Phrenic Nerve
    Accessory phrenic nerve
	Ø Open
	4 Percutaneous Endoscopic
		Z No Device	**1 Cervical Nerve**
			2 Phrenic Nerve

4 Ulnar Nerve
    Cubital nerve
5 Median Nerve
    Anterior interosseous nerve
    Palmar cutaneous nerve
6 Radial Nerve
    Dorsal digital nerve
    Musculospiral nerve
    Palmar cutaneous nerve
    Posterior interosseous nerve
	Ø Open
	4 Percutaneous Endoscopic
		Z No Device	**4 Ulnar Nerve**
			5 Median Nerve
			6 Radial Nerve

8 Thoracic Nerve
    Intercostal nerve
    Intercostobrachial nerve
    Spinal nerve, thoracic
    Subcostal nerve
	Ø Open
	4 Percutaneous Endoscopic
		Z No Device	**8 Thoracic Nerve**

B Lumbar Nerve
    Lumbosacral trunk
    Spinal nerve, lumbar
    Superior clunic (cluneal) nerve
C Pudendal Nerve
    Posterior labial nerve
    Posterior scrotal nerve
	Ø Open
	4 Percutaneous Endoscopic
		Z No Device	**B Lumbar Nerve**
			C Perineal Nerve

D Femoral Nerve
    Anterior crural nerve
    Saphenous nerve
F Sciatic Nerve
    Ischiatic nerve
G Tibial Nerve
    Lateral plantar nerve
    Medial plantar nerve
    Medial popliteal nerve
    Medial sural cutaneous nerve
H Peroneal Nerve
    Common fibular nerve
    Common peroneal nerve
    External popliteal nerve
    Lateral sural cutaneous nerve
	Ø Open
	4 Percutaneous Endoscopic
		Z No Device	**D Femoral Nerve**
			F Sciatic Nerve
			G Tibial Nerve
			H Peroneal Nerve

LC Limited Coverage   NC Noncovered   ⊞ Combination Member   HAC associated procedure   Combination Only   DRG Non-OR   Non-OR   New/Revised in GREEN

ICD-10-PCS 2020   **165**

Ø1X–Ø1X

Heart and Great Vessels Ø21–Ø2Y

Character Meanings

This Character Meaning table is provided as a guide to assist the user in the identification of character members that may be found in this section of code tables. It **SHOULD NOT** be used to build a PCS code.

Operation–Character 3	Body Part–Character 4	Approach–Character 5	Device–Character 6	Qualifier–Character 7
1 Bypass	Ø Coronary Artery, One Artery	Ø Open	Ø Monitoring Device, Pressure Sensor	Ø Allogeneic
4 Creation	1 Coronary Artery, Two Arteries	3 Percutaneous	2 Monitoring Device	1 Syngeneic
5 Destruction	2 Coronary Artery, Three Arteries	4 Percutaneous Endoscopic	3 Infusion Device	2 Zooplastic OR Common Atrioventricular Valve
7 Dilation	3 Coronary Artery, Four or More Arteries	X External	4 Intraluminal Device, Drug-eluting	3 Coronary Artery
8 Division	4 Coronary Vein		5 Intraluminal Device, Drug-eluting, Two	4 Coronary Vein
B Excision	5 Atrial Septum		6 Intraluminal Device, Drug-eluting, Three	5 Coronary Circulation
C Extirpation	6 Atrium, Right		7 Intraluminal Device, Drug-eluting, Four or More OR Autologous Tissue Substitute	6 Bifurcation
F Fragmentation	7 Atrium, Left		8 Zooplastic Tissue	7 Atrium, Left
H Insertion	8 Conduction Mechanism		9 Autologous Venous Tissue	8 Internal Mammary, Right
J Inspection	9 Chordae Tendineae		A Autologous Arterial Tissue	9 Internal Mammary, Left
K Map	A Heart		C Extraluminal Device	A Innominate Artery
L Occlusion	B Heart, Right		D Intraluminal Device	B Subclavian
N Release	C Heart, Left		E Intraluminal Device, Two OR Intraluminal Device, Branched or Fenestrated, One or Two Arteries	C Thoracic Artery
P Removal	D Papillary Muscle		F Intraluminal Device, Three OR Intraluminal Device, Branched or Fenestrated, Three or More Arteries	D Carotid
Q Repair	F Aortic Valve		G Intraluminal Device, Four or More	E Atrioventricular Valve, Left
R Replacement	G Mitral Valve		J Synthetic Substitute OR Cardiac Lead, Pacemaker	F Abdominal Artery
S Reposition	H Pulmonary Valve		K Nonautologous Tissue Substitute OR Cardiac Lead, Defibrillator	G Atrioventricular Valve, Right OR Axillary Artery
T Resection	J Tricuspid Valve		M Cardiac Lead	H Transapical OR Brachial Artery
U Supplement	K Ventricle, Right		N Intracardiac Pacemaker	J Truncal Valve OR Temporary OR Intraoperative
V Restriction	L Ventricle, Left		Q Implantable Heart Assist System	K Left Atrial Appendage
W Revision	M Ventricular Septum		R Short-term External Heart Assist System	P Pulmonary Trunk
Y Transplantation	N Pericardium		T Intraluminal Device, Radioactive	Q Pulmonary Artery, Right
	P Pulmonary Trunk		Y Other Device	R Pulmonary Artery, Left
	Q Pulmonary Artery, Right		Z No Device	S Pulmonary Vein, Right OR Biventricular
	R Pulmonary Artery, Left			T Pulmonary Vein, Left OR Ductus Arteriosus
	S Pulmonary Vein, Right			U Pulmonary Vein, Confluence
	T Pulmonary Vein, Left			V Lower Extremity Artery
	V Superior Vena Cava			W Aorta
	W Thoracic Aorta, Descending			X Diagnostic
	X Thoracic Aorta, Ascending/Arch			Z No Qualifier
	Y Great Vessel			

AHA Coding Clinic for table Ø21

2018, 4Q, 45-46	Descending thoracic aorta bypass
2018, 3Q, 8	Coronary artery bypass graft surgery (revision versus total redo)
2018, 3Q, 26	Coronary artery bypass graft surgery with endarterectomy
2017, 4Q, 56	Added approach values - Percutaneous heart valve procedures
2017, 1Q, 19	Norwood Sano procedure
2016, 4Q, 80-81	Thoracic aorta, ascending/arch and descending
2016, 4Q, 82-83	Coronary artery, number of arteries
2016, 4Q, 102-109	Correction of congenital heart defects
2016, 4Q, 144	Repair of atrial septal defect and anomalous pulmonary venous return
2016, 4Q, 145	Modified Warden procedure for repair of septal defect and right partial anomalous pulmonary venous return
2016, 1Q, 27	Aortocoronary bypass graft utilizing Y-graft
2015, 4Q, 22, 24	Congenital heart corrective procedures
2015, 3Q, 16	Revision of previous truncus arteriosus surgery with ventricle to pulmonary artery conduit
2014, 3Q, 3	Blalock-Taussig shunt procedure
2014, 3Q, 8	Coronary artery bypass graft utilizing internal mammary as pedicle graft
2014, 3Q, 20	MAZE procedure performed with coronary artery bypass graft
2014, 3Q, 29	Fontan completion procedure stage II
2014, 3Q, 30	Creation of conduit from right ventricle to pulmonary artery
2014, 1Q, 10	Repair of thoracic aortic aneurysm & coronary artery bypass graft
2013, 2Q, 37	Coronary artery release performed during coronary artery bypass graft

AHA Coding Clinic for table Ø24

2016, 4Q, 101	Root operation Creation
2016, 4Q, 102-109	Correction of congenital heart defects

AHA Coding Clinic for table Ø25

2018, 3Q, 27	Alcohol septal ablation
2016, 4Q, 80-81	Thoracic aorta, ascending/arch and descending
2016, 3Q, 43-44	Peri-pulmonary catheter ablation
2016, 3Q, 44-45	Maze procedure
2016, 2Q, 17	Photodynamic therapy for treatment of malignant mesothelioma
2014, 4Q, 47	Catheter ablation of peripulmonary veins
2014, 3Q, 19	Ablation of ventricular tachycardia with Impella® support
2014, 3Q, 20	MAZE procedure performed with coronary artery bypass graft
2013, 2Q, 38	Catheter ablation to treat atrial fibrillation

AHA Coding Clinic for table Ø27

2018, 3Q, 7	Coronary brachytherapy with angioplasty
2018, 3Q, 10	Disruption of perma-catheter fibrin sheath via angioplasty of superior vena cava
2018, 2Q, 24	Coronary artery bifurcation
2017, 4Q, 32-33	Corrective surgery of left ventricular outflow tract obstruction
2016, 4Q, 80-81	Thoracic aorta, ascending/arch and descending
2016, 4Q, 82-83	Coronary artery, number of arteries
2016, 4Q, 84-85	Coronary Artery, number of stents
2016, 4Q, 86-88	Coronary and peripheral artery bifurcation
2016, 1Q, 16	Pulmonary valvotomy and dilation of annulus
2015, 4Q, 13	New Section X codes—New Technology procedures
2015, 3Q, 9	Failed attempt to treat coronary artery occlusion
2015, 3Q, 10	Coronary angioplasty with unsuccessful stent insertion
2015, 3Q, 16	Revision of previous truncus arteriosus surgery with ventricle to pulmonary artery conduit
2015, 2Q, 3-5	Coronary artery intervention site
2014, 2Q, 4	Coronary angioplasty of bypassed vessel

AHA Coding Clinic for table Ø2B

2017, 1Q, 38	Mitral valve repair and chordae tendineae transfer
2016, 4Q, 80-81	Thoracic aorta, ascending/arch and descending
2015, 2Q, 23	Annuloplasty ring

AHA Coding Clinic for table Ø2C

2018, 3Q, 26	Coronary artery bypass graft surgery with endarterectomy
2018, 2Q, 24	Coronary artery bifurcation
2017, 2Q, 23	Thrombectomy via Fogarty catheter
2016, 4Q, 80-81	Thoracic aorta, ascending/arch and descending
2016, 4Q, 82-83	Coronary artery, number of arteries
2016, 4Q, 86-87	Coronary and peripheral artery bifurcation
2016, 2Q, 24	Repair/decalcification of mitral valve
2016, 2Q, 25	Aortic valve surgery with excision of calcium deposits

AHA Coding Clinic for table Ø2H

2019, 1Q, 24	Replacement of left ventricular assist device with retention of outflow graft
2018, 4Q, 94	Insertion and removal of failed Watchman™ device
2018, 2Q, 3-5	Intra-aortic balloon pump
2018, 2Q, 19	Pacing lead attached to automatic implantable cardioverter defibrillator
2017, 4Q, 42-45	Insertion of external heart assist devices
2017, 4Q, 63-64	Added and revised device values - Vascular access reservoir
2017, 4Q, 104	Placement of Watchman™ left atrial appendage device
2017, 3Q, 11	Placement of peripherally inserted central catheter using 3CG ECG technology
2017, 2Q, 24	Tunneled catheter versus totally implantable catheter
2017, 2Q, 26	Exchange of tunneled catheter
2017, 1Q, 10-11	External heart assist device
2016, 4Q, 80-81	Thoracic aorta, ascending/arch and descending
2016, 4Q, 95	Intracardiac pacemaker
2016, 4Q, 137-138	Heart assist device systems
2016, 2Q, 15	Removal and replacement of tunneled internal jugular catheter
2015, 4Q, 14	New Section X codes—New Technology procedures
2015, 4Q, 26-31	Vascular access devices
2015, 3Q, 35	Swan Ganz catheterization
2015, 2Q, 31	Leadless pacemaker insertion
2015, 2Q, 33	Totally implantable central venous access device (Port-a-Cath)
2013, 3Q, 18	Placement of peripherally inserted central catheter (PICC)

AHA Coding Clinic for table Ø2J

2015, 3Q, 9	Failed attempt to treat coronary artery occlusion

AHA Coding Clinic for table Ø2L

2018, 4Q, 94	Insertion and removal of failed Watchman™ device
2017, 4Q, 31	Resuscitative endovascular balloon occlusion of the aorta
2017, 4Q, 33-34	Occlusion/ligation of pulmonary trunk & right pulmonary artery
2016, 4Q, 102-109	Correction of congenital heart defects
2016, 2Q, 26	Embolization of pulmonary arteriovenous fistula
2015, 4Q, 23	Congenital heart corrective procedures
2014, 3Q, 20	MAZE procedure performed with coronary artery bypass graft

AHA Coding Clinic for table Ø2N

2017, 4Q, 35	Release of myocardial bridge
2016, 4Q, 80-81	Thoracic aorta, ascending/arch and descending
2014, 3Q, 16	Repair of Tetralogy of Fallot

AHA Coding Clinic for table Ø2P

2019, 1Q, 24	Replacement of left ventricular assist device with retention of outflow graft
2018, 4Q, 52-54	Percutaneous extracorporeal membrane oxygenation
2018, 4Q, 85	Externalization of lumboatrial shunt
2018, 4Q, 94	Insertion and removal of failed Watchman™ device
2018, 2Q, 3-5	Intra-aortic balloon pump
2017, 4Q, 42-45	Insertion of external heart assist devices
2017, 4Q, 104	Placement of Watchman™ left atrial appendage device
2017, 3Q, 18	Intra-aortic balloon pump removal
2017, 2Q, 24	Tunneled catheter versus totally implantable catheter
2017, 2Q, 26	Exchange of tunneled catheter
2017, 1Q, 11	External heart assist device
2017, 1Q, 13	SynCardia total artificial heart
2016, 4Q, 95-96	Intracardiac pacemaker
2016, 4Q, 137-139	Heart assist device systems
2016, 3Q, 19	Nonoperative removal of peripherally inserted central catheter
2016, 2Q, 15	Removal and replacement of tunneled internal jugular catheter
2015, 4Q, 31	Vascular access devices
2015, 3Q, 33	Approach values for repositioning and removal of cardiac lead

AHA Coding Clinic for table Ø2Q

2018, 1Q, 12	Percutaneous balloon valvuloplasty & cardiac catheterization with ventriculogram
2017, 1Q, 18	Sutureless repair of pulmonary vein stenosis
2016, 4Q, 80-81	Thoracic aorta, ascending/arch and descending
2016, 4Q, 82-83	Coronary artery, number of arteries
2016, 4Q, 101	Root operation Creation
2016, 4Q, 102-109	Correction of congenital heart defects
2015, 4Q, 23	Congenital heart corrective procedures
2015, 3Q, 16	Vascular ring surgery and double aortic arch
2015, 2Q, 23	Annuloplasty ring
2013, 3Q, 26	Transcatheter replacement of heart valve (TAVR) with measurements

AHA Coding Clinic for table Ø2R

2019, 1Q, 31	Transcatheter aortic valve in valve replacement
2018, 3Q, 11	Transcatheter aortic valve replacement via transaortic approach
2018, 1Q, 12	Percutaneous balloon valvuloplasty & cardiac catheterization with ventriculogram
2017, 4Q, 55-56	Added approach values - Percutaneous heart valve procedures
2017, 1Q, 13	SynCardia total artificial heart
2016, 4Q, 80-81	Thoracic aorta, ascending/arch and descending
2016, 3Q, 32	Transcatheter tricuspid valve replacement
2014, 1Q, 10	Repair of thoracic aortic aneurysm & coronary artery bypass graft

AHA Coding Clinic for table Ø2S

2016, 4Q, 80-81	Thoracic aorta, ascending/arch and descending
2016, 4Q, 82-83	Coronary artery, number of arteries
2016, 4Q, 102-109	Correction of congenital heart defects
2015, 4Q, 23	Congenital heart corrective procedures

AHA Coding Clinic for table Ø2U

2018, 1Q, 12	Percutaneous balloon valvuloplasty & cardiac catheterization with ventriculogram
2017, 4Q, 36	Alfieri stitch procedure
2017, 3Q, 7	Senning procedure (arterial switch)
2017, 1Q, 19	Norwood Sano procedure
2016, 4Q, 80-81	Thoracic aorta, ascending/arch and descending
2016, 4Q, 101	Root operation Creation
2016, 4Q, 102-109	Correction of congenital heart defects
2016, 2Q, 23	Repair of tetralogy of Fallot with autologous pericardial patch graft
2016, 2Q, 26	Aortic valve replacement with aortic root enlargement
2015, 4Q, 22-24	Congenital heart corrective procedures
2015, 3Q, 16	Revision of previous truncus arteriosus surgery with ventricle to pulmonary artery conduit
2015, 2Q, 23	Annuloplasty ring
2014, 3Q, 16	Repair of Tetralogy of Fallot

AHA Coding Clinic for table Ø2V

2017, 4Q, 35-36	Alfieri stitch procedure
2016, 4Q, 80-81	Thoracic aorta, ascending/arch and descending
2016, 4Q, 89-92	Branched and fenestrated endograft repair of aneurysms

AHA Coding Clinic for table Ø2W

2019, 1Q, 24	Replacement of left ventricular assist device with retention of outflow graft
2018, 3Q, 8	Coronary artery bypass graft surgery (revision versus total redo)
2018, 3Q, 9	Fibrin sheath stripping of malfunctioning port-a-cath
2018, 1Q, 17	Repositioning of Impella short-term external heart assist device
2017, 4Q, 42-45	Insertion of external heart assist devices
2017, 4Q, 55-56	Added approach values - Percutaneous heart valve procedures
2016, 4Q, 85	Coronary Artery, number of stents
2016, 4Q, 95-96	Intracardiac pacemaker
2015, 3Q, 32	Approach values for repositioning and removal of cardiac lead
2014, 3Q, 31	Closure of paravalvular leak using Amplatzer® vascular plug

AHA Coding Clinic for table Ø2Y

| 2013, 3Q, 18 | Heart transplant surgery |

Heart and Great Vessels

Coronary Arteries

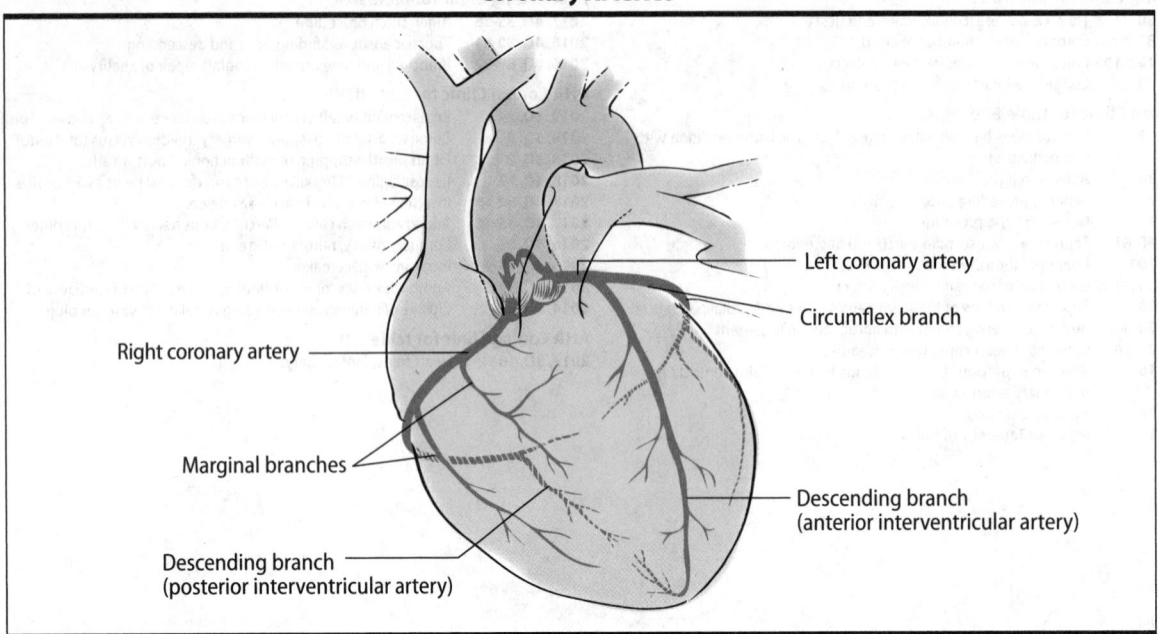

- Left coronary artery
- Circumflex branch
- Right coronary artery
- Marginal branches
- Descending branch (anterior interventricular artery)
- Descending branch (posterior interventricular artery)

Heart Anatomy

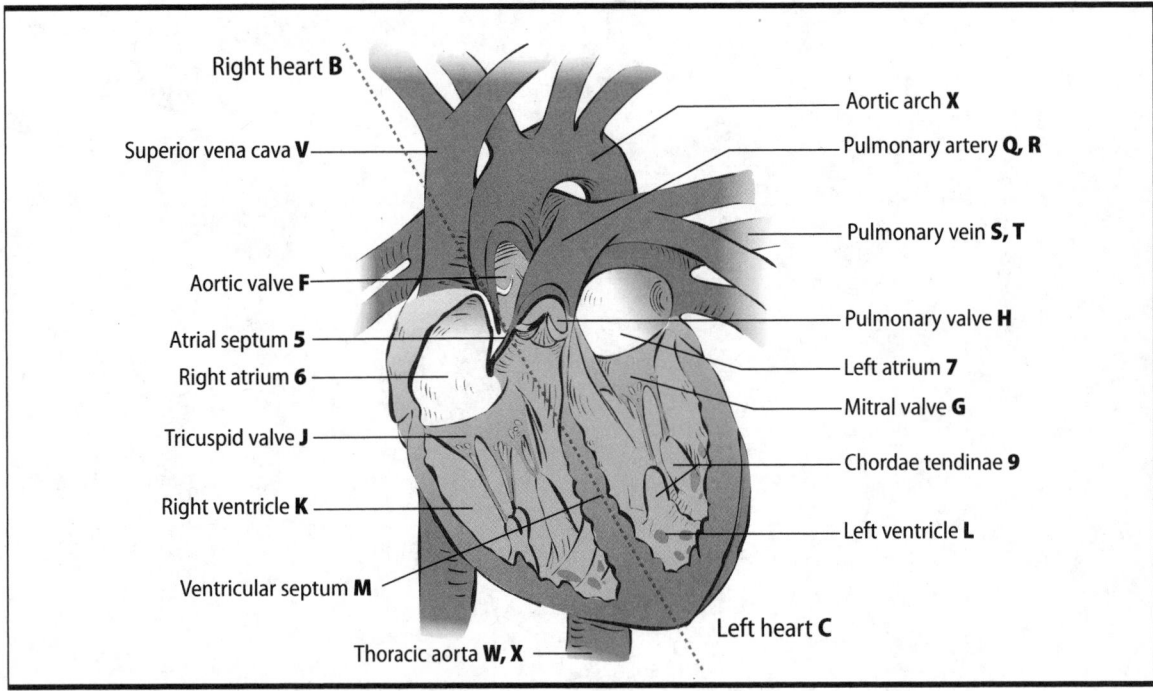

- Right heart **B**
- Superior vena cava **V**
- Aortic valve **F**
- Atrial septum **5**
- Right atrium **6**
- Tricuspid valve **J**
- Right ventricle **K**
- Ventricular septum **M**
- Thoracic aorta **W, X**
- Aortic arch **X**
- Pulmonary artery **Q, R**
- Pulmonary vein **S, T**
- Pulmonary valve **H**
- Left atrium **7**
- Mitral valve **G**
- Chordae tendinae **9**
- Left ventricle **L**
- Left heart **C**

Ø   Medical and Surgical
2   Heart and Great Vessels
1   Bypass   Definition: Altering the route of passage of the contents of a tubular body part

              Explanation: Rerouting contents of a body part to a downstream area of the normal route, to a similar route and body part, or to an abnormal route and dissimilar body part. Includes one or more anastomoses, with or without the use of a device.

Body Part Character 4	Approach Character 5	Device Character 6	Qualifier Character 7
Ø Coronary Artery, One Artery 1 Coronary Artery, Two Arteries 2 Coronary Artery, Three Arteries 3 Coronary Artery, Four or More Arteries	Ø Open	8 Zooplastic Tissue 9 Autologous Venous Tissue A Autologous Arterial Tissue J Synthetic Substitute K Nonautologous Tissue Substitute	3 Coronary Artery 8 Internal Mammary, Right 9 Internal Mammary, Left C Thoracic Artery F Abdominal Artery W Aorta
Ø Coronary Artery, One Artery 1 Coronary Artery, Two Arteries 2 Coronary Artery, Three Arteries 3 Coronary Artery, Four or More Arteries	Ø Open	Z No Device	3 Coronary Artery 8 Internal Mammary, Right 9 Internal Mammary, Left C Thoracic Artery F Abdominal Artery
Ø Coronary Artery, One Artery 1 Coronary Artery, Two Arteries 2 Coronary Artery, Three Arteries 3 Coronary Artery, Four or More Arteries	3 Percutaneous	4 Intraluminal Device, Drug-eluting D Intraluminal Device	4 Coronary Vein
Ø Coronary Artery, One Artery 1 Coronary Artery, Two Arteries 2 Coronary Artery, Three Arteries 3 Coronary Artery, Four or More Arteries	4 Percutaneous Endoscopic	4 Intraluminal Device, Drug-eluting D Intraluminal Device	4 Coronary Vein
Ø Coronary Artery, One Artery 1 Coronary Artery, Two Arteries 2 Coronary Artery, Three Arteries 3 Coronary Artery, Four or More Arteries	4 Percutaneous Endoscopic	8 Zooplastic Tissue 9 Autologous Venous Tissue A Autologous Arterial Tissue J Synthetic Substitute K Nonautologous Tissue Substitute	3 Coronary Artery 8 Internal Mammary, Right 9 Internal Mammary, Left C Thoracic Artery F Abdominal Artery W Aorta
Ø Coronary Artery, One Artery 1 Coronary Artery, Two Arteries 2 Coronary Artery, Three Arteries 3 Coronary Artery, Four or More Arteries	4 Percutaneous Endoscopic	Z No Device	3 Coronary Artery 8 Internal Mammary, Right 9 Internal Mammary, Left C Thoracic Artery F Abdominal Artery

6 Atrium, Right
   Atrium dextrum cordis
   Right auricular appendix
   Sinus venosus
	Ø Open
	4 Percutaneous Endoscopic
		8 Zooplastic Tissue
		9 Autologous Venous Tissue
		A Autologous Arterial Tissue
		J Synthetic Substitute
		K Nonautologous Tissue Substitute
			P Pulmonary Trunk
			Q Pulmonary Artery, Right
			R Pulmonary Artery, Left

6 Atrium, Right
   Atrium dextrum cordis
   Right auricular appendix
   Sinus venosus
	Ø Open
	4 Percutaneous Endoscopic
		Z No Device	7 Atrium, Left
			P Pulmonary Trunk
			Q Pulmonary Artery, Right
			R Pulmonary Artery, Left

6 Atrium, Right
   Atrium dextrum cordis
   Right auricular appendix
   Sinus venosus
	3 Percutaneous	Z No Device	7 Atrium, Left

7 Atrium, Left
   Atrium pulmonale
   Left auricular appendix
V Superior Vena Cava
   Precava
	Ø Open
	4 Percutaneous Endoscopic
		8 Zooplastic Tissue
		9 Autologous Venous Tissue
		A Autologous Arterial Tissue
		J Synthetic Substitute
		K Nonautologous Tissue Substitute
		Z No Device
			P Pulmonary Trunk
			Q Pulmonary Artery, Right
			R Pulmonary Artery, Left
			S Pulmonary Vein, Right
			T Pulmonary Vein, Left
			U Pulmonary Vein, Confluence

K Ventricle, Right Conus arteriosus L Ventricle, Left	Ø Open 4 Percutaneous Endoscopic	8 Zooplastic Tissue 9 Autologous Venous Tissue A Autologous Arterial Tissue J Synthetic Substitute K Nonautologous Tissue Substitute	P Pulmonary Trunk Q Pulmonary Artery, Right R Pulmonary Artery, Left

Ø21 Continued on next page

HAC   Ø21[Ø,1,2,3]Ø[8,9,A,J,K][3,8,9,C,F,W] when reported with SDx J98.51 or J98.59
HAC   Ø21[Ø,1,2,3]ØZ[3,8,9,C,F] when reported with SDx J98.51 or J98.59
HAC   Ø21[Ø,1,2,3]4[8,9,A,J,K][3,8,9,C,F,W] when reported with SDx J98.51 or J98.59
HAC   Ø21[Ø,1,2,3]4Z[3,8,9,C,F] when reported with SDx J98.51 or J98.59

LC Limited Coverage   NC Noncovered   ⊞ Combination Member   HAC associated procedure   Combination Only   DRG Non-OR   Non-OR   New/Revised in GREEN

ICD-10-PCS 2020   171

021 Continued

Ø	Medical and Surgical
2	Heart and Great Vessels
1	Bypass

Definition: Altering the route of passage of the contents of a tubular body part

Explanation: Rerouting contents of a body part to a downstream area of the normal route, to a similar route and body part, or to an abnormal route and dissimilar body part. Includes one or more anastomoses, with or without the use of a device.

Body Part Character 4	Approach Character 5	Device Character 6	Qualifier Character 7
K Ventricle, Right Conus arteriosus L Ventricle, Left	Ø Open 4 Percutaneous Endoscopic	Z No Device	5 Coronary Circulation 8 Internal Mammary, Right 9 Internal Mammary, Left C Thoracic Artery F Abdominal Artery P Pulmonary Trunk Q Pulmonary Artery, Right R Pulmonary Artery, Left W Aorta

P Pulmonary Trunk
Q Pulmonary Artery, Right
R Pulmonary Artery, Left
  Arterial canal (duct)
  Botallo's duct
  Pulmoaortic canal
	Ø Open
	4 Percutaneous Endoscopic
		8 Zooplastic Tissue
		9 Autologous Venous Tissue
		A Autologous Arterial Tissue
		J Synthetic Substitute
		K Nonautologous Tissue Substitute
		Z No Device
			A Innominate Artery
			B Subclavian
			D Carotid

W Thoracic Aorta, Descending	Ø Open	8 Zooplastic Tissue 9 Autologous Venous Tissue A Autologous Arterial Tissue J Synthetic Substitute K Nonautologous Tissue Substitute	A Innominate Artery B Subclavian D Carotid F Abdominal Artery G Axillary Artery H Brachial Artery P Pulmonary Trunk Q Pulmonary Artery, Right R Pulmonary Artery, Left V Lower Extremity Artery
W Thoracic Aorta, Descending	Ø Open	Z No Device	A Innominate Artery B Subclavian D Carotid P Pulmonary Trunk Q Pulmonary Artery, Right R Pulmonary Artery, Left
W Thoracic Aorta, Descending	4 Percutaneous Endoscopic	8 Zooplastic Tissue 9 Autologous Venous Tissue A Autologous Arterial Tissue J Synthetic Substitute K Nonautologous Tissue Substitute Z No Device	A Innominate Artery B Subclavian D Carotid P Pulmonary Trunk Q Pulmonary Artery, Right R Pulmonary Artery, Left

X Thoracic Aorta, Ascending/Arch
  Aortic arch
  Ascending aorta
	Ø Open
	4 Percutaneous Endoscopic
		8 Zooplastic Tissue
		9 Autologous Venous Tissue
		A Autologous Arterial Tissue
		J Synthetic Substitute
		K Nonautologous Tissue Substitute
		Z No Device
			A Innominate Artery
			B Subclavian
			D Carotid
			P Pulmonary Trunk
			Q Pulmonary Artery, Right
			R Pulmonary Artery, Left

Ø	Medical and Surgical
2	Heart and Great Vessels
4	Creation

Definition: Putting in or on biological or synthetic material to form a new body part that to the extent possible replicates the anatomic structure or function of an absent body part

Explanation: Used for gender reassignment surgery and corrective procedures in individuals with congenital anomalies

Body Part Character 4	Approach Character 5	Device Character 6	Qualifier Character 7
F Aortic Valve Aortic annulus	Ø Open	7 Autologous Tissue 8 Zooplastic Tissue J Synthetic Substitute K Nonautologous Tissue Substitute	J Truncal Valve

G Mitral Valve
  Bicuspid valve
  Left atrioventricular valve
  Mitral annulus
J Tricuspid Valve
  Right atrioventricular valve
  Tricuspid annulus
	Ø Open	7 Autologous Tissue
		8 Zooplastic Tissue
		J Synthetic Substitute
		K Nonautologous Tissue Substitute
			2 Common Atrioventricular Valve

🔲 Limited Coverage   🔲 Noncovered   ⊞ Combination Member   HAC associated procedure   Combination Only   DRG Non-OR   Non-OR   New/Revised in GREEN

172   ICD-10-PCS 2020

Ø   **Medical and Surgical**
2   **Heart and Great Vessels**
5   **Destruction**   Definition: Physical eradication of all or a portion of a body part by the direct use of energy, force, or a destructive agent
                        Explanation: None of the body part is physically taken out

Body Part Character 4	Approach Character 5	Device Character 6	Qualifier Character 7
4 **Coronary Vein**	Ø **Open**	Z **No Device**	Z **No Qualifier**
5 **Atrial Septum**	3 **Percutaneous**		
Interatrial septum	4 **Percutaneous Endoscopic**		
6 **Atrium, Right**			
Atrium dextrum cordis			
Right auricular appendix			
Sinus venosus			
8 **Conduction Mechanism**			
Atrioventricular node			
Bundle of His			
Bundle of Kent			
Sinoatrial node			
9 **Chordae Tendineae**			
D **Papillary Muscle**			
F **Aortic Valve**			
Aortic annulus			
G **Mitral Valve**			
Bicuspid valve			
Left atrioventricular valve			
Mitral annulus			
H **Pulmonary Valve**			
Pulmonary annulus			
Pulmonic valve			
J **Tricuspid Valve**			
Right atrioventricular valve			
Tricuspid annulus			
K **Ventricle, Right**			
Conus arteriosus			
L **Ventricle, Left**			
M **Ventricular Septum**			
Interventricular septum			
N **Pericardium**			
P **Pulmonary Trunk**			
Q **Pulmonary Artery, Right**			
R **Pulmonary Artery, Left**			
Arterial canal (duct)			
Botallo's duct			
Pulmoaortic canal			
S **Pulmonary Vein, Right**			
Right inferior pulmonary vein			
Right superior pulmonary vein			
T **Pulmonary Vein, Left**			
Left inferior pulmonary vein			
Left superior pulmonary vein			
V **Superior Vena Cava**			
Precava			
W **Thoracic Aorta, Descending**			
X **Thoracic Aorta, Ascending/Arch**			
Aortic arch			
Ascending aorta			
7 **Atrium, Left**	Ø **Open**	Z **No Device**	K **Left Atrial Appendage**
Atrium pulmonale	3 **Percutaneous**		Z **No Qualifier**
Left auricular appendix	4 **Percutaneous Endoscopic**		

DRG Non-OR   Ø257[Ø,3,4]ZK

LC Limited Coverage **NC** Noncovered ⊞ Combination Member HAC associated procedure Combination Only DRG Non-OR Non-OR New/Revised in GREEN

ICD-1Ø-PCS 2020   173

Ø25–Ø25

Ø   **Medical and Surgical**
2   **Heart and Great Vessels**
7   **Dilation**   Definition: Expanding an orifice or the lumen of a tubular body part

                     Explanation: The orifice can be a natural orifice or an artificially created orifice. Accomplished by stretching a tubular body part using intraluminal pressure or by cutting part of the orifice or wall of the tubular body part.

Body Part Character 4	Approach Character 5	Device Character 6	Qualifier Character 7

Ø Coronary Artery, One Artery
1 Coronary Artery, Two Arteries
2 Coronary Artery, Three Arteries
3 Coronary Artery, Four or More Arteries
	Ø Open
	3 Percutaneous
	4 Percutaneous Endoscopic
		4 Intraluminal Device,
		    Drug-eluting
		5 Intraluminal Device, Drug-eluting,
		    Two
		6 Intraluminal Device, Drug-eluting,
		    Three
		7 Intraluminal Device, Drug-eluting,
		    Four or More
		D Intraluminal Device
		E Intraluminal Device, Two
		F Intraluminal Device, Three
		G Intraluminal Device, Four or More
		T Intraluminal Device, Radioactive
		Z No Device
			6 Bifurcation
			Z No Qualifier

F Aortic Valve
   Aortic annulus
G Mitral Valve
   Bicuspid valve
   Left atrioventricular valve
   Mitral annulus
H Pulmonary Valve
   Pulmonary annulus
   Pulmonic valve
J Tricuspid Valve
   Right atrioventricular valve
   Tricuspid annulus
K Ventricle, Right
   Conus arteriosus
L Ventricle, Left
P Pulmonary Trunk
Q Pulmonary Artery, Right
S Pulmonary Vein, Right
   Right inferior pulmonary vein
   Right superior pulmonary vein
T Pulmonary Vein, Left
   Left inferior pulmonary vein
   Left superior pulmonary vein
V Superior Vena Cava
   Precava
W Thoracic Aorta, Descending
X Thoracic Aorta, Ascending/Arch
   Aortic arch
   Ascending aorta
	Ø Open
	3 Percutaneous
	4 Percutaneous Endoscopic
		4 Intraluminal Device,
		    Drug-eluting
		D Intraluminal Device
		Z No Device
			Z No Qualifier

R Pulmonary Artery, Left
   Arterial canal (duct)
   Botallo's duct
   Pulmoaortic canal
	Ø Open
	3 Percutaneous
	4 Percutaneous Endoscopic
		4 Intraluminal Device,
		    Drug-eluting
		D Intraluminal Device
		Z No Device
			T Ductus Arteriosus
			Z No Qualifier

Ø   **Medical and Surgical**
2   **Heart and Great Vessels**
8   **Division**   Definition: Cutting into a body part, without draining fluids and/or gases from the body part, in order to separate or transect a body part

                     Explanation: All or a portion of the body part is separated into two or more portions

Body Part Character 4	Approach Character 5	Device Character 6	Qualifier Character 7

8 Conduction Mechanism
   Atrioventricular node
   Bundle of His
   Bundle of Kent
   Sinoatrial node
9 Chordae Tendineae
D Papillary Muscle
	Ø Open
	3 Percutaneous
	4 Percutaneous Endoscopic
		Z No Device	**Z** No Qualifier

LC Limited Coverage   **NC** Noncovered   ⊞ Combination Member   HAC associated procedure   Combination Only   DRG Non-OR   Non-OR   New/Revised in **GREEN**

174   ICD-10-PCS 2020

027–028

0   Medical and Surgical
2   Heart and Great Vessels
B   Excision   Definition: Cutting out or off, without replacement, a portion of a body part
                              Explanation: The qualifier DIAGNOSTIC is used to identify excision procedures that are biopsies

Body Part Character 4	Approach Character 5	Device Character 6	Qualifier Character 7
4 Coronary Vein	**0 Open**	**Z No Device**	**X Diagnostic**
5 Atrial Septum	**3 Percutaneous**		**Z No Qualifier**
Interatrial septum	**4 Percutaneous Endoscopic**		
6 Atrium, Right			
Atrium dextrum cordis			
Right auricular appendix			
Sinus venosus			
8 Conduction Mechanism			
Atrioventricular node			
Bundle of His			
Bundle of Kent			
Sinoatrial node			
9 Chordae Tendineae			
D Papillary Muscle			
F Aortic Valve			
Aortic annulus			
G Mitral Valve			
Bicuspid valve			
Left atrioventricular valve			
Mitral annulus			
H Pulmonary Valve			
Pulmonary annulus			
Pulmonic valve			
J Tricuspid Valve			
Right atrioventricular valve			
Tricuspid annulus			
K Ventricle, Right `NC`			
Conus arteriosus			
L Ventricle, Left `NC`			
M Ventricular Septum			
Interventricular septum			
N Pericardium			
P Pulmonary Trunk			
Q Pulmonary Artery, Right			
R Pulmonary Artery, Left			
Arterial canal (duct)			
Botallo's duct			
Pulmoaortic canal			
S Pulmonary Vein, Right			
Right inferior pulmonary vein			
Right superior pulmonary vein			
T Pulmonary Vein, Left			
Left inferior pulmonary vein			
Left superior pulmonary vein			
V Superior Vena Cava			
Precava			
W Thoracic Aorta, Descending			
X Thoracic Aorta, Ascending/Arch			
Aortic arch			
Ascending aorta			
7 Atrium, Left	**0 Open**	**Z No Device**	**K Left Atrial Appendage**
Atrium pulmonale	**3 Percutaneous**		**X Diagnostic**
Left auricular appendix	**4 Percutaneous Endoscopic**		**Z No Qualifier**

DRG Non-OR	02B7[0,3,4]ZK
Non-OR	02B[4,5,6,8,9,D,F,G,H,J,K,L,M][0,3,4]ZX
`NC`	02B[K,L][0,3,4]ZZ

Heart and Great Vessels

Ø   **Medical and Surgical**
2   **Heart and Great Vessels**
C   **Extirpation**   Definition: Taking or cutting out solid matter from a body part

          Explanation: The solid matter may be an abnormal byproduct of a biological function or a foreign body; it may be imbedded in a body part or in the lumen of a tubular body part. The solid matter may or may not have been previously broken into pieces.

Body Part Character 4	Approach Character 5	Device Character 6	Qualifier Character 7
Ø Coronary Artery, One Artery **1 Coronary Artery, Two Arteries** **2 Coronary Artery, Three Arteries** **3 Coronary Artery, Four or More Arteries**	**Ø** Open **3** Percutaneous **4** Percutaneous Endoscopic	**Z** No Device	**6** Bifurcation **Z** No Qualifier

4 Coronary Vein
5 Atrial Septum
    Interatrial septum
6 Atrium, Right
    Atrium dextrum cordis
    Right auricular appendix
    Sinus venosus
7 Atrium, Left
    Atrium pulmonale
    Left auricular appendix
8 Conduction Mechanism
    Atrioventricular node
    Bundle of His
    Bundle of Kent
    Sinoatrial node
9 Chordae Tendineae
D Papillary Muscle
F Aortic Valve
    Aortic annulus
G Mitral Valve
    Bicuspid valve
    Left atrioventricular valve
    Mitral annulus
H Pulmonary Valve
    Pulmonary annulus
    Pulmonic valve
J Tricuspid Valve
    Right atrioventricular valve
    Tricuspid annulus
K Ventricle, Right
    Conus arteriosus
L Ventricle, Left
M Ventricular Septum
    Interventricular septum
N Pericardium
P Pulmonary Trunk
Q Pulmonary Artery, Right
R Pulmonary Artery, Left
    Arterial canal (duct)
    Botallo's duct
    Pulmoaortic canal
S Pulmonary Vein, Right
    Right inferior pulmonary vein
    Right superior pulmonary vein
T Pulmonary Vein, Left
    Left inferior pulmonary vein
    Left superior pulmonary vein
V Superior Vena Cava
    Precava
W Thoracic Aorta, Descending
X Thoracic Aorta, Ascending/Arch
    Aortic arch
    Ascending aorta
	Ø Open
	3 Percutaneous
	4 Percutaneous Endoscopic
		Z No Device	**Z** No Qualifier

Ø   **Medical and Surgical**
2   **Heart and Great Vessels**
F   **Fragmentation**   Definition: Breaking solid matter in a body part into pieces

          Explanation: Physical force (e.g., manual, ultrasonic) applied directly or indirectly is used to break the solid matter into pieces. The solid matter may be an abnormal byproduct of a biological function or a foreign body. The pieces of solid matter are not taken out.

Body Part Character 4	Approach Character 5	Device Character 6	Qualifier Character 7
N Pericardium NC	**Ø** Open **3** Percutaneous **4** Percutaneous Endoscopic **X** External	**Z** No Device	**Z** No Qualifier

Non-OR	02FNXZZ
NC	02FNXZZ

LC Limited Coverage   NC Noncovered   ⊞ Combination Member   HAC associated procedure   Combination Only   DRG Non-OR   Non-OR   New/Revised in GREEN

176   ICD-10-PCS 2020

Ø   Medical and Surgical
2   Heart and Great Vessels
H   Insertion   Definition: Putting in a nonbiological appliance that monitors, assists, performs, or prevents a physiological function but does not physically take the place of a body part
               Explanation: None

Body Part Character 4	Approach Character 5	Device Character 6	Qualifier Character 7
Ø Coronary Artery, One Artery 1 Coronary Artery, Two Arteries 2 Coronary Artery, Three Arteries 3 Coronary Artery, Four or More Arteries	Ø Open 3 Percutaneous 4 Percutaneous Endoscopic	D Intraluminal Device Y Other Device	Z No Qualifier

4 Coronary Vein ⊞
6 Atrium, Right ⊞
   Atrium dextrum cordis
   Right auricular appendix
   Sinus venosus
7 Atrium, Left ⊞
   Atrium pulmonale
   Left auricular appendix
K Ventricle, Right ⊞
   Conus arteriosus
L Ventricle, Left ⊞
	Ø Open
	3 Percutaneous
	4 Percutaneous Endoscopic
		Ø Monitoring Device, Pressure Sensor
		2 Monitoring Device
		3 Infusion Device
		D Intraluminal Device
		J Cardiac Lead, Pacemaker
		K Cardiac Lead, Defibrillator
		M Cardiac Lead
		N Intracardiac Pacemaker
		Y Other Device
			Z No Qualifier

A Heart LC NC	Ø Open 3 Percutaneous 4 Percutaneous Endoscopic	Q Implantable Heart Assist System Y Other Device	Z No Qualifier
A Heart ⊞	Ø Open 3 Percutaneous 4 Percutaneous Endoscopic	R Short-term External Heart Assist System	J Intraoperative S Biventricular Z No Qualifier
N Pericardium ⊞	Ø Open 3 Percutaneous 4 Percutaneous Endoscopic	Ø Monitoring Device, Pressure Sensor 2 Monitoring Device J Cardiac Lead, Pacemaker K Cardiac Lead, Defibrillator M Cardiac Lead Y Other Device	Z No Qualifier

P Pulmonary Trunk
Q Pulmonary Artery, Right
R Pulmonary Artery, Left
   Arterial canal (duct)
   Botallo's duct
   Pulmoaortic canal
S Pulmonary Vein, Right
   Right inferior pulmonary vein
   Right superior pulmonary vein
T Pulmonary Vein, Left
   Left inferior pulmonary vein
   Left superior pulmonary vein
V Superior Vena Cava
   Precava
W Thoracic Aorta, Descending
	Ø Open
	3 Percutaneous
	4 Percutaneous Endoscopic
		Ø Monitoring Device, Pressure Sensor
		2 Monitoring Device
		3 Infusion Device
		D Intraluminal Device
		Y Other Device
			Z No Qualifier

X Thoracic Aorta, Ascending/Arch
   Aortic arch
   Ascending aorta
	Ø Open
	3 Percutaneous
	4 Percutaneous Endoscopic
		Ø Monitoring Device, Pressure Sensor
		2 Monitoring Device
		3 Infusion Device
		D Intraluminal Device
			Z No Qualifier

DRG Non-OR	02H[4,K,L][Ø,3,4][J,M]Z	HAC	02H43[J,K,M]Z when reported with SDx K68.11 or T81.4Ø-T81.49, T82.6-T82.7 with 7th character A
DRG Non-OR	02H[6,7][Ø,4]MZ	HAC	02H[6,K]33Z when reported with SDx J95.811
DRG Non-OR	02H[6,7][3,4]JZ	HAC	02H[6,7]3[J,M]Z when reported with SDx K68.11 or T81.4Ø-T81.49, T82.6-T82.7 with 7th character A
DRG Non-OR	02H70JZ		
DRG Non-OR	02HK32Z	HAC	02H[K,L]3JZ when reported with SDx K68.11 or T81.4Ø-T81.49, T82.6-T82.7 with 7th character A
DRG Non-OR	02HN[Ø,3,4][J,M]Z	HAC	02HN[Ø,3,4][J,M]Z when reported with SDx K68.11 or T81.4Ø-T81.49, T82.6-T82.7 with 7th character A
Non-OR	02H[4,6,7,L]3[2,3]Z	HAC	02H[S,T,V][3,4]3Z when reported with SDx J95.811
Non-OR	02H[6,7]3MZ	LC	02HAØQZ
Non-OR	02HK3[Ø,3]Z	NC	02HA[3,4]QZ
Non-OR	02HN32Z		
Non-OR	02HP[Ø,3,4][Ø,2,3]Z	**See Appendix L for Procedure Combinations**	
Non-OR	02H[Q,R][Ø,3,4][2,3]Z	Combo-only	02H60JZ
Non-OR	02H[S,T,V,W][Ø,3,4]3Z	Combo-only	02H[6,7]3MZ
Non-OR	02H[S,T,V,W]32Z	⊞	02H[4,K,L][Ø,3,4][J,K,M]Z
Non-OR	02HW[Ø,3]ØZ	⊞	02H[6,7][Ø,3,4]KZ
Non-OR	02HX[Ø,3,4][Ø,3]Z	⊞	02H[6,7][Ø,4]MZ
		⊞	02H6[3,4]JZ
		⊞	02H7[Ø,3,4]JZ
		⊞	02HA[Ø,4]R[S,Z]
		⊞	02HA3RS
		⊞	02HN[Ø,3,4][J,K,M]Z

LC Limited Coverage   NC Noncovered   ⊞ Combination Member   HAC associated procedure   Combination Only   DRG Non-OR   Non-OR   New/Revised in GREEN

Heart and Great Vessels

Ø   **Medical and Surgical**
2   **Heart and Great Vessels**
J   **Inspection**   Definition: Visually and/or manually exploring a body part

Explanation: Visual exploration may be performed with or without optical instrumentation. Manual exploration may be performed directly or through intervening body layers.

Body Part Character 4	Approach Character 5	Device Character 6	Qualifier Character 7
A Heart Y Great Vessel	Ø Open 3 Percutaneous 4 Percutaneous Endoscopic	Z No Device	Z No Qualifier

Non-OR   02J[A,Y]3ZZ

Ø   **Medical and Surgical**
2   **Heart and Great Vessels**
K   **Map**   Definition: Locating the route of passage of electrical impulses and/or locating functional areas in a body part

Explanation: Applicable only to the cardiac conduction mechanism and the central nervous system

Body Part Character 4	Approach Character 5	Device Character 6	Qualifier Character 7

8   Conduction Mechanism
    Atrioventricular node
    Bundle of His
    Bundle of Kent
    Sinoatrial node
	Ø Open
	3 Percutaneous
	4 Percutaneous Endoscopic
		Z No Device	Z No Qualifier

DRG Non-OR   02K8[0,3,4]ZZ

Ø   **Medical and Surgical**
2   **Heart and Great Vessels**
L   **Occlusion**   Definition: Completely closing an orifice or the lumen of a tubular body part

Explanation: The orifice can be a natural orifice or an artificially created orifice

Body Part Character 4	Approach Character 5	Device Character 6	Qualifier Character 7

7   Atrium, Left
    Atrium pulmonale
    Left auricular appendix
	Ø Open
	3 Percutaneous
	4 Percutaneous Endoscopic
		C Extraluminal Device
		D Intraluminal Device
		Z No Device
			K Left Atrial Appendage

H   Pulmonary Valve
    Pulmonary annulus
    Pulmonic valve
P   Pulmonary Trunk
Q   Pulmonary Artery, Right
S   Pulmonary Vein, Right
    Right inferior pulmonary vein
    Right superior pulmonary vein
T   Pulmonary Vein, Left
    Left inferior pulmonary vein
    Left superior pulmonary vein
V   Superior Vena Cava
    Precava
	Ø Open
	3 Percutaneous
	4 Percutaneous Endoscopic
		C Extraluminal Device
		D Intraluminal Device
		Z No Device
			Z No Qualifier

R   Pulmonary Artery, Left
    Arterial canal (duct)
    Botallo's duct
    Pulmoaortic canal
	Ø Open
	3 Percutaneous
	4 Percutaneous Endoscopic
		C Extraluminal Device
		D Intraluminal Device
		Z No Device
			T Ductus Arteriosus
			Z No Qualifier

W Thoracic Aorta, Descending	3 Percutaneous	D Intraluminal Device	J Temporary

DRG Non-OR   02L7[0,3,4][C,D,Z]K

LC Limited Coverage   NC Noncovered   ⊞ Combination Member   HAC associated procedure   Combination Only   DRG Non-OR   Non-OR   New/Revised in GREEN

178   ICD-10-PCS 2020

0   **Medical and Surgical**
2   **Heart and Great Vessels**
N   **Release**   Definition: Freeing a body part from an abnormal physical constraint by cutting or by the use of force
                      Explanation: Some of the restraining tissue may be taken out but none of the body part is taken out

Body Part Character 4	Approach Character 5	Device Character 6	Qualifier Character 7
0 **Coronary Artery, One Artery**	**0** Open	**Z** No Device	**Z** No Qualifier
1 **Coronary Artery, Two Arteries**	**3** Percutaneous		
2 **Coronary Artery, Three Arteries**	**4** Percutaneous Endoscopic		
3 **Coronary Artery, Four or More Arteries**			
4 **Coronary Vein**			
5 **Atrial Septum** Interatrial septum			
6 **Atrium, Right** Atrium dextrum cordis Right auricular appendix Sinus venosus			
7 **Atrium, Left** Atrium pulmonale Left auricular appendix			
8 **Conduction Mechanism** Atrioventricular node Bundle of His Bundle of Kent Sinoatrial node			
9 **Chordae Tendineae**			
D **Papillary Muscle**			
F **Aortic Valve** Aortic annulus			
G **Mitral Valve** Bicuspid valve Left atrioventricular valve Mitral annulus			
H **Pulmonary Valve** Pulmonary annulus Pulmonic valve			
J **Tricuspid Valve** Right atrioventricular valve Tricuspid annulus			
K **Ventricle, Right** Conus arteriosus			
L **Ventricle, Left**			
M **Ventricular Septum** Interventricular septum			
N **Pericardium**			
P **Pulmonary Trunk**			
Q **Pulmonary Artery, Right**			
R **Pulmonary Artery, Left** Arterial canal (duct) Botallo's duct Pulmoaortic canal			
S **Pulmonary Vein, Right** Right inferior pulmonary vein Right superior pulmonary vein			
T **Pulmonary Vein, Left** Left inferior pulmonary vein Left superior pulmonary vein			
V **Superior Vena Cava** Precava			
W **Thoracic Aorta, Descending**			
X **Thoracic Aorta, Ascending/Arch** Aortic arch Ascending aorta			

Heart and Great Vessels

0 Medical and Surgical
2 Heart and Great Vessels
P Removal   Definition: Taking out or off a device from a body part

Explanation: If a device is taken out and a similar device put in without cutting or puncturing the skin or mucous membrane, the procedure is coded to the root operation CHANGE. Otherwise, the procedure for taking out a device is coded to the root operation REMOVAL.

Body Part Character 4	Approach Character 5	Device Character 6	Qualifier Character 7
A Heart	0 Open 3 Percutaneous 4 Percutaneous Endoscopic	2 Monitoring Device 3 Infusion Device 7 Autologous Tissue Substitute 8 Zooplastic Tissue C Extraluminal Device D Intraluminal Device J Synthetic Substitute K Nonautologous Tissue Substitute M Cardiac Lead N Intracardiac Pacemaker Q Implantable Heart Assist System Y Other Device	Z No Qualifier
A Heart ⊞	0 Open 3 Percutaneous 4 Percutaneous Endoscopic	R Short-term External Heart Assist System	S Biventricular Z No Qualifier
A Heart	X External	2 Monitoring Device 3 Infusion Device D Intraluminal Device M Cardiac Lead	Z No Qualifier
Y Great Vessel	0 Open 3 Percutaneous 4 Percutaneous Endoscopic	2 Monitoring Device 3 Infusion Device 7 Autologous Tissue Substitute 8 Zooplastic Tissue C Extraluminal Device D Intraluminal Device J Synthetic Substitute K Nonautologous Tissue Substitute Y Other Device	Z No Qualifier
Y Great Vessel	X External	2 Monitoring Device 3 Infusion Device D Intraluminal Device	Z No Qualifier

Non-OR 02PA3[2,3,D]Z
Non-OR 02PA[3,4]YZ
Non-OR 02PAX[2,3,D,M]Z
Non-OR 02PY3[2,3,D]Z
Non-OR 02PY[3,4]YZ
Non-OR 02PYX[2,3,D]Z
HAC 02PA[0,3,4]MZ when reported with SDx K68.11 or T81.40-T81.49, T82.6-T82.7 with 7th character A
HAC 02PAXMZ when reported with SDx K68.11 or T81.40-T81.49, T82.6-T82.7 with 7th character A

See Appendix L for Procedure Combinations
⊞ 02PA[0,3,4]RZ

0   **Medical and Surgical**
2   **Heart and Great Vessels**
Q   **Repair**   Definition: Restoring, to the extent possible, a body part to its normal anatomic structure and function
Explanation: Used only when the method to accomplish the repair is not one of the other root operations

Body Part Character 4	Approach Character 5	Device Character 6	Qualifier Character 7

0 Coronary Artery, One Artery
1 Coronary Artery, Two Arteries
2 Coronary Artery, Three Arteries
3 Coronary Artery, Four or More
    Arteries
4 Coronary Vein
5 Atrial Septum
    Interatrial septum
6 Atrium, Right
    Atrium dextrum cordis
    Right auricular appendix
    Sinus venosus
7 Atrium, Left
    Atrium pulmonale
    Left auricular appendix
8 Conduction Mechanism
    Atrioventricular node
    Bundle of His
    Bundle of Kent
    Sinoatrial node
9 Chordae Tendineae
A Heart
B Heart, Right
    Right coronary sulcus
C Heart, Left
    Left coronary sulcus
    Obtuse margin
D Papillary Muscle
H Pulmonary Valve
    Pulmonary annulus
    Pulmonic valve
K Ventricle, Right
    Conus arteriosus
L Ventricle, Left
M Ventricular Septum
    Interventricular septum
N Pericardium
P Pulmonary Trunk
Q Pulmonary Artery, Right
R Pulmonary Artery, Left
    Arterial canal (duct)
    Botallo's duct
    Pulmoaortic canal
S Pulmonary Vein, Right
    Right inferior pulmonary vein
    Right superior pulmonary vein
T Pulmonary Vein, Left
    Left inferior pulmonary vein
    Left superior pulmonary vein
V Superior Vena Cava
    Precava
W Thoracic Aorta, Descending
X Thoracic Aorta, Ascending/Arch
    Aortic arch
    Ascending aorta
	0 Open
	3 Percutaneous
	4 Percutaneous Endoscopic
		Z No Device	**Z** No Qualifier

F Aortic Valve Aortic annulus	**0** Open **3** Percutaneous **4** Percutaneous Endoscopic	**Z** No Device	**J** Truncal Valve **Z** No Qualifier

G Mitral Valve
    Bicuspid valve
    Left atrioventricular valve
    Mitral annulus
	0 Open
	3 Percutaneous
	4 Percutaneous Endoscopic
		Z No Device	**E** Atrioventricular Valve, Left
			Z No Qualifier

J Tricuspid Valve
    Right atrioventricular valve
    Tricuspid annulus
	0 Open
	3 Percutaneous
	4 Percutaneous Endoscopic
		Z No Device	**G** Atrioventricular Valve, Right
			Z No Qualifier

LC Limited Coverage   **NC** Noncovered   ⊞ Combination Member   HAC associated procedure   Combination Only   DRG Non-OR   Non-OR   New/Revised in GREEN
ICD-10-PCS 2020   181

02Q–02Q

Heart and Great Vessels

Ø   Medical and Surgical
2   Heart and Great Vessels
R   Replacement   Definition: Putting in or on biological or synthetic material that physically takes the place and/or function of all or a portion of a body part
Explanation: The body part may have been taken out or replaced, or may be taken out, physically eradicated, or rendered nonfunctional during the REPLACEMENT procedure. A REMOVAL procedure is coded for taking out the device used in a previous replacement procedure.

Body Part Character 4	Approach Character 5	Device Character 6	Qualifier Character 7

5   Atrial Septum
   Interatrial septum
6   Atrium, Right
   Atrium dextrum cordis
   Right auricular appendix
   Sinus venosus
7   Atrium, Left
   Atrium pulmonale
   Left auricular appendix
9   Chordae Tendineae
D   Papillary Muscle
K   Ventricle, Right LC NC ⊞
   Conus arteriosus
L   Ventricle, Left LC NC ⊞
M   Ventricular Septum
   Interventricular septum
N   Pericardium
P   Pulmonary Trunk
Q   Pulmonary Artery, Right
R   Pulmonary Artery, Left
   Arterial canal (duct)
   Botallo's duct
   Pulmoaortic canal
S   Pulmonary Vein, Right
   Right inferior pulmonary vein
   Right superior pulmonary vein
T   Pulmonary Vein, Left
   Left inferior pulmonary vein
   Left superior pulmonary vein
V   Superior Vena Cava
   Precava
W   Thoracic Aorta, Descending
X   Thoracic Aorta, Ascending/Arch
   Aortic arch
   Ascending aorta
	Ø Open
	4 Percutaneous Endoscopic
		7 Autologous Tissue Substitute
		8 Zooplastic Tissue
		J Synthetic Substitute
		K Nonautologous Tissue Substitute
			Z No Qualifier

F   Aortic Valve
   Aortic annulus
G   Mitral Valve
   Bicuspid valve
   Left atrioventricular valve
   Mitral annulus
H   Pulmonary Valve
   Pulmonary annulus
   Pulmonic valve
J   Tricuspid Valve
   Right atrioventricular valve
   Tricuspid annulus
	Ø Open
	4 Percutaneous Endoscopic
		7 Autologous Tissue Substitute
		8 Zooplastic Tissue
		J Synthetic Substitute
		K Nonautologous Tissue Substitute
			Z No Qualifier

F   Aortic Valve
   Aortic annulus
G   Mitral Valve
   Bicuspid valve
   Left atrioventricular valve
   Mitral annulus
H   Pulmonary Valve
   Pulmonary annulus
   Pulmonic valve
J   Tricuspid Valve
   Right atrioventricular valve
   Tricuspid annulus
	3 Percutaneous	7 Autologous Tissue Substitute
		8 Zooplastic Tissue
		J Synthetic Substitute
		K Nonautologous Tissue Substitute
			H Transapical
			Z No Qualifier

LC   Ø2RKØJZ with Ø2RLØJZ with diagnosis code ZØØ.6
NC   Ø2RKØJZ with Ø2RLØJZ without diagnosis code ZØØ.6

See Appendix L for Procedure Combinations
⊞   Ø2R[K,L]ØJZ

0   Medical and Surgical
2   Heart and Great Vessels
S   Reposition   Definition: Moving to its normal location, or other suitable location, all or a portion of a body part

                   Explanation: The body part is moved to a new location from an abnormal location, or from a normal location where it is not functioning correctly. The body part may or may not be cut out or off to be moved to the new location.

Body Part Character 4	Approach Character 5	Device Character 6	Qualifier Character 7

0   Coronary Artery, One Artery
1   Coronary Artery, Two Arteries
P   Pulmonary Trunk
Q   Pulmonary Artery, Right
R   Pulmonary Artery, Left
     Arterial canal (duct)
     Botallo's duct
     Pulmoaortic canal
S   Pulmonary Vein, Right
     Right inferior pulmonary vein
     Right superior pulmonary vein
T   Pulmonary Vein, Left
     Left inferior pulmonary vein
     Left superior pulmonary vein
V   Superior Vena Cava
     Precava
W   Thoracic Aorta, Descending
X   Thoracic Aorta, Ascending/Arch
     Aortic arch
     Ascending aorta
	0 Open	**Z No Device**	**Z No Qualifier**

0   Medical and Surgical
2   Heart and Great Vessels
T   Resection   Definition: Cutting out or off, without replacement, all of a body part

                   Explanation: None

Body Part Character 4	Approach Character 5	Device Character 6	Qualifier Character 7

5   Atrial Septum
     Interatrial septum
8   Conduction Mechanism
     Atrioventricular node
     Bundle of His
     Bundle of Kent
     Sinoatrial node
9   Chordae Tendineae
D   Papillary Muscle
H   Pulmonary Valve
     Pulmonary annulus
     Pulmonic valve
M   Ventricular Septum
     Interventricular septum
N   Pericardium
	0 Open
	3 Percutaneous
	4 Percutaneous Endoscopic
		Z No Device	**Z No Qualifier**

Heart and Great Vessels

0   Medical and Surgical
2   Heart and Great Vessels
U   Supplement   Definition: Putting in or on biological or synthetic material that physically reinforces and/or augments the function of a portion of a body part
Explanation: The biological material is non-living, or is living and from the same individual. The body part may have been previously replaced, and the SUPPLEMENT procedure is performed to physically reinforce and/or augment the function of the replaced body part.

Body Part Character 4	Approach Character 5	Device Character 6	Qualifier Character 7

0 Coronary Artery, One Artery
1 Coronary Artery, Two Arteries
2 Coronary Artery, Three Arteries
3 Coronary Artery, Four or More
   Arteries
5 **Atrial Septum**
   Interatrial septum
6 **Atrium, Right**
   Atrium dextrum cordis
   Right auricular appendix
   Sinus venosus
7 **Atrium, Left**
   Atrium pulmonale
   Left auricular appendix
9 **Chordae Tendineae**
A **Heart**
D **Papillary Muscle**
H **Pulmonary Valve**
   Pulmonary annulus
   Pulmonic valve
K **Ventricle, Right**
   Conus arteriosus
L **Ventricle, Left**
M **Ventricular Septum**
   Interventricular septum
N **Pericardium**
P **Pulmonary Trunk**
Q **Pulmonary Artery, Right**
R **Pulmonary Artery, Left**
   Arterial canal (duct)
   Botallo's duct
   Pulmoaortic canal
S **Pulmonary Vein, Right**
   Right inferior pulmonary vein
   Right superior pulmonary vein
T **Pulmonary Vein, Left**
   Left inferior pulmonary vein
   Left superior pulmonary vein
V **Superior Vena Cava**
   Precava
W **Thoracic Aorta, Descending**
X **Thoracic Aorta, Ascending/Arch**
   Aortic arch
   Ascending aorta
	0 Open
	3 Percutaneous
	4 Percutaneous Endoscopic
		7 Autologous Tissue Substitute
		8 Zooplastic Tissue
		J Synthetic Substitute
		K Nonautologous Tissue Substitute
			Z No Qualifier

F **Aortic Valve** Aortic annulus	0 Open 3 Percutaneous 4 Percutaneous Endoscopic	7 Autologous Tissue Substitute 8 Zooplastic Tissue J Synthetic Substitute K Nonautologous Tissue Substitute	J Truncal Valve Z No Qualifier

G **Mitral Valve**
   Bicuspid valve
   Left atrioventricular valve
   Mitral annulus
	0 Open
	3 Percutaneous
	4 Percutaneous Endoscopic
		7 Autologous Tissue Substitute
		8 Zooplastic Tissue
		J Synthetic Substitute
		K Nonautologous Tissue Substitute
			E Atrioventricular Valve, Left
			Z No Qualifier

J **Tricuspid Valve**
   Right atrioventricular valve
   Tricuspid annulus
	0 Open
	3 Percutaneous
	4 Percutaneous Endoscopic
		7 Autologous Tissue Substitute
		8 Zooplastic Tissue
		J Synthetic Substitute
		K Nonautologous Tissue Substitute
			G Atrioventricular Valve, Right
			Z No Qualifier

DRG Non-OR   02U7[3,4]JZ

Ø   **Medical and Surgical**
2   **Heart and Great Vessels**
V   **Restriction**   Definition: Partially closing an orifice or the lumen of a tubular body part
                                 Explanation: The orifice can be a natural orifice or an artificially created orifice

Body Part Character 4	Approach Character 5	Device Character 6	Qualifier Character 7
A Heart	**Ø** Open **3** Percutaneous **4** Percutaneous Endoscopic	**C** Extraluminal Device **Z** No Device	**Z** No Qualifier

G   Mitral Valve
      Bicuspid valve
      Left atrioventricular valve
      Mitral annulus
	Ø Open
	3 Percutaneous
	4 Percutaneous Endoscopic
		Z No Device	**Z** No Qualifier

P   Pulmonary Trunk
Q   Pulmonary Artery, Right
S   Pulmonary Vein, Right
      Right inferior pulmonary vein
      Right superior pulmonary vein
T   Pulmonary Vein, Left
      Left inferior pulmonary vein
      Left superior pulmonary vein
V   Superior Vena Cava
      Precava
	Ø Open
	3 Percutaneous
	4 Percutaneous Endoscopic
		C Extraluminal Device
		D Intraluminal Device
		Z No Device
			Z No Qualifier

R   Pulmonary Artery, Left
      Arterial canal (duct)
      Botallo's duct
      Pulmoaortic canal
	Ø Open
	3 Percutaneous
	4 Percutaneous Endoscopic
		C Extraluminal Device
		D Intraluminal Device
		Z No Device
			T Ductus Arteriosus
			Z No Qualifier

W   Thoracic Aorta, Descending
X   Thoracic Aorta, Ascending/Arch
      Aortic arch
      Ascending aorta
	Ø Open
	3 Percutaneous
	4 Percutaneous Endoscopic
		C Extraluminal Device
		D Intraluminal Device
		E Intraluminal Device, Branched or
		      Fenestrated, One or Two Arteries
		F Intraluminal Device, Branched or
		      Fenestrated, Three or More Arteries
		Z No Device
			Z No Qualifier

Heart and Great Vessels

Ø   Medical and Surgical
2   Heart and Great Vessels
W   Revision   Definition: Correcting, to the extent possible, a portion of a malfunctioning device or the position of a displaced device
                Explanation: Revision can include correcting a malfunctioning or displaced device by taking out or putting in components of the device such as a screw or pin

Body Part Character 4	Approach Character 5	Device Character 6	Qualifier Character 7
5 Atrial Septum Interatrial septum **M Ventricular Septum** Interventricular septum	**Ø** Open **4** Percutaneous Endoscopic	**J** Synthetic Substitute	**Z** No Qualifier
A Heart LC NC ⊞	**Ø** Open **3** Percutaneous **4** Percutaneous Endoscopic	**2** Monitoring Device **3** Infusion Device **7** Autologous Tissue Substitute **8** Zooplastic Tissue **C** Extraluminal Device **D** Intraluminal Device **J** Synthetic Substitute **K** Nonautologous Tissue Substitute **M** Cardiac Lead **N** Intracardiac Pacemaker **Q** Implantable Heart Assist System **Y** Other Device	**Z** No Qualifier
A Heart ⊞	**Ø** Open **3** Percutaneous **4** Percutaneous Endoscopic	**R** Short-term External Heart Assist System	**S** Biventricular **Z** No Qualifier
A Heart	**X** External	**2** Monitoring Device **3** Infusion Device **7** Autologous Tissue Substitute **8** Zooplastic Tissue **C** Extraluminal Device **D** Intraluminal Device **J** Synthetic Substitute **K** Nonautologous Tissue Substitute **M** Cardiac Lead **N** Intracardiac Pacemaker **Q** Implantable Heart Assist System	**Z** No Qualifier
A Heart	**X** External	**R** Short-term External Heart Assist System	**S** Biventricular **Z** No Qualifier
F Aortic Valve Aortic annulus **G Mitral Valve** Bicuspid valve Left atrioventricular valve Mitral annulus **H Pulmonary Valve** Pulmonary annulus Pulmonic valve **J Tricuspid Valve** Right atrioventricular valve Tricuspid annulus	**Ø** Open **3** Percutaneous **4** Percutaneous Endoscopic	**7** Autologous Tissue Substitute **8** Zooplastic Tissue **J** Synthetic Substitute **K** Nonautologous Tissue Substitute	**Z** No Qualifier
Y Great Vessel	**Ø** Open **3** Percutaneous **4** Percutaneous Endoscopic	**2** Monitoring Device **3** Infusion Device **7** Autologous Tissue Substitute **8** Zooplastic Tissue **C** Extraluminal Device **D** Intraluminal Device **J** Synthetic Substitute **K** Nonautologous Tissue Substitute **Y** Other Device	**Z** No Qualifier
Y Great Vessel	**X** External	**2** Monitoring Device **3** Infusion Device **7** Autologous Tissue Substitute **8** Zooplastic Tissue **C** Extraluminal Device **D** Intraluminal Device **J** Synthetic Substitute **K** Nonautologous Tissue Substitute	**Z** No Qualifier

Non-OR 02WA3[2,3,D]Z
Non-OR 02WA[3,4]YZ
Non-OR 02WAX[2,3,7,8,C,D,J,K,M,N,Q]Z
Non-OR 02WAXRZ
Non-OR 02WY3[2,3,D]Z
Non-OR 02WY[3,4]YZ
Non-OR 02WYX[2,3,7,8,C,D,J,K]Z

HAC   02WA[Ø,3,4]MZ when reported with T81.4Ø–T81.49, T82.6–T82.7 with 7th character A
LC   02WAØ[J,Q]Z
NC   02WA[3,4]QZ

See Appendix L for Procedure Combinations
⊞   02WA[Ø,3,4]QZ
⊞   02WA[Ø,3,4]RZ

LC Limited Coverage   NC Noncovered   ⊞ Combination Member   HAC associated procedure   Combination Only   DRG Non-OR   Non-OR   New/Revised in GREEN

Ø　Medical and Surgical
2　Heart and Great Vessels
Y　Transplantation　Definition: Putting in or on all or a portion of a living body part taken from another individual or animal to physically take the place and/or
　　　　　　　　　　　　function of all or a portion of a similar body part

　　　　　　　　　　　　Explanation: The native body part may or may not be taken out, and the transplanted body part may take over all or a portion of its function

Body Part Character 4	Approach Character 5	Device Character 6	Qualifier Character 7
A　Heart　　　　　　LC	Ø　Open	Z　No Device	Ø　Allogeneic 1　Syngeneic 2　Zooplastic

LC　Ø2YAØZ[Ø,1,2]

Upper Arteries Ø31–Ø3W

Character Meanings

This Character Meaning table is provided as a guide to assist the user in the identification of character members that may be found in this section of code tables. It **SHOULD NOT** be used to build a PCS code.

Operation–Character 3	Body Part–Character 4	Approach–Character 5	Device–Character 6	Qualifier–Character 7
1 Bypass	Ø Internal Mammary Artery, Right	Ø Open	Ø Drainage Device	Ø Upper Arm Artery, Right
5 Destruction	1 Internal Mammary Artery, Left	3 Percutaneous	2 Monitoring Device	1 Upper Arm Artery, Left OR Drug-Coated Balloon
7 Dilation	2 Innominate Artery	4 Percutaneous Endoscopic	3 Infusion Device	2 Upper Arm Artery, Bilateral
9 Drainage	3 Subclavian Artery, Right	X External	4 Intraluminal Device, Drug-eluting	3 Lower Arm Artery, Right
B Excision	4 Subclavian Artery, Left		5 Intraluminal Device, Drug-eluting, Two	4 Lower Arm Artery, Left
C Extirpation	5 Axillary Artery, Right		6 Intraluminal Device, Drug-eluting, Three	5 Lower Arm Artery, Bilateral
H Insertion	6 Axillary Artery, Left		7 Intraluminal Device, Drug-eluting, Four or More OR Autologous Tissue Substitute	6 Upper Leg Artery, Right
J Inspection	7 Brachial Artery, Right		9 Autologous Venous Tissue	7 Upper Leg Artery, Left OR Stent Retriever
L Occlusion	8 Brachial Artery, Left		A Autologous Arterial Tissue	8 Upper Leg Artery, Bilateral
N Release	9 Ulnar Artery, Right		B Intraluminal Device, Bioactive	9 Lower Leg Artery, Right
P Removal	A Ulnar Artery, Left		C Extraluminal Device	B Lower Leg Artery, Left
Q Repair	B Radial Artery, Right		D Intraluminal Device	C Lower Leg Artery, Bilateral
R Replacement	C Radial Artery, Left		E Intraluminal Device, Two	D Upper Arm Vein
S Reposition	D Hand Artery, Right		F Intraluminal Device, Three	F Lower Arm Vein
U Supplement	F Hand Artery, Left		G Intraluminal Device, Four or More	G Intracranial Artery
V Restriction	G Intracranial Artery		H Intraluminal Device, Flow Diverter	J Extracranial Artery, Right
W Revision	H Common Carotid Artery, Right		J Synthetic Substitute	K Extracranial Artery, Left
	J Common Carotid Artery, Left		K Nonautologous Tissue Substitute	M Pulmonary Artery, Right
	K Internal Carotid Artery, Right		M Stimulator Lead	N Pulmonary Artery, Left
	L Internal Carotid Artery, Left		Y Other Device	T Abdominal Artery
	M External Carotid Artery, Right		Z No Device	V Superior Vena Cava
	N External Carotid Artery, Left			W Lower Extremity Vein
	P Vertebral Artery, Right			X Diagnostic
	Q Vertebral Artery, Left			Y Upper Artery
	R Face Artery			Z No Qualifier
	S Temporal Artery, Right			
	T Temporal Artery, Left			
	U Thyroid Artery, Right			
	V Thyroid Artery, Left			
	Y Upper Artery			

AHA Coding Clinic for table Ø31

2017, 4Q, 64-65	New qualifier values - Left to right carotid bypass
2017, 2Q, 22	Carotid artery to subclavian artery transposition
2017, 1Q, 31	Left to right common carotid artery bypass
2016, 3Q, 37	Insertion of arteriovenous graft using HeRO device
2016, 3Q, 39	Revision of arteriovenous graft
2013, 4Q, 125	Stage II cephalic vein transposition (superficialization) of arteriovenous fistula
2013, 1Q, 27	Creation of radial artery fistula

AHA Coding Clinic for table Ø37

2018, 2Q, 24	Coronary artery bifurcation
2016, 4Q, 86	Peripheral artery, number of stents
2016, 4Q, 86-87	Coronary and peripheral artery bifurcation
2015, 1Q, 32	Deployment of stent for herniated/migrated coil in basilar artery

AHA Coding Clinic for table Ø3B

2016, 2Q, 12	Resection of malignant neoplasm of infratemporal fossa

AHA Coding Clinic for table Ø3C

2018, 4Q, 47-48	Endovascular thrombectomy with stent retriever
2018, 2Q, 24	Coronary artery bifurcation
2017, 4Q, 64-65	New qualifier values - Left to right carotid bypass
2017, 2Q, 23	Thrombectomy via Fogarty catheter
2016, 4Q, 86-87	Coronary and peripheral artery bifurcation
2016, 2Q, 11	Carotid endarterectomy with patch angioplasty
2015, 1Q, 29	Discontinued carotid endarterectomy

AHA Coding Clinic for table Ø3H

2016, 2Q, 32	Arterial catheter placement

AHA Coding Clinic for table Ø3J

2015, 1Q, 29	Discontinued carotid endarterectomy

AHA Coding Clinic for table Ø3L

2016, 2Q, 30	Clipping (occlusion) of cerebral artery, decompressive craniectomy and storage of bone flap in abdominal wall
2014, 4Q, 20	Control of epistaxis
2014, 4Q, 37	Endovascular embolization of arteriovenous malformation using Onyx-18 liquid

AHA Coding Clinic for table Ø3Q

2017, 1Q, 31	Left to right common carotid artery bypass

AHA Coding Clinic for table Ø3S

2017, 2Q, 22	Carotid artery to subclavian artery transposition
2015, 3Q, 27	Moyamoya disease and hemispheric pial synagiosis with craniotomy

AHA Coding Clinic for table Ø3U

2019, 1Q, 22	Cerebral artery fusiform aneurysm repair via wrapping
2016, 2Q, 11	Carotid endarterectomy with patch angioplasty

AHA Coding Clinic for table Ø3V

2019, 1Q, 22	Cerebral artery fusiform aneurysm repair via wrapping
2016, 1Q, 19	Embolization of superior hypophyseal aneurysm using stent-assisted coil

AHA Coding Clinic for table Ø3W

2016, 3Q, 39	Revision of arteriovenous graft
2015, 1Q, 32	Deployment of stent for herniated/migrated coil in basilar artery

Upper Arteries

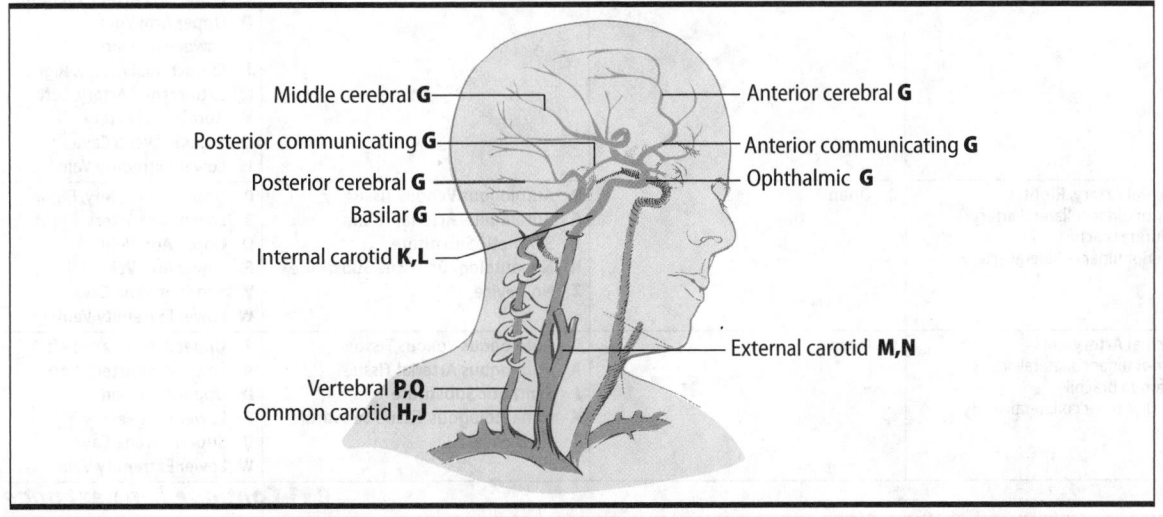

Middle temporal **S, T**
Transverse facial **S, T**
Superficial temporal **S, T**
Face **R**
External carotid **M, N**
Internal carotid **K, L**
Common carotid **H, J**
Superior thyroid **U, V**
Inferior thyroid **U, V**
Vertebral **P, Q**
Subclavian **3, 4**
Innominate **2**
Axillary **5, 6**
Internal thoracic (mammary) **Ø, 1**
Brachial **7, 8**
Radial **B, C**
Ulnar **9, A**
Deep palmar arch **D, F**
Superficial palmar arch **D, F**

Head and Neck Arteries

Middle cerebral **G**
Anterior cerebral **G**
Posterior communicating **G**
Anterior communicating **G**
Posterior cerebral **G**
Ophthalmic **G**
Basilar **G**
Internal carotid **K,L**
External carotid **M,N**
Vertebral **P,Q**
Common carotid **H,J**

Upper Arteries

Ø   **Medical and Surgical**
3   **Upper Arteries**
1   **Bypass**   Definition: Altering the route of passage of the contents of a tubular body part

Explanation: Rerouting contents of a body part to a downstream area of the normal route, to a similar route and body part, or to an abnormal route and dissimilar body part. Includes one or more anastomoses, with or without the use of a device.

Body Part Character 4	Approach Character 5	Device Character 6	Qualifier Character 7

2   **Innominate Artery**
     Brachiocephalic artery
     Brachiocephalic trunk
	Ø Open	9 Autologous Venous Tissue
		A Autologous Arterial Tissue
		J Synthetic Substitute
		K Nonautologous Tissue Substitute
		Z No Device
			Ø Upper Arm Artery, Right
			1 Upper Arm Artery, Left
			2 Upper Arm Artery, Bilateral
			3 Lower Arm Artery, Right
			4 Lower Arm Artery, Left
			5 Lower Arm Artery, Bilateral
			6 Upper Leg Artery, Right
			7 Upper Leg Artery, Left
			8 Upper Leg Artery, Bilateral
			9 Lower Leg Artery, Right
			B Lower Leg Artery, Left
			C Lower Leg Artery, Bilateral
			D Upper Arm Vein
			F Lower Arm Vein
			J Extracranial Artery, Right
			K Extracranial Artery, Left
			W Lower Extremity Vein

3   **Subclavian Artery, Right**
     Costocervical trunk
     Dorsal scapular artery
     Internal thoracic artery
4   **Subclavian Artery, Left**
     See 3 Subclavian Artery, Right
	Ø Open	9 Autologous Venous Tissue
		A Autologous Arterial Tissue
		J Synthetic Substitute
		K Nonautologous Tissue Substitute
		Z No Device
			Ø Upper Arm Artery, Right
			1 Upper Arm Artery, Left
			2 Upper Arm Artery, Bilateral
			3 Lower Arm Artery, Right
			4 Lower Arm Artery, Left
			5 Lower Arm Artery, Bilateral
			6 Upper Leg Artery, Right
			7 Upper Leg Artery, Left
			8 Upper Leg Artery, Bilateral
			9 Lower Leg Artery, Right
			B Lower Leg Artery, Left
			C Lower Leg Artery, Bilateral
			D Upper Arm Vein
			F Lower Arm Vein
			J Extracranial Artery, Right
			K Extracranial Artery, Left
			M Pulmonary Artery, Right
			N Pulmonary Artery, Left
			W Lower Extremity Vein

5   **Axillary Artery, Right**
     Anterior circumflex humeral artery
     Lateral thoracic artery
     Posterior circumflex humeral artery
     Subscapular artery
     Superior thoracic artery
     Thoracoacromial artery
6   **Axillary Artery, Left**
     See 5 Axillary Artery, Right
	Ø Open	9 Autologous Venous Tissue
		A Autologous Arterial Tissue
		J Synthetic Substitute
		K Nonautologous Tissue Substitute
		Z No Device
			Ø Upper Arm Artery, Right
			1 Upper Arm Artery, Left
			2 Upper Arm Artery, Bilateral
			3 Lower Arm Artery, Right
			4 Lower Arm Artery, Left
			5 Lower Arm Artery, Bilateral
			6 Upper Leg Artery, Right
			7 Upper Leg Artery, Left
			8 Upper Leg Artery, Bilateral
			9 Lower Leg Artery, Right
			B Lower Leg Artery, Left
			C Lower Leg Artery, Bilateral
			D Upper Arm Vein
			F Lower Arm Vein
			J Extracranial Artery, Right
			K Extracranial Artery, Left
			T Abdominal Artery
			V Superior Vena Cava
			W Lower Extremity Vein

7   **Brachial Artery, Right**
     Inferior ulnar collateral artery
     Profunda brachii
     Superior ulnar collateral artery
	Ø Open	9 Autologous Venous Tissue
		A Autologous Arterial Tissue
		J Synthetic Substitute
		K Nonautologous Tissue Substitute
		Z No Device
			Ø Upper Arm Artery, Right
			3 Lower Arm Artery, Right
			D Upper Arm Vein
			F Lower Arm Vein
			V Superior Vena Cava
			W Lower Extremity Vein

8   **Brachial Artery, Left**
     Inferior ulnar collateral artery
     Profunda brachii
     Superior ulnar collateral artery
	Ø Open	9 Autologous Venous Tissue
		A Autologous Arterial Tissue
		J Synthetic Substitute
		K Nonautologous Tissue Substitute
		Z No Device
			1 Upper Arm Artery, Left
			4 Lower Arm Artery, Left
			D Upper Arm Vein
			F Lower Arm Vein
			V Superior Vena Cava
			W Lower Extremity Vein

Ø31 Continued on next page

LC Limited Coverage   NC Noncovered   ⊞ Combination Member   HAC associated procedure   Combination Only   DRG Non-OR   Non-OR   New/Revised in GREEN

192   ICD-10-PCS 2020

Ø Medical and Surgical   *Ø31 Continued*
3 Upper Arteries
1 Bypass   Definition: Altering the route of passage of the contents of a tubular body part

Explanation: Rerouting contents of a body part to a downstream area of the normal route, to a similar route and body part, or to an abnormal route and dissimilar body part. Includes one or more anastomoses, with or without the use of a device.

Body Part Character 4	Approach Character 5	Device Character 6	Qualifier Character 7
9 Ulnar Artery, Right Anterior ulnar recurrent artery Common interosseous artery Posterior ulnar recurrent artery **B Radial Artery, Right** Radial recurrent artery	Ø Open	9 Autologous Venous Tissue A Autologous Arterial Tissue J Synthetic Substitute K Nonautologous Tissue Substitute Z No Device	3 Lower Arm Artery, Right F Lower Arm Vein
9 Ulnar Artery, Right Anterior ulnar recurrent artery Common interosseous artery Posterior ulnar recurrent artery **B Radial Artery, Right** Radial recurrent artery	3 Percutaneous	Z No Device	F Lower Arm Vein
A Ulnar Artery, Left Anterior ulnar recurrent artery Common interosseous artery Posterior ulnar recurrent artery **C Radial Artery, Left** Radial recurrent artery	Ø Open	9 Autologous Venous Tissue A Autologous Arterial Tissue J Synthetic Substitute K Nonautologous Tissue Substitute Z No Device	4 Lower Arm Artery, Left F Lower Arm Vein
A Ulnar Artery, Left Anterior ulnar recurrent artery Common interosseous artery Posterior ulnar recurrent artery **C Radial Artery, Left** Radial recurrent artery	3 Percutaneous	Z No Device	F Lower Arm Vein
G Intracranial Artery Anterior cerebral artery Anterior choroidal artery Anterior communicating artery Basilar artery Circle of Willis Internal carotid artery, intracranial portion Middle cerebral artery Ophthalmic artery Posterior cerebral artery Posterior communicating artery Posterior inferior cerebellar artery (PICA) **S Temporal Artery, Right** Middle temporal artery Superficial temporal artery Transverse facial artery **T Temporal Artery, Left** *See S Temporal Artery, Right*	Ø Open	9 Autologous Venous Tissue A Autologous Arterial Tissue J Synthetic Substitute K Nonautologous Tissue Substitute Z No Device	G Intracranial Artery
H Common Carotid Artery, Right **J Common Carotid Artery, Left**	Ø Open	9 Autologous Venous Tissue A Autologous Arterial Tissue J Synthetic Substitute K Nonautologous Tissue Substitute Z No Device	G Intracranial Artery J Extracranial Artery, Right K Extracranial Artery, Left Y Upper Artery
K Internal Carotid Artery, Right Caroticotympanic artery Carotid sinus **L Internal Carotid Artery, Left** Caroticotympanic artery Carotid sinus **M External Carotid Artery, Right** Ascending pharyngeal artery Internal maxillary artery Lingual artery Maxillary artery Occipital artery Posterior auricular artery Superior thyroid artery **N External Carotid Artery, Left** Ascending pharyngeal artery Internal maxillary artery Lingual artery Maxillary artery Occipital artery Posterior auricular artery Superior thyroid artery	Ø Open	9 Autologous Venous Tissue A Autologous Arterial Tissue J Synthetic Substitute K Nonautologous Tissue Substitute Z No Device	J Extracranial Artery, Right K Extracranial Artery, Left

LC Limited Coverage   NC Noncovered   ⊞ Combination Member   HAC associated procedure   Combination Only   DRG Non-OR   Non-OR   New/Revised in GREEN

Upper Arteries (side tab)

Ø   **Medical and Surgical**
3   **Upper Arteries**
5   **Destruction**   Definition: Physical eradication of all or a portion of a body part by the direct use of energy, force, or a destructive agent
                    Explanation: None of the body part is physically taken out

Body Part Character 4	Approach Character 5	Device Character 6	Qualifier Character 7
Ø Internal Mammary Artery, Right Anterior intercostal artery Internal thoracic artery Musculophrenic artery Pericardiophrenic artery Superior epigastric artery **1 Internal Mammary Artery, Left** *See Ø Internal Mammary Artery, Right* **2 Innominate Artery** Brachiocephalic artery Brachiocephalic trunk **3 Subclavian Artery, Right** Costocervical trunk Dorsal scapular artery Internal thoracic artery **4 Subclavian Artery, Left** *See 3 Subclavian Artery, Right* **5 Axillary Artery, Right** Anterior circumflex humeral artery Lateral thoracic artery Posterior circumflex humeral artery Subscapular artery Superior thoracic artery Thoracoacromial artery **6 Axillary Artery, Left** *See 5 Axillary Artery, Right* **7 Brachial Artery, Right** Inferior ulnar collateral artery Profunda brachii Superior ulnar collateral artery **8 Brachial Artery, Left** *See 7 Brachial Artery, Right* **9 Ulnar Artery, Right** Anterior ulnar recurrent artery Common interosseous artery Posterior ulnar recurrent artery **A Ulnar Artery, Left** *See 9 Ulnar Artery, Right* **B Radial Artery, Right** Radial recurrent artery **C Radial Artery, Left** *See B Radial Artery, Right* **D Hand Artery, Right** Deep palmar arch Princeps pollicis artery Radialis indicis Superficial palmar arch **F Hand Artery, Left** *See D Hand Artery, Right* **G Intracranial Artery** Anterior cerebral artery Anterior choroidal artery Anterior communicating artery Basilar artery Circle of Willis Internal carotid artery, intracranial portion Middle cerebral artery Ophthalmic artery Posterior cerebral artery Posterior communicating artery Posterior inferior cerebellar artery (PICA)	**H Common Carotid Artery, Right** **J Common Carotid Artery, Left** **K Internal Carotid Artery, Right** Caroticotympanic artery Carotid sinus **L Internal Carotid Artery, Left** *See K Internal Carotid Artery, Right* **M External Carotid Artery, Right** Ascending pharyngeal artery Internal maxillary artery Lingual artery Maxillary artery Occipital artery Posterior auricular artery Superior thyroid artery **N External Carotid Artery, Left** *See M External Carotid Artery, Right* **P Vertebral Artery, Right** Anterior spinal artery Posterior spinal artery **Q Vertebral Artery, Left** *See P Vertebral Artery, Right* **R Face Artery** Angular artery Ascending palatine artery External maxillary artery Facial artery Inferior labial artery Submental artery Superior labial artery **S Temporal Artery, Right** Middle temporal artery Superficial temporal artery Transverse facial artery **T Temporal Artery, Left** *See S Temporal Artery, Right* **U Thyroid Artery, Right** Cricothyroid artery Hyoid artery Sternocleidomastoid artery Superior laryngeal artery Superior thyroid artery Thyrocervical trunk **V Thyroid Artery, Left** *See U Thyroid Artery, Right* **Y Upper Artery** Aortic intercostal artery Bronchial artery Esophageal artery Subcostal artery	**Ø Open** **3 Percutaneous** **4 Percutaneous Endoscopic**	**Z No Device**	**Z No Qualifier**

Ø   Medical and Surgical
3   Upper Arteries
7   Dilation   Definition: Expanding an orifice or the lumen of a tubular body part

Explanation: The orifice can be a natural orifice or an artificially created orifice. Accomplished by stretching a tubular body part using intraluminal pressure or by cutting part of the orifice or wall of the tubular body part.

Body Part Character 4		Approach Character 5	Device Character 6	Qualifier Character 7
Ø Internal Mammary Artery, Right Anterior intercostal artery Internal thoracic artery Musculophrenic artery Pericardiophrenic artery Superior epigastric artery **1 Internal Mammary Artery, Left** *See Ø Internal Mammary Artery, Right* **2 Innominate Artery** Brachiocephalic artery Brachiocephalic trunk **3 Subclavian Artery, Right** Costocervical trunk Dorsal scapular artery Internal thoracic artery **4 Subclavian Artery, Left** *See 3 Subclavian Artery, Right* **5 Axillary Artery, Right** Anterior circumflex humeral artery Lateral thoracic artery Posterior circumflex humeral artery Subscapular artery Superior thoracic artery Thoracoacromial artery	**6 Axillary Artery, Left** *See 5 Axillary Artery, Right* **7 Brachial Artery, Right** Inferior ulnar collateral artery Profunda brachii Superior ulnar collateral artery **8 Brachial Artery, Left** *See 7 Brachial Artery, Right* **9 Ulnar Artery, Right** Anterior ulnar recurrent artery Common interosseous artery Posterior ulnar recurrent artery **A Ulnar Artery, Left** *See 9 Ulnar Artery, Right* **B Radial Artery, Right** Radial recurrent artery **C Radial Artery, Left** *See B Radial Artery, Right*	**Ø Open** **3 Percutaneous** **4 Percutaneous Endoscopic**	**4 Intraluminal Device, Drug-eluting** **5 Intraluminal Device, Drug-eluting, Two** **6 Intraluminal Device, Drug-eluting, Three** **7 Intraluminal Device, Drug-eluting, Four or More** **E Intraluminal Device, Two** **F Intraluminal Device, Three** **G Intraluminal Device, Four or More**	**Z No Qualifier**
Ø Internal Mammary Artery, Right Anterior intercostal artery Internal thoracic artery Musculophrenic artery Pericardiophrenic artery Superior epigastric artery **1 Internal Mammary Artery, Left** *See Ø Internal Mammary Artery, Right* **2 Innominate Artery** Brachiocephalic artery Brachiocephalic trunk **3 Subclavian Artery, Right** Costocervical trunk Dorsal scapular artery Internal thoracic artery **4 Subclavian Artery, Left** *See 3 Subclavian Artery, Right* **5 Axillary Artery, Right** Anterior circumflex humeral artery Lateral thoracic artery Posterior circumflex humeral artery Subscapular artery Superior thoracic artery Thoracoacromial artery	**6 Axillary Artery, Left** *See 5 Axillary Artery, Right* **7 Brachial Artery, Right** Inferior ulnar collateral artery Profunda brachii Superior ulnar collateral artery **8 Brachial Artery, Left** *See 7 Brachial Artery, Right* **9 Ulnar Artery, Right** Anterior ulnar recurrent artery Common interosseous artery Posterior ulnar recurrent artery **A Ulnar Artery, Left** *See 9 Ulnar Artery, Right* **B Radial Artery, Right** Radial recurrent artery **C Radial Artery, Left** *See B Radial Artery, Right*	**Ø Open** **3 Percutaneous** **4 Percutaneous Endoscopic**	**D Intraluminal Device** **Z No Device**	**1 Drug-Coated Balloon** **Z No Qualifier**

Ø37 Continued on next page

LC Limited Coverage   **NC** Noncovered   ⊞ Combination Member   HAC associated procedure   Combination Only   DRG Non-OR   Non-OR   New/Revised in **GREEN**

ICD-10-PCS 2020   **195**

Ø37–Ø37

0   Medical and Surgical   *037 Continued*
3   Upper Arteries
7   Dilation   Definition: Expanding an orifice or the lumen of a tubular body part

Explanation: The orifice can be a natural orifice or an artificially created orifice. Accomplished by stretching a tubular body part using intraluminal pressure or by cutting part of the orifice or wall of the tubular body part.

Body Part Character 4		Approach Character 5	Device Character 6	Qualifier Character 7

D Hand Artery, Right
Deep palmar arch
Princeps pollicis artery
Radialis indicis
Superficial palmar arch
F Hand Artery, Left
See D Hand Artery, Right
G Intracranial Artery [NC]
Anterior cerebral artery
Anterior choroidal artery
Anterior communicating artery
Basilar artery
Circle of Willis
Internal carotid artery,
   intracranial portion
Middle cerebral artery
Ophthalmic artery
Posterior cerebral artery
Posterior communicating
   artery
Posterior inferior cerebellar
   artery (PICA)
**H Common Carotid Artery,
   Right**
J Common Carotid Artery, Left
K Internal Carotid Artery, Right
Caroticotympanic artery
Carotid sinus
L Internal Carotid Artery, Left
*See K Internal Carotid Artery,
   Right*
M External Carotid Artery, Right
Ascending pharyngeal artery
Internal maxillary artery
Lingual artery
Maxillary artery
Occipital artery
Posterior auricular artery
Superior thyroid artery
	N External Carotid Artery, Left
	*See M External Carotid Artery,
	   Right*
	P Vertebral Artery, Right
	Anterior spinal artery
	Posterior spinal artery
	Q Vertebral Artery, Left
	See P Vertebral Artery, Right
	R Face Artery
	Angular artery
	Ascending palatine artery
	External maxillary artery
	Facial artery
	Inferior labial artery
	Submental artery
	Superior labial artery
	S Temporal Artery, Right
	Middle temporal artery
	Superficial temporal artery
	Transverse facial artery
	T Temporal Artery, Left
	See S Temporal Artery, Right
	U Thyroid Artery, Right
	Cricothyroid artery
	Hyoid artery
	Sternocleidomastoid artery
	Superior laryngeal artery
	Superior thyroid artery
	Thyrocervical trunk
	V Thyroid Artery, Left
	See U Thyroid Artery, Right
	Y Upper Artery
	Aortic intercostal artery
	Bronchial artery
	Esophageal artery
	Subcostal artery
		0 Open
		3 Percutaneous
		4 Percutaneous Endoscopic
			**4 Intraluminal Device,
			   Drug-eluting**
			**5 Intraluminal Device, Drug-
			   eluting, Two**
			**6 Intraluminal Device, Drug-
			   eluting, Three**
			**7 Intraluminal Device, Drug-
			   eluting, Four or More**
			D Intraluminal Device
			E Intraluminal Device, Two
			F Intraluminal Device, Three
			**G Intraluminal Device, Four
			   or More**
			Z No Device
				Z No Qualifier

[NC]   037G[3,4]ZZ

[LC] Limited Coverage [NC] Noncovered ⊞ Combination Member HAC associated procedure Combination Only DRG Non-OR Non-OR New/Revised in GREEN

196   ICD-10-PCS 2020

Ø   **Medical and Surgical**
3   **Upper Arteries**
9   **Drainage**   Definition: Taking or letting out fluids and/or gases from a body part
                    Explanation: The qualifier DIAGNOSTIC is used to identify drainage procedures that are biopsies

Body Part Character 4		Approach Character 5	Device Character 6	Qualifier Character 7
Ø Internal Mammary Artery, Right Anterior intercostal artery Internal thoracic artery Musculophrenic artery Pericardiophrenic artery Superior epigastric artery **1 Internal Mammary Artery, Left** *See Ø Internal Mammary Artery, Right above* **2 Innominate Artery** Brachiocephalic artery Brachiocephalic trunk **3 Subclavian Artery, Right** Costocervical trunk Dorsal scapular artery Internal thoracic artery **4 Subclavian Artery, Left** *See 3 Subclavian Artery, Right* **5 Axillary Artery, Right** Anterior circumflex humeral artery Lateral thoracic artery Posterior circumflex humeral artery Subscapular artery Superior thoracic artery Thoracoacromial artery **6 Axillary Artery, Left** *See 5 Axillary Artery, Right* **7 Brachial Artery, Right** Inferior ulnar collateral artery Profunda brachii Superior ulnar collateral artery **8 Brachial Artery, Left** *See 7 Brachial Artery, Right* **9 Ulnar Artery, Right** Anterior ulnar recurrent artery Common interosseous artery Posterior ulnar recurrent artery **A Ulnar Artery, Left** *See 9 Ulnar Artery, Right* **B Radial Artery, Right** Radial recurrent artery **C Radial Artery, Left** *See B Radial Artery, Right* **D Hand Artery, Right** Deep palmar arch Princeps pollicis artery Radialis indicis Superficial palmar arch **F Hand Artery, Left** *See D Hand Artery, Right* **G Intracranial Artery** Anterior cerebral artery Anterior choroidal artery Anterior communicating artery Basilar artery Circle of Willis Internal carotid artery, intracranial portion Middle cerebral artery Ophthalmic artery Posterior cerebral artery Posterior communicating artery Posterior inferior cerebellar artery (PICA)	**H Common Carotid Artery, Right** **J Common Carotid Artery, Left** **K Internal Carotid Artery, Right** Caroticotympanic artery Carotid sinus **L Internal Carotid Artery, Left** *See K Internal Carotid Artery, Right* **M External Carotid Artery, Right** Ascending pharyngeal artery Internal maxillary artery Lingual artery Maxillary artery Occipital artery Posterior auricular artery Superior thyroid artery **N External Carotid Artery, Left** *See M External Carotid Artery, Right* **P Vertebral Artery, Right** Anterior spinal artery Posterior spinal artery **Q Vertebral Artery, Left** *See P Vertebral Artery, Right* **R Face Artery** Angular artery Ascending palatine artery External maxillary artery Facial artery Inferior labial artery Submental artery Superior labial artery **S Temporal Artery, Right** Middle temporal artery Superficial temporal artery Transverse facial artery **T Temporal Artery, Left** *See S Temporal Artery, Right* **U Thyroid Artery, Right** Cricothyroid artery Hyoid artery Sternocleidomastoid artery Superior laryngeal artery Superior thyroid artery Thyrocervical trunk **V Thyroid Artery, Left** *See U Thyroid Artery, Right* **Y Upper Artery** Aortic intercostal artery Bronchial artery Esophageal artery Subcostal artery	**Ø Open** **3 Percutaneous** **4 Percutaneous Endoscopic**	**Ø Drainage Device**	**Z No Qualifier**

039 Continued on next page

Non-OR   Ø39[Ø,1,2,3,4,5,6,7,8,9,A,B,C,D,F,G,H,J,K,L,M,N,P,Q,R,S,T,U,V,Y][Ø,3,4]ØZ

LC Limited Coverage   NC Noncovered   ⊞ Combination Member   HAC associated procedure   Combination Only   DRG Non-OR   Non-OR   New/Revised in GREEN

0	**Medical and Surgical**			*Ø39 Continued*
3	**Upper Arteries**			
9	**Drainage**	Definition: Taking or letting out fluids and/or gases from a body part		

Explanation: The qualifier DIAGNOSTIC is used to identify drainage procedures that are biopsies

Body Part Character 4		Approach Character 5	Device Character 6	Qualifier Character 7
0 Internal Mammary Artery, Right Anterior intercostal artery Internal thoracic artery Musculophrenic artery Pericardiophrenic artery Superior epigastric artery **1 Internal Mammary Artery, Left** *See Ø Internal Mammary Artery, Right* **2 Innominate Artery** Brachiocephalic artery Brachiocephalic trunk **3 Subclavian Artery, Right** Costocervical trunk Dorsal scapular artery Internal thoracic artery **4 Subclavian Artery, Left** *See 3 Subclavian Artery, Right* **5 Axillary Artery, Right** Anterior circumflex humeral artery Lateral thoracic artery Posterior circumflex humeral artery Subscapular artery Superior thoracic artery Thoracoacromial artery **6 Axillary Artery, Left** *See 5 Axillary Artery, Right* **7 Brachial Artery, Right** Inferior ulnar collateral artery Profunda brachii Superior ulnar collateral artery **8 Brachial Artery, Left** *See 7 Brachial Artery, Right* **9 Ulnar Artery, Right** Anterior ulnar recurrent artery Common interosseous artery Posterior ulnar recurrent artery **A Ulnar Artery, Left** *See 9 Ulnar Artery, Right* **B Radial Artery, Right** Radial recurrent artery **C Radial Artery, Left** *See B Radial Artery, Right* **D Hand Artery, Right** Deep palmar arch Princeps pollicis artery Radialis indicis Superficial palmar arch **F Hand Artery, Left** *See D Hand Artery, Right* **G Intracranial Artery** Anterior cerebral artery Anterior choroidal artery Anterior communicating artery Basilar artery Circle of Willis Internal carotid artery, intracranial portion Middle cerebral artery Ophthalmic artery Posterior cerebral artery Posterior communicating artery Posterior inferior cerebellar artery (PICA)	**H Common Carotid Artery, Right** **J Common Carotid Artery, Left** **K Internal Carotid Artery, Right** Caroticotympanic artery Carotid sinus **L Internal Carotid Artery, Left** *See K Internal Carotid Artery, Right* **M External Carotid Artery, Right** Ascending pharyngeal artery Internal maxillary artery Lingual artery Maxillary artery Occipital artery Posterior auricular artery Superior thyroid artery **N External Carotid Artery, Left** *See M External Carotid Artery, Right* **P Vertebral Artery, Right** Anterior spinal artery Posterior spinal artery **Q Vertebral Artery, Left** *See P Vertebral Artery, Right* **R Face Artery** Angular artery Ascending palatine artery External maxillary artery Facial artery Inferior labial artery Submental artery Superior labial artery **S Temporal Artery, Right** Middle temporal artery Superficial temporal artery Transverse facial artery **T Temporal Artery, Left** *See S Temporal Artery, Right* **U Thyroid Artery, Right** Cricothyroid artery Hyoid artery Sternocleidomastoid artery Superior laryngeal artery Superior thyroid artery Thyrocervical trunk **V Thyroid Artery, Left** *See U Thyroid Artery, Right* **Y Upper Artery** Aortic intercostal artery Bronchial artery Esophageal artery Subcostal artery	**0 Open** **3 Percutaneous** **4 Percutaneous Endoscopic**	**Z No Device**	**X Diagnostic** **Z No Qualifier**

Non-OR Ø39[Ø,1,2,3,4,5,6,7,8,9,A,B,C,D,F,G,H,J,K,L,M,N,P,Q,R,S,T,U,V,Y]3ZX
Non-OR Ø39[Ø,1,2,3,4,5,6,7,8,9,A,B,C,D,F,G,H,J,K,L,M,N,P,Q,R,S,T,U,V,Y][Ø,3,4]ZZ

Ø   Medical and Surgical
3   Upper Arteries
B   Excision   Definition: Cutting out or off, without replacement, a portion of a body part
               Explanation: The qualifier DIAGNOSTIC is used to identify excision procedures that are biopsies

Body Part Character 4		Approach Character 5	Device Character 6	Qualifier Character 7
Ø Internal Mammary Artery, Right Anterior intercostal artery Internal thoracic artery Musculophrenic artery Pericardiophrenic artery Superior epigastric artery **1 Internal Mammary Artery, Left** *See Ø Internal Mammary Artery, Right* **2 Innominate Artery** Brachiocephalic artery Brachiocephalic trunk **3 Subclavian Artery, Right** Costocervical trunk Dorsal scapular artery Internal thoracic artery **4 Subclavian Artery, Left** *See 3 Subclavian Artery, Right* **5 Axillary Artery, Right** Anterior circumflex humeral artery Lateral thoracic artery Posterior circumflex humeral artery Subscapular artery Superior thoracic artery Thoracoacromial artery **6 Axillary Artery, Left** *See 5 Axillary Artery, Right* **7 Brachial Artery, Right** Inferior ulnar collateral artery Profunda brachii Superior ulnar collateral artery **8 Brachial Artery, Left** *See 7 Brachial Artery, Right* **9 Ulnar Artery, Right** Anterior ulnar recurrent artery Common interosseous artery Posterior ulnar recurrent artery **A Ulnar Artery, Left** *See 9 Ulnar Artery, Right* **B Radial Artery, Right** Radial recurrent artery **C Radial Artery, Left** *See B Radial Artery, Right* **D Hand Artery, Right** Deep palmar arch Princeps pollicis artery Radialis indicis Superficial palmar arch **F Hand Artery, Left** *See D Hand Artery, Right* **G Intracranial Artery** Anterior cerebral artery Anterior choroidal artery Anterior communicating artery Basilar artery Circle of Willis Internal carotid artery, intracranial portion Middle cerebral artery Ophthalmic artery Posterior cerebral artery Posterior communicating artery Posterior inferior cerebellar artery (PICA)	**H Common Carotid Artery, Right** **J Common Carotid Artery, Left** **K Internal Carotid Artery, Right** Caroticotympanic artery Carotid sinus **L Internal Carotid Artery, Left** *See K Internal Carotid Artery, Right* **M External Carotid Artery, Right** Ascending pharyngeal artery Internal maxillary artery Lingual artery Maxillary artery Occipital artery Posterior auricular artery Superior thyroid artery **N External Carotid Artery, Left** *See M External Carotid Artery, Right* **P Vertebral Artery, Right** Anterior spinal artery Posterior spinal artery **Q Vertebral Artery, Left** *See P Vertebral Artery, Right* **R Face Artery** Angular artery Ascending palatine artery External maxillary artery Facial artery Inferior labial artery Submental artery Superior labial artery **S Temporal Artery, Right** Middle temporal artery Superficial temporal artery Transverse facial artery **T Temporal Artery, Left** *See S Temporal Artery, Right* **U Thyroid Artery, Right** Cricothyroid artery Hyoid artery Sternocleidomastoid artery Superior laryngeal artery Superior thyroid artery Thyrocervical trunk **V Thyroid Artery, Left** *See U Thyroid Artery, Right* **Y Upper Artery** Aortic intercostal artery Bronchial artery Esophageal artery Subcostal artery	**Ø Open** **3 Percutaneous** **4 Percutaneous Endoscopic**	**Z No Device**	**X Diagnostic** **Z No Qualifier**

0   **Medical and Surgical**
3   **Upper Arteries**
C   **Extirpation**   Definition: Taking or cutting out solid matter from a body part

Explanation: The solid matter may be an abnormal byproduct of a biological function or a foreign body; it may be imbedded in a body part or in the lumen of a tubular body part. The solid matter may or may not have been previously broken into pieces.

Body Part Character 4		Approach Character 5	Device Character 6	Qualifier Character 7
0 **Internal Mammary Artery, Right** Anterior intercostal artery Internal thoracic artery Musculophrenic artery Pericardiophrenic artery Superior epigastric artery **1** **Internal Mammary Artery, Left** *See 0 Internal Mammary Artery, Right* **2** **Innominate Artery** Brachiocephalic artery Brachiocephalic trunk **3** **Subclavian Artery, Right** Costocervical trunk Dorsal scapular artery Internal thoracic artery **4** **Subclavian Artery, Left** *See 3 Subclavian Artery, Right* **5** **Axillary Artery, Right** Anterior circumflex humeral artery Lateral thoracic artery Posterior circumflex humeral artery Subscapular artery Superior thoracic artery Thoracoacromial artery **6** **Axillary Artery, Left** *See 5 Axillary Artery, Right* **7** **Brachial Artery, Right** Inferior ulnar collateral artery Profunda brachii Superior ulnar collateral artery **8** **Brachial Artery, Left** *See 7 Brachial Artery, Right* **9** **Ulnar Artery, Right** Anterior ulnar recurrent artery Common interosseous artery Posterior ulnar recurrent artery	**A** **Ulnar Artery, Left** *See 9 Ulnar Artery, Right* **B** **Radial Artery, Right** Radial recurrent artery **C** **Radial Artery, Left** *See B Radial Artery, Right* **D** **Hand Artery, Right** Deep palmar arch Princeps pollicis artery Radialis indicis Superficial palmar arch **F** **Hand Artery, Left** *See D Hand Artery, Right* **R** **Face Artery** Angular artery Ascending palatine artery External maxillary artery Facial artery Inferior labial artery Submental artery Superior labial artery **S** **Temporal Artery, Right** Middle temporal artery Superficial temporal artery Transverse facial artery **T** **Temporal Artery, Left** *See S Temporal Artery, Right* **U** **Thyroid Artery, Right** Cricothyroid artery Hyoid artery Sternocleidomastoid artery Superior laryngeal artery Superior thyroid artery Thyrocervical trunk **V** **Thyroid Artery, Left** *See U Thyroid Artery, Right* **Y** **Upper Artery** Aortic intercostal artery Bronchial artery Esophageal artery Subcostal artery	**0** Open **3** Percutaneous **4** Percutaneous Endoscopic	**Z** No Device	**Z** No Qualifier
G **Intracranial Artery** Anterior cerebral artery Anterior choroidal artery Anterior communicating artery Basilar artery Circle of Willis Internal carotid artery, intracranial portion Middle cerebral artery Ophthalmic artery Posterior cerebral artery Posterior communicating artery Posterior inferior cerebellar artery (PICA) **H** **Common Carotid Artery, Right** **J** **Common Carotid Artery, Left** **K** **Internal Carotid Artery, Right** Caroticotympanic artery Carotid sinus	**L** **Internal Carotid Artery, Left** *See K Internal Carotid Artery, Right* **M** **External Carotid Artery, Right** Ascending pharyngeal artery Internal maxillary artery Lingual artery Maxillary artery Occipital artery Posterior auricular artery Superior thyroid artery **N** **External Carotid Artery, Left** *See M External Carotid Artery, Right* **P** **Vertebral Artery, Right** Anterior spinal artery Posterior spinal artery **Q** **Vertebral Artery, Left** *See P Vertebral Artery, Right*	**0** Open **4** Percutaneous Endoscopic	**Z** No Device	**Z** No Qualifier

03C Continued on next page

LC Limited Coverage   **NC** Noncovered   ⊞ Combination Member   HAC associated procedure   Combination Only   DRG Non-OR   Non-OR   New/Revised in GREEN

200   ICD-10-PCS 2020

Ø   Medical and Surgical
3   Upper Arteries
C   Extirpation

03C Continued

Definition: Taking or cutting out solid matter from a body part

Explanation: The solid matter may be an abnormal byproduct of a biological function or a foreign body; it may be imbedded in a body part or in the lumen of a tubular body part. The solid matter may or may not have been previously broken into pieces.

Body Part Character 4		Approach Character 5	Device Character 6	Qualifier Character 7

G Intracranial Artery
Anterior cerebral artery
Anterior choroidal artery
Anterior communicating
   artery
Basilar artery
Circle of Willis
Internal carotid artery,
   intracranial portion
Middle cerebral artery
Ophthalmic artery
Posterior cerebral artery
Posterior communicating
   artery
Posterior inferior cerebellar
   artery (PICA)
**H Common Carotid Artery,
Right**
J Common Carotid Artery, Left
K Internal Carotid Artery, Right
Caroticotympanic artery
Carotid sinus
	L Internal Carotid Artery, Left
	*See K Internal Carotid Artery,
	Right*
	M External Carotid Artery, Right
	Ascending pharyngeal artery
	Internal maxillary artery
	Lingual artery
	Maxillary artery
	Occipital artery
	Posterior auricular artery
	Superior thyroid artery
	N External Carotid Artery, Left
	*See M External Carotid Artery,
	Right*
	P Vertebral Artery, Right
	Anterior spinal artery
	Posterior spinal artery
	Q Vertebral Artery, Left
	See P Vertebral Artery, Right
		3 Percutaneous	**Z No Device**	**7 Stent Retriever**
				Z No Qualifier

LC Limited Coverage   **NC** Noncovered   ⊞ Combination Member   HAC associated procedure   Combination Only   DRG Non-OR   Non-OR   New/Revised in GREEN

ICD-10-PCS 2020   **201**

Ø   Medical and Surgical
3   Upper Arteries
H   Insertion

Definition: Putting in a nonbiological appliance that monitors, assists, performs, or prevents a physiological function but does not physically take the place of a body part

Explanation: None

Body Part — Character 4		Approach — Character 5	Device — Character 6	Qualifier — Character 7
Ø Internal Mammary Artery, Right Anterior intercostal artery Internal thoracic artery Musculophrenic artery Pericardiophrenic artery Superior epigastric artery **1 Internal Mammary Artery, Left** *See Ø Internal Mammary Artery, Right* **2 Innominate Artery** Brachiocephalic artery Brachiocephalic trunk **3 Subclavian Artery, Right** Costocervical trunk Dorsal scapular artery Internal thoracic artery **4 Subclavian Artery, Left** *See 3 Subclavian Artery, Right* **5 Axillary Artery, Right** Anterior circumflex humeral artery Lateral thoracic artery Posterior circumflex humeral artery Subscapular artery Superior thoracic artery Thoracoacromial artery **6 Axillary Artery, Left** *See 5 Axillary Artery, Right* **7 Brachial Artery, Right** Inferior ulnar collateral artery Profunda brachii Superior ulnar collateral artery **8 Brachial Artery, Left** *See 7 Brachial Artery, Right* **9 Ulnar Artery, Right** Anterior ulnar recurrent artery Common interosseous artery Posterior ulnar recurrent artery **A Ulnar Artery, Left** *See 9 Ulnar Artery, Right* **B Radial Artery, Right** Radial recurrent artery **C Radial Artery, Left** *See B Radial Artery, Right* **D Hand Artery, Right** Deep palmar arch Princeps pollicis artery Radialis indicis Superficial palmar arch **F Hand Artery, Left** *See D Hand Artery, Right*	**G Intracranial Artery** Anterior cerebral artery Anterior choroidal artery Anterior communicating artery Basilar artery Circle of Willis Internal carotid artery, intracranial portion Middle cerebral artery Ophthalmic artery Posterior cerebral artery Posterior communicating artery Posterior inferior cerebellar artery (PICA) **H Common Carotid Artery, Right** **J Common Carotid Artery, Left** **M External Carotid Artery, Right** Ascending pharyngeal artery Internal maxillary artery Lingual artery Maxillary artery Occipital artery Posterior auricular artery Superior thyroid artery **N External Carotid Artery, Left** *See M External Carotid Artery, Right* **P Vertebral Artery, Right** Anterior spinal artery Posterior spinal artery **Q Vertebral Artery, Left** *See P Vertebral Artery, Right* **R Face Artery** Angular artery Ascending palatine artery External maxillary artery Facial artery Inferior labial artery Submental artery Superior labial artery **S Temporal Artery, Right** Middle temporal artery Superficial temporal artery Transverse facial artery **T Temporal Artery, Left** *See S Temporal Artery, Right* **U Thyroid Artery, Right** Cricothyroid artery Hyoid artery Sternocleidomastoid artery Superior laryngeal artery Superior thyroid artery Thyrocervical trunk **V Thyroid Artery, Left** *See U Thyroid Artery, Right*	**Ø Open** **3 Percutaneous** **4 Percutaneous Endoscopic**	**3 Infusion Device** **D Intraluminal Device**	**Z No Qualifier**
K Internal Carotid Artery, Right Caroticotympanic artery Carotid sinus **L Internal Carotid Artery, Left** *See K Internal Carotid Artery, Right*		**Ø Open** **3 Percutaneous** **4 Percutaneous Endoscope**	**3 Infusion Device** **D Intraluminal Device** **M Stimulator Lead**	**Z No Qualifier**
Y Upper Artery Aortic intercostal artery Bronchial artery Esophageal artery Subcostal artery		**Ø Open** **3 Percutaneous** **4 Percutaneous Endoscopic**	**2 Monitoring Device** **3 Infusion Device** **D Intraluminal Device** **Y Other Device**	**Z No Qualifier**

Non-OR	Ø3H[Ø,1,2,3,4,5,6,7,8,9,A,B,C,D,F,G,H,J,M,N,P,Q,R,S,T,U,V][Ø,3,4]3Z
Non-OR	Ø3H[K,L][Ø,3,4]3Z
Non-OR	Ø3HY[Ø,3,4]3Z
Non-OR	Ø3HY32Z
Non-OR	Ø3HY[3,4]YZ

LC Limited Coverage   NC Noncovered   ⊞ Combination Member   HAC associated procedure   Combination Only   DRG Non-OR   Non-OR   New/Revised in GREEN

202   ICD-10-PCS 2020

Ø Medical and Surgical
3 Upper Arteries
J Inspection   Definition: Visually and/or manually exploring a body part

Explanation: Visual exploration may be performed with or without optical instrumentation. Manual exploration may be performed directly or through intervening body layers.

Body Part Character 4	Approach Character 5	Device Character 6	Qualifier Character 7
Y Upper Artery Aortic intercostal artery Bronchial artery Esophageal artery Subcostal artery	**Ø** Open **3** Percutaneous **4** Percutaneous Endoscopic **X** External	**Z** No Device	**Z** No Qualifier

Non-OR   Ø3JY[3,4,X]ZZ

LC Limited Coverage **NC** Noncovered ⊞ Combination Member HAC associated procedure Combination Only DRG Non-OR Non-OR New/Revised in GREEN

ICD-10-PCS 2020   203

Ø   Medical and Surgical
3   Upper Arteries
L   Occlusion   Definition: Completely closing an orifice or the lumen of a tubular body part
                    Explanation: The orifice can be a natural orifice or an artificially created orifice

Body Part Character 4		Approach Character 5	Device Character 6	Qualifier Character 7
Ø Internal Mammary Artery, Right Anterior intercostal artery Internal thoracic artery Musculophrenic artery Pericardiophrenic artery Superior epigastric artery **1 Internal Mammary Artery, Left** *See Ø Internal Mammary Artery, Left* **2 Innominate Artery** Brachiocephalic artery Brachiocephalic trunk **3 Subclavian Artery, Right** Costocervical trunk Dorsal scapular artery Internal thoracic artery **4 Subclavian Artery, Left** *See 3 Subclavian Artery, Right* **5 Axillary Artery, Right** Anterior circumflex humeral artery Lateral thoracic artery Posterior circumflex humeral artery Subscapular artery Superior thoracic artery Thoracoacromial artery **6 Axillary Artery, Left** *See 5 Axillary Artery, Right* **7 Brachial Artery, Right** Inferior ulnar collateral artery Profunda brachii Superior ulnar collateral artery **8 Brachial Artery, Left** *See 7 Brachial Artery, Right* **9 Ulnar Artery, Right** Anterior ulnar recurrent artery Common interosseous artery Posterior ulnar recurrent artery	**A Ulnar Artery, Left** *See 9 Ulnar Artery, Right* **B Radial Artery, Right** Radial recurrent artery **C Radial Artery, Left** *See B Radial Artery, Right* **D Hand Artery, Right** Deep palmar arch Princeps pollicis artery Radialis indicis Superficial palmar arch **F Hand Artery, Left** *See D Hand Artery, Right* **R Face Artery** Angular artery Ascending palatine artery External maxillary artery Facial artery Inferior labial artery Submental artery Superior labial artery **S Temporal Artery, Right** Middle temporal artery Superficial temporal artery Transverse facial artery **T Temporal Artery, Left** *See S Temporal Artery, Right* **U Thyroid Artery, Right** Cricothyroid artery Hyoid artery Sternocleidomastoid artery Superior laryngeal artery Superior thyroid artery Thyrocervical trunk **V Thyroid Artery, Left** *See U Thyroid Artery, Right* **Y Upper Artery** Aortic intercostal artery Bronchial artery Esophageal artery Subcostal artery	**Ø Open** **3 Percutaneous** **4 Percutaneous Endoscopic**	**C Extraluminal Device** **D Intraluminal Device** **Z No Device**	**Z No Qualifier**
G Intracranial Artery Anterior cerebral artery Anterior choroidal artery Anterior communicating artery Basilar artery Circle of Willis Internal carotid artery, intracranial portion Middle cerebral artery Ophthalmic artery Posterior cerebral artery Posterior communicating artery Posterior inferior cerebellar artery (PICA) **H Common Carotid Artery, Right** **J Common Carotid Artery, Left** **K Internal Carotid Artery, Right** Caroticotympanic artery Carotid sinus	**L Internal Carotid Artery, Left** *See K Internal Carotid Artery, Right* **M External Carotid Artery, Right** Ascending pharyngeal artery Internal maxillary artery Lingual artery Maxillary artery Occipital artery Posterior auricular artery Superior thyroid artery **N External Carotid Artery, Left** *See M External Carotid Artery, Right* **P Vertebral Artery, Right** Anterior spinal artery Posterior spinal artery **Q Vertebral Artery, Left** *See P Vertebral Artery, Right*	**Ø Open** **3 Percutaneous** **4 Percutaneous Endoscopic**	**B Intraluminal Device, Bioactive** **C Extraluminal Device** **D Intraluminal Device** **Z No Device**	**Z No Qualifier**

LC Limited Coverage   **NC** Noncovered   ⊞ Combination Member   HAC associated procedure   Combination Only   DRG Non-OR   Non-OR   New/Revised in GREEN

204
ICD-10-PCS 2020

Upper Arteries

0   **Medical and Surgical**
3   **Upper Arteries**
N   **Release**   Definition: Freeing a body part from an abnormal physical constraint by cutting or by the use of force

                     Explanation: Some of the restraining tissue may be taken out but none of the body part is taken out

Body Part Character 4		Approach Character 5	Device Character 6	Qualifier Character 7
0 **Internal Mammary Artery, Right** Anterior intercostal artery Internal thoracic artery Musculophrenic artery Pericardiophrenic artery Superior epigastric artery	**H** **Common Carotid Artery, Right** **J** **Common Carotid Artery, Left** **K** **Internal Carotid Artery, Right** Caroticotympanic artery Carotid sinus	**0** Open **3** Percutaneous **4** Percutaneous Endoscopic	**Z** No Device	**Z** No Qualifier
1 **Internal Mammary Artery, Left** *See 0 Internal Mammary Artery, Right*	**L** **Internal Carotid Artery, Left** *See K Internal Carotid Artery, Right*			
2 **Innominate Artery** Brachiocephalic artery Brachiocephalic trunk	**M** **External Carotid Artery, Right** Ascending pharyngeal artery Internal maxillary artery Lingual artery Maxillary artery Occipital artery Posterior auricular artery Superior thyroid artery			
3 **Subclavian Artery, Right** Costocervical trunk Dorsal scapular artery Internal thoracic artery	**N** **External Carotid Artery, Left** *See M External Carotid Artery, Right*			
4 **Subclavian Artery, Left** *See 3 Subclavian Artery, Right*	**P** **Vertebral Artery, Right** Anterior spinal artery Posterior spinal artery			
5 **Axillary Artery, Right** Anterior circumflex humeral artery Lateral thoracic artery Posterior circumflex humeral artery Subscapular artery Superior thoracic artery Thoracoacromial artery	**Q** **Vertebral Artery, Left** *See P Vertebral Artery, Right* **R** **Face Artery** Angular artery Ascending palatine artery External maxillary artery Facial artery Inferior labial artery Submental artery Superior labial artery			
6 **Axillary Artery, Left** *See 5 Axillary Artery, Right*				
7 **Brachial Artery, Right** Inferior ulnar collateral artery Profunda brachii Superior ulnar collateral artery	**S** **Temporal Artery, Right** Middle temporal artery Superficial temporal artery Transverse facial artery			
8 **Brachial Artery, Left** *See 7 Brachial Artery, Right*	**T** **Temporal Artery, Left** *See S Temporal Artery, Right*			
9 **Ulnar Artery, Right** Anterior ulnar recurrent artery Common interosseous artery Posterior ulnar recurrent artery	**U** **Thyroid Artery, Right** Cricothyroid artery Hyoid artery Sternocleidomastoid artery Superior laryngeal artery Superior thyroid artery Thyrocervical trunk			
A **Ulnar Artery, Left** *See 9 Ulnar Artery, Right*				
B **Radial Artery, Right** Radial recurrent artery	**V** **Thyroid Artery, Left** *See U Thyroid Artery, Right*			
C **Radial Artery, Left** *See B Radial Artery, Right*	**Y** **Upper Artery** Aortic intercostal artery Bronchial artery Esophageal artery Subcostal artery			
D **Hand Artery, Right** Deep palmar arch Princeps pollicis artery Radialis indicis Superficial palmar arch				
F **Hand Artery, Left** *See D Hand Artery, Right*				
G **Intracranial Artery** Anterior cerebral artery Anterior choroidal artery Anterior communicating artery Basilar artery Circle of Willis Internal carotid artery, intracranial portion Middle cerebral artery Ophthalmic artery Posterior cerebral artery Posterior communicating artery Posterior inferior cerebellar artery (PICA)				

LC Limited Coverage   NC Noncovered   ⊞ Combination Member   HAC associated procedure   Combination Only   DRG Non-OR   Non-OR   New/Revised in GREEN

ICD-10-PCS 2020   205

Ø   **Medical and Surgical**
3   **Upper Arteries**
P   **Removal**   Definition: Taking out or off a device from a body part

Explanation: If a device is taken out and a similar device put in without cutting or puncturing the skin or mucous membrane, the procedure is coded to the root operation CHANGE. Otherwise, the procedure for taking out a device is coded to the root operation REMOVAL.

Body Part Character 4	Approach Character 5	Device Character 6	Qualifier Character 7
Y **Upper Artery** Aortic intercostal artery Bronchial artery Esophageal artery Subcostal artery	**Ø** Open **3** Percutaneous **4** Percutaneous Endoscopic	**Ø** Drainage Device **2** Monitoring Device **3** Infusion Device **7** Autologous Tissue Substitute **C** Extraluminal Device **D** Intraluminal Device **J** Synthetic Substitute **K** Nonautologous Tissue Substitute **M** Stimulator Lead **Y** Other Device	**Z** No Qualifier
Y **Upper Artery** Aortic intercostal artery Bronchial artery Esophageal artery Subcostal artery	**X** External	**Ø** Drainage Device **2** Monitoring Device **3** Infusion Device **D** Intraluminal Device **M** Stimulator Lead	**Z** No Qualifier

Non-OR   Ø3PY3[Ø,2,3,D]Z
Non-OR   Ø3PY[3,4]YZ
Non-OR   Ø3PYX[Ø,2,3,D,M]Z

0   Medical and Surgical
3   Upper Arteries
Q   Repair   Definition: Restoring, to the extent possible, a body part to its normal anatomic structure and function

Explanation: Used only when the method to accomplish the repair is not one of the other root operations

Body Part Character 4		Approach Character 5	Device Character 6	Qualifier Character 7
0 Internal Mammary Artery, Right Anterior intercostal artery Internal thoracic artery Musculophrenic artery Pericardiophrenic artery Superior epigastric artery **1 Internal Mammary Artery, Left** *See 0 Internal Mammary Artery, Right* **2 Innominate Artery** Brachiocephalic artery Brachiocephalic trunk **3 Subclavian Artery, Right** Costocervical trunk Dorsal scapular artery Internal thoracic artery **4 Subclavian Artery, Left** *See 3 Subclavian Artery, Right* **5 Axillary Artery, Right** Anterior circumflex humeral artery Lateral thoracic artery Posterior circumflex humeral artery Subscapular artery Superior thoracic artery Thoracoacromial artery **6 Axillary Artery, Left** *See 5 Axillary Artery, Right* **7 Brachial Artery, Right** Inferior ulnar collateral artery Profunda brachii Superior ulnar collateral artery **8 Brachial Artery, Left** *See 7 Brachial Artery, Right* **9 Ulnar Artery, Right** Anterior ulnar recurrent artery Common interosseous artery Posterior ulnar recurrent artery **A Ulnar Artery, Left** *See 9 Ulnar Artery, Right* **B Radial Artery, Right** Radial recurrent artery **C Radial Artery, Left** *See B Radial Artery, Right* **D Hand Artery, Right** Deep palmar arch Princeps pollicis artery Radialis indicis Superficial palmar arch **F Hand Artery, Left** *See D Hand Artery, Right* **G Intracranial Artery** Anterior cerebral artery Anterior choroidal artery Anterior communicating artery Basilar artery Circle of Willis Internal carotid artery, intracranial portion Middle cerebral artery Ophthalmic artery Posterior cerebral artery Posterior communicating artery Posterior inferior cerebellar artery (PICA)	**H Common Carotid Artery, Right** **J Common Carotid Artery, Left** **K Internal Carotid Artery, Right** Caroticotympanic artery Carotid sinus **L Internal Carotid Artery, Left** *See K Internal Carotid Artery, Right* **M External Carotid Artery, Right** Ascending pharyngeal artery Internal maxillary artery Lingual artery Maxillary artery Occipital artery Posterior auricular artery Superior thyroid artery **N External Carotid Artery, Left** *See M External Carotid Artery, Right* **P Vertebral Artery, Right** Anterior spinal artery Posterior spinal artery **Q Vertebral Artery, Left** *See P Vertebral Artery, Right* **R Face Artery** Angular artery Ascending palatine artery External maxillary artery Facial artery Inferior labial artery Submental artery Superior labial artery **S Temporal Artery, Right** Middle temporal artery Superficial temporal artery Transverse facial artery **T Temporal Artery, Left** *See S Temporal Artery, Right* **U Thyroid Artery, Right** Cricothyroid artery Hyoid artery Sternocleidomastoid artery Superior laryngeal artery Superior thyroid artery Thyrocervical trunk **V Thyroid Artery, Left** *See U Thyroid Artery, Right* **Y Upper Artery** Aortic intercostal artery Bronchial artery Esophageal artery Subcostal artery	**0 Open** **3 Percutaneous** **4 Percutaneous Endoscopic**	**Z No Device**	**Z No Qualifier**

ⓛⓒ Limited Coverage   ⓝⓒ Noncoverced   ⊞ Combination Member   HAC associated procedure   Combination Only   DRG Non-OR   Non-OR   New/Revised in GREEN

ICD-10-PCS 2020   207

03Q–03Q

Upper Arteries

Ø   Medical and Surgical
3   Upper Arteries
R   Replacement   Definition: Putting in or on biological or synthetic material that physically takes the place and/or function of all or a portion of a body part
Explanation: The body part may have been taken out or replaced, or may be taken out, physically eradicated, or rendered nonfunctional during the REPLACEMENT procedure. A REMOVAL procedure is coded for taking out the device used in a previous replacement procedure.

Body Part Character 4		Approach Character 5	Device Character 6	Qualifier Character 7
Ø Internal Mammary Artery, Right Anterior intercostal artery Internal thoracic artery Musculophrenic artery Pericardiophrenic artery Superior epigastric artery **1 Internal Mammary Artery, Left** *See Ø Internal Mammary Artery, Right* **2 Innominate Artery** Brachiocephalic artery Brachiocephalic trunk **3 Subclavian Artery, Right** Costocervical trunk Dorsal scapular artery Internal thoracic artery **4 Subclavian Artery, Left** *See 3 Subclavian Artery, Right* **5 Axillary Artery, Right** Anterior circumflex humeral artery Lateral thoracic artery Posterior circumflex humeral artery Subscapular artery Superior thoracic artery Thoracoacromial artery **6 Axillary Artery, Left** *See 5 Axillary Artery, Right* **7 Brachial Artery, Right** Inferior ulnar collateral artery Profunda brachii Superior ulnar collateral artery **8 Brachial Artery, Left** *See 7 Brachial Artery, Right* **9 Ulnar Artery, Right** Anterior ulnar recurrent artery Common interosseous artery Posterior ulnar recurrent artery **A Ulnar Artery, Left** *See 9 Ulnar Artery, Right* **B Radial Artery, Right** Radial recurrent artery **C Radial Artery, Left** *See B Radial Artery, Right* **D Hand Artery, Right** Deep palmar arch Princeps pollicis artery Radialis indicis Superficial palmar arch **F Hand Artery, Left** *See D Hand Artery, Right* **G Intracranial Artery** Anterior cerebral artery Anterior choroidal artery Anterior communicating artery Basilar artery Circle of Willis Internal carotid artery, intracranial portion Middle cerebral artery Ophthalmic artery Posterior cerebral artery Posterior communicating artery Posterior inferior cerebellar artery (PICA)	**H Common Carotid Artery, Right** **J Common Carotid Artery, Left** **K Internal Carotid Artery, Right** Caroticotympanic artery Carotid sinus **L Internal Carotid Artery, Left** *See K Internal Carotid Artery, Right* **M External Carotid Artery, Right** Ascending pharyngeal artery Internal maxillary artery Lingual artery Maxillary artery Occipital artery Posterior auricular artery Superior thyroid artery **N External Carotid Artery, Left** *See M External Carotid Artery, Right* **P Vertebral Artery, Right** Anterior spinal artery Posterior spinal artery **Q Vertebral Artery, Left** *See P Vertebral Artery, Right* **R Face Artery** Angular artery Ascending palatine artery External maxillary artery Facial artery Inferior labial artery Submental artery Superior labial artery **S Temporal Artery, Right** Middle temporal artery Superficial temporal artery Transverse facial artery **T Temporal Artery, Left** *See S Temporal Artery, Right* **U Thyroid Artery, Right** Cricothyroid artery Hyoid artery Sternocleidomastoid artery Superior laryngeal artery Superior thyroid artery Thyrocervical trunk **V Thyroid Artery, Left** *See U Thyroid Artery, Right* **Y Upper Artery** Aortic intercostal artery Bronchial artery Esophageal artery Subcostal artery	**Ø Open** **4 Percutaneous Endoscopic**	**7 Autologous Tissue Substitute** **J Synthetic Substitute** **K Nonautologous Tissue Substitute**	**Z No Qualifier**

Ø   Medical and Surgical
3   Upper Arteries
S   Reposition   Definition: Moving to its normal location, or other suitable location, all or a portion of a body part

Explanation: The body part is moved to a new location from an abnormal location, or from a normal location where it is not functioning correctly. The body part may or may not be cut out or off to be moved to the new location.

Body Part Character 4		Approach Character 5	Device Character 6	Qualifier Character 7

Ø Internal Mammary Artery, Right
   Anterior intercostal artery
   Internal thoracic artery
   Musculophrenic artery
   Pericardiophrenic artery
   Superior epigastric artery
1 Internal Mammary Artery, Left
   See Ø Internal Mammary Artery, Right
2 Innominate Artery
   Brachiocephalic artery
   Brachiocephalic trunk
3 Subclavian Artery, Right
   Costocervical trunk
   Dorsal scapular artery
   Internal thoracic artery
4 Subclavian Artery, Left
   See 3 Subclavian Artery, Right
5 Axillary Artery, Right
   Anterior circumflex humeral artery
   Lateral thoracic artery
   Posterior circumflex humeral artery
   Subscapular artery
   Superior thoracic artery
   Thoracoacromial artery
6 Axillary Artery, Left
   See 5 Axillary Artery, Right
7 Brachial Artery, Right
   Inferior ulnar collateral artery
   Profunda brachii
   Superior ulnar collateral artery
8 Brachial Artery, Left
   See 7 Brachial Artery, Right
9 Ulnar Artery, Right
   Anterior ulnar recurrent artery
   Common interosseous artery
   Posterior ulnar recurrent artery
A Ulnar Artery, Left
   See 9 Ulnar Artery, Right
B Radial Artery, Right
   Radial recurrent artery
C Radial Artery, Left
   See B Radial Artery, Right
D Hand Artery, Right
   Deep palmar arch
   Princeps pollicis artery
   Radialis indicis
   Superficial palmar arch
F Hand Artery, Left
   See D Hand Artery, Right
G Intracranial Artery
   Anterior cerebral artery
   Anterior choroidal artery
   Anterior communicating artery
   Basilar artery
   Circle of Willis
   Internal carotid artery, intracranial portion
   Middle cerebral artery
   Ophthalmic artery
   Posterior cerebral artery
   Posterior communicating artery
   Posterior inferior cerebellar artery (PICA)
	H Common Carotid Artery, Right
	J Common Carotid Artery, Left
	K Internal Carotid Artery, Right
	   Caroticotympanic artery
	   Carotid sinus
	L Internal Carotid Artery, Left
	   See K Internal Carotid Artery, Right
	M External Carotid Artery, Right
	   Ascending pharyngeal artery
	   Internal maxillary artery
	   Lingual artery
	   Maxillary artery
	   Occipital artery
	   Posterior auricular artery
	   Superior thyroid artery
	N External Carotid Artery, Left
	   See M External Carotid Artery, Right
	P Vertebral Artery, Right
	   Anterior spinal artery
	   Posterior spinal artery
	Q Vertebral Artery, Left
	   See P Vertebral Artery, Right
	R Face Artery
	   Angular artery
	   Ascending palatine artery
	   External maxillary artery
	   Facial artery
	   Inferior labial artery
	   Submental artery
	   Superior labial artery
	S Temporal Artery, Right
	   Middle temporal artery
	   Superficial temporal artery
	   Transverse facial artery
	T Temporal Artery, Left
	   See S Temporal Artery, Right
	U Thyroid Artery, Right
	   Cricothyroid artery
	   Hyoid artery
	   Sternocleidomastoid artery
	   Superior laryngeal artery
	   Superior thyroid artery
	   Thyrocervical trunk
	V Thyroid Artery, Left
	   See U Thyroid Artery, Right
	Y Upper Artery
	   Aortic intercostal artery
	   Bronchial artery
	   Esophageal artery
	   Subcostal artery
		Ø Open
		3 Percutaneous
		4 Percutaneous Endoscopic
			Z No Device	**Z No Qualifier**

LC Limited Coverage   **NC** Noncovered   ⊞ Combination Member   HAC associated procedure   Combination Only   DRG Non-OR   Non-OR   New/Revised in GREEN

ICD-10-PCS 2020   **209**

Ø3S–Ø3S

Ø Medical and Surgical
3 Upper Arteries
U Supplement

Definition: Putting in or on biological or synthetic material that physically reinforces and/or augments the function of a portion of a body part
Explanation: The biological material is non-living, or is living and from the same individual. The body part may have been previously replaced, and the SUPPLEMENT procedure is performed to physically reinforce and/or augment the function of the replaced body part.

Body Part Character 4		Approach Character 5	Device Character 6	Qualifier Character 7
Ø Internal Mammary Artery, Right Anterior intercostal artery Internal thoracic artery Musculophrenic artery Pericardiophrenic artery Superior epigastric artery **1 Internal Mammary Artery, Left** *See Ø Internal Mammary Artery, Right* **2 Innominate Artery** Brachiocephalic artery Brachiocephalic trunk **3 Subclavian Artery, Right** Costocervical trunk Dorsal scapular artery Internal thoracic artery **4 Subclavian Artery, Left** *See 3 Subclavian Artery, Right* **5 Axillary Artery, Right** Anterior circumflex humeral artery Lateral thoracic artery Posterior circumflex humeral artery Subscapular artery Superior thoracic artery Thoracoacromial artery **6 Axillary Artery, Left** *See 5 Axillary Artery, Right* **7 Brachial Artery, Right** Inferior ulnar collateral artery Profunda brachii Superior ulnar collateral artery **8 Brachial Artery, Left** *See 7 Brachial Artery, Right* **9 Ulnar Artery, Right** Anterior ulnar recurrent artery Common interosseous artery Posterior ulnar recurrent artery **A Ulnar Artery, Left** *See 9 Ulnar Artery, Right* **B Radial Artery, Right** Radial recurrent artery **C Radial Artery, Left** *See B Radial Artery, Right* **D Hand Artery, Right** Deep palmar arch Princeps pollicis artery Radialis indicis Superficial palmar arch **F Hand Artery, Left** *See D Hand Artery, Right* **G Intracranial Artery** Anterior cerebral artery Anterior choroidal artery Anterior communicating artery Basilar artery Circle of Willis Internal carotid artery, intracranial portion Middle cerebral artery Ophthalmic artery Posterior cerebral artery Posterior communicating artery Posterior inferior cerebellar artery (PICA)	**H Common Carotid Artery, Right** **J Common Carotid Artery, Left** **K Internal Carotid Artery, Right** Caroticotympanic artery Carotid sinus **L Internal Carotid Artery, Left** *See K Internal Carotid Artery, Right* **M External Carotid Artery, Right** Ascending pharyngeal artery Internal maxillary artery Lingual artery Maxillary artery Occipital artery Posterior auricular artery Superior thyroid artery **N External Carotid Artery, Left** *See M External Carotid Artery, Right* **P Vertebral Artery, Right** Anterior spinal artery Posterior spinal artery **Q Vertebral Artery, Left** *See P Vertebral Artery, Right* **R Face Artery** Angular artery Ascending palatine artery External maxillary artery Facial artery Inferior labial artery Submental artery Superior labial artery **S Temporal Artery, Right** Middle temporal artery Superficial temporal artery Transverse facial artery **T Temporal Artery, Left** *See S Temporal Artery, Right* **U Thyroid Artery, Right** Cricothyroid artery Hyoid artery Sternocleidomastoid artery Superior laryngeal artery Superior thyroid artery Thyrocervical trunk **V Thyroid Artery, Left** *See U Thyroid Artery, Right* **Y Upper Artery** Aortic intercostal artery Bronchial artery Esophageal artery Subcostal artery	**Ø Open** **3 Percutaneous** **4 Percutaneous Endoscopic**	**7 Autologous Tissue Substitute** **J Synthetic Substitute** **K Nonautologous Tissue Substitute**	**Z No Qualifier**

Limited Coverage   Noncovered   Combination Member   HAC associated procedure   Combination Only   DRG Non-OR   Non-OR   New/Revised in GREEN

210   ICD-10-PCS 2020

Ø　Medical and Surgical
3　Upper Arteries
V　Restriction　　Definition: Partially closing an orifice or the lumen of a tubular body part
　　　　　　　　　　　　Explanation: The orifice can be a natural orifice or an artificially created orifice

Body Part Character 4		Approach Character 5	Device Character 6	Qualifier Character 7
Ø Internal Mammary Artery, Right 　Anterior intercostal artery 　Internal thoracic artery 　Musculophrenic artery 　Pericardiophrenic artery 　Superior epigastric artery **1 Internal Mammary Artery, Left** 　*See Ø Internal Mammary Artery,* 　*Right* **2 Innominate Artery** 　Brachiocephalic artery 　Brachiocephalic trunk **3 Subclavian Artery, Right** 　Costocervical trunk 　Dorsal scapular artery 　Internal thoracic artery **4 Subclavian Artery, Left** 　*See 3 Subclavian Artery, Right* **5 Axillary Artery, Right** 　Anterior circumflex humeral artery 　Lateral thoracic artery 　Posterior circumflex humeral artery 　Subscapular artery 　Superior thoracic artery 　Thoracoacromial artery **6 Axillary Artery, Left** 　*See 5 Axillary Artery, Right* **7 Brachial Artery, Right** 　Inferior ulnar collateral artery 　Profunda brachii 　Superior ulnar collateral artery **8 Brachial Artery, Left** 　*See 7 Brachial Artery, Right* **9 Ulnar Artery, Right** 　Anterior ulnar recurrent artery 　Common interosseous artery 　Posterior ulnar recurrent artery **A Ulnar Artery, Left** 　*See 9 Ulnar Artery, Right*	**B Radial Artery, Right** 　Radial recurrent artery **C Radial Artery, Left** 　*See B Radial Artery, Right* **D Hand Artery, Right** 　Deep palmar arch 　Princeps pollicis artery 　Radialis indicis 　Superficial palmar arch **F Hand Artery, Left** 　*See D Hand Artery, Right* **R Face Artery** 　Angular artery 　Ascending palatine artery 　External maxillary artery 　Facial artery 　Inferior labial artery 　Submental artery 　Superior labial artery **S Temporal Artery, Right** 　Middle temporal artery 　Superficial temporal artery 　Transverse facial artery **T Temporal Artery, Left** 　*See S Temporal Artery, Right* **U Thyroid Artery, Right** 　Cricothyroid artery 　Hyoid artery 　Sternocleidomastoid artery 　Superior laryngeal artery 　Superior thyroid artery 　Thyrocervical trunk **V Thyroid Artery, Left** 　*See U Thyroid Artery, Right* **Y Upper Artery** 　Aortic intercostal artery 　Bronchial artery 　Esophageal artery 　Subcostal artery	**Ø Open** **3 Percutaneous** **4 Percutaneous** 　**Endoscopic**	**C Extraluminal Device** **D Intraluminal Device** **Z No Device**	**Z No Qualifier**
G Intracranial Artery 　Anterior cerebral artery 　Anterior choroidal artery 　Anterior communicating artery 　Basilar artery 　Circle of Willis 　Internal carotid artery, 　　intracranial portion 　Middle cerebral artery 　Ophthalmic artery 　Posterior cerebral artery 　Posterior communicating artery 　Posterior inferior cerebellar artery 　　(PICA) **H Common Carotid Artery, Right** **J Common Carotid Artery, Left** **K Internal Carotid Artery, Right** 　Caroticotympanic artery 　Carotid sinus	**L Internal Carotid Artery, Left** 　*See K Internal Carotid Artery, Right* **M External Carotid Artery, Right** 　Ascending pharyngeal artery 　Internal maxillary artery 　Lingual artery 　Maxillary artery 　Occipital artery 　Posterior auricular artery 　Superior thyroid artery **N External Carotid Artery, Left** 　*See M External Carotid Artery, Right* **P Vertebral Artery, Right** 　Anterior spinal artery 　Posterior spinal artery **Q Vertebral Artery, Left** 　*See P Vertebral Artery, Right*	**Ø Open** **3 Percutaneous** **4 Percutaneous** 　**Endoscopic**	**B Intraluminal Device,** 　**Bioactive** **C Extraluminal Device** **D Intraluminal Device** **H Intraluminal Device,** 　**Flow Diverter** **Z No Device**	**Z No Qualifier**

🔳 Limited Coverage　🔳 Noncovered　⊞ Combination Member　HAC associated procedure　Combination Only　DRG Non-OR　Non-OR　New/Revised in GREEN
ICD-10-PCS 2020　　　　　　　　　　　　　　　　　　　　　　　　　　　　　　　　　　　　　　　211

Ø3V–Ø3V

03W–03W   Upper Arteries   ICD-10-PCS 2020

0   Medical and Surgical
3   Upper Arteries
W   Revision   Definition: Correcting, to the extent possible, a portion of a malfunctioning device or the position of a displaced device

Explanation: Revision can include correcting a malfunctioning or displaced device by taking out or putting in components of the device such as a screw or pin

Body Part Character 4	Approach Character 5	Device Character 6	Qualifier Character 7
Y Upper Artery Aortic intercostal artery Bronchial artery Esophageal artery Subcostal artery	**0** Open **3** Percutaneous **4** Percutaneous Endoscopic	**0** Drainage Device **2** Monitoring Device **3** Infusion Device **7** Autologous Tissue Substitute **C** Extraluminal Device **D** Intraluminal Device **J** Synthetic Substitute **K** Nonautologous Tissue Substitute **M** Stimulator Lead **Y** Other Device	**Z** No Qualifier
Y Upper Artery Aortic intercostal artery Bronchial artery Esophageal artery Subcostal artery	**X** External	**0** Drainage Device **2** Monitoring Device **3** Infusion Device **7** Autologous Tissue Substitute **C** Extraluminal Device **D** Intraluminal Device **J** Synthetic Substitute **K** Nonautologous Tissue Substitute **M** Stimulator Lead	**Z** No Qualifier

Non-OR   03WY3[0,2,3,D]Z
Non-OR   03WY[3,4]YZ
Non-OR   03WYX[0,2,3,7,C,D,J,K,M]Z

212   ICD-10-PCS 2020

Lower Arteries Ø41–Ø4W

Character Meanings

This Character Meaning table is provided as a guide to assist the user in the identification of character members that may be found in this section of code tables. It **SHOULD NOT** be used to build a PCS code.

Operation–Character 3	Body Part–Character 4	Approach–Character 5	Device–Character 6	Qualifier–Character 7
1 Bypass	Ø Abdominal Aorta	Ø Open	Ø Drainage Device	Ø Abdominal Aorta
5 Destruction	1 Celiac Artery	3 Percutaneous	1 Radioactive Element	1 Celiac Artery OR Drug-Coated Balloon
7 Dilation	2 Gastric Artery	4 Percutaneous Endoscopic	2 Monitoring Device	2 Mesenteric Artery
9 Drainage	3 Hepatic Artery	X External	3 Infusion Device	3 Renal Artery, Right
B Excision	4 Splenic Artery		4 Intraluminal Device, Drug-eluting	4 Renal Artery, Left
C Extirpation	5 Superior Mesenteric Artery		5 Intraluminal Device, Drug-eluting, Two	5 Renal Artery, Bilateral
H Insertion	6 Colic Artery, Right		6 Intraluminal Device, Drug-eluting, Three	6 Common Iliac Artery, Right
J Inspection	7 Colic Artery, Left		7 Intraluminal Device, Drug-eluting, Four or More OR Autologous Tissue Substitute	7 Common Iliac Artery, Left
L Occlusion	8 Colic Artery, Middle		9 Autologous Venous Tissue	8 Common Iliac Arteries, Bilateral
N Release	9 Renal Artery, Right		A Autologous Arterial Tissue	9 Internal Iliac Artery, Right
P Removal	A Renal Artery, Left		C Extraluminal Device	B Internal Iliac Artery, Left
Q Repair	B Inferior Mesenteric Artery		D Intraluminal Device	C Internal Iliac Arteries, Bilateral
R Replacement	C Common Iliac Artery, Right		E Intraluminal Device, Two OR Intraluminal Device, Branched or Fenestrated, One or Two Arteries	D External Iliac Artery, Right
S Reposition	D Common Iliac Artery, Left		F Intraluminal Device, Three OR Intraluminal Device, Branched or Fenestrated, Three or More Arteries	F External Iliac Artery, Left
U Supplement	E Internal Iliac Artery, Right		G Intraluminal Device, Four or More	G External Iliac Arteries, Bilateral
V Restriction	F Internal Iliac Artery, Left		J Synthetic Substitute	H Femoral Artery, Right
W Revision	H External Iliac Artery, Right		K Nonautologous Tissue Substitute	J Femoral Artery, Left OR Temporary
	J External Iliac Artery, Left		Y Other Device	K Femoral Arteries, Bilateral
	K Femoral Artery, Right		Z No Device	L Popliteal Artery
	L Femoral Artery, Left			M Peroneal Artery
	M Popliteal Artery, Right			N Posterior Tibial Artery
	N Popliteal Artery, Left			P Foot Artery
	P Anterior Tibial Artery, Right			Q Lower Extremity Artery
	Q Anterior Tibial Artery, Left			R Lower Artery
	R Posterior Tibial Artery, Right			S Lower Extremity Vein
	S Posterior Tibial Artery, Left			T Uterine Artery, Right
	T Peroneal Artery, Right			U Uterine Artery, Left
	U Peroneal Artery, Left			X Diagnostic
	V Foot Artery, Right			Z No Qualifier
	W Foot Artery, Left			
	Y Lower Artery			

AHA Coding Clinic for table Ø41

2019, 1Q, 23	Endovascular repair of shaggy aorta and deployment of chimney stent grafts
2018, 3Q, 25	Femoral artery to tibioperoneal trunk bypass
2017, 4Q, 46-47	New and revised body part values - Bypass hepatic artery to renal artery
2017, 3Q, 5	Femoral artery to posterior tibial artery bypass using autologous and synthetic grafts
2017, 3Q, 16	Abdominal aortic debranching with bypass of external iliac artery to bilateral renal arteries and superior mesenteric artery
2017, 1Q, 32	Peroneal artery to dorsalis pedis artery bypass using saphenous vein graft
2016, 2Q, 18	Femoral-tibial artery bypass and saphenous vein graft
2015, 3Q, 28	Bilateral renal artery bypass

AHA Coding Clinic for table Ø47

2018, 2Q, 24	Coronary artery bifurcation
2016, 4Q, 86	Peripheral artery, number of stents
2016, 4Q, 86-88	Coronary and peripheral artery bifurcation
2016, 3Q, 39	Infrarenal abdominal aortic aneurysm repair with iliac graft extension
2015, 4Q, 4-7, 15	Drug-coated balloon angioplasty in peripheral vessels
2015, 3Q, 9	Aborted endovascular stenting of superficial femoral artery

AHA Coding Clinic for table Ø4C

2019, 1Q, 23	Endovascular repair of shaggy aorta and deployment of chimney stent grafts
2018, 2Q, 24	Coronary artery bifurcation
2017, 2Q, 23	Thrombectomy via Fogarty catheter
2016, 4Q, 86-88	Coronary and peripheral artery bifurcation
2016, 1Q, 31	Iliofemoral endarterectomy with patch repair
2015, 1Q, 29	Discontinued carotid endarterectomy
2015, 1Q, 36	Percutaneous mechanical thrombectomy of femoropopliteal bypass graft

AHA Coding Clinic for table Ø4H

2019, 1Q, 23	Endovascular repair of shaggy aorta and deployment of chimney stent grafts
2017, 1Q, 30	Insertion of umbilical artery catheter

AHA Coding Clinic for table Ø4L

2018, 2Q, 18	Transverse rectus abdominis myocutaneous (TRAM) delay
2017, 4Q, 31	Resuscitative endovascular balloon occlusion of the aorta
2015, 2Q, 27	Uterine artery embolization using Gelfoam
2014, 3Q, 26	Coil embolization of gastroduodenal artery with chemoembolization of hepatic artery
2014, 1Q, 24	Endovascular embolization for gastrointestinal bleeding

AHA Coding Clinic for table Ø4N

2015, 2Q, 28	Release and replacement of celiac artery

AHA Coding Clinic for table Ø4Q

2014, 1Q, 21	Repair of femoral artery pseudoaneurysm

AHA Coding Clinic for table Ø4R

2019, 1Q, 22	Abdominal aortic aneurysm repair using tube graft
2015, 2Q, 28	Release and replacement of celiac artery

AHA Coding Clinic for table Ø4U

2019, 1Q, 22	Abdominal aortic aneurysm repair using tube graft
2016, 2Q, 18	Femoral-tibial artery bypass and saphenous vein graft
2016, 1Q, 31	Iliofemoral endarterectomy with patch repair
2014, 4Q, 37	Bovine patch arterioplasty
2014, 1Q, 22	Repair of pseudoaneurysm of femoral-popliteal bypass graft

AHA Coding Clinic for table Ø4V

2019, 1Q, 22	Abdominal aortic aneurysm repair using tube graft
2018, 2Q, 24	Coronary artery bifurcation
2016, 4Q, 86-87	Coronary and peripheral artery bifurcation
2016, 4Q, 89-93	Branched and fenestrated endograft repair of aneurysms
2016, 3Q, 39	Infrarenal abdominal aortic aneurysm repair with iliac graft extension
2014, 1Q, 9	Endovascular repair of abdominal aortic aneurysm

AHA Coding Clinic for table Ø4W

2015, 1Q, 36	Revision of femoropopliteal bypass graft
2014, 1Q, 9	Endovascular repair of endoleak
2014, 1Q, 22	Repair of pseudoaneurysm of femoral-popliteal bypass graft

Lower Arteries

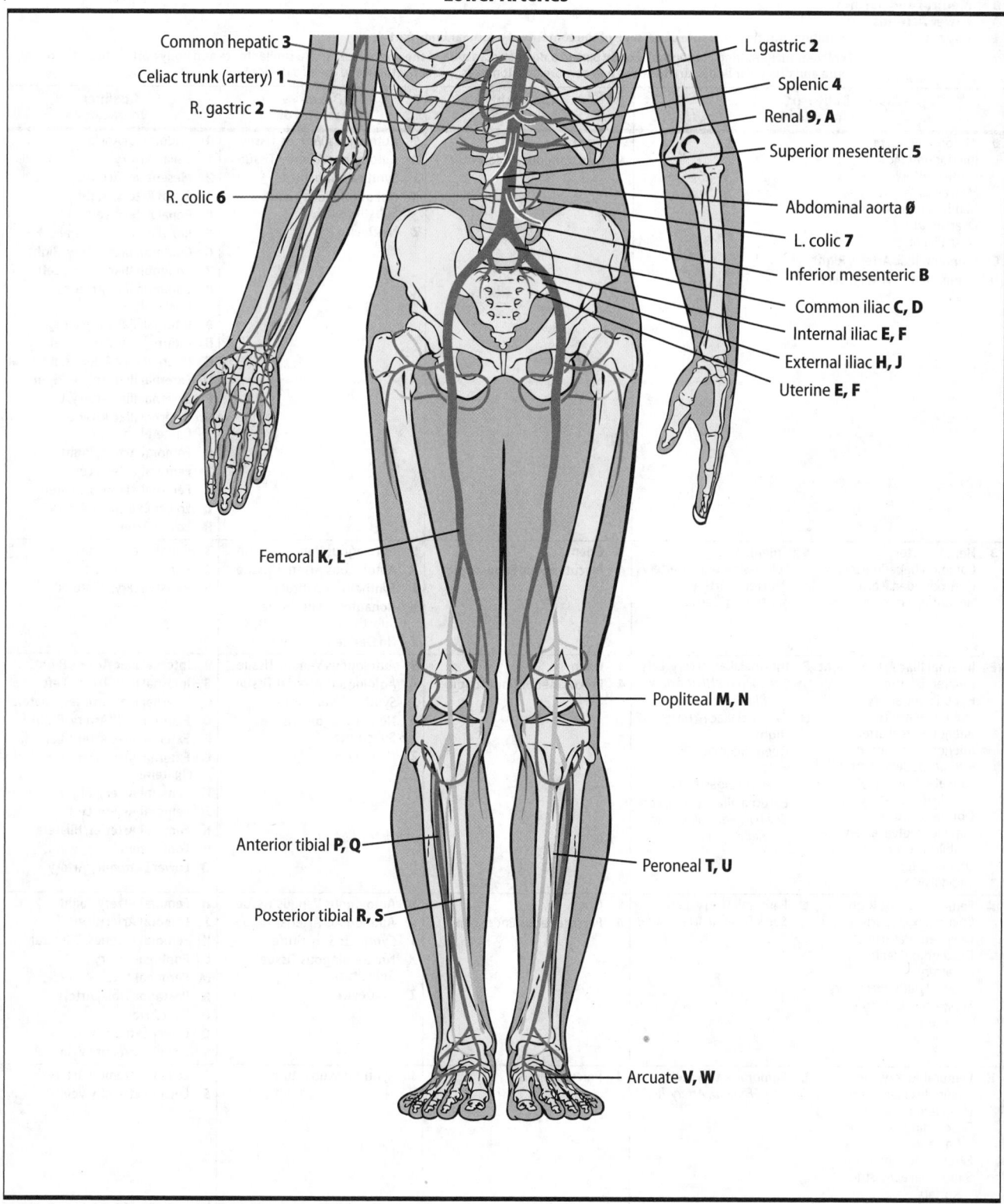

Common hepatic **3**
Celiac trunk (artery) **1**
R. gastric **2**
R. colic **6**

L. gastric **2**
Splenic **4**
Renal **9, A**
Superior mesenteric **5**
Abdominal aorta **Ø**
L. colic **7**
Inferior mesenteric **B**
Common iliac **C, D**
Internal iliac **E, F**
External iliac **H, J**
Uterine **E, F**

Femoral **K, L**

Popliteal **M, N**

Anterior tibial **P, Q**

Peroneal **T, U**

Posterior tibial **R, S**

Arcuate **V, W**

Ø   Medical and Surgical
4   Lower Arteries
1   Bypass   Definition: Altering the route of passage of the contents of a tubular body part

Explanation: Rerouting contents of a body part to a downstream area of the normal route, to a similar route and body part, or to an abnormal route and dissimilar body part. Includes one or more anastomoses, with or without the use of a device.

Body Part Character 4		Approach Character 5	Device Character 6	Qualifier Character 7
Ø **Abdominal Aorta** Inferior phrenic artery Lumbar artery Median sacral artery Middle suprarenal artery Ovarian artery Testicular artery **C** **Common Iliac Artery, Right** **D** **Common Iliac Artery, Left**		**Ø** **Open** **4** **Percutaneous Endoscopic**	**9** **Autologous Venous Tissue** **A** **Autologous Arterial Tissue** **J** **Synthetic Substitute** **K** **Nonautologous Tissue Substitute** **Z** **No Device**	**Ø** **Abdominal Aorta** **1** **Celiac Artery** **2** **Mesenteric Artery** **3** **Renal Artery, Right** **4** **Renal Artery, Left** **5** **Renal Artery, Bilateral** **6** **Common Iliac Artery, Right** **7** **Common Iliac Artery, Left** **8** **Common Iliac Arteries, Bilateral** **9** **Internal Iliac Artery, Right** **B** **Internal Iliac Artery, Left** **C** **Internal Iliac Arteries, Bilateral** **D** **External Iliac Artery, Right** **F** **External Iliac Artery, Left** **G** **External Iliac Arteries, Bilateral** **H** **Femoral Artery, Right** **J** **Femoral Artery, Left** **K** **Femoral Arteries, Bilateral** **Q** **Lower Extremity Artery** **R** **Lower Artery**
3 **Hepatic Artery** Common hepatic artery Gastroduodenal artery Hepatic artery proper	**4** **Splenic Artery** Left gastroepiploic artery Pancreatic artery Short gastric artery	**Ø** **Open** **4** **Percutaneous Endoscopic**	**9** **Autologous Venous Tissue** **A** **Autologous Arterial Tissue** **J** **Synthetic Substitute** **K** **Nonautologous Tissue Substitute** **Z** **No Device**	**3** **Renal Artery, Right** **4** **Renal Artery, Left** **5** **Renal Artery, Bilateral**
E **Internal Iliac Artery, Right** Deferential artery Hypogastric artery Iliolumbar artery Inferior gluteal artery Inferior vesical artery Internal pudendal artery Lateral sacral artery Middle rectal artery Obturator artery Superior gluteal artery Umbilical artery Uterine artery Vaginal artery	**F** **Internal Iliac Artery, Left** *See E Internal Iliac Artery, Right* **H** **External Iliac Artery, Right** Deep circumflex iliac artery Inferior epigastric artery **J** **External Iliac Artery, Left** *See H External Iliac Artery, Right*	**Ø** **Open** **4** **Percutaneous Endoscopic**	**9** **Autologous Venous Tissue** **A** **Autologous Arterial Tissue** **J** **Synthetic Substitute** **K** **Nonautologous Tissue Substitute** **Z** **No Device**	**9** **Internal Iliac Artery, Right** **B** **Internal Iliac Artery, Left** **C** **Internal Iliac Arteries, Bilateral** **D** **External Iliac Artery, Right** **F** **External Iliac Artery, Left** **G** **External Iliac Arteries, Bilateral** **H** **Femoral Artery, Right** **J** **Femoral Artery, Left** **K** **Femoral Arteries, Bilateral** **P** **Foot Artery** **Q** **Lower Extremity Artery**
K **Femoral Artery, Right** Circumflex iliac artery Deep femoral artery Descending genicular artery External pudendal artery Superficial epigastric artery	**L** **Femoral Artery, Left** *See K Femoral Artery, Right*	**Ø** **Open** **4** **Percutaneous Endoscopic**	**9** **Autologous Venous Tissue** **A** **Autologous Arterial Tissue** **J** **Synthetic Substitute** **K** **Nonautologous Tissue Substitute** **Z** **No Device**	**H** **Femoral Artery, Right** **J** **Femoral Artery, Left** **K** **Femoral Arteries, Bilateral** **L** **Popliteal Artery** **M** **Peroneal Artery** **N** **Posterior Tibial Artery** **P** **Foot Artery** **Q** **Lower Extremity Artery** **S** **Lower Extremity Vein**
K **Femoral Artery, Right** Circumflex iliac artery Deep femoral artery Descending genicular artery External pudendal artery Superficial epigastric artery	**L** **Femoral Artery, Left** *See K Femoral Artery, Right*	**3** **Percutaneous**	**J** **Synthetic Substitute**	**Q** **Lower Extremity Artery** **S** **Lower Extremity Vein**
M **Popliteal Artery, Right** Inferior genicular artery Middle genicular artery Superior genicular artery Sural artery Tibioperoneal trunk	**N** **Popliteal Artery, Left** *See M Popliteal Artery, Right*	**Ø** **Open** **4** **Percutaneous Endoscopic**	**9** **Autologous Venous Tissue** **A** **Autologous Arterial Tissue** **J** **Synthetic Substitute** **K** **Nonautologous Tissue Substitute** **Z** **No Device**	**L** **Popliteal Artery** **M** **Peroneal Artery** **P** **Foot Artery** **Q** **Lower Extremity Artery** **S** **Lower Extremity Vein**

Ø41 Continued on next page

LC Limited Coverage   NC Noncovered   ⊞ Combination Member   HAC associated procedure   Combination Only   DRG Non-OR   Non-OR   New/Revised in GREEN

216   ICD-10-PCS 2020

Ø41–Ø41

Ø   Medical and Surgical
4   Lower Arteries
1   Bypass   Definition: Altering the route of passage of the contents of a tubular body part

                   Explanation: Rerouting contents of a body part to a downstream area of the normal route, to a similar route and body part, or to an abnormal route and dissimilar body part. Includes one or more anastomoses, with or without the use of a device.

Body Part Character 4		Approach Character 5	Device Character 6	Qualifier Character 7

M Popliteal Artery, Right
   Inferior genicular artery
   Middle genicular artery
   Superior genicular artery
   Sural artery
   Tibioperoneal trunk
	N Popliteal Artery, Left
	   See M Popliteal Artery, Right
		3 Percutaneous	**J** Synthetic Substitute	**Q** Lower Extremity Artery
				S Lower Extremity Vein

P Anterior Tibial Artery, Right
   Anterior lateral malleolar artery
   Anterior medial malleolar artery
   Anterior tibial recurrent artery
   Dorsalis pedis artery
   Posterior tibial recurrent artery
	Q Anterior Tibial Artery, Left
	   See P Anterior Tibial Artery, Right
	R Posterior Tibial Artery, Right
	S Posterior Tibial Artery, Left
		Ø Open
		3 Percutaneous
		4 Percutaneous Endoscopic
			J Synthetic Substitute	**Q** Lower Extremity Artery
				S Lower Extremity Vein

T Peroneal Artery, Right
   Fibular artery
U Peroneal Artery, Left
   See T Peroneal Artery, Right
	V Foot Artery, Right
	   Arcuate artery
	   Dorsal metatarsal artery
	   Lateral plantar artery
	   Lateral tarsal artery
	   Medial plantar artery
	W Foot Artery, Left
	   See V Foot Artery, Right
		Ø Open
		4 Percutaneous Endoscopic
			9 Autologous Venous Tissue
			A Autologous Arterial Tissue
			J Synthetic Substitute
			K Nonautologous Tissue Substitute
			Z No Device
				P Foot Artery
				Q Lower Extremity Artery
				S Lower Extremity Vein

T Peroneal Artery, Right
   Fibular artery
U Peroneal Artery, Left
   See T Peroneal Artery, Right
	V Foot Artery, Right
	   Arcuate artery
	   Dorsal metatarsal artery
	   Lateral plantar artery
	   Lateral tarsal artery
	   Medial plantar artery
	W Foot Artery, Left
	   See V Foot Artery, Right
		3 Percutaneous	**J** Synthetic Substitute	**Q** Lower Extremity Artery
				S Lower Extremity Vein

Lower Arteries

Ø   **Medical and Surgical**
4   **Lower Arteries**
5   **Destruction**   Definition: Physical eradication of all or a portion of a body part by the direct use of energy, force, or a destructive agent

                             Explanation: None of the body part is physically taken out

Body Part Character 4		Approach Character 5	Device Character 6	Qualifier Character 7

Ø Abdominal Aorta
  Inferior phrenic artery
  Lumbar artery
  Median sacral artery
  Middle suprarenal artery
  Ovarian artery
  Testicular artery
1 Celiac Artery
  Celiac trunk
2 Gastric Artery
  Left gastric artery
  Right gastric artery
3 Hepatic Artery
  Common hepatic artery
  Gastroduodenal artery
  Hepatic artery proper
4 Splenic Artery
  Left gastroepiploic artery
  Pancreatic artery
  Short gastric artery
5 Superior Mesenteric Artery
  Ileal artery
  Ileocolic artery
  Inferior pancreaticoduodenal
    artery
  Jejunal artery
6 Colic Artery, Right
7 Colic Artery, Left
8 Colic Artery, Middle
9 Renal Artery, Right
  Inferior suprarenal artery
  Renal segmental artery
A Renal Artery, Left
  See 9 Renal Artery, Right
B Inferior Mesenteric Artery
  Sigmoid artery
  Superior rectal artery
C Common Iliac Artery, Right
D Common Iliac Artery, Left
E Internal Iliac Artery, Right
  Deferential artery
  Hypogastric artery
  Iliolumbar artery
  Inferior gluteal artery
  Inferior vesical artery
  Internal pudendal artery
  Lateral sacral artery
  Middle rectal artery
  Obturator artery
  Superior gluteal artery
  Umbilical artery
  Uterine artery
  Vaginal artery
	F Internal Iliac Artery, Left
	  See E Internal Iliac Artery, Right
	H External Iliac Artery, Right
	  Deep circumflex iliac artery
	  Inferior epigastric artery
	J External Iliac Artery, Left
	  See H External Iliac Artery, Right
	K Femoral Artery, Right
	  Circumflex iliac artery
	  Deep femoral artery
	  Descending genicular artery
	  External pudendal artery
	  Superficial epigastric artery
	L Femoral Artery, Left
	  See K Femoral Artery, Right
	M Popliteal Artery, Right
	  Inferior genicular artery
	  Middle genicular artery
	  Superior genicular artery
	  Sural artery
	  Tibioperoneal trunk
	N Popliteal Artery, Left
	  See M Popliteal Artery, Right
	P Anterior Tibial Artery, Right
	  Anterior lateral malleolar
	    artery
	  Anterior medial malleolar
	    artery
	  Anterior tibial recurrent artery
	  Dorsalis pedis artery
	  Posterior tibial recurrent artery
	Q Anterior Tibial Artery, Left
	  See P Anterior Tibial Artery,
	    Right
	R Posterior Tibial Artery, Right
	S Posterior Tibial Artery, Left
	T Peroneal Artery, Right
	  Fibular artery
	U Peroneal Artery, Left
	  See T Peroneal Artery, Right
	V Foot Artery, Right
	  Arcuate artery
	  Dorsal metatarsal artery
	  Lateral plantar artery
	  Lateral tarsal artery
	  Medial plantar artery
	W Foot Artery, Left
	  See V Foot Artery, Right
	Y Lower Artery
	  Umbilical artery
		Ø Open
		3 Percutaneous
		4 Percutaneous Endoscopic
			Z No Device	**Z No Qualifier**

Ø   **Medical and Surgical**
4   **Lower Arteries**
7   **Dilation**   Definition: Expanding an orifice or the lumen of a tubular body part

Explanation: The orifice can be a natural orifice or an artificially created orifice. Accomplished by stretching a tubular body part using intraluminal pressure or by cutting part of the orifice or wall of the tubular body part.

Body Part Character 4		Approach Character 5	Device Character 6	Qualifier Character 7

Ø Abdominal Aorta
Inferior phrenic artery
Lumbar artery
Median sacral artery
Middle suprarenal artery
Ovarian artery
Testicular artery
1 Celiac Artery
Celiac trunk
2 Gastric Artery
Left gastric artery
Right gastric artery
3 Hepatic Artery
Common hepatic artery
Gastroduodenal artery
Hepatic artery proper
4 Splenic Artery
Left gastroepiploic artery
Pancreatic artery
Short gastric artery
5 Superior Mesenteric Artery
Ileal artery
Ileocolic artery
Inferior pancreaticoduodenal
    artery
Jejunal artery
6 Colic Artery, Right
7 Colic Artery, Left
8 Colic Artery, Middle
9 Renal Artery, Right
Inferior suprarenal artery
Renal segmental artery
A Renal Artery, Left
See 9 Renal Artery, Right
B Inferior Mesenteric Artery
Sigmoid artery
Superior rectal artery
C Common Iliac Artery, Right
D Common Iliac Artery, Left
E Internal Iliac Artery, Right
Deferential artery
Hypogastric artery
Iliolumbar artery
Inferior gluteal artery
Inferior vesical artery
Internal pudendal artery
Lateral sacral artery
Middle rectal artery
Obturator artery
Superior gluteal artery
Umbilical artery
Uterine artery
Vaginal artery
	F Internal Iliac Artery, Left
	See E Internal Iliac Artery, Right
	H External Iliac Artery, Right
	Deep circumflex iliac artery
	Inferior epigastric artery
	J External Iliac Artery, Left
	See H External Iliac Artery, Right
	K Femoral Artery, Right
	Circumflex iliac artery
	Deep femoral artery
	Descending genicular artery
	External pudendal artery
	Superficial epigastric artery
	L Femoral Artery, Left
	See K Femoral Artery, Right
	M Popliteal Artery, Right
	Inferior genicular artery
	Middle genicular artery
	Superior genicular artery
	Sural artery
	Tibioperoneal trunk
	N Popliteal Artery, Left
	See M Popliteal Artery, Right
	P Anterior Tibial Artery, Right
	Anterior lateral malleolar
	    artery
	Anterior medial malleolar
	    artery
	Anterior tibial recurrent artery
	Dorsalis pedis artery
	Posterior tibial recurrent artery
	Q Anterior Tibial Artery, Left
	See P Anterior Tibial Artery,
	Right
	R Posterior Tibial Artery, Right
	S Posterior Tibial Artery, Left
	T Peroneal Artery, Right
	Fibular artery
	U Peroneal Artery, Left
	See T Peroneal Artery, Right
	V Foot Artery, Right
	Arcuate artery
	Dorsal metatarsal artery
	Lateral plantar artery
	Lateral tarsal artery
	Medial plantar artery
	W Foot Artery, Left
	See V Foot Artery, Right
	Y Lower Artery
	Umbilical artery
		Ø Open
		3 Percutaneous
		4 Percutaneous Endoscopic
			**4 Intraluminal Device,
			   Drug-eluting**
			D Intraluminal Device
			Z No Device
				1 Drug-Coated Balloon
				Z No Qualifier

Ø47 Continued on next page

LC Limited Coverage   NC Noncovered   ⊞ Combination Member   HAC associated procedure   Combination Only   DRG Non-OR   Non-OR   New/Revised in GREEN
ICD-10-PCS 2020   219

Ø47–Ø47

Ø   **Medical and Surgical**
4   **Lower Arteries**
7   **Dilation**   Definition: Expanding an orifice or the lumen of a tubular body part

047 Continued

Explanation: The orifice can be a natural orifice or an artificially created orifice. Accomplished by stretching a tubular body part using intraluminal pressure or by cutting part of the orifice or wall of the tubular body part.

Body Part Character 4		Approach Character 5	Device Character 6	Qualifier Character 7

Ø Abdominal Aorta
Inferior phrenic artery
Lumbar artery
Median sacral artery
Middle suprarenal artery
Ovarian artery
Testicular artery
1 Celiac Artery
Celiac trunk
2 Gastric Artery
Left gastric artery
Right gastric artery
3 Hepatic Artery
Common hepatic artery
Gastroduodenal artery
Hepatic artery proper
4 Splenic Artery
Left gastroepiploic artery
Pancreatic artery
Short gastric artery
5 Superior Mesenteric Artery
Ileal artery
Ileocolic artery
Inferior pancreaticoduodenal
   artery
Jejunal artery
6 Colic Artery, Right
7 Colic Artery, Left
8 Colic Artery, Middle
9 Renal Artery, Right
Inferior suprarenal artery
Renal segmental artery
A Renal Artery, Left
See 9 Renal Artery, Right
B Inferior Mesenteric Artery
Sigmoid artery
Superior rectal artery
C Common Iliac Artery, Right
D Common Iliac Artery, Left
E Internal Iliac Artery, Right
Deferential artery
Hypogastric artery
Iliolumbar artery
Inferior gluteal artery
Inferior vesical artery
Internal pudendal artery
Lateral sacral artery
Middle rectal artery
Obturator artery
Superior gluteal artery
Umbilical artery
Uterine artery
Vaginal artery
	F Internal Iliac Artery, Left
	See E Internal Iliac Artery, Right
	H External Iliac Artery, Right
	Deep circumflex iliac artery
	Inferior epigastric artery
	J External Iliac Artery, Left
	See H External Iliac Artery, Right
	K Femoral Artery, Right
	Circumflex iliac artery
	Deep femoral artery
	Descending genicular artery
	External pudendal artery
	Superficial epigastric artery
	L Femoral Artery, Left
	See K Femoral Artery, Right
	M Popliteal Artery, Right
	Inferior genicular artery
	Middle genicular artery
	Superior genicular artery
	Sural artery
	Tibioperoneal trunk
	N Popliteal Artery, Left
	See M Popliteal Artery, Right
	P Anterior Tibial Artery, Right
	Anterior lateral malleolar
	   artery
	Anterior medial malleolar
	   artery
	Anterior tibial recurrent artery
	Dorsalis pedis artery
	Posterior tibial recurrent artery
	Q Anterior Tibial Artery, Left
	See P Anterior Tibial Artery,
	   Right
	R Posterior Tibial Artery, Right
	S Posterior Tibial Artery, Left
	T Peroneal Artery, Right
	Fibular artery
	U Peroneal Artery, Left
	See T Peroneal Artery, Right
	V Foot Artery, Right
	Arcuate artery
	Dorsal metatarsal artery
	Lateral plantar artery
	Lateral tarsal artery
	Medial plantar artery
	W Foot Artery, Left
	See V Foot Artery, Right
	Y Lower Artery
	Umbilical artery
		Ø Open
		3 Percutaneous
		4 Percutaneous Endoscopic
			5 Intraluminal Device, Drug-
			   eluting, Two
			6 Intraluminal Device, Drug-
			   eluting, Three
			7 Intraluminal Device, Drug-
			   eluting, Four or More
			E Intraluminal Device, Two
			F Intraluminal Device, Three
			G Intraluminal Device, Four
			   or More
				Z No Qualifier

LC Limited Coverage   NC Noncovered   ⊞ Combination Member   HAC associated procedure   Combination Only   DRG Non-OR   Non-OR   New/Revised in GREEN

220   ICD-10-PCS 2020

047–047

0   **Medical and Surgical**
4   **Lower Arteries**
9   **Drainage**   Definition: Taking or letting out fluids and/or gases from a body part
                    Explanation: The qualifier DIAGNOSTIC is used to identify drainage procedures that are biopsies

Body Part Character 4		Approach Character 5	Device Character 6	Qualifier Character 7

0 **Abdominal Aorta**
  Inferior phrenic artery
  Lumbar artery
  Median sacral artery
  Middle suprarenal artery
  Ovarian artery
  Testicular artery
1 **Celiac Artery**
  Celiac trunk
2 **Gastric Artery**
  Left gastric artery
  Right gastric artery
3 **Hepatic Artery**
  Common hepatic artery
  Gastroduodenal artery
  Hepatic artery proper
4 **Splenic Artery**
  Left gastroepiploic artery
  Pancreatic artery
  Short gastric artery
5 **Superior Mesenteric Artery**
  Ileal artery
  Ileocolic artery
  Inferior pancreaticoduodenal
    artery
  Jejunal artery
6 **Colic Artery, Right**
7 **Colic Artery, Left**
8 **Colic Artery, Middle**
9 **Renal Artery, Right**
  Inferior suprarenal artery
  Renal segmental artery
A **Renal Artery, Left**
  See 9 Renal Artery, Right
B **Inferior Mesenteric Artery**
  Sigmoid artery
  Superior rectal artery
C **Common Iliac Artery, Right**
D **Common Iliac Artery, Left**
E **Internal Iliac Artery, Right**
  Deferential artery
  Hypogastric artery
  Iliolumbar artery
  Inferior gluteal artery
  Inferior vesical artery
  Internal pudendal artery
  Lateral sacral artery
  Middle rectal artery
  Obturator artery
  Superior gluteal artery
  Umbilical artery
  Uterine artery
  Vaginal artery
	F **Internal Iliac Artery, Left**
	  See E Internal Iliac Artery, Right
	H **External Iliac Artery, Right**
	  Deep circumflex iliac artery
	  Inferior epigastric artery
	J **External Iliac Artery, Left**
	  See H External Iliac Artery, Right
	K **Femoral Artery, Right**
	  Circumflex iliac artery
	  Deep femoral artery
	  Descending genicular artery
	  External pudendal artery
	  Superficial epigastric artery
	L **Femoral Artery, Left**
	  See K Femoral Artery, Right
	M **Popliteal Artery, Right**
	  Inferior genicular artery
	  Middle genicular artery
	  Superior genicular artery
	  Sural artery
	  Tibioperoneal trunk
	N **Popliteal Artery, Left**
	  See M Popliteal Artery, Right
	P **Anterior Tibial Artery, Right**
	  Anterior lateral malleolar
	    artery
	  Anterior medial malleolar
	    artery
	  Anterior tibial recurrent artery
	  Dorsalis pedis artery
	  Posterior tibial recurrent artery
	Q **Anterior Tibial Artery, Left**
	  See P Anterior Tibial Artery,
	  Right
	R **Posterior Tibial Artery, Right**
	S **Posterior Tibial Artery, Left**
	T **Peroneal Artery, Right**
	  Fibular artery
	U **Peroneal Artery, Left**
	  See T Peroneal Artery, Right
	V **Foot Artery, Right**
	  Arcuate artery
	  Dorsal metatarsal artery
	  Lateral plantar artery
	  Lateral tarsal artery
	  Medial plantar artery
	W **Foot Artery, Left**
	  See V Foot Artery, Right
	Y **Lower Artery**
	  Umbilical artery
		0 Open
		3 Percutaneous
		4 Percutaneous Endoscopic
			0 Drainage Device	**Z** No Qualifier

049 Continued on next page

Non-OR   049[0,1,2,3,4,5,6,7,8,9,A,B,C,D,E,F,H,J,K,L,M,N,P,Q,R,S,T,U,V,W,Y][0,3,4]0Z

🔲 Limited Coverage   🔲 Noncovered   ⊞ Combination Member   HAC associated procedure   Combination Only   DRG Non-OR   Non-OR   New/Revised in GREEN
ICD-10-PCS 2020   221

049–049

Lower Arteries

Ø	Medical and Surgical
4	Lower Arteries
9	Drainage

Ø49 Continued

Definition: Taking or letting out fluids and/or gases from a body part

Explanation: The qualifier DIAGNOSTIC is used to identify drainage procedures that are biopsies

Body Part Character 4		Approach Character 5	Device Character 6	Qualifier Character 7
Ø Abdominal Aorta Inferior phrenic artery Lumbar artery Median sacral artery Middle suprarenal artery Ovarian artery Testicular artery **1 Celiac Artery** Celiac trunk **2 Gastric Artery** Left gastric artery Right gastric artery **3 Hepatic Artery** Common hepatic artery Gastroduodenal artery Hepatic artery proper **4 Splenic Artery** Left gastroepiploic artery Pancreatic artery Short gastric artery **5 Superior Mesenteric Artery** Ileal artery Ileocolic artery Inferior pancreaticoduodenal artery Jejunal artery **6 Colic Artery, Right** **7 Colic Artery, Left** **8 Colic Artery, Middle** **9 Renal Artery, Right** Inferior suprarenal artery Renal segmental artery **A Renal Artery, Left** *See 9 Renal Artery, Right* **B Inferior Mesenteric Artery** Sigmoid artery Superior rectal artery **C Common Iliac Artery, Right** **D Common Iliac Artery, Left** **E Internal Iliac Artery, Right** Deferential artery Hypogastric artery Iliolumbar artery Inferior gluteal artery Inferior vesical artery Internal pudendal artery Lateral sacral artery Middle rectal artery Obturator artery Superior gluteal artery Umbilical artery Uterine artery Vaginal artery	**F Internal Iliac Artery, Left** *See E Internal Iliac Artery, Right* **H External Iliac Artery, Right** Deep circumflex iliac artery Inferior epigastric artery **J External Iliac Artery, Left** *See H External Iliac Artery, Right* **K Femoral Artery, Right** Circumflex iliac artery Deep femoral artery Descending genicular artery External pudendal artery Superficial epigastric artery **L Femoral Artery, Left** *See K Femoral Artery, Right* **M Popliteal Artery, Right** Inferior genicular artery Middle genicular artery Superior genicular artery Sural artery Tibioperoneal trunk **N Popliteal Artery, Left** *See M Popliteal Artery, Right* **P Anterior Tibial Artery, Right** Anterior lateral malleolar artery Anterior medial malleolar artery Anterior tibial recurrent artery Dorsalis pedis artery Posterior tibial recurrent artery **Q Anterior Tibial Artery, Left** *See P Anterior Tibial Artery, Right* **R Posterior Tibial Artery, Right** **S Posterior Tibial Artery, Left** **T Peroneal Artery, Right** Fibular artery **U Peroneal Artery, Left** *See T Peroneal Artery, Right* **V Foot Artery, Right** Arcuate artery Dorsal metatarsal artery Lateral plantar artery Lateral tarsal artery Medial plantar artery **W Foot Artery, Left** *See V Foot Artery, Right* **Y Lower Artery** Umbilical artery	**Ø Open** **3 Percutaneous** **4 Percutaneous Endoscopic**	**Z No Device**	**X Diagnostic** **Z No Qualifier**

Non-OR   Ø49[Ø,1,2,3,4,5,6,7,8,9,A,B,C,D,E,F,H,J,K,L,M,N,P,Q,R,S,T,U,V,W,Y]3ZX
Non-OR   Ø49[Ø,1,2,3,4,5,6,7,8,9,A,B,C,D,E,F,H,J,K,L,M,N,P,Q,R,S,T,U,V,W,Y][Ø,3,4]ZZ

LC Limited Coverage   NC Noncovered   ⊞ Combination Member   HAC associated procedure   Combination Only   DRG Non-OR   Non-OR   New/Revised in GREEN

222   ICD-10-PCS 2020

0   Medical and Surgical
4   Lower Arteries
B   Excision   Definition: Cutting out or off, without replacement, a portion of a body part
                  Explanation: The qualifier DIAGNOSTIC is used to identify excision procedures that are biopsies

Body Part Character 4		Approach Character 5	Device Character 6	Qualifier Character 7

0 Abdominal Aorta
   Inferior phrenic artery
   Lumbar artery
   Median sacral artery
   Middle suprarenal artery
   Ovarian artery
   Testicular artery
1 Celiac Artery
   Celiac trunk
2 Gastric Artery
   Left gastric artery
   Right gastric artery
3 Hepatic Artery
   Common hepatic artery
   Gastroduodenal artery
   Hepatic artery proper
4 Splenic Artery
   Left gastroepiploic artery
   Pancreatic artery
   Short gastric artery
5 Superior Mesenteric Artery
   Ileal artery
   Ileocolic artery
   Inferior pancreaticoduodenal
     artery
   Jejunal artery
6 Colic Artery, Right
7 Colic Artery, Left
8 Colic Artery, Middle
9 Renal Artery, Right
   Inferior suprarenal artery
   Renal segmental artery
A Renal Artery, Left
   See 9 Renal Artery, Right
B Inferior Mesenteric Artery
   Sigmoid artery
   Superior rectal artery
C Common Iliac Artery, Right
D Common Iliac Artery, Left
E Internal Iliac Artery, Right
   Deferential artery
   Hypogastric artery
   Iliolumbar artery
   Inferior gluteal artery
   Inferior vesical artery
   Internal pudendal artery
   Lateral sacral artery
   Middle rectal artery
   Obturator artery
   Superior gluteal artery
   Umbilical artery
   Uterine artery
   Vaginal artery
	F Internal Iliac Artery, Left
	   See E Internal Iliac Artery, Right
	H External Iliac Artery, Right
	   Deep circumflex iliac artery
	   Inferior epigastric artery
	J External Iliac Artery, Left
	   See H External Iliac Artery, Right
	K Femoral Artery, Right
	   Circumflex iliac artery
	   Deep femoral artery
	   Descending genicular artery
	   External pudendal artery
	   Superficial epigastric artery
	L Femoral Artery, Left
	   See K Femoral Artery, Right
	M Popliteal Artery, Right
	   Inferior genicular artery
	   Middle genicular artery
	   Superior genicular artery
	   Sural artery
	   Tibioperoneal trunk
	N Popliteal Artery, Left
	   See M Popliteal Artery, Right
	P Anterior Tibial Artery, Right
	   Anterior lateral malleolar
	     artery
	   Anterior medial malleolar
	     artery
	   Anterior tibial recurrent artery
	   Dorsalis pedis artery
	   Posterior tibial recurrent artery
	Q Anterior Tibial Artery, Left
	   See P Anterior Tibial Artery,
	   Right
	R Posterior Tibial Artery, Right
	S Posterior Tibial Artery, Left
	T Peroneal Artery, Right
	   Fibular artery
	U Peroneal Artery, Left
	   See T Peroneal Artery, Right
	V Foot Artery, Right
	   Arcuate artery
	   Dorsal metatarsal artery
	   Lateral plantar artery
	   Lateral tarsal artery
	   Medial plantar artery
	W Foot Artery, Left
	   See V Foot Artery, Right
	Y Lower Artery
	   Umbilical artery
		0 Open
		3 Percutaneous
		4 Percutaneous Endoscopic
			Z No Device	**X Diagnostic**
				Z No Qualifier

Lower Arteries

0 Medical and Surgical
4 Lower Arteries
C Extirpation   Definition: Taking or cutting out solid matter from a body part

Explanation: The solid matter may be an abnormal byproduct of a biological function or a foreign body; it may be imbedded in a body part or in the lumen of a tubular body part. The solid matter may or may not have been previously broken into pieces.

Body Part Character 4		Approach Character 5	Device Character 6	Qualifier Character 7
0 Abdominal Aorta Inferior phrenic artery Lumbar artery Median sacral artery Middle suprarenal artery Ovarian artery Testicular artery **1 Celiac Artery** Celiac trunk **2 Gastric Artery** Left gastric artery Right gastric artery **3 Hepatic Artery** Common hepatic artery Gastroduodenal artery Hepatic artery proper **4 Splenic Artery** Left gastroepiploic artery Pancreatic artery Short gastric artery **5 Superior Mesenteric Artery** Ileal artery Ileocolic artery Inferior pancreaticoduodenal artery Jejunal artery **6 Colic Artery, Right** **7 Colic Artery, Left** **8 Colic Artery, Middle** **9 Renal Artery, Right** Inferior suprarenal artery Renal segmental artery **A Renal Artery, Left** *See 9 Renal Artery, Right* **B Inferior Mesenteric Artery** Sigmoid artery Superior rectal artery **C Common Iliac Artery, Right** **D Common Iliac Artery, Left** **E Internal Iliac Artery, Right** Deferential artery Hypogastric artery Iliolumbar artery Inferior gluteal artery Inferior vesical artery Internal pudendal artery Lateral sacral artery Middle rectal artery Obturator artery Superior gluteal artery Umbilical artery Uterine artery Vaginal artery	**F Internal Iliac Artery, Left** *See E Internal Iliac Artery, Right* **H External Iliac Artery, Right** Deep circumflex iliac artery Inferior epigastric artery **J External Iliac Artery, Left** *See H External Iliac Artery, Right* **K Femoral Artery, Right** Circumflex iliac artery Deep femoral artery Descending genicular artery External pudendal artery Superficial epigastric artery **L Femoral Artery, Left** *See K Femoral Artery, Right* **M Popliteal Artery, Right** Inferior genicular artery Middle genicular artery Superior genicular artery Sural artery Tibioperoneal trunk **N Popliteal Artery, Left** *See M Popliteal Artery, Right* **P Anterior Tibial Artery, Right** Anterior lateral malleolar artery Anterior medial malleolar artery Anterior tibial recurrent artery Dorsalis pedis artery Posterior tibial recurrent artery **Q Anterior Tibial Artery, Left** *See P Anterior Tibial Artery, Right* **R Posterior Tibial Artery, Right** **S Posterior Tibial Artery, Left** **T Peroneal Artery, Right** Fibular artery **U Peroneal Artery, Left** *See T Peroneal Artery, Right* **V Foot Artery, Right** Arcuate artery Dorsal metatarsal artery Lateral plantar artery Lateral tarsal artery Medial plantar artery **W Foot Artery, Left** *See V Foot Artery, Right* **Y Lower Artery** Umbilical artery	**0 Open** **3 Percutaneous** **4 Percutaneous Endoscopic**	**Z No Device**	**Z No Qualifier**

LC Limited Coverage   NC Noncovered   ⊞ Combination Member   HAC associated procedure   Combination Only   DRG Non-OR   Non-OR   New/Revised in GREEN

224   ICD-10-PCS 2020

Ø   Medical and Surgical
4   Lower Arteries
H   Insertion   Definition: Putting in a nonbiological appliance that monitors, assists, performs, or prevents a physiological function but does not physically take the place of a body part
                Explanation: None

Body Part Character 4		Approach Character 5	Device Character 6	Qualifier Character 7
Ø **Abdominal Aorta** Inferior phrenic artery Lumbar artery Median sacral artery Middle suprarenal artery Ovarian artery Testicular artery		**Ø** Open **3** Percutaneous **4** Percutaneous Endoscopic	**2** Monitoring Device **3** Infusion Device **D** Intraluminal Device	**Z** No Qualifier

1 **Celiac Artery**
Celiac trunk
2 **Gastric Artery**
Left gastric artery
Right gastric artery
3 **Hepatic Artery**
Common hepatic artery
Gastroduodenal artery
Hepatic artery proper
4 **Splenic Artery**
Left gastroepiploic artery
Pancreatic artery
Short gastric artery
5 **Superior Mesenteric Artery**
Ileal artery
Ileocolic artery
Inferior pancreaticoduodenal
   artery
Jejunal artery
6 **Colic Artery, Right**
7 **Colic Artery, Left**
8 **Colic Artery, Middle**
9 **Renal Artery, Right**
Inferior suprarenal artery
Renal segmental artery
A **Renal Artery, Left**
See 9 Renal Artery, Right
B **Inferior Mesenteric Artery**
Sigmoid artery
Superior rectal artery
C **Common Iliac Artery, Right**
D **Common Iliac Artery, Left**
E **Internal Iliac Artery, Right**
Deferential artery
Hypogastric artery
Iliolumbar artery
Inferior gluteal artery
Inferior vesical artery
Internal pudendal artery
Lateral sacral artery
Middle rectal artery
Obturator artery
Superior gluteal artery
Umbilical artery
Uterine artery
Vaginal artery
	F **Internal Iliac Artery, Left**
	See E Internal Iliac Artery, Right
	H **External Iliac Artery, Right**
	Deep circumflex iliac artery
	Inferior epigastric artery
	J **External Iliac Artery, Left**
	See H External Iliac Artery, Right
	K **Femoral Artery, Right**
	Circumflex iliac artery
	Deep femoral artery
	Descending genicular artery
	External pudendal artery
	Superficial epigastric artery
	L **Femoral Artery, Left**
	See K Femoral Artery, Right
	M **Popliteal Artery, Right**
	Inferior genicular artery
	Middle genicular artery
	Superior genicular artery
	Sural artery
	Tibioperoneal trunk
	N **Popliteal Artery, Left**
	See M Popliteal Artery, Right
	P **Anterior Tibial Artery, Right**
	Anterior lateral malleolar artery
	Anterior medial malleolar artery
	Anterior tibial recurrent artery
	Dorsalis pedis artery
	Posterior tibial recurrent artery
	Q **Anterior Tibial Artery, Left**
	See P Anterior Tibial Artery,
	   Right
	R **Posterior Tibial Artery, Right**
	S **Posterior Tibial Artery, Left**
	T **Peroneal Artery, Right**
	Fibular artery
	U **Peroneal Artery, Left**
	See T Peroneal Artery, Right
	V **Foot Artery, Right**
	Arcuate artery
	Dorsal metatarsal artery
	Lateral plantar artery
	Lateral tarsal artery
	Medial plantar artery
	W **Foot Artery, Left**
	See V Foot Artery, Right
		Ø Open
		3 Percutaneous
		4 Percutaneous Endoscopic
			3 Infusion Device
			D Intraluminal Device
				Z No Qualifier

Y **Lower Artery** Umbilical artery		**Ø** Open **3** Percutaneous **4** Percutaneous Endoscopic	**2** Monitoring Device **3** Infusion Device **D** Intraluminal Device **Y** Other Device	**Z** No Qualifier

Non-OR   04HØ[Ø,3,4][2,3]Z
Non-OR   04H[1,2,3,4,5,6,7,8,9,A,B,C,D,E,F,H,J,K,L,M,N,P,Q,R,S,T,U,V,W][Ø,3,4]3Z
Non-OR   04HY32Z
Non-OR   04HY[Ø,3,4]3Z
Non-OR   04HY[3,4]YZ

0   Medical and Surgical
4   Lower Arteries
J   Inspection   Definition: Visually and/or manually exploring a body part

Explanation: Visual exploration may be performed with or without optical instrumentation. Manual exploration may be performed directly or through intervening body layers.

Body Part Character 4	Approach Character 5	Device Character 6	Qualifier Character 7
Y Lower Artery Umbilical artery	0 Open 3 Percutaneous 4 Percutaneous Endoscopic X External	Z No Device	Z No Qualifier

Non-OR   04JY[3,4,X]ZZ

0   Medical and Surgical
4   Lower Arteries
L   Occlusion   Definition: Completely closing an orifice or the lumen of a tubular body part

Explanation: The orifice can be a natural orifice or an artificially created orifice

Body Part Character 4	Approach Character 5	Device Character 6	Qualifier Character 7

0 Abdominal Aorta
   Inferior phrenic artery
   Lumbar artery
   Median sacral artery
   Middle suprarenal artery
   Ovarian artery
   Testicular artery
	0 Open
	4 Percutaneous Endoscopic
		C Extraluminal Device
		D Intraluminal Device
		Z No Device
			Z No Qualifier

0 Abdominal Aorta
   Inferior phrenic artery
   Lumbar artery
   Median sacral artery
   Middle suprarenal artery
   Ovarian artery
   Testicular artery
	3 Percutaneous	C Extraluminal Device
		Z No Device
			Z No Qualifier

0 Abdominal Aorta
   Inferior phrenic artery
   Lumbar artery
   Median sacral artery
   Middle suprarenal artery
   Ovarian artery
   Testicular artery
	3 Percutaneous	D Intraluminal Device	J Temporary
			Z No Qualifier

04L Continued on next page

LC Limited Coverage   NC Noncovered   ⊞ Combination Member   HAC associated procedure   Combination Only   DRG Non-OR   Non-OR   New/Revised in GREEN

226   ICD-10-PCS 2020

0   Medical and Surgical
4   Lower Arteries
L   Occlusion

04L Continued

Definition: Completely closing an orifice or the lumen of a tubular body part
Explanation: The orifice can be a natural orifice or an artificially created orifice

Body Part Character 4		Approach Character 5	Device Character 6	Qualifier Character 7

1 Celiac Artery
  Celiac trunk
2 Gastric Artery
  Left gastric artery
  Right gastric artery
3 Hepatic Artery
  Common hepatic artery
  Gastroduodenal artery
  Hepatic artery proper
4 Splenic Artery
  Left gastroepiploic artery
  Pancreatic artery
  Short gastric artery
5 Superior Mesenteric Artery
  Ileal artery
  Ileocolic artery
  Inferior pancreaticoduodenal
    artery
  Jejunal artery
6 Colic Artery, Right
7 Colic Artery, Left
8 Colic Artery, Middle
9 Renal Artery, Right
  Inferior suprarenal artery
  Renal segmental artery
A Renal Artery, Left
  See 9 Renal Artery, Right
B Inferior Mesenteric Artery
  Sigmoid artery
  Superior rectal artery
C Common Iliac Artery, Right
D Common Iliac Artery, Left
H External Iliac Artery, Right
  Deep circumflex iliac artery
  Inferior epigastric artery
J External Iliac Artery, Left
  See H External Iliac Artery, Right
	K Femoral Artery, Right
	  Circumflex iliac artery
	  Deep femoral artery
	  Descending genicular artery
	  External pudendal artery
	  Superficial epigastric artery
	L Femoral Artery, Left
	  See K Femoral Artery, Right
	M Popliteal Artery, Right
	  Inferior genicular artery
	  Middle genicular artery
	  Superior genicular artery
	  Sural artery
	  Tibioperoneal trunk
	N Popliteal Artery, Left
	  See M Popliteal Artery, Right
	P Anterior Tibial Artery, Right
	  Anterior lateral malleolar
	    artery
	  Anterior medial malleolar
	    artery
	  Anterior tibial recurrent artery
	  Dorsalis pedis artery
	  Posterior tibial recurrent artery
	Q Anterior Tibial Artery, Left
	  See P Anterior Tibial Artery,
	    Right
	R Posterior Tibial Artery, Right
	S Posterior Tibial Artery, Left
	T Peroneal Artery, Right
	  Fibular artery
	U Peroneal Artery, Left
	  See T Peroneal Artery, Right
	V Foot Artery, Right
	  Arcuate artery
	  Dorsal metatarsal artery
	  Lateral plantar artery
	  Lateral tarsal artery
	  Medial plantar artery
	W Foot Artery, Left
	  See V Foot Artery, Right
	Y Lower Artery
	  Umbilical artery
		0 Open
		3 Percutaneous
		4 Percutaneous Endoscopic
			C Extraluminal Device
			D Intraluminal Device
			Z No Device
				Z No Qualifier

E Internal Iliac Artery, Right
  Deferential artery
  Hypogastric artery
  Iliolumbar artery
  Inferior gluteal artery
  Inferior vesical artery
  Internal pudendal artery
  Lateral sacral artery
  Middle rectal artery
  Obturator artery
  Superior gluteal artery
  Umbilical artery
  Uterine artery
  Vaginal artery
		0 Open
		3 Percutaneous
		4 Percutaneous Endoscopic
			C Extraluminal Device
			D Intraluminal Device
			Z No Device
				T Uterine Artery, Right ♀
				Z No Qualifier

F Internal Iliac Artery, Left
  Deferential artery
  Hypogastric artery
  Iliolumbar artery
  Inferior gluteal artery
  Inferior vesical artery
  Internal pudendal artery
  Lateral sacral artery
  Middle rectal artery
  Obturator artery
  Superior gluteal artery
  Umbilical artery
  Uterine Artery
  Vaginal artery
		0 Open
		3 Percutaneous
		4 Percutaneous Endoscopic
			C Extraluminal Device
			D Intraluminal Device
			Z No Device
				U Uterine Artery, Left ♀
				Z No Qualifier

Non-OR   04L23DZ
♀   04LE[0,3,4][C,D,Z]T
♀   04LF[0,3,4][C,D,Z]U

LC Limited Coverage   NC Noncovered   ⊞ Combination Member   HAC associated procedure   Combination Only   DRG Non-OR   Non-OR   New/Revised in GREEN

Lower Arteries

0   Medical and Surgical
4   Lower Arteries
N   Release

Definition: Freeing a body part from an abnormal physical constraint by cutting or by the use of force

Explanation: Some of the restraining tissue may be taken out but none of the body part is taken out

Body Part Character 4		Approach Character 5	Device Character 6	Qualifier Character 7
0 Abdominal Aorta Inferior phrenic artery Lumbar artery Median sacral artery Middle suprarenal artery Ovarian artery Testicular artery	**F Internal Iliac Artery, Left** *See E Internal Iliac Artery,* *Right* **H External Iliac Artery, Right** Deep circumflex iliac artery Inferior epigastric artery	**0 Open** **3 Percutaneous** **4 Percutaneous Endoscopic**	**Z No Device**	**Z No Qualifier**
1 Celiac Artery Celiac trunk	**J External Iliac Artery, Left** *See H External Iliac Artery,* *Right*			
2 Gastric Artery Left gastric artery Right gastric artery	**K Femoral Artery, Right** Circumflex iliac artery Deep femoral artery			
3 Hepatic Artery Common hepatic artery Gastroduodenal artery Hepatic artery proper	Descending genicular artery External pudendal artery Superficial epigastric artery			
4 Splenic Artery Left gastroepiploic artery Pancreatic artery Short gastric artery	**L Femoral Artery, Left** *See K Femoral Artery, Right* **M Popliteal Artery, Right** Inferior genicular artery Middle genicular artery Superior genicular artery			
5 Superior Mesenteric Artery Ileal artery Ileocolic artery Inferior pancreaticoduodenal artery Jejunal artery	Sural artery Tibioperoneal trunk **N Popliteal Artery, Left** *See M Popliteal Artery, Right*			
6 Colic Artery, Right	**P Anterior Tibial Artery, Right** Anterior lateral malleolar artery			
7 Colic Artery, Left	Anterior medial malleolar artery			
8 Colic Artery, Middle	Anterior tibial recurrent artery			
9 Renal Artery, Right Inferior suprarenal artery Renal segmental artery	Dorsalis pedis artery Posterior tibial recurrent artery			
A Renal Artery, Left *See 9 Renal Artery, Right*	**Q Anterior Tibial Artery, Left** *See P Anterior Tibial Artery,* *Right*			
B Inferior Mesenteric Artery Sigmoid artery Superior rectal artery	**R Posterior Tibial Artery,** **Right**			
C Common Iliac Artery, Right	**S Posterior Tibial Artery, Left**			
D Common Iliac Artery, Left	**T Peroneal Artery, Right** Fibular artery			
E Internal Iliac Artery, Right Deferential artery Hypogastric artery Iliolumbar artery Inferior gluteal artery Inferior vesical artery Internal pudendal artery Lateral sacral artery Middle rectal artery Obturator artery Superior gluteal artery Umbilical artery Uterine artery Vaginal artery	**U Peroneal Artery, Left** *See T Peroneal Artery, Right* **V Foot Artery, Right** Arcuate artery Dorsal metatarsal artery Lateral plantar artery Lateral tarsal artery Medial plantar artery **W Foot Artery, Left** *See V Foot Artery, Right* **Y Lower Artery** Umbilical artery			

LC Limited Coverage   **NC** Noncovered   ⊞ Combination Member   HAC associated procedure   Combination Only   DRG Non-OR   Non-OR   New/Revised in **GREEN**

Ø   **Medical and Surgical**
4   **Lower Arteries**
P   **Removal**   Definition: Taking out or off a device from a body part

Explanation: If a device is taken out and a similar device put in without cutting or puncturing the skin or mucous membrane, the procedure is coded to the root operation CHANGE. Otherwise, the procedure for taking out a device is coded to the root operation REMOVAL.

Body Part Character 4	Approach Character 5	Device Character 6	Qualifier Character 7

Y   Lower Artery
      Umbilical artery
	Ø Open
	3 Percutaneous
	4 Percutaneous Endoscopic
		Ø Drainage Device
		2 Monitoring Device
		3 Infusion Device
		7 Autologous Tissue
		      Substitute
		C Extraluminal Device
		D Intraluminal Device
		J Synthetic Substitute
		K Nonautologous Tissue
		      Substitute
		Y Other Device
			Z No Qualifier

Y Lower Artery Umbilical artery	**X** External	**Ø** Drainage Device **1** Radioactive Element **2** Monitoring Device **3** Infusion Device **D** Intraluminal Device	**Z** No Qualifier

Non-OR   Ø4PY3[Ø,2,3,D]Z
Non-OR   Ø4PY[3,4]YZ
Non-OR   Ø4PYX[Ø,1,2,3,D]Z

Ø **Medical and Surgical**
4 **Lower Arteries**
Q **Repair** Definition: Restoring, to the extent possible, a body part to its normal anatomic structure and function

Explanation: Used only when the method to accomplish the repair is not one of the other root operations

Body Part Character 4		Approach Character 5	Device Character 6	Qualifier Character 7
Ø **Abdominal Aorta**	**F** **Internal Iliac Artery, Left**	**Ø** Open	**Z** No Device	**Z** No Qualifier
Inferior phrenic artery	*See E Internal Iliac Artery,*	**3** Percutaneous		
Lumbar artery	*Right*	**4** Percutaneous Endoscopic		
Median sacral artery	**H** **External Iliac Artery, Right**			
Middle suprarenal artery	Deep circumflex iliac artery			
Ovarian artery	Inferior epigastric artery			
Testicular artery	**J** **External Iliac Artery, Left**			
1 **Celiac Artery**	*See H External Iliac Artery,*			
Celiac trunk	*Right*			
2 **Gastric Artery**	**K** **Femoral Artery, Right**			
Left gastric artery	Circumflex iliac artery			
Right gastric artery	Deep femoral artery			
3 **Hepatic Artery**	Descending genicular artery			
Common hepatic artery	External pudendal artery			
Gastroduodenal artery	Superficial epigastric artery			
Hepatic artery proper	**L** **Femoral Artery, Left**			
4 **Splenic Artery**	*See K Femoral Artery, Right*			
Left gastroepiploic artery	**M** **Popliteal Artery, Right**			
Pancreatic artery	Inferior genicular artery			
Short gastric artery	Middle genicular artery			
5 **Superior Mesenteric Artery**	Superior genicular artery			
Ileal artery	Sural artery			
Ileocolic artery	Tibioperoneal trunk			
Inferior pancreaticoduodenal	**N** **Popliteal Artery, Left**			
artery	*See M Popliteal Artery, Right*			
Jejunal artery	**P** **Anterior Tibial Artery, Right**			
6 **Colic Artery, Right**	Anterior lateral malleolar			
7 **Colic Artery, Left**	artery			
8 **Colic Artery, Middle**	Anterior medial malleolar			
9 **Renal Artery, Right**	artery			
Inferior suprarenal artery	Anterior tibial recurrent			
Renal segmental artery	artery			
A **Renal Artery, Left**	Dorsalis pedis artery			
See 9 Renal Artery, Right	Posterior tibial recurrent			
B **Inferior Mesenteric Artery**	artery			
Sigmoid artery	**Q** **Anterior Tibial Artery, Left**			
Superior rectal artery	*See P Anterior Tibial Artery,*			
C **Common Iliac Artery, Right**	*Right*			
D **Common Iliac Artery, Left**	**R** **Posterior Tibial Artery,**			
E **Internal Iliac Artery, Right**	**Right**			
Deferential artery	**S** **Posterior Tibial Artery, Left**			
Hypogastric artery	**T** **Peroneal Artery, Right**			
Iliolumbar artery	Fibular artery			
Inferior gluteal artery	**U** **Peroneal Artery, Left**			
Inferior vesical artery	*See T Peroneal Artery, Right*			
Internal pudendal artery	**V** **Foot Artery, Right**			
Lateral sacral artery	Arcuate artery			
Middle rectal artery	Dorsal metatarsal artery			
Obturator artery	Lateral plantar artery			
Superior gluteal artery	Lateral tarsal artery			
Umbilical artery	Medial plantar artery			
Uterine artery	**W** **Foot Artery, Left**			
Vaginal artery	*See V Foot Artery, Right*			
	Y **Lower Artery**			
	Umbilical artery			

LC Limited Coverage NC Noncovered ⊞ Combination Member HAC associated procedure Combination Only DRG Non-OR Non-OR New/Revised in GREEN

230 ICD-10-PCS 2020

0   Medical and Surgical
4   Lower Arteries
R   Replacement   Definition: Putting in or on biological or synthetic material that physically takes the place and/or function of all or a portion of a body part
Explanation: The body part may have been taken out or replaced, or may be taken out, physically eradicated, or rendered nonfunctional during the REPLACEMENT procedure. A REMOVAL procedure is coded for taking out the device used in a previous replacement procedure.

Body Part Character 4		Approach Character 5	Device Character 6	Qualifier Character 7

0 Abdominal Aorta
   Inferior phrenic artery
   Lumbar artery
   Median sacral artery
   Middle suprarenal artery
   Ovarian artery
   Testicular artery
1 Celiac Artery
   Celiac trunk
2 Gastric Artery
   Left gastric artery
   Right gastric artery
3 Hepatic Artery
   Common hepatic artery
   Gastroduodenal artery
   Hepatic artery proper
4 Splenic Artery
   Left gastroepiploic artery
   Pancreatic artery
   Short gastric artery
5 Superior Mesenteric Artery
   Ileal artery
   Ileocolic artery
   Inferior pancreaticoduodenal
      artery
   Jejunal artery
6 Colic Artery, Right
7 Colic Artery, Left
8 Colic Artery, Middle
9 Renal Artery, Right
   Inferior suprarenal artery
   Renal segmental artery
A Renal Artery, Left
   See 9 Renal Artery, Right
B Inferior Mesenteric Artery
   Sigmoid artery
   Superior rectal artery
C Common Iliac Artery, Right
D Common Iliac Artery, Left
E Internal Iliac Artery, Right
   Deferential artery
   Hypogastric artery
   Iliolumbar artery
   Inferior gluteal artery
   Inferior vesical artery
   Internal pudendal artery
   Lateral sacral artery
   Middle rectal artery
   Obturator artery
   Superior gluteal artery
   Umbilical artery
   Uterine artery
   Vaginal artery
	F Internal Iliac Artery, Left
	   See E Internal Iliac Artery, Right
	H External Iliac Artery, Right
	   Deep circumflex iliac artery
	   Inferior epigastric artery
	J External Iliac Artery, Left
	   See H External Iliac Artery, Right
	K Femoral Artery, Right
	   Circumflex iliac artery
	   Deep femoral artery
	   Descending genicular artery
	   External pudendal artery
	   Superficial epigastric artery
	L Femoral Artery, Left
	   See K Femoral Artery, Right
	M Popliteal Artery, Right
	   Inferior genicular artery
	   Middle genicular artery
	   Superior genicular artery
	   Sural artery
	   Tibioperoneal trunk
	N Popliteal Artery, Left
	   See M Popliteal Artery, Right
	P Anterior Tibial Artery, Right
	   Anterior lateral malleolar
	      artery
	   Anterior medial malleolar
	      artery
	   Anterior tibial recurrent artery
	   Dorsalis pedis artery
	   Posterior tibial recurrent artery
	Q Anterior Tibial Artery, Left
	   See P Anterior Tibial Artery,
	      Right
	R Posterior Tibial Artery, Right
	S Posterior Tibial Artery, Left
	T Peroneal Artery, Right
	   Fibular artery
	U Peroneal Artery, Left
	   See T Peroneal Artery, Right
	V Foot Artery, Right
	   Arcuate artery
	   Dorsal metatarsal artery
	   Lateral plantar artery
	   Lateral tarsal artery
	   Medial plantar artery
	W Foot Artery, Left
	   See V Foot Artery, Right
	Y Lower Artery
	   Umbilical artery
		0 Open
		4 Percutaneous Endoscopic
			7 Autologous Tissue
			   Substitute
			J Synthetic Substitute
			K Nonautologous Tissue
			   Substitute
				Z No Qualifier

Ø   Medical and Surgical
4   Lower Arteries
S   Reposition   Definition: Moving to its normal location, or other suitable location, all or a portion of a body part

Explanation: The body part is moved to a new location from an abnormal location, or from a normal location where it is not functioning correctly. The body part may or may not be cut out or off to be moved to the new location.

Body Part Character 4		Approach Character 5	Device Character 6	Qualifier Character 7

Ø Abdominal Aorta
Inferior phrenic artery
Lumbar artery
Median sacral artery
Middle suprarenal artery
Ovarian artery
Testicular artery
1 Celiac Artery
Celiac trunk
2 Gastric Artery
Left gastric artery
Right gastric artery
3 Hepatic Artery
Common hepatic artery
Gastroduodenal artery
Hepatic artery proper
4 Splenic Artery
Left gastroepiploic artery
Pancreatic artery
Short gastric artery
5 Superior Mesenteric Artery
Ileal artery
Ileocolic artery
Inferior pancreaticoduodenal
    artery
Jejunal artery
6 Colic Artery, Right
7 Colic Artery, Left
8 Colic Artery, Middle
9 Renal Artery, Right
Inferior suprarenal artery
Renal segmental artery
A Renal Artery, Left
See 9 Renal Artery, Right
B Inferior Mesenteric Artery
Sigmoid artery
Superior rectal artery
C Common Iliac Artery, Right
D Common Iliac Artery, Left
E Internal Iliac Artery, Right
Deferential artery
Hypogastric artery
Iliolumbar artery
Inferior gluteal artery
Inferior vesical artery
Internal pudendal artery
Lateral sacral artery
Middle rectal artery
Obturator artery
Superior gluteal artery
Umbilical artery
Uterine artery
Vaginal artery
	F Internal Iliac Artery, Left
	See E Internal Iliac Artery, Right
	H External Iliac Artery, Right
	Deep circumflex iliac artery
	Inferior epigastric artery
	J External Iliac Artery, Left
	See H External Iliac Artery, Right
	K Femoral Artery, Right
	Circumflex iliac artery
	Deep femoral artery
	Descending genicular artery
	External pudendal artery
	Superficial epigastric artery
	L Femoral Artery, Left
	See K Femoral Artery, Right
	M Popliteal Artery, Right
	Inferior genicular artery
	Middle genicular artery
	Superior genicular artery
	Sural artery
	Tibioperoneal trunk
	N Popliteal Artery, Left
	See M Popliteal Artery, Right
	P Anterior Tibial Artery, Right
	Anterior lateral malleolar
	    artery
	Anterior medial malleolar
	    artery
	Anterior tibial recurrent artery
	Dorsalis pedis artery
	Posterior tibial recurrent artery
	Q Anterior Tibial Artery, Left
	See P Anterior Tibial Artery,
	Right
	R Posterior Tibial Artery, Right
	S Posterior Tibial Artery, Left
	T Peroneal Artery, Right
	Fibular artery
	U Peroneal Artery, Left
	See T Peroneal Artery, Right
	V Foot Artery, Right
	Arcuate artery
	Dorsal metatarsal artery
	Lateral plantar artery
	Lateral tarsal artery
	Medial plantar artery
	W Foot Artery, Left
	See V Foot Artery, Right
	Y Lower Artery
	Umbilical artery
		Ø Open
		3 Percutaneous
		4 Percutaneous Endoscopic
			Z No Device	**Z No Qualifier**

0   **Medical and Surgical**
4   **Lower Arteries**
U   **Supplement**

Definition: Putting in or on biological or synthetic material that physically reinforces and/or augments the function of a portion of a body part

Explanation: The biological material is non-living, or is living and from the same individual. The body part may have been previously replaced, and the SUPPLEMENT procedure is performed to physically reinforce and/or augment the function of the replaced body part.

Body Part — Character 4		Approach — Character 5	Device — Character 6	Qualifier — Character 7
0 **Abdominal Aorta** Inferior phrenic artery Lumbar artery Median sacral artery Middle suprarenal artery Ovarian artery Testicular artery **1** **Celiac Artery** Celiac trunk **2** **Gastric Artery** Left gastric artery Right gastric artery **3** **Hepatic Artery** Common hepatic artery Gastroduodenal artery Hepatic artery proper **4** **Splenic Artery** Left gastroepiploic artery Pancreatic artery Short gastric artery **5** **Superior Mesenteric Artery** Ileal artery Ileocolic artery Inferior pancreaticoduodenal artery Jejunal artery **6** **Colic Artery, Right** **7** **Colic Artery, Left** **8** **Colic Artery, Middle** **9** **Renal Artery, Right** Inferior suprarenal artery Renal segmental artery **A** **Renal Artery, Left** *See 9 Renal Artery, Right* **B** **Inferior Mesenteric Artery** Sigmoid artery Superior rectal artery **C** **Common Iliac Artery, Right** **D** **Common Iliac Artery, Left** **E** **Internal Iliac Artery, Right** Deferential artery Hypogastric artery Iliolumbar artery Inferior gluteal artery Inferior vesical artery Internal pudendal artery Lateral sacral artery Middle rectal artery Obturator artery Superior gluteal artery Umbilical artery Uterine artery Vaginal artery	**F** **Internal Iliac Artery, Left** *See E Internal Iliac Artery, Right* **H** **External Iliac Artery, Right** Deep circumflex iliac artery Inferior epigastric artery **J** **External Iliac Artery, Left** *See H External Iliac Artery, Right* **K** **Femoral Artery, Right** Circumflex iliac artery Deep femoral artery Descending genicular artery External pudendal artery Superficial epigastric artery **L** **Femoral Artery, Left** *See K Femoral Artery, Right* **M** **Popliteal Artery, Right** Inferior genicular artery Middle genicular artery Superior genicular artery Sural artery Tibioperoneal trunk **N** **Popliteal Artery, Left** *See M Popliteal Artery, Right* **P** **Anterior Tibial Artery, Right** Anterior lateral malleolar artery Anterior medial malleolar artery Anterior tibial recurrent artery Dorsalis pedis artery Posterior tibial recurrent artery **Q** **Anterior Tibial Artery, Left** *See P Anterior Tibial Artery, Right* **R** **Posterior Tibial Artery, Right** **S** **Posterior Tibial Artery, Left** **T** **Peroneal Artery, Right** Fibular artery **U** **Peroneal Artery, Left** *See T Peroneal Artery, Right* **V** **Foot Artery, Right** Arcuate artery Dorsal metatarsal artery Lateral plantar artery Lateral tarsal artery Medial plantar artery **W** **Foot Artery, Left** *See V Foot Artery, Right* **Y** **Lower Artery** Umbilical artery	**0** Open **3** Percutaneous **4** Percutaneous Endoscopic	**7** Autologous Tissue Substitute **J** Synthetic Substitute **K** Nonautologous Tissue Substitute	**Z** No Qualifier

LC Limited Coverage   **NC** Noncovered   ⊞ Combination Member   HAC associated procedure   Combination Only   DRG Non-OR   Non-OR   New/Revised in GREEN

ICD-10-PCS 2020   233

0 Medical and Surgical
4 Lower Arteries
V Restriction   Definition: Partially closing an orifice or the lumen of a tubular body part
Explanation: The orifice can be a natural orifice or an artificially created orifice

Body Part Character 4		Approach Character 5	Device Character 6	Qualifier Character 7
0 Abdominal Aorta Inferior phrenic artery Lumbar artery Median sacral artery Middle suprarenal artery Ovarian artery Testicular artery		**0 Open** **3 Percutaneous** **4 Percutaneous Endoscopic**	**C Extraluminal Device** **E Intraluminal Device, Branched or Fenestrated, One or Two Arteries** **F Intraluminal Device, Branched or Fenestrated, Three or More Arteries** **Z No Device**	**Z No Qualifier**
0 Abdominal Aorta Inferior phrenic artery Lumbar artery Median sacral artery Middle suprarenal artery Ovarian artery Testicular artery		**0 Open** **3 Percutaneous** **4 Percutaneous Endoscopic**	**D Intraluminal Device**	**J Temporary** **Z No Qualifier**
1 Celiac Artery Celiac trunk **2 Gastric Artery** Left gastric artery Right gastric artery **3 Hepatic Artery** Common hepatic artery Gastroduodenal artery Hepatic artery proper **4 Splenic Artery** Left gastroepiploic artery Pancreatic artery Short gastric artery **5 Superior Mesenteric Artery** Ileal artery Ileocolic artery Inferior pancreaticoduodenal artery Jejunal artery **6 Colic Artery, Right** **7 Colic Artery, Left** **8 Colic Artery, Middle** **9 Renal Artery, Right** Inferior suprarenal artery Renal segmental artery **A Renal Artery, Left** *See 9 Renal Artery, Right* **B Inferior Mesenteric Artery** Sigmoid artery Superior rectal artery **E Internal Iliac Artery, Right** Deferential artery Hypogastric artery Iliolumbar artery Inferior gluteal artery Inferior vesical artery Internal pudendal artery Lateral sacral artery Middle rectal artery Obturator artery Superior gluteal artery Umbilical artery Uterine artery Vaginal artery **F Internal Iliac Artery, Left** *See E Internal Iliac Artery, Right*	**H External Iliac Artery, Right** Deep circumflex iliac artery Inferior epigastric artery **J External Iliac Artery, Left** *See H External Iliac Artery, Right* **K Femoral Artery, Right** Circumflex iliac artery Deep femoral artery Descending genicular artery External pudendal artery Superficial epigastric artery **L Femoral Artery, Left** *See K Femoral Artery, Right* **M Popliteal Artery, Right** Inferior genicular artery Middle genicular artery Superior genicular artery Sural artery Tibioperoneal trunk **N Popliteal Artery, Left** *See M Popliteal Artery, Right* **P Anterior Tibial Artery, Right** Anterior lateral malleolar artery Anterior medial malleolar artery Anterior tibial recurrent artery Dorsalis pedis artery Posterior tibial recurrent artery **Q Anterior Tibial Artery, Left** *See P Anterior Tibial Artery, Right* **R Posterior Tibial Artery, Right** **S Posterior Tibial Artery, Left** **T Peroneal Artery, Right** Fibular artery **U Peroneal Artery, Left** *See T Peroneal Artery, Right* **V Foot Artery, Right** Arcuate artery Dorsal metatarsal artery Lateral plantar artery Lateral tarsal artery Medial plantar artery **W Foot Artery, Left** *See V Foot Artery, Right* **Y Lower Artery** Umbilical artery	**0 Open** **3 Percutaneous** **4 Percutaneous Endoscopic**	**C Extraluminal Device** **D Intraluminal Device** **Z No Device**	**Z No Qualifier**
C Common Iliac Artery, Right **D Common Iliac Artery, Left**		**0 Open** **3 Percutaneous** **4 Percutaneous Endoscopic**	**C Extraluminal Device** **D Intraluminal Device** **E Intraluminal Device, Branched or Fenestrated, One or Two Arteries** **Z No Device**	**Z No Qualifier**

0   **Medical and Surgical**
4   **Lower Arteries**
W   **Revision**   Definition: Correcting, to the extent possible, a portion of a malfunctioning device or the position of a displaced device

Explanation: Revision can include correcting a malfunctioning or displaced device by taking out or putting in components of the device such as a screw or pin

Body Part Character 4	Approach Character 5	Device Character 6	Qualifier Character 7
Y Lower Artery Umbilical artery	**0** Open **3** Percutaneous **4** Percutaneous Endoscopic	**0** Drainage Device **2** Monitoring Device **3** Infusion Device **7** Autologous Tissue Substitute **C** Extraluminal Device **D** Intraluminal Device **J** Synthetic Substitute **K** Nonautologous Tissue Substitute **Y** Other Device	**Z** No Qualifier
Y Lower Artery Umbilical artery	**X** External	**0** Drainage Device **2** Monitoring Device **3** Infusion Device **7** Autologous Tissue Substitute **C** Extraluminal Device **D** Intraluminal Device **J** Synthetic Substitute **K** Nonautologous Tissue Substitute	**Z** No Qualifier

Non-OR   04WY3[0,2,3,D]Z
Non-OR   04WY[3,4]YZ
Non-OR   04WYX[0,2,3,7,C,D,J,K]Z

Upper Veins Ø51–Ø5W

Character Meanings

This Character Meaning table is provided as a guide to assist the user in the identification of character members that may be found in this section of code tables. It **SHOULD NOT** be used to build a PCS code.

Operation–Character 3		Body Part–Character 4		Approach–Character 5		Device–Character 6		Qualifier–Character 7	
1	Bypass	Ø	Azygos Vein	Ø	Open	Ø	Drainage Device	1	Drug-Coated Balloon
5	Destruction	1	Hemiazygos Vein	3	Percutaneous	2	Monitoring Device	X	Diagnostic
7	Dilation	3	Innominate Vein, Right	4	Percutaneous Endoscopic	3	Infusion Device	Y	Upper Vein
9	Drainage	4	Innominate Vein, Left	X	External	7	Autologous Tissue Substitute	Z	No Qualifier
B	Excision	5	Subclavian Vein, Right			9	Autologous Venous Tissue		
C	Extirpation	6	Subclavian Vein, Left			A	Autologous Arterial Tissue		
D	Extraction	7	Axillary Vein, Right			C	Extraluminal Device		
H	Insertion	8	Axillary Vein, Left			D	Intraluminal Device		
J	Inspection	9	Brachial Vein, Right			J	Synthetic Substitute		
L	Occlusion	A	Brachial Vein, Left			K	Nonautologous Tissue Substitute		
N	Release	B	Basilic Vein, Right			M	Neurostimulator Lead		
P	Removal	C	Basilic Vein, Left			Y	Other Device		
Q	Repair	D	Cephalic Vein, Right			Z	No Device		
R	Replacement	F	Cephalic Vein, Left						
S	Reposition	G	Hand Vein, Right						
U	Supplement	H	Hand Vein, Left						
V	Restriction	L	Intracranial Vein						
W	Revision	M	Internal Jugular Vein, Right						
		N	Internal Jugular Vein, Left						
		P	External Jugular Vein, Right						
		Q	External Jugular Vein, Left						
		R	Vertebral Vein, Right						
		S	Vertebral Vein, Left						
		T	Face Vein, Right						
		V	Face Vein, Left						
		Y	Upper Vein						

AHA Coding Clinic for table Ø51
2017, 3Q, 15   Bypass of innominate vein to atrial appendage

AHA Coding Clinic for table Ø59
2018, 3Q, 7   Catheter placement for treatment of congestive heart failure

AHA Coding Clinic for table Ø5B
2016, 2Q, 12   Resection of malignant neoplasm of infratemporal fossa

AHA Coding Clinic for table Ø5H
2016, 4Q, 97-98   Phrenic neurostimulator

AHA Coding Clinic for table Ø5P
2016, 4Q, 97-98   Phrenic neurostimulator

AHA Coding Clinic for table Ø5Q
2017, 3Q, 15   Bypass of innominate vein to atrial appendage

AHA Coding Clinic for table Ø5S
2013, 4Q, 125   Stage II cephalic vein transposition (superficialization) of arteriovenous fistula

AHA Coding Clinic for table Ø5W
2016, 4Q, 97-98   Phrenic neurostimulator

Head and Neck Veins

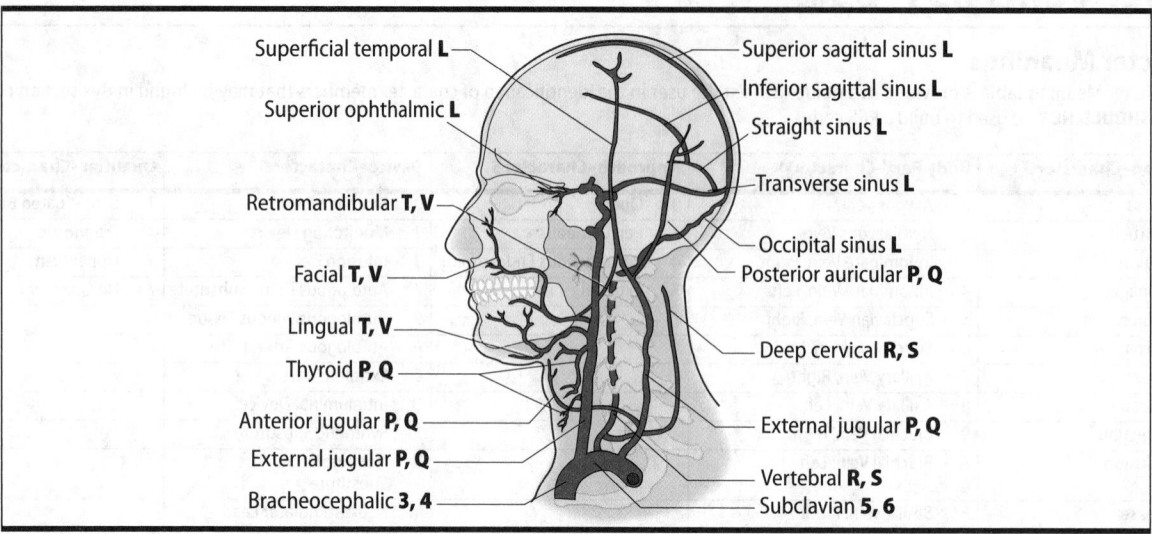

Superficial temporal **L**
Superior ophthalmic **L**
Retromandibular **T, V**
Facial **T, V**
Lingual **T, V**
Thyroid **P, Q**
Anterior jugular **P, Q**
External jugular **P, Q**
Bracheocephalic **3, 4**

Superior sagittal sinus **L**
Inferior sagittal sinus **L**
Straight sinus **L**
Transverse sinus **L**
Occipital sinus **L**
Posterior auricular **P, Q**
Deep cervical **R, S**
External jugular **P, Q**
Vertebral **R, S**
Subclavian **5, 6**

Upper Veins

Superficial temporal **L**
Vertebral **R, S**
Internal jugular **M, N**
External jugular **P, Q**
Subclavian **5, 6**
Innominate **3, 4**
Azygos **Ø**
Axillary **7,8**
Hemiazygos **1**
Brachial **9, A**
Cephalic **D, F**
Basilic **B, C**
Radial **9, A**
Ulnar **9, A**
Digital **G, H**

Ø Medical and Surgical
5 Upper Veins
1 Bypass

Definition: Altering the route of passage of the contents of a tubular body part

Explanation: Rerouting contents of a body part to a downstream area of the normal route, to a similar route and body part, or to an abnormal route and dissimilar body part. Includes one or more anastomoses, with or without the use of a device.

Body Part Character 4		Approach Character 5	Device Character 6	Qualifier Character 7
Ø Azygos Vein Right ascending lumbar vein Right subcostal vein **1 Hemiazygos Vein** Left ascending lumbar vein Left subcostal vein **3 Innominate Vein, Right** Brachiocephalic vein Inferior thyroid vein **4 Innominate Vein, Left** *See 3 Innominate Vein, Right* **5 Subclavian Vein, Right** **6 Subclavian Vein, Left** **7 Axillary Vein, Right** **8 Axillary Vein, Left** **9 Brachial Vein, Right** Radial vein Ulnar vein **A Brachial Vein, Left** *See 9 Brachial Vein, Right* **B Basilic Vein, Right** Median antebrachial vein Median cubital vein **C Basilic Vein, Left** *See B Basilic Vein, Right* **D Cephalic Vein, Right** Accessory cephalic vein **F Cephalic Vein, Left** *See D Cephalic Vein, Right* **G Hand Vein, Right** Dorsal metacarpal vein Palmar (volar) digital vein Palmar (volar) metacarpal vein Superficial palmar venous arch Volar (palmar) digital vein Volar (palmar) metacarpal vein	**H Hand Vein, Left** *See G Hand Vein, Right* **L Intracranial Vein** Anterior cerebral vein Basal (internal) cerebral vein Dural venous sinus Great cerebral vein Inferior cerebellar vein Inferior cerebral vein Internal (basal) cerebral vein Middle cerebral vein Ophthalmic vein Superior cerebellar vein Superior cerebral vein **M Internal Jugular Vein, Right** **N Internal Jugular Vein, Left** **P External Jugular Vein, Right** Posterior auricular vein **Q External Jugular Vein, Left** *See P External Jugular Vein, Right* **R Vertebral Vein, Right** Deep cervical vein Suboccipital venous plexus **S Vertebral Vein, Left** *See R Vertebral Vein, Right* **T Face Vein, Right** Angular vein Anterior facial vein Common facial vein Deep facial vein Frontal vein Posterior facial (retromandibular) vein Supraorbital vein **V Face Vein, Left** *See T Face Vein, Right*	**Ø Open** **4 Percutaneous Endoscopic**	**7 Autologous Tissue Substitute** **9 Autologous Venous Tissue** **A Autologous Arterial Tissue** **J Synthetic Substitute** **K Nonautologous Tissue Substitute** **Z No Device**	**Y Upper Vein**

LC Limited Coverage   NC Noncovered   ⊞ Combination Member   HAC associated procedure   Combination Only   DRG Non-OR   Non-OR   New/Revised in GREEN

ICD-10-PCS 2020   239

Ø51–Ø51

Upper Veins

Ø   **Medical and Surgical**
5   **Upper Veins**
5   **Destruction**   Definition: Physical eradication of all or a portion of a body part by the direct use of energy, force, or a destructive agent
                        Explanation: None of the body part is physically taken out

Body Part Character 4		Approach Character 5	Device Character 6	Qualifier Character 7
Ø **Azygos Vein** Right ascending lumbar vein Right subcostal vein **1** **Hemiazygos Vein** Left ascending lumbar vein Left subcostal vein **3** **Innominate Vein, Right** Brachiocephalic vein Inferior thyroid vein **4** **Innominate Vein, Left** *See 3 Innominate Vein, Right* **5** **Subclavian Vein, Right** **6** **Subclavian Vein, Left** **7** **Axillary Vein, Right** **8** **Axillary Vein, Left** **9** **Brachial Vein, Right** Radial vein Ulnar vein **A** **Brachial Vein, Left** *See 9 Brachial Vein, Right* **B** **Basilic Vein, Right** Median antebrachial vein Median cubital vein **C** **Basilic Vein, Left** *See B Basilic Vein, Right* **D** **Cephalic Vein, Right** Accessory cephalic vein **F** **Cephalic Vein, Left** *See D Cephalic Vein, Right* **G** **Hand Vein, Right** Dorsal metacarpal vein Palmar (volar) digital vein Palmar (volar) metacarpal vein Superficial palmar venous arch Volar (palmar) digital vein Volar (palmar) metacarpal vein	**H** **Hand Vein, Left** *See G Hand Vein, Right* **L** **Intracranial Vein** Anterior cerebral vein Basal (internal) cerebral vein Dural venous sinus Great cerebral vein Inferior cerebellar vein Inferior cerebral vein Internal (basal) cerebral vein Middle cerebral vein Ophthalmic vein Superior cerebellar vein Superior cerebral vein **M** **Internal Jugular Vein, Right** **N** **Internal Jugular Vein, Left** **P** **External Jugular Vein, Right** Posterior auricular vein **Q** **External Jugular Vein, Left** *See P External Jugular Vein, Right* **R** **Vertebral Vein, Right** Deep cervical vein Suboccipital venous plexus **S** **Vertebral Vein, Left** *See R Vertebral Vein, Right* **T** **Face Vein, Right** Angular vein Anterior facial vein Common facial vein Deep facial vein Frontal vein Posterior facial (retromandibular) vein Supraorbital vein **V** **Face Vein, Left** *See T Face Vein, Right* **Y** **Upper Vein**	**Ø** Open **3** Percutaneous **4** Percutaneous Endoscopic	**Z** No Device	**Z** No Qualifier

Ø   **Medical and Surgical**
5   **Upper Veins**
7   **Dilation**   Definition: Expanding an orifice or the lumen of a tubular body part

                       Explanation: The orifice can be a natural orifice or an artificially created orifice. Accomplished by stretching a tubular body part using intraluminal pressure or by cutting part of the orifice or wall of the tubular body part.

Body Part Character 4		Approach Character 5	Device Character 6	Qualifier Character 7

Ø Azygos Vein
  Right ascending lumbar vein
  Right subcostal vein
1 Hemiazygos Vein
  Left ascending lumbar vein
  Left subcostal vein
G Hand Vein, Right
  Dorsal metacarpal vein
  Palmar (volar) digital vein
  Palmar (volar) metacarpal vein
  Superficial palmar venous arch
  Volar (palmar) digital vein
  Volar (palmar) metacarpal vein
H Hand Vein, Left
  See G Hand Vein, Right
L Intracranial Vein NC
  Anterior cerebral vein
  Basal (internal) cerebral vein
  Dural venous sinus
  Great cerebral vein
  Inferior cerebellar vein
  Inferior cerebral vein
  Internal (basal) cerebral vein
  Middle cerebral vein
  Ophthalmic vein
  Superior cerebellar vein
  Superior cerebral vein
	M Internal Jugular Vein, Right
	N Internal Jugular Vein, Left
	P External Jugular Vein, Right
	  Posterior auricular vein
	Q External Jugular Vein, Left
	  See P External Jugular Vein, Right
	R Vertebral Vein, Right
	  Deep cervical vein
	  Suboccipital venous plexus
	S Vertebral Vein, Left
	  See R Vertebral Vein, Right
	T Face Vein, Right
	  Angular vein
	  Anterior facial vein
	  Common facial vein
	  Deep facial vein
	  Frontal vein
	  Posterior facial
	    (retromandibular) vein
	  Supraorbital vein
	V Face Vein, Left
	  See T Face Vein, Right
	Y Upper Vein
		Ø Open
		3 Percutaneous
		4 Percutaneous Endoscopic
			D Intraluminal Device
			Z No Device
				Z No Qualifier

3 Innominate Vein, Right
  Brachiocephalic vein
  Inferior thyroid vein
4 Innominate Vein, Left
  See 3 Innominate Vein, Right
5 Subclavian Vein, Right
6 Subclavian Vein, Left
7 Axillary Vein, Right
8 Axillary Vein, Left
9 Brachial Vein, Right
  Radial vein
  Ulnar vein
	A Brachial Vein, Left
	  See 9 Brachial Vein, Right
	B Basilic Vein, Right
	  Median antebrachial vein
	  Median cubital vein
	C Basilic Vein, Left
	  See B Basilic Vein, Right
	D Cephalic Vein, Right
	  Accessory cephalic vein
	F Cephalic Vein, Left
	  See D Cephalic Vein, Right
		Ø Open
		3 Percutaneous
		4 Percutaneous Endoscopic
			D Intraluminal Device
			Z No Device
				1 Drug-Coated Balloon
				Z No Qualifier

NC   Ø57L[3,4]ZZ

LC Limited Coverage   NC Noncovered   ⊞ Combination Member   HAC associated procedure   Combination Only   DRG Non-OR   Non-OR   New/Revised in GREEN

ICD-10-PCS 2020   241

Ø Medical and Surgical
5 Upper Veins
9 Drainage   Definition: Taking or letting out fluids and/or gases from a body part
             Explanation: The qualifier DIAGNOSTIC is used to identify drainage procedures that are biopsies

Body Part Character 4		Approach Character 5	Device Character 6	Qualifier Character 7
Ø Azygos Vein Right ascending lumbar vein Right subcostal vein **1 Hemiazygos Vein** Left ascending lumbar vein Left subcostal vein **3 Innominate Vein, Right** Brachiocephalic vein Inferior thyroid vein **4 Innominate Vein, Left** *See 3 Innominate Vein, Right* **5 Subclavian Vein, Right** **6 Subclavian Vein, Left** **7 Axillary Vein, Right** **8 Axillary Vein, Left** **9 Brachial Vein, Right** Radial vein Ulnar vein **A Brachial Vein, Left** *See 9 Brachial Vein, Right* **B Basilic Vein, Right** Median antebrachial vein Median cubital vein **C Basilic Vein, Left** *See B Basilic Vein, Right* **D Cephalic Vein, Right** Accessory cephalic vein **F Cephalic Vein, Left** *See D Cephalic Vein, Right* **G Hand Vein, Right** Dorsal metacarpal vein Palmar (volar) digital vein Palmar (volar) metacarpal vein Superficial palmar venous arch Volar (palmar) digital vein Volar (palmar) metacarpal vein	**H Hand Vein, Left** *See G Hand Vein, Right* **L Intracranial Vein** Anterior cerebral vein Basal (internal) cerebral vein Dural venous sinus Great cerebral vein Inferior cerebellar vein Inferior cerebral vein Internal (basal) cerebral vein Middle cerebral vein Ophthalmic vein Superior cerebellar vein Superior cerebral vein **M Internal Jugular Vein, Right** **N Internal Jugular Vein, Left** **P External Jugular Vein, Right** Posterior auricular vein **Q External Jugular Vein, Left** *See P External Jugular Vein, Right* **R Vertebral Vein, Right** Deep cervical vein Suboccipital venous plexus **S Vertebral Vein, Left** *See R Vertebral Vein, Right* **T Face Vein, Right** Angular vein Anterior facial vein Common facial vein Deep facial vein Frontal vein Posterior facial (retromandibular) vein Supraorbital vein **V Face Vein, Left** *See T Face Vein, Right* **Y Upper Vein**	**Ø Open** **3 Percutaneous** **4 Percutaneous Endoscopic**	**Ø Drainage Device**	**Z No Qualifier**
Ø Azygos Vein Right ascending lumbar vein Right subcostal vein **1 Hemiazygos Vein** Left ascending lumbar vein Left subcostal vein **3 Innominate Vein, Right** Brachiocephalic vein Inferior thyroid vein **4 Innominate Vein, Left** *See 3 Innominate Vein, Right* **5 Subclavian Vein, Right** **6 Subclavian Vein, Left** **7 Axillary Vein, Right** **8 Axillary Vein, Left** **9 Brachial Vein, Right** Radial vein Ulnar vein **A Brachial Vein, Left** *See 9 Brachial Vein, Right* **B Basilic Vein, Right** Median antebrachial vein Median cubital vein **C Basilic Vein, Left** *See B Basilic Vein, Right* **D Cephalic Vein, Right** Accessory cephalic vein **F Cephalic Vein, Left** *See D Cephalic Vein, Right* **G Hand Vein, Right** Dorsal metacarpal vein Palmar (volar) digital vein Palmar (volar) metacarpal vein Superficial palmar venous arch Volar (palmar) digital vein Volar (palmar) metacarpal vein	**H Hand Vein, Left** *See G Hand Vein, Right* **L Intracranial Vein** Anterior cerebral vein Basal (internal) cerebral vein Dural venous sinus Great cerebral vein Inferior cerebellar vein Inferior cerebral vein Internal (basal) cerebral vein Middle cerebral vein Ophthalmic vein Superior cerebellar vein Superior cerebral vein **M Internal Jugular Vein, Right** **N Internal Jugular Vein, Left** **P External Jugular Vein, Right** Posterior auricular vein **Q External Jugular Vein, Left** *See P External Jugular Vein, Right* **R Vertebral Vein, Right** Deep cervical vein Suboccipital venous plexus **S Vertebral Vein, Left** *See R Vertebral Vein, Right* **T Face Vein, Right** Angular vein Anterior facial vein Common facial vein Deep facial vein Frontal vein Posterior facial (retromandibular) vein Supraorbital vein **V Face Vein, Left** *See T Face Vein, Right* **Y Upper Vein**	**Ø Open** **3 Percutaneous** **4 Percutaneous Endoscopic**	**Z No Device**	**X Diagnostic** **Z No Qualifier**

Non-OR   Ø59[Ø,1,3,4,5,6,7,8,9,A,B,C,D,F,G,H,L,M,N,P,Q,R,S,T,V,Y][Ø,3,4]ØZ
Non-OR   Ø59[Ø,1,3,4,5,6,7,8,9,A,B,C,D,F,G,H,L,M,N,P,Q,R,S,T,V,Y]3ZX
Non-OR   Ø59[Ø,1,3,4,5,6,7,8,9,A,B,C,D,F,G,H,L,M,N,P,Q,R,S,T,V,Y][Ø,3,4]ZZ

LC Limited Coverage   **NC** Noncovered   ⊞ Combination Member   HAC associated procedure   Combination Only   DRG Non-OR   Non-OR   New/Revised in GREEN

242   ICD-10-PCS 2020

Ø   Medical and Surgical
5   Upper Veins
B   Excision   Definition: Cutting out or off, without replacement, a portion of a body part

                     Explanation: The qualifier DIAGNOSTIC is used to identify excision procedures that are biopsies

Body Part Character 4		Approach Character 5	Device Character 6	Qualifier Character 7
Ø Azygos Vein Right ascending lumbar vein Right subcostal vein **1 Hemiazygos Vein** Left ascending lumbar vein Left subcostal vein **3 Innominate Vein, Right** Brachiocephalic vein Inferior thyroid vein **4 Innominate Vein, Left** *See 3 Innominate Vein, Right* **5 Subclavian Vein, Right** **6 Subclavian Vein, Left** **7 Axillary Vein, Right** **8 Axillary Vein, Left** **9 Brachial Vein, Right** Radial vein Ulnar vein **A Brachial Vein, Left** *See 9 Brachial Vein, Right* **B Basilic Vein, Right** Median antebrachial vein Median cubital vein **C Basilic Vein, Left** *See B Basilic Vein, Right* **D Cephalic Vein, Right** Accessory cephalic vein **F Cephalic Vein, Left** *See D Cephalic Vein, Right* **G Hand Vein, Right** Dorsal metacarpal vein Palmar (volar) digital vein Palmar (volar) metacarpal vein Superficial palmar venous arch Volar (palmar) digital vein Volar (palmar) metacarpal vein	**H Hand Vein, Left** *See G Hand Vein, Right* **L Intracranial Vein** Anterior cerebral vein Basal (internal) cerebral vein Dural venous sinus Great cerebral vein Inferior cerebellar vein Inferior cerebral vein Internal (basal) cerebral vein Middle cerebral vein Ophthalmic vein Superior cerebellar vein Superior cerebral vein **M Internal Jugular Vein, Right** **N Internal Jugular Vein, Left** **P External Jugular Vein, Right** Posterior auricular vein **Q External Jugular Vein, Left** *See P External Jugular Vein, Right* **R Vertebral Vein, Right** Deep cervical vein Suboccipital venous plexus **S Vertebral Vein, Left** *See R Vertebral Vein, Right* **T Face Vein, Right** Angular vein Anterior facial vein Common facial vein Deep facial vein Frontal vein Posterior facial (retromandibular) vein Supraorbital vein **V Face Vein, Left** *See T Face Vein, Right* **Y Upper Vein**	**Ø Open** **3 Percutaneous** **4 Percutaneous Endoscopic**	**Z No Device**	**X Diagnostic** **Z No Qualifier**

Upper Veins

0   **Medical and Surgical**
5   **Upper Veins**
C   **Extirpation**   Definition: Taking or cutting out solid matter from a body part

Explanation: The solid matter may be an abnormal byproduct of a biological function or a foreign body; it may be imbedded in a body part or in the lumen of a tubular body part. The solid matter may or may not have been previously broken into pieces.

Body Part Character 4		Approach Character 5	Device Character 6	Qualifier Character 7
0 **Azygos Vein** Right ascending lumbar vein Right subcostal vein **1** **Hemiazygos Vein** Left ascending lumbar vein Left subcostal vein **3** **Innominate Vein, Right** Brachiocephalic vein Inferior thyroid vein **4** **Innominate Vein, Left** *See 3 Innominate Vein, Right* **5** **Subclavian Vein, Right** **6** **Subclavian Vein, Left** **7** **Axillary Vein, Right** **8** **Axillary Vein, Left** **9** **Brachial Vein, Right** Radial vein Ulnar vein **A** **Brachial Vein, Left** *See 9 Brachial Vein, Right* **B** **Basilic Vein, Right** Median antebrachial vein Median cubital vein **C** **Basilic Vein, Left** *See B Basilic Vein, Right* **D** **Cephalic Vein, Right** Accessory cephalic vein **F** **Cephalic Vein, Left** *See D Cephalic Vein, Right* **G** **Hand Vein, Right** Dorsal metacarpal vein Palmar (volar) digital vein Palmar (volar) metacarpal vein Superficial palmar venous arch Volar (palmar) digital vein Volar (palmar) metacarpal vein	**H** **Hand Vein, Left** *See G Hand Vein, Right* **L** **Intracranial Vein** Anterior cerebral vein Basal (internal) cerebral vein Dural venous sinus Great cerebral vein Inferior cerebellar vein Inferior cerebral vein Internal (basal) cerebral vein Middle cerebral vein Ophthalmic vein Superior cerebellar vein Superior cerebral vein **M** **Internal Jugular Vein, Right** **N** **Internal Jugular Vein, Left** **P** **External Jugular Vein, Right** Posterior auricular vein **Q** **External Jugular Vein, Left** *See P External Jugular Vein,* *Right* **R** **Vertebral Vein, Right** Deep cervical vein Suboccipital venous plexus **S** **Vertebral Vein, Left** *See R Vertebral Vein, Right* **T** **Face Vein, Right** Angular vein Anterior facial vein Common facial vein Deep facial vein Frontal vein Posterior facial (retromandibular) vein Supraorbital vein **V** **Face Vein, Left** *See T Face Vein, Right* **Y** **Upper Vein**	**0** Open **3** Percutaneous **4** Percutaneous Endoscopic	**Z** No Device	**Z** No Qualifier

0   **Medical and Surgical**
5   **Upper Veins**
D   **Extraction**   Definition: Pulling or stripping out or off all or a portion of a body part by the use of force

Explanation: The qualifier DIAGNOSTIC is used to identify extraction procedures that are biopsies

Body Part Character 4		Approach Character 5	Device Character 6	Qualifier Character 7
9 **Brachial Vein, Right** Radial vein Ulnar vein **A** **Brachial Vein, Left** *See 9 Brachial Vein, Right* **B** **Basilic Vein, Right** Median antebrachial vein Median cubital vein **C** **Basilic Vein, Left** *See B Basilic Vein, Right* **D** **Cephalic Vein, Right** Accessory cephalic vein	**F** **Cephalic Vein, Left** *See D Cephalic Vein, Right* **G** **Hand Vein, Right** Dorsal metacarpal vein Palmar (volar) digital vein Palmar (volar) metacarpal vein Superficial palmar venous arch Volar (palmar) digital vein Volar (palmar) metacarpal vein **H** **Hand Vein, Left** *See G Hand Vein, Right* **Y** **Upper Vein**	**0** Open **3** Percutaneous	**Z** No Device	**Z** No Qualifier

LC Limited Coverage   **NC** Noncovered   ⊞ Combination Member   HAC associated procedure   Combination Only   DRG Non-OR   Non-OR   New/Revised in GREEN

244   ICD-10-PCS 2020

Ø   Medical and Surgical
5   Upper Veins
H   Insertion   Definition: Putting in a nonbiological appliance that monitors, assists, performs, or prevents a physiological function but does not physically take the place of a body part
                    Explanation: None

Body Part — Character 4		Approach — Character 5	Device — Character 6	Qualifier — Character 7
Ø Azygos Vein ⊞ Right ascending lumbar vein Right subcostal vein		**Ø** Open **3** Percutaneous **4** Percutaneous Endoscopic	**2** Monitoring Device **3** Infusion Device **D** Intraluminal Device **M** Neurostimulator Lead	**Z** No Qualifier
1 Hemiazygos Vein Left ascending lumbar vein Left subcostal vein **5 Subclavian Vein, Right** **6 Subclavian Vein, Left** **7 Axillary Vein, Right** **8 Axillary Vein, Left** **9 Brachial Vein, Right** Radial vein Ulnar vein **A Brachial Vein, Left** *See 9 Brachial Vein, Right* **B Basilic Vein, Right** Median antebrachial vein Median cubital vein **C Basilic Vein, Left** *See B Basilic Vein, Right* **D Cephalic Vein, Right** Accessory cephalic vein **F Cephalic Vein, Left** *See D Cephalic Vein, Right* **G Hand Vein, Right** Dorsal metacarpal vein Palmar (volar) digital vein Palmar (volar) metacarpal vein Superficial palmar venous arch Volar (palmar) digital vein Volar (palmar) metacarpal vein **H Hand Vein, Left** *See G Hand Vein, Right*	**L Intracranial Vein** Anterior cerebral vein Basal (internal) cerebral vein Dural venous sinus Great cerebral vein Inferior cerebellar vein Inferior cerebral vein Internal (basal) cerebral vein Middle cerebral vein Ophthalmic vein Superior cerebellar vein Superior cerebral vein **M Internal Jugular Vein, Right** **N Internal Jugular Vein, Left** **P External Jugular Vein, Right** Posterior auricular vein **Q External Jugular Vein, Left** *See P External Jugular Vein, Right* **R Vertebral Vein, Right** Deep cervical vein Suboccipital venous plexus **S Vertebral Vein, Left** *See R Vertebral Vein, Right* **T Face Vein, Right** Angular vein Anterior facial vein Common facial vein Deep facial vein Frontal vein Posterior facial (retromandibular) vein Supraorbital vein **V Face Vein, Left** *See T Face Vein, Right*	**Ø** Open **3** Percutaneous **4** Percutaneous Endoscopic	**3** Infusion Device **D** Intraluminal Device	**Z** No Qualifier
3 Innominate Vein, Right ⊞ Brachiocephalic vein Inferior thyroid vein **4 Innominate Vein, Left** ⊞ *See 3 Innominate Vein, Right*		**Ø** Open **3** Percutaneous **4** Percutaneous Endoscopic	**3** Infusion Device **D** Intraluminal Device **M** Neurostimulator Lead	**Z** No Qualifier
Y Upper Vein		**Ø** Open **3** Percutaneous **4** Percutaneous Endoscopic	**2** Monitoring Device **3** Infusion Device **D** Intraluminal Device **Y** Other Device	**Z** No Qualifier

Non-OR Ø5HØ[Ø,3,4]3Z	
Non-OR Ø5H[1,5,6,7,8,9,A,B,C,D,F,G,H,L,M,N,P,Q,R,S,T,V][Ø,3,4]3Z	
Non-OR Ø5H[3,4][Ø,3,4]3Z	
Non-OR Ø5HY[Ø,3,4]3Z	
Non-OR Ø5HY32Z	
Non-OR Ø5HY[3,4]YZ	
HAC Ø5HØ[3,4]3Z when reported with SDx J95.811	
HAC Ø5H[1,5,6][3,4]3Z when reported with SDx J95.811	
HAC Ø5H[M,N,P,Q]33Z when reported with SDx J95.811	
HAC Ø5H[3,4][3,4]3Z when reported with SDx J95.811	

See Appendix L for Procedure Combinations
⊞   Ø5HØ[Ø,3,4]MZ
⊞   Ø5H[3,4][Ø,3,4]MZ

LC Limited Coverage   **NC** Noncovered   ⊞ Combination Member   HAC associated procedure   Combination Only   DRG Non-OR   Non-OR   New/Revised in GREEN

Ø Medical and Surgical
5 Upper Veins
J Inspection   Definition: Visually and/or manually exploring a body part

Explanation: Visual exploration may be performed with or without optical instrumentation. Manual exploration may be performed directly or through intervening body layers.

Body Part Character 4	Approach Character 5	Device Character 6	Qualifier Character 7
Y Upper Vein	Ø Open 3 Percutaneous 4 Percutaneous Endoscopic X External	Z No Device	Z No Qualifier

Non-OR   Ø5JY[3,X]ZZ

Ø Medical and Surgical
5 Upper Veins
L Occlusion   Definition: Completely closing an orifice or the lumen of a tubular body part

Explanation: The orifice can be a natural orifice or an artificially created orifice

Body Part Character 4	Approach Character 5	Device Character 6	Qualifier Character 7
Ø **Azygos Vein** Right ascending lumbar vein Right subcostal vein 1 **Hemiazygos Vein** Left ascending lumbar vein Left subcostal vein 3 **Innominate Vein, Right** Brachiocephalic vein Inferior thyroid vein 4 **Innominate Vein, Left** *See 3 Innominate Vein, Right* 5 **Subclavian Vein, Right** 6 **Subclavian Vein, Left** 7 **Axillary Vein, Right** 8 **Axillary Vein, Left** 9 **Brachial Vein, Right** Radial vein Ulnar vein A **Brachial Vein, Left** *See 9 Brachial Vein, Right* B **Basilic Vein, Right** Median antebrachial vein Median cubital vein C **Basilic Vein, Left** *See B Basilic Vein, Right* D **Cephalic Vein, Right** Accessory cephalic vein F **Cephalic Vein, Left** *See D Cephalic Vein, Right* G **Hand Vein, Right** Dorsal metacarpal vein Palmar (volar) digital vein Palmar (volar) metacarpal vein Superficial palmar venous arch Volar (palmar) digital vein Volar (palmar) metacarpal vein	H **Hand Vein, Left** *See G Hand Vein, Right* L **Intracranial Vein** Anterior cerebral vein Basal (internal) cerebral vein Dural venous sinus Great cerebral vein Inferior cerebellar vein Inferior cerebral vein Internal (basal) cerebral vein Middle cerebral vein Ophthalmic vein Superior cerebellar vein Superior cerebral vein M **Internal Jugular Vein, Right** N **Internal Jugular Vein, Left** P **External Jugular Vein, Right** Posterior auricular vein Q **External Jugular Vein, Left** *See P External Jugular Vein,* *Right* R **Vertebral Vein, Right** Deep cervical vein Suboccipital venous plexus S **Vertebral Vein, Left** *See R Vertebral Vein, Right* T **Face Vein, Right** Angular vein Anterior facial vein Common facial vein Deep facial vein Frontal vein Posterior facial (retromandibular) vein Supraorbital vein V **Face Vein, Left** *See T Face Vein, Right* Y **Upper Vein**	Ø Open 3 Percutaneous 4 Percutaneous Endoscopic	C Extraluminal Device D Intraluminal Device Z No Device	Z No Qualifier

---

LC Limited Coverage   **NC** Noncovered   ⊞ Combination Member   HAC associated procedure   Combination Only   DRG Non-OR   Non-OR   New/Revised in GREEN

246   ICD-10-PCS 2020

Ø5J–Ø5L

Ø   Medical and Surgical
5   Upper Veins
N   Release   Definition: Freeing a body part from an abnormal physical constraint by cutting or by the use of force
                   Explanation: Some of the restraining tissue may be taken out but none of the body part is taken out

Body Part Character 4		Approach Character 5	Device Character 6	Qualifier Character 7
Ø Azygos Vein Right ascending lumbar vein Right subcostal vein **1 Hemiazygos Vein** Left ascending lumbar vein Left subcostal vein **3 Innominate Vein, Right** Brachiocephalic vein Inferior thyroid vein **4 Innominate Vein, Left** *See 3 Innominate Vein, Right* **5 Subclavian Vein, Right** **6 Subclavian Vein, Left** **7 Axillary Vein, Right** **8 Axillary Vein, Left** **9 Brachial Vein, Right** Radial vein Ulnar vein **A Brachial Vein, Left** *See 9 Brachial Vein, Right* **B Basilic Vein, Right** Median antebrachial vein Median cubital vein **C Basilic Vein, Left** *See B Basilic Vein, Right* **D Cephalic Vein, Right** Accessory cephalic vein **F Cephalic Vein, Left** *See D Cephalic Vein, Right* **G Hand Vein, Right** Dorsal metacarpal vein Palmar (volar) digital vein Palmar (volar) metacarpal vein Superficial palmar venous arch Volar (palmar) digital vein Volar (palmar) metacarpal vein	**H Hand Vein, Left** *See G Hand Vein, Right* **L Intracranial Vein** Anterior cerebral vein Basal (internal) cerebral vein Dural venous sinus Great cerebral vein Inferior cerebellar vein Inferior cerebral vein Internal (basal) cerebral vein Middle cerebral vein Ophthalmic vein Superior cerebellar vein Superior cerebral vein **M Internal Jugular Vein, Right** **N Internal Jugular Vein, Left** **P External Jugular Vein, Right** Posterior auricular vein **Q External Jugular Vein, Left** *See P External Jugular Vein,* *Right* **R Vertebral Vein, Right** Deep cervical vein Suboccipital venous plexus **S Vertebral Vein, Left** *See R Vertebral Vein, Right* **T Face Vein, Right** Angular vein Anterior facial vein Common facial vein Deep facial vein Frontal vein Posterior facial (retromandibular) vein Supraorbital vein **V Face Vein, Left** *See T Face Vein, Right* **Y Upper Vein**	**Ø Open** **3 Percutaneous** **4 Percutaneous Endoscopic**	**Z No Device**	**Z No Qualifier**

Ø   Medical and Surgical
5   Upper Veins
P   Removal   Definition: Taking out or off a device from a body part

Explanation: If a device is taken out and a similar device put in without cutting or puncturing the skin or mucous membrane, the procedure is coded to the root operation CHANGE. Otherwise, the procedure for taking out a device is coded to the root operation REMOVAL.

Body Part Character 4	Approach Character 5	Device Character 6	Qualifier Character 7
Ø **Azygos Vein** Right ascending lumbar vein Right subcostal vein	**Ø** Open **3** Percutaneous **4** Percutaneous Endoscopic **X** External	**2** Monitoring Device **M** Neurostimulator Lead	**Z** No Qualifier
3 **Innominate Vein, Right** Brachiocephalic vein Inferior thyroid vein **4** **Innominate Vein, Left** *See 3 Innominate Vein, Right*	**Ø** Open **3** Percutaneous **4** Percutaneous Endoscopic **X** External	**M** Neurostimulator Lead	**Z** No Qualifier
Y **Upper Vein**	**Ø** Open **3** Percutaneous **4** Percutaneous Endoscopic	**Ø** Drainage Device **2** Monitoring Device **3** Infusion Device **7** Autologous Tissue Substitute **C** Extraluminal Device **D** Intraluminal Device **J** Synthetic Substitute **K** Nonautologous Tissue Substitute **Y** Other Device	**Z** No Qualifier
Y **Upper Vein**	**X** External	**Ø** Drainage Device **2** Monitoring Device **3** Infusion Device **D** Intraluminal Device	**Z** No Qualifier

Non-OR   Ø5PØ[Ø,3,4,X]2Z
Non-OR   Ø5PY3[Ø,2,3]Z
Non-OR   Ø5PY[3,4]YZ
Non-OR   Ø5PYX[Ø,2,3,D]Z

LC Limited Coverage   **NC** Noncovered   ⊞ Combination Member   HAC associated procedure   Combination Only   DRG Non-OR   Non-OR   New/Revised in GREEN

248   ICD-10-PCS 2020

Ø   Medical and Surgical
5   Upper Veins
Q   Repair   Definition: Restoring, to the extent possible, a body part to its normal anatomic structure and function
                  Explanation: Used only when the method to accomplish the repair is not one of the other root operations

Body Part Character 4		Approach Character 5	Device Character 6	Qualifier Character 7
Ø Azygos Vein Right ascending lumbar vein Right subcostal vein **1 Hemiazygos Vein** Left ascending lumbar vein Left subcostal vein **3 Innominate Vein, Right** Brachiocephalic vein Inferior thyroid vein **4 Innominate Vein, Left** *See 3 Innominate Vein, Right* **5 Subclavian Vein, Right** **6 Subclavian Vein, Left** **7 Axillary Vein, Right** **8 Axillary Vein, Left** **9 Brachial Vein, Right** Radial vein Ulnar vein **A Brachial Vein, Left** *See 9 Brachial Vein, Right* **B Basilic Vein, Right** Median antebrachial vein Median cubital vein **C Basilic Vein, Left** *See B Basilic Vein, Right* **D Cephalic Vein, Right** Accessory cephalic vein **F Cephalic Vein, Left** *See D Cephalic Vein, Right* **G Hand Vein, Right** Dorsal metacarpal vein Palmar (volar) digital vein Palmar (volar) metacarpal vein Superficial palmar venous arch Volar (palmar) digital vein Volar (palmar) metacarpal vein	**H Hand Vein, Left** *See G Hand Vein, Right* **L Intracranial Vein** Anterior cerebral vein Basal (internal) cerebral vein Dural venous sinus Great cerebral vein Inferior cerebellar vein Inferior cerebral vein Internal (basal) cerebral vein Middle cerebral vein Ophthalmic vein Superior cerebellar vein Superior cerebral vein **M Internal Jugular Vein, Right** **N Internal Jugular Vein, Left** **P External Jugular Vein, Right** Posterior auricular vein **Q External Jugular Vein, Left** *See P External Jugular Vein, Right* **R Vertebral Vein, Right** Deep cervical vein Suboccipital venous plexus **S Vertebral Vein, Left** *See R Vertebral Vein, Right* **T Face Vein, Right** Angular vein Anterior facial vein Common facial vein Deep facial vein Frontal vein Posterior facial (retromandibular) vein Supraorbital vein **V Face Vein, Left** *See T Face Vein, Right* **Y Upper Vein**	**Ø Open** **3 Percutaneous** **4 Percutaneous Endoscopic**	**Z No Device**	**Z No Qualifier**

LC Limited Coverage   NC Noncovered   ⊞ Combination Member   HAC associated procedure   Combination Only   DRG Non-OR   Non-OR   New/Revised in GREEN

ICD-10-PCS 2020   **249**

05Q–05Q

Ø   **Medical and Surgical**
5   **Upper Veins**
R   **Replacement**   Definition: Putting in or on biological or synthetic material that physically takes the place and/or function of all or a portion of a body part

Explanation: The body part may have been taken out or replaced, or may be taken out, physically eradicated, or rendered nonfunctional during the REPLACEMENT procedure. A REMOVAL procedure is coded for taking out the device used in a previous replacement procedure.

Body Part Character 4		Approach Character 5	Device Character 6	Qualifier Character 7

Ø   **Azygos Vein**
   Right ascending lumbar vein
   Right subcostal vein
1   **Hemiazygos Vein**
   Left ascending lumbar vein
   Left subcostal vein
3   **Innominate Vein, Right**
   Brachiocephalic vein
   Inferior thyroid vein
4   **Innominate Vein, Left**
   See 3 Innominate Vein, Right
5   **Subclavian Vein, Right**
6   **Subclavian Vein, Left**
7   **Axillary Vein, Right**
8   **Axillary Vein, Left**
9   **Brachial Vein, Right**
   Radial vein
   Ulnar vein
A   **Brachial Vein, Left**
   See 9 Brachial Vein, Right
B   **Basilic Vein, Right**
   Median antebrachial vein
   Median cubital vein
C   **Basilic Vein, Left**
   See B Basilic Vein, Right
D   **Cephalic Vein, Right**
   Accessory cephalic vein
F   **Cephalic Vein, Left**
   See D Cephalic Vein, Right
G   **Hand Vein, Right**
   Dorsal metacarpal vein
   Palmar (volar) digital vein
   Palmar (volar) metacarpal vein
   Superficial palmar venous arch
   Volar (palmar) digital vein
   Volar (palmar) metacarpal vein
	H **Hand Vein, Left**
	   See G Hand Vein, Right
	L **Intracranial Vein**
	   Anterior cerebral vein
	   Basal (internal) cerebral vein
	   Dural venous sinus
	   Great cerebral vein
	   Inferior cerebellar vein
	   Inferior cerebral vein
	   Internal (basal) cerebral vein
	   Middle cerebral vein
	   Ophthalmic vein
	   Superior cerebellar vein
	   Superior cerebral vein
	M **Internal Jugular Vein, Right**
	N **Internal Jugular Vein, Left**
	P **External Jugular Vein, Right**
	   Posterior auricular vein
	Q **External Jugular Vein, Left**
	   See P External Jugular Vein,
	   Right
	R **Vertebral Vein, Right**
	   Deep cervical vein
	   Suboccipital venous plexus
	S **Vertebral Vein, Left**
	   See R Vertebral Vein, Right
	T **Face Vein, Right**
	   Angular vein
	   Anterior facial vein
	   Common facial vein
	   Deep facial vein
	   Frontal vein
	   Posterior facial
	     (retromandibular) vein
	   Supraorbital vein
	V **Face Vein, Left**
	   See T Face Vein, Right
	Y **Upper Vein**
		Ø **Open**
		4 **Percutaneous Endoscopic**
			7 **Autologous Tissue**
			   Substitute
			J **Synthetic Substitute**
			K **Nonautologous Tissue**
			   Substitute
				Z **No Qualifier**

Ø   **Medical and Surgical**
5   **Upper Veins**
S   **Reposition**   Definition: Moving to its normal location, or other suitable location, all or a portion of a body part

Explanation: The body part is moved to a new location from an abnormal location, or from a normal location where it is not functioning correctly. The body part may or may not be cut out or off to be moved to the new location.

Body Part Character 4		Approach Character 5	Device Character 6	Qualifier Character 7

Ø   **Azygos Vein**
    Right ascending lumbar vein
    Right subcostal vein
	H **Hand Vein, Left**
	    See G Hand Vein, Right
		Ø Open
		3 Percutaneous
		4 Percutaneous Endoscopic
			Z No Device	**Z** No Qualifier

1   **Hemiazygos Vein**
    Left ascending lumbar vein
    Left subcostal vein
	L **Intracranial Vein**
	    Anterior cerebral vein
	    Basal (internal) cerebral vein			

3   **Innominate Vein, Right**
    Brachiocephalic vein
    Inferior thyroid vein
	Dural venous sinus
	    Great cerebral vein
	    Inferior cerebellar vein			

4   **Innominate Vein, Left**
    See 3 Innominate Vein, Right
	Inferior cerebral vein
	    Internal (basal) cerebral vein
	    Middle cerebral vein			

5 **Subclavian Vein, Right**	Ophthalmic vein Superior cerebellar vein			
6 **Subclavian Vein, Left**	Superior cerebral vein			
7 **Axillary Vein, Right**	**M** **Internal Jugular Vein, Right**			
8 **Axillary Vein, Left**	**N** **Internal Jugular Vein, Left**			

9   **Brachial Vein, Right**
    Radial vein
    Ulnar vein
	P **External Jugular Vein, Right**
	    Posterior auricular vein			

A   **Brachial Vein, Left**
    See 9 Brachial Vein, Right
	Q **External Jugular Vein, Left**
	    See P External Jugular Vein,
	    Right			

B   **Basilic Vein, Right**
    Median antebrachial vein
    Median cubital vein
	R **Vertebral Vein, Right**
	    Deep cervical vein
	    Suboccipital venous plexus			

C   **Basilic Vein, Left**
    See B Basilic Vein, Right
	S **Vertebral Vein, Left**
	    See R Vertebral Vein, Right			

D   **Cephalic Vein, Right**
    Accessory cephalic vein
	T **Face Vein, Right**
	    Angular vein
	    Anterior facial vein			

F   **Cephalic Vein, Left**
    See D Cephalic Vein, Right
	Common facial vein
	    Deep facial vein
	    Frontal vein			

G   **Hand Vein, Right**
    Dorsal metacarpal vein
    Palmar (volar) digital vein
    Palmar (volar) metacarpal vein
    Superficial palmar venous arch
    Volar (palmar) digital vein
    Volar (palmar) metacarpal vein
	Posterior facial
	      (retromandibular) vein
	    Supraorbital vein
	V **Face Vein, Left**
	    See T Face Vein, Right
	Y **Upper Vein**			

LG Limited Coverage   NC Noncovered   ⊞ Combination Member   HAC associated procedure   Combination Only   DRG Non-OR   Non-OR   New/Revised in GREEN

Upper Veins

Ø   **Medical and Surgical**
5   **Upper Veins**
U   **Supplement**   Definition: Putting in or on biological or synthetic material that physically reinforces and/or augments the function of a portion of a body part
                     Explanation: The biological material is non-living, or is living and from the same individual. The body part may have been previously replaced,
                     and the SUPPLEMENT procedure is performed to physically reinforce and/or augment the function of the replaced body part.

Body Part Character 4		Approach Character 5	Device Character 6	Qualifier Character 7

Ø   Azygos Vein
    Right ascending lumbar vein
    Right subcostal vein
	H Hand Vein, Left
	    See G Hand Vein, Right
	L Intracranial Vein
	    Anterior cerebral vein
		Ø Open
		3 Percutaneous
		4 Percutaneous Endoscopic
			**7 Autologous Tissue
			    Substitute**
			J Synthetic Substitute
			K Nonautologous Tissue
				Z No Qualifier

1   Hemiazygos Vein
    Left ascending lumbar vein
    Left subcostal vein
	Basal (internal) cerebral vein
	    Dural venous sinus
	    Great cerebral vein
			** Substitute**	

3   Innominate Vein, Right
    Brachiocephalic vein
    Inferior thyroid vein
	Inferior cerebellar vein
	    Inferior cerebral vein
	    Internal (basal) cerebral vein			

4   Innominate Vein, Left
    See 3 Innominate Vein, Right
	Middle cerebral vein
	    Ophthalmic vein			

5 Subclavian Vein, Right	Superior cerebellar vein Superior cerebral vein			
6 Subclavian Vein, Left	**M Internal Jugular Vein, Right**			
7 Axillary Vein, Right	**N Internal Jugular Vein, Left**			
8 Axillary Vein, Left	**P External Jugular Vein, Right**			

9   Brachial Vein, Right
    Radial vein
    Ulnar vein
	Posterior auricular vein
	Q External Jugular Vein, Left
	    See P External Jugular Vein,			

A Brachial Vein, Left *See 9 Brachial Vein, Right*	* Right* **R Vertebral Vein, Right**			

B   Basilic Vein, Right
    Median antebrachial vein
    Median cubital vein
	Deep cervical vein
	    Suboccipital venous plexus
	S Vertebral Vein, Left			

C Basilic Vein, Left *See B Basilic Vein, Right*	*See R Vertebral Vein, Right* **T Face Vein, Right**			

D   Cephalic Vein, Right
    Accessory cephalic vein
	Angular vein
	    Anterior facial vein			

F   Cephalic Vein, Left
    See D Cephalic Vein, Right
	Common facial vein
	    Deep facial vein			

G   Hand Vein, Right
    Dorsal metacarpal vein
	Frontal vein
	    Posterior facial			

Palmar (volar) digital vein
    Palmar (volar) metacarpal vein
	(retromandibular) vein
	    Supraorbital vein			

Superficial palmar venous arch
    Volar (palmar) digital vein
	V Face Vein, Left
	    See T Face Vein, Right			

Volar (palmar) metacarpal vein	**Y Upper Vein**			

Ø   **Medical and Surgical**
5   **Upper Veins**
V   **Restriction**   Definition: Partially closing an orifice or the lumen of a tubular body part
                         Explanation: The orifice can be a natural orifice or an artificially created orifice

Body Part Character 4		Approach Character 5	Device Character 6	Qualifier Character 7

Ø Azygos Vein
  Right ascending lumbar vein
  Right subcostal vein
1 Hemiazygos Vein
  Left ascending lumbar vein
  Left subcostal vein
3 Innominate Vein, Right
  Brachiocephalic vein
  Inferior thyroid vein
4 Innominate Vein, Left
  See 3 Innominate Vein, Right
5 Subclavian Vein, Right
6 Subclavian Vein, Left
7 Axillary Vein, Right
8 Axillary Vein, Left
9 Brachial Vein, Right
  Radial vein
  Ulnar vein
A Brachial Vein, Left
  See 9 Brachial Vein, Right
B Basilic Vein, Right
  Median antebrachial vein
  Median cubital vein
C Basilic Vein, Left
  See B Basilic Vein, Right
D Cephalic Vein, Right
  Accessory cephalic vein
F Cephalic Vein, Left
  See D Cephalic Vein, Right
G Hand Vein, Right
  Dorsal metacarpal vein
  Palmar (volar) digital vein
  Palmar (volar) metacarpal vein
  Superficial palmar venous arch
  Volar (palmar) digital vein
  Volar (palmar) metacarpal vein
	H Hand Vein, Left
	  See G Hand Vein, Right
	L Intracranial Vein
	  Anterior cerebral vein
	  Basal (internal) cerebral vein
	  Dural venous sinus
	  Great cerebral vein
	  Inferior cerebellar vein
	  Inferior cerebral vein
	  Internal (basal) cerebral vein
	  Middle cerebral vein
	  Ophthalmic vein
	  Superior cerebellar vein
	  Superior cerebral vein
	M Internal Jugular Vein, Right
	N Internal Jugular Vein, Left
	P External Jugular Vein, Right
	  Posterior auricular vein
	Q External Jugular Vein, Left
	  See P External Jugular Vein,
	    Right
	R Vertebral Vein, Right
	  Deep cervical vein
	  Suboccipital venous plexus
	S Vertebral Vein, Left
	  See R Vertebral Vein, Right
	T Face Vein, Right
	  Angular vein
	  Anterior facial vein
	  Common facial vein
	  Deep facial vein
	  Frontal vein
	  Posterior facial
	    (retromandibular) vein
	  Supraorbital vein
	V Face Vein, Left
	  See T Face Vein, Right
	Y Upper Vein
		Ø Open
		3 Percutaneous
		4 Percutaneous Endoscopic
			C Extraluminal Device
			D Intraluminal Device
			Z No Device
				Z No Qualifier

Ø   **Medical and Surgical**
5   **Upper Veins**
W   **Revision**   Definition: Correcting, to the extent possible, a portion of a malfunctioning device or the position of a displaced device

                    Explanation: Revision can include correcting a malfunctioning or displaced device by taking out or putting in components of the device such as a screw or pin

Body Part Character 4	Approach Character 5	Device Character 6	Qualifier Character 7

Ø **Azygos Vein**
  Right ascending lumbar vein
  Right subcostal vein
	Ø Open
	3 Percutaneous
	4 Percutaneous Endoscopic
	X External
		2 Monitoring Device
		M Neurostimulator Lead
			Z No Qualifier

3 **Innominate Vein, Right**
  Brachiocephalic vein
  Inferior thyroid vein
4 **Innominate Vein, Left**
  See 3 Innominate Vein, Right
	Ø Open
	3 Percutaneous
	4 Percutaneous Endoscopic
	X External
		M Neurostimulator Lead	**Z** No Qualifier

Y **Upper Vein**	**Ø** Open **3** Percutaneous **4** Percutaneous Endoscopic	**Ø** Drainage Device **2** Monitoring Device **3** Infusion Device **7** Autologous Tissue Substitute **C** Extraluminal Device **D** Intraluminal Device **J** Synthetic Substitute **K** Nonautologous Tissue Substitute **Y** Other Device	**Z** No Qualifier
Y **Upper Vein**	**X** External	**Ø** Drainage Device **2** Monitoring Device **3** Infusion Device **7** Autologous Tissue Substitute **C** Extraluminal Device **D** Intraluminal Device **J** Synthetic Substitute **K** Nonautologous Tissue Substitute	**Z** No Qualifier

Non-OR	Ø5WØXMZ
Non-OR	Ø5W[3,4]XMZ
Non-OR	Ø5WY3[Ø,2,3,D]Z
Non-OR	Ø5WY[3,4]YZ
Non-OR	Ø5WYX[Ø,2,3,7,C,D,J,K]Z

🔲 Limited Coverage   🔲 Noncovered   ⊞ Combination Member   HAC associated procedure   Combination Only   DRG Non-OR   Non-OR   New/Revised in GREEN

254   ICD-10-PCS 2020

Ø5W–Ø5W

Lower Veins Ø61–Ø6W

Character Meanings

This Character Meaning table is provided as a guide to assist the user in the identification of character members that may be found in this section of code tables. It **SHOULD NOT** be used to build a PCS code.

Operation–Character 3	Body Part–Character 4	Approach–Character 5	Device–Character 6	Qualifier–Character 7
1 Bypass	Ø Inferior Vena Cava	Ø Open	Ø Drainage Device	4 Hepatic Vein
5 Destruction	1 Splenic Vein	3 Percutaneous	2 Monitoring Device	5 Superior Mesenteric Vein
7 Dilation	2 Gastric Vein	4 Percutaneous Endoscopic	3 Infusion Device	6 Inferior Mesenteric Vein
9 Drainage	3 Esophageal Vein	7 Via Natural or Artificial Opening	7 Autologous Tissue Substitute	9 Renal Vein, Right
B Excision	4 Hepatic Vein	8 Via Natural or Artificial Opening Endoscopic	9 Autologous Venous Tissue	B Renal Vein, Left
C Extirpation	5 Superior Mesenteric Vein	X External	A Autologous Arterial Tissue	C Hemorrhoidal Plexus
D Extraction	6 Inferior Mesenteric Vein		C Extraluminal Device	P Pulmonary Trunk
H Insertion	7 Colic Vein		D Intraluminal Device	Q Pulmonary Artery, Right
J Inspection	8 Portal Vein		J Synthetic Substitute	R Pulmonary Artery, Left
L Occlusion	9 Renal Vein, Right		K Nonautologous Tissue Substitute	T Via Umbilical Vein
N Release	B Renal Vein, Left		Y Other Device	X Diagnostic
P Removal	C Common Iliac Vein, Right		Z No Device	Y Lower Vein
Q Repair	D Common Iliac Vein, Left			Z No Qualifier
R Replacement	F External Iliac Vein, Right			
S Reposition	G External Iliac Vein, Left			
U Supplement	H Hypogastric Vein, Right			
V Restriction	J Hypogastric Vein, Left			
W Revision	M Femoral Vein, Right			
	N Femoral Vein, Left			
	P Saphenous Vein, Right			
	Q Saphenous Vein, Left			
	T Foot Vein, Right			
	V Foot Vein, Left			
	Y Lower Vein			

AHA Coding Clinic for table Ø61
2017, 4Q, 36-38	Fontan completion procedure
2017, 4Q, 66-67	New qualifier values - Portal to hepatic shunt

AHA Coding Clinic for table Ø6B
2017, 3Q, 5	Femoral artery to posterior tibial artery bypass using autologous and synthetic grafts
2017, 1Q, 31	Left to right common carotid artery bypass
2017, 1Q, 32	Peroneal artery to dorsalis pedis artery bypass using saphenous vein graft
2016, 3Q, 31	Femoral to peroneal artery bypass with in-situ saphenous vein graft and lysis of valves
2016, 2Q, 18	Femoral-tibial artery bypass and saphenous vein graft
2016, 1Q, 27	Aortocoronary bypass graft utilizing Y-graft
2014, 3Q, 8	Excision of saphenous vein for coronary artery bypass graft
2014, 3Q, 20	MAZE procedure performed with coronary artery bypass graft
2014, 1Q, 10	Repair of thoracic aortic aneurysm & coronary artery bypass graft

AHA Coding Clinic for table Ø6H
2017, 3Q, 11	Placement of peripherally inserted central catheter using 3CG ECG technology
2017, 1Q, 31	Umbilical vein catheterization
2017, 1Q, 31	Central catheter placement in femoral vein
2013, 3Q, 18	Heart transplant surgery

AHA Coding Clinic for table Ø6L
2018, 2Q, 18	Transverse rectus abdominis myocutaneous (TRAM) delay
2017, 4Q, 57-58	Added approach values - Transorifice esophageal vein banding
2013, 4Q, 112	Endoscopic banding of esophageal varices

AHA Coding Clinic for table Ø6V
2018, 3Q, 11	Transvenous transcatheter placement of valve in inferior vena cava
2018, 1Q, 10	Revision of transjugular intrahepatic portosystemic shunt

AHA Coding Clinic for table Ø6W
2018, 1Q, 10	Revision of transjugular intrahepatic portosystemic shunt
2014, 3Q, 25	Revision of transjugular intrahepatic portosystemic shunt (TIPS)

Lower Veins

Inferior vena cava **Ø**

Common hepatic **4**

Portal **B**

Colic **7**

Internal pudendal **H, J**

Femoral **M, N**

Greater saphenous **P, Q**

Lesser saphenous **P, Q**

Anterior tibial **M, N**

Posterior tibial **M, N**

Digital **T, V**

Esophageal **3**

Gastric **2**

Splenic **1**

Renal **9, B**

Inferior mesenteric **6**

Superior mesenteric **5**

Common iliac **C, D**

Internal iliac (Hypogastric) **H, J**

External iliac **F, G**

Rectal venous plexus **H, J**

Popliteal **M, N**

Lesser saphenous **P, Q**

Greater saphenous **P, Q**

Dorsal venous arch **T, V**

Portal Venous Circulation

Inferior vena cava **Ø**

Portal **8**

Gastric **2**

Splenic **1**

Superior mesenteric **5**

Right colic **7**

Ileocolic **7**

Inferior mesenteric **6**

Left colic **7**

Ø   Medical and Surgical
6   Lower Veins
1   Bypass   Definition: Altering the route of passage of the contents of a tubular body part

Explanation: Rerouting contents of a body part to a downstream area of the normal route, to a similar route and body part, or to an abnormal route and dissimilar body part. Includes one or more anastomoses, with or without the use of a device.

Body Part Character 4		Approach Character 5	Device Character 6	Qualifier Character 7
Ø Inferior Vena Cava Postcava Right inferior phrenic vein Right ovarian vein Right second lumbar vein Right suprarenal vein Right testicular vein		**Ø Open** **4 Percutaneous Endoscopic**	**7 Autologous Tissue Substitute** **9 Autologous Venous Tissue** **A Autologous Arterial Tissue** **J Synthetic Substitute** **K Nonautologous Tissue Substitute** **Z No Device**	**5 Superior Mesenteric Vein** **6 Inferior Mesenteric Vein** **P Pulmonary Trunk** **Q Pulmonary Artery, Right** **R Pulmonary Artery, Left** **Y Lower Vein**
1 Splenic Vein Left gastroepiploic vein Pancreatic vein		**Ø Open** **4 Percutaneous Endoscopic**	**7 Autologous Tissue Substitute** **9 Autologous Venous Tissue** **A Autologous Arterial Tissue** **J Synthetic Substitute** **K Nonautologous Tissue Substitute** **Z No Device**	**9 Renal Vein, Right** **B Renal Vein, Left** **Y Lower Vein**
2 Gastric Vein **3 Esophageal Vein** **4 Hepatic Vein** **5 Superior Mesenteric Vein** Right gastroepiploic vein **6 Inferior Mesenteric Vein** Sigmoid vein Superior rectal vein **7 Colic Vein** Ileocolic vein Left colic vein Middle colic vein Right colic vein **9 Renal Vein, Right** **B Renal Vein, Left** Left inferior phrenic vein Left ovarian vein Left second lumbar vein Left suprarenal vein Left testicular vein **C Common Iliac Vein, Right** **D Common Iliac Vein, Left** **F External Iliac Vein, Right** **G External Iliac Vein, Left** **H Hypogastric Vein, Right** Gluteal vein Internal iliac vein Internal pudendal vein Lateral sacral vein Middle hemorrhoidal vein Obturator vein Uterine vein Vaginal vein Vesical vein	**J Hypogastric Vein, Left** *See H Hypogastric Vein, Right* **M Femoral Vein, Right** Deep femoral (profunda femoris) vein Popliteal vein Profunda femoris (deep femoral) vein **N Femoral Vein, Left** *See M Femoral Vein, Right* **P Saphenous Vein, Right** External pudendal vein Great(er) saphenous vein Lesser saphenous vein Small saphenous vein Superficial circumflex iliac vein Superficial epigastric vein **Q Saphenous Vein, Left** *See P Saphenous Vein, Right* **T Foot Vein, Right** Common digital vein Dorsal metatarsal vein Dorsal venous arch Plantar digital vein Plantar metatarsal vein Plantar venous arch **V Foot Vein, Left** *See T Foot Vein, Right*	**Ø Open** **4 Percutaneous Endoscopic**	**7 Autologous Tissue Substitute** **9 Autologous Venous Tissue** **A Autologous Arterial Tissue** **J Synthetic Substitute** **K Nonautologous Tissue Substitute** **Z No Device**	**Y Lower Vein**
8 Portal Vein Hepatic portal vein		**Ø Open**	**7 Autologous Tissue Substitute** **9 Autologous Venous Tissue** **A Autologous Arterial Tissue** **J Synthetic Substitute** **K Nonautologous Tissue Substitute** **Z No Device**	**9 Renal Vein, Right** **B Renal Vein, Left** **Y Lower Vein**
8 Portal Vein Hepatic portal vein		**3 Percutaneous**	**J Synthetic Substitute**	**4 Hepatic Vein** **Y Lower Vein**
8 Portal Vein Hepatic portal vein		**4 Percutaneous Endoscopic**	**7 Autologous Tissue Substitute** **9 Autologous Venous Tissue** **A Autologous Arterial Tissue** **K Nonautologous Tissue Substitute** **Z No Device**	**9 Renal Vein, Right** **B Renal Vein, Left** **Y Lower Vein**
8 Portal Vein Hepatic portal vein		**4 Percutaneous Endoscopic**	**J Synthetic Substitute**	**4 Hepatic Vein** **9 Renal Vein, Right** **B Renal Vein, Left** **Y Lower Vein**

LC Limited Coverage   NC Noncovered   ⊞ Combination Member   HAC associated procedure   Combination Only   DRG Non-OR   Non-OR   New/Revised in GREEN

Lower Veins

Ø   **Medical and Surgical**
6   **Lower Veins**
5   **Destruction**   Definition: Physical eradication of all or a portion of a body part by the direct use of energy, force, or a destructive agent
                            Explanation: None of the body part is physically taken out

Body Part Character 4	Approach Character 5	Device Character 6	Qualifier Character 7
Ø Inferior Vena Cava Postcava Right inferior phrenic vein Right ovarian vein Right second lumbar vein Right suprarenal vein Right testicular vein	**Ø Open** **3 Percutaneous** **4 Percutaneous Endoscopic**	**Z No Device**	**Z No Qualifier**
1 Splenic Vein Left gastroepiploic vein Pancreatic vein			
2 Gastric Vein			
3 Esophageal Vein			
4 Hepatic Vein			
5 Superior Mesenteric Vein Right gastroepiploic vein			
6 Inferior Mesenteric Vein Sigmoid vein Superior rectal vein			
7 Colic Vein Ileocolic vein Left colic vein Middle colic vein Right colic vein			
8 Portal Vein Hepatic portal vein			
9 Renal Vein, Right			
B Renal Vein, Left Left inferior phrenic vein Left ovarian vein Left second lumbar vein Left suprarenal vein Left testicular vein			
C Common Iliac Vein, Right			
D Common Iliac Vein, Left			
F External Iliac Vein, Right			
G External Iliac Vein, Left			
H Hypogastric Vein, Right Gluteal vein Internal iliac vein Internal pudendal vein Lateral sacral vein Middle hemorrhoidal vein Obturator vein Uterine vein Vaginal vein Vesical vein			
J Hypogastric Vein, Left *See H Hypogastric Vein, Right*			
M Femoral Vein, Right Deep femoral (profunda femoris) vein Popliteal vein Profunda femoris (deep femoral) vein			
N Femoral Vein, Left *See M Femoral Vein, Right*			
P Saphenous Vein, Right External pudendal vein Great(er) saphenous vein Lesser saphenous vein Small saphenous vein Superficial circumflex iliac vein Superficial epigastric vein			
Q Saphenous Vein, Left *See P Saphenous Vein, Right*			
T Foot Vein, Right Common digital vein Dorsal metatarsal vein Dorsal venous arch Plantar digital vein Plantar metatarsal vein Plantar venous arch			
V Foot Vein, Left *See T Foot Vein, Right*			
Y Lower Vein	**Ø Open** **3 Percutaneous** **4 Percutaneous Endoscopic**	**Z No Device**	**C Hemorrhoidal Plexus** **Z No Qualifier**

LC Limited Coverage   **NC** Noncovered   ⊞ Combination Member   HAC associated procedure   Combination Only   DRG Non-OR   Non-OR   New/Revised in GREEN

258   ICD-10-PCS 2020

Ø   Medical and Surgical
6   Lower Veins
7   Dilation   Definition: Expanding an orifice or the lumen of a tubular body part

Explanation: The orifice can be a natural orifice or an artificially created orifice. Accomplished by stretching a tubular body part using intraluminal pressure or by cutting part of the orifice or wall of the tubular body part.

Body Part Character 4	Approach Character 5	Device Character 6	Qualifier Character 7
Ø Inferior Vena Cava Postcava Right inferior phrenic vein Right ovarian vein Right second lumbar vein Right suprarenal vein Right testicular vein	**Ø** Open **3** Percutaneous **4** Percutaneous Endoscopic	**D** Intraluminal Device **Z** No Device	**Z** No Qualifier
1 Splenic Vein Left gastroepiploic vein Pancreatic vein			
2 Gastric Vein			
3 Esophageal Vein			
4 Hepatic Vein			
5 Superior Mesenteric Vein Right gastroepiploic vein			
6 Inferior Mesenteric Vein Sigmoid vein Superior rectal vein			
7 Colic Vein Ileocolic vein Left colic vein Middle colic vein Right colic vein			
8 Portal Vein Hepatic portal vein			
9 Renal Vein, Right			
B Renal Vein, Left Left inferior phrenic vein Left ovarian vein Left second lumbar vein Left suprarenal vein Left testicular vein			
C Common Iliac Vein, Right			
D Common Iliac Vein, Left			
F External Iliac Vein, Right			
G External Iliac Vein, Left			
H Hypogastric Vein, Right Gluteal vein Internal iliac vein Internal pudendal vein Lateral sacral vein Middle hemorrhoidal vein Obturator vein Uterine vein Vaginal vein Vesical vein			
J Hypogastric Vein, Left *See H Hypogastric Vein, Right*			
M Femoral Vein, Right Deep femoral (profunda femoris) vein Popliteal vein Profunda femoris (deep femoral) vein			
N Femoral Vein, Left *See M Femoral Vein, Right*			
P Saphenous Vein, Right External pudendal vein Great(er) saphenous vein Lesser saphenous vein Small saphenous vein Superficial circumflex iliac vein Superficial epigastric vein			
Q Saphenous Vein, Left *See P Saphenous Vein, Right*			
T Foot Vein, Right Common digital vein Dorsal metatarsal vein Dorsal venous arch Plantar digital vein Plantar metatarsal vein Plantar venous arch			
V Foot Vein, Left *See T Foot Vein, Right*			
Y Lower Vein			

LC Limited Coverage   NC Noncovered   ⊞ Combination Member   HAC associated procedure   Combination Only   DRG Non-OR   Non-OR   New/Revised in GREEN

ICD-10-PCS 2020   259

067–067

Lower Veins *(side tab)*

Ø   **Medical and Surgical**
6   **Lower Veins**
9   **Drainage**   Definition: Taking or letting out fluids and/or gases from a body part
                   Explanation: The qualifier DIAGNOSTIC is used to identify drainage procedures that are biopsies

Body Part Character 4		Approach Character 5	Device Character 6	Qualifier Character 7

Ø Inferior Vena Cava
   Postcava
   Right inferior phrenic vein
   Right ovarian vein
   Right second lumbar vein
   Right suprarenal vein
   Right testicular vein
1 Splenic Vein
   Left gastroepiploic vein
   Pancreatic vein
2 Gastric Vein
3 Esophageal Vein
4 Hepatic Vein
5 Superior Mesenteric Vein
   Right gastroepiploic vein
6 Inferior Mesenteric Vein
   Sigmoid vein
   Superior rectal vein
7 Colic Vein
   Ileocolic vein
   Left colic vein
   Middle colic vein
   Right colic vein
8 Portal Vein
   Hepatic portal vein
9 Renal Vein, Right
B Renal Vein, Left
   Left inferior phrenic vein
   Left ovarian vein
   Left second lumbar vein
   Left suprarenal vein
   Left testicular vein
C Common Iliac Vein, Right
D Common Iliac Vein, Left
F External Iliac Vein, Right
G External Iliac Vein, Left
	H Hypogastric Vein, Right
	   Gluteal vein
	   Internal iliac vein
	   Internal pudendal vein
	   Lateral sacral vein
	   Middle hemorrhoidal vein
	   Obturator vein
	   Uterine vein
	   Vaginal vein
	   Vesical vein
	J Hypogastric Vein, Left
	   See H Hypogastric Vein, Right
	M Femoral Vein, Right
	   Deep femoral (profunda
	     femoris) vein
	   Popliteal vein
	   Profunda femoris (deep
	     femoral) vein
	N Femoral Vein, Left
	   See M Femoral Vein, Right
	P Saphenous Vein, Right
	   External pudendal vein
	   Great(er) saphenous vein
	   Lesser saphenous vein
	   Small saphenous vein
	   Superficial circumflex iliac vein
	   Superficial epigastric vein
	Q Saphenous Vein, Left
	   See P Saphenous Vein, Right
	T Foot Vein, Right
	   Common digital vein
	   Dorsal metatarsal vein
	   Dorsal venous arch
	   Plantar digital vein
	   Plantar metatarsal vein
	   Plantar venous arch
	V Foot Vein, Left
	   See T Foot Vein, Right
	Y Lower Vein
		Ø Open
		3 Percutaneous
		4 Percutaneous Endoscopic
			Ø Drainage Device	**Z No Qualifier**

Ø69 Continued on next page

Non-OR   Ø69[Ø,1,2,4,5,6,7,8,9,B,C,D,F,G,H,J,M,N,P,Q,T,V,Y][Ø,3,4]ØZ
Non-OR   Ø6933ØZ

[LC] Limited Coverage   [NC] Noncovered   ⊞ Combination Member   HAC associated procedure   Combination Only   DRG Non-OR   Non-OR   New/Revised in GREEN
260   ICD-10-PCS 2020

Ø69–Ø69 *(side tab)*

Ø   **Medical and Surgical**   *069 Continued*
6   **Lower Veins**
9   **Drainage**   Definition: Taking or letting out fluids and/or gases from a body part
                          Explanation: The qualifier DIAGNOSTIC is used to identify drainage procedures that are biopsies

Body Part Character 4		Approach Character 5	Device Character 6	Qualifier Character 7
Ø Inferior Vena Cava Postcava Right inferior phrenic vein Right ovarian vein Right second lumbar vein Right suprarenal vein Right testicular vein **1 Splenic Vein** Left gastroepiploic vein Pancreatic vein **2 Gastric Vein** **3 Esophageal Vein** **4 Hepatic Vein** **5 Superior Mesenteric Vein** Right gastroepiploic vein **6 Inferior Mesenteric Vein** Sigmoid vein Superior rectal vein **7 Colic Vein** Ileocolic vein Left colic vein Middle colic vein Right colic vein **8 Portal Vein** Hepatic portal vein **9 Renal Vein, Right** **B Renal Vein, Left** Left inferior phrenic vein Left ovarian vein Left second lumbar vein Left suprarenal vein Left testicular vein **C Common Iliac Vein, Right** **D Common Iliac Vein, Left** **F External Iliac Vein, Right** **G External Iliac Vein, Left**	**H Hypogastric Vein, Right** Gluteal vein Internal iliac vein Internal pudendal vein Lateral sacral vein Middle hemorrhoidal vein Obturator vein Uterine vein Vaginal vein Vesical vein **J Hypogastric Vein, Left** *See H Hypogastric Vein, Right* **M Femoral Vein, Right** Deep femoral (profunda femoris) vein Popliteal vein Profunda femoris (deep femoral) vein **N Femoral Vein, Left** *See M Femoral Vein, Right* **P Saphenous Vein, Right** External pudendal vein Great(er) saphenous vein Lesser saphenous vein Small saphenous vein Superficial circumflex iliac vein Superficial epigastric vein **Q Saphenous Vein, Left** *See P Saphenous Vein, Right* **T Foot Vein, Right** Common digital vein Dorsal metatarsal vein Dorsal venous arch Plantar digital vein Plantar metatarsal vein Plantar venous arch **V Foot Vein, Left** *See T Foot Vein, Right* **Y Lower Vein**	**Ø Open** **3 Percutaneous** **4 Percutaneous Endoscopic**	**Z No Device**	**X Diagnostic** **Z No Qualifier**

Non-OR   069[Ø,1,2,3,4,5,6,7,8,9,B,C,D,F,G,H,J,M,N,P,Q,T,V,Y]3ZX
Non-OR   069[Ø,1,2,4,5,6,7,8,9,B,C,D,F,G,H,J,M,N,P,Q,T,V,Y][Ø,3,4]ZZ
Non-OR   06933ZZ

LC Limited Coverage   NC Noncovered   ⊞ Combination Member   HAC associated procedure   Combination Only   DRG Non-OR   Non-OR   New/Revised in GREEN

0   **Medical and Surgical**
6   **Lower Veins**
B   **Excision**   Definition: Cutting out or off, without replacement, a portion of a body part
                   Explanation: The qualifier DIAGNOSTIC is used to identify excision procedures that are biopsies

Body Part Character 4		Approach Character 5	Device Character 6	Qualifier Character 7

0 **Inferior Vena Cava**
   Postcava
   Right inferior phrenic vein
   Right ovarian vein
   Right second lumbar vein
   Right suprarenal vein
   Right testicular vein
1 **Splenic Vein**
   Left gastroepiploic vein
   Pancreatic vein
2 **Gastric Vein**
3 **Esophageal Vein**
4 **Hepatic Vein**
5 **Superior Mesenteric Vein**
   Right gastroepiploic vein
6 **Inferior Mesenteric Vein**
   Sigmoid vein
   Superior rectal vein
7 **Colic Vein**
   Ileocolic vein
   Left colic vein
   Middle colic vein
   Right colic vein
8 **Portal Vein**
   Hepatic portal vein
9 **Renal Vein, Right**
B **Renal Vein, Left**
   Left inferior phrenic vein
   Left ovarian vein
   Left second lumbar vein
   Left suprarenal vein
   Left testicular vein
C **Common Iliac Vein, Right**
D **Common Iliac Vein, Left**
F **External Iliac Vein, Right**
G **External Iliac Vein, Left**
	H **Hypogastric Vein, Right**
	   Gluteal vein
	   Internal iliac vein
	   Internal pudendal vein
	   Lateral sacral vein
	   Middle hemorrhoidal vein
	   Obturator vein
	   Uterine vein
	   Vaginal vein
	   Vesical vein
	J **Hypogastric Vein, Left**
	   See H Hypogastric Vein, Right
	M **Femoral Vein, Right**
	   Deep femoral (profunda
	     femoris) vein
	   Popliteal vein
	   Profunda femoris (deep
	     femoral) vein
	N **Femoral Vein, Left**
	   See M Femoral Vein, Right
	P **Saphenous Vein, Right**
	   External pudendal vein
	   Great(er) saphenous vein
	   Lesser saphenous vein
	   Small saphenous vein
	   Superficial circumflex iliac vein
	   Superficial epigastric vein
	Q **Saphenous Vein, Left**
	   See P Saphenous Vein, Right
	T **Foot Vein, Right**
	   Common digital vein
	   Dorsal metatarsal vein
	   Dorsal venous arch
	   Plantar digital vein
	   Plantar metatarsal vein
	   Plantar venous arch
	V **Foot Vein, Left**
	   See T Foot Vein, Right
		0 Open
		3 Percutaneous
		4 Percutaneous Endoscopic
			Z No Device	**X** Diagnostic
				Z No Qualifier

Y Lower Vein		**0** Open **3** Percutaneous **4** Percutaneous Endoscopic	**Z** No Device	**C** Hemorrhoidal Plexus **X** Diagnostic **Z** No Qualifier

LC Limited Coverage   **NC** Noncovered   ⊞ Combination Member   HAC associated procedure   Combination Only   DRG Non-OR   Non-OR   New/Revised in **GREEN**

262   ICD-10-PCS 2020

0   **Medical and Surgical**
6   **Lower Veins**
C   **Extirpation**   Definition: Taking or cutting out solid matter from a body part

Explanation: The solid matter may be an abnormal byproduct of a biological function or a foreign body; it may be imbedded in a body part or in the lumen of a tubular body part. The solid matter may or may not have been previously broken into pieces.

Body Part Character 4		Approach Character 5	Device Character 6	Qualifier Character 7

0 **Inferior Vena Cava**
  Postcava
  Right inferior phrenic vein
  Right ovarian vein
  Right second lumbar vein
  Right suprarenal vein
  Right testicular vein
1 **Splenic Vein**
  Left gastroepiploic vein
  Pancreatic vein
2 **Gastric Vein**
3 **Esophageal Vein**
4 **Hepatic Vein**
5 **Superior Mesenteric Vein**
  Right gastroepiploic vein
6 **Inferior Mesenteric Vein**
  Sigmoid vein
  Superior rectal vein
7 **Colic Vein**
  Ileocolic vein
  Left colic vein
  Middle colic vein
  Right colic vein
8 **Portal Vein**
  Hepatic portal vein
9 **Renal Vein, Right**
B **Renal Vein, Left**
  Left inferior phrenic vein
  Left ovarian vein
  Left second lumbar vein
  Left suprarenal vein
  Left testicular vein
C **Common Iliac Vein, Right**
D **Common Iliac Vein, Left**
F **External Iliac Vein, Right**
G **External Iliac Vein, Left**
	H **Hypogastric Vein, Right**
	  Gluteal vein
	  Internal iliac vein
	  Internal pudendal vein
	  Lateral sacral vein
	  Middle hemorrhoidal vein
	  Obturator vein
	  Uterine vein
	  Vaginal vein
	  Vesical vein
	J **Hypogastric Vein, Left**
	  See H Hypogastric Vein, Right
	M **Femoral Vein, Right**
	  Deep femoral (profunda
	    femoris) vein
	  Popliteal vein
	  Profunda femoris (deep
	    femoral) vein
	N **Femoral Vein, Left**
	  See M Femoral Vein, Right
	P **Saphenous Vein, Right**
	  External pudendal vein
	  Great(er) saphenous vein
	  Lesser saphenous vein
	  Small saphenous vein
	  Superficial circumflex iliac vein
	  Superficial epigastric vein
	Q **Saphenous Vein, Left**
	  See P Saphenous Vein, Right
	T **Foot Vein, Right**
	  Common digital vein
	  Dorsal metatarsal vein
	  Dorsal venous arch
	  Plantar digital vein
	  Plantar metatarsal vein
	  Plantar venous arch
	V **Foot Vein, Left**
	  See T Foot Vein, Right
	Y **Lower Vein**
		0 Open
		3 Percutaneous
		4 Percutaneous Endoscopic
			Z No Device	**Z** No Qualifier

0   **Medical and Surgical**
6   **Lower Veins**
D   **Extraction**   Definition: Pulling or stripping out or off all or a portion of a body part by the use of force

Explanation: The qualifier DIAGNOSTIC is used to identify extraction procedures that are biopsies

Body Part Character 4		Approach Character 5	Device Character 6	Qualifier Character 7

M **Femoral Vein, Right**
  Deep femoral (profunda
    femoris) vein
  Popliteal vein
  Profunda femoris (deep
    femoral) vein
N **Femoral Vein, Left**
  See M Femoral Vein, Right
P **Saphenous Vein, Right**
  External pudendal vein
  Great(er) saphenous vein
  Lesser saphenous vein
  Small saphenous vein
  Superficial circumflex iliac vein
  Superficial epigastric vein
Q **Saphenous Vein, Left**
  See P Saphenous Vein, Right
	T **Foot Vein, Right**
	  Common digital vein
	  Dorsal metatarsal vein
	  Dorsal venous arch
	  Plantar digital vein
	  Plantar metatarsal vein
	  Plantar venous arch
	V **Foot Vein, Left**
	  See T Foot Vein, Right
	Y **Lower Vein**
		0 Open
		3 Percutaneous
		4 Percutaneous Endoscopic
			Z No Device	**Z** No Qualifier

LC Limited Coverage   **NC** Noncovered   ⊞ Combination Member   HAC associated procedure   Combination Only   DRG Non-OR   Non-OR   New/Revised in GREEN

ICD-10-PCS 2020   263

06C–06D

Ø   Medical and Surgical
6   Lower Veins
H   Insertion

Definition: Putting in a nonbiological appliance that monitors, assists, performs, or prevents a physiological function but does not physically take the place of a body part

Explanation: None

Body Part Character 4	Approach Character 5	Device Character 6	Qualifier Character 7
Ø Inferior Vena Cava Postcava Right inferior phrenic vein Right ovarian vein Right second lumbar vein Right suprarenal vein Right testicular vein	**Ø** Open **3** Percutaneous	**3** Infusion Device	**T** Via Umbilical Vein **Z** No Qualifier
Ø Inferior Vena Cava Postcava Right inferior phrenic vein Right ovarian vein Right second lumbar vein Right suprarenal vein Right testicular vein	**Ø** Open **3** Percutaneous	**D** Intraluminal Device	**Z** No Qualifier
Ø Inferior Vena Cava Postcava Right inferior phrenic vein Right ovarian vein Right second lumbar vein Right suprarenal vein Right testicular vein	**4** Percutaneous Endoscopic	**3** Infusion Device **D** Intraluminal Device	**Z** No Qualifier
1 Splenic Vein Left gastroepiploic vein Pancreatic vein **2 Gastric Vein** **3 Esophageal Vein** **4 Hepatic Vein** **5 Superior Mesenteric Vein** Right gastroepiploic vein **6 Inferior Mesenteric Vein** Sigmoid vein Superior rectal vein **7 Colic Vein** Ileocolic vein Left colic vein Middle colic vein Right colic vein **8 Portal Vein** Hepatic portal vein **9 Renal Vein, Right** **B Renal Vein, Left** Left inferior phrenic vein Left ovarian vein Left second lumbar vein Left suprarenal vein Left testicular vein **C Common Iliac Vein, Right** **D Common Iliac Vein, Left** **F External Iliac Vein, Right** **G External Iliac Vein, Left** **H Hypogastric Vein, Right** Gluteal vein Internal iliac vein Internal pudendal vein Lateral sacral vein Middle hemorrhoidal vein Obturator vein Uterine vein Vaginal vein Vesical vein **J Hypogastric Vein, Left** *See* H Hypogastric Vein, Right **M Femoral Vein, Right** Deep femoral (profunda femoris) vein Popliteal vein Profunda femoris (deep femoral) vein **N Femoral Vein, Left** *See* M Femoral Vein, Right **P Saphenous Vein, Right** External pudendal vein Great(er) saphenous vein Lesser saphenous vein Small saphenous vein Superficial circumflex iliac vein Superficial epigastric vein **Q Saphenous Vein, Left** *See* P Saphenous Vein, Right **T Foot Vein, Right** Common digital vein Dorsal metatarsal vein Dorsal venous arch Plantar digital vein Plantar metatarsal vein Plantar venous arch **V Foot Vein, Left** *See* T Foot Vein, Right	**Ø** Open **3** Percutaneous **4** Percutaneous Endoscopic	**3** Infusion Device **D** Intraluminal Device	**Z** No Qualifier
Y Lower Vein	**Ø** Open **3** Percutaneous **4** Percutaneous Endoscopic	**2** Monitoring Device **3** Infusion Device **D** Intraluminal Device **Y** Other Device	**Z** No Qualifier

Non-OR	Ø6HØ[Ø,3]3[T,Z]	
Non-OR	Ø6HØ3DZ	
Non-OR	Ø6HØ43Z	
Non-OR	Ø6H[1,2,3,4,5,6,7,8,9,B,C,D,F,G,H,J,M,N,P,Q,T,V][Ø,3,4]3Z	
Non-OR	Ø6HY[Ø,3,4]3Z	
Non-OR	Ø6HY32Z	
Non-OR	Ø6HY[3,4]YZ	

🔳 Limited Coverage   🔳 Noncovered   ⊞ Combination Member   HAC associated procedure   Combination Only   DRG Non-OR   Non-OR   New/Revised in GREEN

264   ICD-10-PCS 2020

Ø   Medical and Surgical
6   Lower Veins
J   Inspection   Definition: Visually and/or manually exploring a body part

Explanation: Visual exploration may be performed with or without optical instrumentation. Manual exploration may be performed directly or through intervening body layers.

Body Part Character 4	Approach Character 5	Device Character 6	Qualifier Character 7
Y Lower Vein	**Ø** Open **3** Percutaneous **4** Percutaneous Endoscopic **X** External	**Z** No Device	**Z** No Qualifier

<u>Non-OR</u>   Ø6JY[3,X]ZZ

Ø   Medical and Surgical
6   Lower Veins
L   Occlusion   Definition: Completely closing an orifice or the lumen of a tubular body part

Explanation: The orifice can be a natural orifice or an artificially created orifice

Body Part Character 4		Approach Character 5	Device Character 6	Qualifier Character 7

Ø   Inferior Vena Cava
    Postcava
    Right inferior phrenic vein
    Right ovarian vein
    Right second lumbar vein
    Right suprarenal vein
    Right testicular vein
1   Splenic Vein
    Left gastroepiploic vein
    Pancreatic vein
4   Hepatic Vein
5   Superior Mesenteric Vein
    Right gastroepiploic vein
6   Inferior Mesenteric Vein
    Sigmoid vein
    Superior rectal vein
7   Colic Vein
    Ileocolic vein
    Left colic vein
    Middle colic vein
    Right colic vein
8   Portal Vein
    Hepatic portal vein
9   Renal Vein, Right
B   Renal Vein, Left
    Left inferior phrenic vein
    Left ovarian vein
    Left second lumbar vein
    Left suprarenal vein
    Left testicular vein
C   Common Iliac Vein, Right
D   Common Iliac Vein, Left
F   External Iliac Vein, Right
G   External Iliac Vein, Left
	H Hypogastric Vein, Right
	    Gluteal vein
	    Internal iliac vein
	    Internal pudendal vein
	    Lateral sacral vein
	    Middle hemorrhoidal vein
	    Obturator vein
	    Uterine vein
	    Vaginal vein
	    Vesical vein
	J Hypogastric Vein, Left
	    See H Hypogastric Vein, Right
	M Femoral Vein, Right
	    Deep femoral (profunda
	      femoris) vein
	    Popliteal vein
	    Profunda femoris (deep
	      femoral) vein
	N Femoral Vein, Left
	    See M Femoral Vein, Right
	P Saphenous Vein, Right
	    External pudendal vein
	    Great(er) saphenous vein
	    Lesser saphenous vein
	    Small saphenous vein
	    Superficial circumflex iliac vein
	    Superficial epigastric vein
	Q Saphenous Vein, Left
	    See P Saphenous Vein, Right
	T Foot Vein, Right
	    Common digital vein
	    Dorsal metatarsal vein
	    Dorsal venous arch
	    Plantar digital vein
	    Plantar metatarsal vein
	    Plantar venous arch
	V Foot Vein, Left
	    See T Foot Vein, Right
		Ø Open
		3 Percutaneous
		4 Percutaneous Endoscopic
			C Extraluminal Device
			D Intraluminal Device
			Z No Device
				Z No Qualifier

2   Gastric Vein
3   Esophageal Vein
		Ø Open
		3 Percutaneous
		4 Percutaneous Endoscopic
		7 Via Natural or Artificial
		      Opening
		8 Via Natural or Artificial
		      Opening Endoscopic
			C Extraluminal Device
			D Intraluminal Device
			Z No Device
				Z No Qualifier

Y Lower Vein		**Ø** Open **3** Percutaneous **4** Percutaneous Endoscopic	**C** Extraluminal Device **D** Intraluminal Device **Z** No Device	**C** Hemorrhoidal Plexus **Z** No Qualifier

<u>Non-OR</u>   Ø6L2[7,8][C,D,Z]Z
<u>Non-OR</u>   Ø6L3[3,4,7,8][C,D,Z]Z

LC Limited Coverage   **NC** Noncovered   ⊞ Combination Member   HAC associated procedure   Combination Only   DRG Non-OR   Non-OR   New/Revised in GREEN

ICD-10-PCS 2020   265

Ø6J–Ø6L

Ø   Medical and Surgical
6   Lower Veins
N   Release   Definition: Freeing a body part from an abnormal physical constraint by cutting or by the use of force

                       Explanation: Some of the restraining tissue may be taken out but none of the body part is taken out

Body Part Character 4		Approach Character 5	Device Character 6	Qualifier Character 7

Ø Inferior Vena Cava
Postcava
Right inferior phrenic vein
Right ovarian vein
Right second lumbar vein
Right suprarenal vein
Right testicular vein
1 Splenic Vein
Left gastroepiploic vein
Pancreatic vein
2 Gastric Vein
3 Esophageal Vein
4 Hepatic Vein
5 Superior Mesenteric Vein
Right gastroepiploic vein
6 Inferior Mesenteric Vein
Sigmoid vein
Superior rectal vein
7 Colic Vein
Ileocolic vein
Left colic vein
Middle colic vein
Right colic vein
8 Portal Vein
Hepatic portal vein
9 Renal Vein, Right
B Renal Vein, Left
Left inferior phrenic vein
Left ovarian vein
Left second lumbar vein
Left suprarenal vein
Left testicular vein
C Common Iliac Vein, Right
D Common Iliac Vein, Left
F External Iliac Vein, Right
G External Iliac Vein, Left
	H Hypogastric Vein, Right
	Gluteal vein
	Internal iliac vein
	Internal pudendal vein
	Lateral sacral vein
	Middle hemorrhoidal vein
	Obturator vein
	Uterine vein
	Vaginal vein
	Vesical vein
	J Hypogastric Vein, Left
	See H Hypogastric Vein, Right
	M Femoral Vein, Right
	Deep femoral (profunda
	  femoris) vein
	Popliteal vein
	Profunda femoris (deep
	  femoral) vein
	N Femoral Vein, Left
	See M Femoral Vein, Right
	P Saphenous Vein, Right
	External pudendal vein
	Great(er) saphenous vein
	Lesser saphenous vein
	Small saphenous vein
	Superficial circumflex iliac vein
	Superficial epigastric vein
	Q Saphenous Vein, Left
	See P Saphenous Vein, Right
	T Foot Vein, Right
	Common digital vein
	Dorsal metatarsal vein
	Dorsal venous arch
	Plantar digital vein
	Plantar metatarsal vein
	Plantar venous arch
	V Foot Vein, Left
	See T Foot Vein, Right
	Y Lower Vein
		Ø Open
		3 Percutaneous
		4 Percutaneous Endoscopic
			Z No Device	**Z No Qualifier**

Ø   Medical and Surgical
6   Lower Veins
P   Removal   Definition: Taking out or off a device from a body part

                       Explanation: If a device is taken out and a similar device put in without cutting or puncturing the skin or mucous membrane, the procedure is coded to the root operation CHANGE. Otherwise, the procedure for taking out a device is coded to the root operation REMOVAL.

Body Part Character 4	Approach Character 5	Device Character 6	Qualifier Character 7
Y Lower Vein	**Ø Open** **3 Percutaneous** **4 Percutaneous Endoscopic**	**Ø Drainage Device** **2 Monitoring Device** **3 Infusion Device** **7 Autologous Tissue Substitute** **C Extraluminal Device** **D Intraluminal Device** **J Synthetic Substitute** **K Nonautologous Tissue Substitute** **Y Other Device**	**Z No Qualifier**
Y Lower Vein	**X External**	**Ø Drainage Device** **2 Monitoring Device** **3 Infusion Device** **D Intraluminal Device**	**Z No Qualifier**

Non-OR   Ø6PY3[Ø,2,3]Z
Non-OR   Ø6PY[3,4]YZ
Non-OR   Ø6PYX[Ø,2,3,D]Z

LC Limited Coverage   NC Noncovered   ⊞ Combination Member   HAC associated procedure   Combination Only   DRG Non-OR   Non-OR   New/Revised in GREEN

266   ICD-10-PCS 2020

Ø   Medical and Surgical
6   Lower Veins
Q   Repair   Definition: Restoring, to the extent possible, a body part to its normal anatomic structure and function
                 Explanation: Used only when the method to accomplish the repair is not one of the other root operations

Body Part Character 4	Approach Character 5	Device Character 6	Qualifier Character 7

Ø Inferior Vena Cava
    Postcava
    Right inferior phrenic vein
    Right ovarian vein
    Right second lumbar vein
    Right suprarenal vein
    Right testicular vein
	Ø Open
	3 Percutaneous
	4 Percutaneous Endoscopic
		Z No Device	**Z No Qualifier**

1 Splenic Vein
    Left gastroepiploic vein
    Pancreatic vein			

2 Gastric Vein			
3 Esophageal Vein			
4 Hepatic Vein			
5 Superior Mesenteric Vein Right gastroepiploic vein			

6 Inferior Mesenteric Vein
    Sigmoid vein
    Superior rectal vein			

7 Colic Vein
    Ileocolic vein
    Left colic vein
    Middle colic vein
    Right colic vein			

8 Portal Vein Hepatic portal vein			
9 Renal Vein, Right			

B Renal Vein, Left
    Left inferior phrenic vein
    Left ovarian vein
    Left second lumbar vein
    Left suprarenal vein
    Left testicular vein			

C Common Iliac Vein, Right			
D Common Iliac Vein, Left			
F External Iliac Vein, Right			
G External Iliac Vein, Left			

H Hypogastric Vein, Right
    Gluteal vein
    Internal iliac vein
    Internal pudendal vein
    Lateral sacral vein
    Middle hemorrhoidal vein
    Obturator vein
    Uterine vein
    Vaginal vein
    Vesical vein			

J Hypogastric Vein, Left *See H Hypogastric Vein, Right*			

M Femoral Vein, Right
    Deep femoral (profunda femoris) vein
    Popliteal vein
    Profunda femoris (deep femoral) vein			

N Femoral Vein, Left *See M Femoral Vein, Right*			

P Saphenous Vein, Right
    External pudendal vein
    Great(er) saphenous vein
    Lesser saphenous vein
    Small saphenous vein
    Superficial circumflex iliac vein
    Superficial epigastric vein			

Q Saphenous Vein, Left *See P Saphenous Vein, Right*			

T Foot Vein, Right
    Common digital vein
    Dorsal metatarsal vein
    Dorsal venous arch
    Plantar digital vein
    Plantar metatarsal vein
    Plantar venous arch			

V Foot Vein, Left *See T Foot Vein, Right*			
Y Lower Vein			

Lower Veins

Ø6R–Ø6R

Ø　Medical and Surgical
6　Lower Veins
R　Replacement　　Definition: Putting in or on biological or synthetic material that physically takes the place and/or function of all or a portion of a body part

Explanation: The body part may have been taken out or replaced, or may be taken out, physically eradicated, or rendered nonfunctional during the REPLACEMENT procedure. A REMOVAL procedure is coded for taking out the device used in a previous replacement procedure.

Body Part Character 4	Approach Character 5	Device Character 6	Qualifier Character 7
Ø　Inferior Vena Cava 　　Postcava 　　Right inferior phrenic vein 　　Right ovarian vein 　　Right second lumbar vein 　　Right suprarenal vein 　　Right testicular vein	**Ø　Open** **4　Percutaneous Endoscopic**	**7　Autologous Tissue Substitute** **J　Synthetic Substitute** **K　Nonautologous Tissue Substitute**	**Z　No Qualifier**
1　Splenic Vein 　　Left gastroepiploic vein 　　Pancreatic vein			
2　Gastric Vein			
3　Esophageal Vein			
4　Hepatic Vein			
5　Superior Mesenteric Vein 　　Right gastroepiploic vein			
6　Inferior Mesenteric Vein 　　Sigmoid vein 　　Superior rectal vein			
7　Colic Vein 　　Ileocolic vein 　　Left colic vein 　　Middle colic vein 　　Right colic vein			
8　Portal Vein 　　Hepatic portal vein			
9　Renal Vein, Right			
B　Renal Vein, Left 　　Left inferior phrenic vein 　　Left ovarian vein 　　Left second lumbar vein 　　Left suprarenal vein 　　Left testicular vein			
C　Common Iliac Vein, Right			
D　Common Iliac Vein, Left			
F　External Iliac Vein, Right			
G　External Iliac Vein, Left			
H　Hypogastric Vein, Right 　　Gluteal vein 　　Internal iliac vein 　　Internal pudendal vein 　　Lateral sacral vein· 　　Middle hemorrhoidal vein 　　Obturator vein 　　Uterine vein 　　Vaginal vein 　　Vesical vein			
J　Hypogastric Vein, Left 　　*See H Hypogastric Vein, Right*			
M　Femoral Vein, Right 　　Deep femoral (profunda femoris) vein 　　Popliteal vein 　　Profunda femoris (deep femoral) vein			
N　Femoral Vein, Left 　　*See M Femoral Vein, Right*			
P　Saphenous Vein, Right 　　External pudendal vein 　　Great(er) saphenous vein 　　Lesser saphenous vein 　　Small saphenous vein 　　Superficial circumflex iliac vein 　　Superficial epigastric vein			
Q　Saphenous Vein, Left 　　*See P Saphenous Vein, Right*			
T　Foot Vein, Right 　　Common digital vein 　　Dorsal metatarsal vein 　　Dorsal venous arch 　　Plantar digital vein 　　Plantar metatarsal vein 　　Plantar venous arch			
V　Foot Vein, Left 　　*See T Foot Vein, Right*			
Y　Lower Vein			

LC Limited Coverage　NC Noncovered　⊞ Combination Member　HAC associated procedure　Combination Only　DRG Non-OR　Non-OR　New/Revised in GREEN

268　　　　　　　　　　　　　　　　　　　　　　　　　　　　　　　　　ICD-10-PCS 2020

Ø Medical and Surgical
6 Lower Veins
S Reposition Definition: Moving to its normal location, or other suitable location, all or a portion of a body part

Explanation: The body part is moved to a new location from an abnormal location, or from a normal location where it is not functioning correctly. The body part may or may not be cut out or off to be moved to the new location.

Body Part Character 4	Approach Character 5	Device Character 6	Qualifier Character 7
Ø Inferior Vena Cava Postcava Right inferior phrenic vein Right ovarian vein Right second lumbar vein Right suprarenal vein Right testicular vein	**Ø Open** **3 Percutaneous** **4 Percutaneous Endoscopic**	**Z No Device**	**Z No Qualifier**
1 Splenic Vein Left gastroepiploic vein Pancreatic vein			
2 Gastric Vein			
3 Esophageal Vein			
4 Hepatic Vein			
5 Superior Mesenteric Vein Right gastroepiploic vein			
6 Inferior Mesenteric Vein Sigmoid vein Superior rectal vein			
7 Colic Vein Ileocolic vein Left colic vein Middle colic vein Right colic vein			
8 Portal Vein Hepatic portal vein			
9 Renal Vein, Right			
B Renal Vein, Left Left inferior phrenic vein Left ovarian vein Left second lumbar vein Left suprarenal vein Left testicular vein			
C Common Iliac Vein, Right			
D Common Iliac Vein, Left			
F External Iliac Vein, Right			
G External Iliac Vein, Left			
H Hypogastric Vein, Right Gluteal vein Internal iliac vein Internal pudendal vein Lateral sacral vein Middle hemorrhoidal vein Obturator vein Uterine vein Vaginal vein Vesical vein			
J Hypogastric Vein, Left *See H Hypogastric Vein, Right*			
M Femoral Vein, Right Deep femoral (profunda femoris) vein Popliteal vein Profunda femoris (deep femoral) vein			
N Femoral Vein, Left *See M Femoral Vein, Right*			
P Saphenous Vein, Right External pudendal vein Great(er) saphenous vein Lesser saphenous vein Small saphenous vein Superficial circumflex iliac vein Superficial epigastric vein			
Q Saphenous Vein, Left *See P Saphenous Vein, Right*			
T Foot Vein, Right Common digital vein Dorsal metatarsal vein Dorsal venous arch Plantar digital vein Plantar metatarsal vein Plantar venous arch			
V Foot Vein, Left *See T Foot Vein, Right*			
Y Lower Vein			

LC Limited Coverage NC Noncovered ⊞ Combination Member HAC associated procedure Combination Only DRG Non-OR Non-OR New/Revised in GREEN

ICD-10-PCS 2020 269

06S–06S

Lower Veins

Ø **Medical and Surgical**
6 **Lower Veins**
U **Supplement** Definition: Putting in or on biological or synthetic material that physically reinforces and/or augments the function of a portion of a body part
Explanation: The biological material is non-living, or is living and from the same individual. The body part may have been previously replaced, and the SUPPLEMENT procedure is performed to physically reinforce and/or augment the function of the replaced body part.

Body Part Character 4	Approach Character 5	Device Character 6	Qualifier Character 7
Ø **Inferior Vena Cava** Postcava Right inferior phrenic vein Right ovarian vein Right second lumbar vein Right suprarenal vein Right testicular vein	Ø Open 3 Percutaneous 4 Percutaneous Endoscopic	7 Autologous Tissue Substitute J Synthetic Substitute K Nonautologous Tissue Substitute	Z No Qualifier
1 **Splenic Vein** Left gastroepiploic vein Pancreatic vein			
2 **Gastric Vein**			
3 **Esophageal Vein**			
4 **Hepatic Vein**			
5 **Superior Mesenteric Vein** Right gastroepiploic vein			
6 **Inferior Mesenteric Vein** Sigmoid vein Superior rectal vein			
7 **Colic Vein** Ileocolic vein Left colic vein Middle colic vein Right colic vein			
8 **Portal Vein** Hepatic portal vein			
9 **Renal Vein, Right**			
B **Renal Vein, Left** Left inferior phrenic vein Left ovarian vein Left second lumbar vein Left suprarenal vein Left testicular vein			
C **Common Iliac Vein, Right**			
D **Common Iliac Vein, Left**			
F **External Iliac Vein, Right**			
G **External Iliac Vein, Left**			
H **Hypogastric Vein, Right** Gluteal vein Internal iliac vein Internal pudendal vein Lateral sacral vein Middle hemorrhoidal vein Obturator vein Uterine vein Vaginal vein Vesical vein			
J **Hypogastric Vein, Left** *See* H Hypogastric Vein, Right			
M **Femoral Vein, Right** Deep femoral (profunda femoris) vein Popliteal vein Profunda femoris (deep femoral) vein			
N **Femoral Vein, Left** *See* M Femoral Vein, Right			
P **Saphenous Vein, Right** External pudendal vein Great(er) saphenous vein Lesser saphenous vein Small saphenous vein Superficial circumflex iliac vein Superficial epigastric vein			
Q **Saphenous Vein, Left** *See* P Saphenous Vein, Right			
T **Foot Vein, Right** Common digital vein Dorsal metatarsal vein Dorsal venous arch Plantar digital vein Plantar metatarsal vein Plantar venous arch			
V **Foot Vein, Left** *See* T Foot Vein, Right			
Y **Lower Vein**			

Ø   Medical and Surgical
6   Lower Veins
V   Restriction   Definition: Partially closing an orifice or the lumen of a tubular body part
                       Explanation: The orifice can be a natural orifice or an artificially created orifice

Body Part Character 4	Approach Character 5	Device Character 6	Qualifier Character 7
Ø Inferior Vena Cava Postcava Right inferior phrenic vein Right ovarian vein Right second lumbar vein Right suprarenal vein Right testicular vein	**Ø Open** **3 Percutaneous** **4 Percutaneous Endoscopic**	**C Extraluminal Device** **D Intraluminal Device** **Z No Device**	**Z No Qualifier**
1 Splenic Vein Left gastroepiploic vein Pancreatic vein			
2 Gastric Vein			
3 Esophageal Vein			
4 Hepatic Vein			
5 Superior Mesenteric Vein Right gastroepiploic vein			
6 Inferior Mesenteric Vein Sigmoid vein Superior rectal vein			
7 Colic Vein Ileocolic vein Left colic vein Middle colic vein Right colic vein			
8 Portal Vein Hepatic portal vein			
9 Renal Vein, Right			
B Renal Vein, Left Left inferior phrenic vein Left ovarian vein Left second lumbar vein Left suprarenal vein Left testicular vein			
C Common Iliac Vein, Right			
D Common Iliac Vein, Left			
F External Iliac Vein, Right			
G External Iliac Vein, Left			
H Hypogastric Vein, Right Gluteal vein Internal iliac vein Internal pudendal vein Lateral sacral vein Middle hemorrhoidal vein Obturator vein Uterine vein Vaginal vein Vesical vein			
J Hypogastric Vein, Left *See H Hypogastric Vein, Right*			
M Femoral Vein, Right Deep femoral (profunda femoris) vein Popliteal vein Profunda femoris (deep femoral) vein			
N Femoral Vein, Left *See M Femoral Vein, Right*			
P Saphenous Vein, Right External pudendal vein Great(er) saphenous vein Lesser saphenous vein Small saphenous vein Superficial circumflex iliac vein Superficial epigastric vein			
Q Saphenous Vein, Left *See P Saphenous Vein, Right*			
T Foot Vein, Right Common digital vein Dorsal metatarsal vein Dorsal venous arch Plantar digital vein Plantar metatarsal vein Plantar venous arch			
V Foot Vein, Left *See T Foot Vein, Right*			
Y Lower Vein			

Ø   Medical and Surgical
6   Lower Veins
W   Revision   Definition: Correcting, to the extent possible, a portion of a malfunctioning device or the position of a displaced device

Explanation: Revision can include correcting a malfunctioning or displaced device by taking out or putting in components of the device such as a screw or pin

Body Part Character 4	Approach Character 5	Device Character 6	Qualifier Character 7
Y Lower Vein	Ø Open 3 Percutaneous 4 Percutaneous Endoscopic	Ø Drainage Device 2 Monitoring Device 3 Infusion Device 7 Autologous Tissue Substitute C Extraluminal Device D Intraluminal Device J Synthetic Substitute K Nonautologous Tissue Substitute Y Other Device	Z No Qualifier
Y Lower Vein	X External	Ø Drainage Device 2 Monitoring Device 3 Infusion Device 7 Autologous Tissue Substitute C Extraluminal Device D Intraluminal Device J Synthetic Substitute K Nonautologous Tissue Substitute	Z No Qualifier

Non-OR   Ø6WY3[Ø,2,3,D]Z
Non-OR   Ø6WY[3,4]YZ
Non-OR   Ø6WYX[Ø,2,3,7,C,D,J,K]Z

LC Limited Coverage   NC Noncovered   ⊞ Combination Member   HAC associated procedure   Combination Only   DRG Non-OR   Non-OR   New/Revised in GREEN

272   ICD-10-PCS 2020

Lymphatic and Hemic Systems Ø72–Ø7Y

Character Meanings*

This Character Meaning table is provided as a guide to assist the user in the identification of character members that may be found in this section of code tables. It **SHOULD NOT** be used to build a PCS code.

Operation–Character 3	Body Part–Character 4	Approach–Character 5	Device–Character 6	Qualifier–Character 7
2 Change	Ø Lymphatic, Head	Ø Open	Ø Drainage Device	Ø Allogeneic
5 Destruction	1 Lymphatic, Right Neck	3 Percutaneous	3 Infusion Device	1 Syngeneic
9 Drainage	2 Lymphatic, Left Neck	4 Percutaneous Endoscopic	7 Autologous Tissue Substitute	2 Zooplastic
B Excision	3 Lymphatic, Right Upper Extremity	8 Via Natural or Artificial Opening Endoscopic	C Extraluminal Device	X Diagnostic
C Extirpation	4 Lymphatic, Left Upper Extremity	X External	D Intraluminal Device	Z No Qualifier
D Extraction	5 Lymphatic, Right Axillary		J Synthetic Substitute	
H Insertion	6 Lymphatic, Left Axillary		K Nonautologous Tissue Substitute	
J Inspection	7 Lymphatic, Thorax		Y Other Device	
L Occlusion	8 Lymphatic, Internal Mammary, Right		Z No Device	
N Release	9 Lymphatic, Internal Mammary, Left			
P Removal	B Lymphatic, Mesenteric			
Q Repair	C Lymphatic, Pelvis			
S Reposition	D Lymphatic, Aortic			
T Resection	F Lymphatic, Right Lower Extremity			
U Supplement	G Lymphatic, Left Lower Extremity			
V Restriction	H Lymphatic, Right Inguinal			
W Revision	J Lymphatic, Left Inguinal			
Y Transplantation	K Thoracic Duct			
	L Cisterna Chyli			
	M Thymus			
	N Lymphatic			
	P Spleen			
	Q Bone Marrow, Sternum			
	R Bone Marrow, Iliac			
	S Bone Marrow, Vertebral			
	T Bone Marrow			

* Includes lymph vessels and lymph nodes.

AHA Coding Clinic for table Ø79

2018, 4Q, 84	Fine needle aspiration biopsy of lymphatic tissue
2017, 1Q, 34	Lymphovenous bypass following mastectomy
2014, 1Q, 26	Transbronchial needle aspiration lymph node biopsy
2013, 4Q, 111	Transbronchial needle aspiration lymph node biopsy

AHA Coding Clinic for table Ø7B

2019, 1Q, 3-8	Whipple procedure
2018, 4Q, 84	Fine needle aspiration biopsy of lymphatic tissue
2018, 1Q, 22	Resection of lymph node chains
2016, 1Q, 30	Axillary lymph node resection with modified radical mastectomy
2014, 3Q, 10	Selective excision of paratracheal lymph nodes
2014, 1Q, 20	Fiducial marker placement
2014, 1Q, 26	Transbronchial endoscopic lymph node aspiration biopsy

AHA Coding Clinic for table Ø7D

| 2018, 4Q, 84 | Fine needle aspiration biopsy of lymphatic tissue |
| 2013, 4Q, 111 | Root operation for bone marrow biopsy |

AHA Coding Clinic for table Ø7Q

| 2017, 1Q, 34 | Lymphovenous bypass following mastectomy |

AHA Coding Clinic for table Ø7T

2018, 1Q, 22	Resection of lymph node chains
2016, 2Q, 12	Resection of malignant neoplasm of infratemporal fossa
2016, 1Q, 30	Axillary lymph node resection with modified radical mastectomy
2015, 4Q, 13	New Section X codes—New Technology procedures
2014, 3Q, 9	Radical resection of level I lymph nodes
2014, 3Q, 16	Repair of Tetralogy of Fallot

Lymphatic System

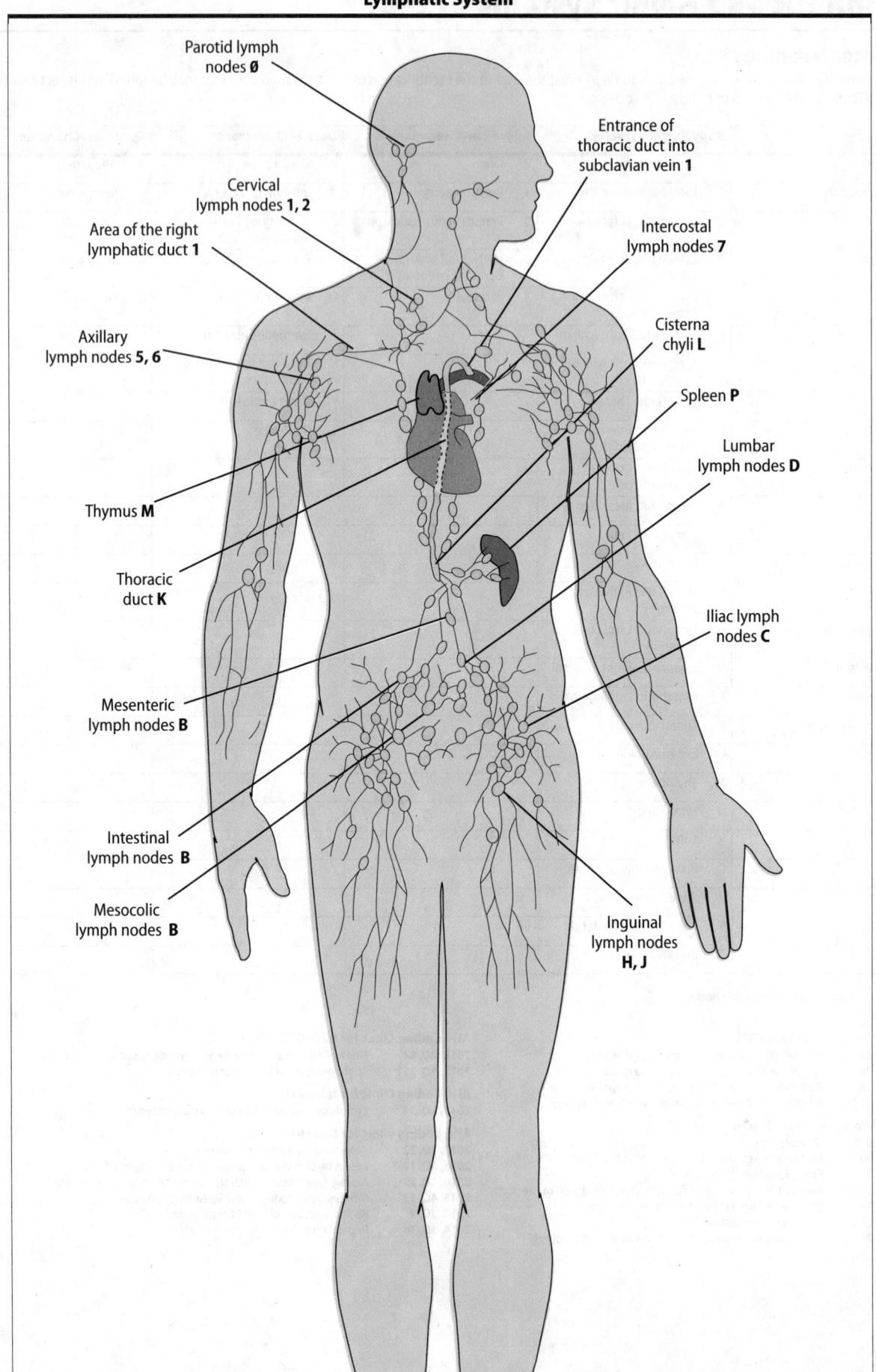

Parotid lymph nodes Ø

Entrance of thoracic duct into subclavian vein 1

Cervical lymph nodes 1, 2

Intercostal lymph nodes 7

Area of the right lymphatic duct 1

Cisterna chyli L

Axillary lymph nodes 5, 6

Spleen P

Lumbar lymph nodes D

Thymus M

Thoracic duct K

Iliac lymph nodes C

Mesenteric lymph nodes B

Intestinal lymph nodes B

Inguinal lymph nodes H, J

Mesocolic lymph nodes B

Ø   Medical and Surgical
7   Lymphatic and Hemic Systems
2   Change   Definition: Taking out or off a device from a body part and putting back an identical or similar device in or on the same body part without cutting or puncturing the skin or a mucous membrane
                 Explanation: All CHANGE procedures are coded using the approach EXTERNAL

Body Part Character 4		Approach Character 5	Device Character 6	Qualifier Character 7

K Thoracic Duct
     Left jugular trunk
     Left subclavian trunk
L Cisterna Chyli
     Intestinal lymphatic trunk
     Lumbar lymphatic trunk
	M Thymus
	     Thymus gland
	N Lymphatic
	P Spleen
	     Accessory spleen
	T Bone Marrow
		X External	**Ø** Drainage Device
			Y Other Device
				Z No Qualifier

Non-OR	All body part, approach, device, and qualifier values

Ø   Medical and Surgical
7   Lymphatic and Hemic Systems
5   Destruction   Definition: Physical eradication of all or a portion of a body part by the direct use of energy, force, or a destructive agent
                 Explanation: None of the body part is physically taken out

Body Part Character 4		Approach Character 5	Device Character 6	Qualifier Character 7

Ø Lymphatic, Head
     Buccinator lymph node
     Infraauricular lymph node
     Infraparotid lymph node
     Parotid lymph node
     Preauricular lymph node
     Submandibular lymph node
     Submaxillary lymph node
     Submental lymph node
     Subparotid lymph node
     Suprahyoid lymph node
1 Lymphatic, Right Neck
     Cervical lymph node
     Jugular lymph node
     Mastoid (postauricular) lymph node
     Occipital lymph node
     Postauricular (mastoid) lymph node
     Retropharyngeal lymph node
     Right jugular trunk
     Right lymphatic duct
     Right subclavian trunk
     Supraclavicular (Virchow's) lymph node
     Virchow's (supraclavicular) lymph node
2 Lymphatic, Left Neck
     Cervical lymph node
     Jugular lymph node
     Mastoid (postauricular) lymph node
     Occipital lymph node
     Postauricular (mastoid) lymph node
     Retropharyngeal lymph node
     Supraclavicular (Virchow's) lymph node
     Virchow's (supraclavicular) lymph node
3 Lymphatic, Right Upper Extremity
     Cubital lymph node
     Deltopectoral (infraclavicular) lymph
         node
     Epitrochlear lymph node
     Infraclavicular (deltopectoral) lymph
         node
     Supratrochlear lymph node
4 Lymphatic, Left Upper Extremity
     See 3 Lymphatic, Right Upper Extremity
5 Lymphatic, Right Axillary
     Anterior (pectoral) lymph node
     Apical (subclavicular) lymph node
     Brachial (lateral) lymph node
     Central axillary lymph node
     Lateral (brachial) lymph node
     Pectoral (anterior) lymph node
     Posterior (subscapular) lymph node
     Subclavicular (apical) lymph node
     Subscapular (posterior) lymph node
	6 Lymphatic, Left Axillary
	     See 5 Lymphatic, Right Axillary
	7 Lymphatic, Thorax
	     Intercostal lymph node
	     Mediastinal lymph node
	     Parasternal lymph node
	     Paratracheal lymph node
	     Tracheobronchial lymph node
	8 Lymphatic, Internal Mammary, Right
	9 Lymphatic, Internal Mammary, Left
	B Lymphatic, Mesenteric
	     Inferior mesenteric lymph node
	     Pararectal lymph node
	     Superior mesenteric lymph node
	C Lymphatic, Pelvis
	     Common iliac (subaortic) lymph node
	     Gluteal lymph node
	     Iliac lymph node
	     Inferior epigastric lymph node
	     Obturator lymph node
	     Sacral lymph node
	     Subaortic (common iliac) lymph node
	     Suprainguinal lymph node
	D Lymphatic, Aortic
	     Celiac lymph node
	     Gastric lymph node
	     Hepatic lymph node
	     Lumbar lymph node
	     Pancreaticosplenic lymph node
	     Paraaortic lymph node
	     Retroperitoneal lymph node
	F Lymphatic, Right Lower Extremity
	     Femoral lymph node
	     Popliteal lymph node
	G Lymphatic, Left Lower Extremity
	     See F Lymphatic, Right Lower Extremity
	H Lymphatic, Right Inguinal
	J Lymphatic, Left Inguinal
	K Thoracic Duct
	     Left jugular trunk
	     Left subclavian trunk
	L Cisterna Chyli
	     Intestinal lymphatic trunk
	     Lumbar lymphatic trunk
	M Thymus
	     Thymus gland
	P Spleen
	     Accessory spleen
		Ø Open
		3 Percutaneous
		4 Percutaneous
		     Endoscopic
			Z No Device	**Z** No Qualifier

Ø   Medical and Surgical
7   Lymphatic and Hemic Systems
9   Drainage   Definition: Taking or letting out fluids and/or gases from a body part
                          Explanation: The qualifier DIAGNOSTIC is used to identify drainage procedures that are biopsies

Body Part Character 4		Approach Character 5	Device Character 6	Qualifier Character 7

Ø   Lymphatic, Head
Buccinator lymph node
Infraauricular lymph node
Infraparotid lymph node
Parotid lymph node
Preauricular lymph node
Submandibular lymph node
Submaxillary lymph node
Submental lymph node
Subparotid lymph node
Suprahyoid lymph node
 	
1   Lymphatic, Right Neck
Cervical lymph node
Jugular lymph node
Mastoid (postauricular) lymph node
Occipital lymph node
Postauricular (mastoid) lymph node
Retropharyngeal lymph node
Right jugular trunk
Right lymphatic duct
Right subclavian trunk
Supraclavicular (Virchow's) lymph
     node
Virchow's (supraclavicular) lymph
     node
 	
2   Lymphatic, Left Neck
Cervical lymph node
Jugular lymph node
Mastoid (postauricular) lymph node
Occipital lymph node
Postauricular (mastoid) lymph node
Retropharyngeal lymph node
Supraclavicular (Virchow's) lymph
     node
Virchow's (supraclavicular) lymph
     node
 	
3   Lymphatic, Right Upper Extremity
Cubital lymph node
Deltopectoral (infraclavicular) lymph
     node
Epitrochlear lymph node
Infraclavicular (deltopectoral) lymph
     node
Supratrochlear lymph node
 	
4   Lymphatic, Left Upper Extremity
See 3 Lymphatic, Right Upper Extremity
 	
5   Lymphatic, Right Axillary
Anterior (pectoral) lymph node
Apical (subclavicular) lymph node
Brachial (lateral) lymph node
Central axillary lymph node
Lateral (brachial) lymph node
Pectoral (anterior) lymph node
Posterior (subscapular) lymph node
Subclavicular (apical) lymph node
Subscapular (posterior) lymph node
	6 Lymphatic, Left Axillary
	See 5 Lymphatic, Right Axillary
	
	7 Lymphatic, Thorax
	Intercostal lymph node
	Mediastinal lymph node
	Parasternal lymph node
	Paratracheal lymph node
	Tracheobronchial lymph node
	
	8 Lymphatic, Internal Mammary, Right
	9 Lymphatic, Internal Mammary, Left
	B Lymphatic, Mesenteric
	Inferior mesenteric lymph node
	Pararectal lymph node
	Superior mesenteric lymph node
	
	C Lymphatic, Pelvis
	Common iliac (subaortic) lymph node
	Gluteal lymph node
	Iliac lymph node
	Inferior epigastric lymph node
	Obturator lymph node
	Sacral lymph node
	Subaortic (common iliac) lymph node
	Suprainguinal lymph node
	
	D Lymphatic, Aortic
	Celiac lymph node
	Gastric lymph node
	Hepatic lymph node
	Lumbar lymph node
	Pancreaticosplenic lymph node
	Paraaortic lymph node
	Retroperitoneal lymph node
	
	F Lymphatic, Right Lower Extremity
	Femoral lymph node
	Popliteal lymph node
	
	G Lymphatic, Left Lower Extremity
	See F Lymphatic, Right Lower Extremity
	
	H Lymphatic, Right Inguinal
	J Lymphatic, Left Inguinal
	K Thoracic Duct
	Left jugular trunk
	Left subclavian trunk
	
	L Cisterna Chyli
	Intestinal lymphatic trunk
	Lumbar lymphatic trunk
		Ø Open
		3 Percutaneous
		**4 Percutaneous
		     Endoscopic**
		**8 Via Natural or
		     Artificial Opening
		     Endoscopic**
			Ø Drainage Device	**Z No Qualifier**

079 Continued on next page

Non-OR	079[Ø,1,2,3,4,5,6,7,8,9,B,C,D,F,G,H,J,K,L][3,8]ØZ

LC Limited Coverage   **NC** Noncovered   ⊞ Combination Member   HAC associated procedure   Combination Only   DRG Non-OR   Non-OR   New/Revised in GREEN

276   ICD-10-PCS 2020

Ø   **Medical and Surgical**   *Ø79 Continued*
7   **Lymphatic and Hemic Systems**
9   **Drainage**   Definition: Taking or letting out fluids and/or gases from a body part

                        Explanation: The qualifier DIAGNOSTIC is used to identify drainage procedures that are biopsies

Body Part Character 4		Approach Character 5	Device Character 6	Qualifier Character 7

Ø Lymphatic, Head
Buccinator lymph node
Infraauricular lymph node
Infraparotid lymph node
Parotid lymph node
Preauricular lymph node
Submandibular lymph node
Submaxillary lymph node
Submental lymph node
Subparotid lymph node
Suprahyoid lymph node
1 Lymphatic, Right Neck
Cervical lymph node
Jugular lymph node
Mastoid (postauricular) lymph node
Occipital lymph node
Postauricular (mastoid) lymph node
Retropharyngeal lymph node
Right jugular trunk
Right lymphatic duct
Right subclavian trunk
Supraclavicular (Virchow's) lymph
   node
Virchow's (supraclavicular) lymph
   node
2 Lymphatic, Left Neck
Cervical lymph node
Jugular lymph node
Mastoid (postauricular) lymph node
Occipital lymph node
Postauricular (mastoid) lymph node
Retropharyngeal lymph node
Supraclavicular (Virchow's) lymph
   node
Virchow's (supraclavicular) lymph
   node
3 Lymphatic, Right Upper Extremity
Cubital lymph node
Deltopectoral (infraclavicular) lymph
   node
Epitrochlear lymph node
Infraclavicular (deltopectoral) lymph
   node
Supratrochlear lymph node
4 Lymphatic, Left Upper Extremity
See 3 Lymphatic, Right Upper Extremity
5 Lymphatic, Right Axillary
Anterior (pectoral) lymph node
Apical (subclavicular) lymph node
Brachial (lateral) lymph node
Central axillary lymph node
Lateral (brachial) lymph node
Pectoral (anterior) lymph node
Posterior (subscapular) lymph node
Subclavicular (apical) lymph node
Subscapular (posterior) lymph node
	6 Lymphatic, Left Axillary
	See 5 Lymphatic, Right Axillary
	7 Lymphatic, Thorax
	Intercostal lymph node
	Mediastinal lymph node
	Parasternal lymph node
	Paratracheal lymph node
	Tracheobronchial lymph node
	8 Lymphatic, Internal Mammary, Right
	9 Lymphatic, Internal Mammary, Left
	B Lymphatic, Mesenteric
	Inferior mesenteric lymph node
	Pararectal lymph node
	Superior mesenteric lymph node
	C Lymphatic, Pelvis
	Common iliac (subaortic) lymph node
	Gluteal lymph node
	Iliac lymph node
	Inferior epigastric lymph node
	Obturator lymph node
	Sacral lymph node
	Subaortic (common iliac) lymph node
	Suprainguinal lymph node
	D Lymphatic, Aortic
	Celiac lymph node
	Gastric lymph node
	Hepatic lymph node
	Lumbar lymph node
	Pancreaticosplenic lymph node
	Paraaortic lymph node
	Retroperitoneal lymph node
	F Lymphatic, Right Lower Extremity
	Femoral lymph node
	Popliteal lymph node
	G Lymphatic, Left Lower Extremity
	See F Lymphatic, Right Lower Extremity
	H Lymphatic, Right Inguinal
	J Lymphatic, Left Inguinal
	K Thoracic Duct
	Left jugular trunk
	Left subclavian trunk
	L Cisterna Chyli
	Intestinal lymphatic trunk
	Lumbar lymphatic trunk
		Ø Open
		3 Percutaneous
		4 Percutaneous
		  Endoscopic
		8 Via Natural or
		  Artificial Opening
		  Endoscopic
			Z No Device	**X Diagnostic**
				Z No Qualifier

M Thymus Thymus gland **P Spleen** Accessory spleen **T Bone Marrow**		**Ø Open** **3 Percutaneous** **4 Percutaneous** **Endoscopic**	**Ø Drainage Device**	**Z No Qualifier**
M Thymus Thymus gland **P Spleen** Accessory spleen **T Bone Marrow**		**Ø Open** **3 Percutaneous** **4 Percutaneous** **Endoscopic**	**Z No Device**	**X Diagnostic** **Z No Qualifier**

Non-OR   Ø79[Ø,1,2,3,4,5,6,7,8,9,B,C,D,F,G,H,J,K,L]8ZX
Non-OR   Ø79[Ø,1,2,3,4,5,6,7,8,9,B,C,D,F,G,H,J,K,L][3,8]ZZ
Non-OR   Ø79M3ØZ
Non-OR   Ø79P[3,4]ØZ
Non-OR   Ø79T[Ø,3,4]ØZ
Non-OR   Ø79M3ZZ
Non-OR   Ø79P[3,4]Z[X,Z]
Non-OR   Ø79T[Ø,3,4]Z[X,Z]

LC Limited Coverage   **NC** Noncovered   ⊞ Combination Member   HAC associated procedure   Combination Only   DRG Non-OR   Non-OR   New/Revised in GREEN

ICD-10-PCS 2020   277

Ø79–Ø79

Lymphatic and Hemic Systems

0   Medical and Surgical
7   Lymphatic and Hemic Systems
B   Excision   Definition: Cutting out or off, without replacement, a portion of a body part
               Explanation: The qualifier DIAGNOSTIC is used to identify excision procedures that are biopsies

Body Part Character 4		Approach Character 5	Device Character 6	Qualifier Character 7

0 Lymphatic, Head
  Buccinator lymph node
  Infraauricular lymph node
  Infraparotid lymph node
  Parotid lymph node
  Preauricular lymph node
  Submandibular lymph node
  Submaxillary lymph node
  Submental lymph node
  Subparotid lymph node
  Suprahyoid lymph node
1 Lymphatic, Right Neck
  Cervical lymph node
  Jugular lymph node
  Mastoid (postauricular) lymph node
  Occipital lymph node
  Postauricular (mastoid) lymph node
  Retropharyngeal lymph node
  Right jugular trunk
  Right lymphatic duct
  Right subclavian trunk
  Supraclavicular (Virchow's) lymph
    node
  Virchow's (supraclavicular) lymph
    node
2 Lymphatic, Left Neck
  Cervical lymph node
  Jugular lymph node
  Mastoid (postauricular) lymph node
  Occipital lymph node
  Postauricular (mastoid) lymph node
  Retropharyngeal lymph node
  Supraclavicular (Virchow's) lymph
    node
  Virchow's (supraclavicular) lymph
    node
3 Lymphatic, Right Upper Extremity
  Cubital lymph node
  Deltopectoral (infraclavicular) lymph
    node
  Epitrochlear lymph node
  Infraclavicular (deltopectoral) lymph
    node
  Supratrochlear lymph node
4 Lymphatic, Left Upper Extremity
  See 3 Lymphatic, Right Upper Extremity
5 Lymphatic, Right Axillary
  Anterior (pectoral) lymph node
  Apical (subclavicular) lymph node
  Brachial (lateral) lymph node
  Central axillary lymph node
  Lateral (brachial) lymph node
  Pectoral (anterior) lymph node
  Posterior (subscapular) lymph node
  Subclavicular (apical) lymph node
  Subscapular (posterior) lymph node
	6 Lymphatic, Left Axillary
	  See 5 Lymphatic, Right Axillary
	7 Lymphatic, Thorax
	  Intercostal lymph node
	  Mediastinal lymph node
	  Parasternal lymph node
	  Paratracheal lymph node
	  Tracheobronchial lymph node
	8 Lymphatic, Internal Mammary, Right
	9 Lymphatic, Internal Mammary, Left
	B Lymphatic, Mesenteric
	  Inferior mesenteric lymph node
	  Pararectal lymph node
	  Superior mesenteric lymph node
	C Lymphatic, Pelvis
	  Common iliac (subaortic) lymph node
	  Gluteal lymph node
	  Iliac lymph node
	  Inferior epigastric lymph node
	  Obturator lymph node
	  Sacral lymph node
	  Subaortic (common iliac) lymph node
	  Suprainguinal lymph node
	D Lymphatic, Aortic
	  Celiac lymph node
	  Gastric lymph node
	  Hepatic lymph node
	  Lumbar lymph node
	  Pancreaticosplenic lymph node
	  Paraaortic lymph node
	  Retroperitoneal lymph node
	F Lymphatic, Right Lower Extremity
	  Femoral lymph node
	  Popliteal lymph node
	G Lymphatic, Left Lower Extremity
	  See F Lymphatic, Right Lower Extremity
	H Lymphatic, Right Inguinal ⊞
	J Lymphatic, Left Inguinal ⊞
	K Thoracic Duct
	  Left jugular trunk
	  Left subclavian trunk
	L Cisterna Chyli
	  Intestinal lymphatic trunk
	  Lumbar lymphatic trunk
	M Thymus
	  Thymus gland
	P Spleen
	  Accessory spleen
		0 Open
		3 Percutaneous
		4 Percutaneous Endoscopic
			Z No Device	**X Diagnostic**
				Z No Qualifier

Non-OR   07BP[3,4]ZX

See Appendix L for Procedure Combinations
     ⊞   07B[H,J][0,4]ZZ

0   **Medical and Surgical**
7   **Lymphatic and Hemic Systems**
C   **Extirpation**   Definition: Taking or cutting out solid matter from a body part

Explanation: The solid matter may be an abnormal byproduct of a biological function or a foreign body; it may be imbedded in a body part or in the lumen of a tubular body part. The solid matter may or may not have been previously broken into pieces.

Body Part Character 4		Approach Character 5	Device Character 6	Qualifier Character 7

0 Lymphatic, Head
Buccinator lymph node
Infraauricular lymph node
Infraparotid lymph node
Parotid lymph node
Preauricular lymph node
Submandibular lymph node
Submaxillary lymph node
Submental lymph node
Subparotid lymph node
Suprahyoid lymph node
1 Lymphatic, Right Neck
Cervical lymph node
Jugular lymph node
Mastoid (postauricular) lymph node
Occipital lymph node
Postauricular (mastoid) lymph node
Retropharyngeal lymph node
Right jugular trunk
Right lymphatic duct
Right subclavian trunk
Supraclavicular (Virchow's) lymph
   node
Virchow's (supraclavicular) lymph
   node
2 Lymphatic, Left Neck
Cervical lymph node
Jugular lymph node
Mastoid (postauricular) lymph node
Occipital lymph node
Postauricular (mastoid) lymph node
Retropharyngeal lymph node
Supraclavicular (Virchow's) lymph
   node
Virchow's (supraclavicular) lymph
   node
3 Lymphatic, Right Upper Extremity
Cubital lymph node
Deltopectoral (infraclavicular) lymph
   node
Epitrochlear lymph node
Infraclavicular (deltopectoral) lymph
   node
Supratrochlear lymph node
4 Lymphatic, Left Upper Extremity
See 3 Lymphatic, Right Upper Extremity
5 Lymphatic, Right Axillary
Anterior (pectoral) lymph node
Apical (subclavicular) lymph node
Brachial (lateral) lymph node
Central axillary lymph node
Lateral (brachial) lymph node
Pectoral (anterior) lymph node
Posterior (subscapular) lymph node
Subclavicular (apical) lymph node
Subscapular (posterior) lymph node
	6 Lymphatic, Left Axillary
	See 5 Lymphatic, Right Axillary
	7 Lymphatic, Thorax
	Intercostal lymph node
	Mediastinal lymph node
	Parasternal lymph node
	Paratracheal lymph node
	Tracheobronchial lymph node
	8 Lymphatic, Internal Mammary, Right
	9 Lymphatic, Internal Mammary, Left
	B Lymphatic, Mesenteric
	Inferior mesenteric lymph node
	Pararectal lymph node
	Superior mesenteric lymph node
	C Lymphatic, Pelvis
	Common iliac (subaortic) lymph node
	Gluteal lymph node
	Iliac lymph node
	Inferior epigastric lymph node
	Obturator lymph node
	Sacral lymph node
	Subaortic (common iliac) lymph node
	Suprainguinal lymph node
	D Lymphatic, Aortic
	Celiac lymph node
	Gastric lymph node
	Hepatic lymph node
	Lumbar lymph node
	Pancreaticosplenic lymph node
	Paraaortic lymph node
	Retroperitoneal lymph node
	F Lymphatic, Right Lower Extremity
	Femoral lymph node
	Popliteal lymph node
	G Lymphatic, Left Lower Extremity
	See F Lymphatic, Right Lower Extremity
	H Lymphatic, Right Inguinal
	J Lymphatic, Left Inguinal
	K Thoracic Duct
	Left jugular trunk
	Left subclavian trunk
	L Cisterna Chyli
	Intestinal lymphatic trunk
	Lumbar lymphatic trunk
	M Thymus
	Thymus gland
	P Spleen
	Accessory spleen
		0 Open
		3 Percutaneous
		**4 Percutaneous
		Endoscopic**
			Z No Device	**Z No Qualifier**

Non-OR   07CP[3,4]ZZ

Ø Medical and Surgical
7 Lymphatic and Hemic Systems
D Extraction   Definition: Pulling or stripping out or off all or a portion of a body part by the use of force
       Explanation: The qualifier DIAGNOSTIC is used to identify extraction procedures that are biopsies

Body Part Character 4		Approach Character 5	Device Character 6	Qualifier Character 7
Ø Lymphatic, Head Buccinator lymph node Infraauricular lymph node Infraparotid lymph node Parotid lymph node Preauricular lymph node Submandibular lymph node Submaxillary lymph node Submental lymph node Subparotid lymph node Suprahyoid lymph node **1 Lymphatic, Right Neck** Cervical lymph node Jugular lymph node Mastoid (postauricular) lymph node Occipital lymph node Postauricular (mastoid) lymph node Retropharyngeal lymph node Right jugular trunk Right lymphatic duct Right subclavian trunk Supraclavicular (Virchow's) lymph node Virchow's (supraclavicular) lymph node **2 Lymphatic, Left Neck** Cervical lymph node Jugular lymph node Mastoid (postauricular) lymph node Occipital lymph node Postauricular (mastoid) lymph node Retropharyngeal lymph node Supraclavicular (Virchow's) lymph node Virchow's (supraclavicular) lymph node **3 Lymphatic, Right Upper Extremity** Cubital lymph node Deltopectoral (infraclavicular) lymph node Epitrochlear lymph node Infraclavicular (deltopectoral) lymph node Supratrochlear lymph node **4 Lymphatic, Left Upper Extremity** *See 3 Lymphatic, Right Upper Extremity* **5 Lymphatic, Right Axillary** Anterior (pectoral) lymph node Apical (subclavicular) lymph node Brachial (lateral) lymph node Central axillary lymph node Lateral (brachial) lymph node Pectoral (anterior) lymph node Posterior (subscapular) lymph node Subclavicular (apical) lymph node Subscapular (posterior) lymph node	**6 Lymphatic, Left Axillary** *See 5 Lymphatic, Right Axillary* **7 Lymphatic, Thorax** Intercostal lymph node Mediastinal lymph node Parasternal lymph node Paratracheal lymph node Tracheobronchial lymph node **8 Lymphatic, Internal Mammary, Right** **9 Lymphatic, Internal Mammary, Left** **B Lymphatic, Mesenteric** Inferior mesenteric lymph node Pararectal lymph node Superior mesenteric lymph node **C Lymphatic, Pelvis** Common iliac (subaortic) lymph node Gluteal lymph node Iliac lymph node Inferior epigastric lymph node Obturator lymph node Sacral lymph node Subaortic (common iliac) lymph node Suprainguinal lymph node **D Lymphatic, Aortic** Celiac lymph node Gastric lymph node Hepatic lymph node Lumbar lymph node Pancreaticosplenic lymph node Paraaortic lymph node Retroperitoneal lymph node **F Lymphatic, Right Lower Extremity** Femoral lymph node Popliteal lymph node **G Lymphatic, Left Lower Extremity** *See F Lymphatic, Right Lower Extremity* **H Lymphatic, Right Inguinal** **J Lymphatic, Left Inguinal** **K Thoracic Duct** Left jugular trunk Left subclavian trunk **L Cisterna Chyli** Intestinal lymphatic trunk Lumbar lymphatic trunk	**3 Percutaneous** **4 Percutaneous Endoscopic** **8 Via Natural or Artificial Opening Endoscopic**	**Z No Device**	**X Diagnostic**
M Thymus Thymus gland **P Spleen** Accessory spleen		**3 Percutaneous** **4 Percutaneous Endoscopic**	**Z No Device**	**X Diagnostic**
Q Bone Marrow, Sternum **R Bone Marrow, Iliac** **S Bone Marrow, Vertebral**		**Ø Open** **3 Percutaneous**	**Z No Device**	**X Diagnostic** **Z No Qualifier**

Non-OR   All body part, approach, device, and qualifier values

0   **Medical and Surgical**
7   **Lymphatic and Hemic Systems**
H   **Insertion**   Definition: Putting in a nonbiological appliance that monitors, assists, performs, or prevents a physiological function but does not physically take the place of a body part
                       Explanation: None

Body Part Character 4	Approach Character 5	Device Character 6	Qualifier Character 7

K **Thoracic Duct**
    Left jugular trunk
    Left subclavian trunk
L **Cisterna Chyli**
    Intestinal lymphatic trunk
    Lumbar lymphatic trunk
M **Thymus**
    Thymus gland
N **Lymphatic**
P **Spleen**
    Accessory spleen
	0 Open
	3 Percutaneous
	4 Percutaneous Endoscopic
		3 Infusion Device
		Y Other Device
			Z No Qualifier

Non-OR	07H[K,L,M,N,P][0,3,4]3Z
Non-OR	07H[K,L,M]3YZ
Non-OR	07H[N,P][3,4]YZ

0   **Medical and Surgical**
7   **Lymphatic and Hemic Systems**
J   **Inspection**   Definition: Visually and/or manually exploring a body part
                       Explanation: Visual exploration may be performed with or without optical instrumentation. Manual exploration may be performed directly or through intervening body layers.

Body Part Character 4	Approach Character 5	Device Character 6	Qualifier Character 7

K **Thoracic Duct**
    Left jugular trunk
    Left subclavian trunk
L **Cisterna Chyli**
    Intestinal lymphatic trunk
    Lumbar lymphatic trunk
M **Thymus**
    Thymus gland
T **Bone Marrow**
	0 Open
	3 Percutaneous
	4 Percutaneous Endoscopic
		Z No Device	**Z** No Qualifier

N Lymphatic	**0** Open **3** Percutaneous **4** Percutaneous Endoscopic **8** Via Natural or Artificial Opening Endoscopic **X** External	**Z** No Device	**Z** No Qualifier
P Spleen Accessory spleen	**0** Open **3** Percutaneous **4** Percutaneous Endoscopic **X** External	**Z** No Device	**Z** No Qualifier

Non-OR	07J[K,L,M]3ZZ
Non-OR	07JT[0,3,4]ZZ
Non-OR	07JN[3,8,X]ZZ
Non-OR	07JP[3,4,X]ZZ

Lymphatic and Hemic Systems

0   **Medical and Surgical**
7   **Lymphatic and Hemic Systems**
L   **Occlusion**   Definition: Completely closing an orifice or the lumen of a tubular body part
                             Explanation: The orifice can be a natural orifice or an artificially created orifice

Body Part Character 4		Approach Character 5	Device Character 6	Qualifier Character 7
0 Lymphatic, Head Buccinator lymph node Infraauricular lymph node Infraparotid lymph node Parotid lymph node Preauricular lymph node Submandibular lymph node Submaxillary lymph node Submental lymph node Subparotid lymph node Suprahyoid lymph node **1 Lymphatic, Right Neck** Cervical lymph node Jugular lymph node Mastoid (postauricular) lymph node Occipital lymph node Postauricular (mastoid) lymph node Retropharyngeal lymph node Right jugular trunk Right lymphatic duct Right subclavian trunk Supraclavicular (Virchow's) lymph node Virchow's (supraclavicular) lymph node **2 Lymphatic, Left Neck** Cervical lymph node Jugular lymph node Mastoid (postauricular) lymph node Occipital lymph node Postauricular (mastoid) lymph node Retropharyngeal lymph node Supraclavicular (Virchow's) lymph node Virchow's (supraclavicular) lymph node **3 Lymphatic, Right Upper Extremity** Cubital lymph node Deltopectoral (infraclavicular) lymph node Epitrochlear lymph node Infraclavicular (deltopectoral) lymph node Supratrochlear lymph node **4 Lymphatic, Left Upper Extremity** *See 3 Lymphatic, Right Upper Extremity* **5 Lymphatic, Right Axillary** Anterior (pectoral) lymph node Apical (subclavicular) lymph node Brachial (lateral) lymph node Central axillary lymph node Lateral (brachial) lymph node Pectoral (anterior) lymph node Posterior (subscapular) lymph node Subclavicular (apical) lymph node Subscapular (posterior) lymph node	**6 Lymphatic, Left Axillary** *See 5 Lymphatic, Right Axillary* **7 Lymphatic, Thorax** Intercostal lymph node Mediastinal lymph node Parasternal lymph node Paratracheal lymph node Tracheobronchial lymph node **8 Lymphatic, Internal Mammary, Right** **9 Lymphatic, Internal Mammary, Left** **B Lymphatic, Mesenteric** Inferior mesenteric lymph node Pararectal lymph node Superior mesenteric lymph node **C Lymphatic, Pelvis** Common iliac (subaortic) lymph node Gluteal lymph node Iliac lymph node Inferior epigastric lymph node Obturator lymph node Sacral lymph node Subaortic (common iliac) lymph node Suprainguinal lymph node **D Lymphatic, Aortic** Celiac lymph node Gastric lymph node Hepatic lymph node Lumbar lymph node Pancreaticosplenic lymph node Paraaortic lymph node Retroperitoneal lymph node **F Lymphatic, Right Lower Extremity** Femoral lymph node Popliteal lymph node **G Lymphatic, Left Lower Extremity** *See F Lymphatic, Right Lower Extremity* **H Lymphatic, Right Inguinal** **J Lymphatic, Left Inguinal** **K Thoracic Duct** Left jugular trunk Left subclavian trunk **L Cisterna Chyli** Intestinal lymphatic trunk Lumbar lymphatic trunk	**0** Open **3** Percutaneous **4** Percutaneous Endoscopic	**C** Extraluminal Device **D** Intraluminal Device **Z** No Device	**Z** No Qualifier

LC Limited Coverage   **NC** Noncovered   ⊞ Combination Member   HAC associated procedure   Combination Only   DRG Non-OR   Non-OR   New/Revised in GREEN

282   ICD-10-PCS 2020

0   **Medical and Surgical**
7   **Lymphatic and Hemic Systems**
N   **Release**   Definition: Freeing a body part from an abnormal physical constraint by cutting or by the use of force
                             Explanation: Some of the restraining tissue may be taken out but none of the body part is taken out

Body Part Character 4		Approach Character 5	Device Character 6	Qualifier Character 7

0 Lymphatic, Head
 Buccinator lymph node
 Infraauricular lymph node
 Infraparotid lymph node
 Parotid lymph node
 Preauricular lymph node
 Submandibular lymph node
 Submaxillary lymph node
 Submental lymph node
 Subparotid lymph node
 Suprahyoid lymph node
 1 Lymphatic, Right Neck
 Cervical lymph node
 Jugular lymph node
 Mastoid (postauricular) lymph node
 Occipital lymph node
 Postauricular (mastoid) lymph node
 Retropharyngeal lymph node
 Right jugular trunk
 Right lymphatic duct
 Right subclavian trunk
 Supraclavicular (Virchow's) lymph
     node
 Virchow's (supraclavicular) lymph
     node
 2 Lymphatic, Left Neck
 Cervical lymph node
 Jugular lymph node
 Mastoid (postauricular) lymph node
 Occipital lymph node
 Postauricular (mastoid) lymph node
 Retropharyngeal lymph node
 Supraclavicular (Virchow's) lymph
     node
 Virchow's (supraclavicular) lymph
     node
 3 Lymphatic, Right Upper Extremity
 Cubital lymph node
 Deltopectoral (infraclavicular) lymph
     node
 Epitrochlear lymph node
 Infraclavicular (deltopectoral) lymph
     node
 Supratrochlear lymph node
 4 Lymphatic, Left Upper Extremity
 See 3 Lymphatic, Right Upper Extremity
 5 Lymphatic, Right Axillary
 Anterior (pectoral) lymph node
 Apical (subclavicular) lymph node
 Brachial (lateral) lymph node
 Central axillary lymph node
 Lateral (brachial) lymph node
 Pectoral (anterior) lymph node
 Posterior (subscapular) lymph node
 Subclavicular (apical) lymph node
 Subscapular (posterior) lymph node
	6 Lymphatic, Left Axillary
	 See 5 Lymphatic, Right Axillary
	 7 Lymphatic, Thorax
	 Intercostal lymph node
	 Mediastinal lymph node
	 Parasternal lymph node
	 Paratracheal lymph node
	 Tracheobronchial lymph node
	 8 Lymphatic, Internal Mammary, Right
	 9 Lymphatic, Internal Mammary, Left
	 B Lymphatic, Mesenteric
	 Inferior mesenteric lymph node
	 Pararectal lymph node
	 Superior mesenteric lymph node
	 C Lymphatic, Pelvis
	 Common iliac (subaortic) lymph node
	 Gluteal lymph node
	 Iliac lymph node
	 Inferior epigastric lymph node
	 Obturator lymph node
	 Sacral lymph node
	 Subaortic (common iliac) lymph node
	 Suprainguinal lymph node
	 D Lymphatic, Aortic
	 Celiac lymph node
	 Gastric lymph node
	 Hepatic lymph node
	 Lumbar lymph node
	 Pancreaticosplenic lymph node
	 Paraaortic lymph node
	 Retroperitoneal lymph node
	 F Lymphatic, Right Lower Extremity
	 Femoral lymph node
	 Popliteal lymph node
	 G Lymphatic, Left Lower Extremity
	 See F Lymphatic, Right Lower Extremity
	 H Lymphatic, Right Inguinal
	 J Lymphatic, Left Inguinal
	 K Thoracic Duct
	 Left jugular trunk
	 Left subclavian trunk
	 L Cisterna Chyli
	 Intestinal lymphatic trunk
	 Lumbar lymphatic trunk
	 M Thymus
	 Thymus gland
	 P Spleen
	 Accessory spleen
		0 Open
		 3 Percutaneous
		 4 Percutaneous Endoscopic
			Z No Device	**Z No Qualifier**

Ø   Medical and Surgical
7   Lymphatic and Hemic Systems
P   Removal   Definition: Taking out or off a device from a body part

Explanation: If a device is taken out and a similar device put in without cutting or puncturing the skin or mucous membrane, the procedure is coded to the root operation CHANGE. Otherwise, the procedure for taking out a device is coded to the root operation REMOVAL.

Body Part Character 4	Approach Character 5	Device Character 6	Qualifier Character 7

K Thoracic Duct
Left jugular trunk
Left subclavian trunk
L Cisterna Chyli
Intestinal lymphatic trunk
Lumbar lymphatic trunk
N Lymphatic
	Ø Open
	3 Percutaneous
	4 Percutaneous Endoscopic
		Ø Drainage Device
		3 Infusion Device
		7 Autologous Tissue
		  Substitute
		C Extraluminal Device
		D Intraluminal Device
		J Synthetic Substitute
		K Nonautologous Tissue
		  Substitute
		Y Other Device
			Z No Qualifier

K Thoracic Duct Left jugular trunk Left subclavian trunk **L Cisterna Chyli** Intestinal lymphatic trunk Lumbar lymphatic trunk **N Lymphatic**	X External	Ø Drainage Device 3 Infusion Device D Intraluminal Device	Z No Qualifier
M Thymus Thymus gland **P Spleen** Accessory spleen	Ø Open 3 Percutaneous 4 Percutaneous Endoscopic	Ø Drainage Device 3 Infusion Device Y Other Device	Z No Qualifier
M Thymus Thymus gland **P Spleen** Accessory spleen	X External	Ø Drainage Device 3 Infusion Device	Z No Qualifier
T Bone Marrow	Ø Open 3 Percutaneous 4 Percutaneous Endoscopic X External	Ø Drainage Device	Z No Qualifier

Non-OR	07P[K,L,N][3,4]YZ
Non-OR	07P[K,L,N]X[Ø,3,D]Z
Non-OR	07P[M,P][3,4]YZ
Non-OR	07P[M,P]X[Ø,3]Z
Non-OR	07PT[Ø,3,4,X]ØZ

Ø   Medical and Surgical
7   Lymphatic and Hemic Systems
Q   Repair   Definition: Restoring, to the extent possible, a body part to its normal anatomic structure and function
                 Explanation: Used only when the method to accomplish the repair is not one of the other root operations

Body Part Character 4		Approach Character 5	Device Character 6	Qualifier Character 7

Ø Lymphatic, Head
Buccinator lymph node
Infraauricular lymph node
Infraparotid lymph node
Parotid lymph node
Preauricular lymph node
Submandibular lymph node
Submaxillary lymph node
Submental lymph node
Subparotid lymph node
Suprahyoid lymph node
1 Lymphatic, Right Neck
Cervical lymph node
Jugular lymph node
Mastoid (postauricular) lymph node
Occipital lymph node
Postauricular (mastoid) lymph node
Retropharyngeal lymph node
Right jugular trunk
Right lymphatic duct
Right subclavian trunk
Supraclavicular (Virchow's) lymph
   node
Virchow's (supraclavicular) lymph
   node
2 Lymphatic, Left Neck
Cervical lymph node
Jugular lymph node
Mastoid (postauricular) lymph node
Occipital lymph node
Postauricular (mastoid) lymph node
Retropharyngeal lymph node
Supraclavicular (Virchow's) lymph
   node
Virchow's (supraclavicular) lymph
   node
3 Lymphatic, Right Upper Extremity
Cubital lymph node
Deltopectoral (infraclavicular) lymph
   node
Epitrochlear lymph node
Infraclavicular (deltopectoral) lymph
   node
Supratrochlear lymph node
4 Lymphatic, Left Upper Extremity
See 3 Lymphatic, Right Upper Extremity
5 Lymphatic, Right Axillary
Anterior (pectoral) lymph node
Apical (subclavicular) lymph node
Brachial (lateral) lymph node
Central axillary lymph node
Lateral (brachial) lymph node
Pectoral (anterior) lymph node
Posterior (subscapular) lymph node
Subclavicular (apical) lymph node
Subscapular (posterior) lymph node
	6 Lymphatic, Left Axillary
	See 5 Lymphatic, Right Axillary
	7 Lymphatic, Thorax
	Intercostal lymph node
	Mediastinal lymph node
	Parasternal lymph node
	Paratracheal lymph node
	Tracheobronchial lymph node
	8 Lymphatic, Internal Mammary, Right
	9 Lymphatic, Internal Mammary, Left
	B Lymphatic, Mesenteric
	Inferior mesenteric lymph node
	Pararectal lymph node
	Superior mesenteric lymph node
	C Lymphatic, Pelvis
	Common iliac (subaortic) lymph node
	Gluteal lymph node
	Iliac lymph node
	Inferior epigastric lymph node
	Obturator lymph node
	Sacral lymph node
	Subaortic (common iliac) lymph node
	Suprainguinal lymph node
	D Lymphatic, Aortic
	Celiac lymph node
	Gastric lymph node
	Hepatic lymph node
	Lumbar lymph node
	Pancreaticosplenic lymph node
	Paraaortic lymph node
	Retroperitoneal lymph node
	F Lymphatic, Right Lower Extremity
	Femoral lymph node
	Popliteal lymph node
	G Lymphatic, Left Lower Extremity
	See F Lymphatic, Right Lower Extremity
	H Lymphatic, Right Inguinal
	J Lymphatic, Left Inguinal
	K Thoracic Duct
	Left jugular trunk
	Left subclavian trunk
	L Cisterna Chyli
	Intestinal lymphatic trunk
	Lumbar lymphatic trunk
		Ø Open
		3 Percutaneous
		**4 Percutaneous
		   Endoscopic**
		**8 Via Natural or
		   Artificial Opening
		   Endoscopic**
			Z No Device	**Z No Qualifier**

M Thymus Thymus gland **P Spleen** Accessory spleen		**Ø Open** **3 Percutaneous** **4 Percutaneous Endoscopic**	**Z No Device**	**Z No Qualifier**

Lymphatic and Hemic Systems (side tab)

0 Medical and Surgical
7 Lymphatic and Hemic Systems
S Reposition   Definition: Moving to its normal location, or other suitable location, all or a portion of a body part

Explanation: The body part is moved to a new location from an abnormal location, or from a normal location where it is not functioning correctly. The body part may or may not be cut out or off to be moved to the new location.

Body Part Character 4	Approach Character 5	Device Character 6	Qualifier Character 7

M Thymus
   Thymus gland
P Spleen
   Accessory spleen
	0 Open	Z No Device	Z No Qualifier

0 Medical and Surgical
7 Lymphatic and Hemic Systems
T Resection   Definition: Cutting out or off, without replacement, all of a body part

Explanation: None

Body Part Character 4		Approach Character 5	Device Character 6	Qualifier Character 7

0 Lymphatic, Head
   Buccinator lymph node
   Infraauricular lymph node
   Infraparotid lymph node
   Parotid lymph node
   Preauricular lymph node
   Submandibular lymph node
   Submaxillary lymph node
   Submental lymph node
   Subparotid lymph node
   Suprahyoid lymph node
1 Lymphatic, Right Neck
   Cervical lymph node
   Jugular lymph node
   Mastoid (postauricular) lymph node
   Occipital lymph node
   Postauricular (mastoid) lymph node
   Retropharyngeal lymph node
   Right jugular trunk
   Right lymphatic duct
   Right subclavian trunk
   Supraclavicular (Virchow's) lymph node
   Virchow's (supraclavicular) lymph node
2 Lymphatic, Left Neck
   Cervical lymph node
   Jugular lymph node
   Mastoid (postauricular) lymph node
   Occipital lymph node
   Postauricular (mastoid) lymph node
   Retropharyngeal lymph node
   Supraclavicular (Virchow's) lymph node
   Virchow's (supraclavicular) lymph node
3 Lymphatic, Right Upper Extremity
   Cubital lymph node
   Deltopectoral (infraclavicular) lymph node
   Epitrochlear lymph node
   Infraclavicular (deltopectoral) lymph node
   Supratrochlear lymph node
4 Lymphatic, Left Upper Extremity
   See 3 Lymphatic, Right Upper Extremity
5 Lymphatic, Right Axillary ⊞
   Anterior (pectoral) lymph node
   Apical (subclavicular) lymph node
   Brachial (lateral) lymph node
   Central axillary lymph node
   Lateral (brachial) lymph node
   Pectoral (anterior) lymph node
   Posterior (subscapular) lymph node
   Subclavicular (apical) lymph node
   Subscapular (posterior) lymph node
	6 Lymphatic, Left Axillary ⊞
	   See 5 Lymphatic, Right Axillary
	7 Lymphatic, Thorax ⊞
	   Intercostal lymph node
	   Mediastinal lymph node
	   Parasternal lymph node
	   Paratracheal lymph node
	   Tracheobronchial lymph node
	8 Lymphatic, Internal Mammary, Right ⊞
	9 Lymphatic, Internal Mammary, Left ⊞
	B Lymphatic, Mesenteric
	   Inferior mesenteric lymph node
	   Pararectal lymph node
	   Superior mesenteric lymph node
	C Lymphatic, Pelvis
	   Common iliac (subaortic) lymph node
	   Gluteal lymph node
	   Iliac lymph node
	   Inferior epigastric lymph node
	   Obturator lymph node
	   Sacral lymph node
	   Subaortic (common iliac) lymph node
	   Suprainguinal lymph node
	D Lymphatic, Aortic
	   Celiac lymph node
	   Gastric lymph node
	   Hepatic lymph node
	   Lumbar lymph node
	   Pancreaticosplenic lymph node
	   Paraaortic lymph node
	   Retroperitoneal lymph node
	F Lymphatic, Right Lower Extremity
	   Femoral lymph node
	   Popliteal lymph node
	G Lymphatic, Left Lower Extremity
	   See F Lymphatic, Right Lower Extremity
	H Lymphatic, Right Inguinal
	J Lymphatic, Left Inguinal
	K Thoracic Duct
	   Left jugular trunk
	   Left subclavian trunk
	L Cisterna Chyli
	   Intestinal lymphatic trunk
	   Lumbar lymphatic trunk
	M Thymus
	   Thymus gland
	P Spleen
	   Accessory spleen
		0 Open
		4 Percutaneous Endoscopic
			Z No Device	Z No Qualifier

See Appendix L for Procedure Combinations
⊞   07T[5,6,7,8,9]0ZZ

LC Limited Coverage   NC Noncovered   ⊞ Combination Member   HAC associated procedure   Combination Only   DRG Non-OR   Non-OR   New/Revised in GREEN

286   ICD-10-PCS 2020

07S–07T (side tab)

0   Medical and Surgical
7   Lymphatic and Hemic Systems
U   Supplement　Definition: Putting in or on biological or synthetic material that physically reinforces and/or augments the function of a portion of a body part
　　　　　　　　Explanation: The biological material is non-living, or is living and from the same individual. The body part may have been previously replaced, and the SUPPLEMENT procedure is performed to physically reinforce and/or augment the function of the replaced body part.

Body Part Character 4		Approach Character 5	Device Character 6	Qualifier Character 7
0 Lymphatic, Head 　Buccinator lymph node 　Infraauricular lymph node 　Infraparotid lymph node 　Parotid lymph node 　Preauricular lymph node 　Submandibular lymph node 　Submaxillary lymph node 　Submental lymph node 　Subparotid lymph node 　Suprahyoid lymph node **1 Lymphatic, Right Neck** 　Cervical lymph node 　Jugular lymph node 　Mastoid (postauricular) lymph node 　Occipital lymph node 　Postauricular (mastoid) lymph node 　Retropharyngeal lymph node 　Right jugular trunk 　Right lymphatic duct 　Right subclavian trunk 　Supraclavicular (Virchow's) lymph 　　node 　Virchow's (supraclavicular) lymph 　　node **2 Lymphatic, Left Neck** 　Cervical lymph node 　Jugular lymph node 　Mastoid (postauricular) lymph node 　Occipital lymph node 　Postauricular (mastoid) lymph node 　Retropharyngeal lymph node 　Supraclavicular (Virchow's) lymph 　　node 　Virchow's (supraclavicular) lymph 　　node **3 Lymphatic, Right Upper Extremity** 　Cubital lymph node 　Deltopectoral (infraclavicular) lymph 　　node 　Epitrochlear lymph node 　Infraclavicular (deltopectoral) lymph 　　node 　Supratrochlear lymph node **4 Lymphatic, Left Upper Extremity** 　*See 3 Lymphatic, Right Upper Extremity* **5 Lymphatic, Right Axillary** 　Anterior (pectoral) lymph node 　Apical (subclavicular) lymph node 　Brachial (lateral) lymph node 　Central axillary lymph node 　Lateral (brachial) lymph node 　Pectoral (anterior) lymph node 　Posterior (subscapular) lymph node 　Subclavicular (apical) lymph node 　Subscapular (posterior) lymph node	**6 Lymphatic, Left Axillary** 　*See 5 Lymphatic, Right Axillary* **7 Lymphatic, Thorax** 　Intercostal lymph node 　Mediastinal lymph node 　Parasternal lymph node 　Paratracheal lymph node 　Tracheobronchial lymph node **8 Lymphatic, Internal Mammary, Right** **9 Lymphatic, Internal Mammary, Left** **B Lymphatic, Mesenteric** 　Inferior mesenteric lymph node 　Pararectal lymph node 　Superior mesenteric lymph node **C Lymphatic, Pelvis** 　Common iliac (subaortic) lymph node 　Gluteal lymph node 　Iliac lymph node 　Inferior epigastric lymph node 　Obturator lymph node 　Sacral lymph node 　Subaortic (common iliac) lymph node 　Suprainguinal lymph node **D Lymphatic, Aortic** 　Celiac lymph node 　Gastric lymph node 　Hepatic lymph node 　Lumbar lymph node 　Pancreaticosplenic lymph node 　Paraaortic lymph node 　Retroperitoneal lymph node **F Lymphatic, Right Lower Extremity** 　Femoral lymph node 　Popliteal lymph node **G Lymphatic, Left Lower Extremity** 　*See F Lymphatic, Right Lower Extremity* **H Lymphatic, Right Inguinal** **J Lymphatic, Left Inguinal** **K Thoracic Duct** 　Left jugular trunk 　Left subclavian trunk **L Cisterna Chyli** 　Intestinal lymphatic trunk 　Lumbar lymphatic trunk	**0 Open** **4 Percutaneous Endoscopic**	**7 Autologous Tissue Substitute** **J Synthetic Substitute** **K Nonautologous Tissue Substitute**	**Z No Qualifier**

Ø Medical and Surgical
7 Lymphatic and Hemic Systems
V Restriction   Definition: Partially closing an orifice or the lumen of a tubular body part
                      Explanation: The orifice can be a natural orifice or an artificially created orifice

Body Part Character 4		Approach Character 5	Device Character 6	Qualifier Character 7

Ø Lymphatic, Head
Buccinator lymph node
Infraauricular lymph node
Infraparotid lymph node
Parotid lymph node
Preauricular lymph node
Submandibular lymph node
Submaxillary lymph node
Submental lymph node
Subparotid lymph node
Suprahyoid lymph node
1 Lymphatic, Right Neck
Cervical lymph node
Jugular lymph node
Mastoid (postauricular) lymph node
Occipital lymph node
Postauricular (mastoid) lymph node
Retropharyngeal lymph node
Right jugular trunk
Right lymphatic duct
Right subclavian trunk
Supraclavicular (Virchow's) lymph
    node
Virchow's (supraclavicular) lymph
    node
2 Lymphatic, Left Neck
Cervical lymph node
Jugular lymph node
Mastoid (postauricular) lymph node
Occipital lymph node
Postauricular (mastoid) lymph node
Retropharyngeal lymph node
Supraclavicular (Virchow's) lymph
    node
Virchow's (supraclavicular) lymph
    node
3 Lymphatic, Right Upper Extremity
Cubital lymph node
Deltopectoral (infraclavicular) lymph
    node
Epitrochlear lymph node
Infraclavicular (deltopectoral) lymph
    node
Supratrochlear lymph node
4 Lymphatic, Left Upper Extremity
See 3 Lymphatic, Right Upper Extremity
5 Lymphatic, Right Axillary
Anterior (pectoral) lymph node
Apical (subclavicular) lymph node
Brachial (lateral) lymph node
Central axillary lymph node
Lateral (brachial) lymph node
Pectoral (anterior) lymph node
Posterior (subscapular) lymph node
Subclavicular (apical) lymph node
Subscapular (posterior) lymph node
	6 Lymphatic, Left Axillary
	See 5 Lymphatic, Right Axillary
	7 Lymphatic, Thorax
	Intercostal lymph node
	Mediastinal lymph node
	Parasternal lymph node
	Paratracheal lymph node
	Tracheobronchial lymph node
	8 Lymphatic, Internal Mammary, Right
	9 Lymphatic, Internal Mammary, Left
	B Lymphatic, Mesenteric
	Inferior mesenteric lymph node
	Pararectal lymph node
	Superior mesenteric lymph node
	C Lymphatic, Pelvis
	Common iliac (subaortic) lymph node
	Gluteal lymph node
	Iliac lymph node
	Inferior epigastric lymph node
	Obturator lymph node
	Sacral lymph node
	Subaortic (common iliac) lymph node
	Suprainguinal lymph node
	D Lymphatic, Aortic
	Celiac lymph node
	Gastric lymph node
	Hepatic lymph node
	Lumbar lymph node
	Pancreaticosplenic lymph node
	Paraaortic lymph node
	Retroperitoneal lymph node
	F Lymphatic, Right Lower Extremity
	Femoral lymph node
	Popliteal lymph node
	G Lymphatic, Left Lower Extremity
	See F Lymphatic, Right Lower Extremity
	H Lymphatic, Right Inguinal
	J Lymphatic, Left Inguinal
	K Thoracic Duct
	Left jugular trunk
	Left subclavian trunk
	L Cisterna Chyli
	Intestinal lymphatic trunk
	Lumbar lymphatic trunk
		Ø Open
		3 Percutaneous
		**4 Percutaneous
		Endoscopic**
			C Extraluminal Device
			D Intraluminal Device
			Z No Device
				Z No Qualifier

Ø   Medical and Surgical
7   Lymphatic and Hemic Systems
W   Revision   Definition: Correcting, to the extent possible, a portion of a malfunctioning device or the position of a displaced device

                  Explanation: Revision can include correcting a malfunctioning or displaced device by taking out or putting in components of the device such as a screw or pin

Body Part Character 4	Approach Character 5	Device Character 6	Qualifier Character 7

K Thoracic Duct
Left jugular trunk
Left subclavian trunk
L Cisterna Chyli
Intestinal lymphatic trunk
Lumbar lymphatic trunk
N Lymphatic
	Ø Open
	3 Percutaneous
	4 Percutaneous Endoscopic
		Ø Drainage Device
		3 Infusion Device
		7 Autologous Tissue
		    Substitute
		C Extraluminal Device
		D Intraluminal Device
		J Synthetic Substitute
		K Nonautologous Tissue
		    Substitute
		Y Other Device
			Z No Qualifier

K Thoracic Duct
Left jugular trunk
Left subclavian trunk
L Cisterna Chyli
Intestinal lymphatic trunk
Lumbar lymphatic trunk
N Lymphatic
	X External	**Ø** Drainage Device
		3 Infusion Device
		7 Autologous Tissue
		    Substitute
		C Extraluminal Device
		D Intraluminal Device
		J Synthetic Substitute
		K Nonautologous Tissue
		    Substitute
			Z No Qualifier

M Thymus Thymus gland **P Spleen** Accessory spleen	**Ø** Open **3** Percutaneous **4** Percutaneous Endoscopic	**Ø** Drainage Device **3** Infusion Device **Y** Other Device	**Z** No Qualifier
M Thymus Thymus gland **P Spleen** Accessory spleen	**X** External	**Ø** Drainage Device **3** Infusion Device	**Z** No Qualifier
T Bone Marrow	**Ø** Open **3** Percutaneous **4** Percutaneous Endoscopic **X** External	**Ø** Drainage Device	**Z** No Qualifier

Non-OR	Ø7W[K,L,N][3,4]YZ
Non-OR	Ø7W[K,L,N]X[Ø,3,7,C,D,J,K]Z
Non-OR	Ø7W[M,P][3,4]YZ
Non-OR	Ø7W[M,P]X[Ø,3]Z
Non-OR	Ø7WT[Ø,3,4,X]ØZ

Ø   Medical and Surgical
7   Lymphatic and Hemic Systems
Y   Transplantation   Definition: Putting in or on all or a portion of a living body part taken from another individual or animal to physically take the place and/or function of all or a portion of a similar body part

                  Explanation: The native body part may or may not be taken out, and the transplanted body part may take over all or a portion of its function

Body Part Character 4	Approach Character 5	Device Character 6	Qualifier Character 7
M Thymus Thymus gland **P Spleen** Accessory spleen	**Ø** Open	**Z** No Device	**Ø** Allogeneic **1** Syngeneic **2** Zooplastic

🅛🅒 Limited Coverage   🅝🅒 Noncovered   ⊞ Combination Member   HAC associated procedure   Combination Only   DRG Non-OR   Non-OR   New/Revised in GREEN

ICD-10-PCS 2020   **289**

Eye Ø8Ø–Ø8X

Character Meanings

This Character Meaning table is provided as a guide to assist the user in the identification of character members that may be found in this section of code tables. It **SHOULD NOT** be used to build a PCS code.

Operation–Character 3		Body Part–Character 4		Approach–Character 5		Device–Character 6		Qualifier–Character 7	
Ø	Alteration	Ø	Eye, Right	Ø	Open	Ø	Drainage Device OR Synthetic Substitute, Intraocular Telescope	3	Nasal Cavity
1	Bypass	1	Eye, Left	3	Percutaneous	1	Radioactive Element	4	Sclera
2	Change	2	Anterior Chamber, Right	7	Via Natural or Artificial Opening	3	Infusion Device	X	Diagnostic
5	Destruction	3	Anterior Chamber, Left	8	Via Natural or Artificial Opening Endoscopic	5	Epiretinal Visual Prosthesis	Z	No Qualifier
7	Dilation	4	Vitreous, Right	X	External	7	Autologous Tissue Substitute		
9	Drainage	5	Vitreous, Left			C	Extraluminal Device		
B	Excision	6	Sclera, Right			D	Intraluminal Device		
C	Extirpation	7	Sclera, Left			J	Synthetic Substitute		
D	Extraction	8	Cornea, Right			K	Nonautologous Tissue Substitute		
F	Fragmentation	9	Cornea, Left			Y	Other Device		
H	Insertion	A	Choroid, Right			Z	No Device		
J	Inspection	B	Choroid, Left						
L	Occlusion	C	Iris, Right						
M	Reattachment	D	Iris, Left						
N	Release	E	Retina, Right						
P	Removal	F	Retina, Left						
Q	Repair	G	Retinal Vessel, Right						
R	Replacement	H	Retinal Vessel, Left						
S	Reposition	J	Lens, Right						
T	Resection	K	Lens, Left						
U	Supplement	L	Extraocular Muscle, Right						
V	Restriction	M	Extraocular Muscle, Left						
W	Revision	N	Upper Eyelid, Right						
X	Transfer	P	Upper Eyelid, Left						
		Q	Lower Eyelid, Right						
		R	Lower Eyelid, Left						
		S	Conjunctiva, Right						
		T	Conjunctiva, Left						
		V	Lacrimal Gland, Right						
		W	Lacrimal Gland, Left						
		X	Lacrimal Duct, Right						
		Y	Lacrimal Duct, Left						

AHA Coding Clinic for table Ø81
2019, 1Q, 27   Glaucoma tube shunt

AHA Coding Clinic for table Ø89
2016, 2Q, 21   Laser trabeculoplasty

AHA Coding Clinic for table Ø8B
2014, 4Q, 35   Vitrectomy with air/fluid exchange
2014, 4Q, 36   Pars plans vitrectomy without mention of instillation of oil, air or fluid

AHA Coding Clinic for table Ø8J
2015, 1Q, 35   Attempted removal of foreign body from cornea

AHA Coding Clinic for table Ø8N
2015, 2Q, 24   Penetrating keratoplasty and anterior segment reconstruction

AHA Coding Clinic for table Ø8Q
2018, 3Q, 13   Repair of ruptured globe

AHA Coding Clinic for table Ø8R
2015, 2Q, 24   Penetrating keratoplasty and anterior segment reconstruction
2015, 2Q, 25   Penetrating keratoplasty and placement of viscoelastic eye with paracentesis

AHA Coding Clinic for table Ø8T
2015, 2Q, 12   Orbital exenteration

AHA Coding Clinic for table Ø8U
2014, 3Q, 31   Corneal amniotic membrane transplantation

Eye

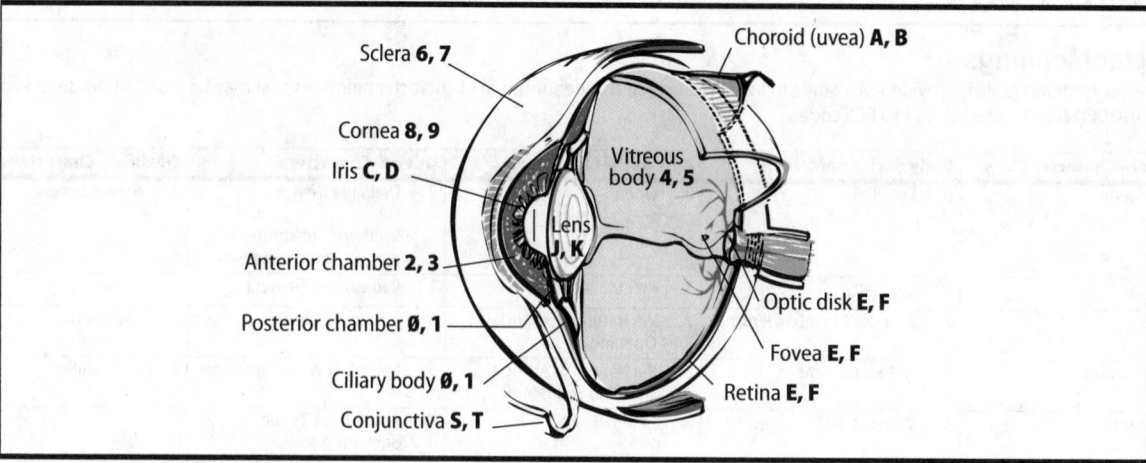

Sclera **6, 7**
Cornea **8, 9**
Iris **C, D**
Anterior chamber **2, 3**
Posterior chamber **Ø, 1**
Ciliary body **Ø, 1**
Conjunctiva **S, T**

Choroid (uvea) **A, B**
Vitreous body **4, 5**
Lens **J, K**
Optic disk **E, F**
Fovea **E, F**
Retina **E, F**

Eye Musculature

Superior rectus
Superior oblique
Lateral rectus
Medial rectus
Inferior oblique
Inferior rectus

Muscles and actions (right eye) **L, M**

Lacrimal System

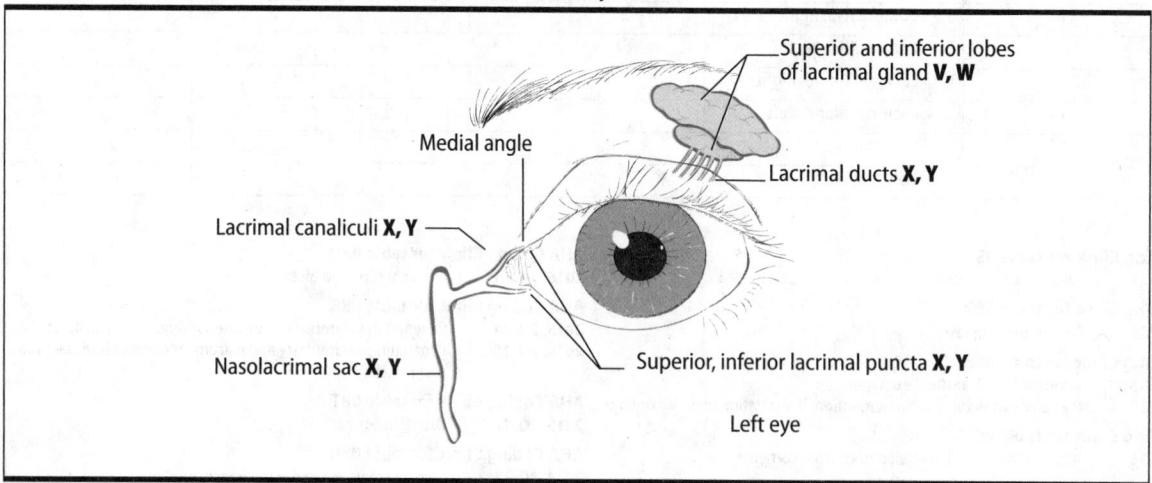

Superior and inferior lobes of lacrimal gland **V, W**
Medial angle
Lacrimal ducts **X, Y**
Lacrimal canaliculi **X, Y**
Nasolacrimal sac **X, Y**
Superior, inferior lacrimal puncta **X, Y**

Left eye

Ø   **Medical and Surgical**
8   **Eye**
Ø   **Alteration**   Definition: Modifying the anatomic structure of a body part without affecting the function of the body part

                         Explanation: Principal purpose is to improve appearance

Body Part Character 4	Approach Character 5	Device Character 6	Qualifier Character 7

N Upper Eyelid, Right
  Lateral canthus
  Levator palpebrae superioris muscle
  Orbicularis oculi muscle
  Superior tarsal plate
P Upper Eyelid, Left
  See N Upper Eyelid, Right
Q Lower Eyelid, Right
  Inferior tarsal plate
  Medial canthus
R Lower Eyelid, Left
  See Q Lower Eyelid, Right
	Ø Open
	3 Percutaneous
	X External
		7 Autologous Tissue Substitute
		J Synthetic Substitute
		K Nonautologous Tissue Substitute
		Z No Device
			Z No Qualifier

Non-OR   All body part, approach, device, and qualifier values

Ø   **Medical and Surgical**
8   **Eye**
1   **Bypass**   Definition: Altering the route of passage of the contents of a tubular body part

                         Explanation: Rerouting contents of a body part to a downstream area of the normal route, to a similar route and body part, or to an abnormal route and dissimilar body part. Includes one or more anastomoses, with or without the use of a device.

Body Part Character 4	Approach Character 5	Device Character 6	Qualifier Character 7

2 Anterior Chamber, Right
  Aqueous humour
3 Anterior Chamber, Left
  See 2 Anterior Chamber, Right
	3 Percutaneous	**J** Synthetic Substitute
		K Nonautologous Tissue Substitute
		Z No Device
			4 Sclera

X Lacrimal Duct, Right
  Lacrimal canaliculus
  Lacrimal punctum
  Lacrimal sac
  Nasolacrimal duct
Y Lacrimal Duct, Left
  See X Lacrimal Duct, Right
	Ø Open
	3 Percutaneous
		J Synthetic Substitute
		K Nonautologous Tissue Substitute
		Z No Device
			3 Nasal Cavity

Ø   **Medical and Surgical**
8   **Eye**
2   **Change**   Definition: Taking out or off a device from a body part and putting back an identical or similar device in or on the same body part without cutting or puncturing the skin or a mucous membrane

                         Explanation: All CHANGE procedures are coded using the approach EXTERNAL

Body Part Character 4	Approach Character 5	Device Character 6	Qualifier Character 7

Ø Eye, Right
  Ciliary body
  Posterior chamber
1 Eye, Left
  See Ø Eye, Right
	X External	**Ø** Drainage Device
		Y Other Device
			Z No Qualifier

Non-OR   All body part, approach, device, and qualifier values

LC Limited Coverage   NC Noncovered   ⊞ Combination Member   HAC associated procedure   Combination Only   DRG Non-OR   Non-OR   New/Revised in GREEN

ICD-10-PCS 2020   293

080–082

Ø Medical and Surgical
8 Eye
5 Destruction

Definition: Physical eradication of all or a portion of a body part by the direct use of energy, force, or a destructive agent

Explanation: None of the body part is physically taken out

Body Part — Character 4		Approach — Character 5	Device — Character 6	Qualifier — Character 7

Ø Eye, Right
  Ciliary body
  Posterior chamber
1 Eye, Left
  See Ø Eye, Right
6 Sclera, Right
7 Sclera, Left
	8 Cornea, Right
	9 Cornea, Left
	S Conjunctiva, Right
	  Plica semilunaris
	T Conjunctiva, Left
	  See S Conjunctiva, Right
		X External	Z No Device	Z No Qualifier

2 Anterior Chamber, Right
  Aqueous humour
3 Anterior Chamber, Left
  See 2 Anterior Chamber, Right
4 Vitreous, Right
  Vitreous body
5 Vitreous, Left
  See 4 Vitreous, Right
C Iris, Right
D Iris, Left
	E Retina, Right
	  Fovea
	  Macula
	  Optic disc
	F Retina, Left
	  See E Retina, Right
	G Retinal Vessel, Right
	H Retinal Vessel, Left
	J Lens, Right
	  Zonule of Zinn
	K Lens, Left
	  See J Lens, Right
		3 Percutaneous	Z No Device	Z No Qualifier

A Choroid, Right
B Choroid, Left
L Extraocular Muscle, Right
  Inferior oblique muscle
  Inferior rectus muscle
  Lateral rectus muscle
  Medial rectus muscle
  Superior oblique muscle
  Superior rectus muscle
	M Extraocular Muscle, Left
	  See L Extraocular Muscle, Right
	V Lacrimal Gland, Right
	W Lacrimal Gland, Left
		Ø Open
		3 Percutaneous
			Z No Device	Z No Qualifier

N Upper Eyelid, Right
  Lateral canthus
  Levator palpebrae superioris
    muscle
  Orbicularis oculi muscle
  Superior tarsal plate
P Upper Eyelid, Left
  See N Upper Eyelid, Right
	Q Lower Eyelid, Right
	  Inferior tarsal plate
	  Medial canthus
	R Lower Eyelid, Left
	  See Q Lower Eyelid, Right
		Ø Open
		3 Percutaneous
		X External
			Z No Device	Z No Qualifier

X Lacrimal Duct, Right
  Lacrimal canaliculus
  Lacrimal punctum
  Lacrimal sac
  Nasolacrimal duct
	Y Lacrimal Duct, Left
	  See X Lacrimal Duct, Right
		Ø Open
		3 Percutaneous
		7 Via Natural or Artificial Opening
		8 Via Natural or Artificial Opening Endoscopic
			Z No Device	Z No Qualifier

Non-OR   Ø85[E,F]3ZZ

Ø Medical and Surgical
8 Eye
7 Dilation

Definition: Expanding an orifice or the lumen of a tubular body part

Explanation: The orifice can be a natural orifice or an artificially created orifice. Accomplished by stretching a tubular body part using intraluminal pressure or by cutting part of the orifice or wall of the tubular body part.

Body Part — Character 4	Approach — Character 5	Device — Character 6	Qualifier — Character 7

X Lacrimal Duct, Right
  Lacrimal canaliculus
  Lacrimal punctum
  Lacrimal sac
  Nasolacrimal duct
Y Lacrimal Duct, Left
  See X Lacrimal Duct, Right
	Ø Open
	3 Percutaneous
	7 Via Natural or Artificial Opening
	8 Via Natural or Artificial Opening Endoscopic
		D Intraluminal Device
		Z No Device
			Z No Qualifier

LC Limited Coverage   NC Noncovered   ⊞ Combination Member   HAC associated procedure   Combination Only   DRG Non-OR   Non-OR   New/Revised in GREEN

294   ICD-10-PCS 2020

Ø   **Medical and Surgical**
8   **Eye**
9   **Drainage**   Definition: Taking or letting out fluids and/or gases from a body part
                       Explanation: The qualifier DIAGNOSTIC is used to identify drainage procedures that are biopsies

Body Part Character 4		Approach Character 5	Device Character 6	Qualifier Character 7

Ø Eye, Right
  Ciliary body
  Posterior chamber
1 Eye, Left
  See Ø Eye, Right
6 Sclera, Right
7 Sclera, Left
	8 Cornea, Right
	9 Cornea, Left
	S Conjunctiva, Right
	  Plica semilunaris
	T Conjunctiva, Left
	  See S Conjunctiva, Right
		X External	**Ø** Drainage Device	**Z** No Qualifier

Ø Eye, Right
  Ciliary body
  Posterior chamber
1 Eye, Left
  See Ø Eye, Right
6 Sclera, Right
7 Sclera, Left
	8 Cornea, Right
	9 Cornea, Left
	S Conjunctiva, Right
	  Plica semilunaris
	T Conjunctiva, Left
	  See S Conjunctiva, Right
		X External	**Z** No Device	**X** Diagnostic
				Z No Qualifier

2 Anterior Chamber, Right
  Aqueous humour
3 Anterior Chamber, Left
  See 2 Anterior Chamber, Right
4 Vitreous, Right
  Vitreous body
5 Vitreous, Left
  See 4 Vitreous, Right
C Iris, Right
D Iris, Left
	E Retina, Right
	  Fovea
	  Macula
	  Optic disc
	F Retina, Left
	  See E Retina, Right
	G Retinal Vessel, Right
	H Retinal Vessel, Left
	J Lens, Right
	  Zonule of Zinn
	K Lens, Left
	  See J Lens, Right
		3 Percutaneous	**Ø** Drainage Device	**Z** No Qualifier

2 Anterior Chamber, Right
  Aqueous humour
3 Anterior Chamber, Left
  See 2 Anterior Chamber, Right
4 Vitreous, Right
  Vitreous body
5 Vitreous, Left
  See 4 Vitreous, Right
C Iris, Right
D Iris, Left
	E Retina, Right
	  Fovea
	  Macula
	  Optic disc
	F Retina, Left
	  See E Retina, Right
	G Retinal Vessel, Right
	H Retinal Vessel, Left
	J Lens, Right
	  Zonule of Zinn
	K Lens, Left
	  See J Lens, Right
		3 Percutaneous	**Z** No Device	**X** Diagnostic
				Z No Qualifier

A Choroid, Right
B Choroid, Left
L Extraocular Muscle, Right
  Inferior oblique muscle
  Inferior rectus muscle
  Lateral rectus muscle
  Medial rectus muscle
  Superior oblique muscle
  Superior rectus muscle
	M Extraocular Muscle, Left
	  See L Extraocular Muscle, Right
	V Lacrimal Gland, Right
	W Lacrimal Gland, Left
		Ø Open
		3 Percutaneous
			Ø Drainage Device	**Z** No Qualifier

A Choroid, Right
B Choroid, Left
L Extraocular Muscle, Right
  Inferior oblique muscle
  Inferior rectus muscle
  Lateral rectus muscle
  Medial rectus muscle
  Superior oblique muscle
  Superior rectus muscle
	M Extraocular Muscle, Left
	  See L Extraocular Muscle, Right
	V Lacrimal Gland, Right
	W Lacrimal Gland, Left
		Ø Open
		3 Percutaneous
			Z No Device	**X** Diagnostic
				Z No Qualifier

N Upper Eyelid, Right
  Lateral canthus
  Levator palpebrae superioris
    muscle
  Orbicularis oculi muscle
  Superior tarsal plate
P Upper Eyelid, Left
  See N Upper Eyelid, Right
	Q Lower Eyelid, Right
	  Inferior tarsal plate
	  Medial canthus
	R Lower Eyelid, Left
	  See Q Lower Eyelid, Right
		Ø Open
		3 Percutaneous
		X External
			Ø Drainage Device	**Z** No Qualifier

Ø89 Continued on next page

Non-OR   Ø89[Ø,1,6,7,8,9,S,T]XZ[X,Z]
Non-OR   Ø89[N,P,Q,R][Ø,3,X]ØZ

Ø   Medical and Surgical   *Ø89 Continued*
8   Eye
9   Drainage   Definition: Taking or letting out fluids and/or gases from a body part

Explanation: The qualifier DIAGNOSTIC is used to identify drainage procedures that are biopsies

Body Part Character 4		Approach Character 5	Device Character 6	Qualifier Character 7
N Upper Eyelid, Right Lateral canthus Levator palpebrae superioris 　muscle Orbicularis oculi muscle Superior tarsal plate **P Upper Eyelid, Left** *See N Upper Eyelid, Right*	**Q Lower Eyelid, Right** Inferior tarsal plate Medial canthus **R Lower Eyelid, Left** *See Q Lower Eyelid, Right*	**Ø Open** **3 Percutaneous** **X External**	**Z No Device**	**X Diagnostic** **Z No Qualifier**
X Lacrimal Duct, Right Lacrimal canaliculus Lacrimal punctum Lacrimal sac Nasolacrimal duct	**Y Lacrimal Duct, Left** *See X Lacrimal Duct, Right*	**Ø Open** **3 Percutaneous** **7 Via Natural or Artificial 　Opening** **8 Via Natural or Artificial 　Opening Endoscopic**	**Ø Drainage Device**	**Z No Qualifier**
X Lacrimal Duct, Right Lacrimal canaliculus Lacrimal punctum Lacrimal sac Nasolacrimal duct	**Y Lacrimal Duct, Left** *See X Lacrimal Duct, Right*	**Ø Open** **3 Percutaneous** **7 Via Natural or Artificial 　Opening** **8 Via Natural or Artificial 　Opening Endoscopic**	**Z No Device**	**X Diagnostic** **Z No Qualifier**

Non-OR   Ø89[N,P,Q,R]ØZZ
Non-OR   Ø89[N,P,Q,R][3,X]Z[X,Z]

Ø   Medical and Surgical
8   Eye
B   Excision   Definition: Cutting out or off, without replacement, a portion of a body part

Explanation: The qualifier DIAGNOSTIC is used to identify excision procedures that are biopsies

Body Part Character 4		Approach Character 5	Device Character 6	Qualifier Character 7
Ø Eye, Right Ciliary body Posterior chamber **1 Eye, Left** *See Ø Eye, Right* **N Upper Eyelid, Right** Lateral canthus Levator palpebrae superioris 　muscle Orbicularis oculi muscle Superior tarsal plate	**P Upper Eyelid, Left** *See N Upper Eyelid, Right* **Q Lower Eyelid, Right** Inferior tarsal plate Medial canthus **R Lower Eyelid, Left** *See Q Lower Eyelid, Right*	**Ø Open** **3 Percutaneous** **X External**	**Z No Device**	**X Diagnostic** **Z No Qualifier**
4 Vitreous, Right Vitreous body **5 Vitreous, Left** *See 4 Vitreous, Right* **C Iris, Right** **D Iris, Left** **E Retina, Right** Fovea Macula Optic disc	**F Retina, Left** *See E Retina, Right* **J Lens, Right** Zonule of Zinn **K Lens, Left** *See J Lens, Right*	**3 Percutaneous**	**Z No Device**	**X Diagnostic** **Z No Qualifier**
6 Sclera, Right **7 Sclera, Left** **8 Cornea, Right** **9 Cornea, Left**	**S Conjunctiva, Right** Plica semilunaris **T Conjunctiva, Left** *See S Conjunctiva, Right*	**X External**	**Z No Device**	**X Diagnostic** **Z No Qualifier**
A Choroid, Right **B Choroid, Left** **L Extraocular Muscle, Right** Inferior oblique muscle Inferior rectus muscle Lateral rectus muscle Medial rectus muscle Superior oblique muscle Superior rectus muscle	**M Extraocular Muscle, Left** *See L Extraocular Muscle, Right* **V Lacrimal Gland, Right** **W Lacrimal Gland, Left**	**Ø Open** **3 Percutaneous**	**Z No Device**	**X Diagnostic** **Z No Qualifier**
X Lacrimal Duct, Right Lacrimal canaliculus Lacrimal punctum Lacrimal sac Nasolacrimal duct	**Y Lacrimal Duct, Left** *See X Lacrimal Duct, Right*	**Ø Open** **3 Percutaneous** **7 Via Natural or Artificial 　Opening** **8 Via Natural or Artificial 　Opening Endoscopic**	**Z No Device**	**X Diagnostic** **Z No Qualifier**

LC Limited Coverage   NC Noncovered   ⊞ Combination Member   HAC associated procedure   Combination Only   DRG Non-OR   Non-OR   New/Revised in GREEN

296   ICD-10-PCS 2020

Ø89–Ø8B

Ø   Medical and Surgical
8   Eye
C   Extirpation   Definition: Taking or cutting out solid matter from a body part

Explanation: The solid matter may be an abnormal byproduct of a biological function or a foreign body; it may be imbedded in a body part or in the lumen of a tubular body part. The solid matter may or may not have been previously broken into pieces.

Body Part Character 4	Approach Character 5	Device Character 6	Qualifier Character 7
Ø Eye, Right Ciliary body Posterior chamber **1 Eye, Left** *See Ø Eye, Right* **6 Sclera, Right** **7 Sclera, Left** **8 Cornea, Right** **9 Cornea, Left** **S Conjunctiva, Right** Plica semilunaris **T Conjunctiva, Left** *See S Conjunctiva, Right*	**X** External	**Z** No Device	**Z** No Qualifier
2 Anterior Chamber, Right Aqueous humour **3 Anterior Chamber, Left** *See 2 Anterior Chamber, Right* **4 Vitreous, Right** Vitreous body **5 Vitreous, Left** *See 4 Vitreous, Right* **C Iris, Right** **D Iris, Left** **E Retina, Right** Fovea Macula Optic disc **F Retina, Left** *See E Retina, Right* **G Retinal Vessel, Right** **H Retinal Vessel, Left** **J Lens, Right** Zonule of Zinn **K Lens, Left** *See J Lens, Right*	**3** Percutaneous **X** External	**Z** No Device	**Z** No Qualifier
A Choroid, Right **B Choroid, Left** **L Extraocular Muscle, Right** Inferior oblique muscle Inferior rectus muscle Lateral rectus muscle Medial rectus muscle Superior oblique muscle Superior rectus muscle **M Extraocular Muscle, Left** *See L Extraocular Muscle, Right* **N Upper Eyelid, Right** Lateral canthus Levator palpebrae superioris muscle Orbicularis oculi muscle Superior tarsal plate **P Upper Eyelid, Left** *See N Upper Eyelid, Right* **Q Lower Eyelid, Right** Inferior tarsal plate Medial canthus **R Lower Eyelid, Left** *See Q Lower Eyelid, Right* **V Lacrimal Gland, Right** **W Lacrimal Gland, Left**	**Ø** Open **3** Percutaneous **X** External	**Z** No Device	**Z** No Qualifier
X Lacrimal Duct, Right Lacrimal canaliculus Lacrimal punctum Lacrimal sac Nasolacrimal duct **Y Lacrimal Duct, Left** *See X Lacrimal Duct, Right*	**Ø** Open **3** Percutaneous **7** Via Natural or Artificial Opening **8** Via Natural or Artificial Opening Endoscopic	**Z** No Device	**Z** No Qualifier

Non-OR   08C[Ø,1,6,7,S,T]XZZ
Non-OR   08C[2,3]XZZ
Non-OR   08C[N,P,Q,R][Ø,3,X]ZZ

LC Limited Coverage   **NC** Noncovered   ⊞ Combination Member   HAC associated procedure   Combination Only   DRG Non-OR   Non-OR   New/Revised in GREEN

Ø   **Medical and Surgical**
8   **Eye**
D   **Extraction**   Definition: Pulling or stripping out or off all or a portion of a body part by the use of force
           Explanation: The qualifier DIAGNOSTIC is used to identify extraction procedures that are biopsies

Body Part Character 4	Approach Character 5	Device Character 6	Qualifier Character 7
8 Cornea, Right 9 Cornea, Left	X External	Z No Device	X Diagnostic Z No Qualifier

J   Lens, Right
     Zonule of Zinn
K   Lens, Left
     See J Lens, Right
	3 Percutaneous	Z No Device	Z No Qualifier

Ø   **Medical and Surgical**
8   **Eye**
F   **Fragmentation**   Definition: Breaking solid matter in a body part into pieces
           Explanation: Physical force (e.g., manual, ultrasonic) applied directly or indirectly is used to break the solid matter into pieces. The solid matter may be an abnormal byproduct of a biological function or a foreign body. The pieces of solid matter are not taken out.

Body Part Character 4	Approach Character 5	Device Character 6	Qualifier Character 7

4   Vitreous, Right   NC
     Vitreous body
5   Vitreous, Left   NC
     See 4 Vitreous, Right
	3 Percutaneous
	X External
		Z No Device	Z No Qualifier

Non-OR   Ø8F[4,5]XZZ
NC   Ø8F[4,5]XZZ

Ø   **Medical and Surgical**
8   **Eye**
H   **Insertion**   Definition: Putting in a nonbiological appliance that monitors, assists, performs, or prevents a physiological function but does not physically take the place of a body part
           Explanation: None

Body Part Character 4	Approach Character 5	Device Character 6	Qualifier Character 7

Ø   Eye, Right
     Ciliary body
     Posterior chamber
1   Eye, Left
     See Ø Eye, Right
	Ø Open	5 Epiretinal Visual Prosthesis
		Y Other Device
			Z No Qualifier

Ø   Eye, Right
     Ciliary body
     Posterior chamber
1   Eye, Left
     See Ø Eye, Right
	3 Percutaneous	1 Radioactive Element
		3 Infusion Device
		Y Other Device
			Z No Qualifier

Ø   Eye, Right
     Ciliary body
     Posterior chamber
1   Eye, Left
     See Ø Eye, Right
	7 Via Natural or Artificial Opening
	8 Via Natural or Artificial Opening Endoscopic
		Y Other Device	Z No Qualifier

Ø   Eye, Right
     Ciliary body
     Posterior chamber
1   Eye, Left
     See Ø Eye, Right
	X External	1 Radioactive Element
		3 Infusion Device
			Z No Qualifier

Non-OR   Ø8H[Ø,1]3YZ
Non-OR   Ø8H[Ø,1][7,8]YZ

Ø　Medical and Surgical
8　Eye
J　Inspection　　Definition: Visually and/or manually exploring a body part

Explanation: Visual exploration may be performed with or without optical instrumentation. Manual exploration may be performed directly or through intervening body layers.

Body Part Character 4	Approach Character 5	Device Character 6	Qualifier Character 7
Ø **Eye, Right** 　Ciliary body 　Posterior chamber 1 **Eye, Left** 　*See Ø Eye, Right* J **Lens, Right** 　Zonule of Zinn K **Lens, Left** 　*See J Lens, Right*	X　External	Z　No Device	Z　No Qualifier
L **Extraocular Muscle, Right** 　Inferior oblique muscle 　Inferior rectus muscle 　Lateral rectus muscle 　Medial rectus muscle 　Superior oblique muscle 　Superior rectus muscle M **Extraocular Muscle, Left** 　*See L Extraocular Muscle, Right*	Ø　Open X　External	Z　No Device	Z　No Qualifier

Non-OR　08J[Ø,1,J,K]XZZ
Non-OR　08J[L,M]XZZ

Ø　Medical and Surgical
8　Eye
L　Occlusion　　Definition: Completely closing an orifice or the lumen of a tubular body part

Explanation: The orifice can be a natural orifice or an artificially created orifice

Body Part Character 4	Approach Character 5	Device Character 6	Qualifier Character 7
X **Lacrimal Duct, Right** 　Lacrimal canaliculus 　Lacrimal punctum 　Lacrimal sac 　Nasolacrimal duct Y **Lacrimal Duct, Left** 　*See X Lacrimal Duct, Right*	Ø　Open 3　Percutaneous	C　Extraluminal Device D　Intraluminal Device Z　No Device	Z　No Qualifier
X **Lacrimal Duct, Right** 　Lacrimal canaliculus 　Lacrimal punctum 　Lacrimal sac 　Nasolacrimal duct Y **Lacrimal Duct, Left** 　*See X Lacrimal Duct, Right*	7　Via Natural or Artificial Opening 8　Via Natural or Artificial Opening Endoscopic	D　Intraluminal Device Z　No Device	Z　No Qualifier

Ø　Medical and Surgical
8　Eye
M　Reattachment　　Definition: Putting back in or on all or a portion of a separated body part to its normal location or other suitable location

Explanation: Vascular circulation and nervous pathways may or may not be reestablished

Body Part Character 4	Approach Character 5	Device Character 6	Qualifier Character 7
N **Upper Eyelid, Right** 　Lateral canthus 　Levator palpebrae superioris muscle 　Orbicularis oculi muscle 　Superior tarsal plate P **Upper Eyelid, Left** 　*See N Upper Eyelid, Right* Q **Lower Eyelid, Right** 　Inferior tarsal plate 　Medial canthus R **Lower Eyelid, Left** 　*See Q Lower Eyelid, Right*	X　External	Z　No Device	Z　No Qualifier

Ø   Medical and Surgical
8   Eye
N   Release   Definition: Freeing a body part from an abnormal physical constraint by cutting or by the use of force
                    Explanation: Some of the restraining tissue may be taken out but none of the body part is taken out

Body Part Character 4	Approach Character 5	Device Character 6	Qualifier Character 7
Ø Eye, Right Ciliary body Posterior chamber **1 Eye, Left** *See Ø Eye, Right* **6 Sclera, Right** **7 Sclera, Left** **8 Cornea, Right** **9 Cornea, Left** **S Conjunctiva, Right** Plica semilunaris **T Conjunctiva, Left** *See S Conjunctiva, Right*	**X External**	**Z No Device**	**Z No Qualifier**
2 Anterior Chamber, Right Aqueous humour **3 Anterior Chamber, Left** *See 2 Anterior Chamber, Right* **4 Vitreous, Right** Vitreous body **5 Vitreous, Left** *See 4 Vitreous, Right* **C Iris, Right** **D Iris, Left** **E Retina, Right** Fovea Macula Optic disc **F Retina, Left** *See E Retina, Right* **G Retinal Vessel, Right** **H Retinal Vessel, Left** **J Lens, Right** Zonule of Zinn **K Lens, Left** *See J Lens, Right*	**3 Percutaneous**	**Z No Device**	**Z No Qualifier**
A Choroid, Right **B Choroid, Left** **L Extraocular Muscle, Right** Inferior oblique muscle Inferior rectus muscle Lateral rectus muscle Medial rectus muscle Superior oblique muscle Superior rectus muscle **M Extraocular Muscle, Left** *See L Extraocular Muscle, Right* **V Lacrimal Gland, Right** **W Lacrimal Gland, Left**	**Ø Open** **3 Percutaneous**	**Z No Device**	**Z No Qualifier**
N Upper Eyelid, Right Lateral canthus Levator palpebrae superioris muscle Orbicularis oculi muscle Superior tarsal plate **P Upper Eyelid, Left** *See N Upper Eyelid, Right* **Q Lower Eyelid, Right** Inferior tarsal plate Medial canthus **R Lower Eyelid, Left** *See Q Lower Eyelid, Right*	**Ø Open** **3 Percutaneous** **X External**	**Z No Device**	**Z No Qualifier**
X Lacrimal Duct, Right Lacrimal canaliculus Lacrimal punctum Lacrimal sac Nasolacrimal duct **Y Lacrimal Duct, Left** *See X Lacrimal Duct, Right*	**Ø Open** **3 Percutaneous** **7 Via Natural or Artificial Opening** **8 Via Natural or Artificial Opening Endoscopic**	**Z No Device**	**Z No Qualifier**

LC Limited Coverage   NC Noncovered   ⊞ Combination Member   HAC associated procedure   Combination Only   DRG Non-OR   Non-OR   New/Revised in GREEN
300   ICD-10-PCS 2020

Ø8N–Ø8N

Ø   Medical and Surgical
8   Eye
P   Removal   Definition: Taking out or off a device from a body part

Explanation: If a device is taken out and a similar device put in without cutting or puncturing the skin or mucous membrane, the procedure is coded to the root operation CHANGE. Otherwise, the procedure for taking out a device is coded to the root operation REMOVAL.

Body Part Character 4	Approach Character 5	Device Character 6	Qualifier Character 7

Ø   Eye, Right
   Ciliary body
   Posterior chamber
1   Eye, Left
   See Ø Eye, Right
	Ø Open
	3 Percutaneous
	7 Via Natural or Artificial Opening
	**8 Via Natural or Artificial Opening
	    Endoscopic**
		Ø Drainage Device
		1 Radioactive Element
		3 Infusion Device
		7 Autologous Tissue Substitute
		C Extraluminal Device
		D Intraluminal Device
		J Synthetic Substitute
		K Nonautologous Tissue Substitute
		Y Other Device
			Z No Qualifier

Ø   Eye, Right
   Ciliary body
   Posterior chamber
1   Eye, Left
   See Ø Eye, Right
	X External	**Ø Drainage Device**
		1 Radioactive Element
		3 Infusion Device
		7 Autologous Tissue Substitute
		C Extraluminal Device
		D Intraluminal Device
		J Synthetic Substitute
		K Nonautologous Tissue Substitute
			Z No Qualifier

J   Lens, Right
   Zonule of Zinn
K   Lens, Left
   See J Lens, Right
	3 Percutaneous	**J Synthetic Substitute**
		Y Other Device
			Z No Qualifier

L   Extraocular Muscle, Right
   Inferior oblique muscle
   Inferior rectus muscle
   Lateral rectus muscle
   Medial rectus muscle
   Superior oblique muscle
   Superior rectus muscle
M   Extraocular Muscle, Left
   See L Extraocular Muscle, Right
	Ø Open
	3 Percutaneous
		Ø Drainage Device
		7 Autologous Tissue Substitute
		J Synthetic Substitute
		K Nonautologous Tissue Substitute
		Y Other Device
			Z No Qualifier

Non-OR	Ø8P[Ø,1]3YZ
Non-OR	Ø8P[Ø,1][7,8][Ø,3,D,Y]Z
Non-OR	Ø8P[Ø,1]X[Ø,1,3,C,D,J]Z
Non-OR	Ø8P[J,K]3YZ
Non-OR	Ø8P[L,M]3YZ

LC Limited Coverage   **NC** Noncovered   ⊞ Combination Member   HAC associated procedure   Combination Only   DRG Non-OR   Non-OR   New/Revised in GREEN

ICD-10-PCS 2020   301

Ø8P–Ø8P

Ø   Medical and Surgical
8   Eye
Q   Repair   Definition: Restoring, to the extent possible, a body part to its normal anatomic structure and function
               Explanation: Used only when the method to accomplish the repair is not one of the other root operations

Body Part Character 4	Approach Character 5	Device Character 6	Qualifier Character 7

Ø   **Eye, Right**
    Ciliary body
    Posterior chamber
1   **Eye, Left**
    See Ø Eye, Right
6   **Sclera, Right**
7   **Sclera, Left**
8   **Cornea, Right**   NC
9   **Cornea, Left**   NC
S   **Conjunctiva, Right**
    Plica semilunaris
T   **Conjunctiva, Left**
    See S Conjunctiva, Right
	X External	**Z** No Device	**Z** No Qualifier

2   **Anterior Chamber, Right**
    Aqueous humour
3   **Anterior Chamber, Left**
    See 2 Anterior Chamber, Right
4   **Vitreous, Right**
    Vitreous body
5   **Vitreous, Left**
    See 4 Vitreous, Right
C   **Iris, Right**
D   **Iris, Left**
E   **Retina, Right**
    Fovea
    Macula
    Optic disc
F   **Retina, Left**
    See E Retina, Right
G   **Retinal Vessel, Right**
H   **Retinal Vessel, Left**
J   **Lens, Right**
    Zonule of Zinn
K   **Lens, Left**
    See J Lens, Right
	3 Percutaneous	**Z** No Device	**Z** No Qualifier

A   **Choroid, Right**
B   **Choroid, Left**
L   **Extraocular Muscle, Right**
    Inferior oblique muscle
    Inferior rectus muscle
    Lateral rectus muscle
    Medial rectus muscle
    Superior oblique muscle
    Superior rectus muscle
M   **Extraocular Muscle, Left**
    See L Extraocular Muscle, Right
V   **Lacrimal Gland, Right**
W   **Lacrimal Gland, Left**
	Ø Open
	3 Percutaneous
		Z No Device	**Z** No Qualifier

N   **Upper Eyelid, Right**
    Lateral canthus
    Levator palpebrae superioris muscle
    Orbicularis oculi muscle
    Superior tarsal plate
P   **Upper Eyelid, Left**
    See N Upper Eyelid, Right
Q   **Lower Eyelid, Right**
    Inferior tarsal plate
    Medial canthus
R   **Lower Eyelid, Left**
    See Q Lower Eyelid, Right
	Ø Open
	3 Percutaneous
	X External
		Z No Device	**Z** No Qualifier

X   **Lacrimal Duct, Right**
    Lacrimal canaliculus
    Lacrimal punctum
    Lacrimal sac
    Nasolacrimal duct
Y   **Lacrimal Duct, Left**
    See X Lacrimal Duct, Right
	Ø Open
	3 Percutaneous
	7 Via Natural or Artificial Opening
	8 Via Natural or Artificial Opening
	     Endoscopic
		Z No Device	**Z** No Qualifier

Non-OR   Ø8Q[N,P,Q,R][Ø,3,X]ZZ
NC   Ø8Q[8,9]XZZ

LC Limited Coverage   NC Noncovered   ⊞ Combination Member   HAC associated procedure   Combination Only   DRG Non-OR   Non-OR   New/Revised in GREEN

Ø   Medical and Surgical
8   Eye
R   Replacement   Definition: Putting in or on biological or synthetic material that physically takes the place and/or function of all or a portion of a body part
                   Explanation: The body part may have been taken out or replaced, or may be taken out, physically eradicated, or rendered nonfunctional during the REPLACEMENT procedure. A REMOVAL procedure is coded for taking out the device used in a previous replacement procedure.

Body Part Character 4	Approach Character 5	Device Character 6	Qualifier Character 7

Ø   **Eye, Right**
     Ciliary body
     Posterior chamber
1   **Eye, Left**
     See Ø Eye, Right
A   **Choroid, Right**
B   **Choroid, Left**
	Ø Open
	3 Percutaneous
		7 Autologous Tissue Substitute
		J Synthetic Substitute
		K Nonautologous Tissue Substitute
			Z No Qualifier

4   **Vitreous, Right**
     Vitreous body
5   **Vitreous, Left**
     See 4 Vitreous, Right
C   **Iris, Right**
D   **Iris, Left**
G   **Retinal Vessel, Right**
H   **Retinal Vessel, Left**
	3 Percutaneous	**7** Autologous Tissue Substitute
		J Synthetic Substitute
		K Nonautologous Tissue Substitute
			Z No Qualifier

6   **Sclera, Right**
7   **Sclera, Left**
S   **Conjunctiva, Right**
     Plica semilunaris
T   **Conjunctiva, Left**
     See S Conjunctiva, Right
	X External	**7** Autologous Tissue Substitute
		J Synthetic Substitute
		K Nonautologous Tissue Substitute
			Z No Qualifier

8 **Cornea, Right** **9** **Cornea, Left**	**3** Percutaneous **X** External	**7** Autologous Tissue Substitute **J** Synthetic Substitute **K** Nonautologous Tissue Substitute	**Z** No Qualifier

J   **Lens, Right**
     Zonule of Zinn
K   **Lens, Left**
     See J Lens, Right
	3 Percutaneous	**Ø** Synthetic Substitute, Intraocular Telescope
		7 Autologous Tissue Substitute
		J Synthetic Substitute
		K Nonautologous Tissue Substitute
			Z No Qualifier

N   **Upper Eyelid, Right**
     Lateral canthus
     Levator palpebrae superioris muscle
     Orbicularis oculi muscle
     Superior tarsal plate
P   **Upper Eyelid, Left**
     See N Upper Eyelid, Right
Q   **Lower Eyelid, Right**
     Inferior tarsal plate
     Medial canthus
R   **Lower Eyelid, Left**
     See Q Lower Eyelid, Right
	Ø Open
	3 Percutaneous
	X External
		7 Autologous Tissue Substitute
		J Synthetic Substitute
		K Nonautologous Tissue Substitute
			Z No Qualifier

X   **Lacrimal Duct, Right**
     Lacrimal canaliculus
     Lacrimal punctum
     Lacrimal sac
     Nasolacrimal duct
Y   **Lacrimal Duct, Left**
     See X Lacrimal Duct, Right
	Ø Open
	3 Percutaneous
	7 Via Natural or Artificial Opening
	8 Via Natural or Artificial Opening Endoscopic
		7 Autologous Tissue Substitute
		J Synthetic Substitute
		K Nonautologous Tissue Substitute
			Z No Qualifier

LC Limited Coverage   NC Noncovered   ⊞ Combination Member   HAC associated procedure   Combination Only   DRG Non-OR   Non-OR   New/Revised in GREEN

ICD-10-PCS 2020   303

Ø8R–Ø8R

0   **Medical and Surgical**
8   **Eye**
S   **Reposition**   Definition: Moving to its normal location, or other suitable location, all or a portion of a body part

                         Explanation: The body part is moved to a new location from an abnormal location, or from a normal location where it is not functioning correctly. The body part may or may not be cut out or off to be moved to the new location.

Body Part Character 4	Approach Character 5	Device Character 6	Qualifier Character 7

C   **Iris, Right**
D   **Iris, Left**
G   **Retinal Vessel, Right**
H   **Retinal Vessel, Left**
J   **Lens, Right**
     Zonule of Zinn
K   **Lens, Left**
     See J Lens, Right
	3 Percutaneous	**Z** No Device	**Z** No Qualifier

L   **Extraocular Muscle, Right**
     Inferior oblique muscle
     Inferior rectus muscle
     Lateral rectus muscle
     Medial rectus muscle
     Superior oblique muscle
     Superior rectus muscle
M   **Extraocular Muscle, Left**
     See L Extraocular Muscle, Right
V   **Lacrimal Gland, Right**
W   **Lacrimal Gland, Left**
	0 Open
	3 Percutaneous
		Z No Device	**Z** No Qualifier

N   **Upper Eyelid, Right**
     Lateral canthus
     Levator palpebrae superioris muscle
     Orbicularis oculi muscle
     Superior tarsal plate
P   **Upper Eyelid, Left**
     See N Upper Eyelid, Right
Q   **Lower Eyelid, Right**
     Inferior tarsal plate
     Medial canthus
R   **Lower Eyelid, Left**
     See Q Lower Eyelid, Right
	0 Open
	3 Percutaneous
	X External
		Z No Device	**Z** No Qualifier

X   **Lacrimal Duct, Right**
     Lacrimal canaliculus
     Lacrimal punctum
     Lacrimal sac
     Nasolacrimal duct
Y   **Lacrimal Duct, Left**
     See X Lacrimal Duct, Right
	0 Open
	3 Percutaneous
	7 Via Natural or Artificial Opening
	8 Via Natural or Artificial Opening Endoscopic
		Z No Device	**Z** No Qualifier

LC Limited Coverage   NC Noncovered   ⊞ Combination Member   HAC associated procedure   Combination Only   DRG Non-OR   Non-OR   New/Revised in GREEN

304   ICD-10-PCS 2020

Ø   Medical and Surgical
8   Eye
T   Resection   Definition: Cutting out or off, without replacement, all of a body part
                   Explanation: None

Body Part Character 4	Approach Character 5	Device Character 6	Qualifier Character 7
Ø Eye, Right Ciliary body Posterior chamber **1 Eye, Left** *See Ø Eye, Right* **8 Cornea, Right** **9 Cornea, Left**	**X External**	**Z No Device**	**Z No Qualifier**
4 Vitreous, Right Vitreous body **5 Vitreous, Left** *See 4 Vitreous, Right* **C Iris, Right** **D Iris, Left** **J Lens, Right** Zonule of Zinn **K Lens, Left** *See J Lens, Right*	**3 Percutaneous**	**Z No Device**	**Z No Qualifier**
L Extraocular Muscle, Right Inferior oblique muscle Inferior rectus muscle Lateral rectus muscle Medial rectus muscle Superior oblique muscle Superior rectus muscle **M Extraocular Muscle, Left** *See L Extraocular Muscle, Right* **V Lacrimal Gland, Right** **W Lacrimal Gland, Left**	**Ø Open** **3 Percutaneous**	**Z No Device**	**Z No Qualifier**
N Upper Eyelid, Right Lateral canthus Levator palpebrae superioris muscle Orbicularis oculi muscle Superior tarsal plate **P Upper Eyelid, Left** *See N Upper Eyelid, Right* **Q Lower Eyelid, Right** Inferior tarsal plate Medial canthus **R Lower Eyelid, Left** *See Q Lower Eyelid, Right*	**Ø Open** **X External**	**Z No Device**	**Z No Qualifier**
X Lacrimal Duct, Right Lacrimal canaliculus Lacrimal punctum Lacrimal sac Nasolacrimal duct **Y Lacrimal Duct, Left** *See X Lacrimal Duct, Right*	**Ø Open** **3 Percutaneous** **7 Via Natural or Artificial Opening** **8 Via Natural or Artificial Opening Endoscopic**	**Z No Device**	**Z No Qualifier**

Ø   **Medical and Surgical**
8   **Eye**
U   **Supplement**   Definition: Putting in or on biological or synthetic material that physically reinforces and/or augments the function of a portion of a body part

           Explanation: The biological material is non-living, or is living and from the same individual. The body part may have been previously replaced, and the SUPPLEMENT procedure is performed to physically reinforce and/or augment the function of the replaced body part.

Body Part Character 4	Approach Character 5	Device Character 6	Qualifier Character 7

Ø **Eye, Right**
    Ciliary body
    Posterior chamber
1 **Eye, Left**
    See Ø Eye, Right
C **Iris, Right**
D **Iris, Left**
E **Retina, Right**
    Fovea
    Macula
    Optic disc
F **Retina, Left**
    See E Retina, Right
G **Retinal Vessel, Right**
H **Retinal Vessel, Left**
L **Extraocular Muscle, Right**
    Inferior oblique muscle
    Inferior rectus muscle
    Lateral rectus muscle
    Medial rectus muscle
    Superior oblique muscle
    Superior rectus muscle
M **Extraocular Muscle, Left**
    See L Extraocular Muscle, Right
	Ø **Open**
	3 **Percutaneous**
		7 **Autologous Tissue Substitute**
		J **Synthetic Substitute**
		K **Nonautologous Tissue Substitute**
			Z **No Qualifier**

8 **Cornea, Right**   `NC`
9 **Cornea, Left**   `NC`
N **Upper Eyelid, Right**
    Lateral canthus
    Levator palpebrae superioris muscle
    Orbicularis oculi muscle
    Superior tarsal plate
P **Upper Eyelid, Left**
    See N Upper Eyelid, Right
Q **Lower Eyelid, Right**
    Inferior tarsal plate
    Medial canthus
R **Lower Eyelid, Left**
    See Q Lower Eyelid, Right
	Ø **Open**
	3 **Percutaneous**
	X **External**
		7 **Autologous Tissue Substitute**
		J **Synthetic Substitute**
		K **Nonautologous Tissue Substitute**
			Z **No Qualifier**

X **Lacrimal Duct, Right**
    Lacrimal canaliculus
    Lacrimal punctum
    Lacrimal sac
    Nasolacrimal duct
Y **Lacrimal Duct, Left**
    See X Lacrimal Duct, Right
	Ø **Open**
	3 **Percutaneous**
	7 **Via Natural or Artificial Opening**
	8 **Via Natural or Artificial Opening
	    Endoscopic**
		7 **Autologous Tissue Substitute**
		J **Synthetic Substitute**
		K **Nonautologous Tissue Substitute**
			Z **No Qualifier**

    `NC`   Ø8U[8,9][Ø,3,X]KZ

Ø   **Medical and Surgical**
8   **Eye**
V   **Restriction**   Definition: Partially closing an orifice or the lumen of a tubular body part

           Explanation: The orifice can be a natural orifice or an artificially created orifice

Body Part Character 4	Approach Character 5	Device Character 6	Qualifier Character 7

X **Lacrimal Duct, Right**
    Lacrimal canaliculus
    Lacrimal punctum
    Lacrimal sac
    Nasolacrimal duct
Y **Lacrimal Duct, Left**
    See X Lacrimal Duct, Right
	Ø **Open**
	3 **Percutaneous**
		C **Extraluminal Device**
		D **Intraluminal Device**
		Z **No Device**
			Z **No Qualifier**

X **Lacrimal Duct, Right**
    Lacrimal canaliculus
    Lacrimal punctum
    Lacrimal sac
    Nasolacrimal duct
Y **Lacrimal Duct, Left**
    See X Lacrimal Duct, Right
	7 **Via Natural or Artificial Opening**
	8 **Via Natural or Artificial Opening
	    Endoscopic**
		D **Intraluminal Device**
		Z **No Device**
			Z **No Qualifier**

`LC` Limited Coverage   `NC` Noncovered   ⊞ Combination Member   HAC associated procedure   Combination Only   DRG Non-OR   Non-OR   New/Revised in GREEN

306   ICD-10-PCS 2020

Ø **Medical and Surgical**
8 **Eye**
W **Revision**　　Definition: Correcting, to the extent possible, a portion of a malfunctioning device or the position of a displaced device
　　　　　　　　Explanation: Revision can include correcting a malfunctioning or displaced device by taking out or putting in components of the device such as a screw or pin

Body Part Character 4	Approach Character 5	Device Character 6	Qualifier Character 7
Ø Eye, Right 　Ciliary body 　Posterior chamber **1** Eye, Left 　*See Ø Eye, Right*	**Ø** Open **3** Percutaneous **7** Via Natural or Artificial Opening **8** Via Natural or Artificial Opening Endoscopic	**Ø** Drainage Device **3** Infusion Device **7** Autologous Tissue Substitute **C** Extraluminal Device **D** Intraluminal Device **J** Synthetic Substitute **K** Nonautologous Tissue Substitute **Y** Other Device	**Z** No Qualifier
Ø Eye, Right 　Ciliary body 　Posterior chamber **1** Eye, Left 　*See Ø Eye, Right*	**X** External	**Ø** Drainage Device **3** Infusion Device **7** Autologous Tissue Substitute **C** Extraluminal Device **D** Intraluminal Device **J** Synthetic Substitute **K** Nonautologous Tissue Substitute	**Z** No Qualifier
J Lens, Right 　Zonule of Zinn **K** Lens, Left 　*See J Lens, Right*	**3** Percutaneous	**J** Synthetic Substitute **Y** Other Device	**Z** No Qualifier
J Lens, Right 　Zonule of Zinn **K** Lens, Left 　*See J Lens, Right*	**X** External	**J** Synthetic Substitute	**Z** No Qualifier
L Extraocular Muscle, Right 　Inferior oblique muscle 　Inferior rectus muscle 　Lateral rectus muscle 　Medial rectus muscle 　Superior oblique muscle 　Superior rectus muscle **M** Extraocular Muscle, Left 　*See L Extraocular Muscle, Right*	**Ø** Open **3** Percutaneous	**Ø** Drainage Device **7** Autologous Tissue Substitute **J** Synthetic Substitute **K** Nonautologous Tissue Substitute **Y** Other Device	**Z** No Qualifier

Non-OR	Ø8W[Ø,1][3,7,8]YZ
Non-OR	Ø8W[Ø,1]X[Ø,3,7,C,D,J,K]Z
Non-OR	Ø8W[J,K]3YZ
Non-OR	Ø8W[J,K]XJZ
Non-OR	Ø8W[L,M]3YZ

Ø **Medical and Surgical**
8 **Eye**
X **Transfer**　　Definition: Moving, without taking out, all or a portion of a body part to another location to take over the function of all or a portion of a body part
　　　　　　　Explanation: The body part transferred remains connected to its vascular and nervous supply

Body Part Character 4	Approach Character 5	Device Character 6	Qualifier Character 7
L Extraocular Muscle, Right 　Inferior oblique muscle 　Inferior rectus muscle 　Lateral rectus muscle 　Medial rectus muscle 　Superior oblique muscle 　Superior rectus muscle **M** Extraocular Muscle, Left 　*See L Extraocular Muscle, Right*	**Ø** Open **3** Percutaneous	**Z** No Device	**Z** No Qualifier

Ear, Nose, Sinus Ø9Ø–Ø9W

Character Meanings*

This Character Meaning table is provided as a guide to assist the user in the identification of character members that may be found in this section of code tables. It **SHOULD NOT** be used to build a PCS code.

Operation–Character 3	Body Part–Character 4	Approach–Character 5	Device–Character 6	Qualifier–Character 7
Ø Alteration	Ø . External Ear, Right	Ø Open	Ø Drainage Device	Ø Endolymphatic
1 Bypass	1 External Ear, Left	3 Percutaneous	4 Hearing Device, Bone Conduction	X Diagnostic
2 Change	2 External Ear, Bilateral	4 Percutaneous Endoscopic	5 Hearing Device, Single Channel Cochlear Prosthesis	Z No Qualifier
3 Control	3 External Auditory Canal, Right	7 Via Natural or Artificial Opening	6 Hearing Device, Multiple Channel Cochlear Prosthesis	
5 Destruction	4 External Auditory Canal, Left	8 Via Natural or Artificial Opening Endoscopic	7 Autologous Tissue Substitute	
7 Dilation	5 Middle Ear, Right	X External	B Intraluminal Device, Airway	
8 Division	6 Middle Ear, Left		D Intraluminal Device	
9 Drainage	7 Tympanic Membrane, Right		J Synthetic Substitute	
B Excision	8 Tympanic Membrane, Left		K Nonautologous Tissue Substitute	
C Extirpation	9 Auditory Ossicle, Right		S Hearing Device	
D Extraction	A Auditory Ossicle, Left		Y Other Device	
H Insertion	B Mastoid Sinus, Right		Z No Device	
J Inspection	C Mastoid Sinus, Left			
M Reattachment	D Inner Ear, Right			
N Release	E Inner Ear, Left			
P Removal	F Eustachian Tube, Right			
Q Repair	G Eustachian Tube, Left			
R Replacement	H Ear, Right			
S Reposition	J Ear, Left			
T Resection	K Nasal Mucosa and Soft Tissue			
U Supplement	L Nasal Turbinate			
W Revision	M Nasal Septum			
	N Nasopharynx			
	P Accessory Sinus			
	Q Maxillary Sinus, Right			
	R Maxillary Sinus, Left			
	S Frontal Sinus, Right			
	T Frontal Sinus, Left			
	U Ethmoid Sinus, Right			
	V Ethmoid Sinus, Left			
	W Sphenoid Sinus, Right			
	X Sphenoid Sinus, Left			
	Y Sinus			

* Includes sinus ducts.

AHA Coding Clinic for table Ø93
2018, 4Q, 38   Control of epistaxis

AHA Coding Clinic for table Ø95
2018, 1Q, 19   Control of epistaxis via silver nitrate cauterization

AHA Coding Clinic for table Ø9Q
2018, 1Q, 19   Control of epistaxis via silver nitrate cauterization
2017, 4Q, 106   Control of bleeding of external naris using suture
2014, 4Q, 20   Control of epistaxis
2014, 3Q, 22   Transsphenoidal removal of pituitary tumor and fat graft placement
2013, 4Q, 114   Balloon sinuplasty

Ear Anatomy

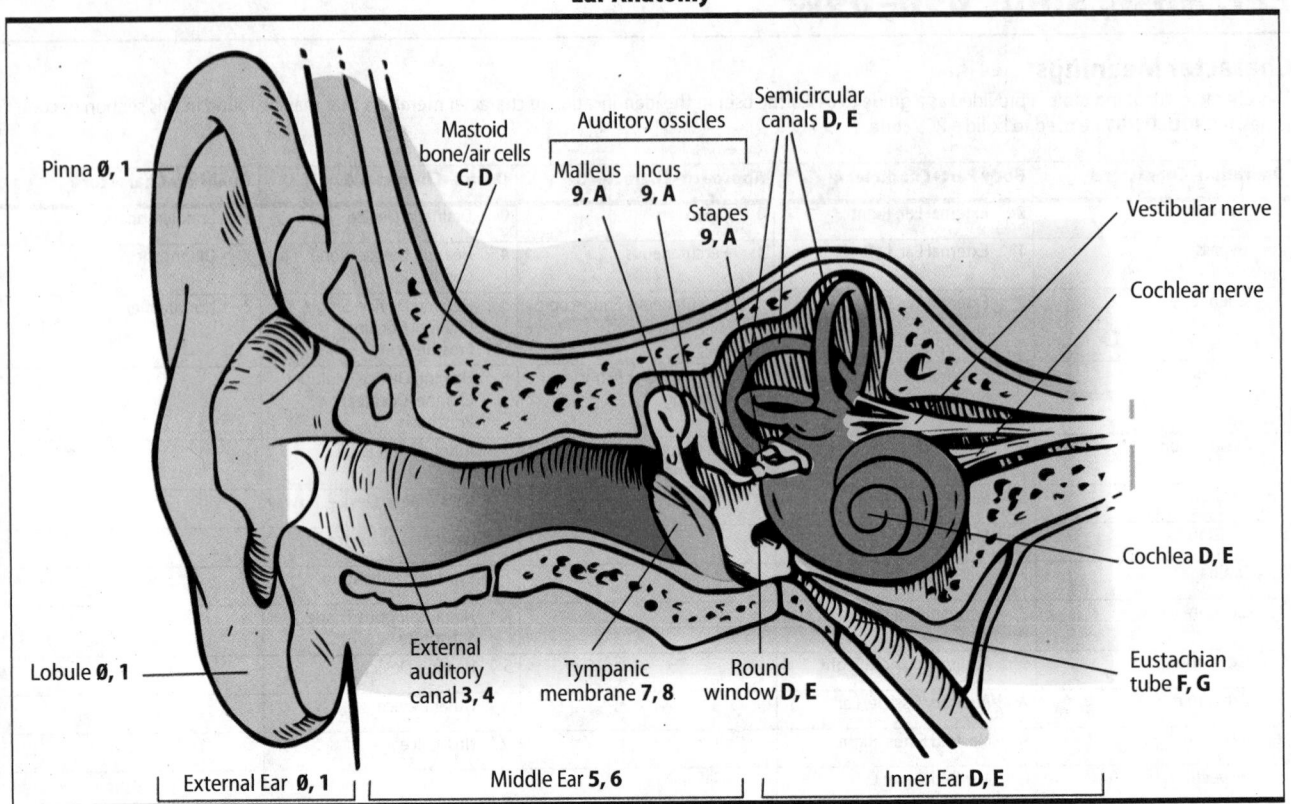

Pinna Ø, 1

Lobule Ø, 1

Mastoid bone/air cells C, D

Auditory ossicles

Malleus 9, A Incus 9, A

Stapes 9, A

Semicircular canals D, E

Vestibular nerve

Cochlear nerve

Cochlea D, E

Eustachian tube F, G

External auditory canal 3, 4

Tympanic membrane 7, 8

Round window D, E

External Ear Ø, 1   Middle Ear 5, 6   Inner Ear D, E

Nasal Turbinates

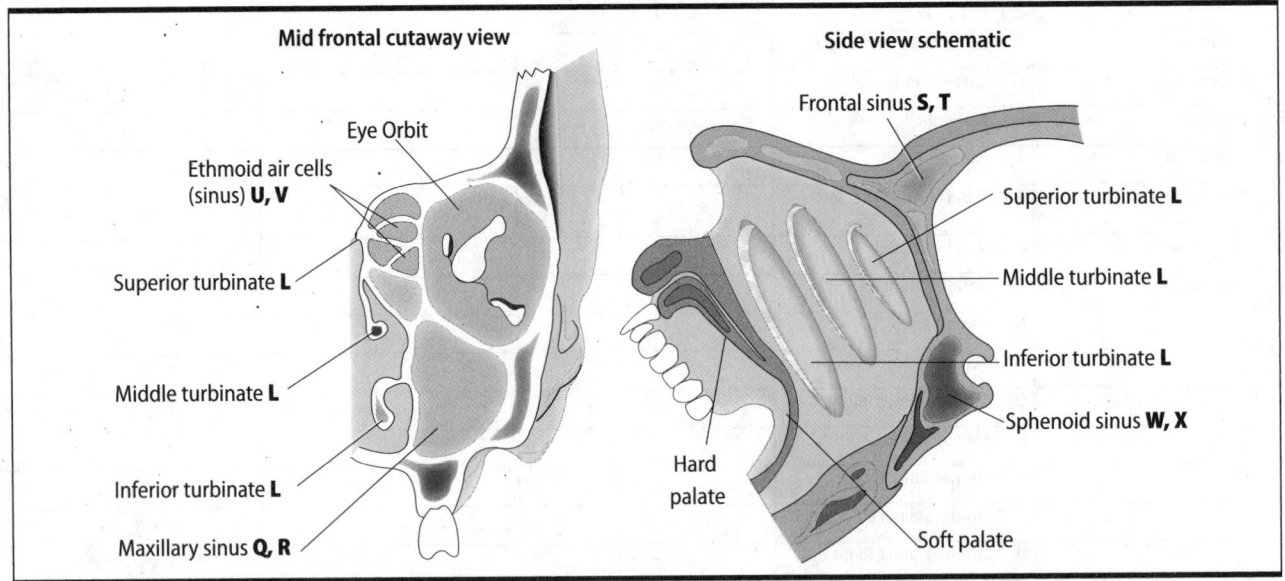

Mid frontal cutaway view

Ethmoid air cells (sinus) U, V

Eye Orbit

Superior turbinate L

Middle turbinate L

Inferior turbinate L

Maxillary sinus Q, R

Side view schematic

Frontal sinus S, T

Superior turbinate L

Middle turbinate L

Inferior turbinate L

Sphenoid sinus W, X

Hard palate

Soft palate

Paranasal Sinuses

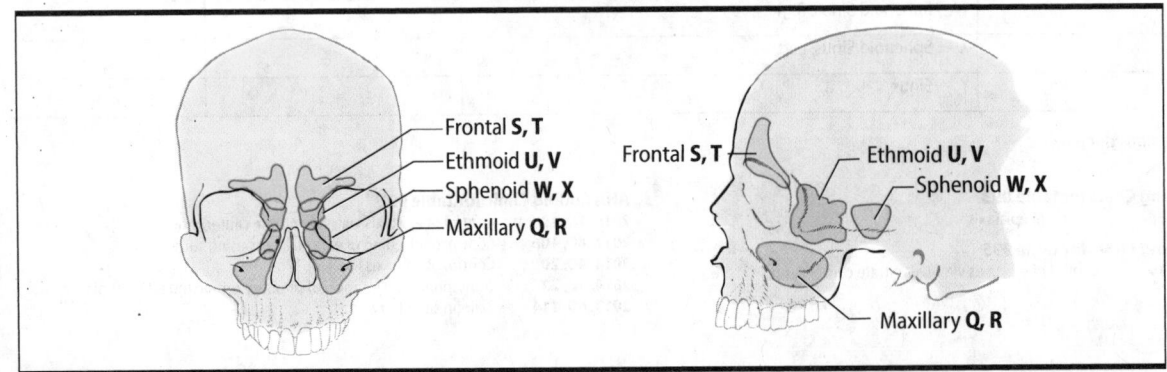

Frontal S, T
Ethmoid U, V
Sphenoid W, X
Maxillary Q, R

Frontal S, T
Ethmoid U, V
Sphenoid W, X

Maxillary Q, R

Ø   Medical and Surgical
9   Ear, Nose, Sinus
Ø   Alteration   Definition: Modifying the anatomic structure of a body part without affecting the function of the body part
           Explanation: Principal purpose is to improve appearance

Body Part Character 4		Approach Character 5	Device Character 6	Qualifier Character 7
Ø **External Ear, Right** Antihelix Antitragus Auricle Earlobe Helix Pinna Tragus 1 **External Ear, Left** *See Ø External Ear, Right*	2 **External Ear, Bilateral** *See Ø External Ear, Right* K **Nasal Mucosa and Soft Tissue** Columella External naris Greater alar cartilage Internal naris Lateral nasal cartilage Lesser alar cartilage Nasal cavity Nostril	Ø **Open** 3 **Percutaneous** 4 **Percutaneous Endoscopic** X **External**	7 **Autologous Tissue Substitute** J **Synthetic Substitute** K **Nonautologous Tissue Substitute** Z **No Device**	Z **No Qualifier**

Ø   Medical and Surgical
9   Ear, Nose, Sinus
1   Bypass   Definition: Altering the route of passage of the contents of a tubular body part
           Explanation: Rerouting contents of a body part to a downstream area of the normal route, to a similar route and body part, or to an abnormal route and dissimilar body part. Includes one or more anastomoses, with or without the use of a device.

Body Part Character 4	Approach Character 5	Device Character 6	Qualifier Character 7
D **Inner Ear, Right** Bony labyrinth Bony vestibule Cochlea Round window Semicircular canal E **Inner Ear, Left** *See D Inner Ear, Right*	Ø **Open**	7 **Autologous Tissue Substitute** J **Synthetic Substitute** K **Nonautologous Tissue Substitute** Z **No Device**	Ø **Endolymphatic**

Ø   Medical and Surgical
9   Ear, Nose, Sinus
2   Change   Definition: Taking out or off a device from a body part and putting back an identical or similar device in or on the same body part without cutting or puncturing the skin or a mucous membrane
           Explanation: All CHANGE procedures are coded using the approach EXTERNAL

Body Part Character 4	Approach Character 5	Device Character 6	Qualifier Character 7
H **Ear, Right** J **Ear, Left** K **Nasal Mucosa and Soft Tissue** Columella External naris Greater alar cartilage Internal naris Lateral nasal cartilage Lesser alar cartilage Nasal cavity Nostril Y **Sinus**	X **External**	Ø **Drainage Device** Y **Other Device**	Z **No Qualifier**

Non-OR   All body part, approach, device, and qualifier values

Ø   Medical and Surgical
9   Ear, Nose, Sinus
3   Control   Definition: Stopping, or attempting to stop, postprocedural or other acute bleeding
           Explanation: None

Body Part Character 4	Approach Character 5	Device Character 6	Qualifier Character 7
K **Nasal Mucosa and Soft Tissue** Columella External naris Greater alar cartilage Internal naris Lateral nasal cartilage Lesser alar cartilage Nasal cavity Nostril	7 **Via Natural or Artificial Opening** 8 **Via Natural or Artificial Opening Endoscopic**	Z **No Device**	Z **No Qualifier**

Non-OR   Ø93K[7,8]ZZ

Ear, Nose, Sinus

Ø   **Medical and Surgical**
9   **Ear, Nose, Sinus**
5   **Destruction**   Definition: Physical eradication of all or a portion of a body part by the direct use of energy, force, or a destructive agent

                             Explanation: None of the body part is physically taken out

Body Part Character 4		Approach Character 5	Device Character 6	Qualifier Character 7
Ø **External Ear, Right** Antihelix Antitragus Auricle Earlobe Helix Pinna Tragus	**1** **External Ear, Left** *See Ø External Ear, Right*	**Ø** Open **3** Percutaneous **4** Percutaneous Endoscopic **X** External	**Z** No Device	**Z** No Qualifier
3 **External Auditory Canal, Right** External auditory meatus	**4** **External Auditory Canal, Left** *See 3 External Auditory Canal, Right*	**Ø** Open **3** Percutaneous **4** Percutaneous Endoscopic **7** Via Natural or Artificial Opening **8** Via Natural or Artificial Opening Endoscopic **X** External	**Z** No Device	**Z** No Qualifier
5 **Middle Ear, Right** Oval window Tympanic cavity **6** **Middle Ear, Left** *See 5 Middle Ear, Right* **9** **Auditory Ossicle, Right** Incus Malleus Stapes **A** **Auditory Ossicle, Left** *See 9 Auditory Ossicle, Right*	**D** **Inner Ear, Right** Bony labyrinth Bony vestibule Cochlea Round window Semicircular canal **E** **Inner Ear, Left** *See D Inner Ear, Right*	**Ø** Open **8** Via Natural or Artificial Opening Endoscopic	**Z** No Device	**Z** No Qualifier
7 **Tympanic Membrane, Right** Pars flaccida **8** **Tympanic Membrane, Left** *See 7 Tympanic Membrane, Right* **F** **Eustachian Tube, Right** Auditory tube Pharyngotympanic tube **G** **Eustachian Tube, Left** *See F Eustachian Tube, Right*	**L** **Nasal Turbinate** Inferior turbinate Middle turbinate Nasal concha Superior turbinate **N** **Nasopharynx** Choana Fossa of Rosenmuller Pharyngeal recess Rhinopharynx	**Ø** Open **3** Percutaneous **4** Percutaneous Endoscopic **7** Via Natural or Artificial Opening **8** Via Natural or Artificial Opening Endoscopic	**Z** No Device	**Z** No Qualifier
B **Mastoid Sinus, Right** Mastoid air cells **C** **Mastoid Sinus, Left** *See B Mastoid Sinus, Right* **M** **Nasal Septum** Quadrangular cartilage Septal cartilage Vomer bone **P** **Accessory Sinus** **Q** **Maxillary Sinus, Right** Antrum of Highmore	**R** **Maxillary Sinus, Left** *See Q Maxillary Sinus, Right* **S** **Frontal Sinus, Right** **T** **Frontal Sinus, Left** **U** **Ethmoid Sinus, Right** Ethmoidal air cell **V** **Ethmoid Sinus, Left** *See U Ethmoid Sinus, Right* **W** **Sphenoid Sinus, Right** **X** **Sphenoid Sinus, Left**	**Ø** Open **3** Percutaneous **4** Percutaneous Endoscopic **8** Via Natural or Artificial Opening Endoscopic	**Z** No Device	**Z** No Qualifier
K **Nasal Mucosa and Soft Tissue** Columella External naris Greater alar cartilage Internal naris Lateral nasal cartilage Lesser alar cartilage Nasal cavity Nostril		**Ø** Open **3** Percutaneous **4** Percutaneous Endoscopic **8** Via Natural or Artificial Opening Endoscopic **X** External	**Z** No Device	**Z** No Qualifier

Non-OR	Ø95[Ø,1][Ø,3,4,X]ZZ	
Non-OR	Ø95[3,4][Ø,3,4,7,8,X]ZZ	
Non-OR	Ø95[F,G][Ø,3,4,7,8]ZZ	
Non-OR	Ø95M[Ø,3,4,8]ZZ	
Non-OR	Ø95K[Ø,3,4,8,X]ZZ	

LC Limited Coverage   **NC** Noncovered   ⊞ Combination Member   HAC associated procedure   Combination Only   DRG Non-OR   Non-OR   New/Revised in GREEN

312   ICD-10-PCS 2020

Ø   Medical and Surgical
9   Ear, Nose, Sinus
7   Dilation   Definition: Expanding an orifice or the lumen of a tubular body part

Explanation: The orifice can be a natural orifice or an artificially created orifice. Accomplished by stretching a tubular body part using intraluminal pressure or by cutting part of the orifice or wall of the tubular body part.

Body Part Character 4	Approach Character 5	Device Character 6	Qualifier Character 7
F Eustachian Tube, Right Auditory tube Pharyngotympanic tube **G** Eustachian Tube, Left *See F Eustachian Tube, Right*	**Ø** Open **7** Via Natural or Artificial Opening **8** Via Natural or Artificial Opening Endoscopic	**D** Intraluminal Device **Z** No Device	**Z** No Qualifier
F Eustachian Tube, Right Auditory tube Pharyngotympanic tube **G** Eustachian Tube, Left *See F Eustachian Tube, Right*	**3** Percutaneous **4** Percutaneous Endoscopic	**Z** No Device	**Z** No Qualifier

Non-OR   All body part, approach, device, and qualifier values

Ø   Medical and Surgical
9   Ear, Nose, Sinus
8   Division   Definition: Cutting into a body part, without draining fluids and/or gases from the body part, in order to separate or transect a body part

Explanation: All or a portion of the body part is separated into two or more portions

Body Part Character 4	Approach Character 5	Device Character 6	Qualifier Character 7
L Nasal Turbinate Inferior turbinate Middle turbinate Nasal concha Superior turbinate	**Ø** Open **3** Percutaneous **4** Percutaneous Endoscopic **7** Via Natural or Artificial Opening **8** Via Natural or Artificial Opening Endoscopic	**Z** No Device	**Z** No Qualifier

LC Limited Coverage   NC Noncovered   ⊞ Combination Member   HAC associated procedure   Combination Only   DRG Non-OR   Non-OR   New/Revised in GREEN

ICD-1Ø-PCS 2020   313

Ear, Nose, Sinus *(side margin)*

Ø　**Medical and Surgical**
9　**Ear, Nose, Sinus**
9　**Drainage**　　Definition: Taking or letting out fluids and/or gases from a body part
　　　　　　　　　　Explanation: The qualifier DIAGNOSTIC is used to identify drainage procedures that are biopsies

Body Part Character 4		Approach Character 5	Device Character 6	Qualifier Character 7
Ø　**External Ear, Right**　 Antihelix Antitragus Auricle Earlobe Helix Pinna Tragus	1　**External Ear, Left**　 *See Ø External Ear, Right*	Ø　Open 3　Percutaneous 4　Percutaneous Endoscopic X　External	Ø　Drainage Device	Z　No Qualifier
Ø　**External Ear, Right**　 Antihelix Antitragus Auricle Earlobe Helix Pinna Tragus	1　**External Ear, Left**　 *See Ø External Ear, Right*	Ø　Open 3　Percutaneous 4　Percutaneous Endoscopic X　External	Z　No Device	X　Diagnostic Z　No Qualifier
3　**External Auditory Canal, Right**　 External auditory meatus 4　**External Auditory Canal, Left**　 *See 3 External Auditory Canal, Right*	K　**Nasal Mucosa and Soft Tissue**　 Columella External naris Greater alar cartilage Internal naris Lateral nasal cartilage Lesser alar cartilage Nasal cavity Nostril	Ø　Open 3　Percutaneous 4　Percutaneous Endoscopic 7　Via Natural or Artificial Opening 8　Via Natural or Artificial Opening Endoscopic X　External	Ø　Drainage Device	Z　No Qualifier
3　**External Auditory Canal, Right**　 External auditory meatus 4　**External Auditory Canal, Left**　 *See 3 External Auditory Canal, Right*	K　**Nasal Mucosa and Soft Tissue**　 Columella External naris Greater alar cartilage Internal naris Lateral nasal cartilage Lesser alar cartilage Nasal cavity Nostril	Ø　Open 3　Percutaneous 4　Percutaneous Endoscopic 7　Via Natural or Artificial Opening 8　Via Natural or Artificial Opening Endoscopic X　External	Z　No Device	X　Diagnostic Z　No Qualifier
5　**Middle Ear, Right**　 Oval window Tympanic cavity 6　**Middle Ear, Left**　 *See 5 Middle Ear, Right* 9　**Auditory Ossicle, Right**　 Incus Malleus Stapes	A　**Auditory Ossicle, Left**　 *See 9 Auditory Ossicle, Right* D　**Inner Ear, Right**　 Bony labyrinth Bony vestibule Cochlea Round window Semicircular canal E　**Inner Ear, Left**　 *See D Inner Ear, Right*	Ø　Open 7　Via Natural or Artificial Opening 8　Via Natural or Artificial Opening Endoscopic	Ø　Drainage Device	Z　No Qualifier
5　**Middle Ear, Right**　 Oval window Tympanic cavity 6　**Middle Ear, Left**　 *See 5 Middle Ear, Right* 9　**Auditory Ossicle, Right**　 Incus Malleus Stapes	A　**Auditory Ossicle, Left**　 *See 9 Auditory Ossicle, Right* D　**Inner Ear, Right**　 Bony labyrinth Bony vestibule Cochlea Round window Semicircular canal E　**Inner Ear, Left**　 *See D Inner Ear, Right*	Ø　Open 7　Via Natural or Artificial Opening 8　Via Natural or Artificial Opening Endoscopic	Z　No Device	X　Diagnostic Z　No Qualifier

Ø99 Continued on next page

Non-OR	Ø99[Ø,1][Ø,3,4,X]ØZ
Non-OR	Ø99[Ø,1][Ø,3,4,X]Z[X,Z]
Non-OR	Ø99[3,4,K][Ø,3,4,7,8,X]ØZ
Non-OR	Ø99[3,4,K][Ø,3,4,7,8,X]Z[X,Z]
Non-OR	Ø99580Z
Non-OR	Ø99[6,9,A,D,E][7,8]ØZ
Non-OR	Ø99[5,6]ØZZ
Non-OR	Ø99[5,6,9,A,D,E][7,8]Z[X,Z]

Ø   **Medical and Surgical**   *Ø99 Continued*
9   **Ear, Nose, Sinus**
9   **Drainage**   Definition: Taking or letting out fluids and/or gases from a body part
                             Explanation: The qualifier DIAGNOSTIC is used to identify drainage procedures that are biopsies

Body Part Character 4		Approach Character 5	Device Character 6	Qualifier Character 7
7 Tympanic Membrane, Right Pars flaccida **8 Tympanic Membrane, Left** *See 7 Tympanic Membrane, Right* **B Mastoid Sinus, Right** Mastoid air cells **C Mastoid Sinus, Left** *See B Mastoid Sinus, Right* **F Eustachian Tube, Right** Auditory tube Pharyngotympanic tube **G Eustachian Tube, Left** *See F Eustachian Tube, Right* **L Nasal Turbinate** Inferior turbinate Middle turbinate Nasal concha Superior turbinate **M Nasal Septum** Quadrangular cartilage Septal cartilage Vomer bone	**N Nasopharynx** Choana Fossa of Rosenmuller Pharyngeal recess Rhinopharynx **P Accessory Sinus** **Q Maxillary Sinus, Right** Antrum of Highmore **R Maxillary Sinus, Left** *See Q Maxillary Sinus, Right* **S Frontal Sinus, Right** **T Frontal Sinus, Left** **U Ethmoid Sinus, Right** Ethmoidal air cell **V Ethmoid Sinus, Left** *See U Ethmoid Sinus, Right* **W Sphenoid Sinus, Right** **X Sphenoid Sinus, Left**	**Ø Open** **3 Percutaneous** **4 Percutaneous Endoscopic** **7 Via Natural or Artificial Opening** **8 Via Natural or Artificial Opening Endoscopic**	**Ø Drainage Device**	**Z No Qualifier**
7 Tympanic Membrane, Right Pars flaccida **8 Tympanic Membrane, Left** *See 7 Tympanic Membrane, Right* **B Mastoid Sinus, Right** Mastoid air cells **C Mastoid Sinus, Left** *See B Mastoid Sinus, Right* **F Eustachian Tube, Right** Auditory tube Pharyngotympanic tube **G Eustachian Tube, Left** *See F Eustachian Tube, Right* **L Nasal Turbinate** Inferior turbinate Middle turbinate Nasal concha Superior turbinate **M Nasal Septum** Quadrangular cartilage Septal cartilage Vomer bone	**N Nasopharynx** Choana Fossa of Rosenmuller Pharyngeal recess Rhinopharynx **P Accessory Sinus** **Q Maxillary Sinus, Right** Antrum of Highmore **R Maxillary Sinus, Left** *See Q Maxillary Sinus, Right* **S Frontal Sinus, Right** **T Frontal Sinus, Left** **U Ethmoid Sinus, Right** Ethmoidal air cell **V Ethmoid Sinus, Left** *See U Ethmoid Sinus, Right* **W Sphenoid Sinus, Right** **X Sphenoid Sinus, Left**	**Ø Open** **3 Percutaneous** **4 Percutaneous Endoscopic** **7 Via Natural or Artificial Opening** **8 Via Natural or Artificial Opening Endoscopic**	**Z No Device**	**X Diagnostic** **Z No Qualifier**

Non-OR	Ø99[B,C][3,7,8]ØZ
Non-OR	Ø99[F,G,L,M][Ø,3,4,7,8]ØZ
Non-OR	Ø99N3ØZ
Non-OR	Ø99[P,Q,R,S,T,U,V,W,X][3,4,7,8]ØZ
Non-OR	Ø99[7,8][Ø,3,4,7,8]ZZ
Non-OR	Ø99[7,8][7,8]ZX
Non-OR	Ø99[B,C]3ZZ
Non-OR	Ø99[B,C][7,8]Z[X,Z]
Non-OR	Ø99[F,G][Ø,3,4,7,8]ZZ
Non-OR	Ø99[F,G][7,8]ZX
Non-OR	Ø99[L,M][Ø,3,4,7,8]Z[X,Z]
Non-OR	Ø99N[Ø,3,4,7,8]ZX
Non-OR	Ø99N3ZZ
Non-OR	Ø99[P,Q,R,S,T,U,V,W,X][3,4,7,8]Z[X,Z]

LC Limited Coverage   NC Noncovered   ⊞ Combination Member   HAC associated procedure   Combination Only   DRG Non-OR   Non-OR   New/Revised in GREEN

ICD-10-PCS 2020   315

Ø99–Ø99

0 Medical and Surgical
9 Ear, Nose, Sinus
B Excision Definition: Cutting out or off, without replacement, a portion of a body part
Explanation: The qualifier DIAGNOSTIC is used to identify excision procedures that are biopsies

Body Part Character 4		Approach Character 5	Device Character 6	Qualifier Character 7
0 External Ear, Right Antihelix Antitragus Auricle Earlobe Helix Pinna Tragus	**1 External Ear, Left** *See 0 External Ear, Right*	**0** Open **3** Percutaneous **4** Percutaneous Endoscopic **X** External	**Z** No Device	**X** Diagnostic **Z** No Qualifier
3 External Auditory Canal, Right External auditory meatus	**4 External Auditory Canal, Left** *See 3 External Auditory Canal, Right*	**0** Open **3** Percutaneous **4** Percutaneous Endoscopic **7** Via Natural or Artificial Opening **8** Via Natural or Artificial Opening Endoscopic **X** External	**Z** No Device	**X** Diagnostic **Z** No Qualifier
5 Middle Ear, Right Oval window Tympanic cavity **6 Middle Ear, Left** *See 5 Middle Ear, Right* **9 Auditory Ossicle, Right** Incus Malleus Stapes	**A Auditory Ossicle, Left** *See 9 Auditory Ossicle, Right* **D Inner Ear, Right** Bony labyrinth Bony vestibule Cochlea Round window Semicircular canal **E Inner Ear, Left** *See D Inner Ear, Right*	**0** Open **8** Via Natural or Artificial Opening Endoscopic	**Z** No Device	**X** Diagnostic **Z** No Qualifier
7 Tympanic Membrane, Right Pars flaccida **8 Tympanic Membrane, Left** *See 7 Tympanic Membrane, Right* **F Eustachian Tube, Right** Auditory tube Pharyngotympanic tube **G Eustachian Tube, Left** *See F Eustachian Tube, Right*	**L Nasal Turbinate** Inferior turbinate Middle turbinate Nasal concha Superior turbinate **N Nasopharynx** Choana Fossa of Rosenmuller Pharyngeal recess Rhinopharynx	**0** Open **3** Percutaneous **4** Percutaneous Endoscopic **7** Via Natural or Artificial Opening **8** Via Natural or Artificial Opening Endoscopic	**Z** No Device	**X** Diagnostic **Z** No Qualifier
B Mastoid Sinus, Right Mastoid air cells **C Mastoid Sinus, Left** *See B Mastoid Sinus, Right* **M Nasal Septum** Quadrangular cartilage Septal cartilage Vomer bone **P Accessory Sinus** **Q Maxillary Sinus, Right** Antrum of Highmore	**R Maxillary Sinus, Left** *See Q Maxillary Sinus, Right* **S Frontal Sinus, Right** **T Frontal Sinus, Left** **U Ethmoid Sinus, Right** Ethmoidal air cell **V Ethmoid Sinus, Left** *See U Ethmoid Sinus, Right* **W Sphenoid Sinus, Right** **X Sphenoid Sinus, Left**	**0** Open **3** Percutaneous **4** Percutaneous Endoscopic **8** Via Natural or Artificial Opening Endoscopic	**Z** No Device	**X** Diagnostic **Z** No Qualifier
K Nasal Mucosa and Soft Tissue Columella External naris Greater alar cartilage Internal naris Lateral nasal cartilage Lesser alar cartilage Nasal cavity Nostril		**0** Open **3** Percutaneous **4** Percutaneous Endoscopic **8** Via Natural or Artificial Opening Endoscopic **X** External	**Z** No Device	**X** Diagnostic **Z** No Qualifier

Non-OR 09B[0,1][0,3,4,X]Z[X,Z]
Non-OR 09B[3,4][0,3,4,7,8,X]Z[X,Z]
Non-OR 09B[F,G,L,N][0,3,4,7,8]Z[X,Z]
Non-OR 09BM[0,3,4,8]ZX
Non-OR 09B[P,Q,R,S,T,U,V,W,X][3,4,8]ZX
Non-OR 09BK8Z[X,Z]

Ø   **Medical and Surgical**
9   **Ear, Nose, Sinus**
C   **Extirpation**   Definition: Taking or cutting out solid matter from a body part

Explanation: The solid matter may be an abnormal byproduct of a biological function or a foreign body; it may be imbedded in a body part or in the lumen of a tubular body part. The solid matter may or may not have been previously broken into pieces.

Body Part Character 4		Approach Character 5	Device Character 6	Qualifier Character 7
Ø **External Ear, Right** Antihelix Antitragus Auricle Earlobe Helix Pinna Tragus	**1** **External Ear, Left** *See Ø External Ear, Right*	**Ø** Open **3** Percutaneous **4** Percutaneous Endoscopic **X** External	**Z** No Device	**Z** No Qualifier
3 **External Auditory Canal, Right** External auditory meatus	**4** **External Auditory Canal, Left** *See 3 External Auditory Canal, Right*	**Ø** Open **3** Percutaneous **4** Percutaneous Endoscopic **7** Via Natural or Artificial Opening **8** Via Natural or Artificial Opening Endoscopic **X** External	**Z** No Device	**Z** No Qualifier
5 **Middle Ear, Right** Oval window Tympanic cavity **6** **Middle Ear, Left** *See 5 Middle Ear, Right* **9** **Auditory Ossicle, Right** Incus Malleus Stapes	**A** **Auditory Ossicle, Left** *See 9 Auditory Ossicle, Right* **D** **Inner Ear, Right** Bony labyrinth Bony vestibule Cochlea Round window Semicircular canal **E** **Inner Ear, Left** *See D Inner Ear, Right*	**Ø** Open **8** Via Natural or Artificial Opening Endoscopic	**Z** No Device	**Z** No Qualifier
7 **Tympanic Membrane, Right** Pars flaccida **8** **Tympanic Membrane, Left** *See 7 Tympanic Membrane, Right* **F** **Eustachian Tube, Right** Auditory tube Pharyngotympanic tube **G** **Eustachian Tube, Left** *See F Eustachian Tube, Right*	**L** **Nasal Turbinate** Inferior turbinate Middle turbinate Nasal concha Superior turbinate **N** **Nasopharynx** Choana Fossa of Rosenmuller Pharyngeal recess Rhinopharynx	**Ø** Open **3** Percutaneous **4** Percutaneous Endoscopic **7** Via Natural or Artificial Opening **8** Via Natural or Artificial Opening Endoscopic	**Z** No Device	**Z** No Qualifier
B **Mastoid Sinus, Right** Mastoid air cells **C** **Mastoid Sinus, Left** *See B Mastoid Sinus, Right* **M** **Nasal Septum** Quadrangular cartilage Septal cartilage Vomer bone **P** **Accessory Sinus** **Q** **Maxillary Sinus, Right** Antrum of Highmore	**R** **Maxillary Sinus, Left** *See Q Maxillary Sinus, Right* **S** **Frontal Sinus, Right** **T** **Frontal Sinus, Left** **U** **Ethmoid Sinus, Right** Ethmoidal air cell **V** **Ethmoid Sinus, Left** *See U Ethmoid Sinus, Right* **W** **Sphenoid Sinus, Right** **X** **Sphenoid Sinus, Left**	**Ø** Open **3** Percutaneous **4** Percutaneous Endoscopic **8** Via Natural or Artificial Opening Endoscopic	**Z** No Device	**Z** No Qualifier
K **Nasal Mucosa and Soft Tissue** Columella External naris Greater alar cartilage Internal naris Lateral nasal cartilage Lesser alar cartilage Nasal cavity Nostril		**Ø** Open **3** Percutaneous **4** Percutaneous Endoscopic **8** Via Natural or Artificial Opening Endoscopic **X** External	**Z** No Device	**Z** No Qualifier

Non-OR   Ø9C[Ø,1][Ø,3,4,X]ZZ
Non-OR   Ø9C[3,4][Ø,3,4,7,8,X]ZZ
Non-OR   Ø9C[7,8,F,G,L][Ø,3,4,7,8]ZZ
Non-OR   Ø9CM[Ø,3,4,8]ZZ
Non-OR   Ø9CK8ZZ

LC Limited Coverage   **NC** Noncovered   ⊞ Combination Member   HAC associated procedure   Combination Only   DRG Non-OR   Non-OR   New/Revised in GREEN

ICD-10-PCS 2020   317

09C–09C

Ø   **Medical and Surgical**
9   **Ear, Nose, Sinus**
D   **Extraction**   Definition: Pulling or stripping out or off all or a portion of a body part by the use of force
                           Explanation: The qualifier DIAGNOSTIC is used to identify extraction procedures that are biopsies

Body Part Character 4	Approach Character 5	Device Character 6	Qualifier Character 7

7 **Tympanic Membrane, Right**
   Pars flaccida
8 **Tympanic Membrane, Left**
   See 7 Tympanic Membrane, Right
L **Nasal Turbinate**
   Inferior turbinate
   Middle turbinate
   Nasal concha
   Superior turbinate
	Ø Open
	3 Percutaneous
	4 Percutaneous Endoscopic
	7 Via Natural or Artificial Opening
	8 Via Natural or Artificial Opening
	   Endoscopic
		Z No Device	**Z** No Qualifier

9 **Auditory Ossicle, Right**
   Incus
   Malleus
   Stapes
A **Auditory Ossicle, Left**
   See 9 Auditory Ossicle, Right
	Ø Open	**Z** No Device	**Z** No Qualifier

B **Mastoid Sinus, Right**
   Mastoid air cells
C **Mastoid Sinus, Left**
   See B Mastoid Sinus, Right
M **Nasal Septum**
   Quadrangular cartilage
   Septal cartilage
   Vomer bone
P **Accessory Sinus**
Q **Maxillary Sinus, Right**
   Antrum of Highmore
R **Maxillary Sinus, Left**
   See Q Maxillary Sinus, Right
S **Frontal Sinus, Right**
T **Frontal Sinus, Left**
U **Ethmoid Sinus, Right**
   Ethmoidal air cell
V **Ethmoid Sinus, Left**
   See U Ethmoid Sinus, Right
W **Sphenoid Sinus, Right**
X **Sphenoid Sinus, Left**
	Ø Open
	3 Percutaneous
	4 Percutaneous Endoscopic
		Z No Device	**Z** No Qualifier

Ø   **Medical and Surgical**
9   **Ear, Nose, Sinus**
H   **Insertion**   Definition: Putting in a nonbiological appliance that monitors, assists, performs, or prevents a physiological function but does not physically
                           take the place of a body part
                           Explanation: None

Body Part Character 4	Approach Character 5	Device Character 6	Qualifier Character 7

D **Inner Ear, Right**
   Bony labyrinth
   Bony vestibule
   Cochlea
   Round window
   Semicircular canal
E **Inner Ear, Left**
   See D Inner Ear, Right
	Ø Open
	3 Percutaneous
	4 Percutaneous Endoscopic
		4 Hearing Device, Bone Conduction
		5 Hearing Device, Single Channel
		   Cochlear Prosthesis
		6 Hearing Device, Multiple Channel
		   Cochlear Prosthesis
		S Hearing Device
			Z No Qualifier

H **Ear, Right**
J **Ear, Left**
K **Nasal Mucosa and Soft Tissue**
   Columella
   External naris
   Greater alar cartilage
   Internal naris
   Lateral nasal cartilage
   Lesser alar cartilage
   Nasal cavity
   Nostril
Y **Sinus**
	Ø Open
	3 Percutaneous
	4 Percutaneous Endoscopic
	7 Via Natural or Artificial Opening
	8 Via Natural or Artificial Opening
	   Endoscopic
		Y Other Device	**Z** No Qualifier

N **Nasopharynx**
   Choana
   Fossa of Rosenmuller
   Pharyngeal recess
   Rhinopharynx
	7 Via Natural or Artificial Opening
	8 Via Natural or Artificial Opening
	   Endoscopic
		B Intraluminal Device, Airway	**Z** No Qualifier

Non-OR   Ø9H[H,J][3,4,7,8]YZ
Non-OR   Ø9H[K,Y][Ø,3,4,7,8]YZ
Non-OR   Ø9HN[7,8]BZ

Ø   **Medical and Surgical**
9   **Ear, Nose, Sinus**
J   **Inspection**   Definition: Visually and/or manually exploring a body part

Explanation: Visual exploration may be performed with or without optical instrumentation. Manual exploration may be performed directly or through intervening body layers.

Body Part Character 4	Approach Character 5	Device Character 6	Qualifier Character 7

7 Tympanic Membrane, Right
  Pars flaccida
8 Tympanic Membrane, Left
  See 7 Tympanic Membrane, Right
H Ear, Right
J Ear, Left
	Ø Open
	3 Percutaneous
	4 Percutaneous Endoscopic
	7 Via Natural or Artificial Opening
	**8 Via Natural or Artificial Opening
	   Endoscopic**
	X External
		Z No Device	**Z No Qualifier**

D Inner Ear, Right
  Bony labyrinth
  Bony vestibule
  Cochlea
  Round window
  Semicircular canal
E Inner Ear, Left
  See D Inner Ear, Right
K Nasal Mucosa and Soft Tissue
  Columella
  External naris
  Greater alar cartilage
  Internal naris
  Lateral nasal cartilage
  Lesser alar cartilage
  Nasal cavity
  Nostril
Y Sinus
	Ø Open
	3 Percutaneous
	4 Percutaneous Endoscopic
	**8 Via Natural or Artificial Opening
	   Endoscopic**
	X External
		Z No Device	**Z No Qualifier**

Non-OR   09J[7,8][3,7,8,X]ZZ
Non-OR   09J[H,J][Ø,3,4,7,8,X]ZZ
Non-OR   09J[D,E][3,8,X]ZZ
Non-OR   09J[K,Y][Ø,3,4,8,X]ZZ

Ø   **Medical and Surgical**
9   **Ear, Nose, Sinus**
M   **Reattachment**   Definition: Putting back in or on all or a portion of a separated body part to its normal location or other suitable location

Explanation: Vascular circulation and nervous pathways may or may not be reestablished

Body Part Character 4	Approach Character 5	Device Character 6	Qualifier Character 7

Ø External Ear, Right
  Antihelix
  Antitragus
  Auricle
  Earlobe
  Helix
  Pinna
  Tragus
1 External Ear, Left
  See Ø External Ear, Right
K Nasal Mucosa and Soft Tissue
  Columella
  External naris
  Greater alar cartilage
  Internal naris
  Lateral nasal cartilage
  Lesser alar cartilage
  Nasal cavity
  Nostril
	X External	**Z No Device**	**Z No Qualifier**

Ear, Nose, Sinus

Ø   **Medical and Surgical**
9   **Ear, Nose, Sinus**
N   **Release**   Definition: Freeing a body part from an abnormal physical constraint by cutting or by the use of force
                      Explanation: Some of the restraining tissue may be taken out but none of the body part is taken out

Body Part Character 4		Approach Character 5	Device Character 6	Qualifier Character 7
Ø **External Ear, Right** Antihelix Antitragus Auricle Earlobe Helix Pinna Tragus	**1** **External Ear, Left** *See Ø External Ear, Right*	**Ø** Open **3** Percutaneous **4** Percutaneous Endoscopic **X** External	**Z** No Device	**Z** No Qualifier
3 **External Auditory Canal, Right** External auditory meatus	**4** **External Auditory Canal, Left** *See 3 External Auditory Canal, Right*	**Ø** Open **3** Percutaneous **4** Percutaneous Endoscopic **7** Via Natural or Artificial Opening **8** Via Natural or Artificial Opening Endoscopic **X** External	**Z** No Device	**Z** No Qualifier
5 **Middle Ear, Right** Oval window Tympanic cavity **6** **Middle Ear, Left** *See 5 Middle Ear, Right* **9** **Auditory Ossicle, Right** Incus Malleus Stapes	**A** **Auditory Ossicle, Left** *See 9 Auditory Ossicle, Right* **D** **Inner Ear, Right** Bony labyrinth Bony vestibule Cochlea Round window Semicircular canal **E** **Inner Ear, Left** *See D Inner Ear, Right*	**Ø** Open **8** Via Natural or Artificial Opening Endoscopic	**Z** No Device	**Z** No Qualifier
7 **Tympanic Membrane, Right** Pars flaccida **8** **Tympanic Membrane, Left** *See 7 Tympanic Membrane, Right* **F** **Eustachian Tube, Right** Auditory tube Pharyngotympanic tube **G** **Eustachian Tube, Left** *See F Eustachian Tube, Right*	**L** **Nasal Turbinate** Inferior turbinate Middle turbinate Nasal concha Superior turbinate **N** **Nasopharynx** Choana Fossa of Rosenmuller Pharyngeal recess Rhinopharynx	**Ø** Open **3** Percutaneous **4** Percutaneous Endoscopic **7** Via Natural or Artificial Opening **8** Via Natural or Artificial Opening Endoscopic	**Z** No Device	**Z** No Qualifier
B **Mastoid Sinus, Right** Mastoid air cells **C** **Mastoid Sinus, Left** *See B Mastoid Sinus, Right* **M** **Nasal Septum** Quadrangular cartilage Septal cartilage Vomer bone **P** **Accessory Sinus** **Q** **Maxillary Sinus, Right** Antrum of Highmore	**R** **Maxillary Sinus, Left** *See Q Maxillary Sinus, Right* **S** **Frontal Sinus, Right** **T** **Frontal Sinus, Left** **U** **Ethmoid Sinus, Right** Ethmoidal air cell **V** **Ethmoid Sinus, Left** *See U Ethmoid Sinus, Right* **W** **Sphenoid Sinus, Right** **X** **Sphenoid Sinus, Left**	**Ø** Open **3** Percutaneous **4** Percutaneous Endoscopic **8** Via Natural or Artificial Opening Endoscopic	**Z** No Device	**Z** No Qualifier
K **Nasal Mucosa and Soft Tissue** Columella External naris Greater alar cartilage Internal naris Lateral nasal cartilage Lesser alar cartilage Nasal cavity Nostril		**Ø** Open **3** Percutaneous **4** Percutaneous Endoscopic **8** Via Natural or Artificial Opening Endoscopic **X** External	**Z** No Device	**Z** No Qualifier

Non-OR   Ø9N[Ø,1]XZZ
Non-OR   Ø9N[3,4]XZZ
Non-OR   Ø9N[F,G,L][Ø,3,4,7,8]ZZ
Non-OR   Ø9NM[Ø,3,4,8]ZZ
Non-OR   Ø9NK[Ø,3,4,8,X]ZZ

Ø   Medical and Surgical
9   Ear, Nose, Sinus
P   Removal   Definition: Taking out or off a device from a body part

           Explanation: If a device is taken out and a similar device put in without cutting or puncturing the skin or mucous membrane, the procedure is coded to the root operation CHANGE. Otherwise, the procedure for taking out a device is coded to the root operation REMOVAL.

Body Part Character 4	Approach Character 5	Device Character 6	Qualifier Character 7
7 Tympanic Membrane, Right Pars flaccida **8 Tympanic Membrane, Left** *See 7 Tympanic Membrane, Right*	**Ø Open** **7 Via Natural or Artificial Opening** **8 Via Natural or Artificial Opening Endoscopic** **X External**	**Ø Drainage Device**	**Z No Qualifier**
D Inner Ear, Right Bony labyrinth Bony vestibule Cochlea Round window Semicircular canal **E Inner Ear, Left** *See D Inner Ear, Right*	**Ø Open** **7 Via Natural or Artificial Opening** **8 Via Natural or Artificial Opening Endoscopic**	**S Hearing Device**	**Z No Qualifier**
H Ear, Right **J Ear, Left** **K Nasal Mucosa and Soft Tissue** Columella External naris Greater alar cartilage Internal naris Lateral nasal cartilage Lesser alar cartilage Nasal cavity Nostril	**Ø Open** **3 Percutaneous** **4 Percutaneous Endoscopic** **7 Via Natural or Artificial Opening** **8 Via Natural or Artificial Opening Endoscopic**	**Ø Drainage Device** **7 Autologous Tissue Substitute** **D Intraluminal Device** **J Synthetic Substitute** **K Nonautologous Tissue Substitute** **Y Other Device**	**Z No Qualifier**
H Ear, Right **J Ear, Left** **K Nasal Mucosa and Soft Tissue** Columella External naris Greater alar cartilage Internal naris Lateral nasal cartilage Lesser alar cartilage Nasal cavity Nostril	**X External**	**Ø Drainage Device** **7 Autologous Tissue Substitute** **D Intraluminal Device** **J Synthetic Substitute** **K Nonautologous Tissue Substitute**	**Z No Qualifier**
Y Sinus	**Ø Open** **3 Percutaneous** **4 Percutaneous Endoscopic**	**Ø Drainage Device** **Y Other Device**	**Z No Qualifier**
Y Sinus	**7 Via Natural or Artificial Opening** **8 Via Natural or Artificial Opening Endoscopic**	**Y Other Device**	**Z No Qualifier**
Y Sinus	**X External**	**Ø Drainage Device**	**Z No Qualifier**

Non-OR   Ø9P[7,8][Ø,7,8,X]ØZ
Non-OR   Ø9P[H,J][3,4][Ø,J,K,Y]Z
Non-OR   Ø9P[H,J][7,8][Ø,D,Y]Z
Non-OR   Ø9PK[Ø,3,4,7,8][Ø,7,D,J,K,Y]Z
Non-OR   Ø9P[H,J]X[Ø,7,D,J,K]Z
Non-OR   Ø9PKX[Ø,7,D,J,K]Z
Non-OR   Ø9PY[3,4]YZ
Non-OR   Ø9PY[7,8]YZ
Non-OR   Ø9PYXØZ

Ø   Medical and Surgical
9   Ear, Nose, Sinus
Q   Repair   Definition: Restoring, to the extent possible, a body part to its normal anatomic structure and function
                          Explanation: Used only when the method to accomplish the repair is not one of the other root operations

Body Part Character 4		Approach Character 5	Device Character 6	Qualifier Character 7
Ø External Ear, Right Antihelix Antitragus Auricle Earlobe Helix Pinna Tragus	**1 External Ear, Left** *See Ø External Ear, Right* **2 External Ear, Bilateral** *See Ø External Ear, Right*	**Ø** Open **3** Percutaneous **4** Percutaneous Endoscopic **X** External	**Z** No Device	**Z** No Qualifier
3 External Auditory Canal, Right External auditory meatus **4 External Auditory Canal, Left** *See 3 External Auditory Canal, Right*	**F Eustachian Tube, Right** Auditory tube Pharyngotympanic tube **G Eustachian Tube, Left** *See F Eustachian Tube, Right*	**Ø** Open **3** Percutaneous **4** Percutaneous Endoscopic **7** Via Natural or Artificial Opening **8** Via Natural or Artificial Opening Endoscopic **X** External	**Z** No Device	**Z** No Qualifier
5 Middle Ear, Right Oval window Tympanic cavity **6 Middle Ear, Left** *See 5 Middle Ear, Right* **9 Auditory Ossicle, Right** Incus Malleus Stapes	**A Auditory Ossicle, Left** *See 9 Auditory Ossicle, Right* **D Inner Ear, Right** Bony labyrinth Bony vestibule Cochlea Round window Semicircular canal **E Inner Ear, Left** *See D Inner Ear, Right*	**Ø** Open **8** Via Natural or Artificial Opening Endoscopic	**Z** No Device	**Z** No Qualifier
7 Tympanic Membrane, Right Pars flaccida **8 Tympanic Membrane, Left** *See 7 Tympanic Membrane, Right* **L Nasal Turbinate** Inferior turbinate Middle turbinate Nasal concha Superior turbinate	**N Nasopharynx** Choana Fossa of Rosenmuller Pharyngeal recess Rhinopharynx	**Ø** Open **3** Percutaneous **4** Percutaneous Endoscopic **7** Via Natural or Artificial Opening **8** Via Natural or Artificial Opening Endoscopic	**Z** No Device	**Z** No Qualifier
B Mastoid Sinus, Right Mastoid air cells **C Mastoid Sinus, Left** *See B Mastoid Sinus, Right* **M Nasal Septum** Quadrangular cartilage Septal cartilage Vomer bone **P Accessory Sinus** **Q Maxillary Sinus, Right** Antrum of Highmore	**R Maxillary Sinus, Left** *See Q Maxillary Sinus, Right* **S Frontal Sinus, Right** **T Frontal Sinus, Left** **U Ethmoid Sinus, Right** Ethmoidal air cell **V Ethmoid Sinus, Left** *See U Ethmoid Sinus, Right* **W Sphenoid Sinus, Right** **X Sphenoid Sinus, Left**	**Ø** Open **3** Percutaneous **4** Percutaneous Endoscopic **8** Via Natural or Artificial Opening Endoscopic	**Z** No Device	**Z** No Qualifier
K Nasal Mucosa and Soft Tissue Columella External naris Greater alar cartilage Internal naris Lateral nasal cartilage Lesser alar cartilage Nasal cavity Nostril		**Ø** Open **3** Percutaneous **4** Percutaneous Endoscopic **8** Via Natural or Artificial Opening Endoscopic **X** External	**Z** No Device	**Z** No Qualifier

Non-OR   09Q[Ø,1,2]XZZ
Non-OR   09Q[3,4]XZZ
Non-OR   09Q[F,G][Ø,3,4,7,8,X]ZZ
Non-OR   09QKXZZ

Ø   Medical and Surgical
9   Ear, Nose, Sinus
R   Replacement   Definition: Putting in or on biological or synthetic material that physically takes the place and/or function of all or a portion of a body part
                          Explanation: The body part may have been taken out or replaced, or may be taken out, physically eradicated, or rendered nonfunctional during the REPLACEMENT procedure. A REMOVAL procedure is coded for taking out the device used in a previous replacement procedure.

Body Part Character 4	Approach Character 5	Device Character 6	Qualifier Character 7
Ø External Ear, Right Antihelix Antitragus Auricle Earlobe Helix Pinna Tragus **1 External Ear, Left** *See Ø External Ear, Right* **2 External Ear, Bilateral** *See Ø External Ear, Right* **K Nasal Mucosa and Soft Tissue** Columella External naris Greater alar cartilage Internal naris Lateral nasal cartilage Lesser alar cartilage Nasal cavity Nostril	**Ø Open** **X External**	**7 Autologous Tissue Substitute** **J Synthetic Substitute** **K Nonautologous Tissue Substitute**	**Z No Qualifier**
5 Middle Ear, Right Oval window Tympanic cavity **6 Middle Ear, Left** *See 5 Middle Ear, Right* **9 Auditory Ossicle, Right** Incus Malleus Stapes **A Auditory Ossicle, Left** *See 9 Auditory Ossicle, Right* **D Inner Ear, Right** Bony labyrinth Bony vestibule Cochlea Round window Semicircular canal **E Inner Ear, Left** *See D Inner Ear, Right*	**Ø Open**	**7 Autologous Tissue Substitute** **J Synthetic Substitute** **K Nonautologous Tissue Substitute**	**Z No Qualifier**
7 Tympanic Membrane, Right Pars flaccida **8 Tympanic Membrane, Left** *See 7 Tympanic Membrane, Right* **N Nasopharynx** Choana Fossa of Rosenmuller Pharyngeal recess Rhinopharynx	**Ø Open** **7 Via Natural or Artificial Opening** **8 Via Natural or Artificial Opening Endoscopic**	**7 Autologous Tissue Substitute** **J Synthetic Substitute** **K Nonautologous Tissue Substitute**	**Z No Qualifier**
L Nasal Turbinate Inferior turbinate Middle turbinate Nasal concha Superior turbinate	**Ø Open** **3 Percutaneous** **4 Percutaneous Endoscopic** **7 Via Natural or Artificial Opening** **8 Via Natural or Artificial Opening Endoscopic**	**7 Autologous Tissue Substitute** **J Synthetic Substitute** **K Nonautologous Tissue Substitute**	**Z No Qualifier**
M Nasal Septum Quadrangular cartilage Septal cartilage Vomer bone	**Ø Open** **3 Percutaneous** **4 Percutaneous Endoscopic**	**7 Autologous Tissue Substitute** **J Synthetic Substitute** **K Nonautologous Tissue Substitute**	**Z No Qualifier**

LC Limited Coverage NC Noncovered ⊞ Combination Member HAC associated procedure Combination Only DRG Non-OR Non-OR New/Revised in GREEN
ICD-10-PCS 2020   323

Ø9R–Ø9R

0 Medical and Surgical
9 Ear, Nose, Sinus
S Reposition　Definition: Moving to its normal location, or other suitable location, all or a portion of a body part

Explanation: The body part is moved to a new location from an abnormal location, or from a normal location where it is not functioning correctly. The body part may or may not be cut out or off to be moved to the new location.

Body Part Character 4	Approach Character 5	Device Character 6	Qualifier Character 7
0 External Ear, Right Antihelix Antitragus Auricle Earlobe Helix Pinna Tragus **1 External Ear, Left** *See 0 External Ear, Right* **2 External Ear, Bilateral** *See 0 External Ear, Right* **K Nasal Mucosa and Soft Tissue** Columella External naris Greater alar cartilage Internal naris Lateral nasal cartilage Lesser alar cartilage Nasal cavity Nostril	**0 Open** **4 Percutaneous Endoscopic** **X External**	**Z No Device**	**Z No Qualifier**
7 Tympanic Membrane, Right Pars flaccida **8 Tympanic Membrane, Left** *See 7 Tympanic Membrane, Right* **F Eustachian Tube, Right** Auditory tube Pharyngotympanic tube **G Eustachian Tube, Left** *See F Eustachian Tube, Right* **L Nasal Turbinate** Inferior turbinate Middle turbinate Nasal concha Superior turbinate	**0 Open** **4 Percutaneous Endoscopic** **7 Via Natural or Artificial Opening** **8 Via Natural or Artificial Opening Endoscopic**	**Z No Device**	**Z No Qualifier**
9 Auditory Ossicle, Right Incus Malleus Stapes **A Auditory Ossicle, Left** *See 9 Auditory Ossicle, Right* **M Nasal Septum** Quadrangular cartilage Septal cartilage Vomer bone	**0 Open** **4 Percutaneous Endoscopic**	**Z No Device**	**Z No Qualifier**

Non-OR　09S[F,G][0,4,7,8]ZZ

Ø Medical and Surgical
9 Ear, Nose, Sinus
T Resection   Definition: Cutting out or off, without replacement, all of a body part
                Explanation: None

Body Part Character 4		Approach Character 5	Device Character 6	Qualifier Character 7
Ø External Ear, Right Antihelix Antitragus Auricle Earlobe Helix Pinna Tragus	**1 External Ear, Left** *See Ø External Ear, Right*	**Ø Open** **4 Percutaneous Endoscopic** **X External**	**Z No Device**	**Z No Qualifier**
5 Middle Ear, Right Oval window Tympanic cavity **6 Middle Ear, Left** *See 5 Middle Ear, Right* **9 Auditory Ossicle, Right** Incus Malleus Stapes	**A Auditory Ossicle, Left** *See 9 Auditory Ossicle, Right* **D Inner Ear, Right** Bony labyrinth Bony vestibule Cochlea Round window Semicircular canal **E Inner Ear, Left** *See D Inner Ear, Right*	**Ø Open** **8 Via Natural or Artificial Opening Endoscopic**	**Z No Device**	**Z No Qualifier**
7 Tympanic Membrane, Right Pars flaccida **8 Tympanic Membrane, Left** *See 7 Tympanic Membrane, Right* **F Eustachian Tube, Right** Auditory tube Pharyngotympanic tube **G Eustachian Tube, Left** *See F Eustachian Tube, Right*	**L Nasal Turbinate** Inferior turbinate Middle turbinate Nasal concha Superior turbinate **N Nasopharynx** Choana Fossa of Rosenmuller Pharyngeal recess Rhinopharynx	**Ø Open** **4 Percutaneous Endoscopic** **7 Via Natural or Artificial Opening** **8 Via Natural or Artificial Opening Endoscopic**	**Z No Device**	**Z No Qualifier**
B Mastoid Sinus, Right Mastoid air cells **C Mastoid Sinus, Left** *See B Mastoid Sinus, Right* **M Nasal Septum** Quadrangular cartilage Septal cartilage Vomer bone **P Accessory Sinus** **Q Maxillary Sinus, Right** Antrum of Highmore	**R Maxillary Sinus, Left** *See Q Maxillary Sinus, Right* **S Frontal Sinus, Right** **T Frontal Sinus, Left** **U Ethmoid Sinus, Right** Ethmoidal air cell **V Ethmoid Sinus, Left** *See U Ethmoid Sinus, Right* **W Sphenoid Sinus, Right** **X Sphenoid Sinus, Left**	**Ø Open** **4 Percutaneous Endoscopic** **8 Via Natural or Artificial Opening Endoscopic**	**Z No Device**	**Z No Qualifier**
K Nasal Mucosa and Soft Tissue Columella External naris Greater alar cartilage Internal naris Lateral nasal cartilage Lesser alar cartilage Nasal cavity Nostril		**Ø Open** **4 Percutaneous Endoscopic** **8 Via Natural or Artificial Opening Endoscopic** **X External**	**Z No Device**	**Z No Qualifier**

Non-OR   Ø9T[F,G][Ø,4,7,8]ZZ

🔲 Limited Coverage   🔲 Noncovered   ⊞ Combination Member   HAC associated procedure   Combination Only   DRG Non-OR   Non-OR   New/Revised in GREEN

ICD-10-PCS 2020   325

Ø   **Medical and Surgical**
9   **Ear, Nose, Sinus**
U   **Supplement**   Definition: Putting in or on biological or synthetic material that physically reinforces and/or augments the function of a portion of a body part

Explanation: The biological material is non-living, or is living and from the same individual. The body part may have been previously replaced, and the SUPPLEMENT procedure is performed to physically reinforce and/or augment the function of the replaced body part.

Body Part Character 4		Approach Character 5	Device Character 6	Qualifier Character 7
Ø **External Ear, Right** Antihelix Antitragus Auricle Earlobe Helix Pinna Tragus	**1** **External Ear, Left** *See Ø External Ear, Right* **2** **External Ear, Bilateral** *See Ø External Ear, Right*	**Ø** Open **X** External	**7** Autologous Tissue Substitute **J** Synthetic Substitute **K** Nonautologous Tissue Substitute	**Z** No Qualifier
5 **Middle Ear, Right** Oval window Tympanic cavity **6** **Middle Ear, Left** *See 5 Middle Ear, Right* **9** **Auditory Ossicle, Right** Incus Malleus Stapes **A** **Auditory Ossicle, Left** *See 9 Auditory Ossicle, Right*	**D** **Inner Ear, Right** Bony labyrinth Bony vestibule Cochlea Round window Semicircular canal **E** **Inner Ear, Left** *See D Inner Ear, Right*	**Ø** Open **8** Via Natural or Artificial Opening Endoscopic	**7** Autologous Tissue Substitute **J** Synthetic Substitute **K** Nonautologous Tissue Substitute	**Z** No Qualifier
7 **Tympanic Membrane, Right** Pars flaccida **8** **Tympanic Membrane, Left** *See 7 Tympanic Membrane, Right*	**N** Nasopharynx Choana Fossa of Rosenmuller Pharyngeal recess Rhinopharynx	**Ø** Open **7** Via Natural or Artificial Opening **8** Via Natural or Artificial Opening Endoscopic	**7** Autologous Tissue Substitute **J** Synthetic Substitute **K** Nonautologous Tissue Substitute	**Z** No Qualifier
B Mastoid Sinus, Right Mastoid air cells **C** Mastoid Sinus, Left *See B Mastoid Sinus, Right* **L** Nasal Turbinate Inferior turbinate Middle turbinate Nasal concha Superior turbinate **P** Accessory Sinus **Q** Maxillary Sinus, Right Antrum of Highmore	**R** Maxillary Sinus, Left *See Q Maxillary Sinus, Right* **S** Frontal Sinus, Right **T** Frontal Sinus, Left **U** Ethmoid Sinus, Right Ethmoidal air cell **V** Ethmoid Sinus, Left *See U Ethmoid Sinus, Right* **W** Sphenoid Sinus, Right **X** Sphenoid Sinus, Left	**Ø** Open **3** Percutaneous **4** Percutaneous Endoscopic **7** Via Natural or Artificial Opening **8** Via Natural or Artificial Opening Endoscopic	**7** Autologous Tissue Substitute **J** Synthetic Substitute **K** Nonautologous Tissue Substitute	**Z** No Qualifier
K Nasal Mucosa and Soft Tissue Columella External naris Greater alar cartilage Internal naris Lateral nasal cartilage Lesser alar cartilage Nasal cavity Nostril		**Ø** Open **8** Via Natural or Artificial Opening Endoscopic **X** External	**7** Autologous Tissue Substitute **J** Synthetic Substitute **K** Nonautologous Tissue Substitute	**Z** No Qualifier
M Nasal Septum Quadrangular cartilage Septal cartilage Vomer bone		**Ø** Open **3** Percutaneous **4** Percutaneous Endoscopic **8** Via Natural or Artificial Opening Endoscopic	**7** Autologous Tissue Substitute **J** Synthetic Substitute **K** Nonautologous Tissue Substitute	**Z** No Qualifier

LC Limited Coverage   **NC** Noncovered   ⊞ Combination Member   HAC associated procedure   Combination Only   DRG Non-OR   Non-OR   New/Revised in GREEN

326   ICD-10-PCS 2020

Ø   **Medical and Surgical**
9   **Ear, Nose, Sinus**
W   **Revision**   Definition: Correcting, to the extent possible, a portion of a malfunctioning device or the position of a displaced device

Explanation: Revision can include correcting a malfunctioning or displaced device by taking out or putting in components of the device such as a screw or pin

Body Part Character 4	Approach Character 5	Device Character 6	Qualifier Character 7
7 Tympanic Membrane, Right Pars flaccida **8 Tympanic Membrane, Left** *See 7 Tympanic Membrane, Right* **9 Auditory Ossicle, Right** Incus Malleus Stapes **A Auditory Ossicle, Left** *See 9 Auditory Ossicle, Right*	**Ø Open** **7 Via Natural or Artificial Opening** **8 Via Natural or Artificial Opening Endoscopic**	**7 Autologous Tissue Substitute** **J Synthetic Substitute** **K Nonautologous Tissue Substitute**	**Z No Qualifier**
D Inner Ear, Right Bony labyrinth Bony vestibule Cochlea Round window Semicircular canal **E Inner Ear, Left** *See D Inner Ear, Right*	**Ø Open** **7 Via Natural or Artificial Opening** **8 Via Natural or Artificial Opening Endoscopic**	**S Hearing Device**	**Z No Qualifier**
H Ear, Right **J Ear, Left** **K Nasal Mucosa and Soft Tissue** Columella External naris Greater alar cartilage Internal naris Lateral nasal cartilage Lesser alar cartilage Nasal cavity Nostril	**Ø Open** **3 Percutaneous** **4 Percutaneous Endoscopic** **7 Via Natural or Artificial Opening** **8 Via Natural or Artificial Opening Endoscopic**	**Ø Drainage Device** **7 Autologous Tissue Substitute** **D Intraluminal Device** **J Synthetic Substitute** **K Nonautologous Tissue Substitute** **Y Other Device**	**Z No Qualifier**
H Ear, Right **J Ear, Left** **K Nasal Mucosa and Soft Tissue** Columella External naris Greater alar cartilage Internal naris Lateral nasal cartilage Lesser alar cartilage Nasal cavity Nostril	**X External**	**Ø Drainage Device** **7 Autologous Tissue Substitute** **D Intraluminal Device** **J Synthetic Substitute** **K Nonautologous Tissue Substitute**	**Z No Qualifier**
Y Sinus	**Ø Open** **3 Percutaneous** **4 Percutaneous Endoscopic**	**Ø Drainage Device** **Y Other Device**	**Z No Qualifier**
Y Sinus	**7 Via Natural or Artificial Opening** **8 Via Natural or Artificial Opening Endoscopic**	**Y Other Device**	**Z No Qualifier**
Y Sinus	**X External**	**Ø Drainage Device**	**Z No Qualifier**

Non-OR   09W[H,J][3,4][J,K,Y]Z
Non-OR   09W[H,J][7,8][D,Y]Z
Non-OR   09WK[Ø,3,4,7,8][Ø,7,D,J,K,Y]Z
Non-OR   09W[H,J,K]X[Ø,7,D,J,K]Z
Non-OR   09WY[3,4]YZ
Non-OR   09WY[7,8]YZ
Non-OR   09WYXØZ

Respiratory System ØB1–ØBY

Character Meanings

This Character Meaning table is provided as a guide to assist the user in the identification of character members that may be found in this section of code tables. It **SHOULD NOT** be used to build a PCS code.

Operation–Character 3		Body Part–Character 4		Approach–Character 5		Device–Character 6		Qualifier–Character 7	
1	Bypass	Ø	Tracheobronchial Tree	Ø	Open	Ø	Drainage Device	Ø	Allogeneic
2	Change	1	Trachea	3	Percutaneous	1	Radioactive Element	1	Syngeneic
5	Destruction	2	Carina	4	Percutaneous Endoscopic	2	Monitoring Device	2	Zooplastic
7	Dilation	3	Main Bronchus, Right	7	Via Natural or Artificial Opening	3	Infusion Device	4	Cutaneous
9	Drainage	4	Upper Lobe Bronchus, Right	8	Via Natural or Artificial Opening Endoscopic	7	Autologous Tissue Substitute	6	Esophagus
B	Excision	5	Middle Lobe Bronchus, Right	X	External	C	Extraluminal Device	X	Diagnostic
C	Extirpation	6	Lower Lobe Bronchus, Right			D	Intraluminal Device	Z	No Qualifier
D	Extraction	7	Main Bronchus, Left			E	Intraluminal Device, Endotracheal Airway		
F	Fragmentation	8	Upper Lobe Bronchus, Left			F	Tracheostomy Device		
H	Insertion	9	Lingula Bronchus			G	Intraluminal Device, Endobronchial Valve		
J	Inspection	B	Lower Lobe Bronchus, Left			J	Synthetic Substitute		
L	Occlusion	C	Upper Lung Lobe, Right			K	Nonautologous Tissue Substitute		
M	Reattachment	D	Middle Lung Lobe, Right			M	Diaphragmatic Pacemaker Lead		
N	Release	F	Lower Lung Lobe, Right			Y	Other Device		
P	Removal	G	Upper Lung Lobe, Left			Z	No Device		
Q	Repair	H	Lung Lingula						
R	Replacement	J	Lower Lung Lobe, Left						
S	Reposition	K	Lung, Right						
T	Resection	L	Lung, Left						
U	Supplement	M	Lungs, Bilateral						
V	Restriction	N	Pleura, Right						
W	Revision	P	Pleura, Left						
Y	Transplantation	Q	Pleura						
		T	Diaphragm						

AHA Coding Clinic for table ØB5
| 2016, 2Q, 17 | Photodynamic therapy for treatment of malignant mesothelioma |
| 2015, 2Q, 31 | Thoracoscopic talc pleurodesis |

AHA Coding Clinic for table ØB9
2017, 3Q, 15	Bronchoscopy with suctioning for removal of retained secretions
2017, 1Q, 51	Bronchoalveolar lavage
2016, 1Q, 26	Bronchoalveolar lavage, endobronchial biopsy and transbronchial biopsy
2016, 1Q, 27	Fiberoptic bronchoscopy with brushings and bronchoalveolar lavage

AHA Coding Clinic for table ØBB
2016, 1Q, 26	Bronchoalveolar lavage, endobronchial biopsy and transbronchial biopsy
2016, 1Q, 27	Fiberoptic bronchoscopy with brushings and bronchoalveolar lavage
2014, 1Q, 20	Fiducial marker placement

AHA Coding Clinic for table ØBC
| 2017, 3Q, 14 | Bronchoscopy with suctioning and washings for removal of mucus plug |

AHA Coding Clinic for table ØBD
| 2018, 3Q, 28 | Lung decortication for empyema |

AHA Coding Clinic for table ØBH
| 2014, 4Q, 3-10 | Mechanical ventilation |

AHA Coding Clinic for table ØBJ
| 2015, 2Q, 31 | Thoracoscopic talc pleurodesis |
| 2014, 1Q, 20 | Fiducial marker placement |

AHA Coding Clinic for table ØBN
2018, 3Q, 28	Lung decortication
2018, 3Q, 28	Lung decortication for empyema
2015, 3Q, 15	Vascular ring surgery with release of esophagus and trachea

AHA Coding Clinic for table ØBQ
| 2016, 2Q, 22 | Esophageal lengthening Collis gastroplasty with Nissen fundoplication and hiatal hernia |
| 2014, 3Q, 28 | Laparoscopic Nissen fundoplication and diaphragmatic hernia repair |

AHA Coding Clinic for table ØBU
| 2015, 1Q, 28 | Repair of bronchopleural fistula using omental pedicle graft |

Respiratory System

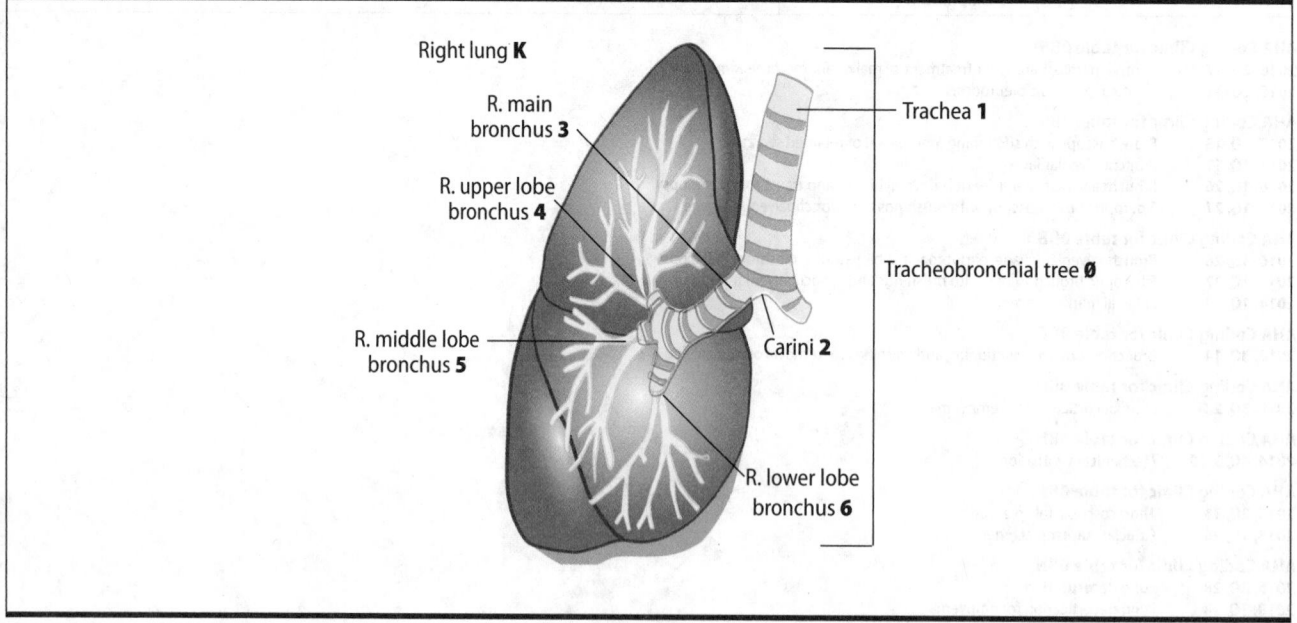

Trachea **1**

Right lung **K**

Right main/
primary
bronchus **3**

Diaphragm **T**

Pleura **N, P, Q**

Left lung **L**

Carina of trachea **2**

Left main/
primary
bronchus **7**

Right Lung Bronchi

Right lung **K**

R. main
bronchus **3**

R. upper lobe
bronchus **4**

R. middle lobe
bronchus **5**

R. lower lobe
bronchus **6**

Trachea **1**

Tracheobronchial tree **Ø**

Carini **2**

Ø   Medical and Surgical
B   Respiratory System
1   Bypass   Definition: Altering the route of passage of the contents of a tubular body part

Explanation: Rerouting contents of a body part to a downstream area of the normal route, to a similar route and body part, or to an abnormal route and dissimilar body part. Includes one or more anastomoses, with or without the use of a device.

Body Part Character 4	Approach Character 5	Device Character 6	Qualifier Character 7
1 Trachea Cricoid cartilage	Ø Open	D Intraluminal Device	6 Esophagus
1 Trachea Cricoid cartilage	Ø Open	F Tracheostomy Device Z No Device	4 Cutaneous
1 Trachea Cricoid cartilage	3 Percutaneous 4 Percutaneous Endoscopic	F Tracheostomy Device Z No Device	4 Cutaneous

DRG Non-OR   ØB113[F,Z]4
Non-OR   ØB11ØD6

Ø   Medical and Surgical
B   Respiratory System
2   Change   Definition: Taking out or off a device from a body part and putting back an identical or similar device in or on the same body part without cutting or puncturing the skin or a mucous membrane

Explanation: All CHANGE procedures are coded using the approach EXTERNAL

Body Part Character 4	Approach Character 5	Device Character 6	Qualifier Character 7
Ø Tracheobronchial Tree K Lung, Right L Lung, Left Q Pleura T Diaphragm	X External	Ø Drainage Device Y Other Device	Z No Qualifier
1 Trachea Cricoid cartilage	X External	Ø Drainage Device E Intraluminal Device, Endotracheal Airway F Tracheostomy Device Y Other Device	Z No Qualifier

Non-OR   All body part, approach, device, and qualifier values

Ø   Medical and Surgical
B   Respiratory System
5   Destruction   Definition: Physical eradication of all or a portion of a body part by the direct use of energy, force, or a destructive agent

Explanation: None of the body part is physically taken out

Body Part Character 4	Approach Character 5	Device Character 6	Qualifier Character 7

1   Trachea
    Cricoid cartilage
2   Carina
3   Main Bronchus, Right
    Bronchus intermedius
    Intermediate bronchus
4   Upper Lobe Bronchus, Right
5   Middle Lobe Bronchus, Right
6   Lower Lobe Bronchus, Right
7   Main Bronchus, Left
8   Upper Lobe Bronchus, Left
9   Lingula Bronchus
B   Lower Lobe Bronchus, Left
C   Upper Lung Lobe, Right
D   Middle Lung Lobe, Right
F   Lower Lung Lobe, Right
G   Upper Lung Lobe, Left
H   Lung Lingula
J   Lower Lung Lobe, Left
K   Lung, Right
L   Lung, Left
M   Lungs, Bilateral
	Ø Open
	3 Percutaneous
	4 Percutaneous Endoscopic
	7 Via Natural or Artificial Opening
	8 Via Natural or Artificial Opening Endoscopic
		Z No Device	Z No Qualifier

N Pleura, Right P Pleura, Left T Diaphragm	Ø Open 3 Percutaneous 4 Percutaneous Endoscopic	Z No Device	Z No Qualifier

Non-OR   ØB5[3,4,5,6,7,8,9,B][4,8]ZZ
Non-OR   ØB5[C,D,F,G,H,J,K,L,M]8ZZ

LG Limited Coverage   NC Noncovered   ⊞ Combination Member   HAC associated procedure   Combination Only   DRG Non-OR   Non-OR   New/Revised in GREEN

Ø **Medical and Surgical**
B **Respiratory System**
7 **Dilation** Definition: Expanding an orifice or the lumen of a tubular body part

Explanation: The orifice can be a natural orifice or an artificially created orifice. Accomplished by stretching a tubular body part using intraluminal pressure or by cutting part of the orifice or wall of the tubular body part.

Body Part Character 4	Approach Character 5	Device Character 6	Qualifier Character 7

1 Trachea
  Cricoid cartilage
2 Carina
3 Main Bronchus, Right
  Bronchus intermedius
  Intermediate bronchus
4 Upper Lobe Bronchus, Right
5 Middle Lobe Bronchus, Right
6 Lower Lobe Bronchus, Right
7 Main Bronchus, Left
8 Upper Lobe Bronchus, Left
9 Lingula Bronchus
B Lower Lobe Bronchus, Left
	Ø Open
	3 Percutaneous
	4 Percutaneous Endoscopic
	7 Via Natural or Artificial
	  Opening
	8 Via Natural or Artificial
	  Opening Endoscopic
		D Intraluminal Device
		Z No Device
			Z No Qualifier

Non-OR ØB7[3,4,5,6,7,8,9,B][Ø,3,4,7,8][D,Z]Z

Ø **Medical and Surgical**
B **Respiratory System**
9 **Drainage** Definition: Taking or letting out fluids and/or gases from a body part

Explanation: The qualifier DIAGNOSTIC is used to identify drainage procedures that are biopsies

Body Part Character 4		Approach Character 5	Device Character 6	Qualifier Character 7

1 Trachea
  Cricoid cartilage
2 Carina
3 Main Bronchus, Right
  Bronchus intermedius
  Intermediate bronchus
4 Upper Lobe Bronchus,
  Right
5 Middle Lobe Bronchus,
  Right
6 Lower Lobe Bronchus,
  Right
7 Main Bronchus, Left
	8 Upper Lobe Bronchus, Left
	9 Lingula Bronchus
	B Lower Lobe Bronchus, Left
	C Upper Lung Lobe, Right
	D Middle Lung Lobe, Right
	F Lower Lung Lobe, Right
	G Upper Lung Lobe, Left
	H Lung Lingula
	J Lower Lung Lobe, Left
	K Lung, Right
	L Lung, Left
	M Lungs, Bilateral
		Ø Open
		3 Percutaneous
		4 Percutaneous Endoscopic
		7 Via Natural or Artificial
		  Opening
		8 Via Natural or Artificial
		  Opening Endoscopic
			Ø Drainage Device	Z No Qualifier

1 Trachea
  Cricoid cartilage
2 Carina
3 Main Bronchus, Right
  Bronchus intermedius
  Intermediate bronchus
4 Upper Lobe Bronchus,
  Right
5 Middle Lobe Bronchus,
  Right
6 Lower Lobe Bronchus, Right
7 Main Bronchus, Left
	8 Upper Lobe Bronchus, Left
	9 Lingula Bronchus
	B Lower Lobe Bronchus, Left
	C Upper Lung Lobe, Right
	D Middle Lung Lobe, Right
	F Lower Lung Lobe, Right
	G Upper Lung Lobe, Left
	H Lung Lingula
	J Lower Lung Lobe, Left
	K Lung, Right
	L Lung, Left
	M Lungs, Bilateral
		Ø Open
		3 Percutaneous
		4 Percutaneous Endoscopic
		7 Via Natural or Artificial
		  Opening
		8 Via Natural or Artificial
		  Opening Endoscopic
			Z No Device	X Diagnostic
				Z No Qualifier

N Pleura, Right P Pleura, Left		Ø Open 3 Percutaneous 4 Percutaneous Endoscopic 8 Via Natural or Artificial Opening Endoscopic	Ø Drainage Device	Z No Qualifier
N Pleura, Right P Pleura, Left		Ø Open 3 Percutaneous 4 Percutaneous Endoscopic 8 Via Natural or Artificial Opening Endoscopic	Z No Device	X Diagnostic Z No Qualifier
T Diaphragm		Ø Open 3 Percutaneous 4 Percutaneous Endoscopic	Ø Drainage Device	Z No Qualifier
T Diaphragm		Ø Open 3 Percutaneous 4 Percutaneous Endoscopic	Z No Device	X Diagnostic Z No Qualifier

Non-OR ØB9[1,2,3,4,5,6,7,8,9,B][7,8]ØZ
Non-OR ØB9[1,2,3,4,5,6,7,8,9,B][3,4]ZX
Non-OR ØB9[1,2,3,4,5,6,7,8,9,B][7,8]Z[X,Z]
Non-OR ØB9[C,D,F,G,J][3,4,7,8]ZX
Non-OR ØB9[H,K,L,M][3,4,7]ZX

Non-OR ØB9[N,P][Ø,3,8]ØZ
Non-OR ØB9[N,P][Ø,3,8]Z[X,Z]
Non-OR ØB9[N,P]4ZX
Non-OR ØB9T[3,4]ØZ
Non-OR ØB9T[3,4]Z[X,Z]

Ø Medical and Surgical
B Respiratory System
B Excision   Definition: Cutting out or off, without replacement, a portion of a body part
              Explanation: The qualifier DIAGNOSTIC is used to identify excision procedures that are biopsies

Body Part Character 4	Approach Character 5	Device Character 6	Qualifier Character 7

1 Trachea
    Cricoid cartilage
2 Carina
3 Main Bronchus, Right
    Bronchus intermedius
    Intermediate bronchus
4 Upper Lobe Bronchus, Right
5 Middle Lobe Bronchus, Right
6 Lower Lobe Bronchus, Right
7 Main Bronchus, Left
8 Upper Lobe Bronchus, Left
9 Lingula Bronchus
B Lower Lobe Bronchus, Left
C Upper Lung Lobe, Right
D Middle Lung Lobe, Right
F Lower Lung Lobe, Right
G Upper Lung Lobe, Left
H Lung Lingula
J Lower Lung Lobe, Left
K Lung, Right
L Lung, Left
M Lungs, Bilateral
	Ø Open
	3 Percutaneous
	4 Percutaneous Endoscopic
	7 Via Natural or Artificial Opening
	8 Via Natural or Artificial Opening
	    Endoscopic
		Z No Device	**X** Diagnostic
			Z No Qualifier

N Pleura, Right **P** Pleura, Left	**Ø** Open **3** Percutaneous **4** Percutaneous Endoscopic **8** Via Natural or Artificial Opening Endoscopic	**Z** No Device	**X** Diagnostic **Z** No Qualifier
T Diaphragm	**Ø** Open **3** Percutaneous **4** Percutaneous Endoscopic	**Z** No Device	**X** Diagnostic **Z** No Qualifier

Non-OR ØBB[1,2,3,4,5,6,7,8,9,B][3,4,7,8]ZX
Non-OR ØBB[3,4,5,6,7,8,9,B,M][4,8]ZZ   **Non-OR** ØBB[C,D,F,G,H,J,K,L]8ZZ
Non-OR ØBB[C,D,F,G,H,J,K,L,M]3ZX   **Non-OR** ØBB[N,P][Ø,3]ZX

Ø Medical and Surgical
B Respiratory System
C Extirpation   Definition: Taking or cutting out solid matter from a body part
              Explanation: The solid matter may be an abnormal byproduct of a biological function or a foreign body; it may be imbedded in a body part or in the lumen of a tubular body part. The solid matter may or may not have been previously broken into pieces.

Body Part Character 4	Approach Character 5	Device Character 6	Qualifier Character 7

1 Trachea
    Cricoid cartilage
2 Carina
3 Main Bronchus, Right
    Bronchus intermedius
    Intermediate bronchus
4 Upper Lobe Bronchus, Right
5 Middle Lobe Bronchus, Right
6 Lower Lobe Bronchus, Right
7 Main Bronchus, Left
8 Upper Lobe Bronchus, Left
9 Lingula Bronchus
B Lower Lobe Bronchus, Left
C Upper Lung Lobe, Right
D Middle Lung Lobe, Right
F Lower Lung Lobe, Right
G Upper Lung Lobe, Left
H Lung Lingula
J Lower Lung Lobe, Left
K Lung, Right
L Lung, Left
M Lungs, Bilateral
	Ø Open
	3 Percutaneous
	4 Percutaneous Endoscopic
	7 Via Natural or Artificial Opening
	8 Via Natural or Artificial Opening
	    Endoscopic
		Z No Device	**Z** No Qualifier

N Pleura, Right **P** Pleura, Left **T** Diaphragm	**Ø** Open **3** Percutaneous **4** Percutaneous Endoscopic	**Z** No Device	**Z** No Qualifier

Non-OR ØBC[1,2,3,4,5,6,7,8,9,B][7,8]ZZ
Non-OR ØBC[N,P]3ZZ

LC Limited Coverage   NC Noncovered   ⊞ Combination Member   HAC associated procedure   Combination Only   DRG Non-OR   Non-OR   New/Revised in GREEN

Respiratory System

Ø **Medical and Surgical**
B **Respiratory System**
D **Extraction**　　Definition: Pulling or stripping out or off all or a portion of a body part by the use of force

　　　　　　　　Explanation: The qualifier DIAGNOSTIC is used to identify extraction procedures that are biopsies

Body Part Character 4	Approach Character 5	Device Character 6	Qualifier Character 7
1 Trachea 　Cricoid cartilage 2 Carina 3 Main Bronchus, Right 　Bronchus intermedius 　Intermediate bronchus 4 Upper Lobe Bronchus, Right 5 Middle Lobe Bronchus, Right 6 Lower Lobe Bronchus, Right 7 Main Bronchus, Left 8 Upper Lobe Bronchus, Left 9 Lingula Bronchus B Lower Lobe Bronchus, Left C Upper Lung Lobe, Right D Middle Lung Lobe, Right F Lower Lung Lobe, Right G Upper Lung Lobe, Left H Lung Lingula J Lower Lung Lobe, Left K Lung, Right L Lung, Left M Lungs, Bilateral	4 Percutaneous Endoscopic 8 Via Natural or Artificial Opening 　Endoscopic	Z No Device	X Diagnostic
N Pleura, Right P Pleura, Left	Ø Open 3 Percutaneous 4 Percutaneous Endoscopic	Z No Device	X Diagnostic Z No Qualifier

Non-OR　ØBD[1,2,3,4,5,6,7,8,9,B,C,D,F,G,H,J,K,L,M][4,8]ZX

Ø **Medical and Surgical**
B **Respiratory System**
F **Fragmentation**　　Definition: Breaking solid matter in a body part into pieces

　　　　　　　　Explanation: Physical force (e.g., manual, ultrasonic) applied directly or indirectly is used to break the solid matter into pieces. The solid matter may be an abnormal byproduct of a biological function or a foreign body. The pieces of solid matter are not taken out.

Body Part Character 4	Approach Character 5	Device Character 6	Qualifier Character 7
1 Trachea　NC 　Cricoid cartilage 2 Carina　NC 3 Main Bronchus, Right　NC 　Bronchus intermedius 　Intermediate bronchus 4 Upper Lobe Bronchus, Right　NC 5 Middle Lobe Bronchus, Right　NC 6 Lower Lobe Bronchus, Right　NC 7 Main Bronchus, Left　NC 8 Upper Lobe Bronchus, Left　NC 9 Lingula Bronchus　NC B Lower Lobe Bronchus, Left　NC	Ø Open 3 Percutaneous 4 Percutaneous Endoscopic 7 Via Natural or Artificial Opening 8 Via Natural or Artificial Opening 　Endoscopic X External	Z No Device	Z No Qualifier

Non-OR　ØBF[1,2,3,4,5,6,7,8,9,B]XZZ
Non-OR　ØBF[3,4,5,6,7,8,9,B][7,8]ZZ
NC　　ØBF[1,2,3,4,5,6,7,8,9,B]XZZ

Ø   Medical and Surgical
B   Respiratory System
H   Insertion   Definition: Putting in a nonbiological appliance that monitors, assists, performs, or prevents a physiological function but does not physically take the place of a body part
                Explanation: None

Body Part Character 4	Approach Character 5	Device Character 6	Qualifier Character 7
Ø Tracheobronchial Tree	Ø Open 3 Percutaneous 4 Percutaneous Endoscopic 7 Via Natural or Artificial Opening 8 Via Natural or Artificial Opening Endoscopic	1 Radioactive Element 2 Monitoring Device 3 Infusion Device D Intraluminal Device Y Other Device	Z No Qualifier
1 Trachea Cricoid cartilage	Ø Open	2 Monitoring Device D Intraluminal Device Y Other Device	Z No Qualifier
1 Trachea Cricoid cartilage	3 Percutaneous	D Intraluminal Device E Intraluminal Device, Endotracheal Airway Y Other Device	Z No Qualifier
1 Trachea Cricoid cartilage	4 Percutaneous Endoscopic	D Intraluminal Device Y Other Device	Z No Qualifier
1 Trachea Cricoid cartilage	7 Via Natural or Artificial Opening 8 Via Natural or Artificial Opening Endoscopic	2 Monitoring Device D Intraluminal Device E Intraluminal Device, Endotracheal Airway Y Other Device	Z No Qualifier

3   Main Bronchus, Right
     Bronchus intermedius
     Intermediate bronchus
4   Upper Lobe Bronchus, Right
5   Middle Lobe Bronchus, Right
6   Lower Lobe Bronchus, Right
7   Main Bronchus, Left
8   Upper Lobe Bronchus, Left
9   Lingula Bronchus
B   Lower Lobe Bronchus, Left
	Ø Open
	3 Percutaneous
	4 Percutaneous Endoscopic
	7 Via Natural or Artificial Opening
	8 Via Natural or Artificial Opening Endoscopic
		G Intraluminal Device, Endobronchial Valve	Z No Qualifier

K Lung, Right L Lung, Left	Ø Open 3 Percutaneous 4 Percutaneous Endoscopic 7 Via Natural or Artificial Opening 8 Via Natural or Artificial Opening Endoscopic	1 Radioactive Element 2 Monitoring Device 3 Infusion Device Y Other Device	Z No Qualifier
Q Pleura	Ø Open 3 Percutaneous 4 Percutaneous Endoscopic 7 Via Natural or Artificial Opening 8 Via Natural or Artificial Opening Endoscopic	Y Other Device	Z No Qualifier
T Diaphragm	Ø Open 3 Percutaneous 4 Percutaneous Endoscopic	2 Monitoring Device M Diaphragmatic Pacemaker Lead Y Other Device	Z No Qualifier
T Diaphragm	7 Via Natural or Artificial Opening 8 Via Natural or Artificial Opening Endoscopic	Y Other Device	Z No Qualifier

Non-OR	ØBHØ3YZ
Non-OR	ØBHØ[7,8][2,3,D,Y]Z
Non-OR	ØBH13[E,Y]Z
Non-OR	ØBH1[7,8][2,D,E,Y]Z
Non-OR	ØBH[3,4,5,6,7,8,9,B]8GZ
Non-OR	ØBH[K,L]3YZ
Non-OR	ØBH[K,L]7[2,3,Y]Z
Non-OR	ØBH[K,L]8[2,3]Z
Non-OR	ØBHQ[3,7]YZ
Non-OR	ØBHT3YZ
Non-OR	ØBHT[7,8]YZ

LC Limited Coverage   NC Noncovered   ⊞ Combination Member   HAC associated procedure   Combination Only   DRG Non-OR   Non-OR   New/Revised in GREEN

ICD-10-PCS 2020   335

ØBH–ØBH

Ø   Medical and Surgical
B   Respiratory System
J   Inspection   Definition: Visually and/or manually exploring a body part

Explanation: Visual exploration may be performed with or without optical instrumentation. Manual exploration may be performed directly or through intervening body layers.

Body Part Character 4	Approach Character 5	Device Character 6	Qualifier Character 7
Ø Tracheobronchial Tree 1 Trachea Cricoid cartilage K Lung, Right L Lung, Left Q Pleura T Diaphragm	Ø Open 3 Percutaneous 4 Percutaneous Endoscopic 7 Via Natural or Artificial Opening 8 Via Natural or Artificial Opening Endoscopic X External	Z No Device	Z No Qualifier

Non-OR   ØBJ[Ø,K,L,Q,T][3,7,8,X]ZZ
Non-OR   ØBJ1[3,4,7,8,X]ZZ

Ø   Medical and Surgical
B   Respiratory System
L   Occlusion   Definition: Completely closing an orifice or the lumen of a tubular body part

Explanation: The orifice can be a natural orifice or an artificially created orifice

Body Part Character 4	Approach Character 5	Device Character 6	Qualifier Character 7

1   Trachea
     Cricoid cartilage
2   Carina
3   Main Bronchus, Right
     Bronchus intermedius
     Intermediate bronchus
4   Upper Lobe Bronchus, Right
5   Middle Lobe Bronchus, Right
6   Lower Lobe Bronchus, Right
7   Main Bronchus, Left
8   Upper Lobe Bronchus, Left
9   Lingula Bronchus
B   Lower Lobe Bronchus, Left
	Ø Open
	3 Percutaneous
	4 Percutaneous Endoscopic
		C Extraluminal Device
		D Intraluminal Device
		Z No Device
			Z No Qualifier

1   Trachea
     Cricoid cartilage
2   Carina
3   Main Bronchus, Right
     Bronchus intermedius
     Intermediate bronchus
4   Upper Lobe Bronchus, Right
5   Middle Lobe Bronchus, Right
6   Lower Lobe Bronchus, Right
7   Main Bronchus, Left
8   Upper Lobe Bronchus, Left
9   Lingula Bronchus
B   Lower Lobe Bronchus, Left
	7 Via Natural or Artificial Opening
	8 Via Natural or Artificial Opening Endoscopic
		D Intraluminal Device
		Z No Device
			Z No Qualifier

Ø   Medical and Surgical
B   Respiratory System
M   Reattachment   Definition: Putting back in or on all or a portion of a separated body part to its normal location or other suitable location
                       Explanation: Vascular circulation and nervous pathways may or may not be reestablished

Body Part Character 4	Approach Character 5	Device Character 6	Qualifier Character 7

1   Trachea
     Cricoid cartilage
2   Carina
3   Main Bronchus, Right
     Bronchus intermedius
     Intermediate bronchus
4   Upper Lobe Bronchus, Right
5   Middle Lobe Bronchus, Right
6   Lower Lobe Bronchus, Right
7   Main Bronchus, Left
8   Upper Lobe Bronchus, Left
9   Lingula Bronchus
B   Lower Lobe Bronchus, Left
C   Upper Lung Lobe, Right
D   Middle Lung Lobe, Right
F   Lower Lung Lobe, Right
G   Upper Lung Lobe, Left
H   Lung Lingula
J   Lower Lung Lobe, Left
K   Lung, Right
L   Lung, Left
T   Diaphragm
	Ø Open	Z No Device	Z No Qualifier

Ø   Medical and Surgical
B   Respiratory System
N   Release   Definition: Freeing a body part from an abnormal physical constraint by cutting or by the use of force
               Explanation: Some of the restraining tissue may be taken out but none of the body part is taken out

Body Part Character 4	Approach Character 5	Device Character 6	Qualifier Character 7

1   Trachea
     Cricoid cartilage
2   Carina
3   Main Bronchus, Right
     Bronchus intermedius
     Intermediate bronchus
4   Upper Lobe Bronchus, Right
5   Middle Lobe Bronchus, Right
6   Lower Lobe Bronchus, Right
7   Main Bronchus, Left
8   Upper Lobe Bronchus, Left
9   Lingula Bronchus
B   Lower Lobe Bronchus, Left
C   Upper Lung Lobe, Right
D   Middle Lung Lobe, Right
F   Lower Lung Lobe, Right
G   Upper Lung Lobe, Left
H   Lung Lingula
J   Lower Lung Lobe, Left
K   Lung, Right
L   Lung, Left
M   Lungs, Bilateral
	Ø Open
	3 Percutaneous
	4 Percutaneous Endoscopic
	7 Via Natural or Artificial Opening
	8 Via Natural or Artificial Opening
	     Endoscopic
		Z No Device	Z No Qualifier

N Pleura, Right P Pleura, Left T Diaphragm	Ø Open 3 Percutaneous 4 Percutaneous Endoscopic	Z No Device	Z No Qualifier

Ø   Medical and Surgical
B   Respiratory System
P   Removal   Definition: Taking out or off a device from a body part

Explanation: If a device is taken out and a similar device put in without cutting or puncturing the skin or mucous membrane, the procedure is coded to the root operation CHANGE. Otherwise, the procedure for taking out a device is coded to the root operation REMOVAL.

Body Part Character 4	Approach Character 5	Device Character 6	Qualifier Character 7
Ø Tracheobronchial Tree	Ø Open 3 Percutaneous 4 Percutaneous Endoscopic 7 Via Natural or Artificial Opening 8 Via Natural or Artificial Opening Endoscopic	Ø Drainage Device 1 Radioactive Element 2 Monitoring Device 3 Infusion Device 7 Autologous Tissue Substitute C Extraluminal Device D Intraluminal Device J Synthetic Substitute K Nonautologous Tissue Substitute Y Other Device	Z No Qualifier
Ø Tracheobronchial Tree	X External	Ø Drainage Device 1 Radioactive Element 2 Monitoring Device 3 Infusion Device D Intraluminal Device	Z No Qualifier
1 Trachea Cricoid cartilage	Ø Open 3 Percutaneous 4 Percutaneous Endoscopic 7 Via Natural or Artificial Opening 8 Via Natural or Artificial Opening Endoscopic	Ø Drainage Device 2 Monitoring Device 7 Autologous Tissue Substitute C Extraluminal Device D Intraluminal Device F Tracheostomy Device J Synthetic Substitute K Nonautologous Tissue Substitute	Z No Qualifier
1 Trachea Cricoid cartilage	X External	Ø Drainage Device 2 Monitoring Device D Intraluminal Device F Tracheostomy Device	Z No Qualifier
K Lung, Right L Lung, Left	Ø Open 3 Percutaneous 4 Percutaneous Endoscopic 7 Via Natural or Artificial Opening 8 Via Natural or Artificial Opening Endoscopic	Ø Drainage Device 1 Radioactive Element 2 Monitoring Device 3 Infusion Device Y Other Device	Z No Qualifier
K Lung, Right L Lung, Left	X External	Ø Drainage Device 1 Radioactive Element 2 Monitoring Device 3 Infusion Device	Z No Qualifier
Q Pleura	Ø Open 3 Percutaneous 4 Percutaneous Endoscopic 7 Via Natural or Artificial Opening 8 Via Natural or Artificial Opening Endoscopic	Ø Drainage Device 1 Radioactive Element 2 Monitoring Device Y Other Device	Z No Qualifier
Q Pleura	X External	Ø Drainage Device 1 Radioactive Element 2 Monitoring Device	Z No Qualifier
T Diaphragm	Ø Open 3 Percutaneous 4 Percutaneous Endoscopic 7 Via Natural or Artificial Opening 8 Via Natural or Artificial Opening Endoscopic	Ø Drainage Device 2 Monitoring Device 7 Autologous Tissue Substitute J Synthetic Substitute K Nonautologous Tissue Substitute M Diaphragmatic Pacemaker Lead Y Other Device	Z No Qualifier
T Diaphragm	X External	Ø Drainage Device 2 Monitoring Device M Diaphragmatic Pacemaker Lead	Z No Qualifier

Non-OR	ØBPØ[3,4]YZ	Non-OR	ØBPL7[Ø,2,3,Y]Z
Non-OR	ØBPØ[7,8][Ø,2,3,D,Y]Z	Non-OR	ØBPL8[Ø,2,3]Z
Non-OR	ØBPØX[Ø,1,2,3,D]Z	Non-OR	ØBP[K,L]X[Ø,1,2,3]Z
Non-OR	ØBP1[Ø,3,4]FZ	Non-OR	ØBPQ[Ø,3,4,7,8][Ø,1,2,]Z
Non-OR	ØBP1[7,8][Ø,2,D,F]Z	Non-OR	ØBPQ[3,7]YZ
Non-OR	ØBP1X[Ø,2,D,F]Z	Non-OR	ØBPQX[Ø,1,2]Z
Non-OR	ØBP[K,L]3YZ	Non-OR	ØBPT3YZ
Non-OR	ØBPK7[Ø,1,2,3,Y]Z	Non-OR	ØBPT[7,8][Ø,2,Y]Z
Non-OR	ØBPK8[Ø,1,2,3]Z	Non-OR	ØBPTX[Ø,2,M]Z

Ø   **Medical and Surgical**
B   **Respiratory System**
Q   **Repair**   Definition: Restoring, to the extent possible, a body part to its normal anatomic structure and function
                         Explanation: Used only when the method to accomplish the repair is not one of the other root operations

Body Part Character 4	Approach Character 5	Device Character 6	Qualifier Character 7

1 Trachea
    Cricoid cartilage
2 Carina
3 Main Bronchus, Right
    Bronchus intermedius
    Intermediate bronchus
4 Upper Lobe Bronchus, Right
5 Middle Lobe Bronchus, Right
6 Lower Lobe Bronchus, Right
7 Main Bronchus, Left
8 Upper Lobe Bronchus, Left
9 Lingula Bronchus
B Lower Lobe Bronchus, Left
C Upper Lung Lobe, Right
D Middle Lung Lobe, Right
F Lower Lung Lobe, Right
G Upper Lung Lobe, Left
H Lung Lingula
J Lower Lung Lobe, Left
K Lung, Right
L Lung, Left
M Lungs, Bilateral
	Ø Open
	3 Percutaneous
	4 Percutaneous Endoscopic
	7 Via Natural or Artificial Opening
	8 Via Natural or Artificial Opening
	    Endoscopic
		Z No Device	**Z** No Qualifier

N Pleura, Right **P** Pleura, Left **T** Diaphragm	**Ø** Open **3** Percutaneous **4** Percutaneous Endoscopic	**Z** No Device	**Z** No Qualifier

LC Limited Coverage   **NC** Noncovered   ⊞ Combination Member   HAC associated procedure   Combination Only   DRG Non-OR   Non-OR   New/Revised in GREEN

ICD-10-PCS 2020   339

Ø   Medical and Surgical
B   Respiratory System
R   Replacement   Definition: Putting in or on biological or synthetic material that physically takes the place and/or function of all or a portion of a body part

Explanation: The body part may have been taken out or replaced, or may be taken out, physically eradicated, or rendered nonfunctional during the REPLACEMENT procedure. A REMOVAL procedure is coded for taking out the device used in a previous replacement procedure.

Body Part Character 4	Approach Character 5	Device Character 6	Qualifier Character 7
1 Trachea Cricoid cartilage **2 Carina** **3 Main Bronchus, Right** Bronchus intermedius Intermediate bronchus **4 Upper Lobe Bronchus, Right** **5 Middle Lobe Bronchus, Right** **6 Lower Lobe Bronchus, Right** **7 Main Bronchus, Left** **8 Upper Lobe Bronchus, Left** **9 Lingula Bronchus** **B Lower Lobe Bronchus, Left** **T Diaphragm**	**Ø Open** **4 Percutaneous Endoscopic**	**7 Autologous Tissue Substitute** **J Synthetic Substitute** **K Nonautologous Tissue Substitute**	**Z No Qualifier**

Ø   Medical and Surgical
B   Respiratory System
S   Reposition   Definition: Moving to its normal location, or other suitable location, all or a portion of a body part

Explanation: The body part is moved to a new location from an abnormal location, or from a normal location where it is not functioning correctly. The body part may or may not be cut out or off to be moved to the new location.

Body Part Character 4	Approach Character 5	Device Character 6	Qualifier Character 7
1 Trachea Cricoid cartilage **2 Carina** **3 Main Bronchus, Right** Bronchus intermedius Intermediate bronchus **4 Upper Lobe Bronchus, Right** **5 Middle Lobe Bronchus, Right** **6 Lower Lobe Bronchus, Right** **7 Main Bronchus, Left** **8 Upper Lobe Bronchus, Left** **9 Lingula Bronchus** **B Lower Lobe Bronchus, Left** **C Upper Lung Lobe, Right** **D Middle Lung Lobe, Right** **F Lower Lung Lobe, Right** **G Upper Lung Lobe, Left** **H Lung Lingula** **J Lower Lung Lobe, Left** **K Lung, Right** **L Lung, Left** **T Diaphragm**	**Ø Open**	**Z No Device**	**Z No Qualifier**

LC Limited Coverage   **NC** Noncovered   ⊞ Combination Member   HAC associated procedure   Combination Only   DRG Non-OR   Non-OR   New/Revised in GREEN

340   ICD-10-PCS 2020

ØBR–ØBS

Ø   **Medical and Surgical**
B   **Respiratory System**
T   **Resection**   Definition: Cutting out or off, without replacement, all of a body part
                  Explanation: None

Body Part Character 4	Approach Character 5	Device Character 6	Qualifier Character 7

1 Trachea
    Cricoid cartilage
2 Carina
3 Main Bronchus, Right
    Bronchus intermedius
    Intermediate bronchus
4 Upper Lobe Bronchus, Right
5 Middle Lobe Bronchus, Right
6 Lower Lobe Bronchus, Right
7 Main Bronchus, Left
8 Upper Lobe Bronchus, Left
9 Lingula Bronchus
B Lower Lobe Bronchus, Left
C Upper Lung Lobe, Right
D Middle Lung Lobe, Right
F Lower Lung Lobe, Right
G Upper Lung Lobe, Left
H Lung Lingula
J Lower Lung Lobe, Left
K Lung, Right
L Lung, Left
M Lungs, Bilateral
T Diaphragm
	Ø Open
	4 Percutaneous Endoscopic
		Z No Device	**Z** No Qualifier

Ø   **Medical and Surgical**
B   **Respiratory System**
U   **Supplement**   Definition: Putting in or on biological or synthetic material that physically reinforces and/or augments the function of a portion of a body part
                  Explanation: The biological material is non-living, or is living and from the same individual. The body part may have been previously replaced, and the SUPPLEMENT procedure is performed to physically reinforce and/or augment the function of the replaced body part.

Body Part Character 4	Approach Character 5	Device Character 6	Qualifier Character 7

1 Trachea
    Cricoid cartilage
2 Carina
3 Main Bronchus, Right
    Bronchus intermedius
    Intermediate bronchus
4 Upper Lobe Bronchus, Right
5 Middle Lobe Bronchus, Right
6 Lower Lobe Bronchus, Right
7 Main Bronchus, Left
8 Upper Lobe Bronchus, Left
9 Lingula Bronchus
B Lower Lobe Bronchus, Left
	Ø Open
	4 Percutaneous Endoscopic
	8 Via Natural or Artificial Opening
	    Endoscopic
		7 Autologous Tissue Substitute
		J Synthetic Substitute
		K Nonautologous Tissue Substitute
			Z No Qualifier

T Diaphragm	**Ø** Open **4** Percutaneous Endoscopic	**7** Autologous Tissue Substitute **J** Synthetic Substitute **K** Nonautologous Tissue Substitute	**Z** No Qualifier

LC Limited Coverage   **NC** Noncovered   ⊞ Combination Member   HAC associated procedure   Combination Only   DRG Non-OR   Non-OR   New/Revised in GREEN

ICD-10-PCS 2020   341

Ø Medical and Surgical
B Respiratory System
V Restriction Definition: Partially closing an orifice or the lumen of a tubular body part

Explanation: The orifice can be a natural orifice or an artificially created orifice

Body Part Character 4	Approach Character 5	Device Character 6	Qualifier Character 7
1 Trachea Cricoid cartilage **2 Carina** **3 Main Bronchus, Right** Bronchus intermedius Intermediate bronchus **4 Upper Lobe Bronchus, Right** **5 Middle Lobe Bronchus, Right** **6 Lower Lobe Bronchus, Right** **7 Main Bronchus, Left** **8 Upper Lobe Bronchus, Left** **9 Lingula Bronchus** **B Lower Lobe Bronchus, Left**	**Ø Open** **3 Percutaneous** **4 Percutaneous Endoscopic**	**C Extraluminal Device** **D Intraluminal Device** **Z No Device**	**Z No Qualifier**
1 Trachea Cricoid cartilage **2 Carina** **3 Main Bronchus, Right** Bronchus intermedius Intermediate bronchus **4 Upper Lobe Bronchus, Right** **5 Middle Lobe Bronchus, Right** **6 Lower Lobe Bronchus, Right** **7 Main Bronchus, Left** **8 Upper Lobe Bronchus, Left** **9 Lingula Bronchus** **B Lower Lobe Bronchus, Left**	**7 Via Natural or Artificial Opening** **8 Via Natural or Artificial Opening Endoscopic**	**D Intraluminal Device** **Z No Device**	**Z No Qualifier**

Ø   Medical and Surgical
B   Respiratory System
W   Revision   Definition: Correcting, to the extent possible, a portion of a malfunctioning device or the position of a displaced device

         Explanation: Revision can include correcting a malfunctioning or displaced device by taking out or putting in components of the device such as a screw or pin

Body Part Character 4	Approach Character 5	Device Character 6	Qualifier Character 7
Ø Tracheobronchial Tree	Ø Open 3 Percutaneous 4 Percutaneous Endoscopic 7 Via Natural or Artificial Opening 8 Via Natural or Artificial Opening Endoscopic	Ø Drainage Device 2 Monitoring Device 3 Infusion Device 7 Autologous Tissue Substitute C Extraluminal Device D Intraluminal Device J Synthetic Substitute K Nonautologous Tissue Substitute Y Other Device	Z No Qualifier
Ø Tracheobronchial Tree	X External	Ø Drainage Device 2 Monitoring Device 3 Infusion Device 7 Autologous Tissue Substitute C Extraluminal Device D Intraluminal Device J Synthetic Substitute K Nonautologous Tissue Substitute	Z No Qualifier

1   Trachea
    Cricoid cartilage
	Ø Open
	3 Percutaneous
	4 Percutaneous Endoscopic
	7 Via Natural or Artificial Opening
	8 Via Natural or Artificial Opening
	    Endoscopic
	X External
		Ø Drainage Device
		2 Monitoring Device
		7 Autologous Tissue Substitute
		C Extraluminal Device
		D Intraluminal Device
		F Tracheostomy Device
		J Synthetic Substitute
		K Nonautologous Tissue Substitute
			Z No Qualifier

K Lung, Right L Lung, Left	Ø Open 3 Percutaneous 4 Percutaneous Endoscopic 7 Via Natural or Artificial Opening 8 Via Natural or Artificial Opening Endoscopic	Ø Drainage Device 2 Monitoring Device 3 Infusion Device Y Other Device	Z No Qualifier
K Lung, Right L Lung, Left	X External	Ø Drainage Device 2 Monitoring Device 3 Infusion Device	Z No Qualifier
Q Pleura	Ø Open 3 Percutaneous 4 Percutaneous Endoscopic 7 Via Natural or Artificial Opening 8 Via Natural or Artificial Opening Endoscopic	Ø Drainage Device 2 Monitoring Device Y Other Device	Z No Qualifier
Q Pleura	X External	Ø Drainage Device 2 Monitoring Device	Z No Qualifier
T Diaphragm	Ø Open 3 Percutaneous 4 Percutaneous Endoscopic 7 Via Natural or Artificial Opening 8 Via Natural or Artificial Opening Endoscopic	Ø Drainage Device 2 Monitoring Device 7 Autologous Tissue Substitute J Synthetic Substitute K Nonautologous Tissue Substitute M Diaphragmatic Pacemaker Lead Y Other Device	Z No Qualifier
T Diaphragm	X External	Ø Drainage Device 2 Monitoring Device 7 Autologous Tissue Substitute J Synthetic Substitute K Nonautologous Tissue Substitute M Diaphragmatic Pacemaker Lead	Z No Qualifier

Non-OR   ØBWØ[3,4]YZ
Non-OR   ØBWØ[7,8][2,3,D,Y]Z
Non-OR   ØBWØX[Ø,2,3,7,C,D,J,K]Z
Non-OR   ØBW1X[Ø,2,7,C,D,F,J,K]Z
Non-OR   ØBW[K,L]3YZ
Non-OR   ØBW[K,L]7[Ø,2,3,Y]Z
Non-OR   ØBW[K,L]8[Ø,2,3]Z
Non-OR   ØBW[K,L]X[Ø,2,3]Z
Non-OR   ØBWQ[Ø,3,4,7,8][Ø,2]Z
Non-OR   ØBWQ[Ø,3,7]YZ
Non-OR   ØBWQX[Ø,2]Z
Non-OR   ØBWT[3,7,8]YZ
Non-OR   ØBWTX[Ø,2,7,J,K,M]Z

Respiratory System

Ø   **Medical and Surgical**
B   **Respiratory System**
Y   **Transplantation**   Definition: Putting in or on all or a portion of a living body part taken from another individual or animal to physically take the place and/or function of all or a portion of a similar body part

           Explanation: The native body part may or may not be taken out, and the transplanted body part may take over all or a portion of its function

Body Part Character 4	Approach Character 5	Device Character 6	Qualifier Character 7
C Upper Lung Lobe, Right LC D Middle Lung Lobe, Right LC F Lower Lung Lobe, Right LC G Upper Lung Lobe, Left LC H Lung Lingula LC J Lower Lung Lobe, Left LC K Lung, Right LC L Lung, Left LC M Lungs, Bilateral LC	Ø Open	Z No Device	Ø Allogeneic 1 Syngeneic 2 Zooplastic

LC   ØBY[C,D,F,G,H,J,K,L,M]ØZ[Ø,1,2]

LC Limited Coverage   NC Noncovered   ⊞ Combination Member   HAC associated procedure   Combination Only   DRG Non-OR   Non-OR   New/Revised in GREEN

344   ICD-10-PCS 2020

Mouth and Throat 0C0–0CX

Character Meanings

This Character Meaning table is provided as a guide to assist the user in the identification of character members that may be found in this section of code tables. It **SHOULD NOT** be used to build a PCS code.

Operation–Character 3	Body Part–Character 4	Approach–Character 5	Device–Character 6	Qualifier–Character 7
0 Alteration	0 Upper Lip	0 Open	0 Drainage Device	0 Single
2 Change	1 Lower Lip	3 Percutaneous	1 Radioactive Element	1 Multiple
5 Destruction	2 Hard Palate	4 Percutaneous Endoscopic	5 External Fixation Device	2 All
7 Dilation	3 Soft Palate	7 Via Natural or Artificial Opening	7 Autologous Tissue Substitute	X Diagnostic
9 Drainage	4 Buccal Mucosa	8 Via Natural or Artificial Opening Endoscopic	B Intraluminal Device, Airway	Z No Qualifier
B Excision	5 Upper Gingiva	X External	C Extraluminal Device	
C Extirpation	6 Lower Gingiva		D Intraluminal Device	
D Extraction	7 Tongue		J Synthetic Substitute	
F Fragmentation	8 Parotid Gland, Right		K Nonautologous Tissue Substitute	
H Insertion	9 Parotid Gland, Left		Y Other Device	
J Inspection	A Salivary Gland		Z No Device	
L Occlusion	B Parotid Duct, Right			
M Reattachment	C Parotid Duct, Left			
N Release	D Sublingual Gland, Right			
P Removal	F Sublingual Gland, Left			
Q Repair	G Submaxillary Gland, Right			
R Replacement	H Submaxillary Gland, Left			
S Reposition	J Minor Salivary Gland			
T Resection	M Pharynx			
U Supplement	N Uvula			
V Restriction	P Tonsils			
W Revision	Q Adenoids			
X Transfer	R Epiglottis			
	S Larynx			
	T Vocal Cord, Right			
	V Vocal Cord, Left			
	W Upper Tooth			
	X Lower Tooth			
	Y Mouth and Throat			

AHA Coding Clinic for table 0C9
2017, 2Q, 16   Incision and drainage of floor of mouth

AHA Coding Clinic for table 0CB
2017, 2Q, 16   Excision of floor of mouth
2016, 3Q, 28   Lingual tonsillectomy, tongue base excision and epiglottopexy
2016, 2Q, 19   Biopsy of the base of tongue
2014, 3Q, 21   Superficial parotidectomy

AHA Coding Clinic for table 0CC
2016, 2Q, 20   Sialendoscopy with stone removal

AHA Coding Clinic for table 0CQ
2017, 1Q, 20   Preparatory nasal adhesion repair before definitive cleft palate repair

AHA Coding Clinic for table 0CR
2014, 3Q, 25   Excision of soft palate with placement of surgical obturator
2014, 2Q, 5   Oasis acellular matrix graft
2014, 2Q, 6   Composite grafting (synthetic versus nonautologous tissue substitute)

AHA Coding Clinic for table 0CS
2016, 3Q, 28   Lingual tonsillectomy, tongue base excision and epiglottopexy

AHA Coding Clinic for table 0CT
2016, 2Q, 12   Resection of malignant neoplasm of infratemporal fossa
2014, 3Q, 21   Superficial parotidectomy
2014, 3Q, 23   Le Fort I osteotomy

Mouth and Throat

Salivary Glands

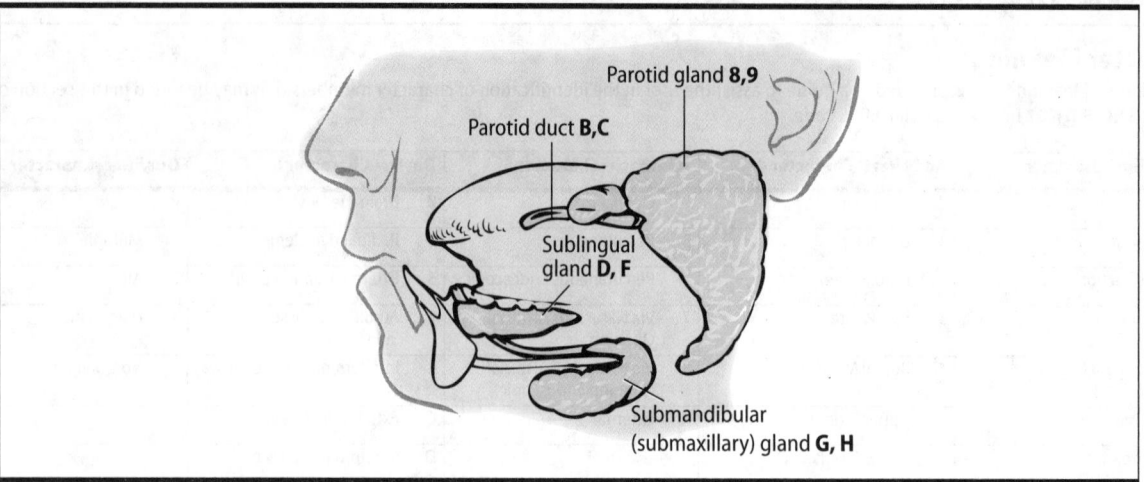

Parotid gland **8,9**

Parotid duct **B,C**

Sublingual gland **D, F**

Submandibular (submaxillary) gland **G, H**

Oral Anatomy

Nasal cavity

Soft palate **3**

Hard palate **2**

Tongue **7**

Pharynx **M**

Epiglottis **R**

Nasopharynx region **M**

Larynx **S**

Oropharynx region **M**

Hypopharynx region **M**

Vocal cords **T,V**

Mouth Frontal View (Upper)

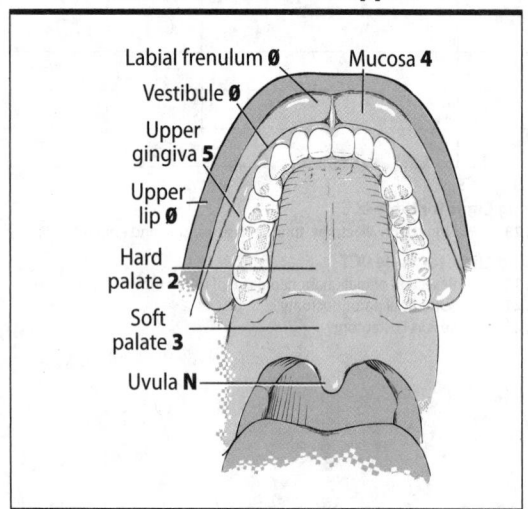

Labial frenulum **Ø**

Mucosa **4**

Vestibule **Ø**

Upper gingiva **5**

Upper lip **Ø**

Hard palate **2**

Soft palate **3**

Uvula **N**

Mouth Frontal View (Lower)

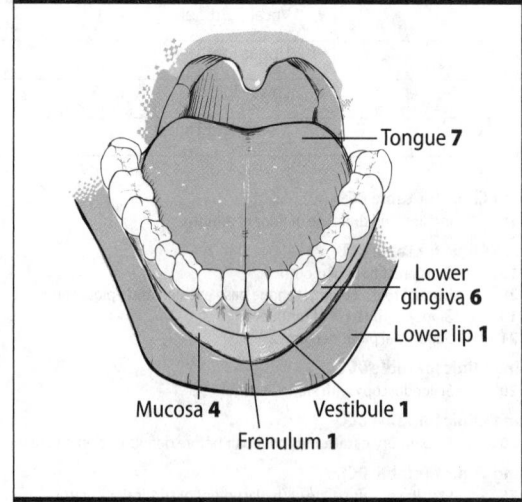

Tongue **7**

Lower gingiva **6**

Lower lip **1**

Mucosa **4**

Vestibule **1**

Frenulum **1**

0　**Medical and Surgical**
C　**Mouth and Throat**
0　**Alteration**　　Definition: Modifying the anatomic structure of a body part without affecting the function of the body part
　　　　　　　　　　　Explanation: Principal purpose is to improve appearance

Body Part Character 4	Approach Character 5	Device Character 6	Qualifier Character 7
0　**Upper Lip** 　　Frenulum labii superioris 　　Labial gland 　　Vermilion border **1**　**Lower Lip** 　　Frenulum labii inferioris 　　Labial gland 　　Vermilion border	**X**　External	**7**　Autologous Tissue Substitute **J**　Synthetic Substitute **K**　Nonautologous Tissue Substitute **Z**　No Device	**Z**　No Qualifier

0　**Medical and Surgical**
C　**Mouth and Throat**
2　**Change**　　Definition: Taking out or off a device from a body part and putting back an identical or similar device in or on the same body part without cutting or puncturing the skin or a mucous membrane
　　　　　　　　　Explanation: All CHANGE procedures are coded using the approach EXTERNAL

Body Part Character 4	Approach Character 5	Device Character 6	Qualifier Character 7
A　Salivary Gland **S**　Larynx 　　Aryepiglottic fold 　　Arytenoid cartilage 　　Corniculate cartilage 　　Cuneiform cartilage 　　False vocal cord 　　Glottis 　　Rima glottidis 　　Thyroid cartilage 　　Ventricular fold **Y**　Mouth and Throat	**X**　External	**0**　Drainage Device **Y**　Other Device	**Z**　No Qualifier

Non-OR　All body part, approach, device, and qualifier values

LC Limited Coverage　**NC** Noncovered　⊞ Combination Member　HAC associated procedure　Combination Only　DRG Non-OR　Non-OR　New/Revised in GREEN
ICD-10-PCS 2020　　　**347**

0C0–0C2

Mouth and Throat

Ø Medical and Surgical
C Mouth and Throat
5 Destruction Definition: Physical eradication of all or a portion of a body part by the direct use of energy, force, or a destructive agent

Explanation: None of the body part is physically taken out

Body Part — Character 4		Approach — Character 5	Device — Character 6	Qualifier — Character 7
Ø Upper Lip Frenulum labii superioris Labial gland Vermilion border **1 Lower Lip** Frenulum labii inferioris Labial gland Vermilion border **2 Hard Palate** **3 Soft Palate** **4 Buccal Mucosa** Buccal gland Molar gland Palatine gland	**5 Upper Gingiva** **6 Lower Gingiva** **7 Tongue** Frenulum linguae **N Uvula** Palatine uvula **P Tonsils** Palatine tonsil **Q Adenoids** Pharyngeal tonsil	**Ø Open** **3 Percutaneous** **X External**	**Z No Device**	**Z No Qualifier**
8 Parotid Gland, Right **9 Parotid Gland, Left** **B Parotid Duct, Right** Stensen's duct **C Parotid Duct, Left** *See B Parotid Duct, Right* **D Sublingual Gland, Right**	**F Sublingual Gland, Left** **G Submaxillary Gland, Right** Submandibular gland **H Submaxillary Gland, Left** *See G Submaxillary Gland, Right* **J Minor Salivary Gland** Anterior lingual gland	**Ø Open** **3 Percutaneous**	**Z No Device**	**Z No Qualifier**
M Pharynx Base of tongue Hypopharynx Laryngopharynx Lingual tonsil Oropharynx Piriform recess (sinus) Tongue, base of **R Epiglottis** Glossoepiglottic fold	**S Larynx** Aryepiglottic fold Arytenoid cartilage Corniculate cartilage Cuneiform cartilage False vocal cord Glottis Rima glottidis Thyroid cartilage Ventricular fold **T Vocal Cord, Right** Vocal fold **V Vocal Cord, Left** *See T Vocal Cord, Right*	**Ø Open** **3 Percutaneous** **4 Percutaneous Endoscopic** **7 Via Natural or Artificial Opening** **8 Via Natural or Artificial Opening Endoscopic**	**Z No Device**	**Z No Qualifier**
W Upper Tooth **X Lower Tooth**		**Ø Open** **X External**	**Z No Device**	**Ø Single** **1 Multiple** **2 All**

Non-OR ØC5[5,6][Ø,3,X]ZZ
Non-OR ØC5[W,X][Ø,X]Z[Ø,1,2]

Ø Medical and Surgical
C Mouth and Throat
7 Dilation Definition: Expanding an orifice or the lumen of a tubular body part

Explanation: The orifice can be a natural orifice or an artificially created orifice. Accomplished by stretching a tubular body part using intraluminal pressure or by cutting part of the orifice or wall of the tubular body part.

Body Part — Character 4	Approach — Character 5	Device — Character 6	Qualifier — Character 7
B Parotid Duct, Right Stensen's duct **C Parotid Duct, Left** *See B Parotid Duct, Right*	**Ø Open** **3 Percutaneous** **7 Via Natural or Artificial Opening**	**D Intraluminal Device** **Z No Device**	**Z No Qualifier**
M Pharynx Base of tongue Hypopharynx Laryngopharynx Lingual tonsil Oropharynx Piriform recess (sinus) Tongue, base of	**7 Via Natural or Artificial Opening** **8 Via Natural or Artificial Opening Endoscopic**	**D Intraluminal Device** **Z No Device**	**Z No Qualifier**
S Larynx Aryepiglottic fold Arytenoid cartilage Corniculate cartilage Cuneiform cartilage False vocal cord Glottis Rima glottidis Thyroid cartilage Ventricular fold	**Ø Open** **3 Percutaneous** **4 Percutaneous Endoscopic** **7 Via Natural or Artificial Opening** **8 Via Natural or Artificial Opening Endoscopic**	**D Intraluminal Device** **Z No Device**	**Z No Qualifier**

Non-OR ØC7[B,C][Ø,3,7][D,Z]Z
Non-OR ØC7M[7,8][D,Z]Z

LC Limited Coverage NC Noncovered ⊞ Combination Member HAC associated procedure Combination Only DRG Non-OR Non-OR New/Revised in GREEN

0   **Medical and Surgical**
C   **Mouth and Throat**
9   **Drainage**   Definition: Taking or letting out fluids and/or gases from a body part
                     Explanation: The qualifier DIAGNOSTIC is used to identify drainage procedures that are biopsies

Body Part Character 4		Approach Character 5	Device Character 6	Qualifier Character 7

0 Upper Lip
  Frenulum labii superioris
  Labial gland
  Vermilion border
1 Lower Lip
  Frenulum labii inferioris
  Labial gland
  Vermilion border
2 Hard Palate
3 Soft Palate
4 Buccal Mucosa
  Buccal gland
  Molar gland
  Palatine gland
	5 Upper Gingiva
	6 Lower Gingiva
	7 Tongue
	  Frenulum linguae
	N Uvula
	  Palatine uvula
	P Tonsils
	  Palatine tonsil
	Q Adenoids
	  Pharyngeal tonsil
		0 Open
		3 Percutaneous
		X External
			0 Drainage Device	**Z** No Qualifier

0 Upper Lip
  Frenulum labii superioris
  Labial gland
  Vermilion border
1 Lower Lip
  Frenulum labii inferioris
  Labial gland
  Vermilion border
2 Hard Palate
3 Soft Palate
4 Buccal Mucosa
  Buccal gland
  Molar gland
  Palatine gland
	5 Upper Gingiva
	6 Lower Gingiva
	7 Tongue
	  Frenulum linguae
	N Uvula
	  Palatine uvula
	P Tonsils
	  Palatine tonsil
	Q Adenoids
	  Pharyngeal tonsil
		0 Open
		3 Percutaneous
		X External
			Z No Device	**X** Diagnostic
				Z No Qualifier

8 Parotid Gland, Right
9 Parotid Gland, Left
B Parotid Duct, Right
  Stensen's duct
C Parotid Duct, Left
  See B Parotid Duct, Right
D Sublingual Gland, Right
	F Sublingual Gland, Left
	G Submaxillary Gland, Right
	  Submandibular gland
	H Submaxillary Gland, Left
	  See G Submaxillary Gland, Right
	J Minor Salivary Gland
	  Anterior lingual gland
		0 Open
		3 Percutaneous
			0 Drainage Device	**Z** No Qualifier

8 Parotid Gland, Right
9 Parotid Gland, Left
B Parotid Duct, Right
  Stensen's duct
C Parotid Duct, Left
  See B Parotid Duct, Right
	D Sublingual Gland, Right
	F Sublingual Gland, Left
	G Submaxillary Gland, Right
	  Submandibular gland
	H Submaxillary Gland, Left
	  See G Submaxillary Gland, Right
	J Minor Salivary Gland
	  Anterior lingual gland
		0 Open
		3 Percutaneous
			Z No Device	**X** Diagnostic
				Z No Qualifier

M Pharynx
  Base of tongue
  Hypopharynx
  Laryngopharynx
  Lingual tonsil
  Oropharynx
  Piriform recess (sinus)
  Tongue, base of
R Epiglottis
  Glossoepiglottic fold
	S Larynx
	  Aryepiglottic fold
	  Arytenoid cartilage
	  Corniculate cartilage
	  Cuneiform cartilage
	  False vocal cord
	  Glottis
	  Rima glottidis
	  Thyroid cartilage
	  Ventricular fold
	T Vocal Cord, Right
	  Vocal fold
	V Vocal Cord, Left
	  See T Vocal Cord, Right
		0 Open
		3 Percutaneous
		4 Percutaneous Endoscopic
		7 Via Natural or Artificial Opening
		8 Via Natural or Artificial Opening Endoscopic
			0 Drainage Device	**Z** No Qualifier

0C9 Continued on next page

Non-OR	0C9[0,1,2,3,4,7,N,P,Q]30Z
Non-OR	0C9[5,6][0,3,X]0Z
Non-OR	0C9[0,1,4][0,3,X]ZX
Non-OR	0C9[0,1,2,3,4,7,N,P,Q]3ZZ
Non-OR	0C9[5,6][0,3,X]Z[X,Z]
Non-OR	0C97[3,X]ZX
Non-OR	0C9[8,9,B,C,D,F,G,H,J][0,3]0Z
Non-OR	0C9[8,9,B,C,D,F,G,H,J]3ZX
Non-OR	0C9[8,9,G,H]3ZZ
Non-OR	0C9[B,C,D, F,J][0,3]ZZ
Non-OR	0C9[M,R,S,T,V]30Z

LC Limited Coverage   **NC** Noncovered   ⊞ Combination Member   HAC associated procedure   Combination Only   DRG Non-OR   Non-OR   New/Revised in GREEN

ICD-10-PCS 2020   **349**

0C9–0C9

0C9 Continued

0	**Medical and Surgical**
C	**Mouth and Throat**
9	**Drainage**

Definition: Taking or letting out fluids and/or gases from a body part

Explanation: The qualifier DIAGNOSTIC is used to identify drainage procedures that are biopsies

Body Part Character 4		Approach Character 5	Device Character 6	Qualifier Character 7

M Pharynx
  Base of tongue
  Hypopharynx
  Laryngopharynx
  Lingual tonsil
  Oropharynx
  Piriform recess (sinus)
  Tongue, base of
R **Epiglottis**
  Glossoepiglottic fold
	S Larynx
	  Aryepiglottic fold
	  Arytenoid cartilage
	  Corniculate cartilage
	  Cuneiform cartilage
	  False vocal cord
	  Glottis
	  Rima glottidis
	  Thyroid cartilage
	  Ventricular fold
	T **Vocal Cord, Right**
	  Vocal fold
	V **Vocal Cord, Left**
	  See T Vocal Cord, Right
		0 Open
		3 Percutaneous
		4 Percutaneous Endoscopic
		7 Via Natural or Artificial Opening
		8 Via Natural or Artificial Opening Endoscopic
			Z No Device	**X** Diagnostic
				Z No Qualifier

W Upper Tooth **X** Lower Tooth		**0** Open **X** External	**0** Drainage Device **Z** No Device	**0** Single **1** Multiple **2** All

Non-OR	0C9M[0,3,4,7,8]ZX
Non-OR	0C9[M,R,S,T,V]3ZZ
Non-OR	0C9[R,S,T,V][3,4,7,8]ZX
Non-OR	0C9[W,X][0,X][0,Z][0,1,2]

0	**Medical and Surgical**
C	**Mouth and Throat**
B	**Excision**

Definition: Cutting out or off, without replacement, a portion of a body part

Explanation: The qualifier DIAGNOSTIC is used to identify excision procedures that are biopsies

Body Part Character 4		Approach Character 5	Device Character 6	Qualifier Character 7

0 Upper Lip
  Frenulum labii superioris
  Labial gland
  Vermilion border
1 Lower Lip
  Frenulum labii inferioris
  Labial gland
  Vermilion border
2 Hard Palate
3 Soft Palate
4 Buccal Mucosa
  Buccal gland
  Molar gland
  Palatine gland
	5 Upper Gingiva
	6 Lower Gingiva
	7 Tongue
	  Frenulum linguae
	N Uvula
	  Palatine uvula
	P Tonsils
	  Palatine tonsil
	Q Adenoids
	  Pharyngeal tonsil
		0 Open
		3 Percutaneous
		X External
			Z No Device	**X** Diagnostic
				Z No Qualifier

8 Parotid Gland, Right
9 Parotid Gland, Left
B Parotid Duct, Right
  Stensen's duct
C Parotid Duct, Left
  See B Parotid Duct, Right
D Sublingual Gland, Right
	F Sublingual Gland, Left
	G Submaxillary Gland, Right
	  Submandibular gland
	H Submaxillary Gland, Left
	  See G Submaxillary Gland, Right
	J Minor Salivary Gland
	  Anterior lingual gland
		0 Open
		3 Percutaneous
			Z No Device	**X** Diagnostic
				Z No Qualifier

M Pharynx
  Base of tongue
  Hypopharynx
  Laryngopharynx
  Lingual tonsil
  Oropharynx
  Piriform recess (sinus)
  Tongue, base of
R **Epiglottis**
  Glossoepiglottic fold
	S Larynx
	  Aryepiglottic fold
	  Arytenoid cartilage
	  Corniculate cartilage
	  Cuneiform cartilage
	  False vocal cord
	  Glottis
	  Rima glottidis
	  Thyroid cartilage
	  Ventricular fold
	T **Vocal Cord, Right**
	  Vocal fold
	V **Vocal Cord, Left**
	  See T Vocal Cord, Right
		0 Open
		3 Percutaneous
		4 Percutaneous Endoscopic
		7 Via Natural or Artificial Opening
		8 Via Natural or Artificial Opening Endoscopic
			Z No Device	**X** Diagnostic
				Z No Qualifier

W Upper Tooth **X** Lower Tooth		**0** Open **X** External	**Z** No Device	**0** Single **1** Multiple **2** All

Non-OR	0CB[0,1,4][0,3,X]ZX	Non-OR	0CBM[0,3,4,7,8]ZX
Non-OR	0CB[5,6][0,3,X]Z[X,Z]	Non-OR	0CB[R,S,T,V][3,4,7,8]ZX
Non-OR	0CB7[3,X]ZX	Non-OR	0CB[W,X][0,X]Z[0,1,2]
Non-OR	0CB[8,9,B,C,D,F,G,H,J]3ZX		

LC Limited Coverage   **NC** Noncovered   ⊞ Combination Member   HAC associated procedure   Combination Only   DRG Non-OR   Non-OR   New/Revised in GREEN

350   ICD-10-PCS 2020

Ø   Medical and Surgical
C   Mouth and Throat
C   Extirpation   Definition: Taking or cutting out solid matter from a body part

Explanation: The solid matter may be an abnormal byproduct of a biological function or a foreign body; it may be imbedded in a body part or in the lumen of a tubular body part. The solid matter may or may not have been previously broken into pieces.

Body Part Character 4		Approach Character 5	Device Character 6	Qualifier Character 7
Ø Upper Lip Frenulum labii superioris Labial gland Vermilion border **1** Lower Lip Frenulum labii inferioris Labial gland Vermilion border **2** Hard Palate **3** Soft Palate **4** Buccal Mucosa Buccal gland Molar gland Palatine gland	**5** Upper Gingiva **6** Lower Gingiva **7** Tongue Frenulum linguae **N** Uvula Palatine uvula **P** Tonsils Palatine tonsil **Q** Adenoids Pharyngeal tonsil	**Ø** Open **3** Percutaneous **X** External	**Z** No Device	**Z** No Qualifier
8 Parotid Gland, Right **9** Parotid Gland, Left **B** Parotid Duct, Right Stensen's duct **C** Parotid Duct, Left *See B Parotid Duct, Right* **D** Sublingual Gland, Right	**F** Sublingual Gland, Left **G** Submaxillary Gland, Right Submandibular gland **H** Submaxillary Gland, Left *See G Submaxillary Gland, Right* **J** Minor Salivary Gland Anterior lingual gland	**Ø** Open **3** Percutaneous	**Z** No Device	**Z** No Qualifier
M Pharynx Base of tongue Hypopharynx Laryngopharynx Lingual tonsil Oropharynx Piriform recess (sinus) Tongue, base of **R** Epiglottis Glossoepiglottic fold	**S** Larynx Aryepiglottic fold Arytenoid cartilage Corniculate cartilage Cuneiform cartilage False vocal cord Glottis Rima glottidis Thyroid cartilage Ventricular fold **T** Vocal Cord, Right Vocal fold **V** Vocal Cord, Left *See T Vocal Cord, Right*	**Ø** Open **3** Percutaneous **4** Percutaneous Endoscopic **7** Via Natural or Artificial Opening **8** Via Natural or Artificial Opening Endoscopic	**Z** No Device	**Z** No Qualifier
W Upper Tooth **X** Lower Tooth		**Ø** Open **X** External	**Z** No Device	**Ø** Single **1** Multiple **2** All

Non-OR	ØCC[Ø,1,2,3,4,7,N,P,Q]XZZ
Non-OR	ØCC[5,6][Ø,3,X]ZZ
Non-OR	ØCC[8,9,G,H]3ZZ
Non-OR	ØCC[B,C,D, F,J][Ø,3]ZZ
Non-OR	ØCC[M,S][7,8]ZZ
Non-OR	ØCC[W,X][Ø,X]Z[Ø,1,2]

Ø   Medical and Surgical
C   Mouth and Throat
D   Extraction   Definition: Pulling or stripping out or off all or a portion of a body part by the use of force

Explanation: The qualifier DIAGNOSTIC is used to identify extraction procedures that are biopsies

Body Part Character 4	Approach Character 5	Device Character 6	Qualifier Character 7
T Vocal Cord, Right Vocal fold **V** Vocal Cord, Left *See T Vocal Cord, Right*	**Ø** Open **3** Percutaneous **4** Percutaneous Endoscopic **7** Via Natural or Artificial Opening **8** Via Natural or Artificial Opening Endoscopic	**Z** No Device	**Z** No Qualifier
W Upper Tooth **X** Lower Tooth	**X** External	**Z** No Device	**Ø** Single **1** Multiple **2** All

Non-OR	ØCD[W,X]XZ[Ø,1,2]

LC Limited Coverage   **NC** Noncovered   ⊞ Combination Member   HAC associated procedure   Combination Only   DRG Non-OR   Non-OR   New/Revised in GREEN

ICD-10-PCS 2020   351

Ø Medical and Surgical
C Mouth and Throat
F Fragmentation Definition: Breaking solid matter in a body part into pieces

Explanation: Physical force (e.g., manual, ultrasonic) applied directly or indirectly is used to break the solid matter into pieces. The solid matter may be an abnormal byproduct of a biological function or a foreign body. The pieces of solid matter are not taken out.

Body Part Character 4	Approach Character 5	Device Character 6	Qualifier Character 7
B Parotid Duct, Right NC Stensen's duct C Parotid Duct, Left NC *See B Parotid Duct, Right*	Ø Open 3 Percutaneous 7 Via Natural or Artificial Opening X External	Z No Device	Z No Qualifier

Non-OR All body part, approach, device, and qualifier values
NC ØCF[B,C]XZZ

Ø Medical and Surgical
C Mouth and Throat
H Insertion Definition: Putting in a nonbiological appliance that monitors, assists, performs, or prevents a physiological function but does not physically take the place of a body part

Explanation: None

Body Part Character 4	Approach Character 5	Device Character 6	Qualifier Character 7
7 Tongue Frenulum linguae	Ø Open 3 Percutaneous X External	1 Radioactive Element	Z No Qualifier
A Salivary Gland S Larynx Aryepiglottic fold Arytenoid cartilage Corniculate cartilage Cuneiform cartilage False vocal cord Glottis Rima glottidis Thyroid cartilage Ventricular fold	Ø Open 3 Percutaneous 7 Via Natural or Artificial Opening 8 Via Natural or Artificial Opening Endoscopic	Y Other Device	Z No Qualifier
Y Mouth and Throat	Ø Open 3 Percutaneous	Y Other Device	Z No Qualifier
Y Mouth and Throat	7 Via Natural or Artificial Opening 8 Via Natural or Artificial Opening Endoscopic	B Intraluminal Device, Airway Y Other Device	Z No Qualifier

Non-OR ØCH[A,S][3,7,8]YZ
Non-OR ØCHSØYZ
Non-OR ØCHY[Ø,3]YZ
Non-OR ØCHY[7,8][B,Y]Z

Ø Medical and Surgical
C Mouth and Throat
J Inspection Definition: Visually and/or manually exploring a body part

Explanation: Visual exploration may be performed with or without optical instrumentation. Manual exploration may be performed directly or through intervening body layers.

Body Part Character 4	Approach Character 5	Device Character 6	Qualifier Character 7
A Salivary Gland	Ø Open 3 Percutaneous X External	Z No Device	Z No Qualifier
S Larynx Aryepiglottic fold Arytenoid cartilage Corniculate cartilage Cuneiform cartilage False vocal cord Glottis Rima glottidis Thyroid cartilage Ventricular fold Y Mouth and Throat	Ø Open 3 Percutaneous 4 Percutaneous Endoscopic 7 Via Natural or Artificial Opening 8 Via Natural or Artificial Opening Endoscopic X External	Z No Device	Z No Qualifier

Non-OR All body part, approach, device, and qualifier values

Ø **Medical and Surgical**
C **Mouth and Throat**
L **Occlusion** Definition: Completely closing an orifice or the lumen of a tubular body part
　　　　　　　　Explanation: The orifice can be a natural orifice or an artificially created orifice

Body Part Character 4	Approach Character 5	Device Character 6	Qualifier Character 7
B Parotid Duct, Right Stensen's duct **C** Parotid Duct, Left *See B Parotid Duct, Right*	**Ø** Open **3** Percutaneous **4** Percutaneous Endoscopic	**C** Extraluminal Device **D** Intraluminal Device **Z** No Device	**Z** No Qualifier
B Parotid Duct, Right Stensen's duct **C** Parotid Duct, Left *See B Parotid Duct, Right*	**7** Via Natural or Artificial Opening **8** Via Natural or Artificial Opening 　　Endoscopic	**D** Intraluminal Device **Z** No Device	**Z** No Qualifier

Ø **Medical and Surgical**
C **Mouth and Throat**
M **Reattachment** Definition: Putting back in or on all or a portion of a separated body part to its normal location or other suitable location
　　　　　　　　　Explanation: Vascular circulation and nervous pathways may or may not be reestablished

Body Part Character 4	Approach Character 5	Device Character 6	Qualifier Character 7
Ø Upper Lip 　Frenulum labii superioris 　Labial gland 　Vermilion border **1** Lower Lip 　Frenulum labii inferioris 　Labial gland 　Vermilion border **3** Soft Palate **7** Tongue 　Frenulum linguae **N** Uvula 　Palatine uvula	**Ø** Open	**Z** No Device	**Z** No Qualifier
W Upper Tooth **X** Lower Tooth	**Ø** Open **X** External	**Z** No Device	**Ø** Single **1** Multiple **2** All

Non-OR ØCM[W,X][Ø,X]Z[Ø,1,2]

LC Limited Coverage　**NC** Noncovered　⊞ Combination Member　HAC associated procedure　Combination Only　DRG Non-OR　Non-OR　New/Revised in GREEN

ICD-10-PCS 2020　　　　　　　　　　　　　　　　　　　　　　　　　　　　　　　　　　　353

Mouth and Throat

Ø   **Medical and Surgical**
C   **Mouth and Throat**
N   **Release**   Definition: Freeing a body part from an abnormal physical constraint by cutting or by the use of force
                     Explanation: Some of the restraining tissue may be taken out but none of the body part is taken out

Body Part Character 4	Approach Character 5	Device Character 6	Qualifier Character 7

Ø   **Upper Lip**
    Frenulum labii superioris
    Labial gland
    Vermilion border
1   **Lower Lip**
    Frenulum labii inferioris
    Labial gland
    Vermilion border
2   **Hard Palate**
3   **Soft Palate**
4   **Buccal Mucosa**
    Buccal gland
    Molar gland
    Palatine gland
5   **Upper Gingiva**
6   **Lower Gingiva**
7   **Tongue**
    Frenulum linguae
N   **Uvula**
    Palatine uvula
P   **Tonsils**
    Palatine tonsil
Q   **Adenoids**
    Pharyngeal tonsil
	Ø **Open**
	3 **Percutaneous**
	X **External**
		Z **No Device**	Z **No Qualifier**

8   **Parotid Gland, Right**
9   **Parotid Gland, Left**
B   **Parotid Duct, Right**
    Stensen's duct
C   **Parotid Duct, Left**
    See B Parotid Duct, Right
D   **Sublingual Gland, Right**
F   **Sublingual Gland, Left**
G   **Submaxillary Gland, Right**
    Submandibular gland
H   **Submaxillary Gland, Left**
    See G Submaxillary Gland, Right
J   **Minor Salivary Gland**
    Anterior lingual gland
	Ø **Open**
	3 **Percutaneous**
		Z **No Device**	Z **No Qualifier**

M   **Pharynx**
    Base of tongue
    Hypopharynx
    Laryngopharynx
    Lingual tonsil
    Oropharynx
    Piriform recess (sinus)
    Tongue, base of
R   **Epiglottis**
    Glossoepiglottic fold
S   **Larynx**
    Aryepiglottic fold
    Arytenoid cartilage
    Corniculate cartilage
    Cuneiform cartilage
    False vocal cord
    Glottis
    Rima glottidis
    Thyroid cartilage
    Ventricular fold
T   **Vocal Cord, Right**
    Vocal fold
V   **Vocal Cord, Left**
    See T Vocal Cord, Right
	Ø **Open**
	3 **Percutaneous**
	4 **Percutaneous Endoscopic**
	7 **Via Natural or Artificial Opening**
	8 **Via Natural or Artificial Opening Endoscopic**
		Z **No Device**	Z **No Qualifier**

W **Upper Tooth** X **Lower Tooth**	Ø **Open** X **External**	Z **No Device**	Ø **Single** 1 **Multiple** 2 **All**

Non-OR   ØCN[Ø,1,5,6,7][Ø,3,X]ZZ
Non-OR   ØCN[W,X][Ø,X]Z[Ø,1,2]

Ø Medical and Surgical
C Mouth and Throat
P Removal   Definition: Taking out or off a device from a body part

Explanation: If a device is taken out and a similar device put in without cutting or puncturing the skin or mucous membrane, the procedure is coded to the root operation CHANGE. Otherwise, the procedure for taking out a device is coded to the root operation REMOVAL.

Body Part Character 4	Approach Character 5	Device Character 6	Qualifier Character 7
A Salivary Gland	**Ø** Open **3** Percutaneous	**Ø** Drainage Device **C** Extraluminal Device **Y** Other Device	**Z** No Qualifier
A Salivary Gland	**7** Via Natural or Artificial Opening **8** Via Natural or Artificial Opening Endoscopic	**Y** Other Device	**Z** No Qualifier
S Larynx Aryepiglottic fold Arytenoid cartilage Corniculate cartilage Cuneiform cartilage False vocal cord Glottis Rima glottidis Thyroid cartilage Ventricular fold	**Ø** Open **3** Percutaneous **7** Via Natural or Artificial Opening **8** Via Natural or Artificial Opening Endoscopic	**Ø** Drainage Device **7** Autologous Tissue Substitute **D** Intraluminal Device **J** Synthetic Substitute **K** Nonautologous Tissue Substitute **Y** Other Device	**Z** No Qualifier
S Larynx Aryepiglottic fold Arytenoid cartilage Corniculate cartilage Cuneiform cartilage False vocal cord Glottis Rima glottidis Thyroid cartilage Ventricular fold	**X** External	**Ø** Drainage Device **7** Autologous Tissue Substitute **D** Intraluminal Device **J** Synthetic Substitute **K** Nonautologous Tissue Substitute	**Z** No Qualifier
Y Mouth and Throat	**Ø** Open **3** Percutaneous **7** Via Natural or Artificial Opening **8** Via Natural or Artificial Opening Endoscopic	**Ø** Drainage Device **1** Radioactive Element **7** Autologous Tissue Substitute **D** Intraluminal Device **J** Synthetic Substitute **K** Nonautologous Tissue Substitute **Y** Other Device	**Z** No Qualifier
Y Mouth and Throat	**X** External	**Ø** Drainage Device **1** Radioactive Element **7** Autologous Tissue Substitute **D** Intraluminal Device **J** Synthetic Substitute **K** Nonautologous Tissue Substitute	**Z** No Qualifier

Non-OR ØCPA[Ø,3][Ø,C,Y]Z
Non-OR ØCPA[7,8]YZ
Non-OR ØCPS3YZ
Non-OR ØCPS[7,8][Ø,D,Y]Z
Non-OR ØCPSX[Ø,7,D,J,K]Z
Non-OR ØCPY3YZ
Non-OR ØCPY[7,8][Ø,D,Y]Z
Non-OR ØCPYX[Ø,1,7,D,J,K]Z

LC Limited Coverage   NC Noncovered   ⊞ Combination Member   HAC associated procedure   Combination Only   DRG Non-OR   Non-OR   New/Revised in GREEN

ICD-10-PCS 2020   355

ØCP–ØCP

Mouth and Throat

Ø   **Medical and Surgical**
C   **Mouth and Throat**
Q   **Repair**   Definition: Restoring, to the extent possible, a body part to its normal anatomic structure and function

                     Explanation: Used only when the method to accomplish the repair is not one of the other root operations

Body Part Character 4	Approach Character 5	Device Character 6	Qualifier Character 7

Ø   **Upper Lip**
    Frenulum labii superioris
    Labial gland
    Vermilion border
1   **Lower Lip**
    Frenulum labii inferioris
    Labial gland
    Vermilion border
2   **Hard Palate**
3   **Soft Palate**
4   **Buccal Mucosa**
    Buccal gland
    Molar gland
    Palatine gland
5   **Upper Gingiva**
6   **Lower Gingiva**
7   **Tongue**
    Frenulum linguae
N   **Uvula**
    Palatine uvula
P   **Tonsils**
    Palatine tonsil
Q   **Adenoids**
    Pharyngeal tonsil
	Ø Open
	3 Percutaneous
	X External
		Z No Device	**Z** No Qualifier

8   **Parotid Gland, Right**
9   **Parotid Gland, Left**
B   **Parotid Duct, Right**
    Stensen's duct
C   **Parotid Duct, Left**
    See B Parotid Duct, Right
D   **Sublingual Gland, Right**
F   **Sublingual Gland, Left**
G   **Submaxillary Gland, Right**
    Submandibular gland
H   **Submaxillary Gland, Left**
    See G Submaxillary Gland, Right
J   **Minor Salivary Gland**
    Anterior lingual gland
	Ø Open
	3 Percutaneous
		Z No Device	**Z** No Qualifier

M   **Pharynx**
    Base of tongue
    Hypopharynx
    Laryngopharynx
    Lingual tonsil
    Oropharynx
    Piriform recess (sinus)
    Tongue, base of
R   **Epiglottis**
    Glossoepiglottic fold
S   **Larynx**
    Aryepiglottic fold
    Arytenoid cartilage
    Corniculate cartilage
    Cuneiform cartilage
    False vocal cord
    Glottis
    Rima glottidis
    Thyroid cartilage
    Ventricular fold
T   **Vocal Cord, Right**
    Vocal fold
V   **Vocal Cord, Left**
    See T Vocal Cord, Right
	Ø Open
	3 Percutaneous
	4 Percutaneous Endoscopic
	7 Via Natural or Artificial Opening
	8 Via Natural or Artificial Opening Endoscopic
		Z No Device	**Z** No Qualifier

W **Upper Tooth** **X** **Lower Tooth**	**Ø** Open **X** External	**Z** No Device	**Ø** Single **1** Multiple **2** All

Non-OR   ØCQ[Ø,1,4,7]XZZ
Non-OR   ØCQ[5,6][Ø,3,X]ZZ
Non-OR   ØCQ[W,X][Ø,X]Z[Ø,1,2]

LC Limited Coverage   **NC** Noncovered   ⊞ Combination Member   HAC associated procedure   Combination Only   DRG Non-OR   Non-OR   New/Revised in **GREEN**

356   ICD-10-PCS 2020

Ø   **Medical and Surgical**
C   **Mouth and Throat**
R   **Replacement**   Definition: Putting in or on biological or synthetic material that physically takes the place and/or function of all or a portion of a body part

Explanation: The body part may have been taken out or replaced, or may be taken out, physically eradicated, or rendered nonfunctional during the REPLACEMENT procedure. A REMOVAL procedure is coded for taking out the device used in a previous replacement procedure.

Body Part Character 4	Approach Character 5	Device Character 6	Qualifier Character 7

Ø **Upper Lip**
   Frenulum labii superioris
   Labial gland
   Vermilion border
1 **Lower Lip**
   Frenulum labii inferioris
   Labial gland
   Vermilion border
2 **Hard Palate**
3 **Soft Palate**
4 **Buccal Mucosa**
   Buccal gland
   Molar gland
   Palatine gland
5 **Upper Gingiva**
6 **Lower Gingiva**
7 **Tongue**
   Frenulum linguae
N **Uvula**
   Palatine uvula
	Ø Open
	3 Percutaneous
	X External
		7 Autologous Tissue Substitute
		J Synthetic Substitute
		K Nonautologous Tissue Substitute
			Z No Qualifier

B **Parotid Duct, Right**
   Stensen's duct
C **Parotid Duct, Left**
   See B Parotid Duct, Right
	Ø Open
	3 Percutaneous
		7 Autologous Tissue Substitute
		J Synthetic Substitute
		K Nonautologous Tissue Substitute
			Z No Qualifier

M **Pharynx**
   Base of tongue
   Hypopharynx
   Laryngopharynx
   Lingual tonsil
   Oropharynx
   Piriform recess (sinus)
   Tongue, base of
R **Epiglottis**
   Glossoepiglottic fold
S **Larynx**
   Aryepiglottic fold
   Arytenoid cartilage
   Corniculate cartilage
   Cuneiform cartilage
   False vocal cord
   Glottis
   Rima glottidis
   Thyroid cartilage
   Ventricular fold
T **Vocal Cord, Right**
   Vocal fold
V **Vocal Cord, Left**
   See T Vocal Cord, Right
	Ø Open
	7 Via Natural or Artificial Opening
	8 Via Natural or Artificial Opening Endoscopic
		7 Autologous Tissue Substitute
		J Synthetic Substitute
		K Nonautologous Tissue Substitute
			Z No Qualifier

W **Upper Tooth** **X** **Lower Tooth**	**Ø** Open **X** External	**7** Autologous Tissue Substitute **J** Synthetic Substitute **K** Nonautologous Tissue Substitute	**Ø** Single **1** Multiple **2** All

Non-OR   ØCR[W,X][Ø,X][7,J,K][Ø,1,2]

LC Limited Coverage   **NC** Noncovered   ⊞ Combination Member   HAC associated procedure   Combination Only   DRG Non-OR   Non-OR   New/Revised in GREEN

ICD-10-PCS 2020　　　　　　　　　　　　　　　　　　　　　　　　　　　　　　　　　　　　　**357**

ØCR–ØCR

Ø   Medical and Surgical
C   Mouth and Throat
S   Reposition   Definition: Moving to its normal location, or other suitable location, all or a portion of a body part

                Explanation: The body part is moved to a new location from an abnormal location, or from a normal location where it is not functioning correctly. The body part may or may not be cut out or off to be moved to the new location.

Body Part Character 4	Approach Character 5	Device Character 6	Qualifier Character 7

Ø   Upper Lip
    Frenulum labii superioris
    Labial gland
    Vermilion border
1   Lower Lip
    Frenulum labii inferioris
    Labial gland
    Vermilion border
2   Hard Palate
3   Soft Palate
7   Tongue
    Frenulum linguae
N   Uvula
    Palatine uvula
	Ø Open
	X External
		Z No Device	**Z No Qualifier**

B   Parotid Duct, Right
    Stensen's duct
C   Parotid Duct, Left
    See B Parotid Duct, Right
	Ø Open
	3 Percutaneous
		Z No Device	**Z No Qualifier**

R   Epiglottis
    Glossoepiglottic fold
T   Vocal Cord, Right
    Vocal fold
V   Vocal Cord, Left
    See T Vocal Cord, Right
	Ø Open
	7 Via Natural or Artificial Opening
	**8 Via Natural or Artificial Opening
	    Endoscopic**
		Z No Device	**Z No Qualifier**

W Upper Tooth **X Lower Tooth**	**Ø Open** **X External**	**5 External Fixation Device** **Z No Device**	**Ø Single** **1 Multiple** **2 All**

Non-OR   ØCS[W,X][Ø,X][5,Z][Ø,1,2]

LC Limited Coverage   NC Noncovered   ⊞ Combination Member   HAC associated procedure   Combination Only   DRG Non-OR   Non-OR   New/Revised in GREEN

358   ICD-10-PCS 2020

0   **Medical and Surgical**
C   **Mouth and Throat**
T   **Resection**   Definition: Cutting out or off, without replacement, all of a body part
                    Explanation: None

Body Part Character 4	Approach Character 5	Device Character 6	Qualifier Character 7

0   **Upper Lip**
    Frenulum labii superioris
    Labial gland
    Vermilion border
1   **Lower Lip**
    Frenulum labii inferioris
    Labial gland
    Vermilion border
2   **Hard Palate**
3   **Soft Palate**
7   **Tongue**
    Frenulum linguae
N   **Uvula**
    Palatine uvula
P   **Tonsils**
    Palatine tonsil
Q   **Adenoids**
    Pharyngeal tonsil
	0 Open
	X External
		Z No Device	**Z** No Qualifier

8   **Parotid Gland, Right**
9   **Parotid Gland, Left**
B   **Parotid Duct, Right**
    Stensen's duct
C   **Parotid Duct, Left**
    See B Parotid Duct, Right
D   **Sublingual Gland, Right**
F   **Sublingual Gland, Left**
G   **Submaxillary Gland, Right**
    Submandibular gland
H   **Submaxillary Gland, Left**
    See G Submaxillary Gland, Right
J   **Minor Salivary Gland**
    Anterior lingual gland
	0 Open	**Z** No Device	**Z** No Qualifier

M   **Pharynx**
    Base of tongue
    Hypopharynx
    Laryngopharynx
    Lingual tonsil
    Oropharynx
    Piriform recess (sinus)
    Tongue, base of
R   **Epiglottis**
    Glossoepiglottic fold
S   **Larynx**
    Aryepiglottic fold
    Arytenoid cartilage
    Corniculate cartilage
    Cuneiform cartilage
    False vocal cord
    Glottis
    Rima glottidis
    Thyroid cartilage
    Ventricular fold
T   **Vocal Cord, Right**
    Vocal fold
V   **Vocal Cord, Left**
    See T Vocal Cord, Right
	0 Open
	4 Percutaneous Endoscopic
	7 Via Natural or Artificial Opening
	8 Via Natural or Artificial Opening
	    Endoscopic
		Z No Device	**Z** No Qualifier

W **Upper Tooth** **X** **Lower Tooth**	**0** Open	**Z** No Device	**0** Single **1** Multiple **2** All

Non-OR   0CT[W,X]0Z[0,1,2]

LC Limited Coverage   NC Noncovered   ⊞ Combination Member   HAC associated procedure   Combination Only   DRG Non-OR   Non-OR   New/Revised in GREEN

ICD-10-PCS 2020   359

Mouth and Throat

Ø Medical and Surgical
C Mouth and Throat
U Supplement Definition: Putting in or on biological or synthetic material that physically reinforces and/or augments the function of a portion of a body part

Explanation: The biological material is non-living, or is living and from the same individual. The body part may have been previously replaced, and the SUPPLEMENT procedure is performed to physically reinforce and/or augment the function of the replaced body part.

Body Part Character 4	Approach Character 5	Device Character 6	Qualifier Character 7

Ø Upper Lip
  Frenulum labii superioris
  Labial gland
  Vermilion border
1 Lower Lip
  Frenulum labii inferioris
  Labial gland
  Vermilion border
2 Hard Palate
3 Soft Palate
4 Buccal Mucosa
  Buccal gland
  Molar gland
  Palatine gland
5 Upper Gingiva
6 Lower Gingiva
7 Tongue
  Frenulum linguae
N Uvula
  Palatine uvula
	Ø Open
	3 Percutaneous
	X External
		7 Autologous Tissue Substitute
		J Synthetic Substitute
		K Nonautologous Tissue Substitute
			Z No Qualifier

M Pharynx
  Base of tongue
  Hypopharynx
  Laryngopharynx
  Lingual tonsil
  Oropharynx
  Piriform recess (sinus)
  Tongue, base of
R Epiglottis
  Glossoepiglottic fold
S Larynx
  Aryepiglottic fold
  Arytenoid cartilage
  Corniculate cartilage
  Cuneiform cartilage
  False vocal cord
  Glottis
  Rima glottidis
  Thyroid cartilage
  Ventricular fold
T Vocal Cord, Right
  Vocal fold
V Vocal Cord, Left
  See T Vocal Cord, Right
	Ø Open
	7 Via Natural or Artificial Opening
	8 Via Natural or Artificial Opening Endoscopic
		7 Autologous Tissue Substitute
		J Synthetic Substitute
		K Nonautologous Tissue Substitute
			Z No Qualifier

Non-OR ØCU2[Ø,3]JZ

Ø Medical and Surgical
C Mouth and Throat
V Restriction Definition: Partially closing an orifice or the lumen of a tubular body part

Explanation: The orifice can be a natural orifice or an artificially created orifice

Body Part Character 4	Approach Character 5	Device Character 6	Qualifier Character 7

B Parotid Duct, Right
  Stensen's duct
C Parotid Duct, Left
  See B Parotid Duct, Right
	Ø Open
	3 Percutaneous
		C Extraluminal Device
		D Intraluminal Device
		Z No Device
			Z No Qualifier

B Parotid Duct, Right
  Stensen's duct
C Parotid Duct, Left
  See B Parotid Duct, Right
	7 Via Natural or Artificial Opening
	8 Via Natural or Artificial Opening Endoscopic
		D Intraluminal Device
		Z No Device
			Z No Qualifier

Ø   Medical and Surgical
C   Mouth and Throat
W   Revision   Definition: Correcting, to the extent possible, a portion of a malfunctioning device or the position of a displaced device
                Explanation: Revision can include correcting a malfunctioning or displaced device by taking out or putting in components of the device such as a screw or pin

Body Part Character 4	Approach Character 5	Device Character 6	Qualifier Character 7
A Salivary Gland	**Ø** Open **3** Percutaneous	**Ø** Drainage Device **C** Extraluminal Device **Y** Other Device	**Z** No Qualifier
A Salivary Gland	**7** Via Natural or Artificial Opening **8** Via Natural or Artificial Opening Endoscopic	**Y** Other Device	**Z** No Qualifier
A Salivary Gland	**X** External	**Ø** Drainage Device **C** Extraluminal Device	**Z** No Qualifier

S   Larynx
     Aryepiglottic fold
     Arytenoid cartilage
     Corniculate cartilage
     Cuneiform cartilage
     False vocal cord
     Glottis
     Rima glottidis
     Thyroid cartilage
     Ventricular fold
	Ø Open
	3 Percutaneous
	7 Via Natural or Artificial Opening
	8 Via Natural or Artificial Opening
	     Endoscopic
		Ø Drainage Device
		7 Autologous Tissue Substitute
		D Intraluminal Device
		J Synthetic Substitute
		K Nonautologous Tissue Substitute
		Y Other Device
			Z No Qualifier

S   Larynx
     Aryepiglottic fold
     Arytenoid cartilage
     Corniculate cartilage
     Cuneiform cartilage
     False vocal cord
     Glottis
     Rima glottidis
     Thyroid cartilage
     Ventricular fold
	X External	**Ø** Drainage Device
		7 Autologous Tissue Substitute
		D Intraluminal Device
		J Synthetic Substitute
		K Nonautologous Tissue Substitute
			Z No Qualifier

Y Mouth and Throat	**Ø** Open **3** Percutaneous **7** Via Natural or Artificial Opening **8** Via Natural or Artificial Opening Endoscopic	**Ø** Drainage Device **1** Radioactive Element **7** Autologous Tissue Substitute **D** Intraluminal Device **J** Synthetic Substitute **K** Nonautologous Tissue Substitute **Y** Other Device	**Z** No Qualifier
Y Mouth and Throat	**X** External	**Ø** Drainage Device **1** Radioactive Element **7** Autologous Tissue Substitute **D** Intraluminal Device **J** Synthetic Substitute **K** Nonautologous Tissue Substitute	**Z** No Qualifier

Non-OR   ØCWA[Ø,3][Ø,C,Y]Z
Non-OR   ØCWA[7,8]YZ
Non-OR   ØCWAX[Ø,C]Z
Non-OR   ØCWS[3,7,8]YZ
Non-OR   ØCWSX[Ø,7,D,J,K]Z
Non-OR   ØCWYØ7Z
Non-OR   ØCWY[3,7,8]YZ
Non-OR   ØCWYX[Ø,1,7,D,J,K]Z

Mouth and Throat

Ø   **Medical and Surgical**
C   **Mouth and Throat**
X   **Transfer**   Definition: Moving, without taking out, all or a portion of a body part to another location to take over the function of all or a portion of a body part
                                     Explanation: The body part transferred remains connected to its vascular and nervous supply

Body Part Character 4	Approach Character 5	Device Character 6	Qualifier Character 7

Ø Upper Lip
   Frenulum labii superioris
   Labial gland
   Vermilion border
1 Lower Lip
   Frenulum labii inferioris
   Labial gland
   Vermilion border
3 Soft Palate
4 Buccal Mucosa
   Buccal gland
   Molar gland
   Palatine gland
5 Upper Gingiva
6 Lower Gingiva
7 Tongue
   Frenulum linguae
	Ø Open
	X External
		Z No Device	**Z No Qualifier**

LC Limited Coverage   **NC** Noncovered   ⊞ Combination Member   HAC associated procedure   Combination Only   DRG Non-OR   Non-OR   New/Revised in GREEN

362   ICD-10-PCS 2020

Gastrointestinal System ØD1–ØDY

Character Meanings

This Character Meaning table is provided as a guide to assist the user in the identification of character members that may be found in this section of code tables. It **SHOULD NOT** be used to build a PCS code.

Operation–Character 3		Body Part–Character 4		Approach–Character 5		Device–Character 6		Qualifier–Character 7	
1	Bypass	Ø	Upper Intestinal Tract	Ø	Open	Ø	Drainage Device	Ø	Allogeneic
2	Change	1	Esophagus, Upper	3	Percutaneous	1	Radioactive Element	1	Syngeneic
5	Destruction	2	Esophagus, Middle	4	Percutaneous Endoscopic	2	Monitoring Device	2	Zooplastic
7	Dilation	3	Esophagus, Lower	7	Via Natural or Artificial Opening	3	Infusion Device	3	Vertical
8	Division	4	Esophagogastric Junction	8	Via Natural or Artificial Opening Endoscopic	7	Autologous Tissue Substitute	4	Cutaneous
9	Drainage	5	Esophagus	F	Via Natural or Artificial Opening with Percutaneous Endoscopic Assistance	B	Intraluminal Device, Airway	5	Esophagus
B	Excision	6	Stomach	X	External	C	Extraluminal Device	6	Stomach
C	Extirpation	7	Stomach, Pylorus			D	Intraluminal Device	7	Vagina
D	Extraction	8	Small Intestine			J	Synthetic Substitute	8	Small Intestine
F	Fragmentation	9	Duodenum			K	Nonautologous Tissue Substitute	9	Duodenum
H	Insertion	A	Jejunum			L	Artificial Sphincter	A	Jejunum
J	Inspection	B	Ileum			M	Stimulator Lead	B	Ileum
L	Occlusion	C	Ileocecal Valve			U	Feeding Device	E	Large Intestine
M	Reattachment	D	Lower Intestinal Tract			Y	Other Device	H	Cecum
N	Release	E	Large Intestine			Z	No Device	K	Ascending Colon
P	Removal	F	Large Intestine, Right					L	Transverse Colon
Q	Repair	G	Large Intestine, Left					M	Descending Colon
R	Replacement	H	Cecum					N	Sigmoid Colon
S	Reposition	J	Appendix					P	Rectum
T	Resection	K	Ascending Colon					Q	Anus
U	Supplement	L	Transverse Colon					X	Diagnostic
V	Restriction	M	Descending Colon					Z	No Qualifier
W	Revision	N	Sigmoid Colon						
X	Transfer	P	Rectum						
Y	Transplantation	Q	Anus						
		R	Anal Sphincter						
		U	Omentum						
		V	Mesentery						
		W	Peritoneum						

AHA Coding Clinic for table ØD1

2017, 2Q, 17	Billroth II (distal gastrectomy and gastrojejunostomy)
2016, 2Q, 31	Laparoscopic biliopancreatic diversion with duodenal switch
2014, 4Q, 41	Abdominoperineal resection (APR) with flap closure of perineum and colostomy

AHA Coding Clinic for table ØD2

2019, 1Q, 26	Exchange of clogged gastrojejunostomy tube

AHA Coding Clinic for table ØD5

2017, 1Q, 34	Debulking of tumor and peritoneum ablation

AHA Coding Clinic for table ØD7

2017, 3Q, 23	Laparoscopic pyloromyotomy
2014, 4Q, 40	Dilation of gastrojejunostomy anastomosis stricture

AHA Coding Clinic for table ØD8

2017, 3Q, 22	Laparoscopic esophagomyotomy (Heller type) and Toupet fundoplication
2017, 3Q, 23	Laparoscopic pyloromyotomy

AHA Coding Clinic for table ØD9

2015, 2Q, 29	Insertion of nasogastric tube for drainage and feeding

AHA Coding Clinic for table ØDB

2019, 1Q, 3-8	Whipple procedure
2019, 1Q, 27	Excision of pelvic sidewall mass
2017, 2Q, 17	Billroth II (distal gastrectomy and gastrojejunostomy)
2017, 1Q, 16	Hepatic flexure versus transverse colon
2016, 3Q, 3-7	Stoma creation & takedown procedures
2016, 2Q, 31	Laparoscopic biliopancreatic diversion with duodenal switch
2016, 1Q, 22	Perineal proctectomy
2016, 1Q, 24	Endoscopic brush biopsy of esophagus
2014, 4Q, 40	Abdominoperineal resection (APR) with flap closure of perineum and colostomy
2014, 3Q, 28	Ileostomy takedown and parastomal hernia repair
2014, 3Q, 32	Pyloric-sparing Whipple procedure

AHA Coding Clinic for table ØDD

2017, 4Q, 41-42	Extraction procedures

AHA Coding Clinic for table ØDH

2016, 3Q, 26	Insertion of gastrostomy tube
2013, 4Q, 117	Percutaneous endoscopic placement of gastrostomy tube

AHA Coding Clinic for table ØDJ

2019, 1Q, 25	Laparoscopic appendectomy converted to open procedure
2019, 1Q, 25	Milking of inspissated material from ileum to colon
2017, 2Q, 15	Low anterior resection with sigmoidoscopy
2016, 2Q, 20	Capsule endoscopy of small intestine
2015, 3Q, 24	Esophagogastroduodenoscopy with epinephrine injection for control of bleeding

AHA Coding Clinic for table ØDL

2013, 4Q, 112	Endoscopic banding of esophageal varices

AHA Coding Clinic for table ØDN

2017, 4Q, 49-50	New and revised body part values - Repositioning of the intestine
2017, 1Q, 35	Lysis of omental and peritoneal adhesions
2015, 3Q, 15	Vascular ring surgery with release of esophagus and trachea
2015, 3Q, 16	Vascular ring surgery and double aortic arch

AHA Coding Clinic for table ØDQ

2018, 2Q, 25	Third and fourth degree obstetric lacerations
2018, 1Q, 11	Repair of internal hernia at Petersen space
2017, 3Q, 17	Posterior sagittal anorectoplasty
2016, 3Q, 3-7	Stoma creation & takedown procedures
2016, 3Q, 26	Insertion of gastrostomy tube
2016, 1Q, 7	Obstetrical perineal laceration repair
2016, 1Q, 8	Obstetrical perineal laceration repair
2014, 4Q, 20	Control of bleeding duodenal ulcer

AHA Coding Clinic for table ØDS

2019, 1Q, 30	Laparoscopic-assisted rectopexy with manual reduction of prolapse
2017, 4Q, 49-50	New and revised body part values - Repositioning of the intestine
2017, 3Q, 9	Ileocolic intussusception reduction via air enema
2017, 3Q, 17	Posterior sagittal anorectoplasty
2016, 3Q, 3-5	Stoma creation & takedown procedures

AHA Coding Clinic for table ØDT

2019, 1Q, 3-8	Whipple procedure
2019, 1Q, 14	Esophagectomy with colon interposition
2017, 4Q, 49-50	New and revised body part values - Repositioning of the intestine
2014, 4Q, 40	Abdominoperineal resection (APR) with flap closure of perineum and colostomy
2014, 4Q, 42	Right colectomy with side-to-side functional end-to-end anastomosis
2014, 3Q, 6	Ileocecectomy including cecum, terminal ileum and appendix
2014, 3Q, 6	Right colectomy

AHA Coding Clinic for table ØDU

2019, 1Q, 30	Laparoscopic-assisted rectopexy with manual reduction of prolapse

AHA Coding Clinic for table ØDV

2017, 3Q, 22	Laparoscopic esophagomyotomy (Heller type) and Toupet fundoplication
2016, 2Q, 22	Esophageal lengthening Collis gastroplasty with Nissen fundoplication and hiatal hernia
2014, 3Q, 28	Laparoscopic Nissen fundoplication and diaphragmatic hernia repair

AHA Coding Clinic for table ØDW

2018, 1Q, 20	Adjustment of gastric band

AHA Coding Clinic for table ØDX

2019, 1Q, 14	Esophagectomy with colon interposition
2017, 2Q, 18	Esophagectomy and esophagogastrectomy with cervical esophagogastrostomy
2016, 2Q, 22	Esophageal lengthening Collis gastroplasty with Nissen fundoplication and hiatal hernia
2015, 1Q, 28	Repair of bronchopleural fistula using omental pedicle graft

Upper Intestinal Tract (Ø) and Lower Intestinal Tract (D)

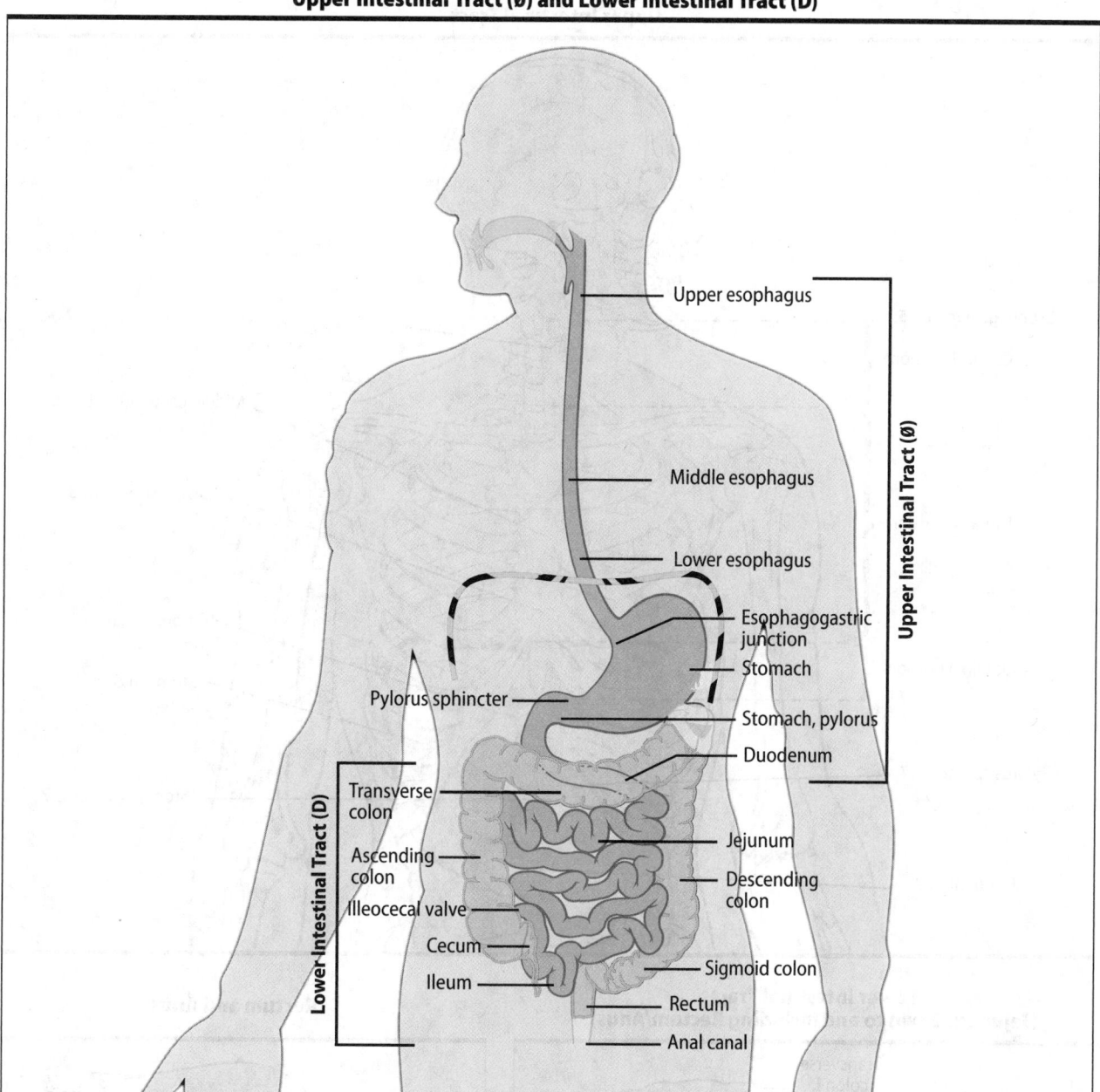

Upper Intestinal Tract

Esophageal region **5**:

Cervical portion

Thoracic portion

Abdominal portion

Pylorus sphincter **7**

Duodenum **9**

Upper esophagus **1**

Middle esophagus **2**

Lower esophagus **3**

Esophagogastric junction **4**

Stomach **6**

Stomach, pylorus **7**

Lower Intestinal Tract
(Jejunum Down to and Including Rectum/Anus)

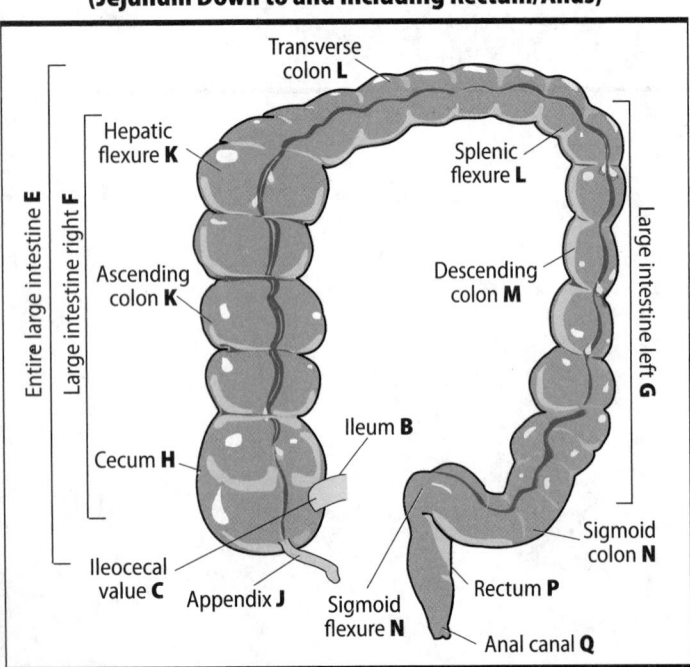

Transverse colon **L**

Hepatic flexure **K**

Splenic flexure **L**

Ascending colon **K**

Descending colon **M**

Cecum **H**

Ileum **B**

Ileocecal value **C**

Appendix **J**

Sigmoid flexure **N**

Rectum **P**

Sigmoid colon **N**

Anal canal **Q**

Entire large intestine **E**

Large intestine right **F**

Large intestine left **G**

Rectum and Anus

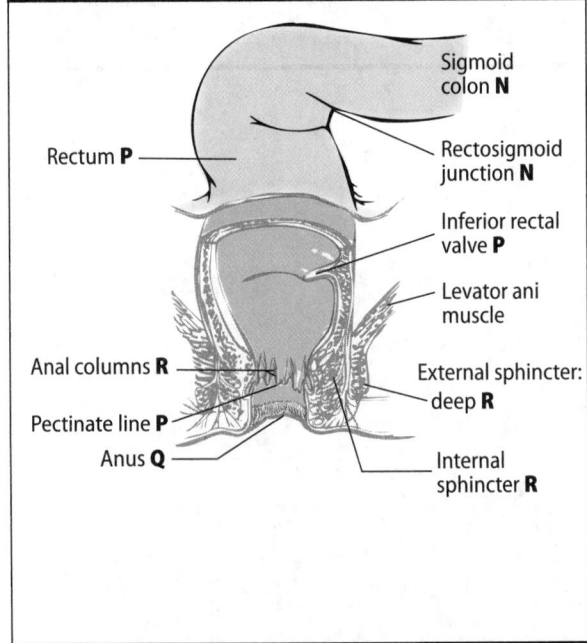

Sigmoid colon **N**

Rectosigmoid junction **N**

Inferior rectal valve **P**

Levator ani muscle

External sphincter: deep **R**

Internal sphincter **R**

Rectum **P**

Anal columns **R**

Pectinate line **P**

Anus **Q**

Ø   **Medical and Surgical**
D   **Gastrointestinal System**
1   **Bypass**   Definition: Altering the route of passage of the contents of a tubular body part

                 Explanation: Rerouting contents of a body part to a downstream area of the normal route, to a similar route and body part, or to an abnormal route and dissimilar body part. Includes one or more anastomoses, with or without the use of a device.

Body Part Character 4	Approach Character 5	Device Character 6	Qualifier Character 7
1 Esophagus, Upper Cervical esophagus **2 Esophagus, Middle** Thoracic esophagus **3 Esophagus, Lower** Abdominal esophagus **5 Esophagus**	**Ø Open** **4 Percutaneous Endoscopic** **8 Via Natural or Artificial Opening Endoscopic**	**7 Autologous Tissue Substitute** **J Synthetic Substitute** **K Nonautologous Tissue Substitute** **Z No Device**	**4 Cutaneous** **6 Stomach** **9 Duodenum** **A Jejunum** **B Ileum**
1 Esophagus, Upper Cervical esophagus **2 Esophagus, Middle** Thoracic esophagus **3 Esophagus, Lower** Abdominal esophagus **5 Esophagus**	**3 Percutaneous**	**J Synthetic Substitute**	**4 Cutaneous**
6 Stomach **9 Duodenum**	**Ø Open** **4 Percutaneous Endoscopic** **8 Via Natural or Artificial Opening Endoscopic**	**7 Autologous Tissue Substitute** **J Synthetic Substitute** **K Nonautologous Tissue Substitute** **Z No Device**	**4 Cutaneous** **9 Duodenum** **A Jejunum** **B Ileum** **L Transverse Colon**
6 Stomach **9 Duodenum**	**3 Percutaneous**	**J Synthetic Substitute**	**4 Cutaneous**
8 Small Intestine	**Ø Open** **4 Percutaneous Endoscopic** **8 Via Natural or Artificial Opening Endoscopic**	**7 Autologous Tissue Substitute** **J Synthetic Substitute** **K Nonautologous Tissue Substitute** **Z No Device**	**4 Cutaneous** **8 Small Intestine** **H Cecum** **K Ascending Colon** **L Transverse Colon** **M Descending Colon** **N Sigmoid Colon** **P Rectum** **Q Anus**
A Jejunum Duodenojejunal flexure	**Ø Open** **4 Percutaneous Endoscopic** **8 Via Natural or Artificial Opening Endoscopic**	**7 Autologous Tissue Substitute** **J Synthetic Substitute** **K Nonautologous Tissue Substitute** **Z No Device**	**4 Cutaneous** **A Jejunum** **B Ileum** **H Cecum** **K Ascending Colon** **L Transverse Colon** **M Descending Colon** **N Sigmoid Colon** **P Rectum** **Q Anus**
A Jejunum Duodenojejunal flexure	**3 Percutaneous**	**J Synthetic Substitute**	**4 Cutaneous**
B Ileum	**Ø Open** **4 Percutaneous Endoscopic** **8 Via Natural or Artificial Opening Endoscopic**	**7 Autologous Tissue Substitute** **J Synthetic Substitute** **K Nonautologous Tissue Substitute** **Z No Device**	**4 Cutaneous** **B Ileum** **H Cecum** **K Ascending Colon** **L Transverse Colon** **M Descending Colon** **N Sigmoid Colon** **P Rectum** **Q Anus**
B Ileum	**3 Percutaneous**	**J Synthetic Substitute**	**4 Cutaneous**
E Large Intestine	**Ø Open** **4 Percutaneous Endoscopic** **8 Via Natural or Artificial Opening Endoscopic**	**7 Autologous Tissue Substitute** **J Synthetic Substitute** **K Nonautologous Tissue Substitute** **Z No Device**	**4 Cutaneous** **E Large Intestine** **P Rectum**
H Cecum	**Ø Open** **4 Percutaneous Endoscopic** **8 Via Natural or Artificial Opening Endoscopic**	**7 Autologous Tissue Substitute** **J Synthetic Substitute** **K Nonautologous Tissue Substitute** **Z No Device**	**4 Cutaneous** **H Cecum** **K Ascending Colon** **L Transverse Colon** **M Descending Colon** **N Sigmoid Colon** **P Rectum**
H Cecum	**3 Percutaneous**	**J Synthetic Substitute**	**4 Cutaneous**

ØD1 Continued on next page

Non-OR   ØD16[Ø,4,8][7,J,K,Z]4
Non-OR   ØD163J4
HAC   ØD16[Ø,4,8][7,J,K,Z][9,A,B,L] when reported with PDx E66.Ø1 and SDx K68.11, K95.Ø1, K95.81 or T81.4Ø–T81.49
            with7th character A

LC Limited Coverage   **NC** Noncovered   ⊞ Combination Member   HAC associated procedure   Combination Only   DRG Non-OR   Non-OR   New/Revised in GREEN
ICD-10-PCS 2020   367

ØD1–ØD1

Gastrointestinal System

ØD1 Continued

Ø **Medical and Surgical**
D **Gastrointestinal System**
1 **Bypass**   Definition: Altering the route of passage of the contents of a tubular body part

Explanation: Rerouting contents of a body part to a downstream area of the normal route, to a similar route and body part, or to an abnormal route and dissimilar body part. Includes one or more anastomoses, with or without the use of a device.

Body Part Character 4	Approach Character 5	Device Character 6	Qualifier Character 7
K Ascending Colon	Ø Open 4 Percutaneous Endoscopic 8 Via Natural or Artificial Opening Endoscopic	7 Autologous Tissue Substitute J Synthetic Substitute K Nonautologous Tissue Substitute Z No Device	4 Cutaneous K Ascending Colon L Transverse Colon M Descending Colon N Sigmoid Colon P Rectum
K Ascending Colon	3 Percutaneous	J Synthetic Substitute	4 Cutaneous

L Transverse Colon
   Hepatic flexure
   Splenic flexure
	Ø Open
	4 Percutaneous Endoscopic
	8 Via Natural or Artificial Opening Endoscopic
		7 Autologous Tissue Substitute
		J Synthetic Substitute
		K Nonautologous Tissue Substitute
		Z No Device
			4 Cutaneous
			L Transverse Colon
			M Descending Colon
			N Sigmoid Colon
			P Rectum

L Transverse Colon
   Hepatic flexure
   Splenic flexure
	3 Percutaneous	J Synthetic Substitute	4 Cutaneous

M Descending Colon	Ø Open 4 Percutaneous Endoscopic 8 Via Natural or Artificial Opening Endoscopic	7 Autologous Tissue Substitute J Synthetic Substitute K Nonautologous Tissue Substitute Z No Device	4 Cutaneous M Descending Colon N Sigmoid Colon P Rectum
M Descending Colon	3 Percutaneous	J Synthetic Substitute	4 Cutaneous

N Sigmoid Colon
   Rectosigmoid junction
   Sigmoid flexure
	Ø Open
	4 Percutaneous Endoscopic
	8 Via Natural or Artificial Opening Endoscopic
		7 Autologous Tissue Substitute
		J Synthetic Substitute
		K Nonautologous Tissue Substitute
		Z No Device
			4 Cutaneous
			N Sigmoid Colon
			P Rectum

N Sigmoid Colon
   Rectosigmoid junction
   Sigmoid flexure
	3 Percutaneous	J Synthetic Substitute	4 Cutaneous

Ø **Medical and Surgical**
D **Gastrointestinal System**
2 **Change**   Definition: Taking out or off a device from a body part and putting back an identical or similar device in or on the same body part without cutting or puncturing the skin or a mucous membrane

Explanation: All CHANGE procedures are coded using the approach EXTERNAL

Body Part Character 4	Approach Character 5	Device Character 6	Qualifier Character 7
Ø Upper Intestinal Tract D Lower Intestinal Tract	X External	Ø Drainage Device U Feeding Device Y Other Device	Z No Qualifier

U Omentum
   Gastrocolic ligament
   Gastrocolic omentum
   Gastrohepatic omentum
   Gastrophrenic ligament
   Gastrosplenic ligament
   Greater Omentum
   Hepatogastric ligament
   Lesser Omentum
V Mesentery
   Mesoappendix
   Mesocolon
W Peritoneum
   Epiploic foramen
	X External	Ø Drainage Device
		Y Other Device
			Z No Qualifier

Non-OR   All body part, approach, device, and qualifier values

Ø　Medical and Surgical
D　Gastrointestinal System
5　Destruction　　Definition: Physical eradication of all or a portion of a body part by the direct use of energy, force, or a destructive agent
　　　　　　　　　　　Explanation: None of the body part is physically taken out

Body Part Character 4	Approach Character 5	Device Character 6	Qualifier Character 7
1　Esophagus, Upper 　　Cervical esophagus **2　Esophagus, Middle** 　　Thoracic esophagus **3　Esophagus, Lower** 　　Abdominal esophagus **4　Esophagogastric Junction** 　　Cardia 　　Cardioesophageal junction 　　Gastroesophageal (GE) junction **5　Esophagus** **6　Stomach** **7　Stomach, Pylorus** 　　Pyloric antrum 　　Pyloric canal 　　Pyloric sphincter **8　Small Intestine** **9　Duodenum** **A　Jejunum** 　　Duodenojejunal flexure **B　Ileum** **C　Ileocecal Valve** **E　Large Intestine** **F　Large Intestine, Right** **G　Large Intestine, Left** **H　Cecum** **J　Appendix** 　　Vermiform appendix **K　Ascending Colon** **L　Transverse Colon** 　　Hepatic flexure 　　Splenic flexure **M　Descending Colon** **N　Sigmoid Colon** 　　Rectosigmoid junction 　　Sigmoid flexure **P　Rectum** 　　Anorectal junction	**Ø　Open** **3　Percutaneous** **4　Percutaneous Endoscopic** **7　Via Natural or Artificial Opening** **8　Via Natural or Artificial Opening 　　Endoscopic**	**Z　No Device**	**Z　No Qualifier**
Q　Anus 　　Anal orifice	**Ø　Open** **3　Percutaneous** **4　Percutaneous Endoscopic** **7　Via Natural or Artificial Opening** **8　Via Natural or Artificial Opening 　　Endoscopic** **X　External**	**Z　No Device**	**Z　No Qualifier**
R　Anal Sphincter 　　External anal sphincter 　　Internal anal sphincter **U　Omentum** 　　Gastrocolic ligament 　　Gastrocolic omentum 　　Gastrohepatic omentum 　　Gastrophrenic ligament 　　Gastrosplenic ligament 　　Greater Omentum 　　Hepatogastric ligament 　　Lesser Omentum **V　Mesentery** 　　Mesoappendix 　　Mesocolon **W　Peritoneum** 　　Epiploic foramen	**Ø　Open** **3　Percutaneous** **4　Percutaneous Endoscopic**	**Z　No Device**	**Z　No Qualifier**

Non-OR　ØD5[1,2,3,4,5,6,7,9,E,F,G,H,K,L,M,N][4,8]ZZ
Non-OR　ØD5[8,A,B,C]8ZZ
Non-OR　ØD5P[Ø,3,4,7,8]ZZ
Non-OR　ØD5Q[4,8]ZZ
Non-OR　ØD5R4ZZ

LC Limited Coverage　**NC** Noncovered　⊞ Combination Member　HAC associated procedure　Combination Only　DRG Non-OR　Non-OR　New/Revised in GREEN
ICD-10-PCS 2020　　　　　　　　　　　　　　　　　　　　　　　　　　　　　　　　　　　　　　369

ØD5–ØD5

Ø   Medical and Surgical
D   Gastrointestinal System
7   Dilation   Definition: Expanding an orifice or the lumen of a tubular body part

Explanation: The orifice can be a natural orifice or an artificially created orifice. Accomplished by stretching a tubular body part using intraluminal pressure or by cutting part of the orifice or wall of the tubular body part.

Body Part Character 4	Approach Character 5	Device Character 6	Qualifier Character 7

1 **Esophagus, Upper**
  Cervical esophagus
2 **Esophagus, Middle**
  Thoracic esophagus
3 **Esophagus, Lower**
  Abdominal esophagus
4 **Esophagogastric Junction**
  Cardia
  Cardioesophageal junction
  Gastroesophageal (GE) junction
5 **Esophagus**
6 **Stomach**
7 **Stomach, Pylorus**
  Pyloric antrum
  Pyloric canal
  Pyloric sphincter
8 **Small Intestine**
9 **Duodenum**
A **Jejunum**
  Duodenojejunal flexure
B **Ileum**
C **Ileocecal Valve**
E **Large Intestine**
F **Large Intestine, Right**
G **Large Intestine, Left**
H **Cecum**
K **Ascending Colon**
L **Transverse Colon**
  Hepatic flexure
  Splenic flexure
M **Descending Colon**
N **Sigmoid Colon**
  Rectosigmoid junction
  Sigmoid flexure
P **Rectum**
  Anorectal junction
Q **Anus**
  Anal orifice
	Ø **Open**
	3 **Percutaneous**
	4 **Percutaneous Endoscopic**
	7 **Via Natural or Artificial Opening**
	8 **Via Natural or Artificial Opening Endoscopic**
		D **Intraluminal Device**
		Z **No Device**
			Z **No Qualifier**

Non-OR   ØD7[1,2,3,4,5,6,8,9,A,B,C,E,F,G,H,K,L,M,N,P,Q][7,8][D,Z]Z
Non-OR   ØD77[4,8]DZ
Non-OR   ØD777[D,Z]Z
Non-OR   ØD7[8,9,A,B,C,E,F,G,H,K,L,M,N][Ø,3,4]DZ

Ø   Medical and Surgical
D   Gastrointestinal System
8   Division   Definition: Cutting into a body part, without draining fluids and/or gases from the body part, in order to separate or transect a body part

Explanation: All or a portion of the body part is separated into two or more portions

Body Part Character 4	Approach Character 5	Device Character 6	Qualifier Character 7

4 **Esophagogastric Junction**
  Cardia
  Cardioesophageal junction
  Gastroesophageal (GE) junction
7 **Stomach, Pylorus**
  Pyloric antrum
  Pyloric canal
  Pyloric sphincter
	Ø **Open**
	3 **Percutaneous**
	4 **Percutaneous Endoscopic**
	7 **Via Natural or Artificial Opening**
	8 **Via Natural or Artificial Opening Endoscopic**
		Z **No Device**	Z **No Qualifier**

R **Anal Sphincter**
  External anal sphincter
  Internal anal sphincter
	Ø **Open**
	3 **Percutaneous**
		Z **No Device**	Z **No Qualifier**

Ø   Medical and Surgical
D   Gastrointestinal System
9   Drainage   Definition: Taking or letting out fluids and/or gases from a body part
                Explanation: The qualifier DIAGNOSTIC is used to identify drainage procedures that are biopsies

Body Part — Character 4		Approach — Character 5	Device — Character 6	Qualifier — Character 7

1 Esophagus, Upper
  Cervical esophagus
2 Esophagus, Middle
  Thoracic esophagus
3 Esophagus, Lower
  Abdominal esophagus
4 Esophagogastric Junction
  Cardia
  Cardioesophageal junction
  Gastroesophageal (GE) junction
5 Esophagus
6 Stomach
7 Stomach, Pylorus
  Pyloric antrum
  Pyloric canal
  Pyloric sphincter
8 Small Intestine
9 Duodenum
	A Jejunum
	  Duodenojejunal flexure
	B Ileum
	C Ileocecal Valve
	E Large Intestine
	F Large Intestine, Right
	G Large Intestine, Left
	H Cecum
	J Appendix
	  Vermiform appendix
	K Ascending Colon
	L Transverse Colon
	  Hepatic flexure
	  Splenic flexure
	M Descending Colon
	N Sigmoid Colon
	  Rectosigmoid junction
	  Sigmoid flexure
	P Rectum
	  Anorectal junction
		Ø Open
		3 Percutaneous
		4 Percutaneous Endoscopic
		7 Via Natural or Artificial Opening
		8 Via Natural or Artificial Opening Endoscopic
			Ø Drainage Device	Z No Qualifier

1 Esophagus, Upper
  Cervical esophagus
2 Esophagus, Middle
  Thoracic esophagus
3 Esophagus, Lower
  Abdominal esophagus
4 Esophagogastric Junction
  Cardia
  Cardioesophageal junction
  Gastroesophageal (GE) junction
5 Esophagus
6 Stomach
7 Stomach, Pylorus
  Pyloric antrum
  Pyloric canal
  Pyloric sphincter
8 Small Intestine
9 Duodenum
	A Jejunum
	  Duodenojejunal flexure
	B Ileum
	C Ileocecal Valve
	E Large Intestine
	F Large Intestine, Right
	G Large Intestine, Left
	H Cecum
	J Appendix
	  Vermiform appendix
	K Ascending Colon
	L Transverse Colon
	  Hepatic flexure
	  Splenic flexure
	M Descending Colon
	N Sigmoid Colon
	  Rectosigmoid junction
	  Sigmoid flexure
	P Rectum
	  Anorectal junction
		Ø Open
		3 Percutaneous
		4 Percutaneous Endoscopic
		7 Via Natural or Artificial Opening
		8 Via Natural or Artificial Opening Endoscopic
			Z No Device	X Diagnostic
				Z No Qualifier

Q Anus Anal orifice		Ø Open 3 Percutaneous 4 Percutaneous Endoscopic 7 Via Natural or Artificial Opening 8 Via Natural or Artificial Opening Endoscopic X External	Ø Drainage Device	Z No Qualifier
Q Anus Anal orifice		Ø Open 3 Percutaneous 4 Percutaneous Endoscopic 7 Via Natural or Artificial Opening 8 Via Natural or Artificial Opening Endoscopic X External	Z No Device	X Diagnostic Z No Qualifier

ØD9 Continued on next page

Non-OR	ØD9[1,2,3,4,5,C,J]3ØZ
Non-OR	ØD9[6,7,8,9,A,B,E,F,G,H,K,L,M,N,P][3,7,8]ØZ
Non-OR	ØD9[1,2,3,4,5,6,7,8,9,A,B,C,E,F,G,H,K,L,M,N,P][3,4,7,8]ZX
Non-OR	ØD9[1,2,3,4,5,6,7,8,9,A,B,C,E,F,G,H,J,K,L,M,N,P]3ZZ
Non-OR	ØD9Q3ØZ
Non-OR	ØD9Q[Ø,4,7,8,X]ZX
Non-OR	ØD9Q3Z[X,Z]

LC Limited Coverage   NC Noncovered   ⊞ Combination Member   HAC associated procedure   Combination Only   DRG Non-OR   Non-OR   New/Revised in GREEN

ICD-10-PCS 2020   371

ØD9–ØD9

Ø   Medical and Surgical   *ØD9 Continued*
D   Gastrointestinal System
9   Drainage   Definition: Taking or letting out fluids and/or gases from a body part
                          Explanation: The qualifier DIAGNOSTIC is used to identify drainage procedures that are biopsies

Body Part Character 4	Approach Character 5	Device Character 6	Qualifier Character 7
R Anal Sphincter 　External anal sphincter 　Internal anal sphincter **U** **Omentum** 　Gastrocolic ligament 　Gastrocolic omentum 　Gastrohepatic omentum 　Gastrophrenic ligament 　Gastrosplenic ligament 　Greater Omentum 　Hepatogastric ligament 　Lesser Omentum **V** **Mesentery** 　Mesoappendix 　Mesocolon **W** **Peritoneum** 　Epiploic foramen	**Ø** Open **3** Percutaneous **4** Percutaneous Endoscopic	**Ø** Drainage Device	**Z** No Qualifier
R Anal Sphincter 　External anal sphincter 　Internal anal sphincter **U** **Omentum** 　Gastrocolic ligament 　Gastrocolic omentum 　Gastrohepatic omentum 　Gastrophrenic ligament 　Gastrosplenic ligament 　Greater Omentum 　Hepatogastric ligament 　Lesser Omentum **V** **Mesentery** 　Mesoappendix 　Mesocolon **W** **Peritoneum** 　Epiploic foramen	**Ø** Open **3** Percutaneous **4** Percutaneous Endoscopic	**Z** No Device	**X** Diagnostic **Z** No Qualifier

Non-OR	ØD9R3ØZ
Non-OR	ØD9[U,V,W][3,4]ØZ
Non-OR	ØD9R[Ø,4]ZX
Non-OR	ØD9[R,U,V,W]3Z[X,Z]
Non-OR	ØD9[U,V,W]4ZZ

Ø   **Medical and Surgical**
D   **Gastrointestinal System**
B   **Excision**   Definition: Cutting out or off, without replacement, a portion of a body part
                      Explanation: The qualifier DIAGNOSTIC is used to identify excision procedures that are biopsies

Body Part Character 4		Approach Character 5	Device Character 6	Qualifier Character 7

1 **Esophagus, Upper**
   Cervical esophagus
2 **Esophagus, Middle**
   Thoracic esophagus
3 **Esophagus, Lower**
   Abdominal esophagus
4 **Esophagogastric**
   Junction
   Cardia
   Cardioesophageal
     junction
   Gastroesophageal (GE)
     junction
5 **Esophagus**
7 **Stomach, Pylorus**
   Pyloric antrum
   Pyloric canal
   Pyloric sphincter
	8 **Small Intestine**
	9 **Duodenum**
	A **Jejunum**
	   Duodenojejunal flexure
	B **Ileum**
	C **Ileocecal Valve**
	E **Large Intestine**
	F **Large Intestine, Right**
	H **Cecum**
	J **Appendix**
	   Vermiform appendix
	K **Ascending Colon**
	P **Rectum**
	   Anorectal junction
		Ø Open
		3 Percutaneous
		4 Percutaneous Endoscopic
		7 Via Natural or Artificial
		   Opening
		8 Via Natural or Artificial
		   Opening Endoscopic
			Z No Device	X Diagnostic
				Z No Qualifier

6 **Stomach**		Ø Open
		3 Percutaneous
		4 Percutaneous Endoscopic
		7 Via Natural or Artificial
		   Opening
		8 Via Natural or Artificial
		   Opening Endoscopic
			Z No Device	3 Vertical
				X Diagnostic
				Z No Qualifier

G **Large Intestine, Left**
L **Transverse Colon**
   Hepatic flexure
   Splenic flexure
M **Descending Colon**
N **Sigmoid Colon**
   Rectosigmoid junction
   Sigmoid flexure
		Ø Open
		3 Percutaneous
		4 Percutaneous Endoscopic
		7 Via Natural or Artificial
		   Opening
		8 Via Natural or Artificial
		   Opening Endoscopic
			Z No Device	X Diagnostic
				Z No Qualifier

G **Large Intestine, Left**
L **Transverse Colon**
   Hepatic flexure
   Splenic flexure
M **Descending Colon**
N **Sigmoid Colon**
   Rectosigmoid junction
   Sigmoid flexure
		F Via Natural or Artificial
		   Opening with Percutaneous
		   Endoscopic Assistance
			Z No Device	Z No Qualifier

Q **Anus**
   Anal orifice
		Ø Open
		3 Percutaneous
		4 Percutaneous Endoscopic
		7 Via Natural or Artificial
		   Opening
		8 Via Natural or Artificial
		   Opening Endoscopic
		X External
			Z No Device	X Diagnostic
				Z No Qualifier

R **Anal Sphincter**
   External anal sphincter
   Internal anal sphincter
U **Omentum**
   Gastrocolic ligament
   Gastrocolic omentum
   Gastrohepatic omentum
   Gastrophrenic ligament
   Gastrosplenic ligament
   Greater Omentum
   Hepatogastric ligament
   Lesser Omentum
V **Mesentery**
   Mesoappendix
   Mesocolon
W **Peritoneum**
   Epiploic foramen
		Ø Open
		3 Percutaneous
		4 Percutaneous Endoscopic
			Z No Device	X Diagnostic
				Z No Qualifier

Non-OR	ØDB[1,2,3,4,5,7,8,9,A,B,C,E,F,H,K,P][3,4,7,8]ZX		**Non-OR**	ØDB[G,L,M,N]8ZZ
Non-OR	ØDB[1,2,3,5,7,9][4,8]ZZ		**Non-OR**	ØDBQ[Ø,3,4,7,8,X]ZX
Non-OR	ØDB[4,E,F,H,K,P]8ZZ		**Non-OR**	ØDBQ8ZZ
Non-OR	ØDB6[3,4,7,8]ZX		**Non-OR**	ØDBR[Ø,3,4]ZX
Non-OR	ØDB6[4,8]ZZ		**Non-OR**	ØDB[U,V,W][3,4]ZX
Non-OR	ØDB[G,L,M,N][3,4,7,8]ZX			

🔲 Limited Coverage 🔲 Noncovered ⊞ Combination Member   HAC associated procedure   Combination Only   DRG Non-OR   Non-OR   New/Revised in GREEN
ICD-10-PCS 2020   373

ØDB–ØDB

Ø   Medical and Surgical
D   Gastrointestinal System
C   Extirpation   Definition: Taking or cutting out solid matter from a body part

Explanation: The solid matter may be an abnormal byproduct of a biological function or a foreign body; it may be imbedded in a body part or in the lumen of a tubular body part. The solid matter may or may not have been previously broken into pieces.

Body Part Character 4	Approach Character 5	Device Character 6	Qualifier Character 7

1 Esophagus, Upper
    Cervical esophagus
2 Esophagus, Middle
    Thoracic esophagus
3 Esophagus, Lower
    Abdominal esophagus
4 Esophagogastric Junction
    Cardia
    Cardioesophageal junction
    Gastroesophageal (GE) junction
5 Esophagus
6 Stomach
7 Stomach, Pylorus
    Pyloric antrum
    Pyloric canal
    Pyloric sphincter
8 Small Intestine
9 Duodenum
A Jejunum
    Duodenojejunal flexure
B Ileum
C Ileocecal Valve
E Large Intestine
F Large Intestine, Right
G Large Intestine, Left
H Cecum
J Appendix
    Vermiform appendix
K Ascending Colon
L Transverse Colon
    Hepatic flexure
    Splenic flexure
M Descending Colon
N Sigmoid Colon
    Rectosigmoid junction
    Sigmoid flexure
P Rectum
    Anorectal junction
	Ø Open
	3 Percutaneous
	4 Percutaneous Endoscopic
	7 Via Natural or Artificial Opening
	**8 Via Natural or Artificial Opening
	    Endoscopic**
		Z No Device	**Z No Qualifier**

Q Anus
    Anal orifice
	Ø Open
	3 Percutaneous
	4 Percutaneous Endoscopic
	7 Via Natural or Artificial Opening
	**8 Via Natural or Artificial Opening
	    Endoscopic**
	X External
		Z No Device	**Z No Qualifier**

R Anal Sphincter
    External anal sphincter
    Internal anal sphincter
U Omentum
    Gastrocolic ligament
    Gastrocolic omentum
    Gastrohepatic omentum
    Gastrophrenic ligament
    Gastrosplenic ligament
    Greater Omentum
    Hepatogastric ligament
    Lesser Omentum
V Mesentery
    Mesoappendix
    Mesocolon
W Peritoneum
    Epiploic foramen
	Ø Open
	3 Percutaneous
	4 Percutaneous Endoscopic
		Z No Device	**Z No Qualifier**

Non-OR   ØDC[1,2,3,4,5,6,7,8,9,A,B,C,E,F,G,H,K,L,M,N,P][7,8]ZZ
Non-OR   ØDCQ[7,8,X]ZZ

LC Limited Coverage   **NC** Noncovered   ⊞ Combination Member   HAC associated procedure   Combination Only   DRG Non-OR   Non-OR   New/Revised in GREEN

374   ICD-10-PCS 2020

Ø   Medical and Surgical
D   Gastrointestinal System
D   Extraction   Definition: Pulling or stripping out or off all or a portion of a body part by the use of force
                    Explanation: The qualifier DIAGNOSTIC is used to identify extraction procedures that are biopsies

Body Part Character 4	Approach Character 5	Device Character 6	Qualifier Character 7

1   **Esophagus, Upper**
     Cervical esophagus
2   **Esophagus, Middle**
     Thoracic esophagus
3   **Esophagus, Lower**
     Abdominal esophagus
4   **Esophagogastric Junction**
     Cardia
     Cardioesophageal junction
     Gastroesophageal (GE) junction
5   **Esophagus**
6   **Stomach**
7   **Stomach, Pylorus**
     Pyloric antrum
     Pyloric canal
     Pyloric sphincter
8   **Small Intestine**
9   **Duodenum**
A   **Jejunum**
     Duodenojejunal flexure
B   **Ileum**
C   **Ileocecal Valve**
E   **Large Intestine**
F   **Large Intestine, Right**
G   **Large Intestine, Left**
H   **Cecum**
J   **Appendix**
     Vermiform appendix
K   **Ascending Colon**
L   **Transverse Colon**
     Hepatic flexure
     Splenic flexure
M   **Descending Colon**
N   **Sigmoid Colon**
     Rectosigmoid junction
     Sigmoid flexure
P   **Rectum**
     Anorectal junction
	3 **Percutaneous**
	4 **Percutaneous Endoscopic**
	8 **Via Natural or Artificial Opening**
	     Endoscopic
		Z **No Device**	**X** **Diagnostic**

Q   **Anus**
     Anal orifice
	3 **Percutaneous**
	4 **Percutaneous Endoscopic**
	8 **Via Natural or Artificial Opening**
	     Endoscopic
	X **External**
		Z **No Device**	**X** **Diagnostic**

Non-OR   ØDD[1,2,3,4,5,6,7,8,9,A,B,C,E,F,G,H,K,L,M,N,P][3,4,8]ZX
Non-OR   ØDDQ[3,4,8,X]ZX

Ø   Medical and Surgical
D   Gastrointestinal System
F   Fragmentation   Definition: Breaking solid matter in a body part into pieces

               Explanation: Physical force (e.g., manual, ultrasonic) applied directly or indirectly is used to break the solid matter into pieces. The solid matter may be an abnormal byproduct of a biological function or a foreign body. The pieces of solid matter are not taken out.

Body Part Character 4	Approach Character 5	Device Character 6	Qualifier Character 7

5   Esophagus   NC
6   Stomach   NC
8   Small Intestine   NC
9   Duodenum   NC
A   Jejunum   NC
     Duodenojejunal flexure
B   Ileum   NC
E   Large Intestine   NC
F   Large Intestine, Right   NC
G   Large Intestine, Left   NC
H   Cecum   NC
J   Appendix   NC
     Vermiform appendix
K   Ascending Colon   NC
L   Transverse Colon   NC
     Hepatic flexure
     Splenic flexure
M   Descending Colon   NC
N   Sigmoid Colon   NC
     Rectosigmoid junction
     Sigmoid flexure
P   Rectum   NC
     Anorectal junction
Q   Anus   NC
     Anal orifice
	Ø Open
	3 Percutaneous
	4 Percutaneous Endoscopic
	7 Via Natural or Artificial Opening
	8 Via Natural or Artificial Opening
	     Endoscopic
	X External
		Z No Device	Z No Qualifier

Non-OR   ØDF[5,6,8,9,A,B,E,F,G,H,J,K,L,M,N,P,Q]XZZ
NC   ØDF[5,6,8,9,A,B,E,F,G,H,J,K,L,M,N,P,Q]XZZ

LC Limited Coverage   NC Noncovered   ⊞ Combination Member   HAC associated procedure   Combination Only   DRG Non-OR   Non-OR   New/Revised in GREEN

376   ICD-10-PCS 2020

Ø   Medical and Surgical
D   Gastrointestinal System
H   Insertion   Definition: Putting in a nonbiological appliance that monitors, assists, performs, or prevents a physiological function but does not physically take the place of a body part
         Explanation: None

Body Part Character 4	Approach Character 5	Device Character 6	Qualifier Character 7
Ø Upper Intestinal Tract D Lower Intestinal Tract	Ø Open 3 Percutaneous 4 Percutaneous Endoscopic 7 Via Natural or Artificial Opening 8 Via Natural or Artificial Opening Endoscopic	Y Other Device	Z No Qualifier
5 Esophagus	Ø Open 3 Percutaneous 4 Percutaneous Endoscopic	1 Radioactive Element 2 Monitoring Device 3 Infusion Device D Intraluminal Device U Feeding Device Y Other Device	Z No Qualifier
5 Esophagus	7 Via Natural or Artificial Opening 8 Via Natural or Artificial Opening Endoscopic	1 Radioactive Element 2 Monitoring Device 3 Infusion Device B Intraluminal Device, Airway D Intraluminal Device U Feeding Device Y Other Device	Z No Qualifier
6 Stomach ⊞	Ø Open 3 Percutaneous 4 Percutaneous Endoscopic	2 Monitoring Device 3 Infusion Device D Intraluminal Device M Stimulator Lead U Feeding Device Y Other Device	Z No Qualifier
6 Stomach	7 Via Natural or Artificial Opening 8 Via Natural or Artificial Opening Endoscopic	2 Monitoring Device 3 Infusion Device D Intraluminal Device U Feeding Device Y Other Device	Z No Qualifier
8 Small Intestine 9 Duodenum A Jejunum Duodenojejunal flexure B Ileum	Ø Open 3 Percutaneous 4 Percutaneous Endoscopic 7 Via Natural or Artificial Opening 8 Via Natural or Artificial Opening Endoscopic	2 Monitoring Device 3 Infusion Device D Intraluminal Device U Feeding Device	Z No Qualifier
E Large Intestine	Ø Open 3 Percutaneous 4 Percutaneous Endoscopic 7 Via Natural or Artificial Opening 8 Via Natural or Artificial Opening Endoscopic	D Intraluminal Device	Z No Qualifier
P Rectum Anorectal junction	Ø Open 3 Percutaneous 4 Percutaneous Endoscopic 7 Via Natural or Artificial Opening 8 Via Natural or Artificial Opening Endoscopic	1 Radioactive Element D Intraluminal Device	Z No Qualifier
Q Anus Anal orifice	Ø Open 3 Percutaneous 4 Percutaneous Endoscopic	D Intraluminal Device L Artificial Sphincter	Z No Qualifier
Q Anus Anal orifice	7 Via Natural or Artificial Opening 8 Via Natural or Artificial Opening Endoscopic	D Intraluminal Device	Z No Qualifier

R Anal Sphincter
   External anal sphincter
   Internal anal sphincter
	Ø Open
	3 Percutaneous
	4 Percutaneous Endoscopic
		M Stimulator Lead	Z No Qualifier

Non-OR   ØDH[Ø,D][Ø,3,4,7,8]YZ
Non-OR   ØDH5[Ø,3,4][D,U]Z
Non-OR   ØDH5[3,4]YZ
Non-OR   ØDH5[7,8][2,3,B,D,U,Y]Z
Non-OR   ØDH6[3,4][U,Y]Z
Non-OR   ØDH6[7,8][2,3,D,U,Y]Z
Non-OR   ØDH[8,9,A,B][Ø,3,4][D,U]Z
Non-OR   ØDH[8,9,A,B][7,8][2,3,D,U]Z
Non-OR   ØDHE[Ø,3,4,7,8]DZ
Non-OR   ØDHP[Ø,3,4,7,8]DZ

See Appendix L for Procedure Combinations
⊞   ØDH6[Ø,3,4]MZ

LC Limited Coverage   NC Noncovered   ⊞ Combination Member   HAC associated procedure   Combination Only   DRG Non-OR   Non-OR   New/Revised in GREEN

Ø   **Medical and Surgical**
D   **Gastrointestinal System**
J   **Inspection**   Definition: Visually and/or manually exploring a body part

                     Explanation: Visual exploration may be performed with or without optical instrumentation. Manual exploration may be performed directly or through intervening body layers.

Body Part Character 4	Approach Character 5	Device Character 6	Qualifier Character 7
Ø Upper Intestinal Tract **6** Stomach **D** Lower Intestinal Tract	**Ø** Open **3** Percutaneous **4** Percutaneous Endoscopic **7** Via Natural or Artificial Opening **8** Via Natural or Artificial Opening Endoscopic **X** External	**Z** No Device	**Z** No Qualifier

U Omentum
   Gastrocolic ligament
   Gastrocolic omentum
   Gastrohepatic omentum
   Gastrophrenic ligament
   Gastrosplenic ligament
   Greater Omentum
   Hepatogastric ligament
   Lesser Omentum
V Mesentery
   Mesoappendix
   Mesocolon
W Peritoneum
   Epiploic foramen
	Ø Open
	3 Percutaneous
	4 Percutaneous Endoscopic
	X External
		Z No Device	**Z** No Qualifier

Non-OR	ØDJ[Ø,6,D][3,7,8,X]ZZ
Non-OR	ØDJ[U,V,W][3,X]ZZ

LC Limited Coverage   **NC** Noncovered   ⊞ Combination Member   HAC associated procedure   Combination Only   DRG Non-OR   Non-OR   New/Revised in GREEN

378   ICD-10-PCS 2020

Ø   Medical and Surgical
D   Gastrointestinal System
L   Occlusion   Definition: Completely closing an orifice or the lumen of a tubular body part
                       Explanation: The orifice can be a natural orifice or an artificially created orifice

Body Part Character 4		Approach Character 5	Device Character 6	Qualifier Character 7

1 **Esophagus, Upper**
  Cervical esophagus
2 **Esophagus, Middle**
  Thoracic esophagus
3 **Esophagus, Lower**
  Abdominal esophagus
4 **Esophagogastric**
  Junction
  Cardia
  Cardioesophageal
    junction
  Gastroesophageal (GE)
    junction
5 **Esophagus**
6 **Stomach**
7 **Stomach, Pylorus**
  Pyloric antrum
  Pyloric canal
  Pyloric sphincter
8 **Small Intestine**
	9 **Duodenum**
	A **Jejunum**
	  Duodenojejunal flexure
	B **Ileum**
	C **Ileocecal Valve**
	E **Large Intestine**
	F **Large Intestine, Right**
	G **Large Intestine, Left**
	H **Cecum**
	K **Ascending Colon**
	L **Transverse Colon**
	  Hepatic flexure
	  Splenic flexure
	M **Descending Colon**
	N **Sigmoid Colon**
	  Rectosigmoid junction
	  Sigmoid flexure
	P **Rectum**
	  Anorectal junction
		Ø **Open**
		3 **Percutaneous**
		4 **Percutaneous Endoscopic**
			C **Extraluminal Device**
			D **Intraluminal Device**
			Z **No Device**
				Z **No Qualifier**

1 **Esophagus, Upper**
  Cervical esophagus
2 **Esophagus, Middle**
  Thoracic esophagus
3 **Esophagus, Lower**
  Abdominal esophagus
4 **Esophagogastric**
  Junction
  Cardia
  Cardioesophageal
    junction
  Gastroesophageal (GE)
    junction
5 **Esophagus**
6 **Stomach**
7 **Stomach, Pylorus**
  Pyloric antrum
  Pyloric canal
  Pyloric sphincter
8 **Small Intestine**
	9 **Duodenum**
	A **Jejunum**
	  Duodenojejunal flexure
	B **Ileum**
	C **Ileocecal Valve**
	E **Large Intestine**
	F **Large Intestine, Right**
	G **Large Intestine, Left**
	H **Cecum**
	K **Ascending Colon**
	L **Transverse Colon**
	  Hepatic flexure
	  Splenic flexure
	M **Descending Colon**
	N **Sigmoid Colon**
	  Rectosigmoid junction
	  Sigmoid flexure
	P **Rectum**
	  Anorectal junction
		7 **Via Natural or Artificial Opening**
		8 **Via Natural or Artificial Opening Endoscopic**
			D **Intraluminal Device**
			Z **No Device**
				Z **No Qualifier**

Q **Anus** Anal orifice		Ø **Open** 3 **Percutaneous** 4 **Percutaneous Endoscopic** X **External**	C **Extraluminal Device** D **Intraluminal Device** Z **No Device**	Z **No Qualifier**
Q **Anus** Anal orifice		7 **Via Natural or Artificial Opening** 8 **Via Natural or Artificial Opening Endoscopic**	D **Intraluminal Device** Z **No Device**	Z **No Qualifier**

Non-OR   ØDL[1,2,3,4,5][Ø,3,4][C,D,Z]Z
Non-OR   ØDL[1,2,3,4,5][7,8][D,Z]Z

LC Limited Coverage   NC Noncovered   ⊞ Combination Member   HAC associated procedure   Combination Only   DRG Non-OR   Non-OR   New/Revised in GREEN

ICD-10-PCS 2020   379

Gastrointestinal System

Ø   **Medical and Surgical**
D   **Gastrointestinal System**
M   **Reattachment**   Definition: Putting back in or on all or a portion of a separated body part to its normal location or other suitable location
                          Explanation: Vascular circulation and nervous pathways may or may not be reestablished

Body Part — Character 4	Approach — Character 5	Device — Character 6	Qualifier — Character 7

5 Esophagus
6 Stomach
8 Small Intestine
9 Duodenum
A Jejunum
   Duodenojejunal flexure
B Ileum
E Large Intestine
F Large Intestine, Right
G Large Intestine, Left
H Cecum
K Ascending Colon
L Transverse Colon
   Hepatic flexure
   Splenic flexure
M Descending Colon
N Sigmoid Colon
   Rectosigmoid junction
   Sigmoid flexure
P Rectum
   Anorectal junction
	Ø Open
	4 Percutaneous Endoscopic
		Z No Device	Z No Qualifier

Ø   **Medical and Surgical**
D   **Gastrointestinal System**
N   **Release**   Definition: Freeing a body part from an abnormal physical constraint by cutting or by the use of force
                     Explanation: Some of the restraining tissue may be taken out but none of the body part is taken out

Body Part — Character 4	Approach — Character 5	Device — Character 6	Qualifier — Character 7

1 Esophagus, Upper
   Cervical esophagus
2 Esophagus, Middle
   Thoracic esophagus
3 Esophagus, Lower
   Abdominal esophagus
4 Esophagogastric Junction
   Cardia
   Cardioesophageal junction
   Gastroesophageal (GE) junction
5 Esophagus
6 Stomach
7 Stomach, Pylorus
   Pyloric antrum
   Pyloric canal
   Pyloric sphincter
8 Small Intestine
9 Duodenum
 	
A Jejunum
   Duodenojejunal flexure
B Ileum
C Ileocecal Valve
E Large Intestine
F Large Intestine, Right
G Large Intestine, Left
H Cecum
J Appendix
   Vermiform appendix
K Ascending Colon
L Transverse Colon
   Hepatic flexure
   Splenic flexure
M Descending Colon
N Sigmoid Colon
   Rectosigmoid junction
   Sigmoid flexure
P Rectum
   Anorectal junction
	Ø Open
	3 Percutaneous
	4 Percutaneous Endoscopic
	7 Via Natural or Artificial Opening
	8 Via Natural or Artificial Opening Endoscopic
		Z No Device	Z No Qualifier

Q Anus Anal orifice	Ø Open 3 Percutaneous 4 Percutaneous Endoscopic 7 Via Natural or Artificial Opening 8 Via Natural or Artificial Opening Endoscopic X External	Z No Device	Z No Qualifier

R Anal Sphincter
   External anal sphincter
   Internal anal sphincter
U Omentum
   Gastrocolic ligament
   Gastrocolic omentum
   Gastrohepatic omentum
   Gastrophrenic ligament
   Gastrosplenic ligament
   Greater Omentum
   Hepatogastric ligament
   Lesser Omentum
V Mesentery
   Mesoappendix
   Mesocolon
W Peritoneum
   Epiploic foramen
	Ø Open
	3 Percutaneous
	4 Percutaneous Endoscopic
		Z No Device	Z No Qualifier

Non-OR   ØDN[8,9,A,B,E,F,G,H,K,L,M,N][7,8]ZZ

LC Limited Coverage   NC Noncovered   ⊞ Combination Member   HAC associated procedure   Combination Only   DRG Non-OR   Non-OR   New/Revised in GREEN

Ø   **Medical and Surgical**
D   **Gastrointestinal System**
P   **Removal**   Definition: Taking out or off a device from a body part

         Explanation: If a device is taken out and a similar device put in without cutting or puncturing the skin or mucous membrane, the procedure is coded to the root operation CHANGE. Otherwise, the procedure for taking out a device is coded to the root operation REMOVAL.

Body Part Character 4	Approach Character 5	Device Character 6	Qualifier Character 7
Ø Upper Intestinal Tract D Lower Intestinal Tract	Ø Open 3 Percutaneous 4 Percutaneous Endoscopic 7 Via Natural or Artificial Opening 8 Via Natural or Artificial Opening Endoscopic	Ø Drainage Device 2 Monitoring Device 3 Infusion Device 7 Autologous Tissue Substitute C Extraluminal Device D Intraluminal Device J Synthetic Substitute K Nonautologous Tissue Substitute U Feeding Device Y Other Device	Z No Qualifier
Ø Upper Intestinal Tract D Lower Intestinal Tract	X External	Ø Drainage Device 2 Monitoring Device 3 Infusion Device D Intraluminal Device U Feeding Device	Z No Qualifier
5 Esophagus	Ø Open 3 Percutaneous 4 Percutaneous Endoscopic	1 Radioactive Element 2 Monitoring Device 3 Infusion Device U Feeding Device Y Other Device	Z No Qualifier
5 Esophagus	7 Via Natural or Artificial Opening 8 Via Natural or Artificial Opening Endoscopic	1 Radioactive Element D Intraluminal Device Y Other Device	Z No Qualifier
5 Esophagus	X External	1 Radioactive Element 2 Monitoring Device 3 Infusion Device D Intraluminal Device U Feeding Device	Z No Qualifier
6 Stomach	Ø Open 3 Percutaneous 4 Percutaneous Endoscopic	Ø Drainage Device 2 Monitoring Device 3 Infusion Device 7 Autologous Tissue Substitute C Extraluminal Device D Intraluminal Device J Synthetic Substitute K Nonautologous Tissue Substitute M Stimulator Lead U Feeding Device Y Other Device	Z No Qualifier
6 Stomach	7 Via Natural or Artificial Opening 8 Via Natural or Artificial Opening Endoscopic	Ø Drainage Device 2 Monitoring Device 3 Infusion Device 7 Autologous Tissue Substitute C Extraluminal Device D Intraluminal Device J Synthetic Substitute K Nonautologous Tissue Substitute U Feeding Device Y Other Device	Z No Qualifier
6 Stomach	X External	Ø Drainage Device 2 Monitoring Device 3 Infusion Device D Intraluminal Device U Feeding Device	Z No Qualifier

ØDP Continued on next page

Non-OR	ØDP[Ø,D][3,4]YZ
Non-OR	ØDP[Ø,D][7,8][Ø,2,3,D,U,Y]Z
Non-OR	ØDP[Ø,D]X[Ø,2,3,D,U]Z
Non-OR	ØDP5[3,4]YZ
Non-OR	ØDP5[7,8][1,D,Y]Z
Non-OR	ØDP5X[1,2,3,D,U]Z
Non-OR	ØDP6[3,4]YZ
Non-OR	ØDP6[7,8][Ø,2,3,D,U,Y]Z
Non-OR	ØDP6X[Ø,2,3,D,U]Z

Gastrointestinal System (side tab)

ØDP Continued

Ø   **Medical and Surgical**
D   **Gastrointestinal System**
P   **Removal**   Definition: Taking out or off a device from a body part

Explanation: If a device is taken out and a similar device put in without cutting or puncturing the skin or mucous membrane, the procedure is coded to the root operation CHANGE. Otherwise, the procedure for taking out a device is coded to the root operation REMOVAL.

Body Part Character 4	Approach Character 5	Device Character 6	Qualifier Character 7
P **Rectum** Anorectal junction	**Ø** Open **3** Percutaneous **4** Percutaneous Endoscopic **7** Via Natural or Artificial Opening **8** Via Natural or Artificial Opening Endoscopic **X** External	**1** Radioactive Element	**Z** No Qualifier
Q **Anus** Anal orifice	**Ø** Open **3** Percutaneous **4** Percutaneous Endoscopic **7** Via Natural or Artificial Opening **8** Via Natural or Artificial Opening Endoscopic	**L** Artificial Sphincter	**Z** No Qualifier

R **Anal Sphincter**
   External anal sphincter
   Internal anal sphincter
	Ø Open
	3 Percutaneous
	4 Percutaneous Endoscopic
		M Stimulator Lead	**Z** No Qualifier

U **Omentum**
   Gastrocolic ligament
   Gastrocolic omentum
   Gastrohepatic omentum
   Gastrophrenic ligament
   Gastrosplenic ligament
   Greater Omentum
   Hepatogastric ligament
   Lesser Omentum
V **Mesentery**
   Mesoappendix
   Mesocolon
W **Peritoneum**
   Epiploic foramen
	Ø Open
	3 Percutaneous
	4 Percutaneous Endoscopic
		Ø Drainage Device
		1 Radioactive Element
		7 Autologous Tissue Substitute
		J Synthetic Substitute
		K Nonautologous Tissue Substitute
			Z No Qualifier

Non-OR   ØDPP[7,8,X]1Z

LG Limited Coverage   **NC** Noncovered   ⊞ Combination Member   HAC associated procedure   Combination Only   DRG Non-OR   Non-OR   New/Revised in GREEN

382   ICD-10-PCS 2020

ØDP–ØDP (side tab)

Ø   Medical and Surgical
D   Gastrointestinal System
Q   Repair   Definition: Restoring, to the extent possible, a body part to its normal anatomic structure and function
                    Explanation: Used only when the method to accomplish the repair is not one of the other root operations

Body Part Character 4	Approach Character 5	Device Character 6	Qualifier Character 7

1 Esophagus, Upper
   Cervical esophagus
2 Esophagus, Middle
   Thoracic esophagus
3 Esophagus, Lower
   Abdominal esophagus
4 Esophagogastric Junction
   Cardia
   Cardioesophageal junction
   Gastroesophageal (GE) junction
5 Esophagus
6 Stomach
7 Stomach, Pylorus
   Pyloric antrum
   Pyloric canal
   Pyloric sphincter
8 Small Intestine ⊞
9 Duodenum ⊞
A Jejunum ⊞
   Duodenojejunal flexure
B Ileum ⊞
C Ileocecal Valve
E Large Intestine ⊞
F Large Intestine, Right ⊞
G Large Intestine, Left ⊞
H Cecum ⊞
J Appendix
   Vermiform appendix
K Ascending Colon ⊞
L Transverse Colon ⊞
   Hepatic flexure
   Splenic flexure
M Descending Colon ⊞
N Sigmoid Colon ⊞
   Rectosigmoid junction
   Sigmoid flexure
P Rectum
   Anorectal junction
	Ø Open
	3 Percutaneous
	4 Percutaneous Endoscopic
	7 Via Natural or Artificial Opening
	8 Via Natural or Artificial Opening
	   Endoscopic
		Z No Device	Z No Qualifier

Q Anus
   Anal orifice
	Ø Open
	3 Percutaneous
	4 Percutaneous Endoscopic
	7 Via Natural or Artificial Opening
	8 Via Natural or Artificial Opening
	   Endoscopic
	X External
		Z No Device	Z No Qualifier

R Anal Sphincter
   External anal sphincter
   Internal anal sphincter
U Omentum
   Gastrocolic ligament
   Gastrocolic omentum
   Gastrohepatic omentum
   Gastrophrenic ligament
   Gastrosplenic ligament
   Greater Omentum
   Hepatogastric ligament
   Lesser Omentum
V Mesentery
   Mesoappendix
   Mesocolon
W Peritoneum
   Epiploic foramen
	Ø Open
	3 Percutaneous
	4 Percutaneous Endoscopic
		Z No Device	Z No Qualifier

Non-OR   ØDQU[Ø,3,4]ZZ

See Appendix L for Procedure Combinations
  ⊞   ØDQ[8,9,A,B,E,F,G,H,K,L,M,N]ØZZ

Gastrointestinal System *(left sidebar)*

Ø   **Medical and Surgical**
D   **Gastrointestinal System**
R   **Replacement**   Definition: Putting in or on biological or synthetic material that physically takes the place and/or function of all or a portion of a body part
                Explanation: The body part may have been taken out or replaced, or may be taken out, physically eradicated, or rendered nonfunctional during the REPLACEMENT procedure. A REMOVAL procedure is coded for taking out the device used in a previous replacement procedure.

Body Part Character 4	Approach Character 5	Device Character 6	Qualifier Character 7
5 Esophagus	**Ø** Open **4** Percutaneous Endoscopic **7** Via Natural or Artificial Opening **8** Via Natural or Artificial Opening Endoscopic	**7** Autologous Tissue Substitute **J** Synthetic Substitute **K** Nonautologous Tissue Substitute	**Z** No Qualifier

R Anal Sphincter
   External anal sphincter
   Internal anal sphincter
U Omentum
   Gastrocolic ligament
   Gastrocolic omentum
   Gastrohepatic omentum
   Gastrophrenic ligament
   Gastrosplenic ligament
   Greater Omentum
   Hepatogastric ligament
   Lesser Omentum
V Mesentery
   Mesoappendix
   Mesocolon
W Peritoneum
   Epiploic foramen
	Ø Open
	4 Percutaneous Endoscopic
		7 Autologous Tissue Substitute
		J Synthetic Substitute
		K Nonautologous Tissue Substitute
			Z No Qualifier

Ø   **Medical and Surgical**
D   **Gastrointestinal System**
S   **Reposition**   Definition: Moving to its normal location, or other suitable location, all or a portion of a body part
                Explanation: The body part is moved to a new location from an abnormal location, or from a normal location where it is not functioning correctly. The body part may or may not be cut out or off to be moved to the new location.

Body Part Character 4	Approach Character 5	Device Character 6	Qualifier Character 7

5 Esophagus
6 Stomach
9 Duodenum
A Jejunum
   Duodenojejunal flexure
B Ileum
H Cecum
K Ascending Colon
L Transverse Colon
   Hepatic flexure
   Splenic flexure
M Descending Colon
N Sigmoid Colon
   Rectosigmoid junction
   Sigmoid flexure
P Rectum
   Anorectal junction
Q Anus
   Anal orifice
	Ø Open
	4 Percutaneous Endoscopic
	7 Via Natural or Artificial Opening
	8 Via Natural or Artificial Opening Endoscopic
	X External
		Z No Device	**Z** No Qualifier

8 Small Intestine **E** Large Intestine	**Ø** Open **4** Percutaneous Endoscopic **7** Via Natural or Artificial Opening **8** Via Natural or Artificial Opening Endoscopic	**Z** No Device	**Z** No Qualifier

Non-OR   ØDS[5,6,9,A,B,H,K,L,M,N,P,Q]XZZ

Ø   **Medical and Surgical**
D   **Gastrointestinal System**
T   **Resection**   Definition: Cutting out or off, without replacement, all of a body part
                 Explanation: None

Body Part Character 4	Approach Character 5	Device Character 6	Qualifier Character 7
1 Esophagus, Upper Cervical esophagus **2 Esophagus, Middle** Thoracic esophagus **3 Esophagus, Lower** Abdominal esophagus **4 Esophagogastric Junction** Cardia Cardioesophageal junction Gastroesophageal (GE) junction **5 Esophagus** **6 Stomach** **7 Stomach, Pylorus** Pyloric antrum Pyloric canal Pyloric sphincter **8 Small Intestine** **9 Duodenum** ⊞ **A Jejunum** Duodenojejunal flexure **B Ileum** **C Ileocecal Valve** **E Large Intestine** **F Large Intestine, Right** **H Cecum** **J Appendix** Vermiform appendix **K Ascending Colon** **P Rectum** Anorectal junction **Q Anus** Anal orifice	**Ø Open** **4 Percutaneous Endoscopic** **7 Via Natural or Artificial Opening** **8 Via Natural or Artificial Opening Endoscopic**	**Z No Device**	**Z No Qualifier**
G Large Intestine, Left **L Transverse Colon** Hepatic flexure Splenic flexure **M Descending Colon** **N Sigmoid Colon** Rectosigmoid junction Sigmoid flexure	**Ø Open** **4 Percutaneous Endoscopic** **7 Via Natural or Artificial Opening** **8 Via Natural or Artificial Opening Endoscopic** **F Via Natural or Artificial Opening with Percutaneous Endoscopic Assistance**	**Z No Device**	**Z No Qualifier**
R Anal Sphincter External anal sphincter Internal anal sphincter **U Omentum** Gastrocolic ligament Gastrocolic omentum Gastrohepatic omentum Gastrophrenic ligament Gastrosplenic ligament Greater Omentum Hepatogastric ligament Lesser Omentum	**Ø Open** **4 Percutaneous Endoscopic**	**Z No Device**	**Z No Qualifier**

See Appendix L for Procedure Combinations
   ⊞   ØDT9ØZZ

Gastrointestinal System

Ø   **Medical and Surgical**
D   **Gastrointestinal System**
U   **Supplement**   Definition: Putting in or on biological or synthetic material that physically reinforces and/or augments the function of a portion of a body part
                        Explanation: The biological material is non-living, or is living and from the same individual. The body part may have been previously replaced, and the SUPPLEMENT procedure is performed to physically reinforce and/or augment the function of the replaced body part.

Body Part Character 4	Approach Character 5	Device Character 6	Qualifier Character 7

1 **Esophagus, Upper**
  Cervical esophagus
2 **Esophagus, Middle**
  Thoracic esophagus
3 **Esophagus, Lower**
  Abdominal esophagus
4 **Esophagogastric Junction**
  Cardia
  Cardioesophageal junction
  Gastroesophageal (GE) junction
5 **Esophagus**
6 **Stomach**
7 **Stomach, Pylorus**
  Pyloric antrum
  Pyloric canal
  Pyloric sphincter
8 **Small Intestine**
9 **Duodenum**
A **Jejunum**
  Duodenojejunal flexure
B **Ileum**
C **Ileocecal Valve**
E **Large Intestine**
F **Large Intestine, Right**
G **Large Intestine, Left**
H **Cecum**
K **Ascending Colon**
L **Transverse Colon**
  Hepatic flexure
  Splenic flexure
M **Descending Colon**
N **Sigmoid Colon**
  Rectosigmoid junction
  Sigmoid flexure
P **Rectum**
  Anorectal junction
	Ø **Open**
	4 **Percutaneous Endoscopic**
	7 **Via Natural or Artificial Opening**
	8 **Via Natural or Artificial Opening Endoscopic**
		7 **Autologous Tissue Substitute**
		J **Synthetic Substitute**
		K **Nonautologous Tissue Substitute**
			Z **No Qualifier**

Q **Anus** Anal orifice	Ø **Open** 4 **Percutaneous Endoscopic** 7 **Via Natural or Artificial Opening** 8 **Via Natural or Artificial Opening Endoscopic** X **External**	7 **Autologous Tissue Substitute** J **Synthetic Substitute** K **Nonautologous Tissue Substitute**	Z **No Qualifier**

R **Anal Sphincter**
  External anal sphincter
  Internal anal sphincter
U **Omentum**
  Gastrocolic ligament
  Gastrocolic omentum
  Gastrohepatic omentum
  Gastrophrenic ligament
  Gastrosplenic ligament
  Greater Omentum
  Hepatogastric ligament
  Lesser Omentum
V **Mesentery**
  Mesoappendix
  Mesocolon
W **Peritoneum**
  Epiploic foramen
	Ø **Open**
	4 **Percutaneous Endoscopic**
		7 **Autologous Tissue Substitute**
		J **Synthetic Substitute**
		K **Nonautologous Tissue Substitute**
			Z **No Qualifier**

Ø   **Medical and Surgical**
D   **Gastrointestinal System**
V   **Restriction**   Definition: Partially closing an orifice or the lumen of a tubular body part
                              Explanation: The orifice can be a natural orifice or an artificially created orifice

Body Part Character 4		Approach Character 5	Device Character 6	Qualifier Character 7
1 Esophagus, Upper Cervical esophagus 2 Esophagus, Middle Thoracic esophagus 3 Esophagus, Lower Abdominal esophagus 4 Esophagogastric Junction Cardia Cardioesophageal junction Gastroesophageal (GE) junction 5 Esophagus 6 Stomach 7 Stomach, Pylorus Pyloric antrum Pyloric canal Pyloric sphincter 8 Small Intestine	9 Duodenum A Jejunum Duodenojejunal flexure B Ileum C Ileocecal Valve E Large Intestine F Large Intestine, Right G Large Intestine, Left H Cecum K Ascending Colon L Transverse Colon Hepatic flexure Splenic flexure M Descending Colon N Sigmoid Colon Rectosigmoid junction Sigmoid flexure P Rectum Anorectal junction	Ø Open 3 Percutaneous 4 Percutaneous Endoscopic	C Extraluminal Device D Intraluminal Device Z No Device	Z No Qualifier
1 Esophagus, Upper Cervical esophagus 2 Esophagus, Middle Thoracic esophagus 3 Esophagus, Lower Abdominal esophagus 4 Esophagogastric Junction Cardia Cardioesophageal junction Gastroesophageal (GE) junction 5 Esophagus 6 Stomach NC 7 Stomach, Pylorus Pyloric antrum Pyloric canal Pyloric sphincter 8 Small Intestine	9 Duodenum A Jejunum Duodenojejunal flexure B Ileum C Ileocecal Valve E Large Intestine F Large Intestine, Right G Large Intestine, Left H Cecum K Ascending Colon L Transverse Colon Hepatic flexure Splenic flexure M Descending Colon N Sigmoid Colon Rectosigmoid junction Sigmoid flexure P Rectum Anorectal junction	7 Via Natural or Artificial Opening 8 Via Natural or Artificial Opening Endoscopic	D Intraluminal Device Z No Device	Z No Qualifier
Q Anus Anal orifice		Ø Open 3 Percutaneous 4 Percutaneous Endoscopic X External	C Extraluminal Device D Intraluminal Device Z No Device	Z No Qualifier
Q Anus Anal orifice		7 Via Natural or Artificial Opening 8 Via Natural or Artificial Opening Endoscopic	D Intraluminal Device Z No Device	Z No Qualifier

Non-OR   ØDV6[7,8]DZ
HAC   ØDV64CZ when reported with PDx E66.Ø1 and SDx K68.11, K95.Ø1, K95.81, or T81.4Ø–T81.49 with 7th character A
NC   ØDV6[7,8]DZ

Gastrointestinal System

Ø   **Medical and Surgical**
D   **Gastrointestinal System**
W   **Revision**   Definition: Correcting, to the extent possible, a portion of a malfunctioning device or the position of a displaced device

                      Explanation: Revision can include correcting a malfunctioning or displaced device by taking out or putting in components of the device such as a screw or pin

Body Part Character 4	Approach Character 5	Device Character 6	Qualifier Character 7
Ø Upper Intestinal Tract **D** Lower Intestinal Tract	**Ø** Open **3** Percutaneous **4** Percutaneous Endoscopic **7** Via Natural or Artificial Opening **8** Via Natural or Artificial Opening Endoscopic	**Ø** Drainage Device **2** Monitoring Device **3** Infusion Device **7** Autologous Tissue Substitute **C** Extraluminal Device **D** Intraluminal Device **J** Synthetic Substitute **K** Nonautologous Tissue Substitute **U** Feeding Device **Y** Other Device	**Z** No Qualifier
Ø Upper Intestinal Tract **D** Lower Intestinal Tract	**X** External	**Ø** Drainage Device **2** Monitoring Device **3** Infusion Device **7** Autologous Tissue Substitute **C** Extraluminal Device **D** Intraluminal Device **J** Synthetic Substitute **K** Nonautologous Tissue Substitute **U** Feeding Device	**Z** No Qualifier
5 Esophagus	**Ø** Open **3** Percutaneous **4** Percutaneous Endoscopic	**Y** Other Device	**Z** No Qualifier
5 Esophagus	**7** Via Natural or Artificial Opening **8** Via Natural or Artificial Opening Endoscopic	**D** Intraluminal Device **Y** Other Device	**Z** No Qualifier
5 Esophagus	**X** External	**D** Intraluminal Device	**Z** No Qualifier
6 Stomach	**Ø** Open **3** Percutaneous **4** Percutaneous Endoscopic	**Ø** Drainage Device **2** Monitoring Device **3** Infusion Device **7** Autologous Tissue Substitute **C** Extraluminal Device **D** Intraluminal Device **J** Synthetic Substitute **K** Nonautologous Tissue Substitute **M** Stimulator Lead **U** Feeding Device **Y** Other Device	**Z** No Qualifier
6 Stomach	**7** Via Natural or Artificial Opening **8** Via Natural or Artificial Opening Endoscopic	**Ø** Drainage Device **2** Monitoring Device **3** Infusion Device **7** Autologous Tissue Substitute **C** Extraluminal Device **D** Intraluminal Device **J** Synthetic Substitute **K** Nonautologous Tissue Substitute **U** Feeding Device **Y** Other Device	**Z** No Qualifier
6 Stomach	**X** External	**Ø** Drainage Device **2** Monitoring Device **3** Infusion Device **7** Autologous Tissue Substitute **C** Extraluminal Device **D** Intraluminal Device **J** Synthetic Substitute **K** Nonautologous Tissue Substitute **U** Feeding Device	**Z** No Qualifier

ØDW Continued on next page

Non-OR   ØDW[Ø,D][3,4,7,8]YZ
Non-OR   ØDW[Ø,D]X[Ø,2,3,7,C,D,J,K,U]Z
Non-OR   ØDW5[Ø,3,4]YZ
Non-OR   ØDW5[7,8]YZ
Non-OR   ØDW5XDZ
Non-OR   ØDW6[3,4]YZ
Non-OR   ØDW6[7,8]YZ
Non-OR   ØDW6X[Ø,2,3,7,C,D,J,K,U]Z

LC Limited Coverage   **NC** Noncovered   ⊞ Combination Member   HAC associated procedure   Combination Only   DRG Non-OR   Non-OR   New/Revised in **GREEN**

388   ICD-10-PCS 2020

Ø   **Medical and Surgical**
D   **Gastrointestinal System**
W   **Revision**   Definition: Correcting, to the extent possible, a portion of a malfunctioning device or the position of a displaced device

ØDW Continued

Explanation: Revision can include correcting a malfunctioning or displaced device by taking out or putting in components of the device such as a screw or pin

Body Part Character 4	Approach Character 5	Device Character 6	Qualifier Character 7
8 Small Intestine **E** Large Intestine	**Ø** Open **4** Percutaneous Endoscopic **7** Via Natural or Artificial Opening **8** Via Natural or Artificial Opening Endoscopic	**7** Autologous Tissue Substitute **J** Synthetic Substitute **K** Nonautologous Tissue Substitute	**Z** No Qualifier
Q Anus Anal orifice	**Ø** Open **3** Percutaneous **4** Percutaneous Endoscopic **7** Via Natural or Artificial Opening **8** Via Natural or Artificial Opening Endoscopic	**L** Artificial Sphincter	**Z** No Qualifier

R   Anal Sphincter
     External anal sphincter
     Internal anal sphincter
	Ø Open
	3 Percutaneous
	4 Percutaneous Endoscopic
		M Stimulator Lead	**Z** No Qualifier

U   Omentum
     Gastrocolic ligament
     Gastrocolic omentum
     Gastrohepatic omentum
     Gastrophrenic ligament
     Gastrosplenic ligament
     Greater Omentum
     Hepatogastric ligament
     Lesser Omentum
V   Mesentery
     Mesoappendix
     Mesocolon
W   Peritoneum
     Epiploic foramen
	Ø Open
	3 Percutaneous
	4 Percutaneous Endoscopic
		Ø Drainage Device
		7 Autologous Tissue Substitute
		J Synthetic Substitute
		K Nonautologous Tissue Substitute
			Z No Qualifier

Non-OR   ØDW[U,V,W][Ø,3,4]ØZ

Ø   **Medical and Surgical**
D   **Gastrointestinal System**
X   **Transfer**   Definition: Moving, without taking out, all or a portion of a body part to another location to take over the function of all or a portion of a body part

Explanation: The body part transferred remains connected to its vascular and nervous supply

Body Part Character 4	Approach Character 5	Device Character 6	Qualifier Character 7
6 Stomach **8** Small Intestine	**Ø** Open **4** Percutaneous Endoscopic	**Z** No Device	**5** Esophagus
E Large Intestine	**Ø** Open **4** Percutaneous Endoscopic	**Z** No Device	**5** Esophagus **7** Vagina

---

Ø   **Medical and Surgical**
D   **Gastrointestinal System**
Y   **Transplantation**   Definition: Putting in or on all or a portion of a living body part taken from another individual or animal to physically take the place and/or function of all or a portion of a similar body part

Explanation: The native body part may or may not be taken out, and the transplanted body part may take over all or a portion of its function

Body Part Character 4	Approach Character 5	Device Character 6	Qualifier Character 7
5 Esophagus **6** Stomach **8** Small Intestine [LC] **E** Large Intestine [LC]	**Ø** Open	**Z** No Device	**Ø** Allogeneic **1** Syngeneic **2** Zooplastic

Non-OR   ØDY5ØZ[Ø,1,2]
[LC]   ØDY[8,E]ØZ[Ø,1,2]

[LC] Limited Coverage   [NC] Noncovered   ⊞ Combination Member   HAC associated procedure   Combination Only   DRG Non-OR   Non-OR   New/Revised in GREEN

ICD-10-PCS 2020   389

ØDW–ØDY

Hepatobiliary System and Pancreas ØF1–ØFY

Character Meanings

This Character Meaning table is provided as a guide to assist the user in the identification of character members that may be found in this section of code tables. It **SHOULD NOT** be used to build a PCS code.

Operation–Character 3	Body Part–Character 4	Approach–Character 5	Device–Character 6	Qualifier–Character 7
1 Bypass	Ø Liver	Ø Open	Ø Drainage Device	Ø Allogeneic
2 Change	1 Liver, Right Lobe	3 Percutaneous	1 Radioactive Element	1 Syngeneic
5 Destruction	2 Liver, Left Lobe	4 Percutaneous Endoscopic	2 Monitoring Device	2 Zooplastic
7 Dilation	4 Gallbladder	7 Via Natural or Artificial Opening	3 Infusion Device	3 Duodenum
8 Division	5 Hepatic Duct, Right	8 Via Natural or Artificial Opening Endoscopic	7 Autologous Tissue Substitute	4 Stomach
9 Drainage	6 Hepatic Duct, Left	X External	C Extraluminal Device	5 Hepatic Duct, Right
B Excision	7 Hepatic Duct, Common		D Intraluminal Device	6 Hepatic Duct, Left
C Extirpation	8 Cystic Duct		J Synthetic Substitute	7 Hepatic Duct, Caudate
D Extraction	9 Common Bile Duct		K Nonautologous Tissue Substitute	8 Cystic Duct
F Fragmentation	B Hepatobiliary Duct		Y Other Device	9 Common Bile Duct
H Insertion	C Ampulla of Vater		Z No Device	B Small Intestine
J Inspection	D Pancreatic Duct			C Large Intestine
L Occlusion	F Pancreatic Duct, Accessory			F Irreversible Electroporation
M Reattachment	G Pancreas			X Diagnostic
N Release				Z No Qualifier
P Removal				
Q Repair				
R Replacement				
S Reposition				
T Resection				
U Supplement				
V Restriction				
W Revision				
Y Transplantation				

AHA Coding Clinic for table ØF5
2018, 4Q, 39   Irreversible electroporation

AHA Coding Clinic for table ØF7
2016, 3Q, 27   Endoscopic retrograde cholangiopancreatography with sphincterotomy and insertion of pancreatic stent
2016, 1Q, 25   Endoscopic retrograde cholangiopancreatography with brush biopsy of pancreatic and common bile ducts
2015, 1Q, 32   Percutaneous transhepatic biliary drainage catheter placement
2014, 3Q, 15   Drainage of pancreatic pseudocyst

AHA Coding Clinic for table ØF9
2015, 1Q, 32   Percutaneous transhepatic biliary drainage catheter placement
2014, 3Q, 15   Drainage of pancreatic pseudocyst

AHA Coding Clinic for table ØFB
2019, 1Q, 3-8   Whipple procedure
2016, 3Q, 41   Open cholecystectomy with needle biopsy of liver
2016, 1Q, 23   Endoscopic ultrasound with aspiration biopsy of common hepatic duct
2016, 1Q, 25   Endoscopic retrograde cholangiopancreatography with brush biopsy of pancreatic and common bile ducts
2014, 3Q, 32   Pyloric-sparing Whipple procedure

AHA Coding Clinic for table ØFC
2016, 3Q, 27   Endoscopic retrograde cholangiopancreatography with sphincterotomy and insertion of pancreatic stent

AHA Coding Clinic for table ØFQ
2016, 3Q, 27   Revision of common bile duct anastomosis
2013, 4Q, 109   Separating conjoined twins

AHA Coding Clinic for table ØFT
2019, 1Q, 3-8   Whipple Procedure
2012, 4Q, 99   Domino liver transplant

AHA Coding Clinic for table ØFY
2014, 3Q, 13   Orthotopic liver transplant with end to side cavoplasty
2012, 4Q, 99   Domino liver transplant

Liver

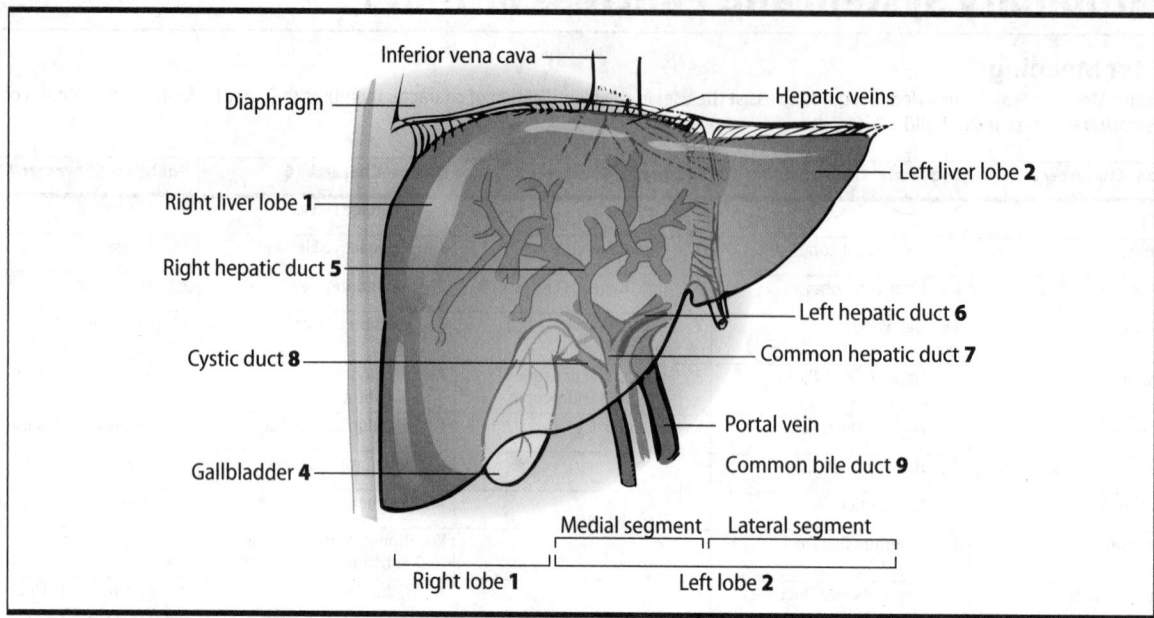

Inferior vena cava
Diaphragm
Hepatic veins
Right liver lobe **1**
Left liver lobe **2**
Right hepatic duct **5**
Left hepatic duct **6**
Common hepatic duct **7**
Cystic duct **8**
Portal vein
Common bile duct **9**
Gallbladder **4**

Medial segment | Lateral segment
Right lobe **1** | Left lobe **2**

Pancreas

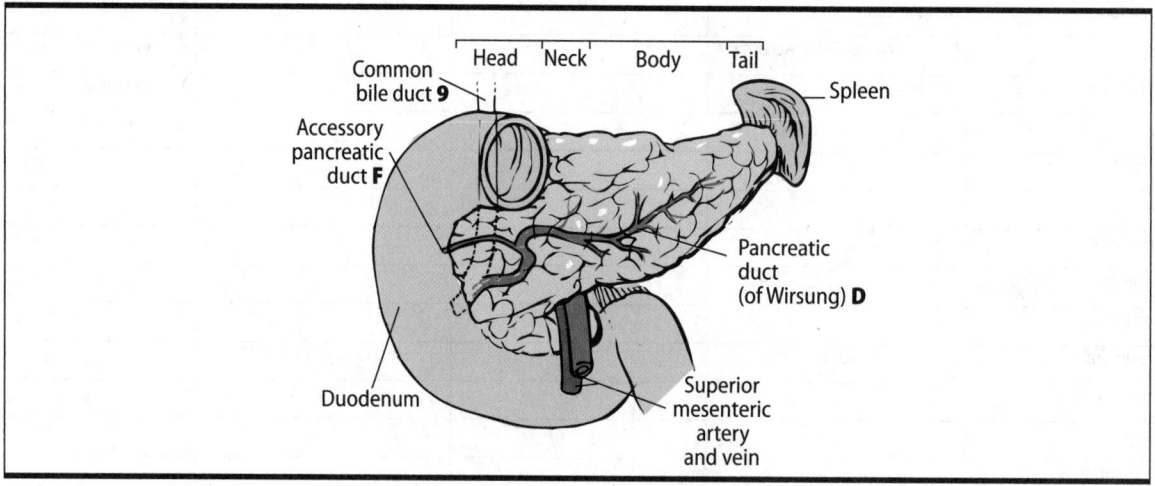

Head | Neck | Body | Tail
Common bile duct **9**
Spleen
Accessory pancreatic duct **F**
Pancreatic duct (of Wirsung) **D**
Duodenum
Superior mesenteric artery and vein

Gallbladder and Ducts

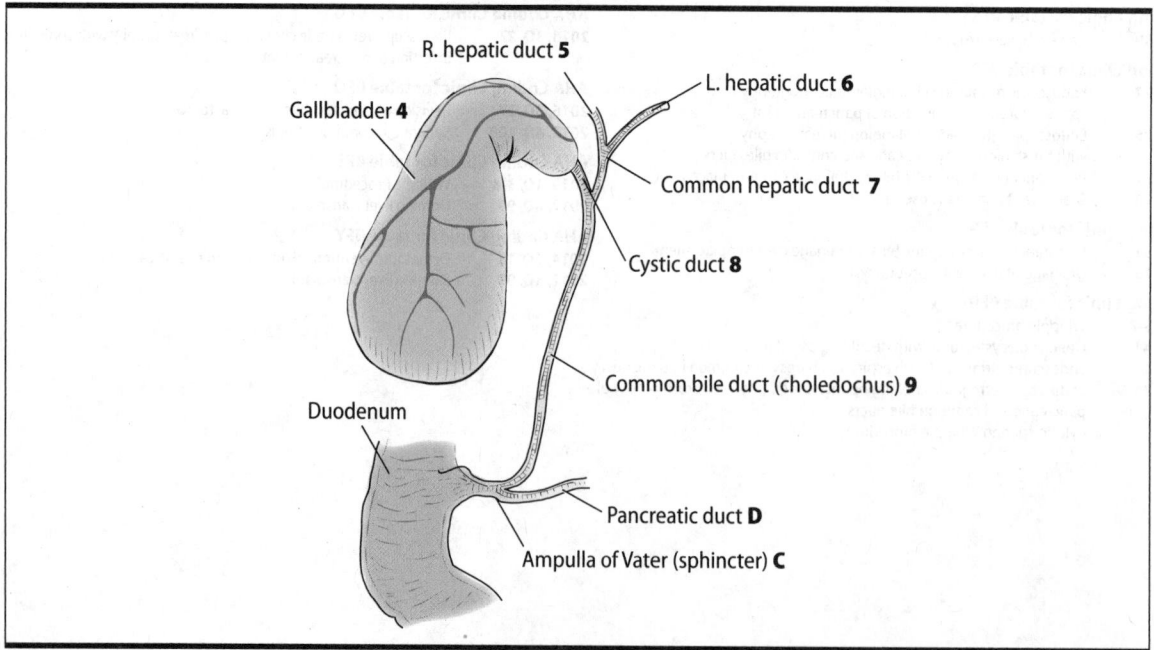

R. hepatic duct **5**
L. hepatic duct **6**
Gallbladder **4**
Common hepatic duct **7**
Cystic duct **8**
Common bile duct (choledochus) **9**
Duodenum
Pancreatic duct **D**
Ampulla of Vater (sphincter) **C**

Ø   **Medical and Surgical**
F   **Hepatobiliary System and Pancreas**
1   **Bypass**   Definition: Altering the route of passage of the contents of a tubular body part

                     Explanation: Rerouting contents of a body part to a downstream area of the normal route, to a similar route and body part, or to an abnormal route and dissimilar body part. Includes one or more anastomoses, with or without the use of a device.

Body Part Character 4	Approach Character 5	Device Character 6	Qualifier Character 7
4 Gallbladder **5** Hepatic Duct, Right **6** Hepatic Duct, Left **7** Hepatic Duct, Common **8** Cystic Duct **9** Common Bile Duct	**Ø** Open **4** Percutaneous Endoscopic	**D** Intraluminal Device **Z** No Device	**3** Duodenum **4** Stomach **5** Hepatic Duct, Right **6** Hepatic Duct, Left **7** Hepatic Duct, Caudate **8** Cystic Duct **9** Common Bile Duct **B** Small Intestine

D Pancreatic Duct
     Duct of Wirsung
F Pancreatic Duct, Accessory
     Duct of Santorini
G Pancreas
	Ø Open
	4 Percutaneous Endoscopic
		D Intraluminal Device
		Z No Device
			3 Duodenum
			B Small Intestine
			C Large Intestine

Ø   **Medical and Surgical**
F   **Hepatobiliary System and Pancreas**
2   **Change**   Definition: Taking out or off a device from a body part and putting back an identical or similar device in or on the same body part without cutting or puncturing the skin or a mucous membrane

                     Explanation: All CHANGE procedures are coded using the approach EXTERNAL

Body Part Character 4	Approach Character 5	Device Character 6	Qualifier Character 7

Ø Liver
     Quadrate lobe
4 Gallbladder
B Hepatobiliary Duct
D Pancreatic Duct
     Duct of Wirsung
G Pancreas
	X External	**Ø** Drainage Device
		Y Other Device
			Z No Qualifier

Non-OR   All body part, approach, device, and qualifier values

Ø   **Medical and Surgical**
F   **Hepatobiliary System and Pancreas**
5   **Destruction**   Definition: Physical eradication of all or a portion of a body part by the direct use of energy, force, or a destructive agent

                     Explanation: None of the body part is physically taken out

Body Part Character 4	Approach Character 5	Device Character 6	Qualifier Character 7
Ø Liver Quadrate lobe **1** Liver, Right Lobe **2** Liver, Left Lobe	**Ø** Open **3** Percutaneous **4** Percutaneous Endoscopic	**Z** No Device	**F** Irreversible Electroporation **Z** No Qualifier
4 Gallbladder	**Ø** Open **3** Percutaneous **4** Percutaneous Endoscopic **8** Via Natural or Artificial Opening Endoscopic	**Z** No Device	**Z** No Qualifier

5 Hepatic Duct, Right
6 Hepatic Duct, Left
7 Hepatic Duct, Common
8 Cystic Duct
9 Common Bile Duct
C Ampulla of Vater
     Duodenal ampulla
     Hepatopancreatic ampulla
D Pancreatic Duct
     Duct of Wirsung
F Pancreatic Duct, Accessory
     Duct of Santorini
	Ø Open
	3 Percutaneous
	4 Percutaneous Endoscopic
	7 Via Natural or Artificial Opening
	8 Via Natural or Artificial Opening Endoscopic
		Z No Device	**Z** No Qualifier

G Pancreas	**Ø** Open **3** Percutaneous **4** Percutaneous Endoscopic	**Z** No Device	**F** Irreversible Electroporation **Z** No Qualifier
G Pancreas	**8** Via Natural or Artificial Opening Endoscopic	**Z** No Device	**Z** No Qualifier

Non-OR   ØF5[5,6,7,8,9,C,D,F][4,8]ZZ
Non-OR   ØF5G4Z[F,Z]
Non-OR   ØF5G8ZZ

LC Limited Coverage   **NC** Noncovered   ⊞ Combination Member   HAC associated procedure   Combination Only   DRG Non-OR   Non-OR   New/Revised in GREEN

ICD-10-PCS 2020   **393**

Ø   Medical and Surgical
F   Hepatobiliary System and Pancreas
7   Dilation   Definition: Expanding an orifice or the lumen of a tubular body part

Explanation: The orifice can be a natural orifice or an artificially created orifice. Accomplished by stretching a tubular body part using intraluminal pressure or by cutting part of the orifice or wall of the tubular body part.

Body Part Character 4	Approach Character 5	Device Character 6	Qualifier Character 7

5   Hepatic Duct, Right
6   Hepatic Duct, Left
7   Hepatic Duct, Common
8   Cystic Duct
9   Common Bile Duct
C   Ampulla of Vater
     Duodenal ampulla
     Hepatopancreatic ampulla
D   Pancreatic Duct
     Duct of Wirsung
F   Pancreatic Duct, Accessory
     Duct of Santorini
	Ø Open
	3 Percutaneous
	4 Percutaneous Endoscopic
	7 Via Natural or Artificial Opening
	8 Via Natural or Artificial Opening
	     Endoscopic
		D Intraluminal Device
		Z No Device
			Z No Qualifier

Non-OR   ØF7[5,6,7,8,9][3,4,8][D,Z]Z
Non-OR   ØF7[5,6,7,8,9,D]]7DZ
Non-OR   ØF7C8[D,Z]Z
Non-OR   ØF7[D,F][4,8][D,Z]Z

Ø   Medical and Surgical
F   Hepatobiliary System and Pancreas
8   Division   Definition: Cutting into a body part, without draining fluids and/or gases from the body part, in order to separate or transect a body part

Explanation: All or a portion of the body part is separated into two or more portions

Body Part Character 4	Approach Character 5	Device Character 6	Qualifier Character 7
G Pancreas	Ø Open 3 Percutaneous 4 Percutaneous Endoscopic	Z No Device	Z No Qualifier

LC Limited Coverage   NC Noncovered   ⊞ Combination Member   HAC associated procedure   Combination Only   DRG Non-OR   Non-OR   New/Revised in GREEN

394   ICD-10-PCS 2020

Ø   Medical and Surgical
F   Hepatobiliary System and Pancreas
9   Drainage   Definition: Taking or letting out fluids and/or gases from a body part

                Explanation: The qualifier DIAGNOSTIC is used to identify drainage procedures that are biopsies

Body Part Character 4	Approach Character 5	Device Character 6	Qualifier Character 7
Ø Liver Quadrate lobe **1 Liver, Right Lobe** **2 Liver, Left Lobe**	**Ø** Open **3** Percutaneous **4** Percutaneous Endoscopic	**Ø** Drainage Device	**Z** No Qualifier
Ø Liver Quadrate lobe **1 Liver, Right Lobe** **2 Liver, Left Lobe**	**Ø** Open **3** Percutaneous **4** Percutaneous Endoscopic	**Z** No Device	**X** Diagnostic **Z** No Qualifier
4 Gallbladder **G Pancreas**	**Ø** Open **3** Percutaneous **4** Percutaneous Endoscopic **8** Via Natural or Artificial Opening Endoscopic	**Ø** Drainage Device	**Z** No Qualifier
4 Gallbladder **G Pancreas**	**Ø** Open **3** Percutaneous **4** Percutaneous Endoscopic **8** Via Natural or Artificial Opening Endoscopic	**Z** No Device	**X** Diagnostic **Z** No Qualifier

5 Hepatic Duct, Right
6 Hepatic Duct, Left
7 Hepatic Duct, Common
8 Cystic Duct
9 Common Bile Duct
C Ampulla of Vater
   Duodenal ampulla
   Hepatopancreatic ampulla
D Pancreatic Duct
   Duct of Wirsung
F Pancreatic Duct, Accessory
   Duct of Santorini
	Ø Open
	3 Percutaneous
	4 Percutaneous Endoscopic
	7 Via Natural or Artificial Opening
	8 Via Natural or Artificial Opening
	   Endoscopic
		Ø Drainage Device	**Z** No Qualifier

5 Hepatic Duct, Right
6 Hepatic Duct, Left
7 Hepatic Duct, Common
8 Cystic Duct
9 Common Bile Duct
C Ampulla of Vater
   Duodenal ampulla
   Hepatopancreatic ampulla
D Pancreatic Duct
   Duct of Wirsung
F Pancreatic Duct, Accessory
   Duct of Santorini
	Ø Open
	3 Percutaneous
	4 Percutaneous Endoscopic
	7 Via Natural or Artificial Opening
	8 Via Natural or Artificial Opening
	   Endoscopic
		Z No Device	**X** Diagnostic
			Z No Qualifier

Non-OR	ØF9[Ø,1,2][3,4]ØZ	**Non-OR**	ØF99[3,8]ØZ
Non-OR	ØF9[Ø,1,2][3,4]Z[X,Z]	**Non-OR**	ØF9C[3,4,8]ØZ
Non-OR	ØF9[4,G]8ØZ	**Non-OR**	ØF9[D,F][3,8]ØZ
Non-OR	ØF9G3ØZ	**Non-OR**	ØF9[5,6,8,9,C,D,F]3Z[X,Z]
Non-OR	ØF9[4,G]8Z[X,Z]	**Non-OR**	ØF9[5,6,8,9,C,D,F][4,7,8]ZX
Non-OR	ØF9G3Z[XZ]	**Non-OR**	ØF9[5,6,8,D,F]8ZZ
Non-OR	ØF9G4ZX	**Non-OR**	ØF97[3,4,7,8]Z[X,Z]
Non-OR	ØF9[5,6,8][3,8]ØZ	**Non-OR**	ØF99[4,7,8]ZZ
Non-OR	ØF97[3,4,7,8]ØZ	**Non-OR**	ØF9C[4,8]ZZ

LC Limited Coverage   **NC** Noncovered   ⊞ Combination Member   HAC associated procedure   Combination Only   DRG Non-OR   Non-OR   New/Revised in GREEN

ICD-10-PCS 2020   395

Ø **Medical and Surgical**
F **Hepatobiliary System and Pancreas**
B **Excision**   Definition: Cutting out or off, without replacement, a portion of a body part

Explanation: The qualifier DIAGNOSTIC is used to identify excision procedures that are biopsies

Body Part Character 4	Approach Character 5	Device Character 6	Qualifier Character 7
Ø Liver Quadrate lobe 1 Liver, Right Lobe 2 Liver, Left Lobe	Ø Open 3 Percutaneous 4 Percutaneous Endoscopic	Z No Device	X Diagnostic Z No Qualifier
4 Gallbladder G Pancreas	Ø Open 3 Percutaneous 4 Percutaneous Endoscopic 8 Via Natural or Artificial Opening Endoscopic	Z No Device	X Diagnostic Z No Qualifier

5 Hepatic Duct, Right
6 Hepatic Duct, Left
7 Hepatic Duct, Common
8 Cystic Duct
9 Common Bile Duct
C Ampulla of Vater
   Duodenal ampulla
   Hepatopancreatic ampulla
D Pancreatic Duct
   Duct of Wirsung
F Pancreatic Duct, Accessory
   Duct of Santorini
	Ø Open
	3 Percutaneous
	4 Percutaneous Endoscopic
	7 Via Natural or Artificial Opening
	8 Via Natural or Artificial Opening
	   Endoscopic
		Z No Device	X Diagnostic
			Z No Qualifier

Non-OR   ØFB[Ø,1,2]3ZX
Non-OR   ØFB[4,G][3,4,8]ZX
Non-OR   ØFB[5,6,7,8,9,C,D,F][3,4,7,8]ZX
Non-OR   ØFB[5,6,7,8,9,C,D,F][4,8]ZZ

Ø **Medical and Surgical**
F **Hepatobiliary System and Pancreas**
C **Extirpation**   Definition: Taking or cutting out solid matter from a body part

Explanation: The solid matter may be an abnormal byproduct of a biological function or a foreign body; it may be imbedded in a body part or in the lumen of a tubular body part. The solid matter may or may not have been previously broken into pieces.

Body Part Character 4	Approach Character 5	Device Character 6	Qualifier Character 7
Ø Liver Quadrate lobe 1 Liver, Right Lobe 2 Liver, Left Lobe	Ø Open 3 Percutaneous 4 Percutaneous Endoscopic	Z No Device	Z No Qualifier
4 Gallbladder G Pancreas	Ø Open 3 Percutaneous 4 Percutaneous Endoscopic 8 Via Natural or Artificial Opening Endoscopic	Z No Device	Z No Qualifier

5 Hepatic Duct, Right
6 Hepatic Duct, Left
7 Hepatic Duct, Common
8 Cystic Duct
9 Common Bile Duct
C Ampulla of Vater
   Duodenal ampulla
   Hepatopancreatic ampulla
D Pancreatic Duct
   Duct of Wirsung
F Pancreatic Duct, Accessory
   Duct of Santorini
	Ø Open
	3 Percutaneous
	4 Percutaneous Endoscopic
	7 Via Natural or Artificial Opening
	8 Via Natural or Artificial Opening
	   Endoscopic
		Z No Device	Z No Qualifier

Non-OR   ØFC[5,6,7,8,9][3,4,7,8]ZZ
Non-OR   ØFCC[4,8]ZZ
Non-OR   ØFC[D,F][3,4,8]ZZ

LC Limited Coverage NC Noncovered ⊞ Combination Member HAC associated procedure Combination Only DRG Non-OR Non-OR New/Revised in GREEN

Ø   Medical and Surgical
F   Hepatobiliary System and Pancreas
D   Extraction   Definition: Pulling or stripping out or off all or a portion of a body part by the use of force

                 Explanation: The qualifier DIAGNOSTIC is used to identify extraction procedures that are biopsies

Body Part Character 4	Approach Character 5	Device Character 6	Qualifier Character 7
Ø Liver Quadrate lobe 1 Liver, Right Lobe 2 Liver, Left Lobe	3 Percutaneous 4 Percutaneous Endoscopic	Z No Device	X Diagnostic

4   Gallbladder
5   Hepatic Duct, Right
6   Hepatic Duct, Left
7   Hepatic Duct, Common
8   Cystic Duct
9   Common Bile Duct
C   Ampulla of Vater
     Duodenal ampulla
     Hepatopancreatic ampulla
D   Pancreatic Duct
     Duct of Wirsung
F   Pancreatic Duct, Accessory
     Duct of Santorini
G   Pancreas
	3 Percutaneous
	4 Percutaneous Endoscopic
	8 Via Natural or Artificial Opening
	     Endoscopic
		Z No Device	X Diagnostic

     Non-OR   ØFD[Ø,1,2]3ZX
     Non-OR   ØFD[4,5,6,7,8,9,C,D,F,G][3,4,8]ZX

Ø   Medical and Surgical
F   Hepatobiliary System and Pancreas
F   Fragmentation   Definition: Breaking solid matter in a body part into pieces

                 Explanation: Physical force (e.g., manual, ultrasonic) applied directly or indirectly is used to break the solid matter into pieces. The solid matter may be an abnormal byproduct of a biological function or a foreign body. The pieces of solid matter are not taken out.

Body Part Character 4	Approach Character 5	Device Character 6	Qualifier Character 7

4   Gallbladder   NC
5   Hepatic Duct, Right   NC
6   Hepatic Duct, Left   NC
7   Hepatic Duct, Common
8   Cystic Duct   NC
9   Common Bile Duct   NC
C   Ampulla of Vater   NC
     Duodenal ampulla
     Hepatopancreatic ampulla
D   Pancreatic Duct   NC
     Duct of Wirsung
F   Pancreatic Duct, Accessory   NC
     Duct of Santorini
	Ø Open
	3 Percutaneous
	4 Percutaneous Endoscopic
	7 Via Natural or Artificial Opening
	8 Via Natural or Artificial Opening
	     Endoscopic
	X External
		Z No Device	Z No Qualifier

     Non-OR   ØFF[4,5,6,7,8,9,C,D,F][8,X]ZZ
     NC   ØFF[4,5,6,8,9,C,D,F]XZZ

Ø   Medical and Surgical
F   Hepatobiliary System and Pancreas
H   Insertion   Definition: Putting in a nonbiological appliance that monitors, assists, performs, or prevents a physiological function but does not physically take the place of a body part

                 Explanation: None

Body Part Character 4	Approach Character 5	Device Character 6	Qualifier Character 7
Ø Liver Quadrate lobe 4 Gallbladder G Pancreas	Ø Open 3 Percutaneous 4 Percutaneous Endoscopic	2 Monitoring Device 3 Infusion Device Y Other Device	Z No Qualifier
1 Liver, Right Lobe 2 Liver, Left Lobe	Ø Open 3 Percutaneous 4 Percutaneous Endoscopic	2 Monitoring Device 3 Infusion Device	Z No Qualifier

B   Hepatobiliary Duct
D   Pancreatic Duct
     Duct of Wirsung
	Ø Open
	3 Percutaneous
	4 Percutaneous Endoscopic
	7 Via Natural or Artificial Opening
	8 Via Natural or Artificial Opening
	     Endoscopic
		1 Radioactive Element
		2 Monitoring Device
		3 Infusion Device
		D Intraluminal Device
		Y Other Device
			Z No Qualifier

     Non-OR   ØFH[Ø,4,G][Ø,3,4]3Z   **Non-OR**   ØFH[B,D]4DZ
     Non-OR   ØFH[Ø,4,G][3,4]YZ   **Non-OR**   ØFH[B,D][7,8][2,3]Z
     Non-OR   ØFH[1,2][Ø,3,4]3Z   **Non-OR**   ØFH[B,D]8DZ
     Non-OR   ØFH[B,D][Ø,3,4]3Z   **Non-OR**   ØFH[B,D][3,4,7,8]YZ

LC Limited Coverage   NC Noncovered   ⊞ Combination Member   HAC associated procedure   Combination Only   DRG Non-OR   Non-OR   New/Revised in GREEN

ICD-10-PCS 2020   397

Ø Medical and Surgical
F Hepatobiliary System and Pancreas
J Inspection Definition: Visually and/or manually exploring a body part

Explanation: Visual exploration may be performed with or without optical instrumentation. Manual exploration may be performed directly or through intervening body layers.

Body Part Character 4	Approach Character 5	Device Character 6	Qualifier Character 7
Ø Liver Quadrate lobe	Ø Open 3 Percutaneous 4 Percutaneous Endoscopic X External	Z No Device	Z No Qualifier
4 Gallbladder G Pancreas	Ø Open 3 Percutaneous 4 Percutaneous Endoscopic 8 Via Natural or Artificial Opening Endoscopic X External	Z No Device	Z No Qualifier
B Hepatobiliary Duct D Pancreatic Duct Duct of Wirsung	Ø Open 3 Percutaneous 4 Percutaneous Endoscopic 7 Via Natural or Artificial Opening 8 Via Natural or Artificial Opening Endoscopic	Z No Device	Z No Qualifier

Non-OR ØFJØ[3,X]ZZ
Non-OR ØFJ[4,G][3,8,X]ZZ
Non-OR ØFJ[B,D][3,7,8]ZZ

Ø Medical and Surgical
F Hepatobiliary System and Pancreas
L Occlusion Definition: Completely closing an orifice or the lumen of a tubular body part

Explanation: The orifice can be a natural orifice or an artificially created orifice

Body Part Character 4	Approach Character 5	Device Character 6	Qualifier Character 7
5 Hepatic Duct, Right 6 Hepatic Duct, Left 7 Hepatic Duct, Common 8 Cystic Duct 9 Common Bile Duct C Ampulla of Vater Duodenal ampulla Hepatopancreatic ampulla D Pancreatic Duct Duct of Wirsung F Pancreatic Duct, Accessory Duct of Santorini	Ø Open 3 Percutaneous 4 Percutaneous Endoscopic	C Extraluminal Device D Intraluminal Device Z No Device	Z No Qualifier
5 Hepatic Duct, Right 6 Hepatic Duct, Left 7 Hepatic Duct, Common 8 Cystic Duct 9 Common Bile Duct C Ampulla of Vater Duodenal ampulla Hepatopancreatic ampulla D Pancreatic Duct Duct of Wirsung F Pancreatic Duct, Accessory Duct of Santorini	7 Via Natural or Artificial Opening 8 Via Natural or Artificial Opening Endoscopic	D Intraluminal Device Z No Device	Z No Qualifier

Non-OR ØFL[5,6,7,8,9][3,4][C,D,Z]Z
Non-OR ØFL[5,6,7,8,9][7,8][D,Z]Z

Ø Medical and Surgical
F Hepatobiliary System and Pancreas
M Reattachment Definition: Putting back in or on all or a portion of a separated body part to its normal location or other suitable location
Explanation: Vascular circulation and nervous pathways may or may not be reestablished

Body Part Character 4	Approach Character 5	Device Character 6	Qualifier Character 7

Ø Liver
  Quadrate lobe
1 Liver, Right Lobe
2 Liver, Left Lobe
4 Gallbladder
5 Hepatic Duct, Right
6 Hepatic Duct, Left
7 Hepatic Duct, Common
8 Cystic Duct
9 Common Bile Duct
C Ampulla of Vater
  Duodenal ampulla
  Hepatopancreatic ampulla
D Pancreatic Duct
  Duct of Wirsung
F Pancreatic Duct, Accessory
  Duct of Santorini
G Pancreas
	Ø Open
	4 Percutaneous Endoscopic
		Z No Device	Z No Qualifier

Non-OR ØFM[4,5,6,7,8,9]4ZZ

Ø Medical and Surgical
F Hepatobiliary System and Pancreas
N Release Definition: Freeing a body part from an abnormal physical constraint by cutting or by the use of force
Explanation: Some of the restraining tissue may be taken out but none of the body part is taken out

Body Part Character 4	Approach Character 5	Device Character 6	Qualifier Character 7
Ø Liver Quadrate lobe 1 Liver, Right Lobe 2 Liver, Left Lobe	Ø Open 3 Percutaneous 4 Percutaneous Endoscopic	Z No Device	Z No Qualifier
4 Gallbladder G Pancreas	Ø Open 3 Percutaneous 4 Percutaneous Endoscopic 8 Via Natural or Artificial Opening Endoscopic	Z No Device	Z No Qualifier

5 Hepatic Duct, Right
6 Hepatic Duct, Left
7 Hepatic Duct, Common
8 Cystic Duct
9 Common Bile Duct
C Ampulla of Vater
  Duodenal ampulla
  Hepatopancreatic ampulla
D Pancreatic Duct
  Duct of Wirsung
F Pancreatic Duct, Accessory
  Duct of Santorini
	Ø Open
	3 Percutaneous
	4 Percutaneous Endoscopic
	7 Via Natural or Artificial Opening
	8 Via Natural or Artificial Opening Endoscopic
		Z No Device	Z No Qualifier

Ø   Medical and Surgical
F   Hepatobiliary System and Pancreas
P   Removal   Definition: Taking out or off a device from a body part

Explanation: If a device is taken out and a similar device put in without cutting or puncturing the skin or mucous membrane, the procedure is coded to the root operation CHANGE. Otherwise, the procedure for taking out a device is coded to the root operation REMOVAL.

Body Part Character 4	Approach Character 5	Device Character 6	Qualifier Character 7
Ø Liver Quadrate lobe	**Ø** Open **3** Percutaneous **4** Percutaneous Endoscopic	**Ø** Drainage Device **2** Monitoring Device **3** Infusion Device **Y** Other Device	**Z** No Qualifier
Ø Liver Quadrate lobe	**X** External	**Ø** Drainage Device **2** Monitoring Device **3** Infusion Device	**Z** No Qualifier
4 Gallbladder **G** Pancreas	**Ø** Open **3** Percutaneous **4** Percutaneous Endoscopic	**Ø** Drainage Device **2** Monitoring Device **3** Infusion Device **D** Intraluminal Device **Y** Other Device	**Z** No Qualifier
4 Gallbladder **G** Pancreas	**X** External	**Ø** Drainage Device **2** Monitoring Device **3** Infusion Device **D** Intraluminal Device	**Z** No Qualifier
B Hepatobiliary Duct **D** Pancreatic Duct Duct of Wirsung	**Ø** Open **3** Percutaneous **4** Percutaneous Endoscopic **7** Via Natural or Artificial Opening **8** Via Natural or Artificial Opening Endoscopic	**Ø** Drainage Device **1** Radioactive Element **2** Monitoring Device **3** Infusion Device **7** Autologous Tissue Substitute **C** Extraluminal Device **D** Intraluminal Device **J** Synthetic Substitute **K** Nonautologous Tissue Substitute **Y** Other Device	**Z** No Qualifier
B Hepatobiliary Duct **D** Pancreatic Duct Duct of Wirsung	**X** External	**Ø** Drainage Device **1** Radioactive Element **2** Monitoring Device **3** Infusion Device **D** Intraluminal Device	**Z** No Qualifier

Non-OR ØFPØ[3,4]YZ	**See Appendix L for Procedure Combinations**
Non-OR ØFPØX[Ø,2,3]Z	**Combo-only** ØFP[B,D]XDZ
Non-OR ØFP[4,G][3,4]YZ	
Non-OR ØFP4X[Ø,2,3,D]Z	
Non-OR ØFPGX[Ø,2,3]Z	
Non-OR ØFP[B,D][3,4]YZ	
Non-OR ØFP[B,D][7,8][Ø,2,3,D,Y]Z	
Non-OR ØFP[B,D]X[Ø,1,2,3,D]Z	

Ø **Medical and Surgical**
F **Hepatobiliary System and Pancreas**
Q **Repair**   Definition: Restoring, to the extent possible, a body part to its normal anatomic structure and function

                      Explanation: Used only when the method to accomplish the repair is not one of the other root operations

Body Part Character 4	Approach Character 5	Device Character 6	Qualifier Character 7
Ø Liver Quadrate lobe 1 Liver, Right Lobe 2 Liver, Left Lobe	Ø Open 3 Percutaneous 4 Percutaneous Endoscopic	Z No Device	Z No Qualifier
4 Gallbladder G Pancreas	Ø Open 3 Percutaneous 4 Percutaneous Endoscopic 8 Via Natural or Artificial Opening Endoscopic	Z No Device	Z No Qualifier

5 Hepatic Duct, Right
6 Hepatic Duct, Left
7 Hepatic Duct, Common
8 Cystic Duct
9 Common Bile Duct
C Ampulla of Vater
   Duodenal ampulla
   Hepatopancreatic ampulla
D Pancreatic Duct
   Duct of Wirsung
F Pancreatic Duct, Accessory
   Duct of Santorini
	Ø Open
	3 Percutaneous
	4 Percutaneous Endoscopic
	7 Via Natural or Artificial Opening
	8 Via Natural or Artificial Opening
	   Endoscopic
		Z No Device	Z No Qualifier

Ø **Medical and Surgical**
F **Hepatobiliary System and Pancreas**
R **Replacement**   Definition: Putting in or on biological or synthetic material that physically takes the place and/or function of all or a portion of a body part

                      Explanation: The body part may have been taken out or replaced, or may be taken out, physically eradicated, or rendered nonfunctional during the REPLACEMENT procedure. A REMOVAL procedure is coded for taking out the device used in a previous replacement procedure.

Body Part Character 4	Approach Character 5	Device Character 6	Qualifier Character 7

5 Hepatic Duct, Right
6 Hepatic Duct, Left
7 Hepatic Duct, Common
8 Cystic Duct
9 Common Bile Duct
C Ampulla of Vater
   Duodenal ampulla
   Hepatopancreatic ampulla
D Pancreatic Duct
   Duct of Wirsung
F Pancreatic Duct, Accessory
   Duct of Santorini
	Ø Open
	4 Percutaneous Endoscopic
	8 Via Natural or Artificial Opening
	   Endoscopic
		7 Autologous Tissue Substitute
		J Synthetic Substitute
		K Nonautologous Tissue Substitute
			Z No Qualifier

Ø **Medical and Surgical**
F **Hepatobiliary System and Pancreas**
S **Reposition**   Definition: Moving to its normal location, or other suitable location, all or a portion of a body part

                      Explanation: The body part is moved to a new location from an abnormal location, or from a normal location where it is not functioning correctly. The body part may or may not be cut out or off to be moved to the new location.

Body Part Character 4	Approach Character 5	Device Character 6	Qualifier Character 7

Ø Liver
   Quadrate lobe
4 Gallbladder
5 Hepatic Duct, Right
6 Hepatic Duct, Left
7 Hepatic Duct, Common
8 Cystic Duct
9 Common Bile Duct
C Ampulla of Vater
   Duodenal ampulla
   Hepatopancreatic ampulla
D Pancreatic Duct
   Duct of Wirsung
F Pancreatic Duct, Accessory
   Duct of Santorini
G Pancreas
	Ø Open
	4 Percutaneous Endoscopic
		Z No Device	Z No Qualifier

LC Limited Coverage   **NC** Noncovered   ⊞ Combination Member   HAC associated procedure   Combination Only   DRG Non-OR   Non-OR   New/Revised in GREEN

ICD-10-PCS 2020   **401**

Ø Medical and Surgical
F Hepatobiliary System and Pancreas
T Resection   Definition: Cutting out or off, without replacement, all of a body part
     Explanation: None

Body Part Character 4	Approach Character 5	Device Character 6	Qualifier Character 7
Ø Liver Quadrate lobe 1 Liver, Right Lobe 2 Liver, Left Lobe 4 Gallbladder G Pancreas ⊞	Ø Open 4 Percutaneous Endoscopic	Z No Device	Z No Qualifier

5 Hepatic Duct, Right
6 Hepatic Duct, Left
7 Hepatic Duct, Common
8 Cystic Duct
9 Common Bile Duct
C Ampulla of Vater
  Duodenal ampulla
  Hepatopancreatic ampulla
D Pancreatic Duct
  Duct of Wirsung
F Pancreatic Duct, Accessory
  Duct of Santorini
	Ø Open
	4 Percutaneous Endoscopic
	7 Via Natural or Artificial Opening
	8 Via Natural or Artificial Opening Endoscopic
		Z No Device	Z No Qualifier

Non-OR ØFT[D,F][4,8]ZZ

See Appendix L for Procedure Combinations
⊞   ØFTGØZZ

Ø Medical and Surgical
F Hepatobiliary System and Pancreas
U Supplement   Definition: Putting in or on biological or synthetic material that physically reinforces and/or augments the function of a portion of a body part
     Explanation: The biological material is non-living, or is living and from the same individual. The body part may have been previously replaced, and the SUPPLEMENT procedure is performed to physically reinforce and/or augment the function of the replaced body part.

Body Part Character 4	Approach Character 5	Device Character 6	Qualifier Character 7

5 Hepatic Duct, Right
6 Hepatic Duct, Left
7 Hepatic Duct, Common
8 Cystic Duct
9 Common Bile Duct
C Ampulla of Vater
  Duodenal ampulla
  Hepatopancreatic ampulla
D Pancreatic Duct
  Duct of Wirsung
F Pancreatic Duct, Accessory
  Duct of Santorini
	Ø Open
	3 Percutaneous
	4 Percutaneous Endoscopic
	8 Via Natural or Artificial Opening Endoscopic
		7 Autologous Tissue Substitute
		J Synthetic Substitute
		K Nonautologous Tissue Substitute
			Z No Qualifier

LC Limited Coverage   NC Noncovered   ⊞ Combination Member   HAC associated procedure   Combination Only   DRG Non-OR   Non-OR   New/Revised in GREEN

402   **ICD-10-PCS 2020**

ØFT–ØFU

Ø Medical and Surgical
F Hepatobiliary System and Pancreas
V Restriction   Definition: Partially closing an orifice or the lumen of a tubular body part

Explanation: The orifice can be a natural orifice or an artificially created orifice

Body Part Character 4	Approach Character 5	Device Character 6	Qualifier Character 7

5 Hepatic Duct, Right
6 Hepatic Duct, Left
7 Hepatic Duct, Common
8 Cystic Duct
9 Common Bile Duct
C Ampulla of Vater
    Duodenal ampulla
    Hepatopancreatic ampulla
D Pancreatic Duct
    Duct of Wirsung
F Pancreatic Duct, Accessory
    Duct of Santorini
	Ø Open
	3 Percutaneous
	4 Percutaneous Endoscopic
		C Extraluminal Device
		D Intraluminal Device
		Z No Device
			Z No Qualifier

5 Hepatic Duct, Right
6 Hepatic Duct, Left
7 Hepatic Duct, Common
8 Cystic Duct
9 Common Bile Duct
C Ampulla of Vater
    Duodenal ampulla
    Hepatopancreatic ampulla
D Pancreatic Duct
    Duct of Wirsung
F Pancreatic Duct, Accessory
    Duct of Santorini
	7 Via Natural or Artificial Opening
	8 Via Natural or Artificial Opening
	    Endoscopic
		D Intraluminal Device
		Z No Device
			Z No Qualifier

Non-OR ØFV[5,6,7,8,9][3,4][C,D,Z]Z
Non-OR ØFV[5,6,7,8,9][7,8][D,Z]Z

Ø   **Medical and Surgical**
F   **Hepatobiliary System and Pancreas**
W   **Revision**   Definition: Correcting, to the extent possible, a portion of a malfunctioning device or the position of a displaced device

         Explanation: Revision can include correcting a malfunctioning or displaced device by taking out or putting in components of the device such as a screw or pin

Body Part Character 4	Approach Character 5	Device Character 6	Qualifier Character 7
Ø **Liver** Quadrate lobe	**Ø** Open **3** Percutaneous **4** Percutaneous Endoscopic	**Ø** Drainage Device **2** Monitoring Device **3** Infusion Device **Y** Other Device	**Z** No Qualifier
Ø **Liver** Quadrate lobe	**X** External	**Ø** Drainage Device **2** Monitoring Device **3** Infusion Device	**Z** No Qualifier
4 **Gallbladder** **G** **Pancreas**	**Ø** Open **3** Percutaneous **4** Percutaneous Endoscopic	**Ø** Drainage Device **2** Monitoring Device **3** Infusion Device **D** Intraluminal Device **Y** Other Device	**Z** No Qualifier
4 **Gallbladder** **G** **Pancreas**	**X** External	**Ø** Drainage Device **2** Monitoring Device **3** Infusion Device **D** Intraluminal Device	**Z** No Qualifier

B   **Hepatobiliary Duct**
D   **Pancreatic Duct**
     Duct of Wirsung
	Ø Open
	3 Percutaneous
	4 Percutaneous Endoscopic
	7 Via Natural or Artificial Opening
	8 Via Natural or Artificial Opening
	     Endoscopic
		Ø Drainage Device
		2 Monitoring Device
		3 Infusion Device
		7 Autologous Tissue Substitute
		C Extraluminal Device
		D Intraluminal Device
		J Synthetic Substitute
		K Nonautologous Tissue Substitute
		Y Other Device
			Z No Qualifier

B **Hepatobiliary Duct** **D** **Pancreatic Duct** Duct of Wirsung	**X** External	**Ø** Drainage Device **2** Monitoring Device **3** Infusion Device **7** Autologous Tissue Substitute **C** Extraluminal Device **D** Intraluminal Device **J** Synthetic Substitute **K** Nonautologous Tissue Substitute	**Z** No Qualifier

Non-OR   ØFWØ[3,4]YZ
Non-OR   ØFWØX[Ø,2,3]Z
Non-OR   ØFW[4,G][3,4]YZ
Non-OR   ØFW[4,G]X[Ø,2,3,D]Z
Non-OR   ØFW[B,D][3,4,7,8]YZ
Non-OR   ØFW[B,D]X[Ø,2,3,7,C,D,J,K]Z

Ø   **Medical and Surgical**
F   **Hepatobiliary System and Pancreas**
Y   **Transplantation**   Definition: Putting in or on all or a portion of a living body part taken from another individual or animal to physically take the place and/or function of all or a portion of a similar body part

         Explanation: The native body part may or may not be taken out, and the transplanted body part may take over all or a portion of its function

Body Part Character 4	Approach Character 5	Device Character 6	Qualifier Character 7
Ø **Liver** LC Quadrate lobe **G** **Pancreas** LC NC ⊞	**Ø** Open	**Z** No Device	**Ø** Allogeneic **1** Syngeneic **2** Zooplastic

LC   ØFYØØZ[Ø,1,2]
LC   ØFYGØZ[Ø,1]
NC   ØFYGØZ2
NC   ØFYGØZ[Ø,1] If reported alone without one of the following procedures
       ØTYØØZ[Ø,1,2], ØTY1ØZ[Ø,1,2] and without one of the following
       diagnoses E1Ø.1Ø-E1Ø.9, E89.1

See Appendix L for Procedure Combinations
    ⊞   ØFYGØZ[Ø,1,2]

Endocrine System 0G2–0GW

Character Meanings

This Character Meaning table is provided as a guide to assist the user in the identification of character members that may be found in this section of code tables. It **SHOULD NOT** be used to build a PCS code.

Operation–Character 3	Body Part–Character 4	Approach–Character 5	Device–Character 6	Qualifier–Character 7
2 Change	0 Pituitary Gland	0 Open	0 Drainage Device	X Diagnostic
5 Destruction	1 Pineal Body	3 Percutaneous	2 Monitoring Device	Z No Qualifier
8 Division	2 Adrenal Gland, Left	4 Percutaneous Endoscopic	3 Infusion Device	
9 Drainage	3 Adrenal Gland, Right	X External	Y Other Device	
B Excision	4 Adrenal Glands, Bilateral		Z No Device	
C Extirpation	5 Adrenal Gland			
H Insertion	6 Carotid Body, Left			
J Inspection	7 Carotid Body, Right			
M Reattachment	8 Carotid Bodies, Bilateral			
N Release	9 Para-aortic Body			
P Removal	B Coccygeal Glomus			
Q Repair	C Glomus Jugulare			
S Reposition	D Aortic Body			
T Resection	F Paraganglion Extremity			
W Revision	G Thyroid Gland Lobe, Left			
	H Thyroid Gland Lobe, Right			
	J Thyroid Gland Isthmus			
	K Thyroid Gland			
	L Superior Parathyroid Gland, Right			
	M Superior Parathyroid Gland, Left			
	N Inferior Parathyroid Gland, Right			
	P Inferior Parathyroid Gland, Left			
	Q Parathyroid Glands, Multiple			
	R Parathyroid Gland			
	S Endocrine Gland			

AHA Coding Clinic for table 0GB
2017, 2Q, 20   Near total thyroidectomy
2014, 3Q, 22   Transsphenoidal removal of pituitary tumor and fat graft placement

AHA Coding Clinic for table 0GT
2017, 2Q, 20   Near total thyroidectomy

Endocrine System

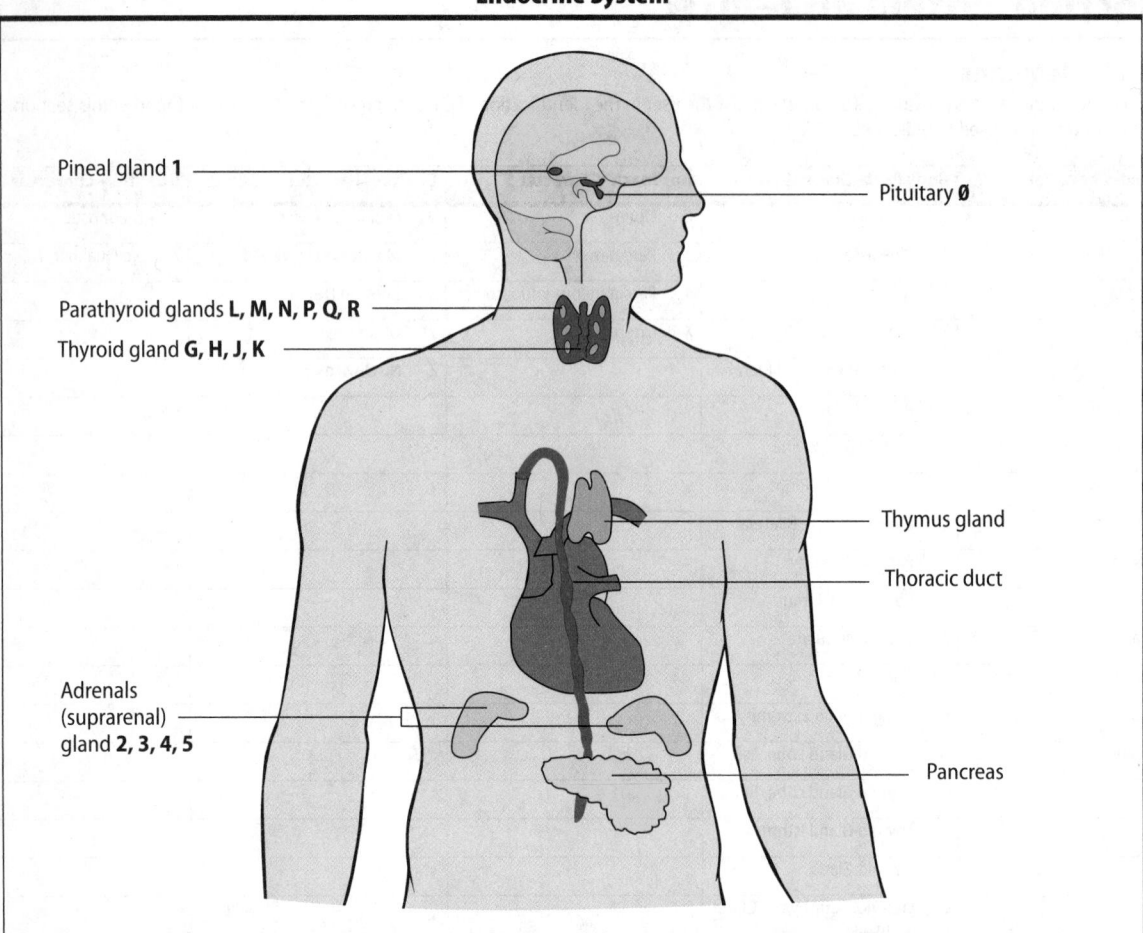

Pineal gland **1**

Pituitary **Ø**

Parathyroid glands **L, M, N, P, Q, R**

Thyroid gland **G, H, J, K**

Thymus gland

Thoracic duct

Adrenals (suprarenal) gland **2, 3, 4, 5**

Pancreas

Left Adrenal Gland

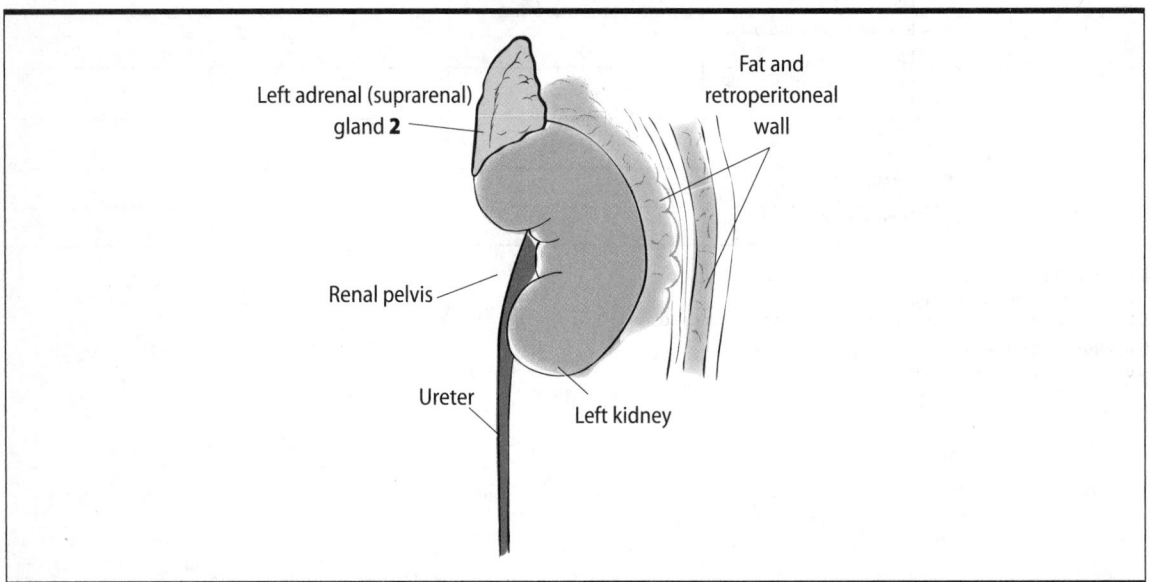

Left adrenal (suprarenal) gland **2**

Fat and retroperitoneal wall

Renal pelvis

Ureter

Left kidney

Thyroid

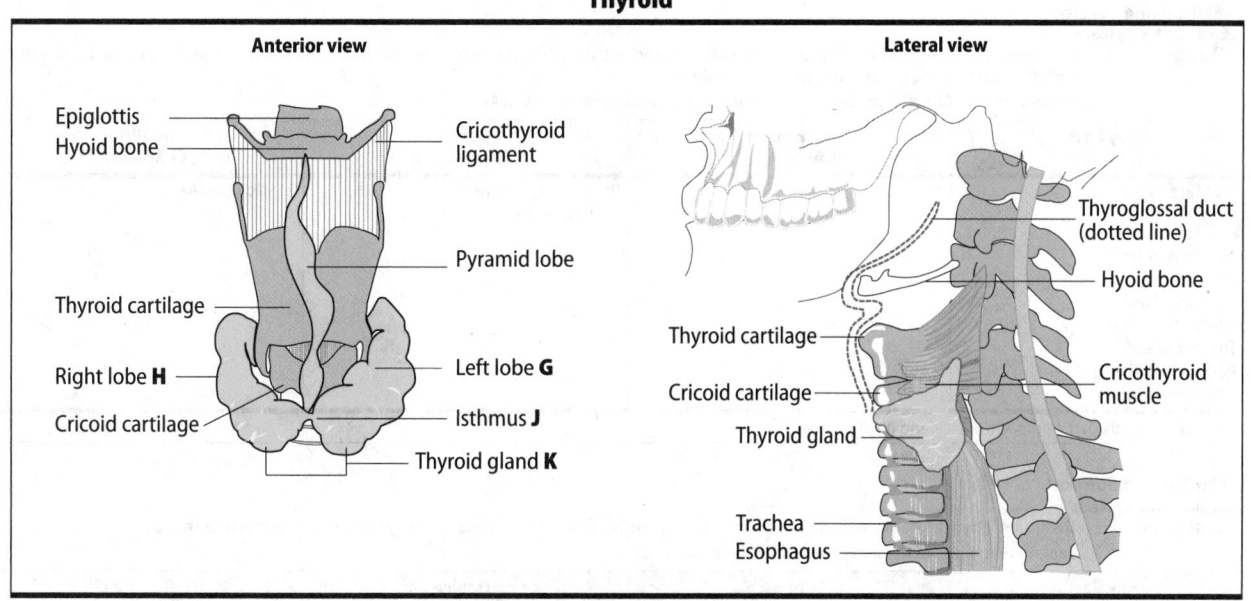

Anterior view

- Epiglottis
- Hyoid bone
- Cricothyroid ligament
- Pyramid lobe
- Thyroid cartilage
- Right lobe **H**
- Left lobe **G**
- Cricoid cartilage
- Isthmus **J**
- Thyroid gland **K**

Lateral view

- Thyroglossal duct (dotted line)
- Hyoid bone
- Thyroid cartilage
- Cricoid cartilage
- Cricothyroid muscle
- Thyroid gland
- Trachea
- Esophagus

Thyroid and Parathyroid Glands

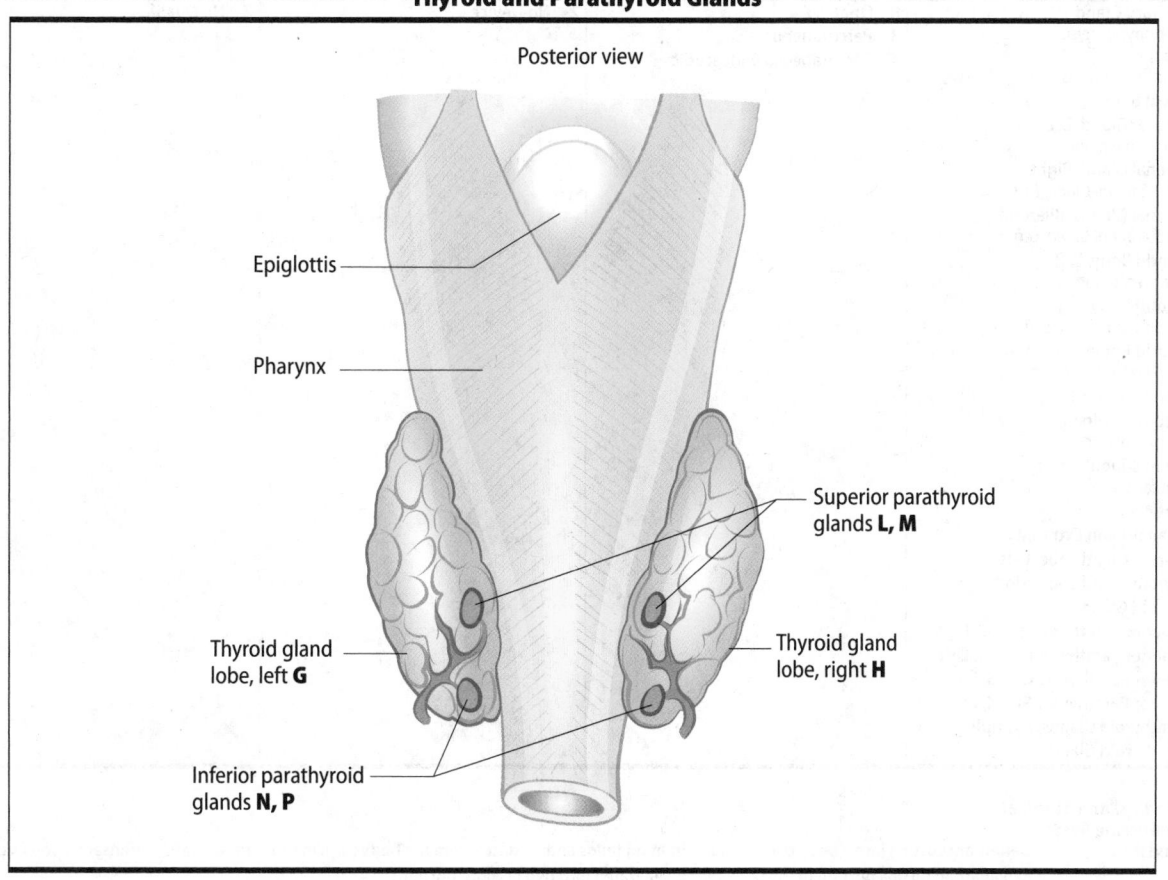

Posterior view

- Epiglottis
- Pharynx
- Thyroid gland lobe, left **G**
- Inferior parathyroid glands **N, P**
- Superior parathyroid glands **L, M**
- Thyroid gland lobe, right **H**

Endocrine System

0   **Medical and Surgical**
G   **Endocrine System**
2   **Change**   Definition: Taking out or off a device from a body part and putting back an identical or similar device in or on the same body part without cutting or puncturing the skin or a mucous membrane

Explanation: All CHANGE procedures are coded using the approach EXTERNAL

Body Part Character 4	Approach Character 5	Device Character 6	Qualifier Character 7

0 Pituitary Gland
    Adenohypophysis
    Hypophysis
    Neurohypophysis
1 Pineal Body
5 Adrenal Gland
    Suprarenal gland
K Thyroid Gland
R Parathyroid Gland
S Endocrine Gland
	X External	**0** Drainage Device
		Y Other Device
			Z No Qualifier

Non-OR   All body part, approach, device, and qualifier values

0   **Medical and Surgical**
G   **Endocrine System**
5   **Destruction**   Definition: Physical eradication of all or a portion of a body part by the direct use of energy, force, or a destructive agent

Explanation: None of the body part is physically taken out

Body Part Character 4	Approach Character 5	Device Character 6	Qualifier Character 7

0 Pituitary Gland
    Adenohypophysis
    Hypophysis
    Neurohypophysis
1 Pineal Body
2 Adrenal Gland, Left
    Suprarenal gland
3 Adrenal Gland, Right
    See 2 Adrenal Gland, Left
4 Adrenal Glands, Bilateral
    See 2 Adrenal Gland, Left
6 Carotid Body, Left
    Carotid glomus
7 Carotid Body, Right
    See 6 Carotid Body, Left
8 Carotid Bodies, Bilateral
    See 6 Carotid Body, Left
9 Para-aortic Body
B Coccygeal Glomus
    Coccygeal body
C Glomus Jugulare
    Jugular body
D Aortic Body
F Paraganglion Extremity
G Thyroid Gland Lobe, Left
H Thyroid Gland Lobe, Right
K Thyroid Gland
L Superior Parathyroid Gland, Right
M Superior Parathyroid Gland, Left
N Inferior Parathyroid Gland, Right
P Inferior Parathyroid Gland, Left
Q Parathyroid Glands, Multiple
R Parathyroid Gland
	0 Open
	3 Percutaneous
	4 Percutaneous Endoscopic
		Z No Device	**Z** No Qualifier

0   **Medical and Surgical**
G   **Endocrine System**
8   **Division**   Definition: Cutting into a body part, without draining fluids and/or gases from the body part, in order to separate or transect a body part

Explanation: All or a portion of the body part is separated into two or more portions

Body Part Character 4	Approach Character 5	Device Character 6	Qualifier Character 7

0 Pituitary Gland
    Adenohypophysis
    Hypophysis
    Neurohypophysis
J Thyroid Gland Isthmus
	0 Open
	3 Percutaneous
	4 Percutaneous Endoscopic
		Z No Device	**Z** No Qualifier

LC Limited Coverage   **NC** Noncovered   ⊞ Combination Member   HAC associated procedure   Combination Only   DRG Non-OR   Non-OR   New/Revised in GREEN

408   ICD-10-PCS 2020

0   **Medical and Surgical**
G   **Endocrine System**
9   **Drainage**   Definition: Taking or letting out fluids and/or gases from a body part
                 Explanation: The qualifier DIAGNOSTIC is used to identify drainage procedures that are biopsies

Body Part Character 4	Approach Character 5	Device Character 6	Qualifier Character 7

0   **Pituitary Gland**
     Adenohypophysis
     Hypophysis
     Neurohypophysis
1   **Pineal Body**
2   **Adrenal Gland, Left**
     Suprarenal gland
3   **Adrenal Gland, Right**
     See 2 Adrenal Gland, Left
4   **Adrenal Glands, Bilateral**
     See 2 Adrenal Gland, Left
6   **Carotid Body, Left**
     Carotid glomus
7   **Carotid Body, Right**
     See 6 Carotid Body, Left
8   **Carotid Bodies, Bilateral**
     See 6 Carotid Body, Left
9   **Para-aortic Body**
B   **Coccygeal Glomus**
     Coccygeal body
C   **Glomus Jugulare**
     Jugular body
D   **Aortic Body**
F   **Paraganglion Extremity**
G   **Thyroid Gland Lobe, Left**
H   **Thyroid Gland Lobe, Right**
K   **Thyroid Gland**
L   **Superior Parathyroid Gland, Right**
M   **Superior Parathyroid Gland, Left**
N   **Inferior Parathyroid Gland, Right**
P   **Inferior Parathyroid Gland, Left**
Q   **Parathyroid Glands, Multiple**
R   **Parathyroid Gland**
	0 Open
	3 Percutaneous
	4 Percutaneous Endoscopic
		0 Drainage Device	**Z** No Qualifier

0   **Pituitary Gland**
     Adenohypophysis
     Hypophysis
     Neurohypophysis
1   **Pineal Body**
2   **Adrenal Gland, Left**
     Suprarenal gland
3   **Adrenal Gland, Right**
     See 2 Adrenal Gland, Left
4   **Adrenal Glands, Bilateral**
     See 2 Adrenal Gland, Left
6   **Carotid Body, Left**
     Carotid glomus
7   **Carotid Body, Right**
     See 6 Carotid Body, Left
8   **Carotid Bodies, Bilateral**
     See 6 Carotid Body, Left
9   **Para-aortic Body**
B   **Coccygeal Glomus**
     Coccygeal body
C   **Glomus Jugulare**
     Jugular body
D   **Aortic Body**
F   **Paraganglion Extremity**
G   **Thyroid Gland Lobe, Left**
H   **Thyroid Gland Lobe, Right**
K   **Thyroid Gland**
L   **Superior Parathyroid Gland, Right**
M   **Superior Parathyroid Gland, Left**
N   **Inferior Parathyroid Gland, Right**
P   **Inferior Parathyroid Gland, Left**
Q   **Parathyroid Glands, Multiple**
R   **Parathyroid Gland**
	0 Open
	3 Percutaneous
	4 Percutaneous Endoscopic
		Z No Device	**X** Diagnostic
			Z No Qualifier

Non-OR   0G9[0,1,2,3,4,6,7,8,9,B,C,D,F,G,H,K,L,M,N,P,Q,R]30Z
Non-OR   0G9[G,H,K,L,M,N,P,Q,R]40Z
Non-OR   0G9[2,3,4,G,H,K][3,4]ZX
Non-OR   0G9[0,1,2,3,4,6,7,8,9,B,C,D,F,G,H,K,L,M,N,P,Q,R]3ZZ
Non-OR   0G9[G,H,K,L,M,N,P,Q,R]4ZZ

LC Limited Coverage   **NC** Noncovered   ⊞ Combination Member   HAC associated procedure   Combination Only   DRG Non-OR   Non-OR   New/Revised in GREEN

ICD-10-PCS 2020   **409**

0G9–0G9

Endocrine System

Ø   **Medical and Surgical**
G   **Endocrine System**
B   **Excision**   Definition: Cutting out or off, without replacement, a portion of a body part
                      Explanation: The qualifier DIAGNOSTIC is used to identify excision procedures that are biopsies

Body Part Character 4	Approach Character 5	Device Character 6	Qualifier Character 7

Ø   **Pituitary Gland**
     Adenohypophysis
     Hypophysis
     Neurohypophysis
1   **Pineal Body**
2   **Adrenal Gland, Left**
     Suprarenal gland
3   **Adrenal Gland, Right**
     See 2 Adrenal Gland, Left
4   **Adrenal Glands, Bilateral**
     See 2 Adrenal Gland, Left
6   **Carotid Body, Left**
     Carotid glomus
7   **Carotid Body, Right**
     See 6 Carotid Body, Left
8   **Carotid Bodies, Bilateral**
     See 6 Carotid Body, Left
9   **Para-aortic Body**
B   **Coccygeal Glomus**
     Coccygeal body
C   **Glomus Jugulare**
     Jugular body
D   **Aortic Body**
F   **Paraganglion Extremity**
G   **Thyroid Gland Lobe, Left**
H   **Thyroid Gland Lobe, Right**
J   **Thyroid Gland Isthmus**
L   **Superior Parathyroid Gland, Right**
M   **Superior Parathyroid Gland, Left**
N   **Inferior Parathyroid Gland, Right**
P   **Inferior Parathyroid Gland, Left**
Q   **Parathyroid Glands, Multiple**
R   **Parathyroid Gland**
	Ø **Open**
	3 **Percutaneous**
	4 **Percutaneous Endoscopic**
		Z **No Device**	**X** **Diagnostic**
			Z **No Qualifier**

Non-OR   ØGB[2,3,4,G,H,J][3,4]ZX

Ø   **Medical and Surgical**
G   **Endocrine System**
C   **Extirpation**   Definition: Taking or cutting out solid matter from a body part
                      Explanation: The solid matter may be an abnormal byproduct of a biological function or a foreign body; it may be imbedded in a body part or in
                      the lumen of a tubular body part. The solid matter may or may not have been previously broken into pieces.

Body Part Character 4	Approach Character 5	Device Character 6	Qualifier Character 7

Ø   **Pituitary Gland**
     Adenohypophysis
     Hypophysis
     Neurohypophysis
1   **Pineal Body**
2   **Adrenal Gland, Left**
     Suprarenal gland
3   **Adrenal Gland, Right**
     See 2 Adrenal Gland, Left
4   **Adrenal Glands, Bilateral**
     See 2 Adrenal Gland, Left
6   **Carotid Body, Left**
     Carotid glomus
7   **Carotid Body, Right**
     See 6 Carotid Body, Left
8   **Carotid Bodies, Bilateral**
     See 6 Carotid Body, Left
9   **Para-aortic Body**
B   **Coccygeal Glomus**
     Coccygeal body
C   **Glomus Jugulare**
     Jugular body
D   **Aortic Body**
F   **Paraganglion Extremity**
G   **Thyroid Gland Lobe, Left**
H   **Thyroid Gland Lobe, Right**
K   **Thyroid Gland**
L   **Superior Parathyroid Gland, Right**
M   **Superior Parathyroid Gland, Left**
N   **Inferior Parathyroid Gland, Right**
P   **Inferior Parathyroid Gland, Left**
Q   **Parathyroid Glands, Multiple**
R   **Parathyroid Gland**
	Ø **Open**
	3 **Percutaneous**
	4 **Percutaneous Endoscopic**
		Z **No Device**	**Z** **No Qualifier**

LC Limited Coverage   **NC** Noncovered   ⊞ Combination Member   HAC associated procedure   Combination Only   DRG Non-OR   Non-OR   New/Revised in GREEN

410   ICD-10-PCS 2020

ØGB–ØGC

0   **Medical and Surgical**
G   **Endocrine System**
H   **Insertion**   Definition: Putting in a nonbiological appliance that monitors, assists, performs, or prevents a physiological function but does not physically take the place of a body part

                      Explanation: None

Body Part Character 4	Approach Character 5	Device Character 6	Qualifier Character 7
S Endocrine Gland	0 Open 3 Percutaneous 4 Percutaneous Endoscopic	2 Monitoring Device 3 Infusion Device Y Other Device	Z No Qualifier

     Non-OR   0GHS[3,4]YZ

0   **Medical and Surgical**
G   **Endocrine System**
J   **Inspection**   Definition: Visually and/or manually exploring a body part

                      Explanation: Visual exploration may be performed with or without optical instrumentation. Manual exploration may be performed directly or through intervening body layers.

Body Part Character 4	Approach Character 5	Device Character 6	Qualifier Character 7

0   Pituitary Gland
     Adenohypophysis
     Hypophysis
     Neurohypophysis
1   Pineal Body
5   Adrenal Gland
     Suprarenal gland
K   Thyroid Gland
R   Parathyroid Gland
S   Endocrine Gland
	0 Open
	3 Percutaneous
	4 Percutaneous Endoscopic
		Z No Device	Z No Qualifier

     Non-OR   0GJ[0,1,5,K,R,S]3ZZ

0   **Medical and Surgical**
G   **Endocrine System**
M   **Reattachment**   Definition: Putting back in or on all or a portion of a separated body part to its normal location or other suitable location

                      Explanation: Vascular circulation and nervous pathways may or may not be reestablished

Body Part Character 4	Approach Character 5	Device Character 6	Qualifier Character 7

2   Adrenal Gland, Left
     Suprarenal gland
3   Adrenal Gland, Right
     See 2 Adrenal Gland, Left
G   Thyroid Gland Lobe, Left
H   Thyroid Gland Lobe, Right
L   Superior Parathyroid Gland, Right
M   Superior Parathyroid Gland, Left
N   Inferior Parathyroid Gland, Right
P   Inferior Parathyroid Gland, Left
Q   Parathyroid Glands, Multiple
R   Parathyroid Gland
	0 Open
	4 Percutaneous Endoscopic
		Z No Device	Z No Qualifier

LC Limited Coverage   NC Noncovered   ⊞ Combination Member   HAC associated procedure   Combination Only   DRG Non-OR   Non-OR   New/Revised in GREEN

ICD-10-PCS 2020   411

Ø Medical and Surgical
G Endocrine System
N Release   Definition: Freeing a body part from an abnormal physical constraint by cutting or by the use of force

                     Explanation: Some of the restraining tissue may be taken out but none of the body part is taken out

Body Part Character 4	Approach Character 5	Device Character 6	Qualifier Character 7
Ø Pituitary Gland Adenohypophysis Hypophysis Neurohypophysis **1 Pineal Body** **2 Adrenal Gland, Left** Suprarenal gland **3 Adrenal Gland, Right** *See 2 Adrenal Gland, Left* **4 Adrenal Glands, Bilateral** *See 2 Adrenal Gland, Left* **6 Carotid Body, Left** Carotid glomus **7 Carotid Body, Right** *See 6 Carotid Body, Left* **8 Carotid Bodies, Bilateral** *See 6 Carotid Body, Left* **9 Para-aortic Body** **B Coccygeal Glomus** Coccygeal body **C Glomus Jugulare** Jugular body **D Aortic Body** **F Paraganglion Extremity** **G Thyroid Gland Lobe, Left** **H Thyroid Gland Lobe, Right** **K Thyroid Gland** **L Superior Parathyroid Gland, Right** **M Superior Parathyroid Gland, Left** **N Inferior Parathyroid Gland, Right** **P Inferior Parathyroid Gland, Left** **Q Parathyroid Glands, Multiple** **R Parathyroid Gland**	**Ø Open** **3 Percutaneous** **4 Percutaneous Endoscopic**	**Z No Device**	**Z No Qualifier**

Non-OR   ØGN[6,7,8,9,B,C,D,F][Ø,3,4]ZZ

Ø Medical and Surgical
G Endocrine System
P Removal   Definition: Taking out or off a device from a body part

                     Explanation: If a device is taken out and a similar device put in without cutting or puncturing the skin or mucous membrane, the procedure is coded to the root operation CHANGE. Otherwise, the procedure for taking out a device is coded to the root operation REMOVAL.

Body Part Character 4	Approach Character 5	Device Character 6	Qualifier Character 7
Ø Pituitary Gland Adenohypophysis Hypophysis Neurohypophysis **1 Pineal Body** **5 Adrenal Gland** Suprarenal gland **K Thyroid Gland** **R Parathyroid Gland**	**Ø Open** **3 Percutaneous** **4 Percutaneous Endoscopic** **X External**	**Ø Drainage Device**	**Z No Qualifier**
S Endocrine Gland	**Ø Open** **3 Percutaneous** **4 Percutaneous Endoscopic**	**Ø Drainage Device** **2 Monitoring Device** **3 Infusion Device** **Y Other Device**	**Z No Qualifier**
S Endocrine Gland	**X External**	**Ø Drainage Device** **2 Monitoring Device** **3 Infusion Device**	**Z No Qualifier**

Non-OR   ØGP[Ø,1,5,K,R]XØZ
Non-OR   ØGPS[3,4]YZ
Non-OR   ØGPSX[Ø,2,3]Z

---

0   **Medical and Surgical**
G   **Endocrine System**
Q   **Repair**   Definition: Restoring, to the extent possible, a body part to its normal anatomic structure and function

           Explanation: Used only when the method to accomplish the repair is not one of the other root operations

Body Part Character 4	Approach Character 5	Device Character 6	Qualifier Character 7

0   **Pituitary Gland**
    Adenohypophysis
    Hypophysis
    Neurohypophysis
1   **Pineal Body**
2   **Adrenal Gland, Left**
    Suprarenal gland
3   **Adrenal Gland, Right**
    See 2 Adrenal Gland, Left
4   **Adrenal Glands, Bilateral**
    See 2 Adrenal Gland, Left
6   **Carotid Body, Left**
    Carotid glomus
7   **Carotid Body, Right**
    See 6 Carotid Body, Left
8   **Carotid Bodies, Bilateral**
    See 6 Carotid Body, Left
9   **Para-aortic Body**
B   **Coccygeal Glomus**
    Coccygeal body
C   **Glomus Jugulare**
    Jugular body
D   **Aortic Body**
F   **Paraganglion Extremity**
G   **Thyroid Gland Lobe, Left**
H   **Thyroid Gland Lobe, Right**
J   **Thyroid Gland Isthmus**
K   **Thyroid Gland**
L   **Superior Parathyroid Gland, Right**
M   **Superior Parathyroid Gland, Left**
N   **Inferior Parathyroid Gland, Right**
P   **Inferior Parathyroid Gland, Left**
Q   **Parathyroid Glands, Multiple**
R   **Parathyroid Gland**
	0 Open
	3 Percutaneous
	4 Percutaneous Endoscopic
		Z No Device	**Z** No Qualifier

0   **Medical and Surgical**
G   **Endocrine System**
S   **Reposition**   Definition: Moving to its normal location, or other suitable location, all or a portion of a body part

           Explanation: The body part is moved to a new location from an abnormal location, or from a normal location where it is not functioning correctly. The body part may or may not be cut out or off to be moved to the new location.

Body Part Character 4	Approach Character 5	Device Character 6	Qualifier Character 7

2   **Adrenal Gland, Left**
    Suprarenal gland
3   **Adrenal Gland, Right**
    See 2 Adrenal Gland, Left
G   **Thyroid Gland Lobe, Left**
H   **Thyroid Gland Lobe, Right**
L   **Superior Parathyroid Gland, Right**
M   **Superior Parathyroid Gland, Left**
N   **Inferior Parathyroid Gland, Right**
P   **Inferior Parathyroid Gland, Left**
Q   **Parathyroid Glands, Multiple**
R   **Parathyroid Gland**
	0 Open
	4 Percutaneous Endoscopic
		Z No Device	**Z** No Qualifier

Ø   Medical and Surgical
G   Endocrine System
T   Resection   Definition: Cutting out or off, without replacement, all of a body part
                            Explanation: None

Body Part Character 4	Approach Character 5	Device Character 6	Qualifier Character 7

Ø **Pituitary Gland**
   Adenohypophysis
   Hypophysis
   Neurohypophysis
1 **Pineal Body**
2 **Adrenal Gland, Left**
   Suprarenal gland
3 **Adrenal Gland, Right**
   See 2 Adrenal Gland, Left
4 **Adrenal Glands, Bilateral**
   See 2 Adrenal Gland, Left
6 **Carotid Body, Left**
   Carotid glomus
7 **Carotid Body, Right**
   See 6 Carotid Body, Left
8 **Carotid Bodies, Bilateral**
   See 6 Carotid Body, Left
9 **Para-aortic Body**
B **Coccygeal Glomus**
   Coccygeal body
C **Glomus Jugulare**
   Jugular body
D **Aortic Body**
F **Paraganglion Extremity**
G **Thyroid Gland Lobe, Left**
H **Thyroid Gland Lobe, Right**
J **Thyroid Gland Isthmus**
K **Thyroid Gland**
L **Superior Parathyroid Gland, Right**
M **Superior Parathyroid Gland, Left**
N **Inferior Parathyroid Gland, Right**
P **Inferior Parathyroid Gland, Left**
Q **Parathyroid Glands, Multiple**
R **Parathyroid Gland**
	Ø Open
	4 Percutaneous Endoscopic
		Z No Device	Z No Qualifier

Non-OR   ØGT[6,7,8,9,B,C,D,F][Ø,4]ZZ

Ø   Medical and Surgical
G   Endocrine System
W   Revision   Definition: Correcting, to the extent possible, a portion of a malfunctioning device or the position of a displaced device
                           Explanation: Revision can include correcting a malfunctioning or displaced device by taking out or putting in components of the device such as a screw or pin

Body Part Character 4	Approach Character 5	Device Character 6	Qualifier Character 7

Ø **Pituitary Gland**
   Adenohypophysis
   Hypophysis
   Neurohypophysis
1 **Pineal Body**
5 **Adrenal Gland**
   Suprarenal gland
K **Thyroid Gland**
R **Parathyroid Gland**
	Ø Open
	3 Percutaneous
	4 Percutaneous Endoscopic
	X External
		Ø Drainage Device	Z No Qualifier

S **Endocrine Gland**	Ø Open 3 Percutaneous 4 Percutaneous Endoscopic	Ø Drainage Device 2 Monitoring Device 3 Infusion Device Y Other Device	Z No Qualifier
S **Endocrine Gland**	X External	Ø Drainage Device 2 Monitoring Device 3 Infusion Device	Z No Qualifier

Non-OR   ØGW[Ø,1,5,K,R]XØZ
Non-OR   ØGWS[3,4]YZ
Non-OR   ØGWSX[Ø,2,3]Z

Skin and Breast ØHØ–ØHX

Character Meanings*

This Character Meaning table is provided as a guide to assist the user in the identification of character members that may be found in this section of code tables. It **SHOULD NOT** be used to build a PCS code.

Operation–Character 3		Body Part–Character 4		Approach–Character 5		Device–Character 6		Qualifier–Character 7	
Ø	Alteration	Ø	Skin, Scalp	Ø	Open	Ø	Drainage Device	2	Cell Suspension Technique
2	Change	1	Skin, Face	3	Percutaneous	1	Radioactive Element	3	Full Thickness
5	Destruction	2	Skin, Right Ear	7	Via Natural or Artificial Opening	7	Autologous Tissue Substitute	4	Partial Thickness
8	Division	3	Skin, Left Ear	8	Via Natural or Artificial Opening Endoscopic	J	Synthetic Substitute	5	Latissimus Dorsi Myocutaneous Flap
9	Drainage	4	Skin, Neck	X	External	K	Nonautologous Tissue Substitute	6	Transverse Rectus Abdominis Myocutaneous Flap
B	Excision	5	Skin, Chest			N	Tissue Expander	7	Deep Inferior Epigastric Artery Perforator Flap
C	Extirpation	6	Skin, Back			Y	Other Device	8	Superficial Inferior Epigastric Artery Flap
D	Extraction	7	Skin, Abdomen			Z	No Device	9	Gluteal Artery Perforator Flap
H	Insertion	8	Skin, Buttock					D	Multiple
J	Inspection	9	Skin, Perineum					X	Diagnostic
M	Reattachment	A	Skin, Inguinal					Z	No Qualifier
N	Release	B	Skin, Right Upper Arm						
P	Removal	C	Skin, Left Upper Arm						
Q	Repair	D	Skin, Right Lower Arm						
R	Replacement	E	Skin, Left Lower Arm						
S	Reposition	F	Skin, Right Hand						
T	Resection	G	Skin, Left Hand						
U	Supplement	H	Skin, Right Upper Leg						
W	Revision	J	Skin, Left Upper Leg						
X	Transfer	K	Skin, Right Lower Leg						
		L	Skin, Left Lower Leg						
		M	Skin, Right Foot						
		N	Skin, Left Foot						
		P	Skin						
		Q	Finger Nail						
		R	Toe Nail						
		S	Hair						
		T	Breast, Right						
		U	Breast, Left						
		V	Breast, Bilateral						
		W	Nipple, Right						
		X	Nipple, Left						
		Y	Supernumerary Breast						

*   Includes skin and breast glands and ducts.

AHA Coding Clinic for table ØHB
2018, 1Q, 14   Excisional debridement of breast tissue and skin
2016, 3Q, 29   Closure of bilateral alveolar clefts
2015, 3Q, 3-8   Excisional and nonexcisional debridement

AHA Coding Clinic for table ØHD
2016, 1Q, 40   Nonexcisional debridement of skin and subcutaneous tissue
2015, 3Q, 3-8   Excisional and nonexcisional debridement

AHA Coding Clinic for table ØHH
2017, 4Q, 67   New qualifier values - Pedicle flap procedures
2014, 2Q, 12   Pedicle latissimus myocutaneous flap with placement of breast tissue expanders
2013, 4Q, 107   Breast tissue expander placement using acellular dermal matrix

AHA Coding Clinic for table ØHP
2018, 3Q, 13   Deep inferior epigastric artery perforator flap breast reconstruction
2016, 2Q, 27   Removal of nonviable transverse rectus abdominis myocutaneous (TRAM) flaps

AHA Coding Clinic for table ØHQ
2018, 2Q, 25   Third and fourth degree obstetric lacerations
2016, 1Q, 7   Obstetrical perineal laceration repair
2014, 4Q, 31   Delayed wound closure following fracture treatment

AHA Coding Clinic for table ØHR
2018, 3Q, 13   Deep inferior epigastric artery perforator flap breast reconstruction
2017, 1Q, 35   Epifix® allograft
2014, 3Q, 14   Application of TheraSkin® and excisional debridement

AHA Coding Clinic for table ØHT
2018, 3Q, 13   Deep inferior epigastric artery perforator flap breast reconstruction
2014, 4Q, 34   Skin-sparing mastectomy

Integumentary Anatomy

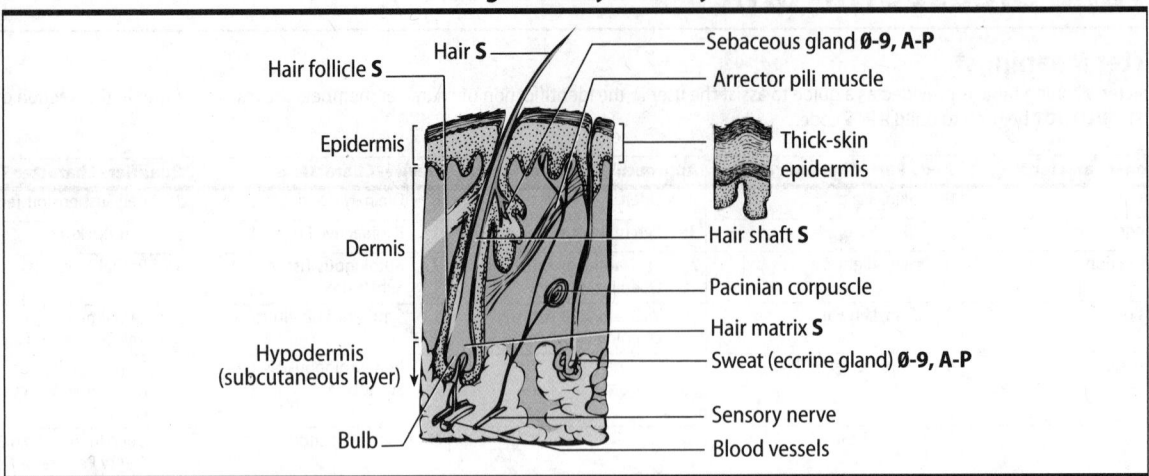

Hair follicle **S**
Hair **S**
Sebaceous gland Ø-9, A-P
Arrector pili muscle
Epidermis
Thick-skin epidermis
Dermis
Hair shaft **S**
Pacinian corpuscle
Hair matrix **S**
Sweat (eccrine gland) Ø-9, A-P
Hypodermis (subcutaneous layer)
Sensory nerve
Bulb
Blood vessels

Nail Anatomy

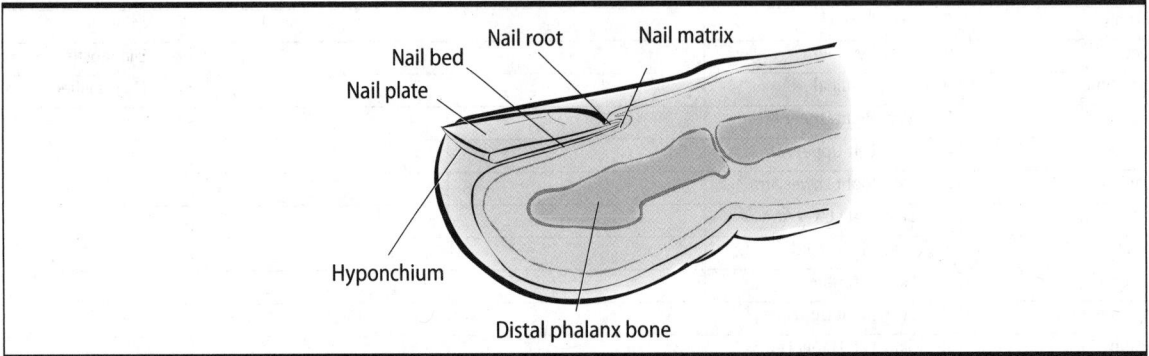

Nail bed
Nail root
Nail matrix
Nail plate
Hyponchium
Distal phalanx bone

Breast

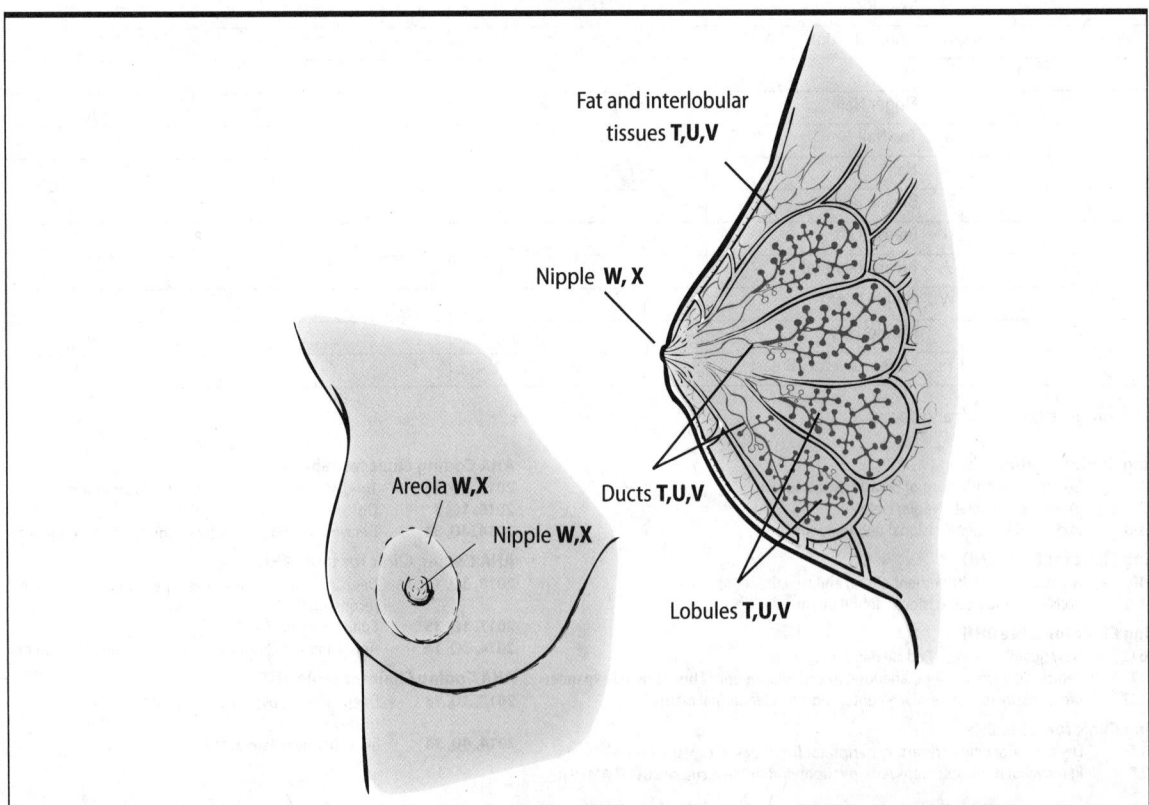

Fat and interlobular tissues **T,U,V**
Nipple **W, X**
Areola **W,X**
Nipple **W,X**
Ducts **T,U,V**
Lobules **T,U,V**

Ø   Medical and Surgical
H   Skin and Breast
Ø   Alteration   Definition: Modifying the anatomic structure of a body part without affecting the function of the body part

Explanation: Principal purpose is to improve appearance

Body Part Character 4	Approach Character 5	Device Character 6	Qualifier Character 7

T Breast, Right
   Mammary duct
   Mammary gland
U Breast, Left
   See T Breast, Right
V Breast, Bilateral
   See T Breast, Right
	Ø Open
	3 Percutaneous
		7 Autologous Tissue
		   Substitute
		J Synthetic Substitute
		K Nonautologous Tissue
		   Substitute
		Z No Device
			Z No Qualifier

Non-OR   ØHØ[T,U,V]3JZ

Ø   Medical and Surgical
H   Skin and Breast
2   Change   Definition: Taking out or off a device from a body part and putting back an identical or similar device in or on the same body part without cutting or puncturing the skin or a mucous membrane

Explanation: All CHANGE procedures are coded using the approach EXTERNAL

Body Part Character 4	Approach Character 5	Device Character 6	Qualifier Character 7

P Skin
   Dermis
   Epidermis
   Sebaceous gland
   Sweat gland
T Breast, Right
   Mammary duct
   Mammary gland
U Breast, Left
   See T Breast, Right
	X External	**Ø** Drainage Device
		Y Other Device
			Z No Qualifier

Non-OR   All body part, approach, device, and qualifier values

Ø   Medical and Surgical
H   Skin and Breast
5   Destruction   Definition: Physical eradication of all or a portion of a body part by the direct use of energy, force, or a destructive agent

Explanation: None of the body part is physically taken out

Body Part Character 4	Approach Character 5	Device Character 6	Qualifier Character 7

Ø Skin, Scalp   **C** Skin, Left Upper Arm
1 Skin, Face   **D** Skin, Right Lower Arm
2 Skin, Right Ear   **E** Skin, Left Lower Arm
3 Skin, Left Ear   **F** Skin, Right Hand
4 Skin, Neck   **G** Skin, Left Hand
5 Skin, Chest   **H** Skin, Right Upper Leg
   Breast procedures, skin   **J** Skin, Left Upper Leg
   only   **K** Skin, Right Lower Leg
6 Skin, Back   **L** Skin, Left Lower Leg
7 Skin, Abdomen   **M** Skin, Right Foot
8 Skin, Buttock   **N** Skin, Left Foot
9 Skin, Perineum
A Skin, Inguinal
B Skin, Right Upper Arm
	X External	**Z** No Device	**D** Multiple
			Z No Qualifier

Q Finger Nail
   Nail bed
   Nail plate
R Toe Nail
   See Q Finger Nail
	X External	**Z** No Device	**Z** No Qualifier

T Breast, Right
   Mammary duct
   Mammary gland
U Breast, Left
   See T Breast, Right
V Breast, Bilateral
   See T Breast, Right
	Ø Open
	3 Percutaneous
	7 Via Natural or Artificial
	   Opening
	8 Via Natural or Artificial
	   Opening Endoscopic
		Z No Device	**Z** No Qualifier

W Nipple, Right
   Areola
X Nipple, Left
   See W Nipple, Right
	Ø Open
	3 Percutaneous
	7 Via Natural or Artificial
	   Opening
	8 Via Natural or Artificial
	   Opening Endoscopic
	X External
		Z No Device	**Z** No Qualifier

DRG Non-OR   ØH5[Ø,1,4,5,6,7,8,9,A,B,C,D,E,F,G,H,J,K,L,M,N]XZ[D,Z]
DRG Non-OR   ØH5[Q,R]XZZ
Non-OR   ØH5[2,3]XZ[D,Z]

LC Limited Coverage   **NC** Noncovered   ⊞ Combination Member   HAC associated procedure   Combination Only   DRG Non-OR   Non-OR   New/Revised in GREEN

ICD-10-PCS 2020   417

Ø **Medical and Surgical**
H **Skin and Breast**
8 **Division**

Definition: Cutting into a body part, without draining fluids and/or gases from the body part, in order to separate or transect a body part

Explanation: All or a portion of the body part is separated into two or more portions

Body Part Character 4	Approach Character 5	Device Character 6	Qualifier Character 7
Ø Skin, Scalp	X External	Z No Device	Z No Qualifier
1 Skin, Face			
2 Skin, Right Ear			
3 Skin, Left Ear			
4 Skin, Neck			
5 Skin, Chest			
Breast procedures, skin only			
6 Skin, Back			
7 Skin, Abdomen			
8 Skin, Buttock			
9 Skin, Perineum			
A Skin, Inguinal			
B Skin, Right Upper Arm			
C Skin, Left Upper Arm			
D Skin, Right Lower Arm			
E Skin, Left Lower Arm			
F Skin, Right Hand			
G Skin, Left Hand			
H Skin, Right Upper Leg			
J Skin, Left Upper Leg			
K Skin, Right Lower Leg			
L Skin, Left Lower Leg			
M Skin, Right Foot			
N Skin, Left Foot			

Non-OR   All body part, approach, device, and qualifier values

---

LC Limited Coverage   NC Noncovered   ⊞ Combination Member   HAC associated procedure   Combination Only   DRG Non-OR   Non-OR   New/Revised in GREEN

418   ICD-10-PCS 2020

Ø   **Medical and Surgical**
H   **Skin and Breast**
9   **Drainage**   Definition: Taking or letting out fluids and/or gases from a body part
                      Explanation: The qualifier DIAGNOSTIC is used to identify drainage procedures that are biopsies

Body Part Character 4	Approach Character 5	Device Character 6	Qualifier Character 7

Ø Skin, Scalp E Skin, Left Lower Arm
1 Skin, Face F Skin, Right Hand
2 Skin, Right Ear G Skin, Left Hand
3 Skin, Left Ear H Skin, Right Upper Leg
4 Skin, Neck J Skin, Left Upper Leg
5 Skin, Chest K Skin, Right Lower Leg
   Breast procedures, skin L Skin, Left Lower Leg
   only M Skin, Right Foot
6 Skin, Back N Skin, Left Foot
7 Skin, Abdomen Q Finger Nail
8 Skin, Buttock Nail bed
9 Skin, Perineum Nail plate
A Skin, Inguinal R Toe Nail
B Skin, Right Upper Arm See Q Finger Nail
C Skin, Left Upper Arm
D Skin, Right Lower Arm
	X External	Ø Drainage Device	Z No Qualifier

Ø Skin, Scalp E Skin, Left Lower Arm
1 Skin, Face F Skin, Right Hand
2 Skin, Right Ear G Skin, Left Hand
3 Skin, Left Ear H Skin, Right Upper Leg
4 Skin, Neck J Skin, Left Upper Leg
5 Skin, Chest K Skin, Right Lower Leg
   Breast procedures, skin L Skin, Left Lower Leg
   only M Skin, Right Foot
6 Skin, Back N Skin, Left Foot
7 Skin, Abdomen Q Finger Nail
8 Skin, Buttock Nail bed
9 Skin, Perineum Nail plate
A Skin, Inguinal R Toe Nail
B Skin, Right Upper Arm See Q Finger Nail
C Skin, Left Upper Arm
D Skin, Right Lower Arm
	X External	Z No Device	X Diagnostic
			Z No Qualifier

T Breast, Right
   Mammary duct
   Mammary gland
U Breast, Left
   See T Breast, Right
V Breast, Bilateral
   See T Breast, Right
	Ø Open
	3 Percutaneous
	7 Via Natural or Artificial Opening
	8 Via Natural or Artificial Opening Endoscopic
		Ø Drainage Device	Z No Qualifier

T Breast, Right
   Mammary duct
   Mammary gland
U Breast, Left
   See T Breast, Right
V Breast, Bilateral
   See T Breast, Right
	Ø Open
	3 Percutaneous
	7 Via Natural or Artificial Opening
	8 Via Natural or Artificial Opening Endoscopic
		Z No Device	X Diagnostic
			Z No Qualifier

W Nipple, Right
   Areola
X Nipple, Left
   See W Nipple, Right
	Ø Open
	3 Percutaneous
	7 Via Natural or Artificial Opening
	8 Via Natural or Artificial Opening Endoscopic
	X External
		Ø Drainage Device	Z No Qualifier

W Nipple, Right
   Areola
X Nipple, Left
   See W Nipple, Right
	Ø Open
	3 Percutaneous
	7 Via Natural or Artificial Opening
	8 Via Natural or Artificial Opening Endoscopic
	X External
		Z No Device	X Diagnostic
			Z No Qualifier

Non-OR   ØH9[Ø,1,2,3,4,5,6,7,8,A,B,C,D,E,F,G,H,J,K,L,M,N,Q,R]XØZ
Non-OR   ØH9[Ø,1,2,3,4,5,6,7,8,A,B,C,D,E,F,G,H,J,K,L,M,N,Q,R]XZ[X,Z]
Non-OR   ØH99XZX
Non-OR   ØH9[T,U,V][Ø,3,7,8]ØZ
Non-OR   ØH9[T,U,V][3,7,8]Z[X,Z]
Non-OR   ØH9[W,X][Ø,3,7,8,X]ØZ
Non-OR   ØH9[W,X][3,7,8,X]Z[X,Z]

LC Limited Coverage NC Noncovered ⊞ Combination Member HAC associated procedure Combination Only DRG Non-OR Non-OR New/Revised in GREEN
ICD-10-PCS 2020   419

ØH9–ØH9

Skin and Breast

Ø **Medical and Surgical**
H **Skin and Breast**
B **Excision**　　　Definition: Cutting out or off, without replacement, a portion of a body part
　　　　　　　　　　　Explanation: The qualifier DIAGNOSTIC is used to identify excision procedures that are biopsies

Body Part Character 4	Approach Character 5	Device Character 6	Qualifier Character 7
Ø Skin, Scalp **1** Skin, Face **2** Skin, Right Ear **3** Skin, Left Ear **4** Skin, Neck **5** Skin, Chest 　　Breast procedures, skin only **6** Skin, Back **7** Skin, Abdomen **8** Skin, Buttock **9** Skin, Perineum **A** Skin, Inguinal **B** Skin, Right Upper Arm **C** Skin, Left Upper Arm **D** Skin, Right Lower Arm **E** Skin, Left Lower Arm **F** Skin, Right Hand **G** Skin, Left Hand **H** Skin, Right Upper Leg **J** Skin, Left Upper Leg **K** Skin, Right Lower Leg **L** Skin, Left Lower Leg **M** Skin, Right Foot **N** Skin, Left Foot **Q** Finger Nail 　　Nail bed 　　Nail plate **R** Toe Nail 　　*See Q Finger Nail*	**X** External	**Z** No Device	**X** Diagnostic **Z** No Qualifier
T Breast, Right 　　Mammary duct 　　Mammary gland **U** Breast, Left 　　*See T Breast, Right* **V** Breast, Bilateral 　　*See T Breast, Right* **Y** Supernumerary Breast	**Ø** Open **3** Percutaneous **7** Via Natural or Artificial Opening **8** Via Natural or Artificial Opening 　　Endoscopic	**Z** No Device	**X** Diagnostic **Z** No Qualifier
W Nipple, Right 　　Areola **X** Nipple, Left 　　*See W Nipple, Right*	**Ø** Open **3** Percutaneous **7** Via Natural or Artificial Opening **8** Via Natural or Artificial Opening 　　Endoscopic **X** External	**Z** No Device	**X** Diagnostic **Z** No Qualifier

DRG Non-OR	ØHB9XZZ
Non-OR	ØHB[Ø,1,2,3,4,5,6,7,8,A,B,C,D,E,F,G,H,J,K,L,M,N,Q,R]XZ[X,Z]
Non-OR	ØHB9XZX
Non-OR	ØHB[T,U,V,Y][3,7,8]ZX
Non-OR	ØHB[W,X][3,7,8,X]ZX

Ø   Medical and Surgical
H   Skin and Breast
C   Extirpation   Definition: Taking or cutting out solid matter from a body part

Explanation: The solid matter may be an abnormal byproduct of a biological function or a foreign body; it may be imbedded in a body part or in the lumen of a tubular body part. The solid matter may or may not have been previously broken into pieces.

Body Part Character 4	Approach Character 5	Device Character 6	Qualifier Character 7

Ø   Skin, Scalp
1   Skin, Face
2   Skin, Right Ear
3   Skin, Left Ear
4   Skin, Neck
5   Skin, Chest
     Breast procedures, skin only
6   Skin, Back
7   Skin, Abdomen
8   Skin, Buttock
9   Skin, Perineum
A   Skin, Inguinal
B   Skin, Right Upper Arm
C   Skin, Left Upper Arm
D   Skin, Right Lower Arm
E   Skin, Left Lower Arm
F   Skin, Right Hand
G   Skin, Left Hand
H   Skin, Right Upper Leg
J   Skin, Left Upper Leg
K   Skin, Right Lower Leg
L   Skin, Left Lower Leg
M   Skin, Right Foot
N   Skin, Left Foot
Q   Finger Nail
     Nail bed
     Nail plate
R   Toe Nail
     See Q Finger Nail
	X External	**Z** No Device	**Z** No Qualifier

T   Breast, Right
     Mammary duct
     Mammary gland
U   Breast, Left
     See T Breast, Right
V   Breast, Bilateral
     See T Breast, Right
	Ø Open
	3 Percutaneous
	7 Via Natural or Artificial Opening
	8 Via Natural or Artificial Opening Endoscopic
		Z No Device	**Z** No Qualifier

W   Nipple, Right
     Areola
X   Nipple, Left
     See W Nipple, Right
	Ø Open
	3 Percutaneous
	7 Via Natural or Artificial Opening
	8 Via Natural or Artificial Opening Endoscopic
	X External
		Z No Device	**Z** No Qualifier

Non-OR   ØHC[Ø,1,2,3,4,5,6,7,8,9,A,B,C,D,E,F,G,H,J,K,L,M,N,Q,R]XZZ
Non-OR   ØHC[T,U,V][3,7,8]ZZ
Non-OR   ØHC[W,X][3,7,8,X]ZZ

Skin and Breast

Ø Medical and Surgical
H Skin and Breast
D Extraction   Definition: Pulling or stripping out or off all or a portion of a body part by the use of force
                      Explanation: The qualifier DIAGNOSTIC is used to identify extraction procedures that are biopsies

Body Part Character 4	Approach Character 5	Device Character 6	Qualifier Character 7

Ø Skin, Scalp
1 Skin, Face
2 Skin, Right Ear
3 Skin, Left Ear
4 Skin, Neck
5 Skin, Chest
   Breast procedures, skin only
6 Skin, Back
7 Skin, Abdomen
8 Skin, Buttock
9 Skin, Perineum
A Skin, Inguinal
B Skin, Right Upper Arm
C Skin, Left Upper Arm
D Skin, Right Lower Arm
E Skin, Left Lower Arm
F Skin, Right Hand
G Skin, Left Hand
H Skin, Right Upper Leg
J Skin, Left Upper Leg
K Skin, Right Lower Leg
L Skin, Left Lower Leg
M Skin, Right Foot
N Skin, Left Foot
Q Finger Nail
   Nail bed
   Nail plate
R Toe Nail
   See Q Finger Nail
S Hair
	X External	Z No Device	Z No Qualifier

T Breast, Right
   Mammary duct
   Mammary gland
U Breast, Left
   See T Breast, Right
V Breast, Bilateral
   See T Breast, Right
Y Supernumerary Breast
	Ø Open	Z No Device	Z No Qualifier

Non-OR   All body part, approach, device, and qualifier values

Ø   Medical and Surgical
H   Skin and Breast
H   Insertion   Definition: Putting in a nonbiological appliance that monitors, assists, performs, or prevents a physiological function but does not physically take the place of a body part
                 Explanation: None

Body Part Character 4	Approach Character 5	Device Character 6	Qualifier Character 7
P Skin	**X** External	**Y** Other Device	**Z** No Qualifier

T   Breast, Right
     Mammary duct
     Mammary gland
U   Breast, Left
     See T Breast, Right
	Ø Open
	3 Percutaneous
	7 Via Natural or Artificial Opening
	8 Via Natural or Artificial Opening Endoscopic
		1 Radioactive Element
		N Tissue Expander
		Y Other Device
			Z No Qualifier

V   Breast, Bilateral
     Mammary duct
     Mammary gland
	Ø Open
	3 Percutaneous
	7 Via Natural or Artificial Opening
	8 Via Natural or Artificial Opening Endoscopic
		1 Radioactive Element
		N Tissue Expander
			Z No Qualifier

W   Nipple, Right
     Areola
X   Nipple, Left
     See W Nipple, Right
	Ø Open
	3 Percutaneous
	7 Via Natural or Artificial Opening
	8 Via Natural or Artificial Opening Endoscopic
		1 Radioactive Element
		N Tissue Expander
			Z No Qualifier

W   Nipple, Right
     Areola
X   Nipple, Left
     See W Nipple, Right
	X External	**1** Radioactive Element	**Z** No Qualifier

Non-OR   ØHHPXYZ
Non-OR   ØHH[T,U][3,7,8]YZ

Ø   Medical and Surgical
H   Skin and Breast
J   Inspection   Definition: Visually and/or manually exploring a body part
                 Explanation: Visual exploration may be performed with or without optical instrumentation. Manual exploration may be performed directly or through intervening body layers.

Body Part Character 4	Approach Character 5	Device Character 6	Qualifier Character 7

P   Skin
     Dermis
     Epidermis
     Sebaceous gland
     Sweat gland
Q   Finger Nail
     Nail bed
     Nail plate
R   Toe Nail
     See Q Finger Nail
	X External	**Z** No Device	**Z** No Qualifier

T   Breast, Right
     Mammary duct
     Mammary gland
U   Breast, Left
     See T Breast, Right
	Ø Open
	3 Percutaneous
	7 Via Natural or Artificial Opening
	8 Via Natural or Artificial Opening Endoscopic
		Z No Device	**Z** No Qualifier

Non-OR   All body part, approach, device and qualifier values

Ø   Medical and Surgical
H   Skin and Breast
M   Reattachment   Definition: Putting back in or on all or a portion of a separated body part to its normal location or other suitable location

                             Explanation: Vascular circulation and nervous pathways may or may not be reestablished

Body Part Character 4	Approach Character 5	Device Character 6	Qualifier Character 7
Ø Skin, Scalp	X External	Z No Device	Z No Qualifier
1 Skin, Face			
2 Skin, Right Ear			
3 Skin, Left Ear			
4 Skin, Neck			
5 Skin, Chest Breast procedures, skin only			
6 Skin, Back			
7 Skin, Abdomen			
8 Skin, Buttock			
9 Skin, Perineum			
A Skin, Inguinal			
B Skin, Right Upper Arm			
C Skin, Left Upper Arm			
D Skin, Right Lower Arm			
E Skin, Left Lower Arm			
F Skin, Right Hand			
G Skin, Left Hand			
H Skin, Right Upper Leg			
J Skin, Left Upper Leg			
K Skin, Right Lower Leg			
L Skin, Left Lower Leg			
M Skin, Right Foot			
N Skin, Left Foot			

T   Breast, Right
     Mammary duct
     Mammary gland			

U Breast, Left *See* T Breast, Right			
V Breast, Bilateral *See* T Breast, Right			
W Nipple, Right Areola			
X Nipple, Left *See* W Nipple, Right			

Non-OR   ØHMØXZZ

LC Limited Coverage   NC Noncovered   ⊞ Combination Member   HAC associated procedure   Combination Only   DRG Non-OR   Non-OR   New/Revised in GREEN

424   ICD-10-PCS 2020

Ø   Medical and Surgical
H   Skin and Breast
N   Release   Definition: Freeing a body part from an abnormal physical constraint by cutting or by the use of force
Explanation: Some of the restraining tissue may be taken out but none of the body part is taken out

Body Part Character 4	Approach Character 5	Device Character 6	Qualifier Character 7

Ø Skin, Scalp
1 Skin, Face
2 Skin, Right Ear
3 Skin, Left Ear
4 Skin, Neck
5 Skin, Chest
    Breast procedures, skin only
6 Skin, Back
7 Skin, Abdomen
8 Skin, Buttock
9 Skin, Perineum
A Skin, Inguinal
B Skin, Right Upper Arm
C Skin, Left Upper Arm
D Skin, Right Lower Arm
E Skin, Left Lower Arm
F Skin, Right Hand
G Skin, Left Hand
H Skin, Right Upper Leg
J Skin, Left Upper Leg
K Skin, Right Lower Leg
L Skin, Left Lower Leg
M Skin, Right Foot
N Skin, Left Foot
Q Finger Nail
    Nail bed
    Nail plate
R Toe Nail
    See Q Finger Nail
	X External	**Z** No Device	**Z** No Qualifier

T Breast, Right
    Mammary duct
    Mammary gland
U Breast, Left
    See T Breast, Right
V Breast, Bilateral
    See T Breast, Right
	Ø Open
	3 Percutaneous
	7 Via Natural or Artificial Opening
	8 Via Natural or Artificial Opening
	    Endoscopic
		Z No Device	**Z** No Qualifier

W Nipple, Right
    Areola
X Nipple, Left
    See W Nipple, Right
	Ø Open
	3 Percutaneous
	7 Via Natural or Artificial Opening
	8 Via Natural or Artificial Opening
	    Endoscopic
	X External
		Z No Device	**Z** No Qualifier

Ø   Medical and Surgical
H   Skin and Breast
P   Removal   Definition: Taking out or off a device from a body part

Explanation: If a device is taken out and a similar device put in without cutting or puncturing the skin or mucous membrane, the procedure is coded to the root operation CHANGE. Otherwise, the procedure for taking out a device is coded to the root operation REMOVAL.

Body Part Character 4	Approach Character 5	Device Character 6	Qualifier Character 7
P Skin Dermis Epidermis Sebaceous gland Sweat gland	**X External**	**Ø Drainage Device** **7 Autologous Tissue Substitute** **J Synthetic Substitute** **K Nonautologous Tissue Substitute** **Y Other Device**	**Z No Qualifier**
Q Finger Nail Nail bed Nail plate **R Toe Nail** *See Q Finger Nail*	**X External**	**Ø Drainage Device** **7 Autologous Tissue Substitute** **J Synthetic Substitute** **K Nonautologous Tissue Substitute**	**Z No Qualifier**
S Hair	**X External**	**7 Autologous Tissue Substitute** **J Synthetic Substitute** **K Nonautologous Tissue Substitute**	**Z No Qualifier**
T Breast, Right Mammary duct Mammary gland **U Breast, Left** *See T Breast, Right*	**Ø Open** **3 Percutaneous** **7 Via Natural or Artificial Opening** **8 Via Natural or Artificial Opening Endoscopic**	**Ø Drainage Device** **1 Radioactive Element** **7 Autologous Tissue Substitute** **J Synthetic Substitute** **K Nonautologous Tissue Substitute** **N Tissue Expander** **Y Other Device**	**Z No Qualifier**

Non-OR   ØHPPX[Ø,7,J,K,Y]Z
Non-OR   ØHP[Q,R]X[Ø,7,J,K]Z
Non-OR   ØHPSX[7,J,K]Z
Non-OR   ØHP[T,U]Ø[Ø,1,7,K]Z
Non-OR   ØHP[T,U]3[Ø,1,7,K,Y]Z
Non-OR   ØHP[T,U][7,8][Ø,1,7,J,K,N,Y]Z

Ø   Medical and Surgical
H   Skin and Breast
Q   Repair   Definition: Restoring, to the extent possible, a body part to its normal anatomic structure and function
                   Explanation: Used only when the method to accomplish the repair is not one of the other root operations

Body Part Character 4	Approach Character 5	Device Character 6	Qualifier Character 7

Ø Skin, Scalp
1 Skin, Face
2 Skin, Right Ear
3 Skin, Left Ear
4 Skin, Neck
5 Skin, Chest
     Breast procedures, skin only
6 Skin, Back
7 Skin, Abdomen
8 Skin, Buttock
9 Skin, Perineum
A Skin, Inguinal
B Skin, Right Upper Arm
C Skin, Left Upper Arm
D Skin, Right Lower Arm
E Skin, Left Lower Arm
F Skin, Right Hand
G Skin, Left Hand
H Skin, Right Upper Leg
J Skin, Left Upper Leg
K Skin, Right Lower Leg
L Skin, Left Lower Leg
M Skin, Right Foot
N Skin, Left Foot
Q Finger Nail
     Nail bed
     Nail plate
R Toe Nail
     See Q Finger Nail
	X External	**Z** No Device	**Z** No Qualifier

T Breast, Right
     Mammary duct
     Mammary gland
U Breast, Left
     See T Breast, Right
V Breast, Bilateral
     See T Breast, Right
Y Supernumerary Breast
	Ø Open
	3 Percutaneous
	7 Via Natural or Artificial Opening
	8 Via Natural or Artificial Opening
	     Endoscopic
		Z No Device	**Z** No Qualifier

W Nipple, Right
     Areola
X Nipple, Left
     See W Nipple, Right
	Ø Open
	3 Percutaneous
	7 Via Natural or Artificial Opening
	8 Via Natural or Artificial Opening
	     Endoscopic
	X External
		Z No Device	**Z** No Qualifier

DRG Non-OR   ØHQ9XZZ
Non-OR   ØHQ[Ø,1,2,3,4,5,6,7,8,A,B,C,D,E,F,G,H,J,K,L,M,N]XZZ

Ø   **Medical and Surgical**
H   **Skin and Breast**
R   **Replacement**

Definition: Putting in or on biological or synthetic material that physically takes the place and/or function of all or a portion of a body part
Explanation: The body part may have been taken out or replaced, or may be taken out, physically eradicated, or rendered nonfunctional during the REPLACEMENT procedure. A REMOVAL procedure is coded for taking out the device used in a previous replacement procedure.

Body Part Character 4		Approach Character 5	Device Character 6	Qualifier Character 7
Ø Skin, Scalp **1** Skin, Face **2** Skin, Right Ear **3** Skin, Left Ear **4** Skin, Neck **5** Skin, Chest Breast procedures, skin only **6** Skin, Back **7** Skin, Abdomen **8** Skin, Buttock **9** Skin, Perineum **A** Skin, Inguinal	**B** Skin, Right Upper Arm **C** Skin, Left Upper Arm **D** Skin, Right Lower Arm **E** Skin, Left Lower Arm **F** Skin, Right Hand **G** Skin, Left Hand **H** Skin, Right Upper Leg **J** Skin, Left Upper Leg **K** Skin, Right Lower Leg **L** Skin, Left Lower Leg **M** Skin, Right Foot **N** Skin, Left Foot	**X** External	**7** Autologous Tissue Substitute	**2** Cell Suspension Technique **3** Full Thickness **4** Partial Thickness
Ø Skin, Scalp **1** Skin, Face **2** Skin, Right Ear **3** Skin, Left Ear **4** Skin, Neck **5** Skin, Chest Breast procedures, skin only **6** Skin, Back **7** Skin, Abdomen **8** Skin, Buttock **9** Skin, Perineum **A** Skin, Inguinal	**B** Skin, Right Upper Arm **C** Skin, Left Upper Arm **D** Skin, Right Lower Arm **E** Skin, Left Lower Arm **F** Skin, Right Hand **G** Skin, Left Hand **H** Skin, Right Upper Leg **J** Skin, Left Upper Leg **K** Skin, Right Lower Leg **L** Skin, Left Lower Leg **M** Skin, Right Foot **N** Skin, Left Foot	**X** External	**J** Synthetic Substitute	**3** Full Thickness **4** Partial Thickness **Z** No Qualifier
Ø Skin, Scalp **1** Skin, Face **2** Skin, Right Ear **3** Skin, Left Ear **4** Skin, Neck **5** Skin, Chest Breast procedures, skin only **6** Skin, Back **7** Skin, Abdomen **8** Skin Buttock **9** Skin, Perineum **A** Skin, Inguinal	**B** Skin, Right Upper Arm **C** Skin, Left Upper Arm **D** Skin, Right Lower Arm **E** Skin, Left Lower Arm **F** Skin, Right Hand **G** Skin, Left Hand **H** Skin, Right Upper Leg **J** Skin, Left Upper Leg **K** Skin, Right Lower Leg **L** Skin, Left Lower Leg **M** Skin, Right Foot **N** Skin, Left Foot	**X** External	**K** Nonautologous Tissue Substitute	**3** Full Thickness **4** Partial Thickness

Q Finger Nail
    Nail bed
    Nail plate
	R Toe Nail
	    See Q Finger Nail
	S Hair
		X External	**7** Autologous Tissue Substitute
			J Synthetic Substitute
			K Nonautologous Tissue Substitute
				Z No Qualifier

T Breast, Right
    Mammary duct
    Mammary gland
	U Breast, Left
	    See T Breast, Right
	V Breast, Bilateral
	    See T Breast, Right
		Ø Open	**7** Autologous Tissue Substitute	**5** Latissimus Dorsi Myocutaneous Flap
				6 Transverse Rectus Abdominis Myocutaneous Flap
				7 Deep Inferior Epigastric Artery Perforator Flap
				8 Superficial Inferior Epigastric Artery Flap
				9 Gluteal Artery Perforator Flap
				Z No Qualifier

T Breast, Right
    Mammary duct
    Mammary gland
	U Breast, Left
	    See T Breast, Right
	V Breast, Bilateral
	    See T Breast, Right
		Ø Open	**J** Synthetic Substitute
			K Nonautologous Tissue Substitute
				Z No Qualifier

T Breast, Right ⊞
    Mammary duct
    Mammary gland
U Breast, Left ⊞
    See T Breast, Right
	V Breast, Bilateral ⊞
	    See T Breast, Right
		3 Percutaneous	**7** Autologous Tissue Substitute
			J Synthetic Substitute
			K Nonautologous Tissue Substitute
				Z No Qualifier

W Nipple, Right
    Areola
	X Nipple, Left
	    See W Nipple, Right
		Ø Open
		3 Percutaneous
		X External
			7 Autologous Tissue Substitute
			J Synthetic Substitute
			K Nonautologous Tissue Substitute
				Z No Qualifier

Non-OR   ØHRSX7Z

See Appendix L for Procedure Combinations
    ⊞   ØHR[T,U,V]37Z

LC Limited Coverage   NC Noncovered   ⊞ Combination Member   HAC associated procedure   Combination Only   DRG Non-OR   Non-OR   New/Revised in GREEN

428   ICD-10-PCS 2020

Ø **Medical and Surgical**
H **Skin and Breast**
S **Reposition**   Definition: Moving to its normal location, or other suitable location, all or a portion of a body part

Explanation: The body part is moved to a new location from an abnormal location, or from a normal location where it is not functioning correctly. The body part may or may not be cut out or off to be moved to the new location.

Body Part Character 4	Approach Character 5	Device Character 6	Qualifier Character 7
S Hair **W** Nipple, Right Areola **X** Nipple, Left *See W Nipple, Right*	**X** External	**Z** No Device	**Z** No Qualifier
T Breast, Right Mammary duct Mammary gland **U** Breast, Left *See T Breast, Right* **V** Breast, Bilateral *See T Breast, Right*	**Ø** Open	**Z** No Device	**Z** No Qualifier

Non-OR ØHSSXZZ

Ø **Medical and Surgical**
H **Skin and Breast**
T **Resection**   Definition: Cutting out or off, without replacement, all of a body part

Explanation: None

Body Part Character 4	Approach Character 5	Device Character 6	Qualifier Character 7
Q Finger Nail Nail bed Nail plate **R** Toe Nail *See Q Finger Nail* **W** Nipple, Right Areola **X** Nipple, Left *See W Nipple, Right*	**X** External	**Z** No Device	**Z** No Qualifier
T Breast, Right ⊞ Mammary duct Mammary gland **U** Breast, Left ⊞ *See T Breast, Right* **V** Breast, Bilateral ⊞ *See T Breast, Right* **Y** Supernumerary Breast	**Ø** Open	**Z** No Device	**Z** No Qualifier

Non-OR ØHT[Q,R]XZZ   **See Appendix L for Procedure Combinations**
                    ⊞   ØHT[T,U,V]ØZZ

Ø **Medical and Surgical**
H **Skin and Breast**
U **Supplement**   Definition: Putting in or on biological or synthetic material that physically reinforces and/or augments the function of a portion of a body part

Explanation: The biological material is non-living, or is living and from the same individual. The body part may have been previously replaced, and the SUPPLEMENT procedure is performed to physically reinforce and/or augment the function of the replaced body part.

Body Part Character 4	Approach Character 5	Device Character 6	Qualifier Character 7
T Breast, Right Mammary duct Mammary gland **U** Breast, Left *See T Breast, Right* **V** Breast, Bilateral *See T Breast, Right*	**Ø** Open **3** Percutaneous **7** Via Natural or Artificial Opening **8** Via Natural or Artificial Opening Endoscopic	**7** Autologous Tissue Substitute **J** Synthetic Substitute **K** Nonautologous Tissue Substitute	**Z** No Qualifier
W Nipple, Right Areola **X** Nipple, Left *See W Nipple, Right*	**Ø** Open **3** Percutaneous **7** Via Natural or Artificial Opening **8** Via Natural or Artificial Opening Endoscopic **X** External	**7** Autologous Tissue Substitute **J** Synthetic Substitute **K** Nonautologous Tissue Substitute	**Z** No Qualifier

Non-OR ØHU[T,U,V]3JZ

LC Limited Coverage   **NC** Noncovered   ⊞ Combination Member   HAC associated procedure   Combination Only   DRG Non-OR   Non-OR   New/Revised in GREEN

ICD-10-PCS 2020   **429**

Skin and Breast

Ø   **Medical and Surgical**
H   **Skin and Breast**
W   **Revision**   Definition: Correcting, to the extent possible, a portion of a malfunctioning device or the position of a displaced device

Explanation: Revision can include correcting a malfunctioning or displaced device by taking out or putting in components of the device such as a screw or pin

Body Part Character 4	Approach Character 5	Device Character 6	Qualifier Character 7
P **Skin** Dermis Epidermis Sebaceous gland Sweat gland	**X** External	**Ø** Drainage Device **7** Autologous Tissue Substitute **J** Synthetic Substitute **K** Nonautologous Tissue Substitute **Y** Other Device	**Z** No Qualifier
Q **Finger Nail** Nail bed Nail plate **R** **Toe Nail** *See Q Finger Nail*	**X** External	**Ø** Drainage Device **7** Autologous Tissue Substitute **J** Synthetic Substitute **K** Nonautologous Tissue Substitute	**Z** No Qualifier
S **Hair**	**X** External	**7** Autologous Tissue Substitute **J** Synthetic Substitute **K** Nonautologous Tissue Substitute	**Z** No Qualifier
T **Breast, Right** Mammary duct Mammary gland **U** **Breast, Left** *See T Breast, Right*	**Ø** Open **3** Percutaneous **7** Via Natural or Artificial Opening **8** Via Natural or Artificial Opening Endoscopic	**Ø** Drainage Device **7** Autologous Tissue Substitute **J** Synthetic Substitute **K** Nonautologous Tissue Substitute **N** Tissue Expander **Y** Other Device	**Z** No Qualifier

Non-OR   ØHWPX[Ø,7,J,K,Y]Z
Non-OR   ØHW[Q,R]X[Ø,7,J,K]Z
Non-OR   ØHWSX[7,J,K]Z
Non-OR   ØHW[T,U]Ø[Ø,7,K,N]Z
Non-OR   ØHW[T,U]3[Ø,7,K,N,Y]Z
Non-OR   ØHW[T,U][7,8][Ø,7,J,K,N,Y]Z

Ø   **Medical and Surgical**
H   **Skin and Breast**
X   **Transfer**   Definition: Moving, without taking out, all or a portion of a body part to another location to take over the function of all or a portion of a body part

Explanation: The body part transferred remains connected to its vascular and nervous supply

Body Part Character 4	Approach Character 5	Device Character 6	Qualifier Character 7
Ø Skin, Scalp **1** Skin, Face **2** Skin, Right Ear **3** Skin, Left Ear **4** Skin, Neck **5** Skin, Chest Breast procedures, skin only **6** Skin, Back **7** Skin, Abdomen **8** Skin, Buttock **9** Skin, Perineum **A** Skin, Inguinal **B** Skin, Right Upper Arm **C** Skin, Left Upper Arm **D** Skin, Right Lower Arm **E** Skin, Left Lower Arm **F** Skin, Right Hand **G** Skin, Left Hand **H** Skin, Right Upper Leg **J** Skin, Left Upper Leg **K** Skin, Right Lower Leg **L** Skin, Left Lower Leg **M** Skin, Right Foot **N** Skin, Left Foot	**X** External	**Z** No Device	**Z** No Qualifier

LC Limited Coverage   **NC** Noncovered   ⊞ Combination Member   HAC associated procedure   Combination Only   DRG Non-OR   Non-OR   New/Revised in GREEN

430   ICD-10-PCS 2020

Subcutaneous Tissue and Fascia ØJØ–ØJX

Character Meanings

This Character Meaning table is provided as a guide to assist the user in the identification of character members that may be found in this section of code tables. It **SHOULD NOT** be used to build a PCS code.

Operation–Character 3	Body Part–Character 4	Approach–Character 5	Device–Character 6	Qualifier–Character 7
Ø Alteration	Ø Subcutaneous Tissue and Fascia, Scalp	Ø Open	Ø Drainage Device OR Monitoring Device, Hemodynamic	B Skin and Subcutaneous Tissue
2 Change	1 Subcutaneous Tissue and Fascia, Face	3 Percutaneous	1 Radioactive Element	C Skin, Subcutaneous Tissue and Fascia
5 Destruction	4 Subcutaneous Tissue and Fascia, Right Neck	X External	2 Monitoring Device	X Diagnostic
8 Division	5 Subcutaneous Tissue and Fascia, Left Neck		3 Infusion Device	Z No Qualifier
9 Drainage	6 Subcutaneous Tissue and Fascia, Chest		4 Pacemaker, Single Chamber	
B Excision	7 Subcutaneous Tissue and Fascia, Back		5 Pacemaker, Single Chamber Rate Responsive	
C Extirpation	8 Subcutaneous Tissue and Fascia, Abdomen		6 Pacemaker, Dual Chamber	
D Extraction	9 Subcutaneous Tissue and Fascia, Buttock		7 Autologous Tissue Substitute OR Cardiac Resynchronization Pacemaker Pulse Generator	
H Insertion	B Subcutaneous Tissue and Fascia, Perineum		8 Defibrillator Generator	
J Inspection	C Subcutaneous Tissue and Fascia, Pelvic Region		9 Cardiac Resynchronization Defibrillator Pulse Generator	
N Release	D Subcutaneous Tissue and Fascia, Right Upper Arm		A Contractility Modulation Device	
P Removal	F Subcutaneous Tissue and Fascia, Left Upper Arm		B Stimulator Generator, Single Array	
Q Repair	G Subcutaneous Tissue and Fascia, Right Lower Arm		C Stimulator Generator, Single Array Rechargeable	
R Replacement	H Subcutaneous Tissue and Fascia, Left Lower Arm		D Stimulator Generator, Multiple Array	
U Supplement	J Subcutaneous Tissue and Fascia, Right Hand		E Stimulator Generator, Multiple Array Rechargeable	
W Revision	K Subcutaneous Tissue and Fascia, Left Hand		F Subcutaneous Defibrillator Lead	
X Transfer	L Subcutaneous Tissue and Fascia, Right Upper Leg		H Contraceptive Device	
	M Subcutaneous Tissue and Fascia, Left Upper Leg		J Synthetic Substitute	
	N Subcutaneous Tissue and Fascia, Right Lower Leg		K Nonautologous Tissue Substitute	
	P Subcutaneous Tissue and Fascia, Left Lower Leg		M Stimulator Generator	
	Q Subcutaneous Tissue and Fascia, Right Foot		N Tissue Expander	
	R Subcutaneous Tissue and Fascia, Left Foot		P Cardiac Rhythm Related Device	
	S Subcutaneous Tissue and Fascia, Head and Neck		V Infusion Device, Pump	
	T Subcutaneous Tissue and Fascia, Trunk		W Vascular Access Device, Totally Implantable	
	V Subcutaneous Tissue and Fascia, Upper Extremity		X Vascular Access Device, Tunneled	
	W Subcutaneous Tissue and Fascia, Lower Extremity		Y Other Device	
			Z No Device	

AHA Coding Clinic for table ØJ2

2018, 3Q, 10	Disruption of perma-catheter fibrin sheath via angioplasty of superior vena cava
2017, 2Q, 26	Exchange of tunneled catheter

AHA Coding Clinic for table ØJ8

2017, 3Q, 11	Bilateral escharotomy of leg, thigh and foot

AHA Coding Clinic for table ØJ9

2018, 3Q, 16	Incision and drainage of submandibular space
2018, 3Q, 16	Incision and drainage of neck abscess
2015, 3Q, 23	Incision and drainage of multiple abscess cavities using vessel loop

AHA Coding Clinic for table ØJB

2018, 3Q, 17	Excisional debridement of periosteum
2018, 1Q, 7	Placement of fat graft following lumbar decompression surgery
2015, 3Q, 3-8	Excisional and nonexcisional debridement
2015, 2Q, 13	Transfer of free flap to reconstruct orbital defect
2015, 1Q, 29	Fistulectomy with placement of seton
2014, 4Q, 38	Abdominoplasty and abdominal wall plication for hernia repair
2014, 3Q, 22	Transsphenoidal removal of pituitary tumor and fat graft placement

AHA Coding Clinic for table ØJC

2017, 3Q, 22	Replacement of native skull bone flap

AHA Coding Clinic for table ØJD

2016, 3Q, 20	VersaJet™ nonexcisional debridement of leg muscle
2016, 3Q, 21	Nonexcisional debridement of infected lumbar wound
2016, 3Q, 21	Nonexcisional pulsed lavage debridement
2016, 3Q, 22	Debridement of bone and tendon using Tenex ultrasound device
2016, 1Q, 40	Nonexcisional debridement of skin and subcutaneous tissue
2015, 3Q, 3-8	Excisional and nonexcisional debridement
2015, 1Q, 23	Non-Excisional debridement with lavage of wound

AHA Coding Clinic for table ØJH

2017, 4Q, 63-64	Added and revised device values - Vascular access reservoir
2017, 2Q, 24	Tunneled catheter versus totally implantable catheter
2017, 2Q, 26	Exchange of tunneled catheter
2016, 4Q, 97-98	Phrenic neurostimulator
2016, 2Q, 14	Insertion of peritoneal totally implantable venous access device
2016, 2Q, 15	Removal and replacement of tunneled internal jugular catheter
2015, 4Q, 14	New Section X codes—New Technology procedures
2015, 4Q, 30-31	Vascular access devices
2015, 2Q, 33	Totally implantable central venous access device (Port-a-Cath)
2014, 3Q, 19	End of life replacement of Baclofen pump
2013, 4Q, 116	Device character for Port-A-Cath placement
2012, 4Q, 104	Placement of subcutaneous implantable cardioverter defibrillator

AHA Coding Clinic for table ØJN

2017, 3Q, 11	Bilateral escharotomy of leg, thigh and foot

AHA Coding Clinic for table ØJP

2018, 4Q, 86	Placement of lumboatrial shunt
2018, 3Q, 29	Decommissioning of left ventricular assist device with exploration of mediastinum
2016, 2Q, 15	Removal and replacement of tunneled internal jugular catheter
2015, 4Q, 31	Vascular access devices
2014, 3Q, 19	End of life replacement of Baclofen pump
2013, 4Q, 109	Separating conjoined twins
2012, 4Q, 104	Placement of subcutaneous implantable cardioverter defibrillator

AHA Coding Clinic for table ØJQ

2017, 3Q, 19	Anterior repair of cystocele
2014, 4Q, 44	Posterior colporrhaphy/rectocele repair

AHA Coding Clinic for table ØJR

2015, 2Q, 13	Transfer of free flap to reconstruct orbital defect

AHA Coding Clinic for table ØJU

2018, 2Q, 20	Prelaminated free flap graft using Alloderm™
2018, 1Q, 7	Placement of fat graft following lumbar decompression surgery

AHA Coding Clinic for table ØJW

2018, 1Q, 8	Ventricular peritoneal shunt ligation
2015, 4Q, 33	Externalization of peritoneal dialysis catheter
2015, 2Q, 9	Revision of ventriculoperitoneal (VP) shunt
2012, 4Q, 104	Placement of subcutaneous implantable cardioverter defibrillator

AHA Coding Clinic for table ØJX

2018, 1Q, 10	Complex wound closure using pericranial flap
2014, 3Q, 18	Placement of reverse sural fasciocutaneous pedicle flap
2013, 4Q, 109	Separating conjoined twins

Ø   **Medical and Surgical**
J   **Subcutaneous Tissue and Fascia**
Ø   **Alteration**   Definition: Modifying the anatomic structure of a body part without affecting the function of the body part
                     Explanation: Principal purpose is to improve appearance

Body Part Character 4		Approach Character 5	Device Character 6	Qualifier Character 7
1 Subcutaneous Tissue and Fascia, Face Masseteric fascia Orbital fascia Submandibular space **4 Subcutaneous Tissue and Fascia, Right Neck** Deep cervical fascia Pretracheal fascia Prevertebral fascia **5 Subcutaneous Tissue and Fascia, Left Neck** *See 4 Subcutaneous Tissue and Fascia, Right Neck* **6 Subcutaneous Tissue and Fascia, Chest** Pectoral fascia **7 Subcutaneous Tissue and Fascia, Back** **8 Subcutaneous Tissue and Fascia, Abdomen** **9 Subcutaneous Tissue and Fascia, Buttock** **D Subcutaneous Tissue and Fascia, Right Upper Arm** Axillary fascia Deltoid fascia Infraspinatus fascia Subscapular aponeurosis Supraspinatus fascia	**F Subcutaneous Tissue and Fascia, Left Upper Arm** *See D Subcutaneous Tissue and Fascia, Right Upper Arm* **G Subcutaneous Tissue and Fascia, Right Lower Arm** Antebrachial fascia Bicipital aponeurosis **H Subcutaneous Tissue and Fascia, Left Lower Arm** *See G Subcutaneous Tissue and Fascia, Right Lower Arm* **L Subcutaneous Tissue and Fascia, Right Upper Leg** Crural fascia Fascia lata Iliac fascia Iliotibial tract (band) **M Subcutaneous Tissue and Fascia, Left Upper Leg** *See L Subcutaneous Tissue and Fascia, Right Upper Leg* **N Subcutaneous Tissue and Fascia, Right Lower Leg** **P Subcutaneous Tissue and Fascia, Left Lower Leg**	**Ø Open** **3 Percutaneous**	**Z No Device**	**Z No Qualifier**

Ø   **Medical and Surgical**
J   **Subcutaneous Tissue and Fascia**
2   **Change**   Definition: Taking out or off a device from a body part and putting back an identical or similar device in or on the same body part without
                     cutting or puncturing the skin or a mucous membrane
                     Explanation: All CHANGE procedures are coded using the approach EXTERNAL

Body Part Character 4	Approach Character 5	Device Character 6	Qualifier Character 7
S Subcutaneous Tissue and Fascia, Head and Neck **T Subcutaneous Tissue and Fascia, Trunk** External oblique aponeurosis Transversalis fascia **V Subcutaneous Tissue and Fascia, Upper Extremity** **W Subcutaneous Tissue and Fascia, Lower Extremity**	**X External**	**Ø Drainage Device** **Y Other Device**	**Z No Qualifier**

Non-OR   All body part, approach, device, and qualifier values

LC Limited Coverage   **NC** Noncovered   ⊞ Combination Member   HAC associated procedure   Combination Only   DRG Non-OR   Non-OR   New/Revised in **GREEN**

ICD-10-PCS 2020   **433**

Ø   Medical and Surgical
J   Subcutaneous Tissue and Fascia
5   Destruction   Definition: Physical eradication of all or a portion of a body part by the direct use of energy, force, or a destructive agent
                         Explanation: None of the body part is physically taken out

Body Part Character 4		Approach Character 5	Device Character 6	Qualifier Character 7
Ø **Subcutaneous Tissue and Fascia, Scalp** Galea aponeurotica **1** **Subcutaneous Tissue and Fascia, Face** Masseteric fascia Orbital fascia Submandibular space **4** **Subcutaneous Tissue and Fascia, Right Neck** Deep cervical fascia Pretracheal fascia Prevertebral fascia **5** **Subcutaneous Tissue and Fascia, Left Neck** *See 4 Subcutaneous Tissue and Fascia, Right Neck* **6** **Subcutaneous Tissue and Fascia, Chest** Pectoral fascia **7** **Subcutaneous Tissue and Fascia, Back** **8** **Subcutaneous Tissue and Fascia, Abdomen** **9** **Subcutaneous Tissue and Fascia, Buttock** **B** **Subcutaneous Tissue and Fascia, Perineum** **C** **Subcutaneous Tissue and Fascia, Pelvic Region** **D** **Subcutaneous Tissue and Fascia, Right Upper Arm** Axillary fascia Deltoid fascia Infraspinatus fascia Subscapular aponeurosis Supraspinatus fascia **F** **Subcutaneous Tissue and Fascia, Left Upper Arm** *See D Subcutaneous Tissue and Fascia, Right Upper Arm*	**G** **Subcutaneous Tissue and Fascia, Right Lower Arm** Antebrachial fascia Bicipital aponeurosis **H** **Subcutaneous Tissue and Fascia, Left Lower Arm** *See G Subcutaneous Tissue and Fascia, Right Lower Arm* **J** **Subcutaneous Tissue and Fascia, Right Hand** Palmar fascia (aponeurosis) **K** **Subcutaneous Tissue and Fascia, Left Hand** *See J Subcutaneous Tissue and Fascia, Right Hand* **L** **Subcutaneous Tissue and Fascia, Right Upper Leg** Crural fascia Fascia lata Iliac fascia Iliotibial tract (band) **M** **Subcutaneous Tissue and Fascia, Left Upper Leg** *See L Subcutaneous Tissue and Fascia, Right Upper Leg* **N** **Subcutaneous Tissue and Fascia, Right Lower Leg** **P** **Subcutaneous Tissue and Fascia, Left Lower Leg** **Q** **Subcutaneous Tissue and Fascia, Right Foot** Plantar fascia (aponeurosis) **R** **Subcutaneous Tissue and Fascia, Left Foot** *See Q Subcutaneous Tissue and Fascia, Right Foot*	**Ø** Open **3** Percutaneous	**Z** No Device	**Z** No Qualifier

DRG Non-OR   All body part, approach, device, and qualifier values

LC Limited Coverage   **NC** Noncovered   ⊞ Combination Member   HAC associated procedure   Combination Only   DRG Non-OR   Non-OR   New/Revised in GREEN

434   ICD-10-PCS 2020

Ø   **Medical and Surgical**
J   **Subcutaneous Tissue and Fascia**
8   **Division**   Definition: Cutting into a body part, without draining fluids and/or gases from the body part, in order to separate or transect a body part
                Explanation: All or a portion of the body part is separated into two or more portions

Body Part Character 4		Approach Character 5	Device Character 6	Qualifier Character 7

Ø **Subcutaneous Tissue and Fascia, Scalp**
   Galea aponeurotica
1 **Subcutaneous Tissue and Fascia, Face**
   Masseteric fascia
   Orbital fascia
   Submandibular space
4 **Subcutaneous Tissue and Fascia, Right Neck**
   Deep cervical fascia
   Pretracheal fascia
   Prevertebral fascia
5 **Subcutaneous Tissue and Fascia, Left Neck**
   See 4 Subcutaneous Tissue and Fascia, Right Neck
6 **Subcutaneous Tissue and Fascia, Chest**
   Pectoral fascia
7 **Subcutaneous Tissue and Fascia, Back**
8 **Subcutaneous Tissue and Fascia, Abdomen**
9 **Subcutaneous Tissue and Fascia, Buttock**
B **Subcutaneous Tissue and Fascia, Perineum**
C **Subcutaneous Tissue and Fascia, Pelvic Region**
D **Subcutaneous Tissue and Fascia, Right Upper Arm**
   Axillary fascia
   Deltoid fascia
   Infraspinatus fascia
   Subscapular aponeurosis
   Supraspinatus fascia
F **Subcutaneous Tissue and Fascia, Left Upper Arm**
   See D Subcutaneous Tissue and Fascia, Right Upper Arm
G **Subcutaneous Tissue and Fascia, Right Lower Arm**
   Antebrachial fascia
   Bicipital aponeurosis
	H **Subcutaneous Tissue and Fascia, Left Lower Arm**
	   See G Subcutaneous Tissue and Fascia, Right Lower Arm
	J **Subcutaneous Tissue and Fascia, Right Hand**
	   Palmar fascia (aponeurosis)
	K **Subcutaneous Tissue and Fascia, Left Hand**
	   See J Subcutaneous Tissue and Fascia, Right Hand
	L **Subcutaneous Tissue and Fascia, Right Upper Leg**
	   Crural fascia
	   Fascia lata
	   Iliac fascia
	   Iliotibial tract (band)
	M **Subcutaneous Tissue and Fascia, Left Upper Leg**
	   See L Subcutaneous Tissue and Fascia, Right Upper Leg
	N **Subcutaneous Tissue and Fascia, Right Lower Leg**
	P **Subcutaneous Tissue and Fascia, Left Lower Leg**
	Q **Subcutaneous Tissue and Fascia, Right Foot**
	   Plantar fascia (aponeurosis)
	R **Subcutaneous Tissue and Fascia, Left Foot**
	   See Q Subcutaneous Tissue and Fascia, Right Foot
	S **Subcutaneous Tissue and Fascia, Head and Neck**
	T **Subcutaneous Tissue and Fascia, Trunk**
	   External oblique aponeurosis
	   Transversalis fascia
	V **Subcutaneous Tissue and Fascia, Upper Extremity**
	W **Subcutaneous Tissue and Fascia, Lower Extremity**
		Ø Open
		3 Percutaneous
			Z No Device	**Z** No Qualifier

Ø   Medical and Surgical
J   Subcutaneous Tissue and Fascia
9   Drainage   Definition: Taking or letting out fluids and/or gases from a body part
                          Explanation: The qualifier DIAGNOSTIC is used to identify drainage procedures that are biopsies

Body Part Character 4		Approach Character 5	Device Character 6	Qualifier Character 7
Ø Subcutaneous Tissue and Fascia, Scalp Galea aponeurotica	**G** Subcutaneous Tissue and Fascia, Right Lower Arm Antebrachial fascia Bicipital aponeurosis	**Ø** Open **3** Percutaneous	**Ø** Drainage Device	**Z** No Qualifier
1 Subcutaneous Tissue and Fascia, Face Masseteric fascia Orbital fascia Submandibular space	**H** Subcutaneous Tissue and Fascia, Left Lower Arm *See G Subcutaneous Tissue and Fascia, Right Lower Arm*			
4 Subcutaneous Tissue and Fascia, Right Neck Deep cervical fascia Pretracheal fascia Prevertebral fascia	**J** Subcutaneous Tissue and Fascia, Right Hand Palmar fascia (aponeurosis)			
5 Subcutaneous Tissue and Fascia, Left Neck *See 4 Subcutaneous Tissue and Fascia, Right Neck*	**K** Subcutaneous Tissue and Fascia, Left Hand *See J Subcutaneous Tissue and Fascia, Right Hand*			
6 Subcutaneous Tissue and Fascia, Chest Pectoral fascia	**L** Subcutaneous Tissue and Fascia, Right Upper Leg Crural fascia Fascia lata Iliac fascia Iliotibial tract (band)			
7 Subcutaneous Tissue and Fascia, Back	**M** Subcutaneous Tissue and Fascia, Left Upper Leg *See L Subcutaneous Tissue and Fascia, Right Upper Leg*			
8 Subcutaneous Tissue and Fascia, Abdomen	**N** Subcutaneous Tissue and Fascia, Right Lower Leg			
9 Subcutaneous Tissue and Fascia, Buttock	**P** Subcutaneous Tissue and Fascia, Left Lower Leg			
B Subcutaneous Tissue and Fascia, Perineum	**Q** Subcutaneous Tissue and Fascia, Right Foot Plantar fascia (aponeurosis)			
C Subcutaneous Tissue and Fascia, Pelvic Region	**R** Subcutaneous Tissue and Fascia, Left Foot *See Q Subcutaneous Tissue and Fascia, Right Foot*			
D Subcutaneous Tissue and Fascia, Right Upper Arm Axillary fascia Deltoid fascia Infraspinatus fascia Subscapular aponeurosis Supraspinatus fascia				
F Subcutaneous Tissue and Fascia, Left Upper Arm *See D Subcutaneous Tissue and Fascia, Right Upper Arm*				

ØJ9 Continued on next page

Non-OR   ØJ9[Ø,1,4,5,6,7,8,9,B,C,D,F,G,H,J,K,L,M,N,P,Q,R][Ø,3]ØZ

Subcutaneous Tissue and Fascia

ØJ9 Continued

Ø   Medical and Surgical
J   Subcutaneous Tissue and Fascia
9   Drainage   Definition: Taking or letting out fluids and/or gases from a body part
                     Explanation: The qualifier DIAGNOSTIC is used to identify drainage procedures that are biopsies

Body Part Character 4		Approach Character 5	Device Character 6	Qualifier Character 7
Ø **Subcutaneous Tissue and Fascia, Scalp** Galea aponeurotica **1** **Subcutaneous Tissue and Fascia, Face** Masseteric fascia Orbital fascia Submandibular space **4** **Subcutaneous Tissue and Fascia, Right Neck** Deep cervical fascia Pretracheal fascia Prevertebral fascia **5** **Subcutaneous Tissue and Fascia, Left Neck** *See 4 Subcutaneous Tissue and Fascia, Right Neck* **6** **Subcutaneous Tissue and Fascia, Chest** Pectoral fascia **7** **Subcutaneous Tissue and Fascia, Back** **8** **Subcutaneous Tissue and Fascia, Abdomen** **9** **Subcutaneous Tissue and Fascia, Buttock** **B** **Subcutaneous Tissue and Fascia, Perineum** **C** **Subcutaneous Tissue and Fascia, Pelvic Region** **D** **Subcutaneous Tissue and Fascia, Right Upper Arm** Axillary fascia Deltoid fascia Infraspinatus fascia Subscapular aponeurosis Supraspinatus fascia **F** **Subcutaneous Tissue and Fascia, Left Upper Arm** *See D Subcutaneous Tissue and Fascia, Right Upper Arm*	**G** **Subcutaneous Tissue and Fascia, Right Lower Arm** Antebrachial fascia Bicipital aponeurosis **H** **Subcutaneous Tissue and Fascia, Left Lower Arm** *See G Subcutaneous Tissue and Fascia, Right Lower Arm* **J** **Subcutaneous Tissue and Fascia, Right Hand** Palmar fascia (aponeurosis) **K** **Subcutaenous Tissue and Fascia, Left Hand** *See J Subcutaneous Tissue and Fascia, Right Hand* **L** **Subcutaneous Tissue and Fascia, Right Upper Leg** Crural fascia Fascia lata Iliac fascia Iliotibial tract (band) **M** **Subcutaneous Tissue and Fascia, Left Upper Leg** *See L Subcutaneous Tissue and Fascia, Right Upper Leg* **N** **Subcutaneous Tissue and Fascia, Right Lower Leg** **P** **Subcutaneous Tissue and Fascia, Left Lower Leg** **Q** **Subcutaneous Tissue and Fascia, Right Foot** Plantar fascia (aponeurosis) **R** **Subcutaneous Tissue and Fascia, Left Foot** *See Q Subcutaneous Tissue and Fascia, Right Foot*	**Ø** Open **3** Percutaneous	**Z** No Device	**X** Diagnostic **Z** No Qualifier

Non-OR   ØJ9[Ø,1,4,5,6,7,8,9,B,C,D,F,G,H,J,K,L,M,N,P,Q,R][Ø,3]ZX
Non-OR   ØJ9[Ø,1,4,5,6,7,8,9,B,C,D,F,G,H,J,K,L,M,N,P,Q,R]3ZZ

Subcutaneous Tissue and Fascia

Ø   **Medical and Surgical**
J   **Subcutaneous Tissue and Fascia**
B   **Excision**   Definition: Cutting out or off, without replacement, a portion of a body part
                       Explanation: The qualifier DIAGNOSTIC is used to identify excision procedures that are biopsies

Body Part Character 4		Approach Character 5	Device Character 6	Qualifier Character 7
Ø Subcutaneous Tissue and Fascia, Scalp Galea aponeurotica	**G Subcutaneous Tissue and Fascia, Right Lower Arm** Antebrachial fascia Bicipital aponeurosis	**Ø Open** **3 Percutaneous**	**Z No Device**	**X Diagnostic** **Z No Qualifier**
1 Subcutaneous Tissue and Fascia, Face Masseteric fascia Orbital fascia Submandibular space	**H Subcutaneous Tissue and Fascia, Left Lower Arm** *See G Subcutaneous Tissue and Fascia, Right Lower Arm*			
4 Subcutaneous Tissue and Fascia, Right Neck Deep cervical fascia Pretracheal fascia Prevertebral fascia	**J Subcutaneous Tissue and Fascia, Right Hand** Palmar fascia (aponeurosis)			
5 Subcutaneous Tissue and Fascia, Left Neck *See 4 Subcutaneous Tissue and Fascia, Right Neck*	**K Subcutaneous Tissue and Fascia, Left Hand** *See J Subcutaneous Tissue and Fascia, Right Hand*			
6 Subcutaneous Tissue and Fascia, Chest Pectoral fascia	**L Subcutaneous Tissue and Fascia, Right Upper Leg** Crural fascia Fascia lata Iliac fascia Iliotibial tract (band)			
7 Subcutaneous Tissue and Fascia, Back	**M Subcutaneous Tissue and Fascia, Left Upper Leg** *See L Subcutaneous Tissue and Fascia, Right Upper Leg*			
8 Subcutaneous Tissue and Fascia, Abdomen	**N Subcutaneous Tissue and Fascia, Right Lower Leg**			
9 Subcutaneous Tissue and Fascia, Buttock	**P Subcutaneous Tissue and Fascia, Left Lower Leg**			
B Subcutaneous Tissue and Fascia, Perineum	**Q Subcutaneous Tissue and Fascia, Right Foot** Plantar fascia (aponeurosis)			
C Subcutaneous Tissue and Fascia, Pelvic Region	**R Subcutaneous Tissue and Fascia, Left Foot** *See Q Subcutaneous Tissue and Fascia, Right Foot*			
D Subcutaneous Tissue and Fascia, Right Upper Arm Axillary fascia Deltoid fascia Infraspinatus fascia Subscapular aponeurosis Supraspinatus fascia				
F Subcutaneous Tissue and Fascia, Left Upper Arm *See D Subcutaneous Tissue and Fascia, Right Upper Arm*				

DRG Non-OR	ØJB[Ø,4,5,6,7,8,9,B,C,D,F,G,H,L,M,N,P,Q,R]3ZZ
Non-OR	ØJB[Ø,1,4,5,6,7,8,9,B,C,D,F,G,H,J,K,L,M,N,P,Q,R][Ø,3]ZX

Subcutaneous Tissue and Fascia

Ø   **Medical and Surgical**
J   **Subcutaneous Tissue and Fascia**
C   **Extirpation**   Definition: Taking or cutting out solid matter from a body part

Explanation: The solid matter may be an abnormal byproduct of a biological function or a foreign body; it may be imbedded in a body part or in the lumen of a tubular body part. The solid matter may or may not have been previously broken into pieces.

Body Part Character 4		Approach Character 5	Device Character 6	Qualifier Character 7

Ø   **Subcutaneous Tissue and Fascia, Scalp**
    Galea aponeurotica
1   **Subcutaneous Tissue and Fascia, Face**
    Masseteric fascia
    Orbital fascia
    Submandibular space
4   **Subcutaneous Tissue and Fascia, Right Neck**
    Deep cervical fascia
    Pretracheal fascia
    Prevertebral fascia
5   **Subcutaneous Tissue and Fascia, Left Neck**
    See 4 *Subcutaneous Tissue and Fascia, Right Neck*
6   **Subcutaneous Tissue and Fascia, Chest**
    Pectoral fascia
7   **Subcutaneous Tissue and Fascia, Back**
8   **Subcutaneous Tissue and Fascia, Abdomen**
9   **Subcutaneous Tissue and Fascia, Buttock**
B   **Subcutaneous Tissue and Fascia, Perineum**
C   **Subcutaneous Tissue and Fascia, Pelvic Region**
D   **Subcutaneous Tissue and Fascia, Right Upper Arm**
    Axillary fascia
    Deltoid fascia
    Infraspinatus fascia
    Subscapular aponeurosis
    Supraspinatus fascia
F   **Subcutaneous Tissue and Fascia, Left Upper Arm**
    See D *Subcutaneous Tissue and Fascia, Right Upper Arm*
	G **Subcutaneous Tissue and Fascia, Right Lower Arm**
	    Antebrachial fascia
	    Bicipital aponeurosis
	H **Subcutaneous Tissue and Fascia, Left Lower Arm**
	    See G *Subcutaneous Tissue and Fascia, Right Lower Arm*
	J **Subcutaneous Tissue and Fascia, Right Hand**
	    Palmar fascia (aponeurosis)
	K **Subcutaneous Tissue and Fascia, Left Hand**
	    See J *Subcutaneous Tissue and Fascia, Right Hand*
	L **Subcutaneous Tissue and Fascia, Right Upper Leg**
	    Crural fascia
	    Fascia lata
	    Iliac fascia
	    Iliotibial tract (band)
	M **Subcutaneous Tissue and Fascia, Left Upper Leg**
	    See L *Subcutaneous Tissue and Fascia, Right Upper Leg*
	N **Subcutaneous Tissue and Fascia, Right Lower Leg**
	P **Subcutaneous Tissue and Fascia, Left Lower Leg**
	Q **Subcutaneous Tissue and Fascia, Right Foot**
	    Plantar fascia (aponeurosis)
	R **Subcutaneous Tissue and Fascia, Left Foot**
	    See Q *Subcutaneous Tissue and Fascia, Right Foot*
		Ø Open
		3 Percutaneous
			Z No Device	**Z** No Qualifier

Non-OR   All body part, approach, device, and qualifier values

Ø Medical and Surgical
J Subcutaneous Tissue and Fascia
D Extraction Definition: Pulling or stripping out or off all or a portion of a body part by the use of force

Explanation: The qualifier DIAGNOSTIC is used to identify extraction procedures that are biopsies

Body Part Character 4		Approach Character 5	Device Character 6	Qualifier Character 7
Ø Subcutaneous Tissue and Fascia, Scalp Galea aponeurotica	**G Subcutaneous Tissue and Fascia, Right Lower Arm** Antebrachial fascia Bicipital aponeurosis	**Ø Open** **3 Percutaneous**	**Z No Device**	**Z No Qualifier**
1 Subcutaneous Tissue and Fascia, Face Masseteric fascia Orbital fascia Submandibular space	**H Subcutaneous Tissue and Fascia, Left Lower Arm** *See G Subcutaneous Tissue and Fascia, Right Lower Arm*			
4 Subcutaneous Tissue and Fascia, Right Neck Deep cervical fascia Pretracheal fascia Prevertebral fascia	**J Subcutaneous Tissue and Fascia, Right Hand** Palmar fascia (aponeurosis)			
5 Subcutaneous Tissue and Fascia, Left Neck *See 4 Subcutaneous Tissue and Fascia, Right Neck*	**K Subcutaneous Tissue and Fascia, Left Hand** *See J Subcutaneous Tissue and Fascia, Right Hand*			
6 Subcutaneous Tissue and Fascia, Chest Pectoral fascia	**L Subcutaneous Tissue and Fascia, Right Upper Leg** Crural fascia Fascia lata Iliac fascia Iliotibial tract (band)			
7 Subcutaneous Tissue and Fascia, Back	**M Subcutaneous Tissue and Fascia, Left Upper Leg** *See L Subcutaneous Tissue and Fascia, Right Upper Leg*			
8 Subcutaneous Tissue and Fascia, Abdomen	**N Subcutaneous Tissue and Fascia, Right Lower Leg**			
9 Subcutaneous Tissue and Fascia, Buttock	**P Subcutaneous Tissue and Fascia, Left Lower Leg**			
B Subcutaneous Tissue and Fascia, Perineum	**Q Subcutaneous Tissue and Fascia, Right Foot** Plantar fascia (aponeurosis)			
C Subcutaneous Tissue and Fascia, Pelvic Region	**R Subcutaneous Tissue and Fascia, Left Foot** *See Q Subcutaneous Tissue and Fascia, Right Foot*			
D Subcutaneous Tissue and Fascia, Right Upper Arm Axillary fascia Deltoid fascia Infraspinatus fascia Subscapular aponeurosis Supraspinatus fascia				
F Subcutaneous Tissue and Fascia, Left Upper Arm *See D Subcutaneous Tissue and Fascia, Right Upper Arm*				

Non-OR ØJD[Ø,1,4,5,B,C,D,F,G,H,J,K,N,P,Q,R]3ZZ

See Appendix L for Procedure Combinations
Combo-only ØJD[6,7,8,9,L,M]3ZZ

Subcutaneous Tissue and Fascia

Ø   **Medical and Surgical**
J   **Subcutaneous Tissue and Fascia**
H   **Insertion**   Definition: Putting in a nonbiological appliance that monitors, assists, performs, or prevents a physiological function but does not physically take the place of a body part
                 Explanation: None

Body Part Character 4		Approach Character 5	Device Character 6	Qualifier Character 7
Ø Subcutaneous Tissue and Fascia, Scalp Galea aponeurotica **1** Subcutaneous Tissue and Fascia, Face Masseteric fascia Orbital fascia Submandibular space **4** Subcutaneous Tissue and Fascia, Right Neck Deep cervical fascia Pretracheal fascia Prevertebral fascia **5** Subcutaneous Tissue and Fascia, Left Neck *See 4 Subcutaneous Tissue and Fascia, Right Neck* **9** Subcutaneous Tissue and Fascia, Buttock **B** Subcutaneous Tissue and Fascia, Perineum	**C** Subcutaneous Tissue and Fascia, Pelvic Region **J** Subcutaneous Tissue and Fascia, Right Hand Palmar fascia (aponeurosis) **K** Subcutaneous Tissue and Fascia, Left Hand *See J Subcutaneous Tissue and Fascia, Right Hand* **Q** Subcutaneous Tissue and Fascia, Right Foot Plantar fascia (aponeurosis) **R** Subcutaneous Tissue and Fascia, Left Foot *See Q Subcutaneous Tissue and Fascia, Right Foot*	**Ø** Open **3** Percutaneous	**N** Tissue Expander	**Z** No Qualifier
6 Subcutaneous Tissue and Fascia, Chest ⊞ Pectoral fascia		**Ø** Open **3** Percutaneous	**Ø** Monitoring Device, Hemodynamic **2** Monitoring Device **4** Pacemaker, Single Chamber **5** Pacemaker, Single Chamber Rate Responsive **6** Pacemaker, Dual Chamber **7** Cardiac Resynchronization Pacemaker Pulse Generator **8** Defibrillator Generator **9** Cardiac Resynchronization Defibrillator Pulse Generator **A** Contractility Modulation Device **B** Stimulator Generator, Single Array **C** Stimulator Generator, Single Array Rechargeable **D** Stimulator Generator, Multiple Array **E** Stimulator Generator, Multiple Array Rechargeable **F** Subcutaneous Defibrillator Lead **H** Contraceptive Device **M** Stimulator Generator **N** Tissue Expander **P** Cardiac Rhythm Related Device **V** Infusion Device, Pump **W** Vascular Access Device, Totally Implantable **X** Vascular Access Device, Tunneled	**Z** No Qualifier
7 Subcutaneous Tissue and Fascia, Back NC ⊞		**Ø** Open **3** Percutaneous	**B** Stimulator Generator, Single Array **C** Stimulator Generator, Single Array Rechargeable **D** Stimulator Generator, Multiple Array **E** Stimulator Generator, Multiple Array Rechargeable **M** Stimulator Generator **N** Tissue Expander **V** Infusion Device, Pump	**Z** No Qualifier

ØJH Continued on next page

DRG Non-OR   ØJH6[Ø,3][4,5,6,7,H,P,X]Z
DRG Non-OR   ØJH63WX

HAC   ØJH6[Ø,3][4,5,6,7,8,9,P]Z when reported with SDx K68.11 or T81.4Ø-T81.49, T82.6-T82.7 with 7th character A
HAC   ØJH63XZ when reported with SDx J95.811
NC   ØJH7[Ø,3]MZ

See Appendix L for Procedure Combinations
⊞   ØJH6[Ø,3][4,5,6,7,8,9,A,B,C,D,E,P]Z
⊞   ØJH7[Ø,3][B,C,D,E]Z

LC Limited Coverage   NC Noncovered   ⊞ Combination Member   HAC associated procedure   ▬ Combination Only   DRG Non-OR   Non-OR   New/Revised in GREEN

Ø **Medical and Surgical**

ØJH Continued

J **Subcutaneous Tissue and Fascia**

H **Insertion**   Definition: Putting in a nonbiological appliance that monitors, assists, performs, or prevents a physiological function but does not physically take the place of a body part

                  Explanation: None

Body Part Character 4		Approach Character 5	Device Character 6	Qualifier Character 7
8 Subcutaneous Tissue and Fascia, Abdomen NC ⊞		**Ø** Open **3** Percutaneous	**Ø** Monitoring Device, Hemodynamic **2** Monitoring Device **4** Pacemaker, Single Chamber **5** Pacemaker, Single Chamber Rate Responsive **6** Pacemaker, Dual Chamber **7** Cardiac Resynchronization Pacemaker Pulse Generator **8** Defibrillator Generator **9** Cardiac Resynchronization Defibrillator Pulse Generator **A** Contractility Modulation Device **B** Stimulator Generator, Single Array **C** Stimulator Generator, Single Array Rechargeable **D** Stimulator Generator, Multiple Array **E** Stimulator Generator, Multiple Array Rechargeable **H** Contraceptive Device **M** Stimulator Generator **N** Tissue Expander **P** Cardiac Rhythm Related Device **V** Infusion Device, Pump **W** Vascular Access Device, Totally Implantable **X** Vascular Access Device, Tunneled	**Z** No Qualifier
D Subcutaneous Tissue and Fascia, Right Upper Arm Axillary fascia Deltoid fascia Infraspinatus fascia Subscapular aponeurosis Supraspinatus fascia **F** Subcutaneous Tissue and Fascia, Left Upper Arm *See D Subcutaneous Tissue and Fascia, Right Upper Arm* **G** Subcutaneous Tissue and Fascia, Right Lower Arm Antebrachial fascia Bicipital aponeurosis **H** Subcutaneous Tissue and Fascia, Left Lower Arm *See G Subcutaneous Tissue and Fascia, Right Lower Arm*	**L** Subcutaneous Tissue and Fascia, Right Upper Leg Crural fascia Fascia lata Iliac fascia Iliotibial tract (band) **M** Subcutaneous Tissue and Fascia, Left Upper Leg *See L Subcutaneous Tissue and Fascia, Right Upper Leg* **N** Subcutaneous Tissue and Fascia, Right Lower Leg **P** Subcutaneous Tissue and Fascia, Left Lower Leg	**Ø** Open **3** Percutaneous	**H** Contraceptive Device **N** Tissue Expander **V** Infusion Device, Pump **W** Vascular Access Device, Totally Implantable **X** Vascular Access Device, Tunneled	**Z** No Qualifier
S Subcutaneous Tissue and Fascia, Head and Neck **V** Subcutaneous Tissue and Fascia, Upper Extremity **W** Subcutaneous Tissue and Fascia, Lower Extremity		**Ø** Open **3** Percutaneous	**1** Radioactive Element **3** Infusion Device **Y** Other Device	**Z** No Qualifier
T Subcutaneous Tissue and Fascia, Trunk External oblique aponeurosis Transversalis fascia		**Ø** Open **3** Percutaneous	**1** Radioactive Element **3** Infusion Device **V** Infusion Device, Pump **Y** Other Device	**Z** No Qualifier

DRG Non-OR ØJH8[Ø,3][4,5,6,7,H,P,X]Z
DRG Non-OR ØJH83WX
DRG Non-OR ØJH8[Ø,3]2Z
DRG Non-OR ØJH[D,F,G,H,L,M,N,P]ØXZ
DRG Non-OR ØJH[D,F,G,H,L,M,N,P]3[W,X]Z
DRG Non-OR ØJHN3HZ
DRG Non-OR ØJHP[Ø,3]HZ

Non-OR ØJH[D,F,G,H,L,M][Ø,3]HZ
Non-OR ØJHNØHZ
Non-OR ØJH[S,V,W]Ø3Z
Non-OR ØJH[S,V,W]3[3,Y]Z
Non-OR ØJHTØ3Z
Non-OR ØJHT3[3,Y]Z

HAC ØJH8[Ø,3][4,5,6,7,8,9,P]Z when reported with SDx K68.11 or T81.4Ø-T81.49, T82.6-T82.7 with 7th character A
NC ØJH8[Ø,3]MZ

See Appendix L for Procedure Combinations
⊞ ØJH8[Ø,3][4,5,6,7,8,9,A,B,C,D,E,P]Z

LC Limited Coverage   NC Noncovered   ⊞ Combination Member   HAC associated procedure   Combination Only   DRG Non-OR   Non-OR   New/Revised in GREEN

Ø   **Medical and Surgical**
J   **Subcutaneous Tissue and Fascia**
J   **Inspection**   Definition: Visually and/or manually exploring a body part

            Explanation: Visual exploration may be performed with or without optical instrumentation. Manual exploration may be performed directly or through intervening body layers.

Body Part Character 4	Approach Character 5	Device Character 6	Qualifier Character 7

S Subcutaneous Tissue and Fascia, Head and Neck
T Subcutaneous Tissue and Fascia, Trunk
   External oblique aponeurosis
   Transversalis fascia
V Subcutaneous Tissue and Fascia, Upper Extremity
W Subcutaneous Tissue and Fascia, Lower Extremity
	Ø Open
	3 Percutaneous
	X External
		Z No Device	**Z** No Qualifier

Non-OR   All body part, approach, device, and qualifier values

Ø   **Medical and Surgical**
J   **Subcutaneous Tissue and Fascia**
N   **Release**   Definition: Freeing a body part from an abnormal physical constraint by cutting or by the use of force

            Explanation: Some of the restraining tissue may be taken out but none of the body part is taken out

Body Part Character 4		Approach Character 5	Device Character 6	Qualifier Character 7

Ø Subcutaneous Tissue and Fascia, Scalp
   Galea aponeurotica
1 Subcutaneous Tissue and Fascia, Face
   Masseteric fascia
   Orbital fascia
   Submandibular space
4 Subcutaneous Tissue and Fascia, Right Neck
   Deep cervical fascia
   Pretracheal fascia
   Prevertebral fascia
5 Subcutaneous Tissue and Fascia, Left Neck
   See 4 Subcutaneous Tissue and Fascia, Right Neck
6 Subcutaneous Tissue and Fascia, Chest
   Pectoral fascia
7 Subcutaneous Tissue and Fascia, Back
8 Subcutaneous Tissue and Fascia, Abdomen
9 Subcutaneous Tissue and Fascia, Buttock
B Subcutaneous Tissue and Fascia, Perineum
C Subcutaneous Tissue and Fascia, Pelvic Region
D Subcutaneous Tissue and Fascia, Right Upper Arm
   Axillary fascia
   Deltoid fascia
   Infraspinatus fascia
   Subscapular aponeurosis
   Supraspinatus fascia
F Subcutaneous Tissue and Fascia, Left Upper Arm
   See D Subcutaneous Tissue and Fascia, Right Upper Arm
	G Subcutaneous Tissue and Fascia, Right Lower Arm
	   Antebrachial fascia
	   Bicipital aponeurosis
	H Subcutaneous Tissue and Fascia, Left Lower Arm
	   See G Subcutaneous Tissue and Fascia, Right Lower Arm
	J Subcutaneous Tissue and Fascia, Right Hand
	   Palmar fascia (aponeurosis)
	K Subcutaneous Tissue and Fascia, Left Hand
	   See J Subcutaneous Tissue and Fascia, Right Hand
	L Subcutaneous Tissue and Fascia, Right Upper Leg
	   Crural fascia
	   Fascia lata
	   Iliac fascia
	   Iliotibial tract (band)
	M Subcutaneous Tissue and Fascia, Left Upper Leg
	   See L Subcutaneous Tissue and Fascia, Right Upper Leg
	N Subcutaneous Tissue and Fascia, Right Lower Leg
	P Subcutaneous Tissue and Fascia, Left Lower Leg
	Q Subcutaneous Tissue and Fascia, Right Foot
	   Plantar fascia (aponeurosis)
	R Subcutaneous Tissue and Fascia, Left Foot
	   See Q Subcutaneous Tissue and Fascia, Right Foot
		Ø Open
		3 Percutaneous
		X External
			Z No Device	**Z** No Qualifier

Non-OR   ØJN[Ø,1,4,5,6,7,8,9,B,C,D,F,G,H,J,K,L,M,N,P,Q,R]XZZ

Subcutaneous Tissue and Fascia

Ø　Medical and Surgical
J　Subcutaneous Tissue and Fascia
P　Removal　　　Definition: Taking out or off a device from a body part

Explanation: If a device is taken out and a similar device put in without cutting or puncturing the skin or mucous membrane, the procedure is coded to the root operation CHANGE. Otherwise, the procedure for taking out a device is coded to the root operation REMOVAL.

Body Part Character 4	Approach Character 5	Device Character 6	Qualifier Character 7
S Subcutaneous Tissue and Fascia, Head and Neck	**Ø** Open **3** Percutaneous	**Ø** Drainage Device **1** Radioactive Element **3** Infusion Device **7** Autologous Tissue Substitute **J** Synthetic Substitute **K** Nonautologous Tissue Substitute **N** Tissue Expander **Y** Other Device	**Z** No Qualifier
S Subcutaneous Tissue and Fascia, Head and Neck	**X** External	**Ø** Drainage Device **1** Radioactive Element **3** Infusion Device	**Z** No Qualifier
T Subcutaneous Tissue and Fascia, Trunk External oblique aponeurosis Transversalis fascia	**Ø** Open **3** Percutaneous	**Ø** Drainage Device **1** Radioactive Element **2** Monitoring Device **3** Infusion Device **7** Autologous Tissue Substitute **F** Subcutaneous Defibrillator Lead **H** Contraceptive Device **J** Synthetic Substitute **K** Nonautologous Tissue Substitute **M** Stimulator Generator **N** Tissue Expander **P** Cardiac Rhythm Related Device **V** Infusion Device, Pump **W** Vascular Access Device, Totally 　Implantable **X** Vascular Access Device, Tunneled **Y** Other Device	**Z** No Qualifier
T Subcutaneous Tissue and Fascia, Trunk External oblique aponeurosis Transversalis fascia	**X** External	**Ø** Drainage Device **1** Radioactive Element **2** Monitoring Device **3** Infusion Device **H** Contraceptive Device **V** Infusion Device, Pump **X** Vascular Access Device, Tunneled	**Z** No Qualifier
V Subcutaneous Tissue and Fascia, Upper Extremity **W** Subcutaneous Tissue and Fascia, Lower Extremity	**Ø** Open **3** Percutaneous	**Ø** Drainage Device **1** Radioactive Element **3** Infusion Device **7** Autologous Tissue Substitute **H** Contraceptive Device **J** Synthetic Substitute **K** Nonautologous Tissue Substitute **N** Tissue Expander **V** Infusion Device, Pump **W** Vascular Access Device, Totally 　Implantable **X** Vascular Access Device, Tunneled **Y** Other Device	**Z** No Qualifier
V Subcutaneous Tissue and Fascia, Upper Extremity **W** Subcutaneous Tissue and Fascia, Lower Extremity	**X** External	**Ø** Drainage Device **1** Radioactive Element **3** Infusion Device **H** Contraceptive Device **V** Infusion Device, Pump **X** Vascular Access Device, Tunneled	**Z** No Qualifier

Non-OR	ØJPS[Ø,3][Ø,1,3,7,J,K,N,Y]Z
Non-OR	ØJPSX[Ø,1,3]Z
Non-OR	ØJPT[Ø,3][Ø,1,2,3,7,H,J,K,M,N,V,W,X,Y]Z
Non-OR	ØJPTX[Ø,1,2,3,H,V,X]Z
Non-OR	ØJP[V,W][Ø,3][Ø,1,3,7,H,J,K,N,V,W,X,Y]Z
Non-OR	ØJP[V,W]X[Ø,1,3,H,V,X]Z
HAC	ØJPT[Ø,3]PZ when reported with SDx K68.11 or T81.4Ø-T81.49, T82.6-T82.7 with 7th character A

Ø Medical and Surgical
J Subcutaneous Tissue and Fascia
Q Repair   Definition: Restoring, to the extent possible, a body part to its normal anatomic structure and function
                    Explanation: Used only when the method to accomplish the repair is not one of the other root operations

Body Part Character 4		Approach Character 5	Device Character 6	Qualifier Character 7
Ø Subcutaneous Tissue and Fascia, Scalp Galea aponeurotica **1 Subcutaneous Tissue and Fascia, Face** Masseteric fascia Orbital fascia Submandibular space **4 Subcutaneous Tissue and Fascia, Right Neck** Deep cervical fascia Pretracheal fascia Prevertebral fascia **5 Subcutaneous Tissue and Fascia, Left Neck** *See 4 Subcutaneous Tissue and Fascia, Right Neck* **6 Subcutaneous Tissue and Fascia, Chest** Pectoral fascia **7 Subcutaneous Tissue and Fascia, Back** **8 Subcutaneous Tissue and Fascia, Abdomen** **9 Subcutaneous Tissue and Fascia, Buttock** **B Subcutaneous Tissue and Fascia, Perineum** **C Subcutaneous Tissue and Fascia, Pelvic Region** **D Subcutaneous Tissue and Fascia, Right Upper Arm** Axillary fascia Deltoid fascia Infraspinatus fascia Subscapular aponeurosis Supraspinatus fascia **F Subcutaneous Tissue and Fascia, Left Upper Arm** *See D Subcutaneous Tissue and Fascia, Right Upper Arm*	**G Subcutaneous Tissue and Fascia, Right Lower Arm** Antebrachial fascia Bicipital aponeurosis **H Subcutaneous Tissue and Fascia, Left Lower Arm** *See G Subcutaneous Tissue and Fascia, Right Lower Arm* **J Subcutaneous Tissue and Fascia, Right Hand** Palmar fascia (aponeurosis) **K Subcutaneous Tissue and Fascia, Left Hand** *See J Subcutaneous Tissue and Fascia, Right Hand* **L Subcutaneous Tissue and Fascia, Right Upper Leg** Crural fascia Fascia lata Iliac fascia Iliotibial tract (band) **M Subcutaneous Tissue and Fascia, Left Upper Leg** *See L Subcutaneous Tissue and Fascia, Right Upper Leg* **N Subcutaneous Tissue and Fascia, Right Lower Leg** **P Subcutaneous Tissue and Fascia, Left Lower Leg** **Q Subcutaneous Tissue and Fascia, Right Foot** Plantar fascia (aponeurosis) **R Subcutaneous Tissue and Fascia, Left Foot** *See Q Subcutaneous Tissue and Fascia, Right Foot*	**Ø** Open **3** Percutaneous	**Z** No Device	**Z** No Qualifier

Non-OR ØJQ[Ø,1,4,5,6,7,8,9,B,C,D,F,G,H,J,K,L,M,N,P,Q,R]3ZZ

Subcutaneous Tissue and Fascia *(left margin)*

Ø   **Medical and Surgical**
J   **Subcutaneous Tissue and Fascia**
R   **Replacement**   Definition: Putting in or on biological or synthetic material that physically takes the place and/or function of all or a portion of a body part
          Explanation: The body part may have been taken out or replaced, or may be taken out, physically eradicated, or rendered nonfunctional during
          the REPLACEMENT procedure. A REMOVAL procedure is coded for taking out the device used in a previous replacement procedure.

Body Part Character 4	Approach Character 5	Device Character 6	Qualifier Character 7

Ø   **Subcutaneous Tissue and Fascia, Scalp**
    Galea aponeurotica
1   **Subcutaneous Tissue and Fascia, Face**
    Masseteric fascia
    Orbital fascia
    Submandibular space
4   **Subcutaneous Tissue and Fascia, Right Neck**
    Deep cervical fascia
    Pretracheal fascia
    Prevertebral fascia
5   **Subcutaneous Tissue and Fascia, Left Neck**
    See 4 Subcutaneous Tissue and Fascia, Right Neck
6   **Subcutaneous Tissue and Fascia, Chest**
    Pectoral fascia
7   **Subcutaneous Tissue and Fascia, Back**
8   **Subcutaneous Tissue and Fascia, Abdomen**
9   **Subcutaneous Tissue and Fascia, Buttock**
B   **Subcutaneous Tissue and Fascia, Perineum**
C   **Subcutaneous Tissue and Fascia, Pelvic Region**
D   **Subcutaneous Tissue and Fascia, Right Upper Arm**
    Axillary fascia
    Deltoid fascia
    Infraspinatus fascia
    Subscapular aponeurosis
    Supraspinatus fascia
F   **Subcutaneous Tissue and Fascia, Left Upper Arm**
    See D Subcutaneous Tissue and Fascia, Right Upper Arm
 	
G   **Subcutaneous Tissue and Fascia, Right Lower Arm**
    Antebrachial fascia
    Bicipital aponeurosis
H   **Subcutaneous Tissue and Fascia, Left Lower Arm**
    See G Subcutaneous Tissue and Fascia, Right Lower Arm
J   **Subcutaneous Tissue and Fascia, Right Hand**
    Palmar fascia (aponeurosis)
K   **Subcutaneous Tissue and Fascia, Left Hand**
    See J Subcutaneous Tissue and Fascia, Right Hand
L   **Subcutaneous Tissue and Fascia, Right Upper Leg**
    Crural fascia
    Fascia lata
    Iliac fascia
    Iliotibial tract (band)
M   **Subcutaneous Tissue and Fascia, Left Upper Leg**
    See L Subcutaneous Tissue and Fascia, Right Upper Leg
N   **Subcutaneous Tissue and Fascia, Right Lower Leg**
P   **Subcutaneous Tissue and Fascia, Left Lower Leg**
Q   **Subcutaneous Tissue and Fascia, Right Foot**
    Plantar fascia (aponeurosis)
R   **Subcutaneous Tissue and Fascia, Left Foot**
    See Q Subcutaneous Tissue and Fascia, Right Foot
	Ø Open
	3 Percutaneous
		7 Autologous Tissue Substitute
		J Synthetic Substitute
		K Nonautologous Tissue Substitute
			Z No Qualifier

[LC] Limited Coverage   [NC] Noncovered   ⊞ Combination Member   HAC associated procedure   Combination Only   DRG Non-OR   Non-OR   New/Revised in GREEN

446   ICD-10-PCS 2020

ØJR–ØJR *(left margin)*

Ø   Medical and Surgical
J   Subcutaneous Tissue and Fascia
U   Supplement: Definition: Putting in or on biological or synthetic material that physically reinforces and/or augments the function of a portion of a body part
                Explanation: The biological material is non-living, or is living and from the same individual. The body part may have been previously replaced, and the SUPPLEMENT procedure is performed to physically reinforce and/or augment the function of the replaced body part.

Body Part Character 4		Approach Character 5	Device Character 6	Qualifier Character 7

Ø   **Subcutaneous Tissue and Fascia, Scalp**
    Galea aponeurotica
1   **Subcutaneous Tissue and Fascia, Face**
    Masseteric fascia
    Orbital fascia
    Submandibular space
4   **Subcutaneous Tissue and Fascia, Right Neck**
    Deep cervical fascia
    Pretracheal fascia
    Prevertebral fascia
5   **Subcutaneous Tissue and Fascia, Left Neck**
    See 4 Subcutaneous Tissue and Fascia, Right Neck
6   **Subcutaneous Tissue and Fascia, Chest**
    Pectoral fascia
7   **Subcutaneous Tissue and Fascia, Back**
8   **Subcutaneous Tissue and Fascia, Abdomen**
9   **Subcutaneous Tissue and Fascia, Buttock**
B   **Subcutaneous Tissue and Fascia, Perineum**
C   **Subcutaneous Tissue and Fascia, Pelvic Region**
D   **Subcutaneous Tissue and Fascia, Right Upper Arm**
    Axillary fascia
    Deltoid fascia
    Infraspinatus fascia
    Subscapular aponeurosis
    Supraspinatus fascia
F   **Subcutaneous Tissue and Fascia, Left Upper Arm**
    See D Subcutaneous Tissue and Fascia, Right Upper Arm
	G **Subcutaneous Tissue and Fascia, Right Lower Arm**
	    Antebrachial fascia
	    Bicipital aponeurosis
	H **Subcutaneous Tissue and Fascia, Left Lower Arm**
	    See G Subcutaneous Tissue and Fascia, Right Lower Arm
	J **Subcutaneous Tissue and Fascia, Right Hand**
	    Palmar fascia (aponeurosis)
	K **Subcutaneous Tissue and Fascia, Left Hand**
	    See J Subcutaneous Tissue and Fascia, Right Hand
	L **Subcutaneous Tissue and Fascia, Right Upper Leg**
	    Crural fascia
	    Fascia lata
	    Iliac fascia
	    Iliotibial tract (band)
	M **Subcutaneous Tissue and Fascia, Left Upper Leg**
	    See L Subcutaneous Tissue and Fascia, Right Upper Leg
	N **Subcutaneous Tissue and Fascia, Right Lower Leg**
	P **Subcutaneous Tissue and Fascia, Left Lower Leg**
	Q **Subcutaneous Tissue and Fascia, Right Foot**
	    Plantar fascia (aponeurosis)
	R **Subcutaneous Tissue and Fascia, Left Foot**
	    See Q Subcutaneous Tissue and Fascia, Right Foot
		Ø Open
		3 Percutaneous
			7 Autologous Tissue Substitute
			J Synthetic Substitute
			K Nonautologous Tissue Substitute
				Z No Qualifier

LG Limited Coverage   NC Noncovered   ⊞ Combination Member   HAC associated procedure   Combination Only   DRG Non-OR   Non-OR   New/Revised in GREEN

ICD-10-PCS 2020   447

Ø   Medical and Surgical
J   Subcutaneous Tissue and Fascia
W   Revision   Definition: Correcting, to the extent possible, a portion of a malfunctioning device or the position of a displaced device

Explanation: Revision can include correcting a malfunctioning or displaced device by taking out or putting in components of the device such as a screw or pin

Body Part Character 4	Approach Character 5	Device Character 6	Qualifier Character 7
S Subcutaneous Tissue and Fascia, Head and Neck	**Ø** Open **3** Percutaneous	**Ø** Drainage Device **3** Infusion Device **7** Autologous Tissue Substitute **J** Synthetic Substitute **K** Nonautologous Tissue Substitute **N** Tissue Expander **Y** Other Device	**Z** No Qualifier
S Subcutaneous Tissue and Fascia, Head and Neck	**X** External	**Ø** Drainage Device **3** Infusion Device **7** Autologous Tissue Substitute **J** Synthetic Substitute **K** Nonautologous Tissue Substitute **N** Tissue Expander	**Z** No Qualifier
T Subcutaneous Tissue and Fascia, Trunk External oblique aponeurosis Transversalis fascia	**Ø** Open **3** Percutaneous	**Ø** Drainage Device **2** Monitoring Device **3** Infusion Device **7** Autologous Tissue Substitute **F** Subcutaneous Defibrillator Lead **H** Contraceptive Device **J** Synthetic Substitute **K** Nonautologous Tissue Substitute **M** Stimulator Generator **N** Tissue Expander **P** Cardiac Rhythm Related Device **V** Infusion Device, Pump **W** Vascular Access Device, Totally Implantable **X** Vascular Access Device, Tunneled **Y** Other Device	**Z** No Qualifier
T Subcutaneous Tissue and Fascia, Trunk External oblique aponeurosis Transversalis fascia	**X** External	**Ø** Drainage Device **2** Monitoring Device **3** Infusion Device **7** Autologous Tissue Substitute **F** Subcutaneous Defibrillator Lead **H** Contraceptive Device **J** Synthetic Substitute **K** Nonautologous Tissue Substitute **M** Stimulator Generator **N** Tissue Expander **P** Cardiac Rhythm Related Device **V** Infusion Device, Pump **W** Vascular Access Device, Totally Implantable **X** Vascular Access Device, Tunneled	**Z** No Qualifier
V Subcutaneous Tissue and Fascia, Upper Extremity **W** Subcutaneous Tissue and Fascia, Lower Extremity	**Ø** Open **3** Percutaneous	**Ø** Drainage Device **3** Infusion Device **7** Autologous Tissue Substitute **H** Contraceptive Device **J** Synthetic Substitute **K** Nonautologous Tissue Substitute **N** Tissue Expander **V** Infusion Device, Pump **W** Vascular Access Device, Totally Implantable **X** Vascular Access Device, Tunneled **Y** Other Device	**Z** No Qualifier
V Subcutaneous Tissue and Fascia, Upper Extremity **W** Subcutaneous Tissue and Fascia, Lower Extremity	**X** External	**Ø** Drainage Device **3** Infusion Device **7** Autologous Tissue Substitute **H** Contraceptive Device **J** Synthetic Substitute **K** Nonautologous Tissue Substitute **N** Tissue Expander **V** Infusion Device, Pump **W** Vascular Access Device, Totally Implantable **X** Vascular Access Device, Tunneled	**Z** No Qualifier

DRG Non-OR   ØJWS[Ø,3][Ø,3,7,J,K,N,Y]Z
DRG Non-OR   ØJWT[Ø,3][Ø,3,7,H,J,K,M,N,V,W,X]Z
DRG Non-OR   ØJWTXMZ
DRG Non-OR   ØJW[V,W][Ø,3][Ø,3,7,H,J,K,N,V,W,X,Y]Z
Non-OR   ØJWSX[Ø,3,7,J,K,N]Z
Non-OR   ØJWT3YZ
Non-OR   ØJWTX[Ø,2,3,7,F,H,J,K,N,P,V,W,X]Z
Non-OR   ØJW[V,W]X[Ø,3,7,H,J,K,N,V,W,X]Z

HAC   ØJWT[Ø,3]PZ when reported with SDx K68.11 or T81.4Ø-T81.49, T82.6-T82.7 with 7th character A

Ø   Medical and Surgical
J   Subcutaneous Tissue and Fascia
X   Transfer   Definition: Moving, without taking out, all or a portion of a body part to another location to take over the function of all or a portion of a body part
                           Explanation: The body part transferred remains connected to its vascular and nervous supply

Body Part Character 4		Approach Character 5	Device Character 6	Qualifier Character 7
Ø Subcutaneous Tissue and Fascia, Scalp Galea aponeurotica **1 Subcutaneous Tissue and Fascia, Face** Masseteric fascia Orbital fascia Submandibular space **4 Subcutaneous Tissue and Fascia, Right Neck** Deep cervical fascia Pretracheal fascia Prevertebral fascia **5 Subcutaneous Tissue and Fascia, Left Neck** *See 4 Subcutaneous Tissue and Fascia, Right Neck* **6 Subcutaneous Tissue and Fascia, Chest** Pectoral fascia **7 Subcutaneous Tissue and Fascia, Back** **8 Subcutaneous Tissue and Fascia, Abdomen** **9 Subcutaneous Tissue and Fascia, Buttock** **B Subcutaneous Tissue and Fascia, Perineum** **C Subcutaneous Tissue and Fascia, Pelvic Region** **D Subcutaneous Tissue and Fascia, Right Upper Arm** Axillary fascia Deltoid fascia Infraspinatus fascia Subscapular aponeurosis Supraspinatus fascia **F Subcutaneous Tissue and Fascia, Left Upper Arm** *See D Subcutaneous Tissue and Fascia, Right Upper Arm*	**G Subcutaneous Tissue and Fascia, Right Lower Arm** Antebrachial fascia Bicipital aponeurosis **H Subcutaneous Tissue and Fascia, Left Lower Arm** *See G Subcutaneous Tissue and Fascia, Right Lower Arm* **J Subcutaneous Tissue and Fascia, Right Hand** Palmar fascia (aponeurosis) **K Subcutaneous Tissue and Fascia, Left Hand** *See J Subcutaneous Tissue and Fascia, Right Hand* **L Subcutaneous Tissue and Fascia, Right Upper Leg** Crural fascia Fascia lata Iliac fascia Iliotibial tract (band) **M Subcutaneous Tissue and Fascia, Left Upper Leg** *See L Subcutaneous Tissue and Fascia, Right Upper Leg* **N Subcutaneous Tissue and Fascia, Right Lower Leg** **P Subcutaneous Tissue and Fascia, Left Lower Leg** **Q Subcutaneous Tissue and Fascia, Right Foot** Plantar fascia (aponeurosis) **R Subcutaneous Tissue and Fascia, Left Foot** *See Q Subcutaneous Tissue and Fascia, Right Foot*	**Ø Open** **3 Percutaneous**	**Z No Device**	**B Skin and Subcutaneous Tissue** **C Skin, Subcutaneous Tissue and Fascia** **Z No Qualifier**

Muscles ØK2–ØKX

Character Meanings

This Character Meaning table is provided as a guide to assist the user in the identification of character members that may be found in this section of code tables. It **SHOULD NOT** be used to build a PCS code.

Operation–Character 3		Body Part–Character 4		Approach–Character 5		Device–Character 6		Qualifier–Character 7	
2	Change	Ø	Head Muscle	Ø	Open	Ø	Drainage Device	Ø	Skin
5	Destruction	1	Facial Muscle	3	Percutaneous	7	Autologous Tissue Substitute	1	Subcutaneous Tissue
8	Division	2	Neck Muscle, Right	4	Percutaneous Endoscopic	J	Synthetic Substitute	2	Skin and Subcutaneous Tissue
9	Drainage	3	Neck Muscle, Left	X	External	K	Nonautologous Tissue Substitute	5	Latissimus Dorsi Myocutaneous Flap
B	Excision	4	Tongue, Palate, Pharynx Muscle			M	Stimulator Lead	6	Transverse Rectus Abdominis Myocutaneous Flap
C	Extirpation	5	Shoulder Muscle, Right			Y	Other Device	7	Deep Inferior Epigastric Artery Perforator Flap
D	Extraction	6	Shoulder Muscle, Left			Z	No Device	8	Superficial Inferior Epigastric Artery Flap
H	Insertion	7	Upper Arm Muscle, Right					9	Gluteal Artery Perforator Flap
J	Inspection	8	Upper Arm Muscle, Left					X	Diagnostic
M	Reattachment	9	Lower Arm and Wrist Muscle, Right					Z	No Qualifier
N	Release	B	Lower Arm and Wrist Muscle, Left						
P	Removal	C	Hand Muscle, Right						
Q	Repair	D	Hand Muscle, Left						
R	Replacement	F	Trunk Muscle, Right						
S	Reposition	G	Trunk Muscle, Left						
T	Resection	H	Thorax Muscle, Right						
U	Supplement	J	Thorax Muscle, Left						
W	Revision	K	Abdomen Muscle, Right						
X	Transfer	L	Abdomen Muscle, Left						
		M	Perineum Muscle						
		N	Hip Muscle, Right						
		P	Hip Muscle, Left						
		Q	Upper Leg Muscle, Right						
		R	Upper Leg Muscle, Left						
		S	Lower Leg Muscle, Right						
		T	Lower Leg Muscle, Left						
		V	Foot Muscle, Right						
		W	Foot Muscle, Left						
		X	Upper Muscle						
		Y	Lower Muscle						

AHA Coding Clinic for table ØKB

2016, 3Q, 20	Excisional debridement of sacrum
2015, 3Q, 3-8	Excisional and nonexcisional debridement

AHA Coding Clinic for table ØKD

2017, 4Q, 41-42	Extraction procedures

AHA Coding Clinic for table ØKN

2017, 2Q, 12	Compartment syndrome and fasciotomy of foot
2017, 2Q, 13	Compartment syndrome and fasciotomy of leg
2015, 2Q, 22	Arthroscopic subacromial decompression
2014, 4Q, 39	Abdominal component release with placement of mesh for hernia repair

AHA Coding Clinic for table ØKQ

2018, 2Q, 25	Third and fourth degree obstetric lacerations
2016, 2Q, 34	Assisted vaginal delivery
2016, 1Q, 7	Obstetrical perineal laceration repair
2014, 4Q, 43	Second degree obstetric perineal laceration
2013, 4Q, 120	Repair of second degree perineum obstetric laceration

AHA Coding Clinic for table ØKS

2017, 1Q, 41	Manual reduction of hernia

AHA Coding Clinic for table ØKT

2016, 2Q, 12	Resection of malignant neoplasm of infratemporal fossa
2015, 1Q, 38	Abdominoperineal resection with flap closure of the perineum and colostomy

AHA Coding Clinic for table ØKX

2018, 2Q, 18	Transverse rectus abdominis myocutaneous (TRAM) delay
2017, 4Q, 67	New qualifier values - Pedicle flap procedures
2016, 3Q, 30	Resection of femur with interposition arthroplasty
2015, 3Q, 33	Cleft lip repair using Millard rotation advancement
2015, 2Q, 26	Pharyngeal flap to soft palate
2014, 4Q, 41	Abdominoperineal resection (APR) with flap closure of perineum and colostomy
2014, 2Q, 10	Transverse abdominomyocutaneous (TRAM) breast reconstruction
2014, 2Q, 12	Pedicle latissimus myocutaneous flap with placement of breast tissue expanders

Muscles

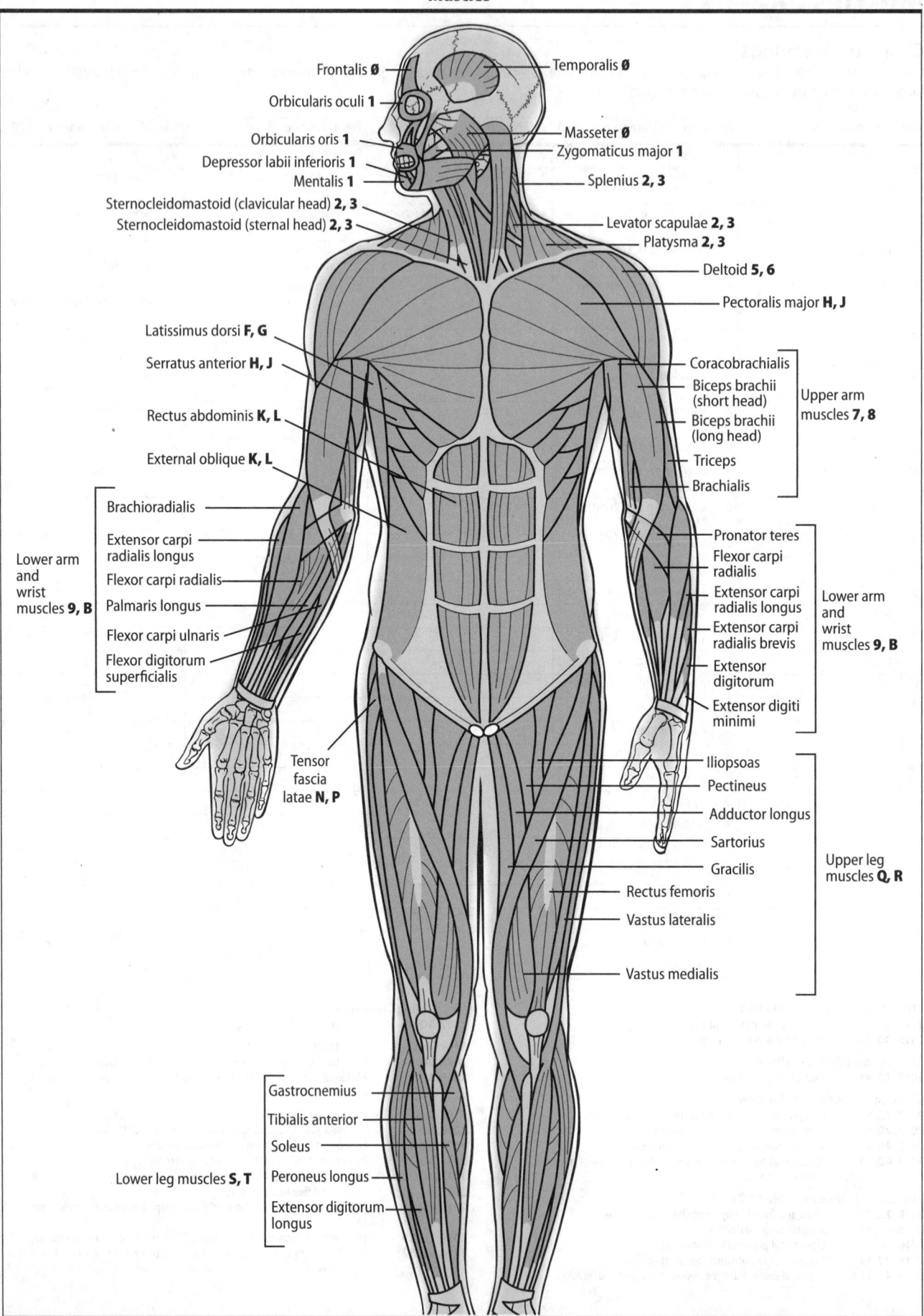

Frontalis **Ø**

Temporalis **Ø**

Orbicularis oculi **1**

Masseter **Ø**

Orbicularis oris **1**

Zygomaticus major **1**

Depressor labii inferioris **1**

Splenius **2, 3**

Mentalis **1**

Sternocleidomastoid (clavicular head) **2, 3**

Sternocleidomastoid (sternal head) **2, 3**

Levator scapulae **2, 3**

Platysma **2, 3**

Deltoid **5, 6**

Pectoralis major **H, J**

Latissimus dorsi **F, G**

Coracobrachialis

Serratus anterior **H, J**

Biceps brachii (short head)

Upper arm muscles **7, 8**

Rectus abdominis **K, L**

Biceps brachii (long head)

External oblique **K, L**

Triceps

Brachialis

Brachioradialis

Pronator teres

Extensor carpi radialis longus

Flexor carpi radialis

Flexor carpi radialis

Extensor carpi radialis longus

Lower arm and wrist muscles **9, B**

Lower arm and wrist muscles **9, B**

Palmaris longus

Extensor carpi radialis brevis

Flexor carpi ulnaris

Extensor digitorum

Flexor digitorum superficialis

Extensor digiti minimi

Iliopsoas

Pectineus

Tensor fascia latae **N, P**

Adductor longus

Sartorius

Gracilis

Upper leg muscles **Q, R**

Rectus femoris

Vastus lateralis

Vastus medialis

Gastrocnemius

Tibialis anterior

Soleus

Lower leg muscles **S, T**

Peroneus longus

Extensor digitorum longus

Ø   **Medical and Surgical**
K   **Muscles**
2   **Change**   Definition: Taking out or off a device from a body part and putting back an identical or similar device in or on the same body part without cutting or puncturing the skin or a mucous membrane

                     Explanation: All CHANGE procedures are coded using the approach EXTERNAL

Body Part Character 4	Approach Character 5	Device Character 6	Qualifier Character 7
X Upper Muscle **Y** Lower Muscle	**X** External	**Ø** Drainage Device **Y** Other Device	**Z** No Qualifier

Non-OR	All body part, approach, device, and qualifier values

Ø   **Medical and Surgical**
K   **Muscles**
5   **Destruction**   Definition: Physical eradication of all or a portion of a body part by the direct use of energy, force, or a destructive agent

                          Explanation: None of the body part is physically taken out

Body Part Character 4			Approach Character 5	Device Character 6	Qualifier Character 7

Ø **Head Muscle**
   Auricularis muscle
   Masseter muscle
   Pterygoid muscle
   Splenius capitis muscle
   Temporalis muscle
   Temporoparietalis muscle
1 **Facial Muscle**
   Buccinator muscle
   Corrugator supercilii muscle
   Depressor anguli oris muscle
   Depressor labii inferioris muscle
   Depressor septi nasi muscle
   Depressor supercilii muscle
   Levator anguli oris muscle
   Levator labii superioris alaeque
     nasi muscle
   Levator labii superioris muscle
   Mentalis muscle
   Nasalis muscle
   Occipitofrontalis muscle
   Orbicularis oris muscle
   Procerus muscle
   Risorius muscle
   Zygomaticus muscle
2 **Neck Muscle, Right**
   Anterior vertebral muscle
   Arytenoid muscle
   Cricothyroid muscle
   Infrahyoid muscle
   Levator scapulae muscle
   Platysma muscle
   Scalene muscle
   Splenius cervicis muscle
   Sternocleidomastoid muscle
   Suprahyoid muscle
   Thyroarytenoid muscle
3 **Neck Muscle, Left**
   See 2 Neck Muscle, Right
4 **Tongue, Palate, Pharynx**
   Muscle
   Chondroglossus muscle
   Genioglossus muscle
   Hyoglossus muscle
   Inferior longitudinal muscle
   Levator veli palatini muscle
   Palatoglossal muscle
   Palatopharyngeal muscle
   Pharyngeal constrictor muscle
   Salpingopharyngeus muscle
   Styloglossus muscle
   Stylopharyngeus muscle
   Superior longitudinal muscle
   Tensor veli palatini muscle
5 **Shoulder Muscle, Right**
   Deltoid muscle
   Infraspinatus muscle
   Subscapularis muscle
   Supraspinatus muscle
   Teres major muscle
   Teres minor muscle
6 **Shoulder Muscle, Left**
   See 5 Shoulder Muscle, Right
	7 **Upper Arm Muscle, Right**
	   Biceps brachii muscle
	   Brachialis muscle
	   Coracobrachialis muscle
	   Triceps brachii muscle
	8 **Upper Arm Muscle, Left**
	   See 7 Upper Arm Muscle, Right
	9 **Lower Arm and Wrist Muscle,**
	   Right
	   Anatomical snuffbox
	   Brachioradialis muscle
	   Extensor carpi radialis muscle
	   Extensor carpi ulnaris muscle
	   Flexor carpi radialis muscle
	   Flexor carpi ulnaris muscle
	   Flexor pollicis longus muscle
	   Palmaris longus muscle
	   Pronator quadratus muscle
	   Pronator teres muscle
	B **Lower Arm and Wrist Muscle,**
	   Left
	   See 9 Lower Arm and Wrist
	   Muscle, Right
	C **Hand Muscle, Right**
	   Hypothenar muscle
	   Palmar interosseous muscle
	   Thenar muscle
	D **Hand Muscle, Left**
	   See C Hand Muscle, Right
	F **Trunk Muscle, Right**
	   Coccygeus muscle
	   Erector spinae muscle
	   Interspinalis muscle
	   Intertransversarius muscle
	   Latissimus dorsi muscle
	   Quadratus lumborum muscle
	   Rhomboid major muscle
	   Rhomboid minor muscle
	   Serratus posterior muscle
	   Transversospinalis muscle
	   Trapezius muscle
	G **Trunk Muscle, Left**
	   See F Trunk Muscle, Right
	H **Thorax Muscle, Right**
	   Intercostal muscle
	   Levatores costarum muscle
	   Pectoralis major muscle
	   Pectoralis minor muscle
	   Serratus anterior muscle
	   Subclavius muscle
	   Subcostal muscle
	   Transverse thoracis muscle
	J **Thorax Muscle, Left**
	   See H Thorax Muscle, Right
	K **Abdomen Muscle, Right**
	   External oblique muscle
	   Internal oblique muscle
	   Pyramidalis muscle
	   Rectus abdominis muscle
	   Transversus abdominis muscle
	L **Abdomen Muscle, Left**
	   See K Abdomen Muscle, Right
		M **Perineum Muscle**
		   Bulbospongiosus muscle
		   Cremaster muscle
		   Deep transverse perineal muscle
		   Ischiocavernosus muscle
		   Levator ani muscle
		   Superficial transverse perineal
		     muscle
		N **Hip Muscle, Right**
		   Gemellus muscle
		   Gluteus maximus muscle
		   Gluteus medius muscle
		   Gluteus minimus muscle
		   Iliacus muscle
		   Obturator muscle
		   Piriformis muscle
		   Psoas muscle
		   Quadratus femoris muscle
		   Tensor fasciae latae muscle
		P **Hip Muscle, Left**
		   See N Hip Muscle, Right
		Q **Upper Leg Muscle, Right**
		   Adductor brevis muscle
		   Adductor longus muscle
		   Adductor magnus muscle
		   Biceps femoris muscle
		   Gracilis muscle
		   Pectineus muscle
		   Quadriceps (femoris)
		   Rectus femoris muscle
		   Sartorius muscle
		   Semimembranosus muscle
		   Semitendinosus muscle
		   Vastus intermedius muscle
		   Vastus lateralis muscle
		   Vastus medialis muscle
		R **Upper Leg Muscle, Left**
		   See Q Upper Leg Muscle, Right
		S **Lower Leg Muscle, Right**
		   Extensor digitorum longus muscle
		   Extensor hallucis longus muscle
		   Fibularis brevis muscle
		   Fibularis longus muscle
		   Flexor digitorum longus muscle
		   Flexor hallucis longus muscle
		   Gastrocnemius muscle
		   Peroneus brevis muscle
		   Peroneus longus muscle
		   Popliteus muscle
		   Soleus muscle
		   Tibialis anterior muscle
		   Tibialis posterior muscle
		T **Lower Leg Muscle, Left**
		   See S Lower Leg Muscle, Right
		V **Foot Muscle, Right**
		   Abductor hallucis muscle
		   Adductor hallucis muscle
		   Extensor digitorum brevis muscle
		   Extensor hallucis brevis muscle
		   Flexor digitorum brevis muscle
		   Flexor hallucis brevis muscle
		   Quadratus plantae muscle
		W **Foot Muscle, Left**
		   See V Foot Muscle, Right
			Ø Open
			3 Percutaneous
			4 Percutaneous
			   Endoscopic
				Z No Device	**Z** No Qualifier

Ø   **Medical and Surgical**
K   **Muscles**
8   **Division**   Definition: Cutting into a body part, without draining fluids and/or gases from the body part, in order to separate or transect a body part
                 Explanation: All or a portion of the body part is separated into two or more portions

Body Part Character 4			Approach Character 5	Device Character 6	Qualifier Character 7
Ø Head Muscle Auricularis muscle Masseter muscle Pterygoid muscle Splenius capitis muscle Temporalis muscle Temporoparietalis muscle **1 Facial Muscle** Buccinator muscle Corrugator supercilii muscle Depressor anguli oris muscle Depressor labii inferioris muscle Depressor septi nasi muscle Depressor supercilii muscle Levator anguli oris muscle Levator labii superioris alaeque nasi muscle Levator labii superioris muscle Mentalis muscle Nasalis muscle Occipitofrontalis muscle Orbicularis oris muscle Procerus muscle Risorius muscle Zygomaticus muscle **2 Neck Muscle, Right** Anterior vertebral muscle Arytenoid muscle Cricothyroid muscle Infrahyoid muscle Levator scapulae muscle Platysma muscle Scalene muscle Splenius cervicis muscle Sternocleidomastoid muscle Suprahyoid muscle Thyroarytenoid muscle **3 Neck Muscle, Left** *See 2 Neck Muscle, Right* **4 Tongue, Palate, Pharynx Muscle** Chondroglossus muscle Genioglossus muscle Hyoglossus muscle Inferior longitudinal muscle Levator veli palatini muscle Palatoglossus muscle Palatopharyngeal muscle Pharyngeal constrictor muscle Salpingopharyngeus muscle Styloglossus muscle Stylopharyngeus muscle Superior longitudinal muscle Tensor veli palatini muscle **5 Shoulder Muscle, Right** Deltoid muscle Infraspinatus muscle Subscapularis muscle Supraspinatus muscle Teres major muscle Teres minor muscle **6 Shoulder Muscle, Left** *See 5 Shoulder Muscle, Right*	**7 Upper Arm Muscle, Right** Biceps brachii muscle Brachialis muscle Coracobrachialis muscle Triceps brachii muscle **8 Upper Arm Muscle, Left** *See 7 Upper Arm Muscle, Right* **9 Lower Arm and Wrist Muscle, Right** Anatomical snuffbox Brachioradialis muscle Extensor carpi radialis muscle Extensor carpi ulnaris muscle Flexor carpi radialis muscle Flexor carpi ulnaris muscle Flexor pollicis longus muscle Palmaris longus muscle Pronator quadratus muscle Pronator teres muscle **B Lower Arm and Wrist Muscle, Left** *See 9 Lower Arm and Wrist Muscle, Right* **C Hand Muscle, Right** Hypothenar muscle Palmar interosseous muscle Thenar muscle **D Hand Muscle, Left** *See C Hand Muscle, Right* **F Trunk Muscle, Right** Coccygeus muscle Erector spinae muscle Interspinalis muscle Intertransversarius muscle Latissimus dorsi muscle Quadratus lumborum muscle Rhomboid major muscle Rhomboid minor muscle Serratus posterior muscle Transversospinalis muscle Trapezius muscle **G Trunk Muscle, Left** *See F Trunk Muscle, Right* **H Thorax Muscle, Right** Intercostal muscle Levatores costarum muscle Pectoralis major muscle Pectoralis minor muscle Serratus anterior muscle Subclavius muscle Subcostal muscle Transverse thoracis muscle **J Thorax Muscle, Left** *See H Thorax Muscle, Right* **K Abdomen Muscle, Right** External oblique muscle Internal oblique muscle Pyramidalis muscle Rectus abdominis muscle Transversus abdominis muscle **L Abdomen Muscle, Left** *See K Abdomen Muscle, Right*	**M Perineum Muscle** Bulbospongiosus muscle Cremaster muscle Deep transverse perineal muscle Ischiocavernosus muscle Levator ani muscle Superficial transverse perineal muscle **N Hip Muscle, Right** Gemellus muscle Gluteus maximus muscle Gluteus medius muscle Gluteus minimus muscle Iliacus muscle Obturator muscle Piriformis muscle Psoas muscle Quadratus femoris muscle Tensor fasciae latae muscle **P Hip Muscle, Left** *See N Hip Muscle, Right* **Q Upper Leg Muscle, Right** Adductor brevis muscle Adductor longus muscle Adductor magnus muscle Biceps femoris muscle Gracilis muscle Pectineus muscle Quadriceps (femoris) Rectus femoris muscle Sartorius muscle Semimembranosus muscle Semitendinosus muscle Vastus intermedius muscle Vastus lateralis muscle Vastus medialis muscle **R Upper Leg Muscle, Left** *See Q Upper Leg Muscle, Right* **S Lower Leg Muscle, Right** Extensor digitorum longus muscle Extensor hallucis longus muscle Fibularis brevis muscle Fibularis longus muscle Flexor digitorum longus muscle Flexor hallucis longus muscle Gastrocnemius muscle Peroneus brevis muscle Peroneus longus muscle Popliteus muscle Soleus muscle Tibialis anterior muscle Tibialis posterior muscle **T Lower Leg Muscle, Left** *See S Lower Leg Muscle, Right* **V Foot Muscle, Right** Abductor hallucis muscle Adductor hallucis muscle Extensor digitorum brevis muscle Extensor hallucis brevis muscle Flexor digitorum brevis muscle Flexor hallucis brevis muscle Quadratus plantae muscle **W Foot Muscle, Left** *See V Foot Muscle, Right*	**Ø Open** **3 Percutaneous** **4 Percutaneous Endoscopic**	**Z No Device**	**Z No Qualifier**

LC Limited Coverage   NC Noncovered   ⊞ Combination Member   HAC associated procedure   Combination Only   DRG Non-OR   Non-OR   New/Revised in GREEN

Ø   Medical and Surgical
K   Muscles
9   Drainage   Definition: Taking or letting out fluids and/or gases from a body part
                     Explanation: The qualifier DIAGNOSTIC is used to identify drainage procedures that are biopsies

Body Part Character 4			Approach Character 5	Device Character 6	Qualifier Character 7
Ø Head Muscle	**7 Upper Arm Muscle, Right**	**M Perineum Muscle**	**Ø** Open	**Ø** Drainage Device	**Z** No Qualifier
Auricularis muscle	Biceps brachii muscle	Bulbospongiosus muscle	**3** Percutaneous		
Masseter muscle	Brachialis muscle	Cremaster muscle	**4** Percutaneous		
Pterygoid muscle	Coracobrachialis muscle	Deep transverse perineal	Endoscopic		
Splenius capitis muscle	Triceps brachii muscle	muscle			
Temporalis muscle	**8 Upper Arm Muscle, Left**	Ischiocavernosus muscle			
Temporoparietalis muscle	*See 7 Upper Arm Muscle,*	Levator ani muscle			
1 Facial Muscle	*Right*	Superficial transverse			
Buccinator muscle	**9 Lower Arm and Wrist**	perineal muscle			
Corrugator supercilii	**Muscle, Right**	**N Hip Muscle, Right**			
muscle	Anatomical snuffbox	Gemellus muscle			
Depressor anguli oris	Brachioradialis muscle	Gluteus maximus muscle			
muscle	Extensor carpi radialis	Gluteus medius muscle			
Depressor labii inferioris	muscle	Gluteus minimus muscle			
muscle	Extensor carpi ulnaris	Iliacus muscle			
Depressor septi nasi	muscle	Obturator muscle			
muscle	Flexor carpi radialis muscle	Piriformis muscle			
Depressor supercilii	Flexor carpi ulnaris muscle	Psoas muscle			
muscle	Flexor pollicis longus	Quadratus femoris muscle			
Levator anguli oris muscle	muscle	Tensor fasciae latae			
Levator labii superioris	Palmaris longus muscle	muscle			
alaeque nasi muscle	Pronator quadratus	**P Hip Muscle, Left**			
Levator labii superioris	muscle	*See N Hip Muscle, Right*			
muscle	Pronator teres muscle	**Q Upper Leg Muscle, Right**			
Mentalis muscle	**B Lower Arm and Wrist**	Adductor brevis muscle			
Nasalis muscle	**Muscle, Left**	Adductor longus muscle			
Occipitofrontalis muscle	*See 9 Lower Arm and Wrist*	Adductor magnus muscle			
Orbicularis oris muscle	*Muscle, Right*	Biceps femoris muscle			
Procerus muscle	**C Hand Muscle, Right**	Gracilis muscle			
Risorius muscle	Hypothenar muscle	Pectineus muscle			
Zygomaticus muscle	Palmar interosseous	Quadriceps (femoris)			
2 Neck Muscle, Right	muscle	Rectus femoris muscle			
Anterior vertebral muscle	Thenar muscle	Sartorius muscle			
Arytenoid muscle	**D Hand Muscle, Left**	Semimembranosus			
Cricothyroid muscle	*See C Hand Muscle, Right*	muscle			
Infrahyoid muscle	**F Trunk Muscle, Right**	Semitendinosus muscle			
Levator scapulae muscle	Coccygeus muscle	Vastus intermedius muscle			
Platysma muscle	Erector spinae muscle	Vastus lateralis muscle			
Scalene muscle	Interspinalis muscle	Vastus medialis muscle			
Splenius cervicis muscle	Intertransversarius muscle	**R Upper Leg Muscle, Left**			
Sternocleidomastoid	Latissimus dorsi muscle	*See Q Upper Leg Muscle,*			
muscle	Quadratus lumborum	*Right*			
Suprahyoid muscle	muscle	**S Lower Leg Muscle, Right**			
Thyroarytenoid muscle	Rhomboid major muscle	Extensor digitorum longus			
3 Neck Muscle, Left	Rhomboid minor muscle	muscle			
See 2 Neck Muscle, Right	Serratus posterior muscle	Extensor hallucis longus			
4 Tongue, Palate, Pharynx	Transversospinalis muscle	muscle			
Muscle	Trapezius muscle	Fibularis brevis muscle			
Chondroglossus muscle	**G Trunk Muscle, Left**	Fibularis longus muscle			
Genioglossus muscle	*See F Trunk Muscle, Right*	Flexor digitorum longus			
Hyoglossus muscle	**H Thorax Muscle, Right**	muscle			
Inferior longitudinal	Intercostal muscle	Flexor hallucis longus			
muscle	Levatores costarum	muscle			
Levator veli palatini	muscle	Gastrocnemius muscle			
muscle	Pectoralis major muscle	Peroneus brevis muscle			
Palatoglossal muscle	Pectoralis minor muscle	Peroneus longus muscle			
Palatopharyngeal muscle	Serratus anterior muscle	Popliteus muscle			
Pharyngeal constrictor	Subclavius muscle	Soleus muscle			
muscle	Subcostal muscle	Tibialis anterior muscle			
Salpingopharyngeus	Transverse thoracis muscle	Tibialis posterior muscle			
muscle	**J Thorax Muscle, Left**	**T Lower Leg Muscle, Left**			
Styloglossus muscle	*See H Thorax Muscle, Right*	*See S Lower Leg Muscle,*			
Stylopharyngeus muscle	**K Abdomen Muscle, Right**	*Right*			
Superior longitudinal	External oblique muscle	**V Foot Muscle, Right**			
muscle	Internal oblique muscle	Abductor hallucis muscle			
Tensor veli palatini muscle	Pyramidalis muscle	Adductor hallucis muscle			
5 Shoulder Muscle, Right	Rectus abdominis muscle	Extensor digitorum brevis			
Deltoid muscle	Transversus abdominis	muscle			
Infraspinatus muscle	muscle	Extensor hallucis brevis			
Subscapularis muscle	**L Abdomen Muscle, Left**	muscle			
Supraspinatus muscle	*See K Abdomen Muscle,*	Flexor digitorum brevis			
Teres major muscle	*Right*	muscle			
Teres minor muscle		Flexor hallucis brevis			
6 Shoulder Muscle, Left		muscle			
See 5 Shoulder Muscle,		Quadratus plantae muscle			
Right		**W Foot Muscle, Left**			
		See V Foot Muscle, Right			

Non-OR   ØK9[Ø,1,2,3,4,5,6,7,8,9,B,C,D,F,G,H,J,K,L,M,N,P,Q,R,S,T,V,W]3ØZ   *ØK9 Continued on next page*

LC Limited Coverage   **NC** Noncovered   ⊞ Combination Member   HAC associated procedure   Combination Only   DRG Non-OR   Non-OR   New/Revised in GREEN

ICD-10-PCS 2020   455

ØK9–ØK9

Ø   Medical and Surgical   *ØK9 Continued*
K   Muscles
9   Drainage   Definition: Taking or letting out fluids and/or gases from a body part
                   Explanation: The qualifier DIAGNOSTIC is used to identify drainage procedures that are biopsies

Body Part Character 4			Approach Character 5	Device Character 6	Qualifier Character 7
Ø Head Muscle	**7 Upper Arm Muscle, Right**	**M Perineum Muscle**	**Ø Open**	**Z No Device**	**X Diagnostic**
Auricularis muscle	Biceps brachii muscle	Bulbospongiosus muscle	**3 Percutaneous**		**Z No Qualifier**
Masseter muscle	Brachialis muscle	Cremaster muscle	**4 Percutaneous**		
Pterygoid muscle	Coracobrachialis muscle	Deep transverse perineal	Endoscopic		
Splenius capitis muscle	Triceps brachii muscle	muscle			
Temporalis muscle	**8 Upper Arm Muscle, Left**	Ischiocavernosus muscle			
Temporoparietalis muscle	*See 7 Upper Arm Muscle,*	Levator ani muscle			
1 Facial Muscle	*Right*	Superficial transverse			
Buccinator muscle	**9 Lower Arm and Wrist**	perineal muscle			
Corrugator supercilii	**Muscle, Right**	**N Hip Muscle, Right**			
muscle	Anatomical snuffbox	Gemellus muscle			
Depressor anguli oris	Brachioradialis muscle	Gluteus maximus muscle			
muscle	Extensor carpi radialis	Gluteus medius muscle			
Depressor labii inferioris	muscle	Gluteus minimus muscle			
muscle	Extensor carpi ulnaris	Iliacus muscle			
Depressor septi nasi	muscle	Obturator muscle			
muscle	Flexor carpi radialis muscle	Piriformis muscle			
Depressor supercilii	Flexor carpi ulnaris muscle	Psoas muscle			
muscle	Flexor pollicis longus	Quadratus femoris muscle			
Levator anguli oris muscle	muscle	Tensor fasciae latae			
Levator labii superioris	Palmaris longus muscle	muscle			
alaeque nasi muscle	Pronator quadratus	**P Hip Muscle, Left**			
Levator labii superioris	muscle	*See N Hip Muscle, Right*			
muscle	Pronator teres muscle	**Q Upper Leg Muscle, Right**			
Mentalis muscle	**B Lower Arm and Wrist**	Adductor brevis muscle			
Nasalis muscle	**Muscle, Left**	Adductor longus muscle			
Occipitofrontalis muscle	*See 9 Lower Arm and Wrist*	Adductor magnus muscle			
Orbicularis oris muscle	*Muscle, Right*	Biceps femoris muscle			
Procerus muscle	**C Hand Muscle, Right**	Gracilis muscle			
Risorius muscle	Hypothenar muscle	Pectineus muscle			
Zygomaticus muscle	Palmar interosseous	Quadriceps (femoris)			
2 Neck Muscle, Right	muscle	Rectus femoris muscle			
Anterior vertebral muscle	Thenar muscle	Sartorius muscle			
Arytenoid muscle	**D Hand Muscle, Left**	Semimembranosus muscle			
Cricothyroid muscle	*See C Hand Muscle, Right*	Semitendinosus muscle			
Infrahyoid muscle	**F Trunk Muscle, Right**	Vastus intermedius muscle			
Levator scapulae muscle	Coccygeus muscle	Vastus lateralis muscle			
Platysma muscle	Erector spinae muscle	Vastus medialis muscle			
Scalene muscle	Interspinalis muscle	**R Upper Leg Muscle, Left**			
Splenius cervicis muscle	Intertransversarius muscle	*See Q Upper Leg Muscle,*			
Sternocleidomastoid	Latissimus dorsi muscle	*Right*			
muscle	Quadratus lumborum	**S Lower Leg Muscle, Right**			
Suprahyoid muscle	muscle	Extensor digitorum longus			
Thyroarytenoid muscle	Rhomboid major muscle	muscle			
3 Neck Muscle, Left	Rhomboid minor muscle	Extensor hallucis longus			
See 2 Neck Muscle, Right	Serratus posterior muscle	muscle			
4 Tongue, Palate, Pharynx	Transversospinalis muscle	Fibularis brevis muscle			
Muscle	Trapezius muscle	Fibularis longus muscle			
Chondroglossus muscle	**G Trunk Muscle, Left**	Flexor digitorum longus			
Genioglossus muscle	*See F Trunk Muscle, Right*	muscle			
Hyoglossus muscle	**H Thorax Muscle, Right**	Flexor hallucis longus			
Inferior longitudinal	Intercostal muscle	muscle			
muscle	Levatores costarum	Gastrocnemius muscle			
Levator veli palatini	muscle	Peroneus brevis muscle			
muscle	Pectoralis major muscle	Peroneus longus muscle			
Palatoglossal muscle	Pectoralis minor muscle	Popliteus muscle			
Palatopharyngeal muscle	Serratus anterior muscle	Soleus muscle			
Pharyngeal constrictor	Subclavius muscle	Tibialis anterior muscle			
muscle	Subcostal muscle	Tibialis posterior muscle			
Salpingopharyngeus	Transverse thoracis muscle	**T Lower Leg Muscle, Left**			
muscle	**J Thorax Muscle, Left**	*See S Lower Leg Muscle,*			
Styloglossus muscle	*See H Thorax Muscle, Right*	*Right*			
Stylopharyngeus muscle	**K Abdomen Muscle, Right**	**V Foot Muscle, Right**			
Superior longitudinal	External oblique muscle	Abductor hallucis muscle			
muscle	Internal oblique muscle	Adductor hallucis muscle			
Tensor veli palatini muscle	Pyramidalis muscle	Extensor digitorum brevis			
5 Shoulder Muscle, Right	Rectus abdominis muscle	muscle			
Deltoid muscle	Transversus abdominis	Extensor hallucis brevis			
Infraspinatus muscle	muscle	muscle			
Subscapularis muscle	**L Abdomen Muscle, Left**	Flexor digitorum brevis			
Supraspinatus muscle	*See K Abdomen Muscle,*	muscle			
Teres major muscle	*Right*	Flexor hallucis brevis			
Teres minor muscle		muscle			
6 Shoulder Muscle, Left		Quadratus plantae muscle			
See 5 Shoulder Muscle,		**W Foot Muscle, Left**			
Right		*See V Foot Muscle, Right*			

Non-OR   ØK9[Ø,1,2,3,4,5,6,7,8,9,B,F,G,H,J,K,L,M,N,P,Q,R,S,T,V,W]3ZZ
Non-OR   ØK9[C,D][3,4]ZZ

LC Limited Coverage   NC Noncovered   ⊞ Combination Member   HAC associated procedure   Combination Only   DRG Non-OR   Non-OR   New/Revised in GREEN

456   ICD-10-PCS 2020

Ø   Medical and Surgical
K   Muscles
B   Excision   Definition: Cutting out or off, without replacement, a portion of a body part

                   Explanation: The qualifier DIAGNOSTIC is used to identify excision procedures that are biopsies

Body Part — Character 4			Approach — Character 5	Device — Character 6	Qualifier — Character 7
Ø Head Muscle Auricularis muscle Masseter muscle Pterygoid muscle Splenius capitis muscle Temporalis muscle Temporoparietalis muscle **1 Facial Muscle** Buccinator muscle Corrugator supercilii muscle Depressor anguli oris muscle Depressor labii inferioris muscle Depressor septi nasi muscle Depressor supercilii muscle Levator anguli oris muscle Levator labii superioris alaeque nasi muscle Levator labii superioris muscle Mentalis muscle Nasalis muscle Occipitofrontalis muscle Orbicularis oris muscle Procerus muscle Risorius muscle Zygomaticus muscle **2 Neck Muscle, Right** Anterior vertebral muscle Arytenoid muscle Cricothyroid muscle Infrahyoid muscle Levator scapulae muscle Platysma muscle Scalene muscle Splenius cervicis muscle Sternocleidomastoid muscle Suprahyoid muscle Thyroarytenoid muscle **3 Neck Muscle, Left** *See 2 Neck Muscle, Right* **4 Tongue, Palate, Pharynx Muscle** Chondroglossus muscle Genioglossus muscle Hyoglossus muscle Inferior longitudinal muscle Levator veli palatini muscle Palatoglossal muscle Palatopharyngeal muscle Pharyngeal constrictor muscle Salpingopharyngeus muscle Styloglossus muscle Stylopharyngeus muscle Superior longitudinal muscle Tensor veli palatini muscle **5 Shoulder Muscle, Right** Deltoid muscle Infraspinatus muscle Subscapularis muscle Supraspinatus muscle Teres major muscle Teres minor muscle **6 Shoulder Muscle, Left** *See 5 Shoulder Muscle, Right*	**7 Upper Arm Muscle, Right** Biceps brachii muscle Brachialis muscle Coracobrachialis muscle Triceps brachii muscle **8 Upper Arm Muscle, Left** *See 7 Upper Arm Muscle, Right* **9 Lower Arm and Wrist Muscle, Right** Anatomical snuffbox Brachioradialis muscle Extensor carpi radialis muscle Extensor carpi ulnaris muscle Flexor carpi radialis muscle Flexor carpi ulnaris muscle Flexor pollicis longus muscle Palmaris longus muscle Pronator quadratus muscle Pronator teres muscle **B Lower Arm and Wrist Muscle, Left** *See 9 Lower Arm and Wrist Muscle, Right* **C Hand Muscle, Right** Hypothenar muscle Palmar interosseous muscle Thenar muscle **D Hand Muscle, Left** *See C Hand Muscle, Right* **F Trunk Muscle, Right** Coccygeus muscle Erector spinae muscle Interspinalis muscle Intertransversarius muscle Latissimus dorsi muscle Quadratus lumborum muscle Rhomboid major muscle Rhomboid minor muscle Serratus posterior muscle Transversospinalis muscle Trapezius muscle **G Trunk Muscle, Left** *See F Trunk Muscle, Right* **H Thorax Muscle, Right** Intercostal muscle Levatores costarum muscle Pectoralis major muscle Pectoralis minor muscle Serratus anterior muscle Subclavius muscle Subcostal muscle Transverse thoracis muscle **J Thorax Muscle, Left** *See H Thorax Muscle, Right* **K Abdomen Muscle, Right** External oblique muscle Internal oblique muscle Pyramidalis muscle Rectus abdominis muscle Transversus abdominis muscle **L Abdomen Muscle, Left** *See K Abdomen Muscle, Right*	**M Perineum Muscle** Bulbospongiosus muscle Cremaster muscle Deep transverse perineal muscle Ischiocavernosus muscle Levator ani muscle Superficial transverse perineal muscle **N Hip Muscle, Right** Gemellus muscle Gluteus maximus muscle Gluteus medius muscle Gluteus minimus muscle Iliacus muscle Obturator muscle Piriformis muscle Psoas muscle Quadratus femoris muscle Tensor fasciae latae muscle **P Hip Muscle, Left** *See N Hip Muscle, Right* **Q Upper Leg Muscle, Right** Adductor brevis muscle Adductor longus muscle Adductor magnus muscle Biceps femoris muscle Gracilis muscle Pectineus muscle Quadriceps (femoris) Rectus femoris muscle Sartorius muscle Semimembranosus muscle Semitendinosus muscle Vastus intermedius muscle Vastus lateralis muscle Vastus medialis muscle **R Upper Leg Muscle, Left** *See Q Upper Leg Muscle, Right* **S Lower Leg Muscle, Right** Extensor digitorum longus muscle Extensor hallucis longus muscle Fibularis brevis muscle Fibularis longus muscle Flexor digitorum longus muscle Flexor hallucis longus muscle Gastrocnemius muscle Peroneus brevis muscle Peroneus longus muscle Popliteus muscle Soleus muscle Tibialis anterior muscle Tibialis posterior muscle **T Lower Leg Muscle, Left** *See S Lower Leg Muscle, Right* **V Foot Muscle, Right** Abductor hallucis muscle Adductor hallucis muscle Extensor digitorum brevis muscle Extensor hallucis brevis muscle Flexor digitorum brevis muscle Flexor hallucis brevis muscle Quadratus plantae muscle **W Foot Muscle, Left** *See V Foot Muscle, Right*	**Ø Open** **3 Percutaneous** **4 Percutaneous Endoscopic**	**Z No Device**	**X Diagnostic** **Z No Qualifier**

LC Limited Coverage   **NC** Noncovered   ⊞ Combination Member   HAC associated procedure   Combination Only   DRG Non-OR   Non-OR   New/Revised in GREEN

ICD-10-PCS 2020   457

ØKB–ØKB

Ø   Medical and Surgical
K   Muscles
C   Extirpation

Definition: Taking or cutting out solid matter from a body part

Explanation: The solid matter may be an abnormal byproduct of a biological function or a foreign body; it may be imbedded in a body part or in the lumen of a tubular body part. The solid matter may or may not have been previously broken into pieces.

Body Part Character 4			Approach Character 5	Device Character 6	Qualifier Character 7
Ø Head Muscle Auricularis muscle Masseter muscle Pterygoid muscle Splenius capitis muscle Temporalis muscle Temporoparietalis muscle **1 Facial Muscle** Buccinator muscle Corrugator supercilii muscle Depressor anguli oris muscle Depressor labii inferioris muscle Depressor septi nasi muscle Depressor supercilii muscle Levator anguli oris muscle Levator labii superioris alaeque nasi muscle Levator labii superioris muscle Mentalis muscle Nasalis muscle Occipitofrontalis muscle Orbicularis oris muscle Procerus muscle Risorius muscle Zygomaticus muscle **2 Neck Muscle, Right** Anterior vertebral muscle Arytenoid muscle Cricothyroid muscle Infrahyoid muscle Levator scapulae muscle Platysma muscle Scalene muscle Splenius cervicis muscle Sternocleidomastoid muscle Suprahyoid muscle Thyroarytenoid muscle **3 Neck Muscle, Left** *See 2 Neck Muscle, Right* **4 Tongue, Palate, Pharynx Muscle** Chondroglossus muscle Genioglossus muscle Hyoglossus muscle Inferior longitudinal muscle Levator veli palatini muscle Palatoglossal muscle Palatopharyngeal muscle Pharyngeal constrictor muscle Salpingopharyngeus muscle Styloglossus muscle Stylopharyngeus muscle Superior longitudinal muscle Tensor veli palatini muscle **5 Shoulder Muscle, Right** Deltoid muscle Infraspinatus muscle Subscapularis muscle Supraspinatus muscle Teres major muscle Teres minor muscle **6 Shoulder Muscle, Left** *See 5 Shoulder Muscle, Right*	**7 Upper Arm Muscle, Right** Biceps brachii muscle Brachialis muscle Coracobrachialis muscle Triceps brachii muscle **8 Upper Arm Muscle, Left** *See 7 Upper Arm Muscle, Right* **9 Lower Arm and Wrist Muscle, Right** Anatomical snuffbox Brachioradialis muscle Extensor carpi radialis muscle Extensor carpi ulnaris muscle Flexor carpi radialis muscle Flexor carpi ulnaris muscle Flexor pollicis longus muscle Palmaris longus muscle Pronator quadratus muscle Pronator teres muscle **B Lower Arm and Wrist Muscle, Left** *See 9 Lower Arm and Wrist Muscle, Right* **C Hand Muscle, Right** Hypothenar muscle Palmar interosseous muscle Thenar muscle **D Hand Muscle, Left** *See C Hand Muscle, Right* **F Trunk Muscle, Right** Coccygeus muscle Erector spinae muscle Interspinalis muscle Intertransversarius muscle Latissimus dorsi muscle Quadratus lumborum muscle Rhomboid major muscle Rhomboid minor muscle Serratus posterior muscle Transversospinalis muscle Trapezius muscle **G Trunk Muscle, Left** *See F Trunk Muscle, Right* **H Thorax Muscle, Right** Intercostal muscle Levatores costarum muscle Pectoralis major muscle Pectoralis minor muscle Serratus anterior muscle Subclavius muscle Subcostal muscle Transverse thoracis muscle **J Thorax Muscle, Left** *See H Thorax Muscle, Right* **K Abdomen Muscle, Right** External oblique muscle Internal oblique muscle Pyramidalis muscle Rectus abdominis muscle Transversus abdominis muscle **L Abdomen Muscle, Left** *See K Abdomen Muscle, Right*	**M Perineum Muscle** Bulbospongiosus muscle Cremaster muscle Deep transverse perineal muscle Ischiocavernosus muscle Levator ani muscle Superficial transverse perineal muscle **N Hip Muscle, Right** Gemellus muscle Gluteus maximus muscle Gluteus medius muscle Gluteus minimus muscle Iliacus muscle Obturator muscle Piriformis muscle Psoas muscle Quadratus femoris muscle Tensor fasciae latae muscle **P Hip Muscle, Left** *See N Hip Muscle, Right* **Q Upper Leg Muscle, Right** Adductor brevis muscle Adductor longus muscle Adductor magnus muscle Biceps femoris muscle Gracilis muscle Pectineus muscle Quadriceps (femoris) Rectus femoris muscle Sartorius muscle Semimembranosus muscle Semitendinosus muscle Vastus intermedius muscle Vastus lateralis muscle Vastus medialis muscle **R Upper Leg Muscle, Left** *See Q Upper Leg Muscle, Right* **S Lower Leg Muscle, Right** Extensor digitorum longus muscle Extensor hallucis longus muscle Fibularis brevis muscle Fibularis longus muscle Flexor digitorum longus muscle Flexor hallucis longus muscle Gastrocnemius muscle Peroneus brevis muscle Peroneus longus muscle Popliteus muscle Soleus muscle Tibialis anterior muscle Tibialis posterior muscle **T Lower Leg Muscle, Left** *See S Lower Leg Muscle, Right* **V Foot Muscle, Right** Abductor hallucis muscle Adductor hallucis muscle Extensor digitorum brevis muscle Extensor hallucis brevis muscle Flexor digitorum brevis muscle Flexor hallucis brevis muscle Quadratus plantae muscle **W Foot Muscle, Left** *See V Foot Muscle, Right*	**Ø Open** **3 Percutaneous** **4 Percutaneous Endoscopic**	**Z No Device**	**Z No Qualifier**

LC Limited Coverage   **NC** Noncovered   ⊞ Combination Member   HAC associated procedure   Combination Only   DRG Non-OR   Non-OR   New/Revised in GREEN

458   ICD-10-PCS 2020

ØKC–ØKC

Ø   **Medical and Surgical**
K   **Muscles**
D   **Extraction**   Definition: Pulling or stripping out or off all or a portion of a body part by the use of force
                              Explanation: The qualifier DIAGNOSTIC is used to identify extraction procedures that are biopsies

Body Part Character 4			Approach Character 5	Device Character 6	Qualifier Character 7

Ø Head Muscle
  Auricularis muscle
  Masseter muscle
  Pterygoid muscle
  Splenius capitis muscle
  Temporalis muscle
  Temporoparietalis muscle
1 Facial Muscle
  Buccinator muscle
  Corrugator supercilii
    muscle
  Depressor anguli oris
    muscle
  Depressor labii inferioris
    muscle
  Depressor septi nasi
    muscle
  Depressor supercilii
    muscle
  Levator anguli oris muscle
  Levator labii superioris
    alaeque nasi muscle
  Levator labii superioris
    muscle
  Mentalis muscle
  Nasalis muscle
  Occipitofrontalis muscle
  Orbicularis oris muscle
  Procerus muscle
  Risorius muscle
  Zygomaticus muscle
2 Neck Muscle, Right
  Anterior vertebral muscle
  Arytenoid muscle
  Cricothyroid muscle
  Infrahyoid muscle
  Levator scapulae muscle
  Platysma muscle
  Scalene muscle
  Splenius cervicis muscle
  Sternocleidomastoid
    muscle
  Suprahyoid muscle
  Thyroarytenoid muscle
3 Neck Muscle, Left
  See 2 Neck Muscle, Right
4 Tongue, Palate, Pharynx
  Muscle
  Chondroglossus muscle
  Genioglossus muscle
  Hyoglossus muscle
  Inferior longitudinal
    muscle
  Levator veli palatini
    muscle
  Palatoglossal muscle
  Palatopharyngeal muscle
  Pharyngeal constrictor
    muscle
  Salpingopharyngeus
    muscle
  Styloglossus muscle
  Stylopharyngeus muscle
  Superior longitudinal
    muscle
  Tensor veli palatini muscle
5 Shoulder Muscle, Right
  Deltoid muscle
  Infraspinatus muscle
  Subscapularis muscle
  Supraspinatus muscle
  Teres major muscle
  Teres minor muscle
6 Shoulder Muscle, Left
  See 5 Shoulder Muscle,
    Right
	7 Upper Arm Muscle, Right
	  Biceps brachii muscle
	  Brachialis muscle
	  Coracobrachialis muscle
	  Triceps brachii muscle
	8 Upper Arm Muscle, Left
	  See 7 Upper Arm Muscle,
	    Right
	9 Lower Arm and Wrist
	  Muscle, Right
	  Anatomical snuffbox
	  Brachioradialis muscle
	  Extensor carpi radialis
	    muscle
	  Extensor carpi ulnaris
	    muscle
	  Flexor carpi radialis muscle
	  Flexor carpi ulnaris muscle
	  Flexor pollicis longus
	    muscle
	  Palmaris longus muscle
	  Pronator quadratus
	    muscle
	  Pronator teres muscle
	B Lower Arm and Wrist
	  Muscle, Left
	  See 9 Lower Arm and Wrist
	    Muscle, Right
	C Hand Muscle, Right
	  Hypothenar muscle
	  Palmar interosseous
	    muscle
	  Thenar muscle
	D Hand Muscle, Left
	  See C Hand Muscle, Right
	F Trunk Muscle, Right
	  Coccygeus muscle
	  Erector spinae muscle
	  Interspinalis muscle
	  Intertransversarius muscle
	  Latissimus dorsi muscle
	  Quadratus lumborum
	    muscle
	  Rhomboid major muscle
	  Rhomboid minor muscle
	  Serratus posterior muscle
	  Transversospinalis muscle
	  Trapezius muscle
	G Trunk Muscle, Left
	  See F Trunk Muscle, Right
	H Thorax Muscle, Right
	  Intercostal muscle
	  Levatores costarum
	    muscle
	  Pectoralis major muscle
	  Pectoralis minor muscle
	  Serratus anterior muscle
	  Subclavius muscle
	  Subcostal muscle
	  Transverse thoracis muscle
	J Thorax Muscle, Left
	  See H Thorax Muscle, Right
	K Abdomen Muscle, Right
	  External oblique muscle
	  Internal oblique muscle
	  Pyramidalis muscle
	  Rectus abdominis muscle
	  Transversus abdominis
	    muscle
	L Abdomen Muscle, Left
	  See K Abdomen Muscle,
	    Right
		M Perineum Muscle
		  Bulbospongiosus muscle
		  Cremaster muscle
		  Deep transverse perineal
		    muscle
		  Ischiocavernosus muscle
		  Levator ani muscle
		  Superficial transverse
		    perineal muscle
		N Hip Muscle, Right
		  Gemellus muscle
		  Gluteus maximus muscle
		  Gluteus medius muscle
		  Gluteus minimus muscle
		  Iliacus muscle
		  Obturator muscle
		  Piriformis muscle
		  Psoas muscle
		  Quadratus femoris muscle
		  Tensor fasciae latae
		    muscle
		P Hip Muscle, Left
		  See N Hip Muscle, Right
		Q Upper Leg Muscle, Right
		  Adductor brevis muscle
		  Adductor longus muscle
		  Adductor magnus muscle
		  Biceps femoris muscle
		  Gracilis muscle
		  Pectineus muscle
		  Quadriceps (femoris)
		  Rectus femoris muscle
		  Sartorius muscle
		  Semimembranosus
		    muscle
		  Semitendinosus muscle
		  Vastus intermedius muscle
		  Vastus lateralis muscle
		  Vastus medialis muscle
		R Upper Leg Muscle, Left
		  See Q Upper Leg Muscle,
		    Right
		S Lower Leg Muscle, Right
		  Extensor digitorum longus
		    muscle
		  Extensor hallucis longus
		    muscle
		  Fibularis brevis muscle
		  Fibularis longus muscle
		  Flexor digitorum longus
		    muscle
		  Flexor hallucis longus
		    muscle
		  Gastrocnemius muscle
		  Peroneus brevis muscle
		  Peroneus longus muscle
		  Popliteus muscle
		  Soleus muscle
		  Tibialis anterior muscle
		  Tibialis posterior muscle
		T Lower Leg Muscle, Left
		  See S Lower Leg Muscle,
		    Right
		V Foot Muscle, Right
		  Abductor hallucis muscle
		  Adductor hallucis muscle
		  Extensor digitorum brevis
		    muscle
		  Extensor hallucis brevis
		    muscle
		  Flexor digitorum brevis
		    muscle
		  Flexor hallucis brevis
		    muscle
		  Quadratus plantae muscle
		W Foot Muscle, Left
		  See V Foot Muscle, Right
			Ø Open	**Z No Device**	**Z No Qualifier**

LC Limited Coverage   NC Noncovered   ⊞ Combination Member   HAC associated procedure   Combination Only   DRG Non-OR   Non-OR   New/Revised in GREEN

ICD-10-PCS 2020   459

ØKD–ØKD

Ø   **Medical and Surgical**
K   **Muscles**
H   **Insertion**   Definition: Putting in a nonbiological appliance that monitors, assists, performs, or prevents a physiological function but does not physically take the place of a body part

                         Explanation: None

Body Part Character 4	Approach Character 5	Device Character 6	Qualifier Character 7
X Upper Muscle **Y** Lower Muscle	**Ø** Open **3** Percutaneous **4** Percutaneous Endoscopic	**M** Stimulator Lead **Y** Other Device	**Z** No Qualifier

Non-OR   ØKH[X,Y][3,4]YZ

Ø   **Medical and Surgical**
K   **Muscles**
J   **Inspection**   Definition: Visually and/or manually exploring a body part

                         Explanation: Visual exploration may be performed with or without optical instrumentation. Manual exploration may be performed directly or through intervening body layers.

Body Part Character 4	Approach Character 5	Device Character 6	Qualifier Character 7
X Upper Muscle **Y** Lower Muscle	**Ø** Open **3** Percutaneous **4** Percutaneous Endoscopic **X** External	**Z** No Device	**Z** No Qualifier

Non-OR   ØKJ[X,Y][3,X]ZZ

LC Limited Coverage   NC Noncovered   ⊞ Combination Member   HAC associated procedure   Combination Only   DRG Non-OR   Non-OR   New/Revised in **GREEN**

460   ICD-10-PCS 2020

Ø   Medical and Surgical
K   Muscles
M   Reattachment   Definition: Putting back in or on all or a portion of a separated body part to its normal location or other suitable location
                       Explanation: Vascular circulation and nervous pathways may or may not be reestablished

Body Part Character 4			Approach Character 5	Device Character 6	Qualifier Character 7

Ø Head Muscle
  Auricularis muscle
  Masseter muscle
  Pterygoid muscle
  Splenius capitis muscle
  Temporalis muscle
  Temporoparietalis muscle
1 Facial Muscle
  Buccinator muscle
  Corrugator supercilii
    muscle
  Depressor anguli oris
    muscle
  Depressor labii inferioris
    muscle
  Depressor septi nasi
    muscle
  Depressor supercilii
    muscle
  Levator anguli oris muscle
  Levator labii superioris
    alaeque nasi muscle
  Levator labii superioris
    muscle
  Mentalis muscle
  Nasalis muscle
  Occipitofrontalis muscle
  Orbicularis oris muscle
  Procerus muscle
  Risorius muscle
  Zygomaticus muscle
2 Neck Muscle, Right
  Anterior vertebral muscle
  Arytenoid muscle
  Cricothyroid muscle
  Infrahyoid muscle
  Levator scapulae muscle
  Platysma muscle
  Scalene muscle
  Splenius cervicis muscle
  Sternocleidomastoid
    muscle
  Suprahyoid muscle
  Thyroarytenoid muscle
3 Neck Muscle, Left
  See 2 Neck Muscle, Right
**4 Tongue, Palate, Pharynx
  Muscle**
  Chondroglossus muscle
  Genioglossus muscle
  Hyoglossus muscle
  Inferior longitudinal
    muscle
  Levator veli palatini
    muscle
  Palatoglossal muscle
  Palatopharyngeal muscle
  Pharyngeal constrictor
    muscle
  Salpingopharyngeus
    muscle
  Styloglossus muscle
  Stylopharyngeus muscle
  Superior longitudinal
    muscle
  Tensor veli palatini muscle
5 Shoulder Muscle, Right
  Deltoid muscle
  Infraspinatus muscle
  Subscapularis muscle
  Supraspinatus muscle
  Teres major muscle
  Teres minor muscle
6 Shoulder Muscle, Left
  *See 5 Shoulder Muscle,
    Right*
	7 Upper Arm Muscle, Right
	  Biceps brachii muscle
	  Brachialis muscle
	  Coracobrachialis muscle
	  Triceps brachii muscle
	8 Upper Arm Muscle, Left
	  *See 7 Upper Arm Muscle,
	    Right*
	**9 Lower Arm and Wrist
	  Muscle, Right**
	  Anatomical snuffbox
	  Brachioradialis muscle
	  Extensor carpi radialis
	    muscle
	  Extensor carpi ulnaris
	    muscle
	  Flexor carpi radialis muscle
	  Flexor carpi ulnaris muscle
	  Flexor pollicis longus
	    muscle
	  Palmaris longus muscle
	  Pronator quadratus
	    muscle
	  Pronator teres muscle
	**B Lower Arm and Wrist
	  Muscle, Left**
	  *See 9 Lower Arm and Wrist
	    Muscle, Right*
	C Hand Muscle, Right
	  Hypothenar muscle
	  Palmar interosseous
	    muscle
	  Thenar muscle
	D Hand Muscle, Left
	  See C Hand Muscle, Right
	F Trunk Muscle, Right
	  Coccygeus muscle
	  Erector spinae muscle
	  Interspinalis muscle
	  Intertransversarius muscle
	  Latissimus dorsi muscle
	  Quadratus lumborum
	    muscle
	  Rhomboid major muscle
	  Rhomboid minor muscle
	  Serratus posterior muscle
	  Transversospinalis muscle
	  Trapezius muscle
	G Trunk Muscle, Left
	  See F Trunk Muscle, Right
	H Thorax Muscle, Right
	  Intercostal muscle
	  Levatores costarum
	    muscle
	  Pectoralis major muscle
	  Pectoralis minor muscle
	  Serratus anterior muscle
	  Subclavius muscle
	  Subcostal muscle
	  Transverse thoracis muscle
	J Thorax Muscle, Left
	  See H Thorax Muscle, Right
	K Abdomen Muscle, Right
	  External oblique muscle
	  Internal oblique muscle
	  Pyramidalis muscle
	  Rectus abdominis muscle
	  Transversus abdominis
	    muscle
	L Abdomen Muscle, Left
	  *See K Abdomen Muscle,
	    Right*
		M Perineum Muscle
		  Bulbospongiosus muscle
		  Cremaster muscle
		  Deep transverse perineal
		    muscle
		  Ischiocavernosus muscle
		  Levator ani muscle
		  Superficial transverse
		    perineal muscle
		N Hip Muscle, Right
		  Gemellus muscle
		  Gluteus maximus muscle
		  Gluteus medius muscle
		  Gluteus minimus muscle
		  Iliacus muscle
		  Obturator muscle
		  Piriformis muscle
		  Psoas muscle
		  Quadratus femoris muscle
		  Tensor fasciae latae
		    muscle
		P Hip Muscle, Left
		  See N Hip Muscle, Right
		Q Upper Leg Muscle, Right
		  Adductor brevis muscle
		  Adductor longus muscle
		  Adductor magnus muscle
		  Biceps femoris muscle
		  Gracilis muscle
		  Pectineus muscle
		  Quadriceps (femoris)
		  Rectus femoris muscle
		  Sartorius muscle
		  Semimembranosus
		    muscle
		  Semitendinosus muscle
		  Vastus intermedius muscle
		  Vastus lateralis muscle
		  Vastus medialis muscle
		R Upper Leg Muscle, Left
		  *See Q Upper Leg Muscle,
		    Right*
		S Lower Leg Muscle, Right
		  Extensor digitorum longus
		    muscle
		  Extensor hallucis longus
		    muscle
		  Fibularis brevis muscle
		  Fibularis longus muscle
		  Flexor digitorum longus
		    muscle
		  Flexor hallucis longus
		    muscle
		  Gastrocnemius muscle
		  Peroneus brevis muscle
		  Peroneus longus muscle
		  Popliteus muscle
		  Soleus muscle
		  Tibialis anterior muscle
		  Tibialis posterior muscle
		T Lower Leg Muscle, Left
		  *See S Lower Leg Muscle,
		    Right*
		V Foot Muscle, Right
		  Abductor hallucis muscle
		  Adductor hallucis muscle
		  Extensor digitorum brevis
		    muscle
		  Extensor hallucis brevis
		    muscle
		  Flexor digitorum brevis
		    muscle
		  Flexor hallucis brevis
		    muscle
		  Quadratus plantae muscle
		W Foot Muscle, Left
		  See V Foot Muscle, Right
			Ø Open
			**4 Percutaneous
			  Endoscopic**
				Z No Device	**Z No Qualifier**

Ø **Medical and Surgical**
K **Muscles**
N **Release**

Definition: Freeing a body part from an abnormal physical constraint by cutting or by the use of force
Explanation: Some of the restraining tissue may be taken out but none of the body part is taken out

Body Part Character 4			Approach Character 5	Device Character 6	Qualifier Character 7
Ø Head Muscle Auricularis muscle Masseter muscle Pterygoid muscle Splenius capitis muscle Temporalis muscle Temporoparietalis muscle **1 Facial Muscle** Buccinator muscle Corrugator supercilii muscle Depressor anguli oris muscle Depressor labii inferioris muscle Depressor septi nasi muscle Depressor supercilii muscle Levator anguli oris muscle Levator labii superioris alaeque nasi muscle Levator labii superioris muscle Mentalis muscle Nasalis muscle Occipitofrontalis muscle Orbicularis oris muscle Procerus muscle Risorius muscle Zygomaticus muscle **2 Neck Muscle, Right** Anterior vertebral muscle Arytenoid muscle Cricothyroid muscle Infrahyoid muscle Levator scapulae muscle Platysma muscle Scalene muscle Splenius cervicis muscle Sternocleidomastoid muscle Suprahyoid muscle Thyroarytenoid muscle **3 Neck Muscle, Left** *See 2 Neck Muscle, Right* **4 Tongue, Palate, Pharynx Muscle** Chondroglossus muscle Genioglossus muscle Hyoglossus muscle Inferior longitudinal muscle Levator veli palatini muscle Palatoglossus muscle Palatopharyngeal muscle Pharyngeal constrictor muscle Salpingopharyngeus muscle Styloglossus muscle Stylopharyngeus muscle Superior longitudinal muscle Tensor veli palatini muscle **5 Shoulder Muscle, Right** Deltoid muscle Infraspinatus muscle Subscapularis muscle Supraspinatus muscle Teres major muscle Teres minor muscle **6 Shoulder Muscle, Left** *See 5 Shoulder Muscle, Right*	**7 Upper Arm Muscle, Right** Biceps brachii muscle Brachialis muscle Coracobrachialis muscle Triceps brachii muscle **8 Upper Arm Muscle, Left** *See 7 Upper Arm Muscle, Right* **9 Lower Arm and Wrist Muscle, Right** Anatomical snuffbox Brachioradialis muscle Extensor carpi radialis muscle Extensor carpi ulnaris muscle Flexor carpi radialis muscle Flexor carpi ulnaris muscle Flexor pollicis longus muscle Palmaris longus muscle Pronator quadratus muscle Pronator teres muscle **B Lower Arm and Wrist Muscle, Left** *See 9 Lower Arm and Wrist Muscle, Right* **C Hand Muscle, Right** Hypothenar muscle Palmar interosseous muscle Thenar muscle **D Hand Muscle, Left** *See C Hand Muscle, Right* **F Trunk Muscle, Right** Coccygeus muscle Erector spinae muscle Interspinalis muscle Intertransversarius muscle Latissimus dorsi muscle Quadratus lumborum muscle Rhomboid major muscle Rhomboid minor muscle Serratus posterior muscle Transversospinalis muscle Trapezius muscle **G Trunk Muscle, Left** *See F Trunk Muscle, Right* **H Thorax Muscle, Right** Intercostal muscle Levatores costarum muscle Pectoralis major muscle Pectoralis minor muscle Serratus anterior muscle Subclavius muscle Subcostal muscle Transverse thoracis muscle **J Thorax Muscle, Left** *See H Thorax Muscle, Right* **K Abdomen Muscle, Right** External oblique muscle Internal oblique muscle Pyramidalis muscle Rectus abdominis muscle Transversus abdominis muscle **L Abdomen Muscle, Left** *See K Abdomen Muscle, Right*	**M Perineum Muscle** Bulbospongiosus muscle Cremaster muscle Deep transverse perineal muscle Ischiocavernosus muscle Levator ani muscle Superficial transverse perineal muscle **N Hip Muscle, Right** Gemellus muscle Gluteus maximus muscle Gluteus medius muscle Gluteus minimus muscle Iliacus muscle Obturator muscle Piriformis muscle Psoas muscle Quadratus femoris muscle Tensor fasciae latae muscle **P Hip Muscle, Left** *See N Hip Muscle, Right* **Q Upper Leg Muscle, Right** Adductor brevis muscle Adductor longus muscle Adductor magnus muscle Biceps femoris muscle Gracilis muscle Pectineus muscle Quadriceps (femoris) Rectus femoris muscle Sartorius muscle Semimembranosus muscle Semitendinosus muscle Vastus intermedius muscle Vastus lateralis muscle Vastus medialis muscle **R Upper Leg Muscle, Left** *See Q Upper Leg Muscle, Right* **S Lower Leg Muscle, Right** Extensor digitorum longus muscle Extensor hallucis longus muscle Fibularis brevis muscle Fibularis longus muscle Flexor digitorum longus muscle Flexor hallucis longus muscle Gastrocnemius muscle Peroneus brevis muscle Peroneus longus muscle Popliteus muscle Soleus muscle Tibialis anterior muscle Tibialis posterior muscle **T Lower Leg Muscle, Left** *See S Lower Leg Muscle, Right* **V Foot Muscle, Right** Abductor hallucis muscle Adductor hallucis muscle Extensor digitorum brevis muscle Extensor hallucis brevis muscle Flexor digitorum brevis muscle Flexor hallucis brevis muscle Quadratus plantae muscle **W Foot Muscle, Left** *See V Foot Muscle, Right*	**Ø** Open **3** Percutaneous **4** Percutaneous Endoscopic **X** External	**Z** No Device	**Z** No Qualifier

Non-OR   ØKN[Ø,1,2,3,4,5,6,7,8,9,B,C,D,F,G,H,J,K,L,M,N,P,Q,R,S,T,V,W]XZZ

LC Limited Coverage   NC Noncovered   ⊞ Combination Member   HAC associated procedure   Combination Only   DRG Non-OR   Non-OR   New/Revised in GREEN

Ø   Medical and Surgical
K   Muscles
P   Removal   Definition: Taking out or off a device from a body part

                  Explanation: If a device is taken out and a similar device put in without cutting or puncturing the skin or mucous membrane, the procedure is coded to the root operation CHANGE. Otherwise, the procedure for taking out a device is coded to the root operation REMOVAL.

Body Part Character 4	Approach Character 5	Device Character 6	Qualifier Character 7
X Upper Muscle **Y** Lower Muscle	**Ø** Open **3** Percutaneous **4** Percutaneous Endoscopic	**Ø** Drainage Device **7** Autologous Tissue Substitute **J** Synthetic Substitute **K** Nonautologous Tissue Substitute **M** Stimulator Lead **Y** Other Device	**Z** No Qualifier
X Upper Muscle **Y** Lower Muscle	**X** External	**Ø** Drainage Device **M** Stimulator Lead	**Z** No Qualifier

    Non-OR   ØKP[X,Y][3,4]YZ
    Non-OR   ØKP[X,Y]X[Ø,M]Z

Ø   **Medical and Surgical**
K   **Muscles**
Q   **Repair**   Definition: Restoring, to the extent possible, a body part to its normal anatomic structure and function
                 Explanation: Used only when the method to accomplish the repair is not one of the other root operations

Body Part Character 4			Approach Character 5	Device Character 6	Qualifier Character 7

Ø **Head Muscle**
  Auricularis muscle
  Masseter muscle
  Pterygoid muscle
  Splenius capitis muscle
  Temporalis muscle
  Temporoparietalis muscle
1 **Facial Muscle**
  Buccinator muscle
  Corrugator supercilii
    muscle
  Depressor anguli oris
    muscle
  Depressor labii inferioris
    muscle
  Depressor septi nasi
    muscle
  Depressor supercilii
    muscle
  Levator anguli oris muscle
  Levator labii superioris
    alaeque nasi muscle
  Levator labii superioris
    muscle
  Mentalis muscle
  Nasalis muscle
  Occipitofrontalis muscle
  Orbicularis oris muscle
  Procerus muscle
  Risorius muscle
  Zygomaticus muscle
2 **Neck Muscle, Right**
  Anterior vertebral muscle
  Arytenoid muscle
  Cricothyroid muscle
  Infrahyoid muscle
  Levator scapulae muscle
  Platysma muscle
  Scalene muscle
  Splenius cervicis muscle
  Sternocleidomastoid
    muscle
  Suprahyoid muscle
  Thyroarytenoid muscle
3 **Neck Muscle, Left**
  See 2 Neck Muscle, Right
4 **Tongue, Palate, Pharynx**
  Muscle
  Chondroglossus muscle
  Genioglossus muscle
  Hyoglossus muscle
  Inferior longitudinal
    muscle
  Levator veli palatini
    muscle
  Palatoglossal muscle
  Palatopharyngeal muscle
  Pharyngeal constrictor
    muscle
  Salpingopharyngeus
    muscle
  Styloglossus muscle
  Stylopharyngeus muscle
  Superior longitudinal
    muscle
  Tensor veli palatini muscle
5 **Shoulder Muscle, Right**
  Deltoid muscle
  Infraspinatus muscle
  Subscapularis muscle
  Supraspinatus muscle
  Teres major muscle
  Teres minor muscle
6 **Shoulder Muscle, Left**
  See 5 Shoulder Muscle,
    Right
	7 **Upper Arm Muscle, Right**
	  Biceps brachii muscle
	  Brachialis muscle
	  Coracobrachialis muscle
	  Triceps brachii muscle
	8 **Upper Arm Muscle, Left**
	  See 7 Upper Arm Muscle,
	    Right
	9 **Lower Arm and Wrist**
	  Muscle, Right
	  Anatomical snuffbox
	  Brachioradialis muscle
	  Extensor carpi radialis
	    muscle
	  Extensor carpi ulnaris
	    muscle
	  Flexor carpi radialis muscle
	  Flexor carpi ulnaris muscle
	  Flexor pollicis longus
	    muscle
	  Palmaris longus muscle
	  Pronator quadratus
	    muscle
	  Pronator teres muscle
	B **Lower Arm and Wrist**
	  Muscle, Left
	  See 9 Lower Arm and Wrist
	    Muscle, Right
	C **Hand Muscle, Right**
	  Hypothenar muscle
	  Palmar interosseous
	    muscle
	  Thenar muscle
	D **Hand Muscle, Left**
	  See C Hand Muscle, Right
	F **Trunk Muscle, Right**
	  Coccygeus muscle
	  Erector spinae muscle
	  Interspinalis muscle
	  Intertransversarius muscle
	  Latissimus dorsi muscle
	  Quadratus lumborum
	    muscle
	  Rhomboid major muscle
	  Rhomboid minor muscle
	  Serratus posterior muscle
	  Transversospinalis muscle
	  Trapezius muscle
	G **Trunk Muscle, Left**
	  See F Trunk Muscle, Right
	H **Thorax Muscle, Right**
	  Intercostal muscle
	  Levatores costarum
	    muscle
	  Pectoralis major muscle
	  Pectoralis minor muscle
	  Serratus anterior muscle
	  Subclavius muscle
	  Subcostal muscle
	  Transverse thoracis muscle
	J **Thorax Muscle, Left**
	  See H Thorax Muscle, Right
	K **Abdomen Muscle, Right**
	  External oblique muscle
	  Internal oblique muscle
	  Pyramidalis muscle
	  Rectus abdominis muscle
	  Transversus abdominis
	    muscle
	L **Abdomen Muscle, Left**
	  See K Abdomen Muscle,
	    Right
		M **Perineum Muscle**
		  Bulbospongiosus muscle
		  Cremaster muscle
		  Deep transverse perineal
		    muscle
		  Ischiocavernosus muscle
		  Levator ani muscle
		  Superficial transverse
		    perineal muscle
		N **Hip Muscle, Right**
		  Gemellus muscle
		  Gluteus maximus muscle
		  Gluteus medius muscle
		  Gluteus minimus muscle
		  Iliacus muscle
		  Obturator muscle
		  Piriformis muscle
		  Psoas muscle
		  Quadratus femoris muscle
		  Tensor fasciae latae
		    muscle
		P **Hip Muscle, Left**
		  See N Hip Muscle, Right
		Q **Upper Leg Muscle, Right**
		  Adductor brevis muscle
		  Adductor longus muscle
		  Adductor magnus muscle
		  Biceps femoris muscle
		  Gracilis muscle
		  Pectineus muscle
		  Quadriceps (femoris)
		  Rectus femoris muscle
		  Sartorius muscle
		  Semimembranosus
		    muscle
		  Semitendinosus muscle
		  Vastus intermedius muscle
		  Vastus lateralis muscle
		  Vastus medialis muscle
		R **Upper Leg Muscle, Left**
		  See Q Upper Leg Muscle,
		    Right
		S **Lower Leg Muscle, Right**
		  Extensor digitorum longus
		    muscle
		  Extensor hallucis longus
		    muscle
		  Fibularis brevis muscle
		  Fibularis longus muscle
		  Flexor digitorum longus
		    muscle
		  Flexor hallucis longus
		    muscle
		  Gastrocnemius muscle
		  Peroneus brevis muscle
		  Peroneus longus muscle
		  Popliteus muscle
		  Soleus muscle
		  Tibialis anterior muscle
		  Tibialis posterior muscle
		T **Lower Leg Muscle, Left**
		  See S Lower Leg Muscle,
		    Right
		V **Foot Muscle, Right**
		  Abductor hallucis muscle
		  Adductor hallucis muscle
		  Extensor digitorum brevis
		    muscle
		  Extensor hallucis brevis
		    muscle
		  Flexor digitorum brevis
		    muscle
		  Flexor hallucis brevis
		    muscle
		  Quadratus plantae muscle
		W **Foot Muscle, Left**
		  See V Foot Muscle, Right
			Ø Open
			3 Percutaneous
			4 Percutaneous
			    Endoscopic
				Z No Device	**Z** No Qualifier

LC Limited Coverage   **NC** Noncovered   ⊞ Combination Member   HAC associated procedure   Combination Only   DRG Non-OR   Non-OR   New/Revised in **GREEN**

464   ICD-10-PCS 2020

ØKQ–ØKQ

Ø Medical and Surgical
K Muscles
R Replacement   Definition: Putting in or on biological or synthetic material that physically takes the place and/or function of all or a portion of a body part

Explanation: The body part may have been taken out or replaced, or may be taken out, physically eradicated, or rendered nonfunctional during the REPLACEMENT procedure. A REMOVAL procedure is coded for taking out the device used in a previous replacement procedure.

Body Part Character 4			Approach Character 5	Device Character 6	Qualifier Character 7
Ø Head Muscle Auricularis muscle Masseter muscle Pterygoid muscle Splenius capitis muscle Temporalis muscle Temporoparietalis muscle **1 Facial Muscle** Buccinator muscle Corrugator supercilii muscle Depressor anguli oris muscle Depressor labii inferioris muscle Depressor septi nasi muscle Depressor supercilii muscle Levator anguli oris muscle Levator labii superioris alaeque nasi muscle Levator labii superioris muscle Mentalis muscle Nasalis muscle Occipitofrontalis muscle Orbicularis oris muscle Procerus muscle Risorius muscle Zygomaticus muscle **2 Neck Muscle, Right** Anterior vertebral muscle Arytenoid muscle Cricothyroid muscle Infrahyoid muscle Levator scapulae muscle Platysma muscle Scalene muscle Splenius cervicis muscle Sternocleidomastoid muscle Suprahyoid muscle Thyroarytenoid muscle **3 Neck Muscle, Left** *See 2 Neck Muscle, Right* **4 Tongue, Palate, Pharynx Muscle** Chondroglossus muscle Genioglossus muscle Hyoglossus muscle Inferior longitudinal muscle Levator veli palatini muscle Palatoglossal muscle Palatopharyngeal muscle Pharyngeal constrictor muscle Salpingopharyngeus muscle Styloglossus muscle Stylopharyngeus muscle Superior longitudinal muscle Tensor veli palatini muscle **5 Shoulder Muscle, Right** Deltoid muscle Infraspinatus muscle Subscapularis muscle Supraspinatus muscle Teres major muscle Teres minor muscle **6 Shoulder Muscle, Left** *See 5 Shoulder Muscle, Right*	**7 Upper Arm Muscle, Right** Biceps brachii muscle Brachialis muscle Coracobrachialis muscle Triceps brachii muscle **8 Upper Arm Muscle, Left** *See 7 Upper Arm Muscle, Right* **9 Lower Arm and Wrist Muscle, Right** Anatomical snuffbox Brachioradialis muscle Extensor carpi radialis muscle Extensor carpi ulnaris muscle Flexor carpi radialis muscle Flexor carpi ulnaris muscle Flexor pollicis longus muscle Palmaris longus muscle Pronator quadratus muscle Pronator teres muscle **B Lower Arm and Wrist Muscle, Left** *See 9 Lower Arm and Wrist Muscle, Right* **C Hand Muscle, Right** Hypothenar muscle Palmar interosseous muscle Thenar muscle **D Hand Muscle, Left** *See C Hand Muscle, Right* **F Trunk Muscle, Right** Coccygeus muscle Erector spinae muscle Interspinalis muscle Intertransversarius muscle Latissimus dorsi muscle Quadratus lumborum muscle Rhomboid major muscle Rhomboid minor muscle Serratus posterior muscle Transversospinalis muscle Trapezius muscle **G Trunk Muscle, Left** *See F Trunk Muscle, Right* **H Thorax Muscle, Right** Intercostal muscle Levatores costarum muscle Pectoralis major muscle Pectoralis minor muscle Serratus anterior muscle Subclavius muscle Subcostal muscle Transverse thoracis muscle **J Thorax Muscle, Left** *See H Thorax Muscle, Right* **K Abdomen Muscle, Right** External oblique muscle Internal oblique muscle Pyramidalis muscle Rectus abdominis muscle Transversus abdominis muscle **L Abdomen Muscle, Left** *See K Abdomen Muscle, Right*	**M Perineum Muscle** Bulbospongiosus muscle Cremaster muscle Deep transverse perineal muscle Ischiocavernosus muscle Levator ani muscle Superficial transverse perineal muscle **N Hip Muscle, Right** Gemellus muscle Gluteus maximus muscle Gluteus medius muscle Gluteus minimus muscle Iliacus muscle Obturator muscle Piriformis muscle Psoas muscle Quadratus femoris muscle Tensor fasciae latae muscle **P Hip Muscle, Left** *See N Hip Muscle, Right* **Q Upper Leg Muscle, Right** Adductor brevis muscle Adductor longus muscle Adductor magnus muscle Biceps femoris muscle Gracilis muscle Pectineus muscle Quadriceps (femoris) Rectus femoris muscle Sartorius muscle Semimembranosus muscle Semitendinosus muscle Vastus intermedius muscle Vastus lateralis muscle Vastus medialis muscle **R Upper Leg Muscle, Left** *See Q Upper Leg Muscle, Right* **S Lower Leg Muscle, Right** Extensor digitorum longus muscle Extensor hallucis longus muscle Fibularis brevis muscle Fibularis longus muscle Flexor digitorum longus muscle Flexor hallucis longus muscle Gastrocnemius muscle Peroneus brevis muscle Peroneus longus muscle Popliteus muscle Soleus muscle Tibialis anterior muscle Tibialis posterior muscle **T Lower Leg Muscle, Left** *See S Lower Leg Muscle, Right* **V Foot Muscle, Right** Abductor hallucis muscle Adductor hallucis muscle Extensor digitorum brevis muscle Extensor hallucis brevis muscle Flexor digitorum brevis muscle Flexor hallucis brevis muscle Quadratus plantae muscle **W Foot Muscle, Left** *See V Foot Muscle, Right*	**Ø Open** **4 Percutaneous Endoscopic**	**7 Autologous Tissue Substitute** **J Synthetic Substitute** **K Nonautologous Tissue Substitute**	**Z No Qualifier**

🔳 Limited Coverage   🆖 Noncovered   ⊞ Combination Member   HAC associated procedure   Combination Only   DRG Non-OR   Non-OR   New/Revised in GREEN

ICD-10-PCS 2020   465

ØKR–ØKR

Ø **Medical and Surgical**
K **Muscles**
S **Reposition** Definition: Moving to its normal location, or other suitable location, all or a portion of a body part

Explanation: The body part is moved to a new location from an abnormal location, or from a normal location where it is not functioning correctly. The body part may or may not be cut out or off to be moved to the new location.

Body Part Character 4			Approach Character 5	Device Character 6	Qualifier Character 7

Ø Head Muscle
Auricularis muscle
Masseter muscle
Pterygoid muscle
Splenius capitis muscle
Temporalis muscle
Temporoparietalis muscle
1 Facial Muscle
Buccinator muscle
Corrugator supercilii
  muscle
Depressor anguli oris
  muscle
Depressor labii inferioris
  muscle
Depressor septi nasi
  muscle
Depressor supercilii
  muscle
Levator anguli oris muscle
Levator labii superioris
  alaeque nasi muscle
Levator labii superioris
  muscle
Mentalis muscle
Nasalis muscle
Occipitofrontalis muscle
Orbicularis oris muscle
Procerus muscle
Risorius muscle
Zygomaticus muscle
2 Neck Muscle, Right
Anterior vertebral muscle
Arytenoid muscle
Cricothyroid muscle
Infrahyoid muscle
Levator scapulae muscle
Platysma muscle
Scalene muscle
Splenius cervicis muscle
Sternocleidomastoid
  muscle
Suprahyoid muscle
Thyroarytenoid muscle
3 Neck Muscle, Left
See 2 Neck Muscle, Right
4 Tongue, Palate, Pharynx
Muscle
Chondroglossus muscle
Genioglossus muscle
Hyoglossus muscle
Inferior longitudinal
  muscle
Levator veli palatini
  muscle
Palatoglossal muscle
Palatopharyngeal muscle
Pharyngeal constrictor
  muscle
Salpingopharyngeus
  muscle
Styloglossus muscle
Stylopharyngeus muscle
Superior longitudinal
  muscle
Tensor veli palatini muscle
5 Shoulder Muscle, Right
Deltoid muscle
Infraspinatus muscle
Subscapularis muscle
Supraspinatus muscle
Teres major muscle
Teres minor muscle
6 Shoulder Muscle, Left
See 5 Shoulder Muscle,
Right
	7 Upper Arm Muscle, Right
	Biceps brachii muscle
	Brachialis muscle
	Coracobrachialis muscle
	Triceps brachii muscle
	8 Upper Arm Muscle, Left
	See 7 Upper Arm Muscle,
	Right
	9 Lower Arm and Wrist
	Muscle, Right
	Anatomical snuffbox
	Brachioradialis muscle
	Extensor carpi radialis
	  muscle
	Extensor carpi ulnaris
	  muscle
	Flexor carpi radialis muscle
	Flexor carpi ulnaris muscle
	Flexor pollicis longus
	  muscle
	Palmaris longus muscle
	Pronator quadratus
	  muscle
	Pronator teres muscle
	B Lower Arm and Wrist
	Muscle, Left
	See 9 Lower Arm and Wrist
	Muscle, Right
	C Hand Muscle, Right
	Hypothenar muscle
	Palmar interosseous
	  muscle
	Thenar muscle
	D Hand Muscle, Left
	See C Hand Muscle, Right
	F Trunk Muscle, Right
	Coccygeus muscle
	Erector spinae muscle
	Interspinalis muscle
	Intertransversarius muscle
	Latissimus dorsi muscle
	Quadratus lumborum
	  muscle
	Rhomboid major muscle
	Rhomboid minor muscle
	Serratus posterior muscle
	Transversospinalis muscle
	Trapezius muscle
	G Trunk Muscle, Left
	See F Trunk Muscle, Right
	H Thorax Muscle, Right
	Intercostal muscle
	Levatores costarum
	  muscle
	Pectoralis major muscle
	Pectoralis minor muscle
	Serratus anterior muscle
	Subclavius muscle
	Subcostal muscle
	Transverse thoracis muscle
	J Thorax Muscle, Left
	See H Thorax Muscle, Right
	K Abdomen Muscle, Right
	External oblique muscle
	Internal oblique muscle
	Pyramidalis muscle
	Rectus abdominis muscle
	Transversus abdominis
	  muscle
	L Abdomen Muscle, Left
	See K Abdomen Muscle,
	Right
		M Perineum Muscle
		Bulbospongiosus muscle
		Cremaster muscle
		Deep transverse perineal
		  muscle
		Ischiocavernosus muscle
		Levator ani muscle
		Superficial transverse
		  perineal muscle
		N Hip Muscle, Right
		Gemellus muscle
		Gluteus maximus muscle
		Gluteus medius muscle
		Gluteus minimus muscle
		Iliacus muscle
		Obturator muscle
		Piriformis muscle
		Psoas muscle
		Quadratus femoris muscle
		Tensor fasciae latae
		  muscle
		P Hip Muscle, Left
		See N Hip Muscle, Right
		Q Upper Leg Muscle, Right
		Adductor brevis muscle
		Adductor longus muscle
		Adductor magnus muscle
		Biceps femoris muscle
		Gracilis muscle
		Pectineus muscle
		Quadriceps (femoris)
		Rectus femoris muscle
		Sartorius muscle
		Semimembranosus
		  muscle
		Semitendinosus muscle
		Vastus intermedius muscle
		Vastus lateralis muscle
		Vastus medialis muscle
		R Upper Leg Muscle, Left
		See Q Upper Leg Muscle,
		Right
		S Lower Leg Muscle, Right
		Extensor digitorum longus
		  muscle
		Extensor hallucis longus
		  muscle
		Fibularis brevis muscle
		Fibularis longus muscle
		Flexor digitorum longus
		  muscle
		Flexor hallucis longus
		  muscle
		Gastrocnemius muscle
		Peroneus brevis muscle
		Peroneus longus muscle
		Popliteus muscle
		Soleus muscle
		Tibialis anterior muscle
		Tibialis posterior muscle
		T Lower Leg Muscle, Left
		See S Lower Leg Muscle,
		Right
		V Foot Muscle, Right
		Abductor hallucis muscle
		Adductor hallucis muscle
		Extensor digitorum brevis
		  muscle
		Extensor hallucis brevis
		  muscle
		Flexor digitorum brevis
		  muscle
		Flexor hallucis brevis
		  muscle
		Quadratus plantae muscle
		W Foot Muscle, Left
		See V Foot Muscle, Right
			Ø Open
			4 Percutaneous
			Endoscopic
				Z No Device	**Z No Qualifier**

LC Limited Coverage   NC Noncovered   ⊞ Combination Member   HAC associated procedure   Combination Only   DRG Non-OR   Non-OR   New/Revised in GREEN

466   ICD-10-PCS 2020

Ø   Medical and Surgical
K   Muscles
T   Resection   Definition: Cutting out or off, without replacement, all of a body part
              Explanation: None

Body Part Character 4			Approach Character 5	Device Character 6	Qualifier Character 7
Ø Head Muscle Auricularis muscle Masseter muscle Pterygoid muscle Splenius capitis muscle Temporalis muscle Temporoparietalis muscle **1 Facial Muscle** Buccinator muscle Corrugator supercilii muscle Depressor anguli oris muscle Depressor labii inferioris muscle Depressor septi nasi muscle Depressor supercilii muscle Levator anguli oris muscle Levator labii superioris alaeque nasi muscle Levator labii superioris muscle Mentalis muscle Nasalis muscle Occipitofrontalis muscle Orbicularis oris muscle Procerus muscle Risorius muscle Zygomaticus muscle **2 Neck Muscle, Right** Anterior vertebral muscle Arytenoid muscle Cricothyroid muscle Infrahyoid muscle Levator scapulae muscle Platysma muscle Scalene muscle Splenius cervicis muscle Sternocleidomastoid muscle Suprahyoid muscle Thyroarytenoid muscle **3 Neck Muscle, Left** *See 2 Neck Muscle, Right* **4 Tongue, Palate, Pharynx Muscle** Chondroglossus muscle Genioglossus muscle Hyoglossus muscle Inferior longitudinal muscle Levator veli palatini muscle Palatoglossal muscle Palatopharyngeal muscle Pharyngeal constrictor muscle Salpingopharyngeus muscle Styloglossus muscle Stylopharyngeus muscle Superior longitudinal muscle Tensor veli palatini muscle **5 Shoulder Muscle, Right** Deltoid muscle Infraspinatus muscle Subscapularis muscle Supraspinatus muscle Teres major muscle Teres minor muscle **6 Shoulder Muscle, Left** *See 5 Shoulder Muscle, Right*	**7 Upper Arm Muscle, Right** Biceps brachii muscle Brachialis muscle Coracobrachialis muscle Triceps brachii muscle **8 Upper Arm Muscle, Left** *See 7 Upper Arm Muscle, Right* **9 Lower Arm and Wrist Muscle, Right** Anatomical snuffbox Brachioradialis muscle Extensor carpi radialis muscle Extensor carpi ulnaris muscle Flexor carpi radialis muscle Flexor carpi ulnaris muscle Flexor pollicis longus muscle Palmaris longus muscle Pronator quadratus muscle Pronator teres muscle **B Lower Arm and Wrist Muscle, Left** *See 9 Lower Arm and Wrist Muscle, Right* **C Hand Muscle, Right** Hypothenar muscle Palmar interosseous muscle Thenar muscle **D Hand Muscle, Left** *See C Hand Muscle, Right* **F Trunk Muscle, Right** Coccygeus muscle Erector spinae muscle Interspinalis muscle Intertransversarius muscle Latissimus dorsi muscle Quadratus lumborum muscle Rhomboid major muscle Rhomboid minor muscle Serratus posterior muscle Transversospinalis muscle Trapezius muscle **G Trunk Muscle, Left** *See F Trunk Muscle, Right* **H Thorax Muscle, Right** ⊞ Intercostal muscle Levatores costarum muscle Pectoralis major muscle Pectoralis minor muscle Serratus anterior muscle Subclavius muscle Subcostal muscle Transverse thoracis muscle **J Thorax Muscle, Left** ⊞ *See H Thorax Muscle, Right* **K Abdomen Muscle, Right** External oblique muscle Internal oblique muscle Pyramidalis muscle Rectus abdominis muscle Transversus abdominis muscle **L Abdomen Muscle, Left** *See K Abdomen Muscle, Right*	**M Perineum Muscle** Bulbospongiosus muscle Cremaster muscle Deep transverse perineal muscle Ischiocavernosus muscle Levator ani muscle Superficial transverse perineal muscle **N Hip Muscle, Right** Gemellus muscle Gluteus maximus muscle Gluteus medius muscle Gluteus minimus muscle Iliacus muscle Obturator muscle Piriformis muscle Psoas muscle Quadratus femoris muscle Tensor fasciae latae muscle **P Hip Muscle, Left** *See N Hip Muscle, Right* **Q Upper Leg Muscle, Right** Adductor brevis muscle Adductor longus muscle Adductor magnus muscle Biceps femoris muscle Gracilis muscle Pectineus muscle Quadriceps (femoris) Rectus femoris muscle Sartorius muscle Semimembranosus muscle Semitendinosus muscle Vastus intermedius muscle Vastus lateralis muscle Vastus medialis muscle **R Upper Leg Muscle, Left** *See Q Upper Leg Muscle, Right* **S Lower Leg Muscle, Right** Extensor digitorum longus muscle Extensor hallucis longus muscle Fibularis brevis muscle Fibularis longus muscle Flexor digitorum longus muscle Flexor hallucis longus muscle Gastrocnemius muscle Peroneus brevis muscle Peroneus longus muscle Popliteus muscle Soleus muscle Tibialis anterior muscle Tibialis posterior muscle **T Lower Leg Muscle, Left** *See S Lower Leg Muscle, Right* **V Foot Muscle, Right** Abductor hallucis muscle Adductor hallucis muscle Extensor digitorum brevis muscle Extensor hallucis brevis muscle Flexor digitorum brevis muscle Flexor hallucis brevis muscle Quadratus plantae muscle **W Foot Muscle, Left** *See V Foot Muscle, Right*	**Ø Open** **4 Percutaneous Endoscopic**	**Z No Device**	**Z No Qualifier**

See Appendix L for Procedure Combinations
     ⊞   ØKT[H,J]ØZZ

Ø Medical and Surgical
K Muscles
U Supplement

Definition: Putting in or on biological or synthetic material that physically reinforces and/or augments the function of a portion of a body part

Explanation: The biological material is non-living, or is living and from the same individual. The body part may have been previously replaced, and the SUPPLEMENT procedure is performed to physically reinforce and/or augment the function of the replaced body part.

Body Part Character 4			Approach Character 5	Device Character 6	Qualifier Character 7
Ø Head Muscle Auricularis muscle Masseter muscle Pterygoid muscle Splenius capitis muscle Temporalis muscle Temporoparietalis muscle **1 Facial Muscle** Buccinator muscle Corrugator supercilii muscle Depressor anguli oris muscle Depressor labii inferioris muscle Depressor septi nasi muscle Depressor supercilii muscle Levator anguli oris muscle Levator labii superioris alaeque nasi muscle Levator labii superioris muscle Mentalis muscle Nasalis muscle Occipitofrontalis muscle Orbicularis oris muscle Procerus muscle Risorius muscle Zygomaticus muscle **2 Neck Muscle, Right** Anterior vertebral muscle Arytenoid muscle Cricothyroid muscle Infrahyoid muscle Levator scapulae muscle Platysma muscle Scalene muscle Splenius cervicis muscle Sternocleidomastoid muscle Suprahyoid muscle Thyroarytenoid muscle **3 Neck Muscle, Left** *See 2 Neck Muscle, Right* **4 Tongue, Palate, Pharynx Muscle** Chondroglossus muscle Genioglossus muscle Hyoglossus muscle Inferior longitudinal muscle Levator veli palatini muscle Palatoglossal muscle Palatopharyngeal muscle Pharyngeal constrictor muscle Salpingopharyngeus muscle Styloglossus muscle Stylopharyngeus muscle Superior longitudinal muscle Tensor veli palatini muscle **5 Shoulder Muscle, Right** Deltoid muscle Infraspinatus muscle Subscapularis muscle Supraspinatus muscle Teres major muscle Teres minor muscle **6 Shoulder Muscle, Left** *See 5 Shoulder Muscle, Right*	**7 Upper Arm Muscle, Right** Biceps brachii muscle Brachialis muscle Coracobrachialis muscle Triceps brachii muscle **8 Upper Arm Muscle, Left** *See 7 Upper Arm Muscle, Right* **9 Lower Arm and Wrist Muscle, Right** Anatomical snuffbox Brachioradialis muscle Extensor carpi radialis muscle Extensor carpi ulnaris muscle Flexor carpi radialis muscle Flexor carpi ulnaris muscle Flexor pollicis longus muscle Palmaris longus muscle Pronator quadratus muscle Pronator teres muscle **B Lower Arm and Wrist Muscle, Left** *See 9 Lower Arm and Wrist Muscle, Right* **C Hand Muscle, Right** Hypothenar muscle Palmar interosseous muscle Thenar muscle **D Hand Muscle, Left** *See C Hand Muscle, Right* **F Trunk Muscle, Right** Coccygeus muscle Erector spinae muscle Interspinalis muscle Intertransversarius muscle Latissimus dorsi muscle Quadratus lumborum muscle Rhomboid major muscle Rhomboid minor muscle Serratus posterior muscle Transversospinalis muscle Trapezius muscle **G Trunk Muscle, Left** *See F Trunk Muscle, Right* **H Thorax Muscle, Right** Intercostal muscle Levatores costarum muscle Pectoralis major muscle Pectoralis minor muscle Serratus anterior muscle Subclavius muscle Subcostal muscle Transverse thoracis muscle **J Thorax Muscle, Left** *See H Thorax Muscle, Right* **K Abdomen Muscle, Right** External oblique muscle Internal oblique muscle Pyramidalis muscle Rectus abdominis muscle Transversus abdominis muscle **L Abdomen Muscle, Left** *See K Abdomen Muscle, Right*	**M Perineum Muscle** Bulbospongiosus muscle Cremaster muscle Deep transverse perineal muscle Ischiocavernosus muscle Levator ani muscle Superficial transverse perineal muscle **N Hip Muscle, Right** Gemellus muscle Gluteus maximus muscle Gluteus medius muscle Gluteus minimus muscle Iliacus muscle Obturator muscle Piriformis muscle Psoas muscle Quadratus femoris muscle Tensor fasciae latae muscle **P Hip Muscle, Left** *See N Hip Muscle, Right* **Q Upper Leg Muscle, Right** Adductor brevis muscle Adductor longus muscle Adductor magnus muscle Biceps femoris muscle Gracilis muscle Pectineus muscle Quadriceps (femoris) Rectus femoris muscle Sartorius muscle Semimembranosus muscle Semitendinosus muscle Vastus intermedius muscle Vastus lateralis muscle Vastus medialis muscle **R Upper Leg Muscle, Left** *See Q Upper Leg Muscle, Right* **S Lower Leg Muscle, Right** Extensor digitorum longus muscle Extensor hallucis longus muscle Fibularis brevis muscle Fibularis longus muscle Flexor digitorum longus muscle Flexor hallucis longus muscle Gastrocnemius muscle Peroneus brevis muscle Peroneus longus muscle Popliteus muscle Soleus muscle Tibialis anterior muscle Tibialis posterior muscle **T Lower Leg Muscle, Left** *See S Lower Leg Muscle, Right* **V Foot Muscle, Right** Abductor hallucis muscle Adductor hallucis muscle Extensor digitorum brevis muscle Extensor hallucis brevis muscle Flexor digitorum brevis muscle Flexor hallucis brevis muscle Quadratus plantae muscle **W Foot Muscle, Left** *See V Foot Muscle, Right*	**Ø Open** **4 Percutaneous Endoscopic**	**7 Autologous Tissue Substitute** **J Synthetic Substitute** **K Nonautologous Tissue Substitute**	**Z No Qualifier**

LC Limited Coverage   **NC** Noncovered   ⊞ Combination Member   HAC associated procedure   Combination Only   DRG Non-OR   Non-OR   New/Revised in GREEN

468

ICD-10-PCS 2020

Ø　Medical and Surgical
K　Muscles
W　Revision　　Definition: Correcting, to the extent possible, a portion of a malfunctioning device or the position of a displaced device
　　　　　　　　Explanation: Revision can include correcting a malfunctioning or displaced device by taking out or putting in components of the device such as a screw or pin

Body Part Character 4	Approach Character 5	Device Character 6	Qualifier Character 7
X　Upper Muscle Y　Lower Muscle	Ø　Open 3　Percutaneous 4　Percutaneous Endoscopic	Ø　Drainage Device 7　Autologous Tissue Substitute J　Synthetic Substitute K　Nonautologous Tissue Substitute M　Stimulator Lead Y　Other Device	Z　No Qualifier
X　Upper Muscle Y　Lower Muscle	X　External	Ø　Drainage Device 7　Autologous Tissue Substitute J　Synthetic Substitute K　Nonautologous Tissue Substitute M　Stimulator Lead	Z　No Qualifier

Non-OR　ØKW[X,Y][3,4]YZ
Non-OR　ØKW[X,Y]X[Ø,7,J,K,M]Z

LC Limited Coverage　NC Noncovered　⊞ Combination Member　HAC associated procedure　Combination Only　DRG Non-OR　Non-OR　New/Revised in GREEN
ICD-10-PCS 2020　　　　　　　　　　　　　　　　　　　　　　　　　　　　　　　　　469

ØKW–ØKW

Ø　**Medical and Surgical**
K　**Muscles**
X　**Transfer**　　Definition: Moving, without taking out, all or a portion of a body part to another location to take over the function of all or a portion of a body part
　　　　　　　　　Explanation: The body part transferred remains connected to its vascular and nervous supply

Body Part Character 4			Approach Character 5	Device Character 6	Qualifier Character 7
Ø Head Muscle Auricularis muscle Masseter muscle Pterygoid muscle Splenius capitis muscle Temporalis muscle Temporoparietalis muscle **1 Facial Muscle** Buccinator muscle Corrugator supercilii muscle Depressor anguli oris muscle Depressor labii inferioris muscle Depressor septi nasi muscle Depressor supercilii muscle Levator anguli oris muscle Levator labii superioris alaeque nasi muscle Levator labii superioris muscle Mentalis muscle Nasalis muscle Occipitofrontalis muscle Orbicularis oris muscle Procerus muscle Risorius muscle Zygomaticus muscle **2 Neck Muscle, Right** Anterior vertebral muscle Arytenoid muscle Cricothyroid muscle Infrahyoid muscle Levator scapulae muscle Platysma muscle Scalene muscle Splenius cervicis muscle Sternocleidomastoid muscle Suprahyoid muscle Thyroarytenoid muscle **3 Neck Muscle, Left** *See 2 Neck Muscle, Right* **4 Tongue, Palate, Pharynx Muscle** Chondroglossus muscle Genioglossus muscle Hyoglossus muscle Inferior longitudinal muscle Levator veli palatini muscle Palatoglossal muscle Palatopharyngeal muscle Pharyngeal constrictor muscle Salpingopharyngeus muscle Styloglossus muscle Stylopharyngeus muscle Superior longitudinal muscle Tensor veli palatini muscle **5 Shoulder Muscle, Right** Deltoid muscle Infraspinatus muscle Subscapularis muscle Supraspinatus muscle Teres major muscle Teres minor muscle	**6 Shoulder Muscle, Left** *See 5 Shoulder Muscle, Right* **7 Upper Arm Muscle, Right** Biceps brachii muscle Brachialis muscle Coracobrachialis muscle Triceps brachii muscle **8 Upper Arm Muscle, Left** *See 7 Upper Arm Muscle, Right* **9 Lower Arm and Wrist Muscle, Right** Anatomical snuffbox Brachioradialis muscle Extensor carpi radialis muscle Extensor carpi ulnaris muscle Flexor carpi radialis muscle Flexor carpi ulnaris muscle Flexor pollicis longus muscle Palmaris longus muscle Pronator quadratus muscle Pronator teres muscle **B Lower Arm and Wrist Muscle, Left** *See 9 Lower Arm and Wrist Muscle, Right* **C Hand Muscle, Right** Hypothenar muscle Palmar interosseous muscle Thenar muscle **D Hand Muscle, Left** *See C Hand Muscle, Right* **H Thorax Muscle, Right** Intercostal muscle Levatores costarum muscle Pectoralis major muscle Pectoralis minor muscle Serratus anterior muscle Subclavius muscle Subcostal muscle Transverse thoracis muscle **J Thorax Muscle, Left** *See H Thorax Muscle, Right* **M Perineum Muscle** Bulbospongiosus muscle Cremaster muscle Deep transverse perineal muscle Ischiocavernosus muscle Levator ani muscle Superficial transverse perineal muscle **N Hip Muscle, Right** Gemellus muscle Gluteus maximus muscle Gluteus medius muscle Gluteus minimus muscle Iliacus muscle Obturator muscle Piriformis muscle Psoas muscle Quadratus femoris muscle Tensor fasciae latae muscle	**P Hip Muscle, Left** *See N Hip Muscle, Right* **Q Upper Leg Muscle, Right** Adductor brevis muscle Adductor longus muscle Adductor magnus muscle Biceps femoris muscle Gracilis muscle Pectineus muscle Quadriceps (femoris) Rectus femoris muscle Sartorius muscle Semimembranosus muscle Semitendinosus muscle Vastus intermedius muscle Vastus lateralis muscle Vastus medialis muscle **R Upper Leg Muscle, Left** *See Q Upper Leg Muscle, Right* **S Lower Leg Muscle, Right** Extensor digitorum longus muscle Extensor hallucis longus muscle Fibularis brevis muscle Fibularis longus muscle Flexor digitorum longus muscle Flexor hallucis longus muscle Gastrocnemius muscle Peroneus brevis muscle Peroneus longus muscle Popliteus muscle Soleus muscle Tibialis anterior muscle Tibialis posterior muscle **T Lower Leg Muscle, Left** *See S Lower Leg Muscle, Right* **V Foot Muscle, Right** Abductor hallucis muscle Adductor hallucis muscle Extensor digitorum brevis muscle Extensor hallucis brevis muscle Flexor digitorum brevis muscle Flexor hallucis brevis muscle Quadratus plantae muscle **W Foot Muscle, Left** *See V Foot Muscle, Right*	**Ø** Open **4** Percutaneous Endoscopic	**Z** No Device	**Ø** Skin **1** Subcutaneous Tissue **2** Skin and Subcutaneous Tissue **Z** No Qualifier

ØKX Continued on next page

Ø   Medical and Surgical
K   Muscles
X   Transfer

ØKX Continued

Definition: Moving, without taking out, all or a portion of a body part to another location to take over the function of all or a portion of a body part

Explanation: The body part transferred remains connected to its vascular and nervous supply

Body Part Character 4	Approach Character 5	Device Character 6	Qualifier Character 7

F   **Trunk Muscle, Right**
   Coccygeus muscle
   Erector spinae muscle
   Interspinalis muscle
   Intertransversarius muscle
   Latissimus dorsi muscle
   Quadratus lumborum muscle
   Rhomboid major muscle
   Rhomboid minor muscle
   Serratus posterior muscle
   Transversospinalis muscle
   Trapezius muscle
G   **Trunk Muscle, Left**
   See F Trunk Muscle, Right
	Ø Open
	4 Percutaneous Endoscopic
		Z No Device	**Ø** Skin
			1 Subcutaneous Tissue
			2 Skin and Subcutaneous Tissue
			5 Latissimus Dorsi Myocutaneous Flap
			7 Deep Inferior Epigastric Artery Perforator Flap
			8 Superficial Inferior Epigastric Artery Flap
			9 Gluteal Artery Perforator Flap
			Z No Qualifier

K   **Abdomen Muscle, Right**
   External oblique muscle
   Internal oblique muscle
   Pyramidalis muscle
   Rectus abdominis muscle
   Transversus abdominis muscle
L   **Abdomen Muscle, Left**
   See K Abdomen Muscle, Right
	Ø Open
	4 Percutaneous Endoscopic
		Z No Device	**Ø** Skin
			1 Subcutaneous Tissue
			2 Skin and Subcutaneous Tissue
			6 Transverse Rectus Abdominis Myocutaneous Flap
			Z No Qualifier

Tendons ØL2–ØLX

Character Meanings*

This Character Meaning table is provided as a guide to assist the user in the identification of character members that may be found in this section of code tables. It **SHOULD NOT** be used to build a PCS code.

Operation–Character 3	Body Part–Character 4	Approach–Character 5	Device–Character 6	Qualifier–Character 7
2 Change	Ø Head and Neck Tendon	Ø Open	Ø Drainage Device	X Diagnostic
5 Destruction	1 Shoulder Tendon, Right	3 Percutaneous	7 Autologous Tissue Substitute	Z No Qualifier
8 Division	2 Shoulder Tendon, Left	4 Percutaneous Endoscopic	J Synthetic Substitute	
9 Drainage	3 Upper Arm Tendon, Right	X External	K Nonautologous Tissue Substitute	
B Excision	4 Upper Arm Tendon, Left		Y Other Device	
C Extirpation	5 Lower Arm and Wrist Tendon, Right		Z No Device	
D Extraction	6 Lower Arm and Wrist Tendon, Left			
H Insertion	7 Hand Tendon, Right			
J Inspection	8 Hand Tendon, Left			
M Reattachment	9 Trunk Tendon, Right			
N Release	B Trunk Tendon, Left			
P Removal	C Thorax Tendon, Right			
Q Repair	D Thorax Tendon, Left			
R Replacement	F Abdomen Tendon, Right			
S Reposition	G Abdomen Tendon, Left			
T Resection	H Perineum Tendon			
U Supplement	J Hip Tendon, Right			
W Revision	K Hip Tendon, Left			
X Transfer	L Upper Leg Tendon, Right			
	M Upper Leg Tendon, Left			
	N Lower Leg Tendon, Right			
	P Lower Leg Tendon, Left			
	Q Knee Tendon, Right			
	R Knee Tendon, Left			
	S Ankle Tendon, Right			
	T Ankle Tendon, Left			
	V Foot Tendon, Right			
	W Foot Tendon, Left			
	X Upper Tendon			
	Y Lower Tendon			

* Includes synovial membrane.

AHA Coding Clinic for table ØL8
2016, 3Q, 30   Resection of femur with interposition arthroplasty

AHA Coding Clinic for table ØLB
2017, 2Q, 21   Arthroscopic anterior cruciate ligament revision using autograft with anterolateral ligament reconstruction
2015, 3Q, 26   Thumb arthroplasty with resection of trapezium
2014, 3Q, 14   Application of TheraSkin® and excisional debridement
2014, 3Q, 18   Placement of reverse sural fasciocutaneous pedicle flap

AHA Coding Clinic for table ØLD
2017, 4Q, 41   Extraction procedures

AHA Coding Clinic for table ØLQ
2016, 3Q, 32   Rotator cuff repair, tenodesis, decompression, acromioplasty and coracoplasty
2015, 2Q, 11   Repair of patellar and quadriceps tendons with allograft
2013, 3Q, 20   Superior labrum anterior posterior (SLAP) repair and subacromial decompression

AHA Coding Clinic for table ØLS
2016, 3Q, 32   Rotator cuff repair, tenodesis, decompression, acromioplasty and coracoplasty
2015, 3Q, 14   Endoprosthetic replacement of humerus and tendon reattachment

AHA Coding Clinic for table ØLU
2015, 2Q, 11   Repair of patellar and quadriceps tendons with allograft

Foot Tendons

Lateral malleolus
of fibula

Medial malleolus
of tibia

Peroneus
brevis **N, P**

Extensor hallucis
longus **N, P**

Extensor digitorum
longus **N, P**

Select extensors
of the foot

Shoulder Tendons

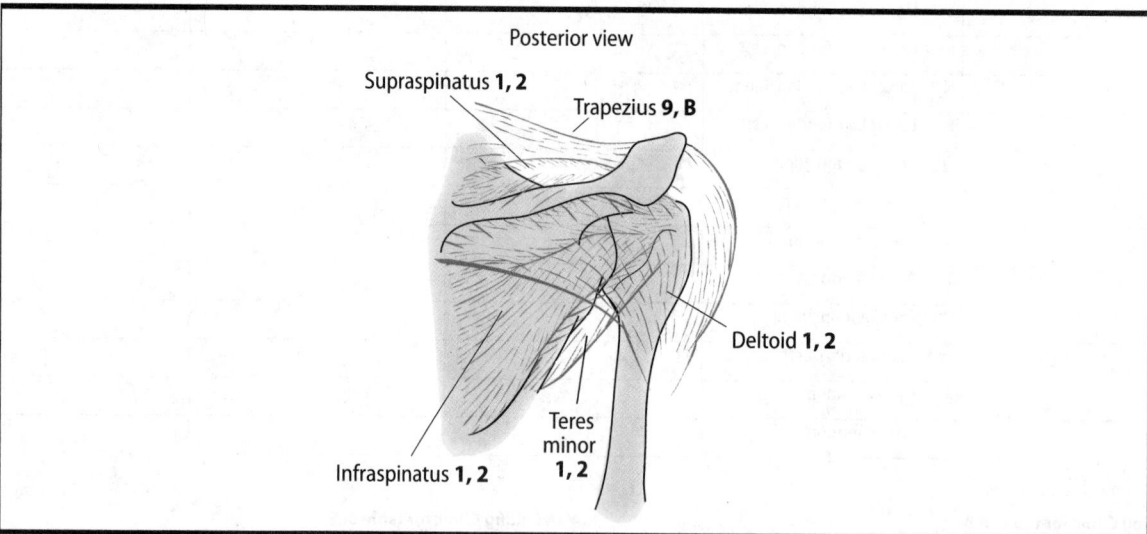

Posterior view

Supraspinatus **1, 2**

Trapezius **9, B**

Deltoid **1, 2**

Infraspinatus **1, 2**

Teres
minor
1, 2

Tendons of Wrist and Hand

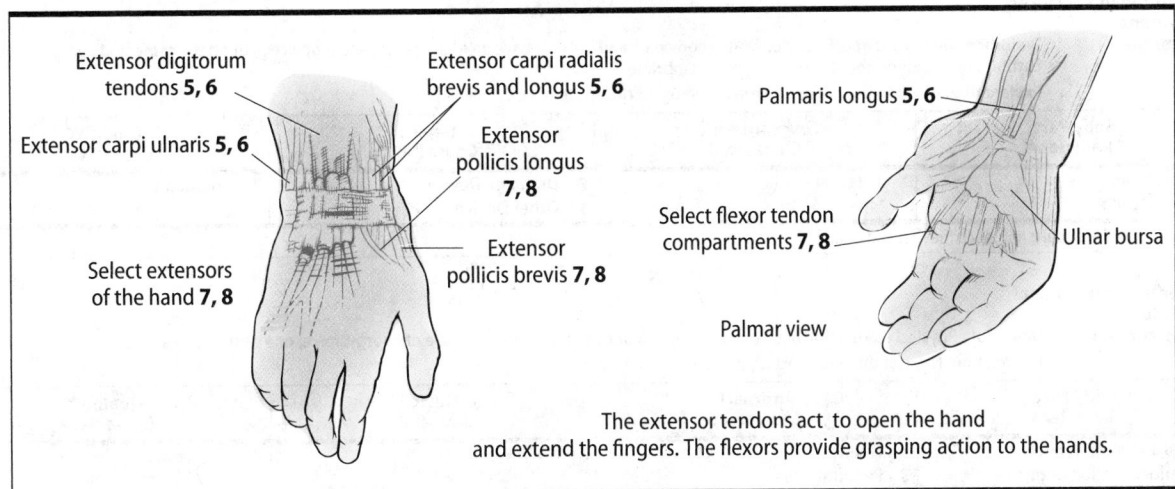

Extensor digitorum tendons **5, 6**

Extensor carpi ulnaris **5, 6**

Select extensors of the hand **7, 8**

Extensor carpi radialis brevis and longus **5, 6**

Extensor pollicis longus **7, 8**

Extensor pollicis brevis **7, 8**

Palmaris longus **5, 6**

Select flexor tendon compartments **7, 8**

Ulnar bursa

Palmar view

The extensor tendons act to open the hand and extend the fingers. The flexors provide grasping action to the hands.

Leg Muscles and Tendons

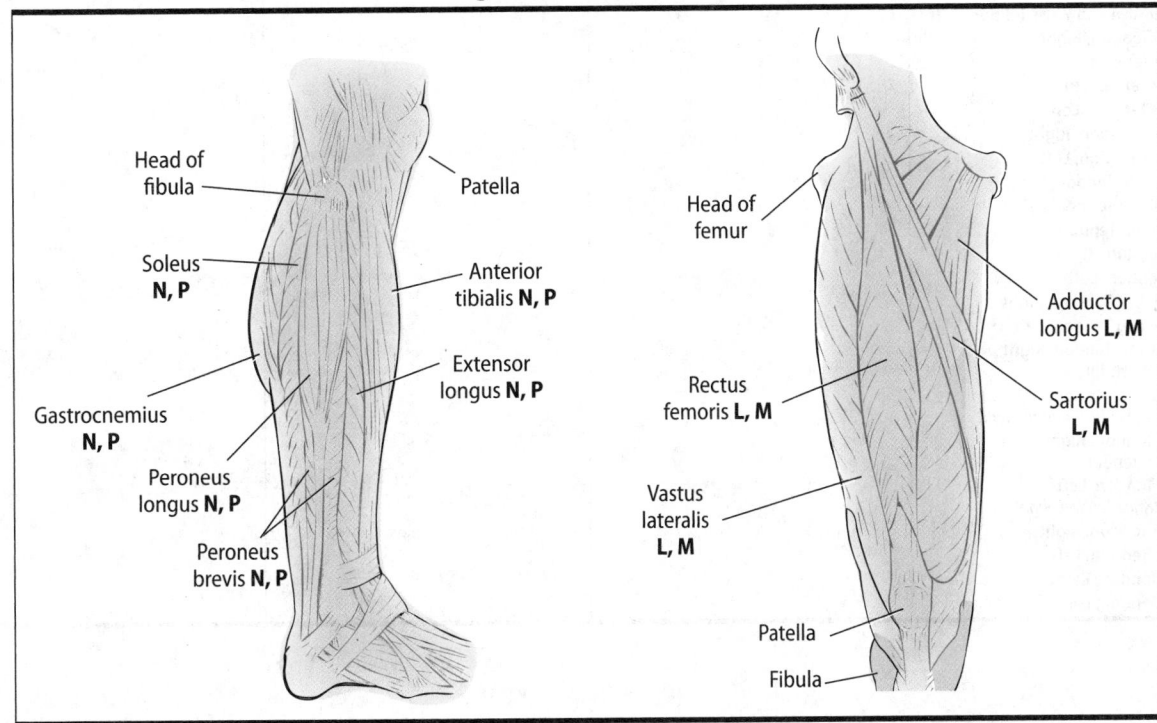

Head of fibula

Soleus **N, P**

Gastrocnemius **N, P**

Peroneus longus **N, P**

Peroneus brevis **N, P**

Patella

Anterior tibialis **N, P**

Extensor longus **N, P**

Head of femur

Rectus femoris **L, M**

Vastus lateralis **L, M**

Patella

Fibula

Adductor longus **L, M**

Sartorius **L, M**

Ø   Medical and Surgical
L   Tendons
2   Change   Definition: Taking out or off a device from a body part and putting back an identical or similar device in or on the same body part without cutting or puncturing the skin or a mucous membrane

Explanation: All CHANGE procedures are coded using the approach EXTERNAL

Body Part Character 4	Approach Character 5	Device Character 6	Qualifier Character 7
X Upper Tendon Y Lower Tendon	X External	Ø Drainage Device Y Other Device	Z No Qualifier

Non-OR	All body part, approach, device, and qualifier values

Ø   Medical and Surgical
L   Tendons
5   Destruction   Definition: Physical eradication of all or a portion of a body part by the direct use of energy, force, or a destructive agent

Explanation: None of the body part is physically taken out

Body Part Character 4	Approach Character 5	Device Character 6	Qualifier Character 7

Ø   Head and Neck Tendon
1   Shoulder Tendon, Right
2   Shoulder Tendon, Left
3   Upper Arm Tendon, Right
4   Upper Arm Tendon, Left
5   Lower Arm and Wrist Tendon, Right
6   Lower Arm and Wrist Tendon, Left
7   Hand Tendon, Right
8   Hand Tendon, Left
9   Trunk Tendon, Right
B   Trunk Tendon, Left
C   Thorax Tendon, Right
D   Thorax Tendon, Left
F   Abdomen Tendon, Right
G   Abdomen Tendon, Left
H   Perineum Tendon
J   Hip Tendon, Right
K   Hip Tendon, Left
L   Upper Leg Tendon, Right
M   Upper Leg Tendon, Left
N   Lower Leg Tendon, Right
     Achilles tendon
P   Lower Leg Tendon, Left
     See N Lower Leg Tendon, Right
Q   Knee Tendon, Right
     Patellar tendon
R   Knee Tendon, Left
     See Q Knee Tendon, Right
S   Ankle Tendon, Right
T   Ankle Tendon, Left
V   Foot Tendon, Right
W   Foot Tendon, Left
	Ø Open
	3 Percutaneous
	4 Percutaneous Endoscopic
		Z No Device	Z No Qualifier

Ø Medical and Surgical
L Tendons
8 Division   Definition: Cutting into a body part, without draining fluids and/or gases from the body part, in order to separate or transect a body part
Explanation: All or a portion of the body part is separated into two or more portions

Body Part Character 4	Approach Character 5	Device Character 6	Qualifier Character 7
Ø Head and Neck Tendon	Ø Open	Z No Device	Z No Qualifier
1 Shoulder Tendon, Right	3 Percutaneous		
2 Shoulder Tendon, Left	4 Percutaneous Endoscopic		
3 Upper Arm Tendon, Right			
4 Upper Arm Tendon, Left			
5 Lower Arm and Wrist Tendon, Right			
6 Lower Arm and Wrist Tendon, Left			
7 Hand Tendon, Right			
8 Hand Tendon, Left			
9 Trunk Tendon, Right			
B Trunk Tendon, Left			
C Thorax Tendon, Right			
D Thorax Tendon, Left			
F Abdomen Tendon, Right			
G Abdomen Tendon, Left			
H Perineum Tendon			
J Hip Tendon, Right			
K Hip Tendon, Left			
L Upper Leg Tendon, Right			
M Upper Leg Tendon, Left			
N Lower Leg Tendon, Right Achilles tendon			
P Lower Leg Tendon, Left See N Lower Leg Tendon, Right			
Q Knee Tendon, Right Patellar tendon			
R Knee Tendon, Left See Q Knee Tendon, Right			
S Ankle Tendon, Right			
T Ankle Tendon, Left			
V Foot Tendon, Right			
W Foot Tendon, Left			

Ø **Medical and Surgical**
L **Tendons**
9 **Drainage** Definition: Taking or letting out fluids and/or gases from a body part
Explanation: The qualifier DIAGNOSTIC is used to identify drainage procedures that are biopsies

Body Part Character 4	Approach Character 5	Device Character 6	Qualifier Character 7

Ø Head and Neck Tendon
1 Shoulder Tendon, Right
2 Shoulder Tendon, Left
3 Upper Arm Tendon, Right
4 Upper Arm Tendon, Left
5 Lower Arm and Wrist Tendon, Right
6 Lower Arm and Wrist Tendon, Left
7 Hand Tendon, Right
8 Hand Tendon, Left
9 Trunk Tendon, Right
B Trunk Tendon, Left
C Thorax Tendon, Right
D Thorax Tendon, Left
F Abdomen Tendon, Right
G Abdomen Tendon, Left
H Perineum Tendon
J Hip Tendon, Right
K Hip Tendon, Left
L Upper Leg Tendon, Right
M Upper Leg Tendon, Left
N Lower Leg Tendon, Right
   Achilles tendon
P Lower Leg Tendon, Left
   See N Lower Leg Tendon, Right
Q Knee Tendon, Right
   Patellar tendon
R Knee Tendon, Left
   See Q Knee Tendon, Right
S Ankle Tendon, Right
T Ankle Tendon, Left
V Foot Tendon, Right
W Foot Tendon, Left
	Ø Open
	3 Percutaneous
	4 Percutaneous Endoscopic
		Ø Drainage Device	**Z** No Qualifier

Ø Head and Neck Tendon
1 Shoulder Tendon, Right
2 Shoulder Tendon, Left
3 Upper Arm Tendon, Right
4 Upper Arm Tendon, Left
5 Lower Arm and Wrist Tendon, Right
6 Lower Arm and Wrist Tendon, Left
7 Hand Tendon, Right
8 Hand Tendon, Left
9 Trunk Tendon, Right
B Trunk Tendon, Left
C Thorax Tendon, Right
D Thorax Tendon, Left
F Abdomen Tendon, Right
G Abdomen Tendon, Left
H Perineum Tendon
J Hip Tendon, Right
K Hip Tendon, Left
L Upper Leg Tendon, Right
M Upper Leg Tendon, Left
N Lower Leg Tendon, Right
   Achilles tendon
P Lower Leg Tendon, Left
   See N Lower Leg Tendon, Right
Q Knee Tendon, Right
   Patellar tendon
R Knee Tendon, Left
   See Q Knee Tendon, Right
S Ankle Tendon, Right
T Ankle Tendon, Left
V Foot Tendon, Right
W Foot Tendon, Left
	Ø Open
	3 Percutaneous
	4 Percutaneous Endoscopic
		Z No Device	**X** Diagnostic
			Z No Qualifier

Non-OR ØL9[Ø,1,2,3,4,5,6,7,8,9,B,C,D,F,G,H,J,K,L,M,N,P,Q,R,S,T,V,W]3ØZ
Non-OR ØL9[Ø,1,2,3,4,5,6,7,8,9,B,C,D,F,G,H,J,K,L,M,N,P,Q,R,S,T,V,W]3ZZ
Non-OR ØL9[7,8]4ZZ

⬛ Limited Coverage ⬛ Noncovered ⊞ Combination Member HAC associated procedure Combination Only DRG Non-OR Non-OR New/Revised in GREEN

478 ICD-10-PCS 2020

ØL9–ØL9

Ø　Medical and Surgical
L　Tendons
B　Excision　　　Definition: Cutting out or off, without replacement, a portion of a body part
　　　　　　　　　　Explanation: The qualifier DIAGNOSTIC is used to identify excision procedures that are biopsies

Body Part Character 4	Approach Character 5	Device Character 6	Qualifier Character 7
Ø Head and Neck Tendon **1** Shoulder Tendon, Right **2** Shoulder Tendon, Left **3** Upper Arm Tendon, Right **4** Upper Arm Tendon, Left **5** Lower Arm and Wrist Tendon, Right **6** Lower Arm and Wrist Tendon, Left **7** Hand Tendon, Right **8** Hand Tendon, Left **9** Trunk Tendon, Right **B** Trunk Tendon, Left **C** Thorax Tendon, Right **D** Thorax Tendon, Left **F** Abdomen Tendon, Right **G** Abdomen Tendon, Left **H** Perineum Tendon **J** Hip Tendon, Right **K** Hip Tendon, Left **L** Upper Leg Tendon, Right **M** Upper Leg Tendon, Left **N** Lower Leg Tendon, Right 　　Achilles tendon **P** Lower Leg Tendon, Left 　　*See* N Lower Leg Tendon, Right **Q** Knee Tendon, Right 　　Patellar tendon **R** Knee Tendon, Left 　　*See* Q Knee Tendon, Right **S** Ankle Tendon, Right **T** Ankle Tendon, Left **V** Foot Tendon, Right **W** Foot Tendon, Left	**Ø** Open **3** Percutaneous **4** Percutaneous Endoscopic	**Z** No Device	**X** Diagnostic **Z** No Qualifier

Ø Medical and Surgical
L Tendons
C Extirpation — Definition: Taking or cutting out solid matter from a body part

Explanation: The solid matter may be an abnormal byproduct of a biological function or a foreign body; it may be imbedded in a body part or in the lumen of a tubular body part. The solid matter may or may not have been previously broken into pieces.

Body Part Character 4	Approach Character 5	Device Character 6	Qualifier Character 7

Ø Head and Neck Tendon
1 Shoulder Tendon, Right
2 Shoulder Tendon, Left
3 Upper Arm Tendon, Right
4 Upper Arm Tendon, Left
5 Lower Arm and Wrist Tendon, Right
6 Lower Arm and Wrist Tendon, Left
7 Hand Tendon, Right
8 Hand Tendon, Left
9 Trunk Tendon, Right
B Trunk Tendon, Left
C Thorax Tendon, Right
D Thorax Tendon, Left
F Abdomen Tendon, Right
G Abdomen Tendon, Left
H Perineum Tendon
J Hip Tendon, Right
K Hip Tendon, Left
L Upper Leg Tendon, Right
M Upper Leg Tendon, Left
N Lower Leg Tendon, Right
   Achilles tendon
P Lower Leg Tendon, Left
   See N Lower Leg Tendon, Right
Q Knee Tendon, Right
   Patellar tendon
R Knee Tendon, Left
   See Q Knee Tendon, Right
S Ankle Tendon, Right
T Ankle Tendon, Left
V Foot Tendon, Right
W Foot Tendon, Left
	Ø Open
	3 Percutaneous
	4 Percutaneous Endoscopic
		Z No Device	Z No Qualifier

Ø   Medical and Surgical
L   Tendons
D   Extraction   Definition: Pulling or stripping out or off all or a portion of a body part by the use of force

Explanation: The qualifier DIAGNOSTIC is used to identify extraction procedures that are biopsies

Body Part Character 4	Approach Character 5	Device Character 6	Qualifier Character 7

Ø   Head and Neck Tendon
1   Shoulder Tendon, Right
2   Shoulder Tendon, Left
3   Upper Arm Tendon, Right
4   Upper Arm Tendon, Left
5   Lower Arm and Wrist Tendon, Right
6   Lower Arm and Wrist Tendon, Left
7   Hand Tendon, Right
8   Hand Tendon, Left
9   Trunk Tendon, Right
B   Trunk Tendon, Left
C   Thorax Tendon, Right
D   Thorax Tendon, Left
F   Abdomen Tendon, Right
G   Abdomen Tendon, Left
H   Perineum Tendon
J   Hip Tendon, Right
K   Hip Tendon, Left
L   Upper Leg Tendon, Right
M   Upper Leg Tendon, Left
N   Lower Leg Tendon, Right
     Achilles tendon
P   Lower Leg Tendon, Left
     See N Lower Leg Tendon, Right
Q   Knee Tendon, Right
     Patellar tendon
R   Knee Tendon, Left
     See Q Knee Tendon, Right
S   Ankle Tendon, Right
T   Ankle Tendon, Left
V   Foot Tendon, Right
W   Foot Tendon, Left
	Ø Open	Z No Device	Z No Qualifier

Ø   Medical and Surgical
L   Tendons
H   Insertion   Definition: Putting in a nonbiological appliance that monitors, assists, performs, or prevents a physiological function but does not physically take the place of a body part

Explanation: None

Body Part Character 4	Approach Character 5	Device Character 6	Qualifier Character 7
X Upper Tendon Y Lower Tendon	Ø Open 3 Percutaneous 4 Percutaneous Endoscopic	Y Other Device	Z No Qualifier

Non-OR   ØLH[X,Y][3,4]YZ

Ø   Medical and Surgical
L   Tendons
J   Inspection   Definition: Visually and/or manually exploring a body part

Explanation: Visual exploration may be performed with or without optical instrumentation. Manual exploration may be performed directly or through intervening body layers.

Body Part Character 4	Approach Character 5	Device Character 6	Qualifier Character 7
X Upper Tendon Y Lower Tendon	Ø Open 3 Percutaneous 4 Percutaneous Endoscopic X External	Z No Device	Z No Qualifier

Non-OR   ØLJ[X,Y][3,X]ZZ

LC Limited Coverage   NC Noncovered   ⊞ Combination Member   HAC associated procedure   Combination Only   DRG Non-OR   Non-OR   New/Revised in GREEN

ICD-10-PCS 2020   481

Ø Medical and Surgical
L Tendons
M Reattachment   Definition: Putting back in or on all or a portion of a separated body part to its normal location or other suitable location
                Explanation: Vascular circulation and nervous pathways may or may not be reestablished

Body Part Character 4	Approach Character 5	Device Character 6	Qualifier Character 7

Ø Head and Neck Tendon
1 Shoulder Tendon, Right
2 Shoulder Tendon, Left
3 Upper Arm Tendon, Right
4 Upper Arm Tendon, Left
5 Lower Arm and Wrist Tendon, Right
6 Lower Arm and Wrist Tendon, Left
7 Hand Tendon, Right
8 Hand Tendon, Left
9 Trunk Tendon, Right
B Trunk Tendon, Left
C Thorax Tendon, Right
D Thorax Tendon, Left
F Abdomen Tendon, Right
G Abdomen Tendon, Left
H Perineum Tendon
J Hip Tendon, Right
K Hip Tendon, Left
L Upper Leg Tendon, Right
M Upper Leg Tendon, Left
N Lower Leg Tendon, Right
    Achilles tendon
P Lower Leg Tendon, Left
    See N Lower Leg Tendon, Right
Q Knee Tendon, Right
    Patellar tendon
R Knee Tendon, Left
    See Q Knee Tendon, Right
S Ankle Tendon, Right
T Ankle Tendon, Left
V Foot Tendon, Right
W Foot Tendon, Left
	Ø Open
	4 Percutaneous Endoscopic
		Z No Device	Z No Qualifier

Ø Medical and Surgical
L Tendons
N Release   Definition: Freeing a body part from an abnormal physical constraint by cutting or by the use of force
                Explanation: Some of the restraining tissue may be taken out but none of the body part is taken out

Body Part Character 4	Approach Character 5	Device Character 6	Qualifier Character 7

Ø Head and Neck Tendon
1 Shoulder Tendon, Right
2 Shoulder Tendon, Left
3 Upper Arm Tendon, Right
4 Upper Arm Tendon, Left
5 Lower Arm and Wrist Tendon, Right
6 Lower Arm and Wrist Tendon, Left
7 Hand Tendon, Right
8 Hand Tendon, Left
9 Trunk Tendon, Right
B Trunk Tendon, Left
C Thorax Tendon, Right
D Thorax Tendon, Left
F Abdomen Tendon, Right
G Abdomen Tendon, Left
H Perineum Tendon
J Hip Tendon, Right
K Hip Tendon, Left
L Upper Leg Tendon, Right
M Upper Leg Tendon, Left
N Lower Leg Tendon, Right
    Achilles tendon
P Lower Leg Tendon, Left
    See N Lower Leg Tendon, Right
Q Knee Tendon, Right
    Patellar tendon
R Knee Tendon, Left
    See Q Knee Tendon, Right
S Ankle Tendon, Right
T Ankle Tendon, Left
V Foot Tendon, Right
W Foot Tendon, Left
	Ø Open
	3 Percutaneous
	4 Percutaneous Endoscopic
	X External
		Z No Device	Z No Qualifier

Non-OR   ØLN[Ø,1,2,3,4,5,6,7,8,9,B,C,D,F,G,H,J,K,L,M,N,P,Q,R,S,T,V,W]XZZ

LC Limited Coverage   NC Noncovered   ⊞ Combination Member   HAC associated procedure   Combination Only   DRG Non-OR   Non-OR   New/Revised in GREEN

482   ICD-10-PCS 2020

Ø   Medical and Surgical
L   Tendons
P   Removal   Definition: Taking out or off a device from a body part

Explanation: If a device is taken out and a similar device put in without cutting or puncturing the skin or mucous membrane, the procedure is coded to the root operation CHANGE. Otherwise, the procedure for taking out a device is coded to the root operation REMOVAL.

Body Part Character 4	Approach Character 5	Device Character 6	Qualifier Character 7
X Upper Tendon **Y** Lower Tendon	**Ø** Open **3** Percutaneous **4** Percutaneous Endoscopic	**Ø** Drainage Device **7** Autologous Tissue Substitute **J** Synthetic Substitute **K** Nonautologous Tissue Substitute **Y** Other Device	**Z** No Qualifier
X Upper Tendon **Y** Lower Tendon	**X** External	**Ø** Drainage Device	**Z** No Qualifier

Non-OR	ØLP[X,Y]3ØZ
Non-OR	ØLP[X,Y][3,4]YZ
Non-OR	ØLP[X,Y]XØZ

Ø   Medical and Surgical
L   Tendons
Q   Repair   Definition: Restoring, to the extent possible, a body part to its normal anatomic structure and function

Explanation: Used only when the method to accomplish the repair is not one of the other root operations

Body Part Character 4	Approach Character 5	Device Character 6	Qualifier Character 7

Ø Head and Neck Tendon
1 Shoulder Tendon, Right
2 Shoulder Tendon, Left
3 Upper Arm Tendon, Right
4 Upper Arm Tendon, Left
5 Lower Arm and Wrist Tendon, Right
6 Lower Arm and Wrist Tendon, Left
7 Hand Tendon, Right
8 Hand Tendon, Left
9 Trunk Tendon, Right
B Trunk Tendon, Left
C Thorax Tendon, Right
D Thorax Tendon, Left
F Abdomen Tendon, Right
G Abdomen Tendon, Left
H Perineum Tendon
J Hip Tendon, Right
K Hip Tendon, Left
L Upper Leg Tendon, Right
M Upper Leg Tendon, Left
N Lower Leg Tendon, Right
   Achilles tendon
P Lower Leg Tendon, Left
   See N Lower Leg Tendon, Right
Q Knee Tendon, Right
   Patellar tendon
R Knee Tendon, Left
   See Q Knee Tendon, Right
S Ankle Tendon, Right
T Ankle Tendon, Left
V Foot Tendon, Right
W Foot Tendon, Left
	Ø Open
	3 Percutaneous
	4 Percutaneous Endoscopic
		Z No Device	**Z** No Qualifier

LC Limited Coverage   **NC** Noncovered   ⊞ Combination Member   HAC associated procedure   Combination Only   DRG Non-OR   Non-OR   New/Revised in GREEN

ICD-10-PCS 2020   483

Ø   **Medical and Surgical**
L   **Tendons**
R   **Replacement**   Definition: Putting in or on biological or synthetic material that physically takes the place and/or function of all or a portion of a body part
                            Explanation: The body part may have been taken out or replaced, or may be taken out, physically eradicated, or rendered nonfunctional during the REPLACEMENT procedure. A REMOVAL procedure is coded for taking out the device used in a previous replacement procedure.

Body Part Character 4	Approach Character 5	Device Character 6	Qualifier Character 7

Ø Head and Neck Tendon
1 Shoulder Tendon, Right
2 Shoulder Tendon, Left
3 Upper Arm Tendon, Right
4 Upper Arm Tendon, Left
5 Lower Arm and Wrist Tendon, Right
6 Lower Arm and Wrist Tendon, Left
7 Hand Tendon, Right
8 Hand Tendon, Left
9 Trunk Tendon, Right
B Trunk Tendon, Left
C Thorax Tendon, Right
D Thorax Tendon, Left
F Abdomen Tendon, Right
G Abdomen Tendon, Left
H Perineum Tendon
J Hip Tendon, Right
K Hip Tendon, Left
L Upper Leg Tendon, Right
M Upper Leg Tendon, Left
N Lower Leg Tendon, Right
    Achilles tendon
P Lower Leg Tendon, Left
    See N Lower Leg Tendon, Right
Q Knee Tendon, Right
    Patellar tendon
R Knee Tendon, Left
    See Q Knee Tendon, Right
S Ankle Tendon, Right
T Ankle Tendon, Left
V Foot Tendon, Right
W Foot Tendon, Left
	Ø Open
	4 Percutaneous Endoscopic
		7 Autologous Tissue Substitute
		J Synthetic Substitute
		K Nonautologous Tissue Substitute
			Z No Qualifier

Ø   **Medical and Surgical**
L   **Tendons**
S   **Reposition**   Definition: Moving to its normal location, or other suitable location, all or a portion of a body part
                          Explanation: The body part is moved to a new location from an abnormal location, or from a normal location where it is not functioning correctly. The body part may or may not be cut out or off to be moved to the new location.

Body Part Character 4	Approach Character 5	Device Character 6	Qualifier Character 7

Ø Head and Neck Tendon
1 Shoulder Tendon, Right
2 Shoulder Tendon, Left
3 Upper Arm Tendon, Right
4 Upper Arm Tendon, Left
5 Lower Arm and Wrist Tendon, Right
6 Lower Arm and Wrist Tendon, Left
7 Hand Tendon, Right
8 Hand Tendon, Left
9 Trunk Tendon, Right
B Trunk Tendon, Left
C Thorax Tendon, Right
D Thorax Tendon, Left
F Abdomen Tendon, Right
G Abdomen Tendon, Left
H Perineum Tendon
J Hip Tendon, Right
K Hip Tendon, Left
L Upper Leg Tendon, Right
M Upper Leg Tendon, Left
N Lower Leg Tendon, Right
    Achilles tendon
P Lower Leg Tendon, Left
    See N Lower Leg Tendon, Right
Q Knee Tendon, Right
    Patellar tendon
R Knee Tendon, Left
    See Q Knee Tendon, Right
S Ankle Tendon, Right
T Ankle Tendon, Left
V Foot Tendon, Right
W Foot Tendon, Left
	Ø Open
	4 Percutaneous Endoscopic
		Z No Device	**Z** No Qualifier

LC Limited Coverage   **NC** Noncovered   ⊞ Combination Member   HAC associated procedure   Combination Only   DRG Non-OR   Non-OR   New/Revised in **GREEN**

484   ICD-10-PCS 2020

Ø   Medical and Surgical
L   Tendons
T   Resection   Definition: Cutting out or off, without replacement, all of a body part
                Explanation: None

Body Part Character 4	Approach Character 5	Device Character 6	Qualifier Character 7

Ø   Head and Neck Tendon
1   Shoulder Tendon, Right
2   Shoulder Tendon, Left
3   Upper Arm Tendon, Right
4   Upper Arm Tendon, Left
5   Lower Arm and Wrist Tendon, Right
6   Lower Arm and Wrist Tendon, Left
7   Hand Tendon, Right
8   Hand Tendon, Left
9   Trunk Tendon, Right
B   Trunk Tendon, Left
C   Thorax Tendon, Right
D   Thorax Tendon, Left
F   Abdomen Tendon, Right
G   Abdomen Tendon, Left
H   Perineum Tendon
J   Hip Tendon, Right
K   Hip Tendon, Left
L   Upper Leg Tendon, Right
M   Upper Leg Tendon, Left
N   Lower Leg Tendon, Right
     Achilles tendon
P   Lower Leg Tendon, Left
     See N Lower Leg Tendon, Right
Q   Knee Tendon, Right
     Patellar tendon
R   Knee Tendon, Left
     See Q Knee Tendon, Right
S   Ankle Tendon, Right
T   Ankle Tendon, Left
V   Foot Tendon, Right
W   Foot Tendon, Left
	Ø Open
	4 Percutaneous Endoscopic
		Z No Device	**Z** No Qualifier

Ø   Medical and Surgical
L   Tendons
U   Supplement   Definition: Putting in or on biological or synthetic material that physically reinforces and/or augments the function of a portion of a body part
                Explanation: The biological material is non-living, or is living and from the same individual. The body part may have been previously replaced, and the SUPPLEMENT procedure is performed to physically reinforce and/or augment the function of the replaced body part.

Body Part Character 4	Approach Character 5	Device Character 6	Qualifier Character 7

Ø   Head and Neck Tendon
1   Shoulder Tendon, Right
2   Shoulder Tendon, Left
3   Upper Arm Tendon, Right
4   Upper Arm Tendon, Left
5   Lower Arm and Wrist Tendon, Right
6   Lower Arm and Wrist Tendon, Left
7   Hand Tendon, Right
8   Hand Tendon, Left
9   Trunk Tendon, Right
B   Trunk Tendon, Left
C   Thorax Tendon, Right
D   Thorax Tendon, Left
F   Abdomen Tendon, Right
G   Abdomen Tendon, Left
H   Perineum Tendon
J   Hip Tendon, Right
K   Hip Tendon, Left
L   Upper Leg Tendon, Right
M   Upper Leg Tendon, Left
N   Lower Leg Tendon, Right
     Achilles tendon
P   Lower Leg Tendon, Left
     See N Lower Leg Tendon, Right
Q   Knee Tendon, Right
     Patellar tendon
R   Knee Tendon, Left
     See Q Knee Tendon, Right
S   Ankle Tendon, Right
T   Ankle Tendon, Left
V   Foot Tendon, Right
W   Foot Tendon, Left
	Ø Open
	4 Percutaneous Endoscopic
		7 Autologous Tissue Substitute
		J Synthetic Substitute
		K Nonautologous Tissue Substitute
			Z No Qualifier

LC Limited Coverage   **NC** Noncovered   ⊞ Combination Member   HAC associated procedure   Combination Only   DRG Non-OR   Non-OR   New/Revised in **GREEN**

Ø   **Medical and Surgical**
L   **Tendons**
W   **Revision**   Definition: Correcting, to the extent possible, a portion of a malfunctioning device or the position of a displaced device

                       Explanation: Revision can include correcting a malfunctioning or displaced device by taking out or putting in components of the device such as a screw or pin

Body Part Character 4	Approach Character 5	Device Character 6	Qualifier Character 7
X Upper Tendon Y Lower Tendon	Ø Open 3 Percutaneous 4 Percutaneous Endoscopic	Ø Drainage Device 7 Autologous Tissue Substitute J Synthetic Substitute K Nonautologous Tissue Substitute Y Other Device	Z No Qualifier
X Upper Tendon Y Lower Tendon	X External	Ø Drainage Device 7 Autologous Tissue Substitute J Synthetic Substitute K Nonautologous Tissue Substitute	Z No Qualifier

Non-OR	ØLW[X,Y][3,4]YZ
Non-OR	ØLW[X,Y]X[Ø,7,J,K]Z

Ø   **Medical and Surgical**
L   **Tendons**
X   **Transfer**   Definition: Moving, without taking out, all or a portion of a body part to another location to take over the function of all or a portion of a body part

                       Explanation: The body part transferred remains connected to its vascular and nervous supply

Body Part Character 4	Approach Character 5	Device Character 6	Qualifier Character 7

Ø   Head and Neck Tendon
1   Shoulder Tendon, Right
2   Shoulder Tendon, Left
3   Upper Arm Tendon, Right
4   Upper Arm Tendon, Left
5   Lower Arm and Wrist Tendon, Right
6   Lower Arm and Wrist Tendon, Left
7   Hand Tendon, Right
8   Hand Tendon, Left
9   Trunk Tendon, Right
B   Trunk Tendon, Left
C   Thorax Tendon, Right
D   Thorax Tendon, Left
F   Abdomen Tendon, Right
G   Abdomen Tendon, Left
H   Perineum Tendon
J   Hip Tendon, Right
K   Hip Tendon, Left
L   Upper Leg Tendon, Right
M   Upper Leg Tendon, Left
N   Lower Leg Tendon, Right
      Achilles tendon
P   Lower Leg Tendon, Left
      See N Lower Leg Tendon, Right
Q   Knee Tendon, Right
      Patellar tendon
R   Knee Tendon, Left
      See Q Knee Tendon, Right
S   Ankle Tendon, Right
T   Ankle Tendon, Left
V   Foot Tendon, Right
W   Foot Tendon, Left
	Ø Open
	4 Percutaneous Endoscopic
		Z No Device	Z No Qualifier

LC Limited Coverage   NC Noncovered   ⊞ Combination Member   HAC associated procedure   Combination Only   DRG Non-OR   Non-OR   New/Revised in GREEN

486   ICD-10-PCS 2020

ØLW–ØLX

Bursae and Ligaments ØM2–ØMX

Character Meanings*

This Character Meaning table is provided as a guide to assist the user in the identification of character members that may be found in this section of code tables. It **SHOULD NOT** be used to build a PCS code.

Operation–Character 3	Body Part–Character 4	Approach–Character 5	Device–Character 6	Qualifier–Character 7
2 Change	Ø Head and Neck Bursa and Ligament	Ø Open	Ø Drainage Device	X Diagnostic
5 Destruction	1 Shoulder Bursa and Ligament, Right	3 Percutaneous	7 Autologous Tissue Substitute	Z No Qualifier
8 Division	2 Shoulder Bursa and Ligament, Left	4 Percutaneous Endoscopic	J Synthetic Substitute	
9 Drainage	3 Elbow Bursa and Ligament, Right	X External	K Nonautologous Tissue Substitute	
B Excision	4 Elbow Bursa and Ligament, Left		Y Other Device	
C Extirpation	5 Wrist Bursa and Ligament, Right		Z No Device	
D Extraction	6 Wrist Bursa and Ligament, Left			
H Insertion	7 Hand Bursa and Ligament, Right			
J Inspection	8 Hand Bursa and Ligament, Left			
M Reattachment	9 Upper Extremity Bursa and Ligament, Right			
N Release	B Upper Extremity Bursa and Ligament, Left			
P Removal	C Upper Spine Bursa and Ligament			
Q Repair	D Lower Spine Bursa and Ligament			
R Replacement	F Sternum Bursa and Ligament			
S Reposition	G Rib(s) Bursa and Ligament			
T Resection	H Abdomen Bursa and Ligament, Right			
U Supplement	J Abdomen Bursa and Ligament, Left			
W Revision	K Perineum Bursa and Ligament			
X Transfer	L Hip Bursa and Ligament, Right			
	M Hip Bursa and Ligament, Left			
	N Knee Bursa and Ligament, Right			
	P Knee Bursa and Ligament, Left			
	Q Ankle Bursa and Ligament, Right			
	R Ankle Bursa and Ligament, Left			
	S Foot Bursa and Ligament, Right			
	T Foot Bursa and Ligament, Left			
	V Lower Extremity Bursa and Ligament, Right			
	W Lower Extremity Bursa and Ligament, Left			
	X Upper Bursa and Ligament			
	Y Lower Bursa and Ligament			

* Includes synovial membrane.

AHA Coding Clinic for table ØMB
2018, 3Q, 17   Excisional debridement of periosteum

AHA Coding Clinic for table ØMM
2013, 3Q, 20   Superior labrum anterior posterior (SLAP) repair and subacromial decompression

AHA Coding Clinic for table ØMQ
2014, 3Q, 9   Interspinous ligamentoplasty

AHA Coding Clinic for table ØMT
2017, 2Q, 21   Arthroscopic anterior cruciate ligament revision using autograft with anterolateral ligament reconstruction

AHA Coding Clinic for table ØMU
2017, 2Q, 21   Arthroscopic anterior cruciate ligament revision using autograft with anterolateral ligament reconstruction

Shoulder Ligaments

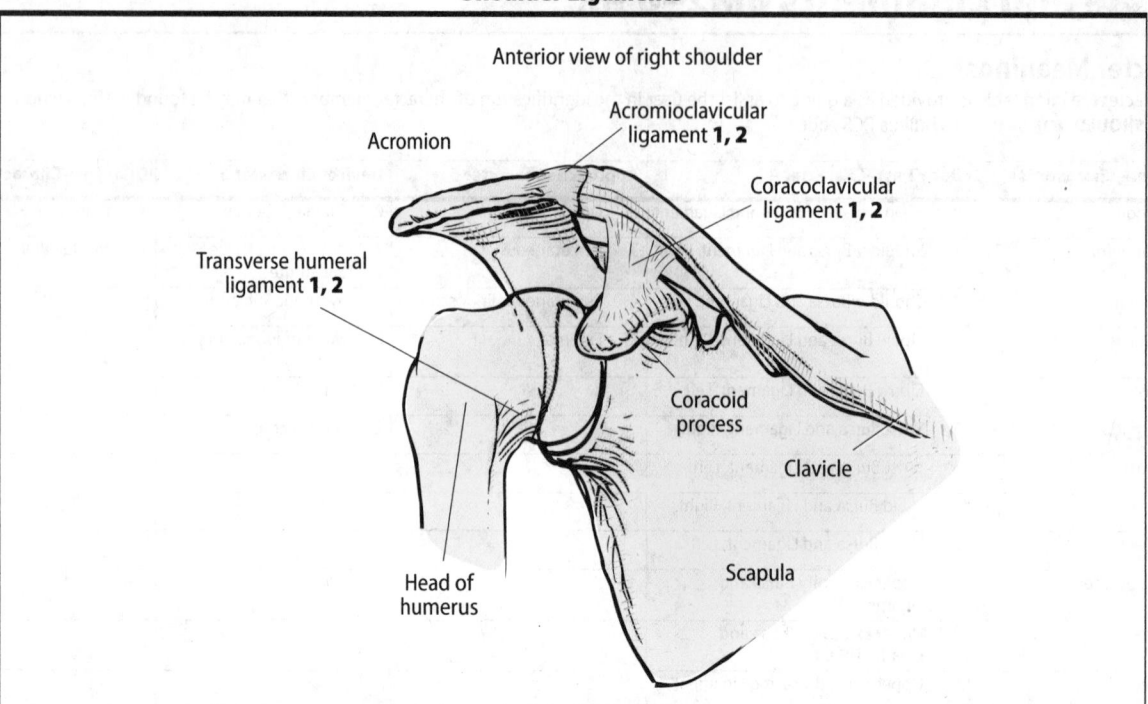

Anterior view of right shoulder

Acromion

Acromioclavicular ligament **1, 2**

Coracoclavicular ligament **1, 2**

Transverse humeral ligament **1, 2**

Coracoid process

Clavicle

Head of humerus

Scapula

Knee Bursae

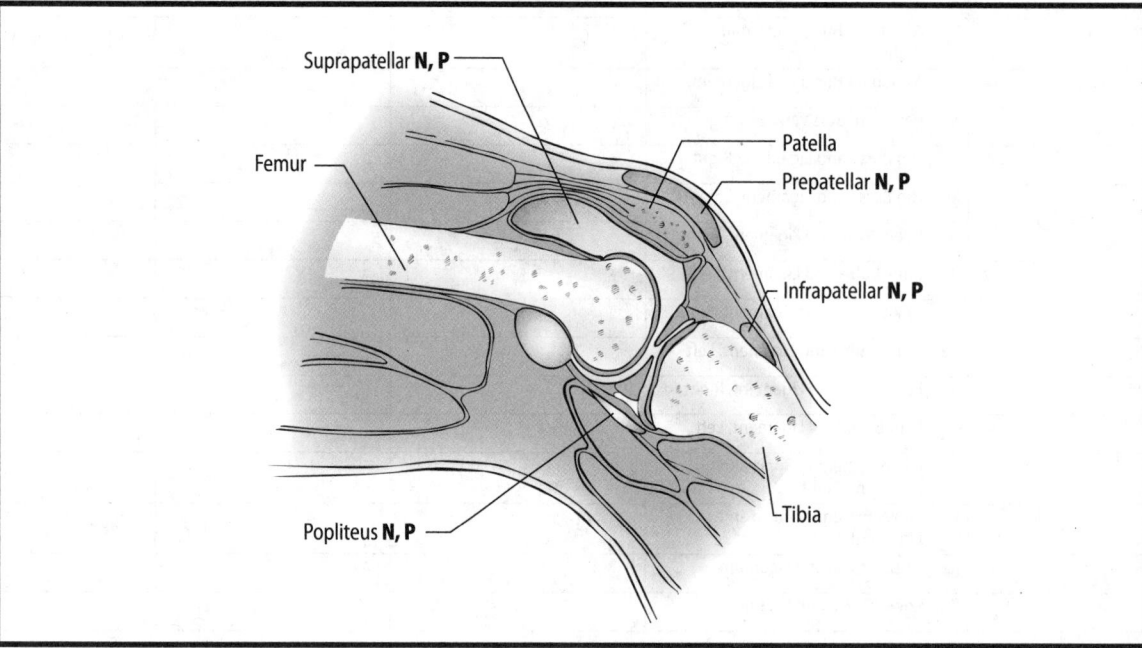

Suprapatellar **N, P**

Femur

Patella

Prepatellar **N, P**

Infrapatellar **N, P**

Popliteus **N, P**

Tibia

Knee Ligaments

Anterior view

Lateral collateral ligament **N, P**

Medial collateral ligament **N, P**

Patella

Posterior cruciate ligament **N, P**
(Behind the Anterior cruciate)

Anterior cruciate ligament **N, P**

Fibula

Tibia

Posterior cruciate
ligament **N, P**

Anterior cruciate ligament **N, P**

Wrist Ligaments

Palmar view

Flexor carpi
ulnaris **5, 6**

Radial collateral
carpal **5, 6**

Ulnar collateral
carpal **5, 6**

Palmar radiocarpal **5, 6**

Dorsal view

Radial collateral
carpal **5, 6**

Ulnar collateral
carpal **5, 6**

Dorsal
radiocarpal **5, 6**

Ulnocarpal **5, 6**

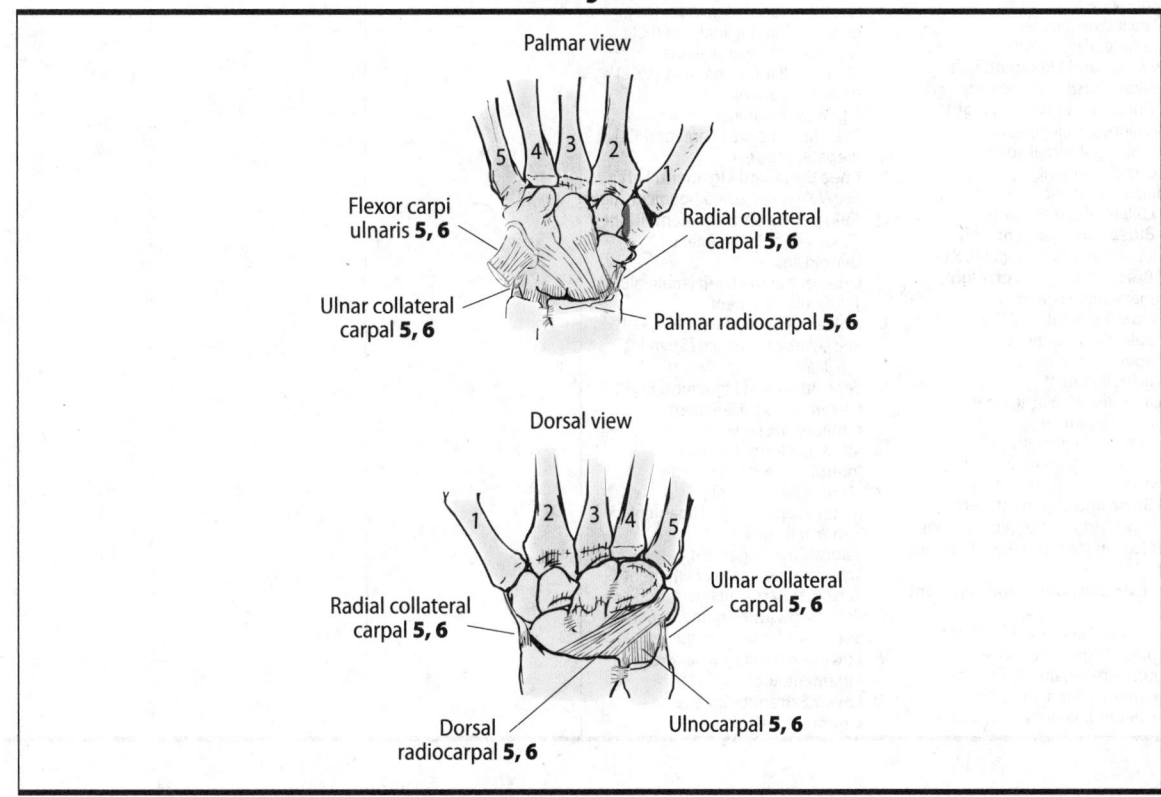

Bursae and Ligaments

Ø   Medical and Surgical
M   Bursae and Ligaments
2   Change   Definition: Taking out or off a device from a body part and putting back an identical or similar device in or on the same body part without cutting or puncturing the skin or a mucous membrane

Explanation: All CHANGE procedures are coded using the approach EXTERNAL

Body Part Character 4	Approach Character 5	Device Character 6	Qualifier Character 7
X Upper Bursa and Ligament Y Lower Bursa and Ligament	X External	Ø Drainage Device Y Other Device	Z No Qualifier

Non-OR   All body part, approach, device, and qualifier values

Ø   Medical and Surgical
M   Bursae and Ligaments
5   Destruction   Definition: Physical eradication of all or a portion of a body part by the direct use of energy, force, or a destructive agent

Explanation: None of the body part is physically taken out

Body Part Character 4		Approach Character 5	Device Character 6	Qualifier Character 7
Ø Head and Neck Bursa and Ligament Alar ligament of axis Cervical interspinous ligament Cervical intertransverse ligament Cervical ligamentum flavum Interspinous ligament, cervical Intertransverse ligament, cervical Lateral temporomandibular ligament Ligamentum flavum, cervical Sphenomandibular ligament Stylomandibular ligament Transverse ligament of atlas **1 Shoulder Bursa and Ligament, Right** Acromioclavicular ligament Coracoacromial ligament Coracoclavicular ligament Coracohumeral ligament Costoclavicular ligament Glenohumeral ligament Interclavicular ligament Sternoclavicular ligament Subacromial bursa Transverse humeral ligament Transverse scapular ligament **2 Shoulder Bursa and Ligament, Left** *See 1 Shoulder Bursa and Ligament, Right* **3 Elbow Bursa and Ligfament, Right** Annular ligament Olecranon bursa Radial collateral ligament Ulnar collateral ligament **4 Elbow Bursa and Ligament, Left** *See 3 Elbow Bursa and Ligament, Right* **5 Wrist Bursa and Ligament, Right** Palmar ulnocarpal ligament Radial collateral carpal ligament Radiocarpal ligament Radioulnar ligament Ulnar collateral carpal ligament **6 Wrist Bursa and Ligament, Left** *See 5 Wrist Bursa and Ligament, Right* **7 Hand Bursa and Ligament, Right** Carpometacarpal ligament Intercarpal ligament Interphalangeal ligament Lunotriquetral ligament Metacarpal ligament Metacarpophalangeal ligament Pisohamate ligament Pisometacarpal ligament Scapholunate ligament Scaphotrapezium ligament **8 Hand Bursa and Ligament, Left** *See 7 Hand Bursa and Ligament, Right* **9 Upper Extremity Bursa and Ligament, Right** **B Upper Extremity Bursa and Ligament, Left** **C Upper Spine Bursa and Ligament** Interspinous ligament, thoracic Intertransverse ligament, thoracic Ligamentum flavum, thoracic Supraspinous ligament	**D Lower Spine Bursa and Ligament** Iliolumbar ligament Interspinous ligament, lumbar Intertransverse ligament, lumbar Ligamentum flavum, lumbar Sacrococcygeal ligament Sacroiliac ligament Sacrospinous ligament Sacrotuberous ligament Supraspinous ligament **F Sternum Bursa and Ligament** Costoxiphoid ligament Sternocostal ligament **G Rib(s) Bursa and Ligament** Costotransverse ligament **H Abdomen Bursa and Ligament, Right** **J Abdomen Bursa and Ligament, Left** **K Perineum Bursa and Ligament** **L Hip Bursa and Ligament, Right** Iliofemoral ligament Ischiofemoral ligament Pubofemoral ligament Transverse acetabular ligament Trochanteric bursa **M Hip Bursa and Ligament, Left** *See L Hip Bursa and Ligament, Right* **N Knee Bursa and Ligament, Right** Anterior cruciate ligament (ACL) Lateral collateral ligament (LCL) Ligament of head of fibula Medial collateral ligament (MCL) Patellar ligament Popliteal ligament Posterior cruciate ligament (PCL) Prepatellar bursa **P Knee Bursa and Ligament, Left** *See N Knee Bursa and Ligament, Right* **Q Ankle Bursa and Ligament, Right** Calcaneofibular ligament Deltoid ligament Ligament of the lateral malleolus Talofibular ligament **R Ankle Bursa and Ligament, Left** *See Q Ankle Bursa and Ligament, Right* **S Foot Bursa and Ligament, Right** Calcaneocuboid ligament Cuneonavicular ligament Intercuneiform ligament Interphalangeal ligament Metatarsal ligament Metatarsophalangeal ligament Subtalar ligament Talocalcaneal ligament Talocalcaneonavicular ligament Tarsometatarsal ligament **T Foot Bursa and Ligament, Left** *See S Foot Bursa and Ligament, Right* **V Lower Extremity Bursa and Ligament, Right** **W Lower Extremity Bursa and Ligament, Left**	Ø Open 3 Percutaneous 4 Percutaneous Endoscopic	Z No Device	Z No Qualifier

LC Limited Coverage   NC Noncovered   ⊞ Combination Member   HAC associated procedure   Combination Only   DRG Non-OR   Non-OR   New/Revised in GREEN

490   ICD-10-PCS 2020

Bursae and Ligaments

Ø   **Medical and Surgical**
M   **Bursae and Ligaments**
8   **Division**   Definition: Cutting into a body part, without draining fluids and/or gases from the body part, in order to separate or transect a body part
                      Explanation: All or a portion of the body part is separated into two or more portions

Body Part Character 4		Approach Character 5	Device Character 6	Qualifier Character 7
Ø Head and Neck Bursa and Ligament Alar ligament of axis Cervical interspinous ligament Cervical intertransverse ligament Cervical ligamentum flavum Interspinous ligament, cervical Intertransverse ligament, cervical Lateral temporomandibular ligament Ligamentum flavum, cervical Sphenomandibular ligament Stylomandibular ligament Transverse ligament of atlas **1 Shoulder Bursa and Ligament, Right** Acromioclavicular ligament Coracoacromial ligament Coracoclavicular ligament Coracohumeral ligament Costoclavicular ligament Glenohumeral ligament Interclavicular ligament Sternoclavicular ligament Subacromial bursa Transverse humeral ligament Transverse scapular ligament **2 Shoulder Bursa and Ligament, Left** *See 1 Shoulder Bursa and Ligament, Right* **3 Elbow Bursa and Ligament, Right** Annular ligament Olecranon bursa Radial collateral ligament Ulnar collateral ligament **4 Elbow Bursa and Ligament, Left** *See 3 Elbow Bursa and Ligament, Right* **5 Wrist Bursa and Ligament, Right** Palmar ulnocarpal ligament Radial collateral carpal ligament Radiocarpal ligament Radioulnar ligament Ulnar collateral carpal ligament **6 Wrist Bursa and Ligament, Left** *See 5 Wrist Bursa and Ligament, Right* **7 Hand Bursa and Ligament, Right** Carpometacarpal ligament Intercarpal ligament Interphalangeal ligament Lunotriquetral ligament Metacarpal ligament Metacarpophalangeal ligament Pisohamate ligament Pisometacarpal ligament Scapholunate ligament Scaphotrapezium ligament **8 Hand Bursa and Ligament, Left** *See 7 Hand Bursa and Ligament, Right* **9 Upper Extremity Bursa and Ligament, Right** **B Upper Extremity Bursa and Ligament, Left** **C Upper Spine Bursa and Ligament** Interspinous ligament, thoracic Intertransverse ligament, thoracic Ligamentum flavum, thoracic Supraspinous ligament	**D Lower Spine Bursa and Ligament** Iliolumbar ligament Interspinous ligament, lumbar Intertransverse ligament, lumbar Ligamentum flavum, lumbar Sacrococcygeal ligament Sacroiliac ligament Sacrospinous ligament Sacrotuberous ligament Supraspinous ligament **F Sternum Bursa and Ligament** Costoxiphoid ligament Sternocostal ligament **G Rib(s) Bursa and Ligament** Costotransverse ligament **H Abdomen Bursa and Ligament, Right** **J Abdomen Bursa and Ligament, Left** **K Perineum Bursa and Ligament** **L Hip Bursa and Ligament, Right** Iliofemoral ligament Ischiofemoral ligament Pubofemoral ligament Transverse acetabular ligament Trochanteric bursa **M Hip Bursa and Ligament, Left** *See L Hip Bursa and Ligament, Right* **N Knee Bursa and Ligament, Right** Anterior cruciate ligament (ACL) Lateral collateral ligament (LCL) Ligament of head of fibula Medial collateral ligament (MCL) Patellar ligament Popliteal ligament Posterior cruciate ligament (PCL) Prepatellar bursa **P Knee Bursa and Ligament, Left** *See N Knee Bursa and Ligament, Right* **Q Ankle Bursa and Ligament, Right** Calcaneofibular ligament Deltoid ligament Ligament of the lateral malleolus Talofibular ligament **R Ankle Bursa and Ligament, Left** *See Q Ankle Bursa and Ligament, Right* **S Foot Bursa and Ligament, Right** Calcaneocuboid ligament Cuneonavicular ligament Intercuneiform ligament Interphalangeal ligament Metatarsal ligament Metatarsophalangeal ligament Subtalar ligament Talocalcaneal ligament Talocalcaneonavicular ligament Tarsometatarsal ligament **T Foot Bursa and Ligament, Left** *See S Foot Bursa and Ligament, Right* **V Lower Extremity Bursa and Ligament, Right** **W Lower Extremity Bursa and Ligament, Left**	**Ø** Open **3** Percutaneous **4** Percutaneous Endoscopic	**Z** No Device	**Z** No Qualifier

Bursae and Ligaments

Ø   **Medical and Surgical**
M   **Bursae and Ligaments**
9   **Drainage**   Definition: Taking or letting out fluids and/or gases from a body part
                   Explanation: The qualifier DIAGNOSTIC is used to identify drainage procedures that are biopsies

Body Part Character 4		Approach Character 5	Device Character 6	Qualifier Character 7
Ø Head and Neck Bursa and Ligament	**D Lower Spine Bursa and Ligament**	**Ø Open**	**Ø Drainage Device**	**Z No Qualifier**
Alar ligament of axis	Iliolumbar ligament	**3 Percutaneous**		
Cervical interspinous ligament	Interspinous ligament, lumbar	**4 Percutaneous Endoscopic**		
Cervical intertransverse ligament	Intertransverse ligament, lumbar			
Cervical ligamentum flavum	Ligamentum flavum, lumbar			
Interspinous ligament, cervical	Sacrococcygeal ligament			
Intertransverse ligament, cervical	Sacroiliac ligament			
Lateral temporomandibular ligament	Sacrospinous ligament			
Ligamentum flavum, cervical	Sacrotuberous ligament			
Sphenomandibular ligament	Supraspinous ligament			
Stylomandibular ligament	**F Sternum Bursa and Ligament**			
Transverse ligament of atlas	Costoxiphoid ligament			
1 Shoulder Bursa and Ligament, Right	Sternocostal ligament			
Acromioclavicular ligament	**G Rib(s) Bursa and Ligament**			
Coracoacromial ligament	Costotransverse ligament			
Coracoclavicular ligament	**H Abdomen Bursa and Ligament, Right**			
Coracohumeral ligament	**J Abdomen Bursa and Ligament, Left**			
Costoclavicular ligament	**K Perineum Bursa and Ligament**			
Glenohumeral ligament	**L Hip Bursa and Ligament, Right**			
Interclavicular ligament	Iliofemoral ligament			
Sternoclavicular ligament	Ischiofemoral ligament			
Subacromial bursa	Pubofemoral ligament			
Transverse humeral ligament	Transverse acetabular ligament			
Transverse scapular ligament	Trochanteric bursa			
2 Shoulder Bursa and Ligament, Left	**M Hip Bursa and Ligament, Left**			
See 1 Shoulder Bursa and Ligament, Right	*See L Hip Bursa and Ligament, Right*			
3 Elbow Bursa and Ligament, Right	**N Knee Bursa and Ligament, Right**			
Annular ligament	Anterior cruciate ligament (ACL)			
Olecranon bursa	Lateral collateral ligament (LCL)			
Radial collateral ligament	Ligament of head of fibula			
Ulnar collateral ligament	Medial collateral ligament (MCL)			
4 Elbow Bursa and Ligament, Left	Patellar ligament			
See 3 Elbow Bursa and Ligament, Right	Popliteal ligament			
5 Wrist Bursa and Ligament, Right	Posterior cruciate ligament (PCL)			
Palmar ulnocarpal ligament	Prepatellar bursa			
Radial collateral carpal ligament	**P Knee Bursa and Ligament, Left**			
Radiocarpal ligament	*See N Knee Bursa and Ligament, Right*			
Radioulnar ligament	**Q Ankle Bursa and Ligament, Right**			
Ulnar collateral carpal ligament	Calcaneofibular ligament			
6 Wrist Bursa and Ligament, Left	Deltoid ligament			
See 5 Wrist Bursa and Ligament, Right	Ligament of the lateral malleolus			
7 Hand Bursa and Ligament, Right	Talofibular ligament			
Carpometacarpal ligament	**R Ankle Bursa and Ligament, Left**			
Intercarpal ligament	*See Q Ankle Bursa and Ligament, Right*			
Interphalangeal ligament	**S Foot Bursa and Ligament, Right**			
Lunotriquetral ligament	Calcaneocuboid ligament			
Metacarpal ligament	Cuneonavicular ligament			
Metacarpophalangeal ligament	Intercuneiform ligament			
Pisohamate ligament	Interphalangeal ligament			
Pisometacarpal ligament	Metatarsal ligament			
Scapholunate ligament	Metatarsophalangeal ligament			
Scaphotrapezium ligament	Subtalar ligament			
8 Hand Bursa and Ligament, Left	Talocalcaneal ligament			
See 7 Hand Bursa and Ligament, Right	Talocalcaneonavicular ligament			
9 Upper Extremity Bursa and Ligament, Right	Tarsometatarsal ligament			
B Upper Extremity Bursa and Ligament, Left	**T Foot Bursa and Ligament, Left**			
C Upper Spine Bursa and Ligament	*See S Foot Bursa and Ligament, Right*			
Interspinous ligament, thoracic	**V Lower Extremity Bursa and Ligament, Right**			
Intertransverse ligament, thoracic	**W Lower Extremity Bursa and Ligament, Left**			
Ligamentum flavum, thoracic				
Supraspinous ligament				

ØM9 Continued on next page

Non-OR   ØM9[Ø,1,2,3,4,5,6,7,8,9,B,C,D,F,G,H,J,K,L,M,N,P,Q,R,S,T,V,W]3ØZ
Non-OR   ØM9[1,2,3,4,7,8,9,B,C,D,F,G,H,J,K,L,M,V,W]4ØZ

Ø　**Medical and Surgical**　　　　　　　　　　　　　　　　　　　　　　　　　　　　*ØM9 Continued*
M　**Bursae and Ligaments**
9　**Drainage**　　　　Definition: Taking or letting out fluids and/or gases from a body part
　　　　　　　　　　　Explanation: The qualifier DIAGNOSTIC is used to identify drainage procedures that are biopsies

Body Part Character 4		Approach Character 5	Device Character 6	Qualifier Character 7
Ø Head and Neck Bursa and Ligament Alar ligament of axis Cervical interspinous ligament Cervical intertransverse ligament Cervical ligamentum flavum Interspinous ligament, cervical Intertransverse ligament, cervical Lateral temporomandibular ligament Ligamentum flavum, cervical Sphenomandibular ligament Stylomandibular ligament Transverse ligament of atlas	**D Lower Spine Bursa and Ligament** Iliolumbar ligament Interspinous ligament, lumbar Intertransverse ligament, lumbar Ligamentum flavum, lumbar Sacrococcygeal ligament Sacroiliac ligament Sacrospinous ligament Sacrotuberous ligament Supraspinous ligament	**Ø** Open **3** Percutaneous **4** Percutaneous Endoscopic	**Z** No Device	**X** Diagnostic **Z** No Qualifier
1 Shoulder Bursa and Ligament, Right Acromioclavicular ligament Coracoacromial ligament Coracoclavicular ligament Coracohumeral ligament Costoclavicular ligament Glenohumeral ligament Interclavicular ligament Sternoclavicular ligament Subacromial bursa Transverse humeral ligament Transverse scapular ligament	**F Sternum Bursa and Ligament** Costoxiphoid ligament Sternocostal ligament **G Rib(s) Bursa and Ligament** Costotransverse ligament **H Abdomen Bursa and Ligament, Right** **J Abdomen Bursa and Ligament, Left** **K Perineum Bursa and Ligament** **L Hip Bursa and Ligament, Right** Iliofemoral ligament Ischiofemoral ligament Pubofemoral ligament Transverse acetabular ligament Trochanteric bursa			
2 Shoulder Bursa and Ligament, Left *See 1 Shoulder Bursa and Ligament, Right*	**M Hip Bursa and Ligament, Left** *See L Hip Bursa and Ligament, Right*			
3 Elbow Bursa and Ligament, Right Annular ligament Olecranon bursa Radial collateral ligament Ulnar collateral ligament	**N Knee Bursa and Ligament, Right** Anterior cruciate ligament (ACL) Lateral collateral ligament (LCL) Ligament of head of fibula Medial collateral ligament (MCL) Patellar ligament Popliteal ligament Posterior cruciate ligament (PCL) Prepatellar bursa			
4 Elbow Bursa and Ligament, Left *See 3 Elbow Bursa and Ligament, Right*	**P Knee Bursa and Ligament, Left** *See N Knee Bursa and Ligament, Right*			
5 Wrist Bursa and Ligament, Right Palmar ulnocarpal ligament Radial collateral carpal ligament Radiocarpal ligament Radioulnar ligament Ulnar collateral carpal ligament	**Q Ankle Bursa and Ligament, Right** Calcaneofibular ligament Deltoid ligament Ligament of the lateral malleolus Talofibular ligament			
6 Wrist Bursa and Ligament, Left *See 5 Wrist Bursa and Ligament, Right*	**R Ankle Bursa and Ligament, Left** *See Q Ankle Bursa and Ligament, Right*			
7 Hand Bursa and Ligament, Right Carpometacarpal ligament Intercarpal ligament Interphalangeal ligament Lunotriquetral ligament Metacarpal ligament Metacarpophalangeal ligament Pisohamate ligament Pisometacarpal ligament Scapholunate ligament Scaphotrapezium ligament	**S Foot Bursa and Ligament, Right** Calcaneocuboid ligament Cuneonavicular ligament Intercuneiform ligament Interphalangeal ligament Metatarsal ligament Metatarsophalangeal ligament Subtalar ligament Talocalcaneal ligament Talocalcaneonavicular ligament Tarsometatarsal ligament			
8 Hand Bursa and Ligament, Left *See 7 Hand Bursa and Ligament, Right*	**T Foot Bursa and Ligament, Left** *See S Foot Bursa and Ligament, Right*			
9 Upper Extremity Bursa and Ligament, Right	**V Lower Extremity Bursa and Ligament, Right**			
B Upper Extremity Bursa and Ligament, Left	**W Lower Extremity Bursa and Ligament, Left**			
C Upper Spine Bursa and Ligament Interspinous ligament, thoracic Intertransverse ligament, thoracic Ligamentum flavum, thoracic Supraspinous ligament				

Non-OR　ØM9[Ø,1,2,3,4,5,6,7,8,C,D,F,G,L,M,N,P,Q,R,S,T][Ø,3,4]ZX
Non-OR　ØM9[Ø,1,2,3,4,5,6,7,8,9,B,C,D,F,G,H,J,K,L,M,N,P,Q,R,S,T,V,W]3ZZ
Non-OR　ØM9[Ø,5,6,7,8,9,B,C,D,F,G,H,J,K,N,P,Q,R,S,T,V,W]4ZZ

LC Limited Coverage　**NC** Noncovered　⊞ Combination Member　HAC associated procedure　Combination Only　DRG Non-OR　Non-OR　New/Revised in GREEN

ICD-10-PCS 2020　　　　　　　　　　　　　　　　　　　　　　　　　　　　　　　　　　　　　　　493

ØM9–ØM9

Ø   **Medical and Surgical**
M   **Bursae and Ligaments**
B   **Excision**   Definition: Cutting out or off, without replacement, a portion of a body part
               Explanation: The qualifier DIAGNOSTIC is used to identify excision procedures that are biopsies

Body Part Character 4		Approach Character 5	Device Character 6	Qualifier Character 7
Ø **Head and Neck Bursa and Ligament** Alar ligament of axis Cervical interspinous ligament Cervical intertransverse ligament Cervical ligamentum flavum Interspinous ligament, cervical Intertransverse ligament, cervical Lateral temporomandibular ligament Ligamentum flavum, cervical Sphenomandibular ligament Stylomandibular ligament Transverse ligament of atlas **1** **Shoulder Bursa and Ligament, Right** Acromioclavicular ligament Coracoacromial ligament Coracoclavicular ligament Coracohumeral ligament Costoclavicular ligament Glenohumeral ligament Interclavicular ligament Sternoclavicular ligament Subacromial bursa Transverse humeral ligament Transverse scapular ligament **2** **Shoulder Bursa and Ligament, Left** *See* 1 Shoulder Bursa and Ligament, Right **3** **Elbow Bursa and Ligament, Right** Annular ligament Olecranon bursa Radial collateral ligament Ulnar collateral ligament **4** **Elbow Bursa and Ligament, Left** *See* 3 Elbow Bursa and Ligament, Right **5** **Wrist Bursa and Ligament, Right** Palmar ulnocarpal ligament Radial collateral carpal ligament Radiocarpal ligament Radioulnar ligament Ulnar collateral carpal ligament **6** **Wrist Bursa and Ligament, Left** *See* 5 Wrist Bursa and Ligament, Right **7** **Hand Bursa and Ligament, Right** Carpometacarpal ligament Intercarpal ligament Interphalangeal ligament Lunotriquetral ligament Metacarpal ligament Metacarpophalangeal ligament Pisohamate ligament Pisometacarpal ligament Scapholunate ligament Scaphotrapezium ligament **8** **Hand Bursa and Ligament, Left** *See* 7 Hand Bursa and Ligament, Right **9** **Upper Extremity Bursa and Ligament, Right** **B** **Upper Extremity Bursa and Ligament, Left** **C** **Upper Spine Bursa and Ligament** Interspinous ligament, thoracic Intertransverse ligament, thoracic Ligamentum flavum, thoracic Supraspinous ligament	**D** **Lower Spine Bursa and Ligament** Iliolumbar ligament Interspinous ligament, lumbar Intertransverse ligament, lumbar Ligamentum flavum, lumbar Sacrococcygeal ligament Sacroiliac ligament Sacrospinous ligament Sacrotuberous ligament Supraspinous ligament **F** **Sternum Bursa and Ligament** Costoxiphoid ligament Sternocostal ligament **G** **Rib(s) Bursa and Ligament** Costotransverse ligament **H** **Abdomen Bursa and Ligament, Right** **J** **Abdomen Bursa and Ligament, Left** **K** **Perineum Bursa and Ligament** **L** **Hip Bursa and Ligament, Right** Iliofemoral ligament Ischiofemoral ligament Pubofemoral ligament Transverse acetabular ligament Trochanteric bursa **M** **Hip Bursa and Ligament, Left** *See* L Hip Bursa and Ligament, Right **N** **Knee Bursa and Ligament, Right** Anterior cruciate ligament (ACL) Lateral collateral ligament (LCL) Ligament of head of fibula Medial collateral ligament (MCL) Patellar ligament Popliteal ligament Posterior cruciate ligament (PCL) Prepatellar bursa **P** **Knee Bursa and Ligament, Left** *See* N Knee Bursa and Ligament, Right **Q** **Ankle Bursa and Ligament, Right** Calcaneofibular ligament Deltoid ligament Ligament of the lateral malleolus Talofibular ligament **R** **Ankle Bursa and Ligament, Left** *See* Q Ankle Bursa and Ligament, Right **S** **Foot Bursa and Ligament, Right** Calcaneocuboid ligament Cuneonavicular ligament Intercuneiform ligament Interphalangeal ligament Metatarsal ligament Metatarsophalangeal ligament Subtalar ligament Talocalcaneal ligament Talocalcaneonavicular ligament Tarsometatarsal ligament **T** **Foot Bursa and Ligament, Left** *See* S Foot Bursa and Ligament, Right **V** **Lower Extremity Bursa and Ligament, Right** **W** **Lower Extremity Bursa and Ligament, Left**	**Ø** Open **3** Percutaneous **4** Percutaneous Endoscopic	**Z** No Device	**X** Diagnostic **Z** No Qualifier

Non-OR   ØMB[Ø,1,2,3,4,5,6,7,8,B,C,D,F,G,L,M,N,P,Q,R,S,T][Ø,3,4]ZX
Non-OR   ØMB94ZX

Ø   Medical and Surgical
M   Bursae and Ligaments
C   Extirpation   Definition: Taking or cutting out solid matter from a body part

Explanation: The solid matter may be an abnormal byproduct of a biological function or a foreign body; it may be imbedded in a body part or in the lumen of a tubular body part. The solid matter may or may not have been previously broken into pieces.

Body Part Character 4		Approach Character 5	Device Character 6	Qualifier Character 7
Ø **Head and Neck Bursa and Ligament** Alar ligament of axis Cervical interspinous ligament Cervical intertransverse ligament Cervical ligamentum flavum Interspinous ligament, cervical Intertransverse ligament, cervical Lateral temporomandibular ligament Ligamentum flavum, cervical Sphenomandibular ligament Stylomandibular ligament Transverse ligament of atlas **1** **Shoulder Bursa and Ligament, Right** Acromioclavicular ligament Coracoacromial ligament Coracoclavicular ligament Coracohumeral ligament Costoclavicular ligament Glenohumeral ligament Interclavicular ligament Sternoclavicular ligament Subacromial bursa Transverse humeral ligament Transverse scapular ligament **2** **Shoulder Bursa and Ligament, Left** *See 1 Shoulder Bursa and Ligament, Right* **3** **Elbow Bursa and Ligament, Right** Annular ligament Olecranon bursa Radial collateral ligament Ulnar collateral ligament **4** **Elbow Bursa and Ligament, Left** *See 3 Elbow Bursa and Ligament, Right* **5** **Wrist Bursa and Ligament, Right** Palmar ulnocarpal ligament Radial collateral carpal ligament Radiocarpal ligament Radioulnar ligament Ulnar collateral carpal ligament **6** **Wrist Bursa and Ligament, Left** *See 5 Wrist Bursa and Ligament, Right* **7** **Hand Bursa and Ligament, Right** Carpometacarpal ligament Intercarpal ligament Interphalangeal ligament Lunotriquetral ligament Metacarpal ligament Metacarpophalangeal ligament Pisohamate ligament Pisometacarpal ligament Scapholunate ligament Scaphotrapezium ligament **8** **Hand Bursa and Ligament, Left** *See 7 Hand Bursa and Ligament, Right* **9** **Upper Extremity Bursa and Ligament, Right** **B** **Upper Extremity Bursa and Ligament, Left** **C** **Upper Spine Bursa and Ligament** Interspinous ligament, thoracic Intertransverse ligament, thoracic Ligamentum flavum, thoracic Supraspinous ligament	**D** **Lower Spine Bursa and Ligament** Iliolumbar ligament Interspinous ligament, lumbar Intertransverse ligament, lumbar Ligamentum flavum, lumbar Sacrococcygeal ligament Sacroiliac ligament Sacrospinous ligament Sacrotuberous ligament Supraspinous ligament **F** **Sternum Bursa and Ligament** Costoxiphoid ligament Sternocostal ligament **G** **Rib(s) Bursa and Ligament** Costotransverse ligament **H** **Abdomen Bursa and Ligament, Right** **J** **Abdomen Bursa and Ligament, Left** **K** **Perineum Bursa and Ligament** **L** **Hip Bursa and Ligament, Right** Iliofemoral ligament Ischiofemoral ligament Pubofemoral ligament Transverse acetabular ligament Trochanteric bursa **M** **Hip Bursa and Ligament, Left** *See L Hip Bursa and Ligament, Right* **N** **Knee Bursa and Ligament, Right** Anterior cruciate ligament (ACL) Lateral collateral ligament (LCL) Ligament of head of fibula Medial collateral ligament (MCL) Patellar ligament Popliteal ligament Posterior cruciate ligament (PCL) Prepatellar bursa **P** **Knee Bursa and Ligament, Left** *See N Knee Bursa and Ligament, Right* **Q** **Ankle Bursa and Ligament, Right** Calcaneofibular ligament Deltoid ligament Ligament of the lateral malleolus Talofibular ligament **R** **Ankle Bursa and Ligament, Left** *See Q Ankle Bursa and Ligament, Right* **S** **Foot Bursa and Ligament, Right** Calcaneocuboid ligament Cuneonavicular ligament Intercuneiform ligament Interphalangeal ligament Metatarsal ligament Metatarsophalangeal ligament Subtalar ligament Talocalcaneal ligament Talocalcaneonavicular ligament Tarsometatarsal ligament **T** **Foot Bursa and Ligament, Left** *See S Foot Bursa and Ligament, Right* **V** **Lower Extremity Bursa and Ligament, Right** **W** **Lower Extremity Bursa and Ligament, Left**	**Ø** Open **3** Percutaneous **4** Percutaneous Endoscopic	**Z** No Device	**Z** No Qualifier

LC Limited Coverage   NC Noncovered   ⊞ Combination Member   HAC associated procedure   Combination Only   DRG Non-OR   Non-OR   New/Revised in GREEN

ICD-10-PCS 2020   495

ØMC–ØMC

Ø **Medical and Surgical**
M **Bursae and Ligaments**
D **Extraction** Definition: Pulling or stripping out or off all or a portion of a body part by the use of force
Explanation: The qualifier DIAGNOSTIC is used to identify extraction procedures that are biopsies

Body Part Character 4		Approach Character 5	Device Character 6	Qualifier Character 7
Ø **Head and Neck Bursa and Ligament** Alar ligament of axis Cervical interspinous ligament Cervical intertransverse ligament Cervical ligamentum flavum Interspinous ligament, cervical Intertransverse ligament, cervical Lateral temporomandibular ligament Ligamentum flavum, cervical Sphenomandibular ligament Stylomandibular ligament Transverse ligament of atlas **1** **Shoulder Bursa and Ligament, Right** Acromioclavicular ligament Coracoacromial ligament Coracoclavicular ligament Coracohumeral ligament Costoclavicular ligament Glenohumeral ligament Interclavicular ligament Sternoclavicular ligament Subacromial bursa Transverse humeral ligament Transverse scapular ligament **2** **Shoulder Bursa and Ligament, Left** *See 1 Shoulder Bursa and Ligament, Right* **3** **Elbow Bursa and Ligament, Right** Annular ligament Olecranon bursa Radial collateral ligament Ulnar collateral ligament **4** **Elbow Bursa and Ligament, Left** *See 3 Elbow Bursa and Ligament, Right* **5** **Wrist Bursa and Ligament, Right** Palmar ulnocarpal ligament Radial collateral carpal ligament Radiocarpal ligament Radioulnar ligament Ulnar collateral carpal ligament **6** **Wrist Bursa and Ligament, Left** *See 5 Wrist Bursa and Ligament, Right* **7** **Hand Bursa and Ligament, Right** Carpometacarpal ligament Intercarpal ligament Interphalangeal ligament Lunotriquetral ligament Metacarpal ligament Metacarpophalangeal ligament Pisohamate ligament Pisometacarpal ligament Scapholunate ligament Scaphotrapezium ligament **8** **Hand Bursa and Ligament, Left** *See 7 Hand Bursa and Ligament, Right* **9** **Upper Extremity Bursa and Ligament, Right** **B** **Upper Extremity Bursa and Ligament, Left** **C** **Upper Spine Bursa and Ligament** Interspinous ligament, thoracic Intertransverse ligament, thoracic Ligamentum flavum, thoracic Supraspinous ligament	**D** **Lower Spine Bursa and Ligament** Iliolumbar ligament Interspinous ligament, lumbar Intertransverse ligament, lumbar Ligamentum flavum, lumbar Sacrococcygeal ligament Sacroiliac ligament Sacrospinous ligament Sacrotuberous ligament Supraspinous ligament **F** **Sternum Bursa and Ligament** Costoxiphoid ligament Sternocostal ligament **G** **Rib(s) Bursa and Ligament** Costotransverse ligament **H** **Abdomen Bursa and Ligament, Right** **J** **Abdomen Bursa and Ligament, Left** **K** **Perineum Bursa and Ligament** **L** **Hip Bursa and Ligament, Right** Iliofemoral ligament Ischiofemoral ligament Pubofemoral ligament Transverse acetabular ligament Trochanteric bursa **M** **Hip Bursa and Ligament, Left** *See L Hip Bursa and Ligament, Right* **N** **Knee Bursa and Ligament, Right** Anterior cruciate ligament (ACL) Lateral collateral ligament (LCL) Ligament of head of fibula Medial collateral ligament (MCL) Patellar ligament Popliteal ligament Posterior cruciate ligament (PCL) Prepatellar bursa **P** **Knee Bursa and Ligament, Left** *See N Knee Bursa and Ligament, Right* **Q** **Ankle Bursa and Ligament, Right** Calcaneofibular ligament Deltoid ligament Ligament of the lateral malleolus Talofibular ligament **R** **Ankle Bursa and Ligament, Left** *See Q Ankle Bursa and Ligament, Right* **S** **Foot Bursa and Ligament, Right** Calcaneocuboid ligament Cuneonavicular ligament Intercuneiform ligament Interphalangeal ligament Metatarsal ligament Metatarsophalangeal ligament Subtalar ligament Talocalcaneal ligament Talocalcaneonavicular ligament Tarsometatarsal ligament **T** **Foot Bursa and Ligament, Left** *See S Foot Bursa and Ligament, Right* **V** **Lower Extremity Bursa and Ligament, Right** **W** **Lower Extremity Bursa and Ligament, Left**	**Ø** Open **3** Percutaneous **4** Percutaneous Endoscopic	**Z** No Device	**Z** No Qualifier

Ø   Medical and Surgical
M   Bursae and Ligaments
H   Insertion   Definition: Putting in a nonbiological appliance that monitors, assists, performs, or prevents a physiological function but does not physically take the place of a body part
                           Explanation: None

Body Part Character 4	Approach Character 5	Device Character 6	Qualifier Character 7
X Upper Bursa and Ligament **Y** Lower Bursa and Ligament	**Ø** Open **3** Percutaneous **4** Percutaneous Endoscopic	**Y** Other Device	**Z** No Qualifier

    Non-OR   ØMH[X,Y][3,4]YZ

Ø   Medical and Surgical
M   Bursae and Ligaments
J   Inspection   Definition: Visually and/or manually exploring a body part
                           Explanation: Visual exploration may be performed with or without optical instrumentation. Manual exploration may be performed directly or through intervening body layers.

Body Part Character 4	Approach Character 5	Device Character 6	Qualifier Character 7
X Upper Bursa and Ligament **Y** Lower Bursa and Ligament	**Ø** Open **3** Percutaneous **4** Percutaneous Endoscopic **X** External	**Z** No Device	**Z** No Qualifier

    Non-OR   ØMJ[X,Y][3,X]ZZ

Ø   Medical and Surgical
M   Bursae and Ligaments
M   Reattachment   Definition: Putting back in or on all or a portion of a separated body part to its normal location or other suitable location
                  Explanation: Vascular circulation and nervous pathways may or may not be reestablished

Body Part Character 4		Approach Character 5	Device Character 6	Qualifier Character 7
Ø Head and Neck Bursa and Ligament Alar ligament of axis Cervical interspinous ligament Cervical intertransverse ligament Cervical ligamentum flavum Interspinous ligament, cervical Intertransverse ligament, cervical Lateral temporomandibular ligament Ligamentum flavum, cervical Sphenomandibular ligament Stylomandibular ligament Transverse ligament of atlas **1 Shoulder Bursa and Ligament, Right** Acromioclavicular ligament Coracoacromial ligament Coracoclavicular ligament Coracohumeral ligament Costoclavicular ligament Glenohumeral ligament Interclavicular ligament Sternoclavicular ligament Subacromial bursa Transverse humeral ligament Transverse scapular ligament **2 Shoulder Bursa and Ligament, Left** *See 1 Shoulder Bursa and Ligament, Right* **3 Elbow Bursa and Ligament, Right** Annular ligament Olecranon bursa Radial collateral ligament Ulnar collateral ligament **4 Elbow Bursa and Ligament, Left** *See 3 Elbow Bursa and Ligament, Right* **5 Wrist Bursa and Ligament, Right** Palmar ulnocarpal ligament Radial collateral carpal ligament Radiocarpal ligament Radioulnar ligament Ulnar collateral carpal ligament **6 Wrist Bursa and Ligament, Left** *See 5 Wrist Bursa and Ligament, Right* **7 Hand Bursa and Ligament, Right** Carpometacarpal ligament Intercarpal ligament Interphalangeal ligament Lunotriquetral ligament Metacarpal ligament Metacarpophalangeal ligament Pisohamate ligament Pisometacarpal ligament Scapholunate ligament Scaphotrapezium ligament **8 Hand Bursa and Ligament, Left** *See 7 Hand Bursa and Ligament, Right* **9 Upper Extremity Bursa and Ligament, Right** **B Upper Extremity Bursa and Ligament, Left** **C Upper Spine Bursa and Ligament** Interspinous ligament, thoracic Intertransverse ligament, thoracic Ligamentum flavum, thoracic Supraspinous ligament	**D Lower Spine Bursa and Ligament** Iliolumbar ligament Interspinous ligament, lumbar Intertransverse ligament, lumbar Ligamentum flavum, lumbar Sacrococcygeal ligament Sacroiliac ligament Sacrospinous ligament Sacrotuberous ligament Supraspinous ligament **F Sternum Bursa and Ligament** Costoxiphoid ligament Sternocostal ligament **G Rib(s) Bursa and Ligament** Costotransverse ligament **H Abdomen Bursa and Ligament, Right** **J Abdomen Bursa and Ligament, Left** **K Perineum Bursa and Ligament** **L Hip Bursa and Ligament, Right** Iliofemoral ligament Ischiofemoral ligament Pubofemoral ligament Transverse acetabular ligament Trochanteric bursa **M Hip Bursa and Ligament, Left** *See L Hip Bursa and Ligament, Right* **N Knee Bursa and Ligament, Right** Anterior cruciate ligament (ACL) Lateral collateral ligament (LCL) Ligament of head of fibula Medial collateral ligament (MCL) Patellar ligament Popliteal ligament Posterior cruciate ligament (PCL) Prepatellar bursa **P Knee Bursa and Ligament, Left** *See N Knee Bursa and Ligament, Right* **Q Ankle Bursa and Ligament, Right** Calcaneofibular ligament Deltoid ligament Ligament of the lateral malleolus Talofibular ligament **R Ankle Bursa and Ligament, Left** *See Q Ankle Bursa and Ligament, Right* **S Foot Bursa and Ligament, Right** Calcaneocuboid ligament Cuneonavicular ligament Intercuneiform ligament Interphalangeal ligament Metatarsal ligament Metatarsophalangeal ligament Subtalar ligament Talocalcaneal ligament Talocalcaneonavicular ligament Tarsometatarsal ligament **T Foot Bursa and Ligament, Left** *See S Foot Bursa and Ligament, Right* **V Lower Extremity Bursa and Ligament, Right** **W Lower Extremity Bursa and Ligament, Left**	**Ø Open** **4 Percutaneous Endoscopic**	**Z No Device**	**Z No Qualifier**

LC Limited Coverage   **NC** Noncovered   ⊞ Combination Member   HAC associated procedure   Combination Only   DRG Non-OR   Non-OR   New/Revised in **GREEN**

498   ICD-10-PCS 2020

Ø   Medical and Surgical
M   Bursae and Ligaments
N   Release   Definition: Freeing a body part from an abnormal physical constraint by cutting or by the use of force
                          Explanation: Some of the restraining tissue may be taken out but none of the body part is taken out

Body Part Character 4		Approach Character 5	Device Character 6	Qualifier Character 7
Ø Head and Neck Bursa and Ligament Alar ligament of axis Cervical interspinous ligament Cervical intertransverse ligament Cervical ligamentum flavum Interspinous ligament, cervical Intertransverse ligament, cervical Lateral temporomandibular ligament Ligamentum flavum, cervical Sphenomandibular ligament Stylomandibular ligament Transverse ligament of atlas **1 Shoulder Bursa and Ligament, Right** Acromioclavicular ligament Coracoacromial ligament Coracoclavicular ligament Coracohumeral ligament Costoclavicular ligament Glenohumeral ligament Interclavicular ligament Sternoclavicular ligament Subacromial bursa Transverse humeral ligament Transverse scapular ligament **2 Shoulder Bursa and Ligament, Left** *See 1 Shoulder Bursa and Ligament, Right* **3 Elbow Bursa and Ligament, Right** Annular ligament Olecranon bursa Radial collateral ligament Ulnar collateral ligament **4 Elbow Bursa and Ligament, Left** *See 3 Elbow Bursa and Ligament, Right* **5 Wrist Bursa and Ligament, Right** Palmar ulnocarpal ligament Radial collateral carpal ligament Radiocarpal ligament Radioulnar ligament Ulnar collateral carpal ligament **6 Wrist Bursa and Ligament, Left** *See 5 Wrist Bursa and Ligament, Right* **7 Hand Bursa and Ligament, Right** Carpometacarpal ligament Intercarpal ligament Interphalangeal ligament Lunotriquetral ligament Metacarpal ligament Metacarpophalangeal ligament Pisohamate ligament Pisometacarpal ligament Scapholunate ligament Scaphotrapezium ligament **8 Hand Bursa and Ligament, Left** *See 7 Hand Bursa and Ligament, Right* **9 Upper Extremity Bursa and Ligament, Right** **B Upper Extremity Bursa and Ligament, Left** **C Upper Spine Bursa and Ligament** Interspinous ligament, thoracic Intertransverse ligament, thoracic Ligamentum flavum, thoracic Supraspinous ligament	**D Lower Spine Bursa and Ligament** Iliolumbar ligament Interspinous ligament, lumbar Intertransverse ligament, lumbar Ligamentum flavum, lumbar Sacrococcygeal ligament Sacroiliac ligament Sacrospinous ligament Sacrotuberous ligament Supraspinous ligament **F Sternum Bursa and Ligament** Costoxiphoid ligament Sternocostal ligament **G Rib(s) Bursa and Ligament** Costotransverse ligament **H Abdomen Bursa and Ligament, Right** **J Abdomen Bursa and Ligament, Left** **K Perineum Bursa and Ligament** **L Hip Bursa and Ligament, Right** Iliofemoral ligament Ischiofemoral ligament Pubofemoral ligament Transverse acetabular ligament Trochanteric bursa **M Hip Bursa and Ligament, Left** *See L Hip Bursa and Ligament, Right* **N Knee Bursa and Ligament, Right** Anterior cruciate ligament (ACL) Lateral collateral ligament (LCL) Ligament of head of fibula Medial collateral ligament (MCL) Patellar ligament Popliteal ligament Posterior cruciate ligament (PCL) Prepatellar bursa **P Knee Bursa and Ligament, Left** *See N Knee Bursa and Ligament, Right* **Q Ankle Bursa and Ligament, Right** Calcaneofibular ligament Deltoid ligament Ligament of the lateral malleolus Talofibular ligament **R Ankle Bursa and Ligament, Left** *See Q Ankle Bursa and Ligament, Right* **S Foot Bursa and Ligament, Right** Calcaneocuboid ligament Cuneonavicular ligament Intercuneiform ligament Interphalangeal ligament Metatarsal ligament Metatarsophalangeal ligament Subtalar ligament Talocalcaneal ligament Talocalcaneonavicular ligament Tarsometatarsal ligament **T Foot Bursa and Ligament, Left** *See S Foot Bursa and Ligament, Right* **V Lower Extremity Bursa and Ligament, Right** **W Lower Extremity Bursa and Ligament, Left**	**Ø** Open **3** Percutaneous **4** Percutaneous Endoscopic **X** External	**Z** No Device	**Z** No Qualifier

Non-OR   ØMN[Ø,1,2,3,4,5,6,7,8,9,B,C,D,F,G,H,J,K,L,M,N,P,Q,R,S,T,V,W]XZZ

LC Limited Coverage   **NC** Noncovered   ⊞ Combination Member   HAC associated procedure   Combination Only   DRG Non-OR   Non-OR   New/Revised in GREEN

ICD-10-PCS 2020   **499**

Ø   Medical and Surgical
M   Bursae and Ligaments
P   Removal   Definition: Taking out or off a device from a body part

Explanation: If a device is taken out and a similar device put in without cutting or puncturing the skin or mucous membrane, the procedure is coded to the root operation CHANGE. Otherwise, the procedure for taking out a device is coded to the root operation REMOVAL.

Body Part Character 4	Approach Character 5	Device Character 6	Qualifier Character 7
X Upper Bursa and Ligament Y Lower Bursa and Ligament	Ø Open 3 Percutaneous 4 Percutaneous Endoscopic	Ø Drainage Device 7 Autologous Tissue Substitute J Synthetic Substitute K Nonautologous Tissue Substitute Y Other Device	Z No Qualifier
X Upper Bursa and Ligament Y Lower Bursa and Ligament	X External	Ø Drainage Device	Z No Qualifier

Non-OR   ØMP[X,Y]3ØZ
Non-OR   ØMP[X,Y][3,4]YZ
Non-OR   ØMP[X,Y]XØZ

ⓁⒸ Limited Coverage   ⓃⒸ Noncovered   ⊞ Combination Member   HAC associated procedure   Combination Only   DRG Non-OR   Non-OR   New/Revised in GREEN

500   ICD-10-PCS 2020

Ø   Medical and Surgical
M   Bursae and Ligaments
Q   Repair   Definition: Restoring, to the extent possible, a body part to its normal anatomic structure and function
                      Explanation: Used only when the method to accomplish the repair is not one of the other root operations

Body Part Character 4		Approach Character 5	Device Character 6	Qualifier Character 7
Ø Head and Neck Bursa and Ligament Alar ligament of axis Cervical interspinous ligament Cervical intertransverse ligament Cervical ligamentum flavum Interspinous ligament, cervical Intertransverse ligament, cervical Lateral temporomandibular ligament Ligamentum flavum, cervical Sphenomandibular ligament Stylomandibular ligament Transverse ligament of atlas **1 Shoulder Bursa and Ligament, Right** Acromioclavicular ligament Coracoacromial ligament Coracoclavicular ligament Coracohumeral ligament Costoclavicular ligament Glenohumeral ligament Interclavicular ligament Sternoclavicular ligament Subacromial bursa Transverse humeral ligament Transverse scapular ligament **2 Shoulder Bursa and Ligament, Left** *See 1 Shoulder Bursa and Ligament, Right* **3 Elbow Bursa and Ligament, Right** Annular ligament Olecranon bursa Radial collateral ligament Ulnar collateral ligament **4 Elbow Bursa and Ligament, Left** *See 3 Elbow Bursa and Ligament, Right* **5 Wrist Bursa and Ligament, Right** Palmar ulnocarpal ligament Radial collateral carpal ligament Radiocarpal ligament Radioulnar ligament Ulnar collateral carpal ligament **6 Wrist Bursa and Ligament, Left** *See 5 Wrist Bursa and Ligament, Right* **7 Hand Bursa and Ligament, Right** Carpometacarpal ligament Intercarpal ligament Interphalangeal ligament Lunotriquetral ligament Metacarpal ligament Metacarpophalangeal ligament Pisohamate ligament Pisometacarpal ligament Scapholunate ligament Scaphotrapezium ligament **8 Hand Bursa and Ligament, Left** *See 7 Hand Bursa and Ligament, Right* **9 Upper Extremity Bursa and Ligament, Right** **B Upper Extremity Bursa and Ligament, Left** **C Upper Spine Bursa and Ligament** Interspinous ligament, thoracic Intertransverse ligament, thoracic Ligamentum flavum, thoracic Supraspinous ligament	**D Lower Spine Bursa and Ligament** Iliolumbar ligament Interspinous ligament, lumbar Intertransverse ligament, lumbar Ligamentum flavum, lumbar Sacrococcygeal ligament Sacroiliac ligament Sacrospinous ligament Sacrotuberous ligament Supraspinous ligament **F Sternum Bursa and Ligament** Costoxiphoid ligament Sternocostal ligament **G Rib(s) Bursa and Ligament** Costotransverse ligament **H Abdomen Bursa and Ligament, Right** **J Abdomen Bursa and Ligament, Left** **K Perineum Bursa and Ligament** **L Hip Bursa and Ligament, Right** Iliofemoral ligament Ischiofemoral ligament Pubofemoral ligament Transverse acetabular ligament Trochanteric bursa **M Hip Bursa and Ligament, Left** *See L Hip Bursa and Ligament, Right* **N Knee Bursa and Ligament, Right** Anterior cruciate ligament (ACL) Lateral collateral ligament (LCL) Ligament of head of fibula Medial collateral ligament (MCL) Patellar ligament Popliteal ligament Posterior cruciate ligament (PCL) Prepatellar bursa **P Knee Bursa and Ligament, Left** *See N Knee Bursa and Ligament, Right* **Q Ankle Bursa and Ligament, Right** Calcaneofibular ligament Deltoid ligament Ligament of the lateral malleolus Talofibular ligament **R Ankle Bursa and Ligament, Left** *See Q Ankle Bursa and Ligament, Right* **S Foot Bursa and Ligament, Right** Calcaneocuboid ligament Cuneonavicular ligament Intercuneiform ligament Interphalangeal ligament Metatarsal ligament Metatarsophalangeal ligament Subtalar ligament Talocalcaneal ligament Talocalcaneonavicular ligament Tarsometatarsal ligament **T Foot Bursa and Ligament, Left** *See S Foot Bursa and Ligament, Right* **V Lower Extremity Bursa and Ligament, Right** **W Lower Extremity Bursa and Ligament, Left**	**Ø** Open **3** Percutaneous **4** Percutaneous Endoscopic	**Z** No Device	**Z** No Qualifier

Bursae and Ligaments (left margin)

Ø Medical and Surgical
M Bursae and Ligaments
R Replacement Definition: Putting in or on biological or synthetic material that physically takes the place and/or function of all or a portion of a body part

Explanation: The body part may have been taken out or replaced, or may be taken out, physically eradicated, or rendered nonfunctional during the REPLACEMENT procedure. A REMOVAL procedure is coded for taking out the device used in a previous replacement procedure.

Body Part Character 4		Approach Character 5	Device Character 6	Qualifier Character 7
Ø Head and Neck Bursa and Ligament Alar ligament of axis Cervical interspinous ligament Cervical intertransverse ligament Cervical ligamentum flavum Interspinous ligament, cervical Intertransverse ligament, cervical Lateral temporomandibular ligament Ligamentum flavum, cervical Sphenomandibular ligament Stylomandibular ligament Transverse ligament of atlas **1 Shoulder Bursa and Ligament, Right** Acromioclavicular ligament Coracoacromial ligament Coracoclavicular ligament Coracohumeral ligament Costoclavicular ligament Glenohumeral ligament Interclavicular ligament Sternoclavicular ligament Subacromial bursa Transverse humeral ligament Transverse scapular ligament **2 Shoulder Bursa and Ligament, Left** *See 1 Shoulder Bursa and Ligament, Right* **3 Elbow Bursa and Ligament, Right** Annular ligament Olecranon bursa Radial collateral ligament Ulnar collateral ligament **4 Elbow Bursa and Ligament, Left** *See 3 Elbow Bursa and Ligament, Right* **5 Wrist Bursa and Ligament, Right** Palmar ulnocarpal ligament Radial collateral carpal ligament Radiocarpal ligament Radioulnar ligament Ulnar collateral carpal ligament **6 Wrist Bursa and Ligament, Left** *See 5 Wrist Bursa and Ligament, Right* **7 Hand Bursa and Ligament, Right** Carpometacarpal ligament Intercarpal ligament Interphalangeal ligament Lunotriquetral ligament Metacarpal ligament Metacarpophalangeal ligament Pisohamate ligament Pisometacarpal ligament Scapholunate ligament Scaphotrapezium ligament **8 Hand Bursa and Ligament, Left** *See 7 Hand Bursa and Ligament, Right* **9 Upper Extremity Bursa and Ligament, Right** **B Upper Extremity Bursa and Ligament, Left** **C Upper Spine Bursa and Ligament** Interspinous ligament, thoracic Intertransverse ligament, thoracic Ligamentum flavum, thoracic Supraspinous ligament	**D Lower Spine Bursa and Ligament** Iliolumbar ligament Interspinous ligament, lumbar Intertransverse ligament, lumbar Ligamentum flavum, lumbar Sacrococcygeal ligament Sacroiliac ligament Sacrospinous ligament Sacrotuberous ligament Supraspinous ligament **F Sternum Bursa and Ligament** Costoxiphoid ligament Sternocostal ligament **G Rib(s) Bursa and Ligament** Costotransverse ligament **H Abdomen Bursa and Ligament, Right** **J Abdomen Bursa and Ligament, Left** **K Perineum Bursa and Ligament** **L Hip Bursa and Ligament, Right** Iliofemoral ligament Ischiofemoral ligament Pubofemoral ligament Transverse acetabular ligament Trochanteric bursa **M Hip Bursa and Ligament, Left** *See L Hip Bursa and Ligament, Right* **N Knee Bursa and Ligament, Right** Anterior cruciate ligament (ACL) Lateral collateral ligament (LCL) Ligament of head of fibula Medial collateral ligament (MCL) Patellar ligament Popliteal ligament Posterior cruciate ligament (PCL) Prepatellar bursa **P Knee Bursa and Ligament, Left** *See N Knee Bursa and Ligament, Right* **Q Ankle Bursa and Ligament, Right** Calcaneofibular ligament Deltoid ligament Ligament of the lateral malleolus Talofibular ligament **R Ankle Bursa and Ligament, Left** *See Q Ankle Bursa and Ligament, Right* **S Foot Bursa and Ligament, Right** Calcaneocuboid ligament Cuneonavicular ligament Intercuneiform ligament Interphalangeal ligament Metatarsal ligament Metatarsophalangeal ligament Subtalar ligament Talocalcaneal ligament Talocalcaneonavicular ligament Tarsometatarsal ligament **T Foot Bursa and Ligament, Left** *See S Foot Bursa and Ligament, Right* **V Lower Extremity Bursa and Ligament, Right** **W Lower Extremity Bursa and Ligament, Left**	**Ø Open** **4 Percutaneous Endoscopic**	**7 Autologous Tissue Substitute** **J Synthetic Substitute** **K Nonautologous Tissue Substitute**	**Z No Qualifier**

LC Limited Coverage NC Noncovered ⊞ Combination Member HAC associated procedure Combination Only DRG Non-OR Non-OR New/Revised in GREEN

Ø   **Medical and Surgical**
M   **Bursae and Ligaments**
S   **Reposition**   Definition: Moving to its normal location, or other suitable location, all or a portion of a body part

Explanation: The body part is moved to a new location from an abnormal location, or from a normal location where it is not functioning correctly. The body part may or may not be cut out or off to be moved to the new location.

Body Part Character 4		Approach Character 5	Device Character 6	Qualifier Character 7
Ø Head and Neck Bursa and Ligament Alar ligament of axis Cervical interspinous ligament Cervical intertransverse ligament Cervical ligamentum flavum Interspinous ligament, cervical Intertransverse ligament, cervical Lateral temporomandibular ligament Ligamentum flavum, cervical Sphenomandibular ligament Stylomandibular ligament Transverse ligament of atlas **1 Shoulder Bursa and Ligament, Right** Acromioclavicular ligament Coracoacromial ligament Coracoclavicular ligament Coracohumeral ligament Costoclavicular ligament Glenohumeral ligament Interclavicular ligament Sternoclavicular ligament Subacromial bursa Transverse humeral ligament Transverse scapular ligament **2 Shoulder Bursa and Ligament, Left** *See 1 Shoulder Bursa and Ligament, Right* **3 Elbow Bursa and Ligament, Right** Annular ligament Olecranon bursa Radial collateral ligament Ulnar collateral ligament **4 Elbow Bursa and Ligament, Left** *See 3 Elbow Bursa and Ligament, Right* **5 Wrist Bursa and Ligament, Right** Palmar ulnocarpal ligament Radial collateral carpal ligament Radiocarpal ligament Radioulnar ligament Ulnar collateral carpal ligament **6 Wrist Bursa and Ligament, Left** *See 5 Wrist Bursa and Ligament, Right* **7 Hand Bursa and Ligament, Right** Carpometacarpal ligament Intercarpal ligament Interphalangeal ligament Lunotriquetral ligament Metacarpal ligament Metacarpophalangeal ligament Pisohamate ligament Pisometacarpal ligament Scapholunate ligament Scaphotrapezium ligament **8 Hand Bursa and Ligament, Left** *See 7 Hand Bursa and Ligament, Right* **9 Upper Extremity Bursa and Ligament, Right** **B Upper Extremity Bursa and Ligament, Left** **C Upper Spine Bursa and Ligament** Interspinous ligament, thoracic Intertransverse ligament, thoracic Ligamentum flavum, thoracic Supraspinous ligament	**D Lower Spine Bursa and Ligament** Iliolumbar ligament Interspinous ligament, lumbar Intertransverse ligament, lumbar Ligamentum flavum, lumbar Sacrococcygeal ligament Sacroiliac ligament Sacrospinous ligament Sacrotuberous ligament Supraspinous ligament **F Sternum Bursa and Ligament** Costoxiphoid ligament Sternocostal ligament **G Rib(s) Bursa and Ligament** Costotransverse ligament **H Abdomen Bursa and Ligament, Right** **J Abdomen Bursa and Ligament, Left** **K Perineum Bursa and Ligament** **L Hip Bursa and Ligament, Right** Iliofemoral ligament Ischiofemoral ligament Pubofemoral ligament Transverse acetabular ligament Trochanteric bursa **M Hip Bursa and Ligament, Left** *See L Hip Bursa and Ligament, Right* **N Knee Bursa and Ligament, Right** Anterior cruciate ligament (ACL) Lateral collateral ligament (LCL) Ligament of head of fibula Medial collateral ligament (MCL) Patellar ligament Popliteal ligament Posterior cruciate ligament (PCL) Prepatellar bursa **P Knee Bursa and Ligament, Left** *See N Knee Bursa and Ligament, Right* **Q Ankle Bursa and Ligament, Right** Calcaneofibular ligament Deltoid ligament Ligament of the lateral malleolus Talofibular ligament **R Ankle Bursa and Ligament, Left** *See Q Ankle Bursa and Ligament, Right* **S Foot Bursa and Ligament, Right** Calcaneocuboid ligament Cuneonavicular ligament Intercuneiform ligament Interphalangeal ligament Metatarsal ligament Metatarsophalangeal ligament Subtalar ligament Talocalcaneal ligament Talocalcaneonavicular ligament Tarsometatarsal ligament **T Foot Bursa and Ligament, Left** *See S Foot Bursa and Ligament, Right* **V Lower Extremity Bursa and Ligament, Right** **W Lower Extremity Bursa and Ligament, Left**	**Ø Open** **4 Percutaneous Endoscopic**	**Z No Device**	**Z No Qualifier**

LC Limited Coverage   **NC** Noncovered   ⊞ Combination Member   HAC associated procedure   Combination Only   DRG Non-OR   Non-OR   New/Revised in GREEN

ICD-10-PCS 2020   503

ØMS–ØMS

Bursae and Ligaments

Ø   Medical and Surgical
M   Bursae and Ligaments
T   Resection   Definition: Cutting out or off, without replacement, all of a body part
               Explanation: None

Body Part Character 4		Approach Character 5	Device Character 6	Qualifier Character 7
Ø Head and Neck Bursa and Ligament Alar ligament of axis Cervical interspinous ligament Cervical intertransverse ligament Cervical ligamentum flavum Interspinous ligament, cervical Intertransverse ligament, cervical Lateral temporomandibular ligament Ligamentum flavum, cervical Sphenomandibular ligament Stylomandibular ligament Transverse ligament of atlas **1 Shoulder Bursa and Ligament, Right** Acromioclavicular ligament Coracoacromial ligament Coracoclavicular ligament Coracohumeral ligament Costoclavicular ligament Glenohumeral ligament Interclavicular ligament Sternoclavicular ligament Subacromial bursa Transverse humeral ligament Transverse scapular ligament **2 Shoulder Bursa and Ligament, Left** *See 1 Shoulder Bursa and Ligament, Right* **3 Elbow Bursa and Ligament, Right** Annular ligament Olecranon bursa Radial collateral ligament Ulnar collateral ligament **4 Elbow Bursa and Ligament, Left** *See 3 Elbow Bursa and Ligament, Right* **5 Wrist Bursa and Ligament, Right** Palmar ulnocarpal ligament Radial collateral carpal ligament Radiocarpal ligament Radioulnar ligament Ulnar collateral carpal ligament **6 Wrist Bursa and Ligament, Left** *See 5 Wrist Bursa and Ligament, Right* **7 Hand Bursa and Ligament, Right** Carpometacarpal ligament Intercarpal ligament Interphalangeal ligament Lunotriquetral ligament Metacarpal ligament Metacarpophalangeal ligament Pisohamate ligament Pisometacarpal ligament Scapholunate ligament Scaphotrapezium ligament **8 Hand Bursa and Ligament, Left** *See 7 Hand Bursa and Ligament, Right* **9 Upper Extremity Bursa and Ligament, Right** **B Upper Extremity Bursa and Ligament, Left** **C Upper Spine Bursa and Ligament** Interspinous ligament, thoracic Intertransverse ligament, thoracic Ligamentum flavum, thoracic Supraspinous ligament	**D Lower Spine Bursa and Ligament** Iliolumbar ligament Interspinous ligament, lumbar Intertransverse ligament, lumbar Ligamentum flavum, lumbar Sacrococcygeal ligament Sacroiliac ligament Sacrospinous ligament Sacrotuberous ligament Supraspinous ligament **F Sternum Bursa and Ligament** Costoxiphoid ligament Sternocostal ligament **G Rib(s) Bursa and Ligament** Costotransverse ligament **H Abdomen Bursa and Ligament, Right** **J Abdomen Bursa and Ligament, Left** **K Perineum Bursa and Ligament** **L Hip Bursa and Ligament, Right** Iliofemoral ligament Ischiofemoral ligament Pubofemoral ligament Transverse acetabular ligament Trochanteric bursa **M Hip Bursa and Ligament, Left** *See L Hip Bursa and Ligament, Right* **N Knee Bursa and Ligament, Right** Anterior cruciate ligament (ACL) Lateral collateral ligament (LCL) Ligament of head of fibula Medial collateral ligament (MCL) Patellar ligament Popliteal ligament Posterior cruciate ligament (PCL) Prepatellar bursa **P Knee Bursa and Ligament, Left** *See N Knee Bursa and Ligament, Right* **Q Ankle Bursa and Ligament, Right** Calcaneofibular ligament Deltoid ligament Ligament of the lateral malleolus Talofibular ligament **R Ankle Bursa and Ligament, Left** *See Q Ankle Bursa and Ligament, Right* **S Foot Bursa and Ligament, Right** Calcaneocuboid ligament Cuneonavicular ligament Intercuneiform ligament Interphalangeal ligament Metatarsal ligament Metatarsophalangeal ligament Subtalar ligament Talocalcaneal ligament Talocalcaneonavicular ligament Tarsometatarsal ligament **T Foot Bursa and Ligament, Left** *See S Foot Bursa and Ligament, Right* **V Lower Extremity Bursa and Ligament, Right** **W Lower Extremity Bursa and Ligament, Left**	**Ø Open** **4 Percutaneous Endoscopic**	**Z No Device**	**Z No Qualifier**

LC Limited Coverage   **NC** Noncovered   ⊞ Combination Member   HAC associated procedure   Combination Only   DRG Non-OR   Non-OR   New/Revised in GREEN

504   ICD-10-PCS 2020

Ø   **Medical and Surgical**
M   **Bursae and Ligaments**
U   **Supplement**   Definition: Putting in or on biological or synthetic material that physically reinforces and/or augments the function of a portion of a body part
         Explanation: The biological material is non-living, or is living and from the same individual. The body part may have been previously replaced, and the SUPPLEMENT procedure is performed to physically reinforce and/or augment the function of the replaced body part.

Body Part Character 4		Approach Character 5	Device Character 6	Qualifier Character 7
Ø **Head and Neck Bursa and Ligament** Alar ligament of axis Cervical interspinous ligament Cervical intertransverse ligament Cervical ligamentum flavum Interspinous ligament, cervical Intertransverse ligament, cervical Lateral temporomandibular ligament Ligamentum flavum, cervical Sphenomandibular ligament Stylomandibular ligament Transverse ligament of atlas **1** **Shoulder Bursa and Ligament, Right** Acromioclavicular ligament Coracoacromial ligament Coracoclavicular ligament Coracohumeral ligament Costoclavicular ligament Glenohumeral ligament Interclavicular ligament Sternoclavicular ligament Subacromial bursa Transverse humeral ligament Transverse scapular ligament **2** **Shoulder Bursa and Ligament, Left** *See 1 Shoulder Bursa and Ligament, Right* **3** **Elbow Bursa and Ligament, Right** Annular ligament Olecranon bursa Radial collateral ligament Ulnar collateral ligament **4** **Elbow Bursa and Ligament, Left** *See 3 Elbow Bursa and Ligament, Right* **5** **Wrist Bursa and Ligament, Right** Palmar ulnocarpal ligament Radial collateral carpal ligament Radiocarpal ligament Radioulnar ligament Ulnar collateral carpal ligament **6** **Wrist Bursa and Ligament, Left** *See 5 Wrist Bursa and Ligament, Right* **7** **Hand Bursa and Ligament, Right** Carpometacarpal ligament Intercarpal ligament Interphalangeal ligament Lunotriquetral ligament Metacarpal ligament Metacarpophalangeal ligament Pisohamate ligament Pisometacarpal ligament Scapholunate ligament Scaphotrapezium ligament **8** **Hand Bursa and Ligament, Left** *See 7 Hand Bursa and Ligament, Right* **9** **Upper Extremity Bursa and Ligament, Right** **B** **Upper Extremity Bursa and Ligament, Left** **C** **Upper Spine Bursa and Ligament** Interspinous ligament, thoracic Intertransverse ligament, thoracic Ligamentum flavum, thoracic Supraspinous ligament	**D** **Lower Spine Bursa and Ligament** Iliolumbar ligament Interspinous ligament, lumbar Intertransverse ligament, lumbar Ligamentum flavum, lumbar Sacrococcygeal ligament Sacroiliac ligament Sacrospinous ligament Sacrotuberous ligament Supraspinous ligament **F** **Sternum Bursa and Ligament** Costoxiphoid ligament Sternocostal ligament **G** **Rib(s) Bursa and Ligament** Costotransverse ligament **H** **Abdomen Bursa and Ligament, Right** **J** **Abdomen Bursa and Ligament, Left** **K** **Perineum Bursa and Ligament** **L** **Hip Bursa and Ligament, Right** Iliofemoral ligament Ischiofemoral ligament Pubofemoral ligament Transverse acetabular ligament Trochanteric bursa **M** **Hip Bursa and Ligament, Left** *See L Hip Bursa and Ligament, Right* **N** **Knee Bursa and Ligament, Right** Anterior cruciate ligament (ACL) Lateral collateral ligament (LCL) Ligament of head of fibula Medial collateral ligament (MCL) Patellar ligament Popliteal ligament Posterior cruciate ligament (PCL) Prepatellar bursa **P** **Knee Bursa and Ligament, Left** *See N Knee Bursa and Ligament, Right* **Q** **Ankle Bursa and Ligament, Right** Calcaneofibular ligament Deltoid ligament Ligament of the lateral malleolus Talofibular ligament **R** **Ankle Bursa and Ligament, Left** *See Q Ankle Bursa and Ligament, Right* **S** **Foot Bursa and Ligament, Right** Calcaneocuboid ligament Cuneonavicular ligament Intercuneiform ligament Interphalangeal ligament Metatarsal ligament Metatarsophalangeal ligament Subtalar ligament Talocalcaneal ligament Talocalcaneonavicular ligament Tarsometatarsal ligament **T** **Foot Bursa and Ligament, Left** *See S Foot Bursa and Ligament, Right* **V** **Lower Extremity Bursa and Ligament, Right** **W** **Lower Extremity Bursa and Ligament, Left**	**Ø** Open **4** Percutaneous Endoscopic	**7** Autologous Tissue Substitute **J** Synthetic Substitute **K** Nonautologous Tissue Substitute	**Z** No Qualifier

LC Limited Coverage   **NC** Noncovered   ⊞ Combination Member   HAC associated procedure   Combination Only   DRG Non-OR   Non-OR   New/Revised in GREEN

ICD-10-PCS 2020   505

Ø   **Medical and Surgical**
M   **Bursae and Ligaments**
W   **Revision**   Definition: Correcting, to the extent possible, a portion of a malfunctioning device or the position of a displaced device

                           Explanation: Revision can include correcting a malfunctioning or displaced device by taking out or putting in components of the device such as a screw or pin

Body Part Character 4	Approach Character 5	Device Character 6	Qualifier Character 7
X Upper Bursa and Ligament Y Lower Bursa and Ligament	Ø Open 3 Percutaneous 4 Percutaneous Endoscopic	Ø Drainage Device 7 Autologous Tissue Substitute J Synthetic Substitute K Nonautologous Tissue Substitute Y Other Device	Z No Qualifier
X Upper Bursa and Ligament Y Lower Bursa and Ligament	X External	Ø Drainage Device 7 Autologous Tissue Substitute J Synthetic Substitute K Nonautologous Tissue Substitute	Z No Qualifier

Non-OR   ØMW[X,Y][3,4]YZ
Non-OR   ØMW[X,Y]X[Ø,7,J,K]Z

LC Limited Coverage   NC Noncovered   ⊞ Combination Member   HAC associated procedure   Combination Only   DRG Non-OR   Non-OR   New/Revised in GREEN

506   ICD-10-PCS 2020

Ø   **Medical and Surgical**
M   **Bursae and Ligaments**
X   **Transfer**   Definition: Moving, without taking out, all or a portion of a body part to another location to take over the function of all or a portion of a body part

Explanation: The body part transferred remains connected to its vascular and nervous supply

Body Part Character 4		Approach Character 5	Device Character 6	Qualifier Character 7
Ø **Head and Neck Bursa and Ligament** Alar ligament of axis Cervical interspinous ligament Cervical intertransverse ligament Cervical ligamentum flavum Interspinous ligament, cervical Intertransverse ligament, cervical Lateral temporomandibular ligament Ligamentum flavum, cervical Sphenomandibular ligament Stylomandibular ligament Transverse ligament of atlas **1** **Shoulder Bursa and Ligament, Right** Acromioclavicular ligament Coracoacromial ligament Coracoclavicular ligament Coracohumeral ligament Costoclavicular ligament Glenohumeral ligament Interclavicular ligament Sternoclavicular ligament Subacromial bursa Transverse humeral ligament Transverse scapular ligament **2** **Shoulder Bursa and Ligament, Left** *See 1 Shoulder Bursa and Ligament, Right* **3** **Elbow Bursa and Ligament, Right** Annular ligament Olecranon bursa Radial collateral ligament Ulnar collateral ligament **4** **Elbow Bursa and Ligament, Left** *See 3 Elbow Bursa and Ligament, Right* **5** **Wrist Bursa and Ligament, Right** Palmar ulnocarpal ligament Radial collateral carpal ligament Radiocarpal ligament Radioulnar ligament Ulnar collateral carpal ligament **6** **Wrist Bursa and Ligament, Left** *See 5 Wrist Bursa and Ligament, Right* **7** **Hand Bursa and Ligament, Right** Carpometacarpal ligament Intercarpal ligament Interphalangeal ligament Lunotriquetral ligament Metacarpal ligament Metacarpophalangeal ligament Pisohamate ligament Pisometacarpal ligament Scapholunate ligament Scaphotrapezium ligament **8** **Hand Bursa and Ligament, Left** *See 7 Hand Bursa and Ligament, Right* **9** **Upper Extremity Bursa and Ligament, Right** **B** **Upper Extremity Bursa and Ligament, Left** **C** **Upper Spine Bursa and Ligament** Interspinous ligament, thoracic Intertransverse ligament, thoracic Ligamentum flavum, thoracic Supraspinous ligament	**D** **Lower Spine Bursa and Ligament** Iliolumbar ligament Interspinous ligament, lumbar Intertransverse ligament, lumbar Ligamentum flavum, lumbar Sacrococcygeal ligament Sacroiliac ligament Sacrospinous ligament Sacrotuberous ligament Supraspinous ligament **F** **Sternum Bursa and Ligament** Costoxiphoid ligament Sternocostal ligament **G** **Rib(s) Bursa and Ligament** Costotransverse ligament **H** **Abdomen Bursa and Ligament, Right** **J** **Abdomen Bursa and Ligament, Left** **K** **Perineum Bursa and Ligament** **L** **Hip Bursa and Ligament, Right** Iliofemoral ligament Ischiofemoral ligament Pubofemoral ligament Transverse acetabular ligament Trochanteric bursa **M** **Hip Bursa and Ligament, Left** *See L Hip Bursa and Ligament, Right* **N** **Knee Bursa and Ligament, Right** Anterior cruciate ligament (ACL) Lateral collateral ligament (LCL) Ligament of head of fibula Medial collateral ligament (MCL) Patellar ligament Popliteal ligament Posterior cruciate ligament (PCL) Prepatellar bursa **P** **Knee Bursa and Ligament, Left** *See N Knee Bursa and Ligament, Right* **Q** **Ankle Bursa and Ligament, Right** Calcaneofibular ligament Deltoid ligament Ligament of the lateral malleolus Talofibular ligament **R** **Ankle Bursa and Ligament, Left** *See Q Ankle Bursa and Ligament, Right* **S** **Foot Bursa and Ligament, Right** Calcaneocuboid ligament Cuneonavicular ligament Intercuneiform ligament Interphalangeal ligament Metatarsal ligament Metatarsophalangeal ligament Subtalar ligament Talocalcaneal ligament Talocalcaneonavicular ligament Tarsometatarsal ligament **T** **Foot Bursa and Ligament, Left** *See S Foot Bursa and Ligament, Right* **V** **Lower Extremity Bursa and Ligament, Right** **W** **Lower Extremity Bursa and Ligament, Left**	**Ø** Open **4** Percutaneous Endoscopic	**Z** No Device	**Z** No Qualifier

LC Limited Coverage   NC Noncovered   ⊞ Combination Member   HAC associated procedure   Combination Only   DRG Non-OR   Non-OR   New/Revised in GREEN

ICD-10-PCS 2020   **507**

Head and Facial Bones ØN2–ØNW

Character Meanings

This Character Meaning table is provided as a guide to assist the user in the identification of character members that may be found in this section of code tables. It **SHOULD NOT** be used to build a PCS code.

Operation–Character 3		Body Part–Character 4		Approach–Character 5		Device–Character 6		Qualifier–Character 7	
2	Change	Ø	Skull	Ø	Open	Ø	Drainage Device	X	Diagnostic
5	Destruction	1	Frontal Bone	3	Percutaneous	4	Internal Fixation Device	Z	No Qualifier
8	Division	3	Parietal Bone, Right	4	Percutaneous Endoscopic	5	External Fixation Device		
9	Drainage	4	Parietal Bone, Left	X	External	7	Autologous Tissue Substitute		
B	Excision	5	Temporal Bone, Right			J	Synthetic Substitute		
C	Extirpation	6	Temporal Bone, Left			K	Nonautologous Tissue Substitute		
D	Extraction	7	Occipital Bone			M	Bone Growth Stimulator		
H	Insertion	B	Nasal Bone			N	Neurostimulator Generator		
J	Inspection	C	Sphenoid Bone			S	Hearing Device		
N	Release	F	Ethmoid Bone, Right			Y	Other Device		
P	Removal	G	Ethmoid Bone, Left			Z	No Device		
Q	Repair	H	Lacrimal Bone, Right						
R	Replacement	J	Lacrimal Bone, Left						
S	Reposition	K	Palatine Bone, Right						
T	Resection	L	Palatine Bone, Left						
U	Supplement	M	Zygomatic Bone, Right						
W	Revision	N	Zygomatic Bone, Left						
		P	Orbit, Right						
		Q	Orbit, Left						
		R	Maxilla						
		T	Mandible, Right						
		V	Mandible, Left						
		W	Facial Bone						
		X	Hyoid Bone						

AHA Coding Clinic for table ØNB
2017, 1Q, 20   Preparatory nasal adhesion repair before definitive cleft palate repair
2015, 3Q, 3-8   Excisional and nonexcisional debridement
2015, 2Q, 12   Orbital exenteration

AHA Coding Clinic for table ØND
2017, 4Q, 41   Extraction procedures

AHA Coding Clinic for table ØNH
2015, 3Q, 13   Nonexcisional debridement of cranial wound with removal and replacement of hardware

AHA Coding Clinic for table ØNP
2015, 3Q, 13   Nonexcisional debridement of cranial wound with removal and replacement of hardware

AHA Coding Clinic for table ØNQ
2016, 3Q, 29   Closure of bilateral alveolar clefts

AHA Coding Clinic for table ØNR
2017, 3Q, 17   Resection of schwannoma and placement of DuraGen and Lorenz cranial plating system
2017, 3Q, 22   Replacement of native skull bone flap
2017, 1Q, 23   Reconstruction of mandible using titanium and bone
2014, 3Q, 7   Hemi-cranioplasty for repair of cranial defect

AHA Coding Clinic for table ØNS
2017, 3Q, 22   Replacement of native skull bone flap
2017, 1Q, 20   Preparatory nasal adhesion repair before definitive cleft palate repair
2016, 2Q, 30   Clipping (occlusion) of cerebral artery, decompressive craniectomy and storage of bone flap in abdominal wall
2015, 3Q, 17   Craniosynostosis with cranial vault reconstruction
2015, 3Q, 27   Moyamoya disease and hemispheric pial synangiosis with craniotomy
2014, 3Q, 23   Le Fort I osteotomy
2013, 3Q, 24   Distraction osteogenesis
2013, 3Q, 25   Fracture of frontal bone with repair and coagulation for hemostasis

AHA Coding Clinic for table ØNU
2016, 3Q, 29   Closure of bilateral alveolar clefts
2013, 3Q, 24   Distraction osteogenesis

Head and Facial Bones

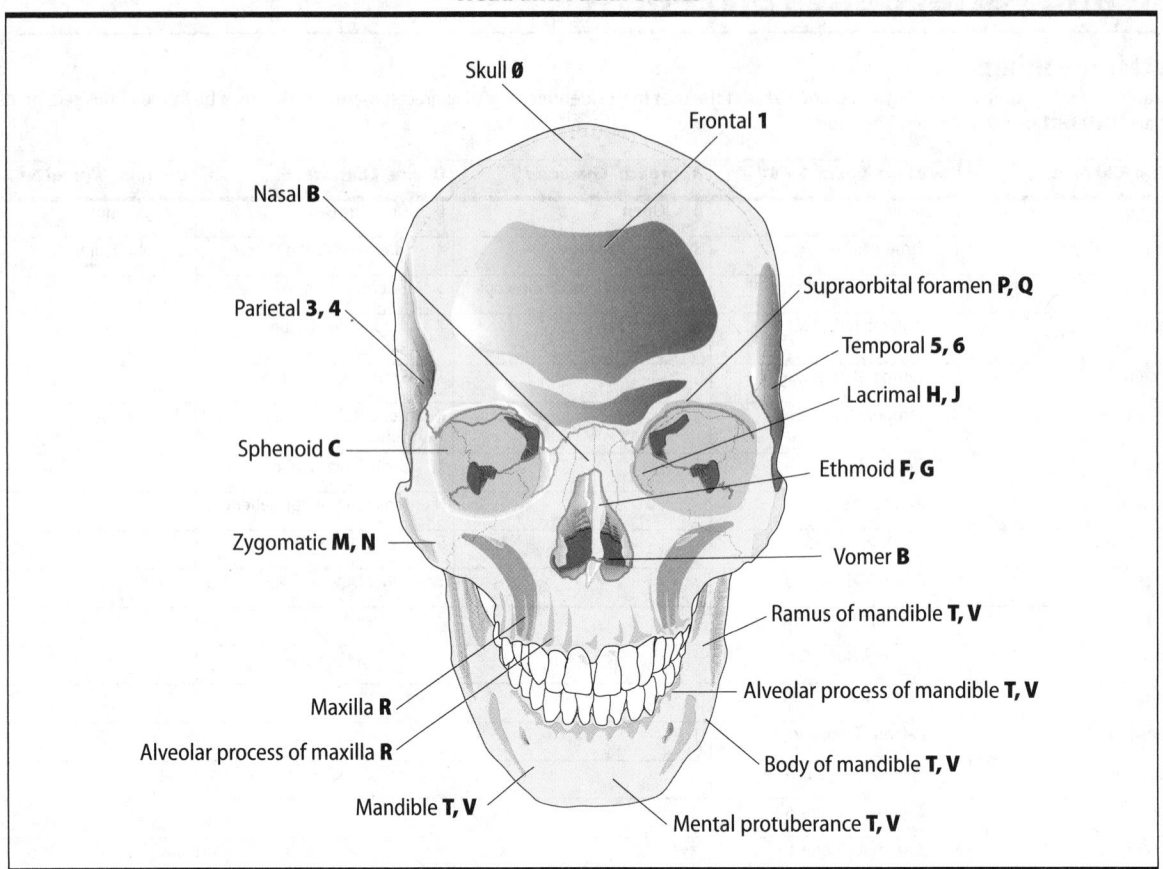

Skull **Ø**

Frontal **1**

Nasal **B**

Supraorbital foramen **P, Q**

Parietal **3, 4**

Temporal **5, 6**

Lacrimal **H, J**

Sphenoid **C**

Ethmoid **F, G**

Zygomatic **M, N**

Vomer **B**

Ramus of mandible **T, V**

Maxilla **R**

Alveolar process of mandible **T, V**

Alveolar process of maxilla **R**

Body of mandible **T, V**

Mandible **T, V**

Mental protuberance **T, V**

Skull Bones

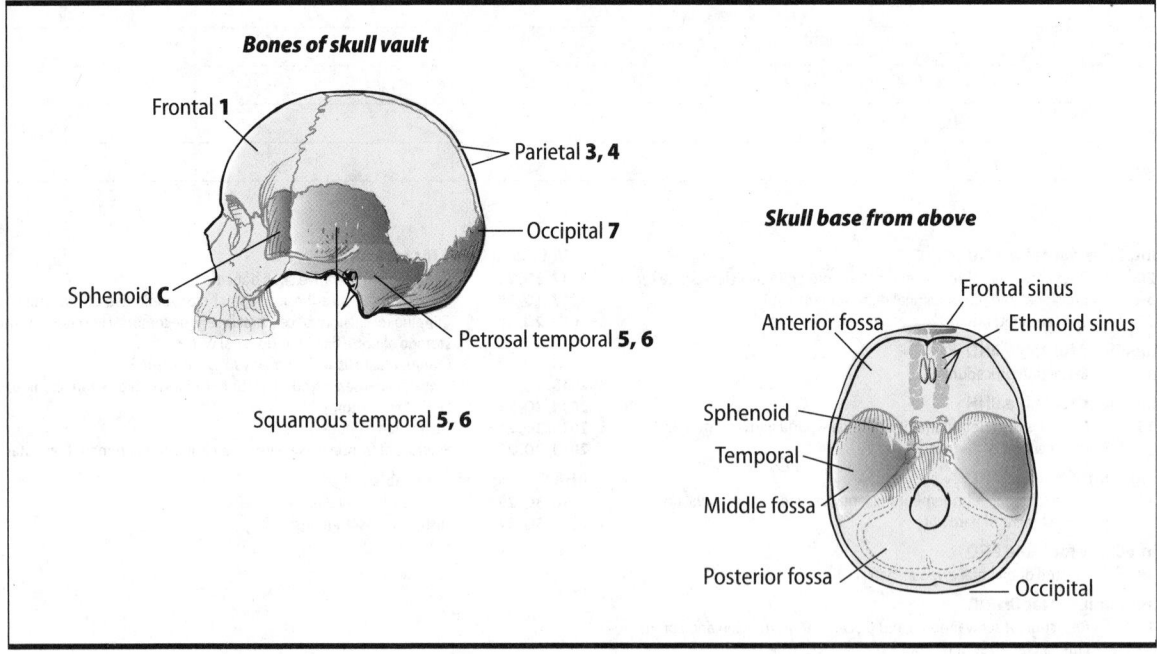

Bones of skull vault

Frontal **1**

Parietal **3, 4**

Occipital **7**

Sphenoid **C**

Petrosal temporal **5, 6**

Squamous temporal **5, 6**

Skull base from above

Frontal sinus

Anterior fossa

Ethmoid sinus

Sphenoid

Temporal

Middle fossa

Posterior fossa

Occipital

Ø	Medical and Surgical
N	Head and Facial Bones
2	Change

Definition: Taking out or off a device from a body part and putting back an identical or similar device in or on the same body part without cutting or puncturing the skin or a mucous membrane

Explanation: All CHANGE procedures are coded using the approach EXTERNAL

Body Part Character 4	Approach Character 5	Device Character 6	Qualifier Character 7
Ø Skull B Nasal Bone 　Vomer of nasal septum W Facial Bone	X External	Ø Drainage Device Y Other Device	Z No Qualifier

Non-OR　All body part, approach, device, and qualifier values

Ø	Medical and Surgical
N	Head and Facial Bones
5	Destruction

Definition: Physical eradication of all or a portion of a body part by the direct use of energy, force, or a destructive agent

Explanation: None of the body part is physically taken out

Body Part Character 4	Approach Character 5	Device Character 6	Qualifier Character 7
Ø Skull 1 Frontal Bone 　Zygomatic process of frontal bone 3 Parietal Bone, Right 4 Parietal Bone, Left 5 Temporal Bone, Right 　Mastoid process 　Petrous part of temporal bone 　Tympanic part of temporal bone 　Zygomatic process of temporal bone 6 Temporal Bone, Left 　See 5 Temporal Bone, Right 7 Occipital Bone 　Foramen magnum B Nasal Bone 　Vomer of nasal septum C Sphenoid Bone 　Greater wing 　Lesser wing 　Optic foramen 　Pterygoid process 　Sella turcica F Ethmoid Bone, Right 　Cribriform plate G Ethmoid Bone, Left 　See F Ethmoid Bone, Right H Lacrimal Bone, Right J Lacrimal Bone, Left K Palatine Bone, Right L Palatine Bone, Left M Zygomatic Bone, Right N Zygomatic Bone, Left P Orbit, Right 　Bony orbit 　Orbital portion of ethmoid bone 　Orbital portion of frontal bone 　Orbital portion of lacrimal bone 　Orbital portion of maxilla 　Orbital portion of palatine bone 　Orbital portion of sphenoid bone 　Orbital portion of zygomatic bone Q Orbit, Left 　See P Orbit, Right R Maxilla 　Alveolar process of maxilla T Mandible, Right 　Alveolar process of mandible 　Condyloid process 　Mandibular notch 　Mental foramen V Mandible, Left 　See T Mandible, Right X Hyoid Bone	Ø Open 3 Percutaneous 4 Percutaneous Endoscopic	Z No Device	Z No Qualifier

Head and Facial Bones

Ø   **Medical and Surgical**
N   **Head and Facial Bones**
8   **Division**   Definition: Cutting into a body part, without draining fluids and/or gases from the body part, in order to separate or transect a body part
                              Explanation: All or a portion of the body part is separated into two or more portions

Body Part Character 4	Approach Character 5	Device Character 6	Qualifier Character 7
Ø **Skull**	**Ø** **Open**	**Z** **No Device**	**Z** **No Qualifier**
1 **Frontal Bone**	**3** **Percutaneous**		
Zygomatic process of frontal bone	**4** **Percutaneous Endoscopic**		
3 **Parietal Bone, Right**			
4 **Parietal Bone, Left**			
5 **Temporal Bone, Right**			
Mastoid process			
Petrous part of temporal bone			
Tympanic part of temporal bone			
Zygomatic process of temporal bone			
6 **Temporal Bone, Left**			
See 5 Temporal Bone, Right			
7 **Occipital Bone**			
Foramen magnum			
B **Nasal Bone**			
Vomer of nasal septum			
C **Sphenoid Bone**			
Greater wing			
Lesser wing			
Optic foramen			
Pterygoid process			
Sella turcica			
F **Ethmoid Bone, Right**			
Cribriform plate			
G **Ethmoid Bone, Left**			
See F Ethmoid Bone, Right			
H **Lacrimal Bone, Right**			
J **Lacrimal Bone, Left**			
K **Palatine Bone, Right**			
L **Palatine Bone, Left**			
M **Zygomatic Bone, Right**			
N **Zygomatic Bone, Left**			
P **Orbit, Right**			
Bony orbit			
Orbital portion of ethmoid bone			
Orbital portion of frontal bone			
Orbital portion of lacrimal bone			
Orbital portion of maxilla			
Orbital portion of palatine bone			
Orbital portion of sphenoid bone			
Orbital portion of zygomatic bone			
Q **Orbit, Left**			
See P Orbit, Right			
R **Maxilla**			
Alveolar process of maxilla			
T **Mandible, Right**			
Alveolar process of mandible			
Condyloid process			
Mandibular notch			
Mental foramen			
V **Mandible, Left**			
See T Mandible, Right			
X **Hyoid Bone**			

Non-OR   ØN8B[Ø,3,4]ZZ

LC Limited Coverage   **NC** Noncovered   ⊞ Combination Member   HAC associated procedure   Combination Only   DRG Non-OR   Non-OR   New/Revised in GREEN

512   ICD-10-PCS 2020

Ø	Medical and Surgical
N	Head and Facial Bones
9	Drainage

Definition: Taking or letting out fluids and/or gases from a body part

Explanation: The qualifier DIAGNOSTIC is used to identify drainage procedures that are biopsies

Body Part Character 4	Approach Character 5	Device Character 6	Qualifier Character 7
Ø Skull	Ø Open	Ø Drainage Device	Z No Qualifier
1 Frontal Bone Zygomatic process of frontal bone	3 Percutaneous 4 Percutaneous Endoscopic		
3 Parietal Bone, Right			
4 Parietal Bone, Left			

5 Temporal Bone, Right
   Mastoid process
   Petrous part of temporal bone
   Tympanic part of temporal bone
   Zygomatic process of temporal bone			

6 Temporal Bone, Left *See* 5 Temporal Bone, Right			
7 Occipital Bone Foramen magnum			
B Nasal Bone Vomer of nasal septum			

C Sphenoid Bone
   Greater wing
   Lesser wing
   Optic foramen
   Pterygoid process
   Sella turcica			

F Ethmoid Bone, Right Cribriform plate			
G Ethmoid Bone, Left *See* F Ethmoid Bone, Right			
H Lacrimal Bone, Right			
J Lacrimal Bone, Left			
K Palatine Bone, Right			
L Palatine Bone, Left			
M Zygomatic Bone, Right			
N Zygomatic Bone, Left			

P Orbit, Right
   Bony orbit
   Orbital portion of ethmoid bone
   Orbital portion of frontal bone
   Orbital portion of lacrimal bone
   Orbital portion of maxilla
   Orbital portion of palatine bone
   Orbital portion of sphenoid bone
   Orbital portion of zygomatic bone			

Q Orbit, Left *See* P Orbit, Right			
R Maxilla Alveolar process of maxilla			

T Mandible, Right
   Alveolar process of mandible
   Condyloid process
   Mandibular notch
   Mental foramen			

V Mandible, Left *See* T Mandible, Right			
X Hyoid Bone			

ØN9 Continued on next page

Non-OR	ØN9[Ø,1,3,4,5,6,7,C,F,G,H,J,K,L,M,N,P,Q,X]3ØZ
Non-OR	ØN9[B,R,T,V][Ø,3,4]ØZ

Head and Facial Bones

ØN9 Continued

Ø   **Medical and Surgical**
N   **Head and Facial Bones**
9   **Drainage**   Definition: Taking or letting out fluids and/or gases from a body part
               Explanation: The qualifier DIAGNOSTIC is used to identify drainage procedures that are biopsies

Body Part Character 4	Approach Character 5	Device Character 6	Qualifier Character 7
Ø Skull	Ø Open	Z No Device	X Diagnostic
1 Frontal Bone	3 Percutaneous		Z No Qualifier
Zygomatic process of frontal bone	4 Percutaneous Endoscopic		
3 Parietal Bone, Right			
4 Parietal Bone, Left			
5 Temporal Bone, Right			
Mastoid process			
Petrous part of temporal bone			
Tympanic part of temporal bone			
Zygomatic process of temporal bone			
6 Temporal Bone, Left			
See 5 Temporal Bone, Right			
7 Occipital Bone			
Foramen magnum			
B Nasal Bone			
Vomer of nasal septum			
C Sphenoid Bone			
Greater wing			
Lesser wing			
Optic foramen			
Pterygoid process			
Sella turcica			
F Ethmoid Bone, Right			
Cribriform plate			
G Ethmoid Bone, Left			
See F Ethmoid Bone, Right			
H Lacrimal Bone, Right			
J Lacrimal Bone, Left			
K Palatine Bone, Right			
L Palatine Bone, Left			
M Zygomatic Bone, Right			
N Zygomatic Bone, Left			
P Orbit, Right			
Bony orbit			
Orbital portion of ethmoid bone			
Orbital portion of frontal bone			
Orbital portion of lacrimal bone			
Orbital portion of maxilla			
Orbital portion of palatine bone			
Orbital portion of sphenoid bone			
Orbital portion of zygomatic bone			
Q Orbit, Left			
See P Orbit, Right			
R Maxilla			
Alveolar process of maxilla			
T Mandible, Right			
Alveolar process of mandible			
Condyloid process			
Mandibular notch			
Mental foramen			
V Mandible, Left			
See T Mandible, Right			
X Hyoid Bone			

Non-OR   ØN9[Ø,1,3,4,5,6,7,C,F,G,H,J,K,L,M,N,P,Q,X]3ZZ
Non-OR   ØN9B[Ø,3,4]Z[X,Z]
Non-OR   ØN9[R,T,V][Ø,3,4]ZZ

Ø   **Medical and Surgical**
N   **Head and Facial Bones**
B   **Excision**   Definition: Cutting out or off, without replacement, a portion of a body part

                  Explanation: The qualifier DIAGNOSTIC is used to identify excision procedures that are biopsies

Body Part Character 4	Approach Character 5	Device Character 6	Qualifier Character 7
Ø **Skull**	**Ø** **Open**	**Z** **No Device**	**X** **Diagnostic**
1 **Frontal Bone**	**3** **Percutaneous**		**Z** **No Qualifier**
Zygomatic process of frontal bone	**4** **Percutaneous Endoscopic**		
3 **Parietal Bone, Right**			
4 **Parietal Bone, Left**			
5 **Temporal Bone, Right**			
Mastoid process			
Petrous part of temporal bone			
Tympanic part of temporal bone			
Zygomatic process of temporal bone			
6 **Temporal Bone, Left**			
See 5 Temporal Bone, Right			
7 **Occipital Bone**			
Foramen magnum			
B **Nasal Bone**			
Vomer of nasal septum			
C **Sphenoid Bone**			
Greater wing			
Lesser wing			
Optic foramen			
Pterygoid process			
Sella turcica			
F **Ethmoid Bone, Right**			
Cribriform plate			
G **Ethmoid Bone, Left**			
See F Ethmoid Bone, Right			
H **Lacrimal Bone, Right**			
J **Lacrimal Bone, Left**			
K **Palatine Bone, Right**			
L **Palatine Bone, Left**			
M **Zygomatic Bone, Right**			
N **Zygomatic Bone, Left**			
P **Orbit, Right**			
Bony orbit			
Orbital portion of ethmoid bone			
Orbital portion of frontal bone			
Orbital portion of lacrimal bone			
Orbital portion of maxilla			
Orbital portion of palatine bone			
Orbital portion of sphenoid bone			
Orbital portion of zygomatic bone			
Q **Orbit, Left**			
See P Orbit, Right			
R **Maxilla**			
Alveolar process of maxilla			
T **Mandible, Right**			
Alveolar process of mandible			
Condyloid process			
Mandibular notch			
Mental foramen			
V **Mandible, Left**			
See T Mandible, Right			
X **Hyoid Bone**			

Non-OR   ØNB[B,R,T,V][Ø,3,4]ZX

LC Limited Coverage   NC Noncovered   ⊞ Combination Member   HAC associated procedure   Combination Only   DRG Non-OR   Non-OR   New/Revised in GREEN

ICD-10-PCS 2020   **515**

ØNB–ØNB

Head and Facial Bones

Ø   **Medical and Surgical**
N   **Head and Facial Bones**
C   **Extirpation**   Definition: Taking or cutting out solid matter from a body part

                         Explanation: The solid matter may be an abnormal byproduct of a biological function or a foreign body; it may be imbedded in a body part or in the lumen of a tubular body part. The solid matter may or may not have been previously broken into pieces.

Body Part Character 4	Approach Character 5	Device Character 6	Qualifier Character 7

1 **Frontal Bone**
    Zygomatic process of frontal bone
3 **Parietal Bone, Right**
4 **Parietal Bone, Left**
5 **Temporal Bone, Right**
    Mastoid process
    Petrous part of temporal bone
    Tympanic part of temporal bone
    Zygomatic process of temporal bone
6 **Temporal Bone, Left**
    See 5 Temporal Bone, Right
7 **Occipital Bone**
    Foramen magnum
B Nasal Bone
    Vomer of nasal septum
C **Sphenoid Bone**
    Greater wing
    Lesser wing
    Optic foramen
    Pterygoid process
    Sella turcica
F **Ethmoid Bone, Right**
    Cribriform plate
G **Ethmoid Bone, Left**
    See F Ethmoid Bone, Right
H **Lacrimal Bone, Right**
J **Lacrimal Bone, Left**
K **Palatine Bone, Right**
L **Palatine Bone, Left**
M **Zygomatic Bone, Right**
N **Zygomatic Bone, Left**
P **Orbit, Right**
    Bony orbit
    Orbital portion of ethmoid bone
    Orbital portion of frontal bone
    Orbital portion of lacrimal bone
    Orbital portion of maxilla
    Orbital portion of palatine bone
    Orbital portion of sphenoid bone
    Orbital portion of zygomatic bone
Q **Orbit, Left**
    See P Orbit, Right
R Maxilla
    Alveolar process of maxilla
T Mandible, Right
    Alveolar process of mandible
    Condyloid process
    Mandibular notch
    Mental foramen
V Mandible, Left
    See T Mandible, Right
X Hyoid Bone
	Ø **Open**
	3 **Percutaneous**
	4 **Percutaneous Endoscopic**
		Z **No Device**	**Z** **No Qualifier**

Non-OR   ØNC[B,R,T,V][Ø,3,4]ZZ

LC Limited Coverage   NC Noncovered   ⊞ Combination Member   HAC associated procedure   Combination Only   DRG Non-OR   Non-OR   New/Revised in GREEN

516   ICD-10-PCS 2020

Ø   **Medical and Surgical**
N   **Head and Facial Bones**
D   **Extraction**   Definition: Pulling or stripping out or off all or a portion of a body part by the use of force
                                Explanation: The qualifier DIAGNOSTIC is used to identify extraction procedures that are biopsies

Body Part Character 4	Approach Character 5	Device Character 6	Qualifier Character 7
Ø **Skull**	Ø Open	Z No Device	Z No Qualifier
1 **Frontal Bone** Zygomatic process of frontal bone			
3 **Parietal Bone, Right**			
4 **Parietal Bone, Left**			

5   **Temporal Bone, Right**
     Mastoid process
     Petrous part of temporal bone
     Tympanic part of temporal bone
     Zygomatic process of temporal bone			

6 **Temporal Bone, Left** *See 5 Temporal Bone, Right*			
7 **Occipital Bone** Foramen magnum			
B **Nasal Bone** Vomer of nasal septum			

C   **Sphenoid Bone**
     Greater wing
     Lesser wing
     Optic foramen
     Pterygoid process
     Sella turcica			

F **Ethmoid Bone, Right** Cribriform plate			
G **Ethmoid Bone, Left** *See F Ethmoid Bone, Right*			
H **Lacrimal Bone, Right**			
J **Lacrimal Bone, Left**			
K **Palatine Bone, Right**			
L **Palatine Bone, Left**			
M **Zygomatic Bone, Right**			
N **Zygomatic Bone, Left**			

P   **Orbit, Right**
     Bony orbit
     Orbital portion of ethmoid bone
     Orbital portion of frontal bone
     Orbital portion of lacrimal bone
     Orbital portion of maxilla
     Orbital portion of palatine bone
     Orbital portion of sphenoid bone
     Orbital portion of zygomatic bone			

Q **Orbit, Left** *See P Orbit, Right*			
R **Maxilla** Alveolar process of maxilla			

T   **Mandible, Right**
     Alveolar process of mandible
     Condyloid process
     Mandibular notch
     Mental foramen			

V **Mandible, Left** *See T Mandible, Right*			
X **Hyoid Bone**			

LC Limited Coverage   **NC** Noncovered   ⊞ Combination Member   HAC associated procedure   Combination Only   DRG Non-OR   Non-OR   New/Revised in GREEN

ICD-10-PCS 2020   517

ØND–ØND

Head and Facial Bones

Ø   **Medical and Surgical**
N   **Head and Facial Bones**
H   **Insertion**   Definition: Putting in a nonbiological appliance that monitors, assists, performs, or prevents a physiological function but does not physically
                    take the place of a body part
                    Explanation: None

Body Part Character 4	Approach Character 5	Device Character 6	Qualifier Character 7
Ø **Skull** ⊞	**Ø** Open	**4** Internal Fixation Device **5** External Fixation Device **M** Bone Growth Stimulator **N** Neurostimulator Generator	**Z** No Qualifier
Ø **Skull**	**3** Percutaneous **4** Percutaneous Endoscopic	**4** Internal Fixation Device **5** External Fixation Device **M** Bone Growth Stimulator	**Z** No Qualifier

1 **Frontal Bone**
    Zygomatic process of frontal bone
3 **Parietal Bone, Right**
4 **Parietal Bone, Left**
7 **Occipital Bone**
    Foramen magnum
C **Sphenoid Bone**
    Greater wing
    Lesser wing
    Optic foramen
    Pterygoid process
    Sella turcica
F **Ethmoid Bone, Right**
    Cribriform plate
G **Ethmoid Bone, Left**
    See F Ethmoid Bone, Right
H **Lacrimal Bone, Right**
J **Lacrimal Bone, Left**
K **Palatine Bone, Right**
L **Palatine Bone, Left**
M **Zygomatic Bone, Right**
N **Zygomatic Bone, Left**
P **Orbit, Right**
    Bony orbit
    Orbital portion of ethmoid bone
    Orbital portion of frontal bone
    Orbital portion of lacrimal bone
    Orbital portion of maxilla
    Orbital portion of palatine bone
    Orbital portion of sphenoid bone
    Orbital portion of zygomatic bone
Q **Orbit, Left**
    See P Orbit, Right
X **Hyoid Bone**
	Ø Open
	3 Percutaneous
	4 Percutaneous Endoscopic
		4 Internal Fixation Device	**Z** No Qualifier

5 **Temporal Bone, Right**
    Mastoid process
    Petrous part of temporal bone
    Tympanic part of temporal bone
    Zygomatic process of temporal bone
6 **Temporal Bone, Left**
    See 5 Temporal Bone, Right
	Ø Open
	3 Percutaneous
	4 Percutaneous Endoscopic
		4 Internal Fixation Device
		S Hearing Device
			Z No Qualifier

B **Nasal Bone** Vomer of nasal septum	**Ø** Open **3** Percutaneous **4** Percutaneous Endoscopic	**4** Internal Fixation Device **M** Bone Growth Stimulator	**Z** No Qualifier

R **Maxilla**
    Alveolar process of maxilla
T **Mandible, Right**
    Alveolar process of mandible
    Condyloid process
    Mandibular notch
    Mental foramen
V **Mandible, Left**
    See T Mandible, Right
	Ø Open
	3 Percutaneous
	4 Percutaneous Endoscopic
		4 Internal Fixation Device
		5 External Fixation Device
			Z No Qualifier

W **Facial Bone**	**Ø** Open **3** Percutaneous **4** Percutaneous Endoscopic	**M** Bone Growth Stimulator	**Z** No Qualifier

Non-OR   ØNHØØ5Z
Non-OR   ØNHØ[3,4]5Z
Non-OR   ØNHB[Ø,3,4][4,M]Z

See Appendix L for Procedure Combinations
⊞   ØNHØØNZ

LC Limited Coverage   NC Noncovered   ⊞ Combination Member   HAC associated procedure   Combination Only   DRG Non-OR   Non-OR   New/Revised in GREEN

518   ICD-10-PCS 2020

Ø   **Medical and Surgical**
N   **Head and Facial Bones**
J   **Inspection**   Definition: Visually and/or manually exploring a body part

Explanation: Visual exploration may be performed with or without optical instrumentation. Manual exploration may be performed directly or through intervening body layers.

Body Part Character 4	Approach Character 5	Device Character 6	Qualifier Character 7
Ø **Skull** **B** **Nasal Bone** Vomer of nasal septum **W** **Facial Bone**	**Ø** Open **3** Percutaneous **4** Percutaneous Endoscopic **X** External	**Z** No Device	**Z** No Qualifier

     Non-OR   ØNJ[Ø,B,W][3,X]ZZ

Ø   **Medical and Surgical**
N   **Head and Facial Bones**
N   **Release**   Definition: Freeing a body part from an abnormal physical constraint by cutting or by the use of force

Explanation: Some of the restraining tissue may be taken out but none of the body part is taken out

Body Part Character 4	Approach Character 5	Device Character 6	Qualifier Character 7

1   **Frontal Bone**
     Zygomatic process of frontal bone
3   **Parietal Bone, Right**
4   **Parietal Bone, Left**
5   **Temporal Bone, Right**
     Mastoid process
     Petrous part of temporal bone
     Tympanic part of temporal bone
     Zygomatic process of temporal bone
6   **Temporal Bone, Left**
     See 5 Temporal Bone, Right
7   **Occipital Bone**
     Foramen magnum
B   **Nasal Bone**
     Vomer of nasal septum
C   **Sphenoid Bone**
     Greater wing
     Lesser wing
     Optic foramen
     Pterygoid process
     Sella turcica
F   **Ethmoid Bone, Right**
     Cribriform plate
G   **Ethmoid Bone, Left**
     See F Ethmoid Bone, Right
H   **Lacrimal Bone, Right**
J   **Lacrimal Bone, Left**
K   **Palatine Bone, Right**
L   **Palatine Bone, Left**
M   **Zygomatic Bone, Right**
N   **Zygomatic Bone, Left**
P   **Orbit, Right**
     Bony orbit
     Orbital portion of ethmoid bone
     Orbital portion of frontal bone
     Orbital portion of lacrimal bone
     Orbital portion of maxilla
     Orbital portion of palatine bone
     Orbital portion of sphenoid bone
     Orbital portion of zygomatic bone
Q   **Orbit, Left**
     See P Orbit, Right
R   **Maxilla**
     Alveolar process of maxilla
T   **Mandible, Right**
     Alveolar process of mandible
     Condyloid process
     Mandibular notch
     Mental foramen
V   **Mandible, Left**
     See T Mandible, Right
X   **Hyoid Bone**
	Ø Open
	3 Percutaneous
	4 Percutaneous Endoscopic
		Z No Device	**Z** No Qualifier

     Non-OR   ØNNB[Ø,3,4]ZZ

Head and Facial Bones

Ø   **Medical and Surgical**
N   **Head and Facial Bones**
P   **Removal**   Definition: Taking out or off a device from a body part

Explanation: If a device is taken out and a similar device put in without cutting or puncturing the skin or mucous membrane, the procedure is coded to the root operation CHANGE. Otherwise, the procedure for taking out a device is coded to the root operation REMOVAL.

Body Part Character 4	Approach Character 5	Device Character 6	Qualifier Character 7
Ø Skull	Ø Open	Ø Drainage Device 4 Internal Fixation Device 5 External Fixation Device 7 Autologous Tissue Substitute J Synthetic Substitute K Nonautologous Tissue Substitute M Bone Growth Stimulator N Neurostimulator Generator S Hearing Device	Z No Qualifier
Ø Skull	3 Percutaneous 4 Percutaneous Endoscopic	Ø Drainage Device 4 Internal Fixation Device 5 External Fixation Device 7 Autologous Tissue Substitute J Synthetic Substitute K Nonautologous Tissue Substitute M Bone Growth Stimulator S Hearing Device	Z No Qualifier
Ø Skull	X External	Ø Drainage Device 4 Internal Fixation Device 5 External Fixation Device M Bone Growth Stimulator S Hearing Device	Z No Qualifier
B Nasal Bone Vomer of nasal septum W Facial Bone	Ø Open 3 Percutaneous 4 Percutaneous Endoscopic	Ø Drainage Device 4 Internal Fixation Device 7 Autologous Tissue Substitute J Synthetic Substitute K Nonautologous Tissue Substitute M Bone Growth Stimulator	Z No Qualifier
B Nasal Bone Vomer of nasal septum W Facial Bone	X External	Ø Drainage Device 4 Internal Fixation Device M Bone Growth Stimulator	Z No Qualifier

Non-OR   ØNPØ[3,4]5Z
Non-OR   ØNPØX[Ø,5]Z
Non-OR   ØNPB[Ø,3,4][Ø,4,7,J,K,M]Z
Non-OR   ØNPBX[Ø,4,M]Z
Non-OR   ØNPWX[Ø,M]Z

Ø   **Medical and Surgical**
N   **Head and Facial Bones**
Q   **Repair**   Definition: Restoring, to the extent possible, a body part to its normal anatomic structure and function

                    Explanation: Used only when the method to accomplish the repair is not one of the other root operations

Body Part Character 4	Approach Character 5	Device Character 6	Qualifier Character 7
Ø **Skull**	**Ø** **Open**	**Z** **No Device**	**Z** **No Qualifier**
1 **Frontal Bone**	**3** **Percutaneous**		
Zygomatic process of frontal bone	**4** **Percutaneous Endoscopic**		
3 **Parietal Bone, Right**	**X** **External**		
4 **Parietal Bone, Left**			
5 **Temporal Bone, Right**			
Mastoid process			
Petrous part of temporal bone			
Tympanic part of temporal bone			
Zygomatic process of temporal bone			
6 **Temporal Bone, Left**			
See 5 Temporal Bone, Right			
7 **Occipital Bone**			
Foramen magnum			
B **Nasal Bone**			
Vomer of nasal septum			
C **Sphenoid Bone**			
Greater wing			
Lesser wing			
Optic foramen			
Pterygoid process			
Sella turcica			
F **Ethmoid Bone, Right**			
Cribriform plate			
G **Ethmoid Bone, Left**			
See F Ethmoid Bone, Right			
H **Lacrimal Bone, Right**			
J **Lacrimal Bone, Left**			
K **Palatine Bone, Right**			
L **Palatine Bone, Left**			
M **Zygomatic Bone, Right**			
N **Zygomatic Bone, Left**			
P **Orbit, Right**			
Bony orbit			
Orbital portion of ethmoid bone			
Orbital portion of frontal bone			
Orbital portion of lacrimal bone			
Orbital portion of maxilla			
Orbital portion of palatine bone			
Orbital portion of sphenoid bone			
Orbital portion of zygomatic bone			
Q **Orbit, Left**			
See P Orbit, Right			
R **Maxilla**			
Alveolar process of maxilla			
T **Mandible, Right**			
Alveolar process of mandible			
Condyloid process			
Mandibular notch			
Mental foramen			
V **Mandible, Left**			
See T Mandible, Right			
X **Hyoid Bone**			

Non-OR   ØNQ[Ø,1,3,4,5,6,7,B,C,F,G,H,J,K,L,M,N,P,Q,R,T,V,X]XZZ

LC Limited Coverage   **NC** Noncovered   ⊞ Combination Member   HAC associated procedure   Combination Only   DRG Non-OR   Non-OR   New/Revised in **GREEN**

ICD-10-PCS 2020   **521**

Head and Facial Bones *(left margin)*

Ø   Medical and Surgical
N   Head and Facial Bones
R   Replacement   Definition: Putting in or on biological or synthetic material that physically takes the place and/or function of all or a portion of a body part
                          Explanation: The body part may have been taken out or replaced, or may be taken out, physically eradicated, or rendered nonfunctional during
                          the REPLACEMENT procedure. A REMOVAL procedure is coded for taking out the device used in a previous replacement procedure.

Body Part Character 4	Approach Character 5	Device Character 6	Qualifier Character 7
Ø Skull	**Ø Open**	**7 Autologous Tissue Substitute**	**Z No Qualifier**
1 Frontal Bone	**3 Percutaneous**	**J Synthetic Substitute**	
Zygomatic process of frontal bone	**4 Percutaneous Endoscopic**	**K Nonautologous Tissue Substitute**	
3 Parietal Bone, Right			
4 Parietal Bone, Left			
5 Temporal Bone, Right			
Mastoid process			
Petrous part of temporal bone			
Tympanic part of temporal bone			
Zygomatic process of temporal bone			
6 Temporal Bone, Left			
See 5 Temporal Bone, Right			
7 Occipital Bone			
Foramen magnum			
B Nasal Bone			
Vomer of nasal septum			
C Sphenoid Bone			
Greater wing			
Lesser wing			
Optic foramen			
Pterygoid process			
Sella turcica			
F Ethmoid Bone, Right			
Cribriform plate			
G Ethmoid Bone, Left			
See F Ethmoid Bone, Right			
H Lacrimal Bone, Right			
J Lacrimal Bone, Left			
K Palatine Bone, Right			
L Palatine Bone, Left			
M Zygomatic Bone, Right			
N Zygomatic Bone, Left			
P Orbit, Right			
Bony orbit			
Orbital portion of ethmoid bone			
Orbital portion of frontal bone			
Orbital portion of lacrimal bone			
Orbital portion of maxilla			
Orbital portion of palatine bone			
Orbital portion of sphenoid bone			
Orbital portion of zygomatic bone			
Q Orbit, Left			
See P Orbit, Right			
R Maxilla			
Alveolar process of maxilla			
T Mandible, Right			
Alveolar process of mandible			
Condyloid process			
Mandibular notch			
Mental foramen			
V Mandible, Left			
See T Mandible, Right			
X Hyoid Bone			

Ø   **Medical and Surgical**
N   **Head and Facial Bones**
S   **Reposition**   Definition: Moving to its normal location, or other suitable location, all or a portion of a body part

                         Explanation: The body part is moved to a new location from an abnormal location, or from a normal location where it is not functioning correctly. The body part may or may not be cut out or off to be moved to the new location.

Body Part Character 4	Approach Character 5	Device Character 6	Qualifier Character 7

Ø **Skull**
R **Maxilla**
    Alveolar process of maxilla
T **Mandible, Right**
    Alveolar process of mandible
    Condyloid process
    Mandibular notch
    Mental foramen
V **Mandible, Left**
    See T Mandible, Right
	Ø **Open**
	3 **Percutaneous**
	4 **Percutaneous Endoscopic**
		4 **Internal Fixation Device**
		5 **External Fixation Device**
		Z **No Device**
			Z **No Qualifier**

Ø **Skull**
R **Maxilla**
    Alveolar process of maxilla
T **Mandible, Right**
    Alveolar process of mandible
    Condyloid process
    Mandibular notch
    Mental foramen
V **Mandible, Left**
    See T Mandible, Right
	X **External**	**Z** **No Device**	**Z** **No Qualifier**

1 **Frontal Bone**
    Zygomatic process of frontal bone
3 **Parietal Bone, Right**
4 **Parietal Bone, Left**
5 **Temporal Bone, Right**
    Mastoid process
    Petrous part of temporal bone
    Tympanic part of temporal bone
    Zygomatic process of temporal bone
6 **Temporal Bone, Left**
    See 5 Temporal Bone, Right
7 **Occipital Bone**
    Foramen magnum
B **Nasal Bone**
    Vomer of nasal septum
C **Sphenoid Bone**
    Greater wing
    Lesser wing
    Optic foramen
    Pterygoid process
    Sella turcica
F **Ethmoid Bone, Right**
    Cribriform plate
G **Ethmoid Bone, Left**
    See F Ethmoid Bone, Right
H **Lacrimal Bone, Right**
J **Lacrimal Bone, Left**
K **Palatine Bone, Right**
L **Palatine Bone, Left**
M **Zygomatic Bone, Right**
N **Zygomatic Bone, Left**
P **Orbit, Right**
    Bony orbit
    Orbital portion of ethmoid bone
    Orbital portion of frontal bone
    Orbital portion of lacrimal bone
    Orbital portion of maxilla
    Orbital portion of palatine bone
    Orbital portion of sphenoid bone
    Orbital portion of zygomatic bone
Q **Orbit, Left**
    See P Orbit, Right
X **Hyoid Bone**
	Ø **Open**
	3 **Percutaneous**
	4 **Percutaneous Endoscopic**
		4 **Internal Fixation Device**
		Z **No Device**
			Z **No Qualifier**

ØNS Continued on next page

Non-OR   ØNS[R,T,V][3,4][4,5,Z]Z
Non-OR   ØNS[Ø,R,T,V]XZZ
Non-OR   ØNS[B,C,F,G,H,J,K,L,M,N,P,Q,X][3,4][4,Z]Z

Head and Facial Bones *(side tab)*

Ø Medical and Surgical
N Head and Facial Bones

ØNS Continued

S Reposition   Definition: Moving to its normal location, or other suitable location, all or a portion of a body part

Explanation: The body part is moved to a new location from an abnormal location, or from a normal location where it is not functioning correctly. The body part may or may not be cut out or off to be moved to the new location.

Body Part Character 4	Approach Character 5	Device Character 6	Qualifier Character 7
1 Frontal Bone Zygomatic process of frontal bone **3 Parietal Bone, Right** **4 Parietal Bone, Left** **5 Temporal Bone, Right** Mastoid process Petrous part of temporal bone Tympanic part of temporal bone Zygomatic process of temporal bone **6 Temporal Bone, Left** *See 5 Temporal Bone, Right* **7 Occipital Bone** Foramen magnum **B Nasal Bone** Vomer of nasal septum **C Sphenoid Bone** Greater wing Lesser wing Optic foramen Pterygoid process Sella turcica **F Ethmoid Bone, Right** Cribriform plate **G Ethmoid Bone, Left** *See F Ethmoid Bone, Right* **H Lacrimal Bone, Right** **J Lacrimal Bone, Left** **K Palatine Bone, Right** **L Palatine Bone, Left** **M Zygomatic Bone, Right** **N Zygomatic Bone, Left** **P Orbit, Right** Bony orbit Orbital portion of ethmoid bone Orbital portion of frontal bone Orbital portion of lacrimal bone Orbital portion of maxilla Orbital portion of palatine bone Orbital portion of sphenoid bone Orbital portion of zygomatic bone **Q Orbit, Left** *See P Orbit, Right* **X Hyoid Bone**	**X External**	**Z No Device**	**Z No Qualifier**

Non-OR   ØNS[1,3,4,5,6,7,B,C,F,G,H,J,K,L,M,N,P,Q,X]XZZ

Ø Medical and Surgical
N Head and Facial Bones
T Resection   Definition: Cutting out or off, without replacement, all of a body part
                 Explanation: None

Body Part Character 4	Approach Character 5	Device Character 6	Qualifier Character 7

1 Frontal Bone
   Zygomatic process of frontal bone
3 Parietal Bone, Right
4 Parietal Bone, Left
5 Temporal Bone, Right
   Mastoid process
   Petrous part of temporal bone
   Tympanic part of temporal bone
   Zygomatic process of temporal bone
6 Temporal Bone, Left
   See 5 Temporal Bone, Right
7 Occipital Bone
   Foramen magnum
B Nasal Bone
   Vomer of nasal septum
C Sphenoid Bone
   Greater wing
   Lesser wing
   Optic foramen
   Pterygoid process
   Sella turcica
F Ethmoid Bone, Right
   Cribriform plate
G Ethmoid Bone, Left
   See F Ethmoid Bone, Right
H Lacrimal Bone, Right
J Lacrimal Bone, Left
K Palatine Bone, Right
L Palatine Bone, Left
M Zygomatic Bone, Right
N Zygomatic Bone, Left
P Orbit, Right
   Bony orbit
   Orbital portion of ethmoid bone
   Orbital portion of frontal bone
   Orbital portion of lacrimal bone
   Orbital portion of maxilla
   Orbital portion of palatine bone
   Orbital portion of sphenoid bone
   Orbital portion of zygomatic bone
Q Orbit, Left
   See P Orbit, Right
R Maxilla
   Alveolar process of maxilla
T Mandible, Right
   Alveolar process of mandible
   Condyloid process
   Mandibular notch
   Mental foramen
V Mandible, Left
   See T Mandible, Right
X Hyoid Bone
	Ø Open	**Z No Device**	**Z No Qualifier**

Head and Facial Bones

Ø **Medical and Surgical**
N **Head and Facial Bones**
U **Supplement** Definition: Putting in or on biological or synthetic material that physically reinforces and/or augments the function of a portion of a body part
Explanation: The biological material is non-living, or is living and from the same individual. The body part may have been previously replaced, and the SUPPLEMENT procedure is performed to physically reinforce and/or augment the function of the replaced body part.

Body Part Character 4	Approach Character 5	Device Character 6	Qualifier Character 7
Ø Skull	**Ø** Open	**7** Autologous Tissue Substitute	**Z** No Qualifier
1 Frontal Bone Zygomatic process of frontal bone	**3** Percutaneous **4** Percutaneous Endoscopic	**J** Synthetic Substitute **K** Nonautologous Tissue Substitute	
3 Parietal Bone, Right			
4 Parietal Bone, Left			
5 Temporal Bone, Right Mastoid process Petrous part of temporal bone Tympanic part of temporal bone Zygomatic process of temporal bone			
6 Temporal Bone, Left *See 5 Temporal Bone, Right*			
7 Occipital Bone Foramen magnum			
B Nasal Bone Vomer of nasal septum			
C Sphenoid Bone Greater wing Lesser wing Optic foramen Pterygoid process Sella turcica			
F Ethmoid Bone, Right Cribriform plate			
G Ethmoid Bone, Left *See F Ethmoid Bone, Right*			
H Lacrimal Bone, Right			
J Lacrimal Bone, Left			
K Palatine Bone, Right			
L Palatine Bone, Left			
M Zygomatic Bone, Right			
N Zygomatic Bone, Left			
P Orbit, Right Bony orbit Orbital portion of ethmoid bone Orbital portion of frontal bone Orbital portion of lacrimal bone Orbital portion of maxilla Orbital portion of palatine bone Orbital portion of sphenoid bone Orbital portion of zygomatic bone			
Q Orbit, Left *See P Orbit, Right*			
R Maxilla Alveolar process of maxilla			
T Mandible, Right Alveolar process of mandible Condyloid process Mandibular notch Mental foramen			
V Mandible, Left *See T Mandible, Right*			
X Hyoid Bone			

Ø   **Medical and Surgical**
N   **Head and Facial Bones**
W   **Revision**   Definition: Correcting, to the extent possible, a portion of a malfunctioning device or the position of a displaced device

                                    Explanation: Revision can include correcting a malfunctioning or displaced device by taking out or putting in components of the device such as a screw or pin

Body Part Character 4	Approach Character 5	Device Character 6	Qualifier Character 7
Ø Skull	Ø Open	Ø Drainage Device 4 Internal Fixation Device 5 External Fixation Device 7 Autologous Tissue Substitute J Synthetic Substitute K Nonautologous Tissue Substitute M Bone Growth Stimulator N Neurostimulator Generator S Hearing Device	Z No Qualifier
Ø Skull	3 Percutaneous 4 Percutaneous Endoscopic X External	Ø Drainage Device 4 Internal Fixation Device 5 External Fixation Device 7 Autologous Tissue Substitute J Synthetic Substitute K Nonautologous Tissue Substitute M Bone Growth Stimulator S Hearing Device	Z No Qualifier
B Nasal Bone Vomer of nasal septum W Facial Bone	Ø Open 3 Percutaneous 4 Percutaneous Endoscopic X External	Ø Drainage Device 4 Internal Fixation Device 7 Autologous Tissue Substitute J Synthetic Substitute K Nonautologous Tissue Substitute M Bone Growth Stimulator	Z No Qualifier

Non-OR   ØNWØX[Ø,4,5,7,J,K,M,S]Z
Non-OR   ØNWB[Ø,3,4,X][Ø,4,7,J,K,M]Z
Non-OR   ØNWWX[Ø,4,7,J,K,M]Z

LC Limited Coverage   NC Noncovered   ⊞ Combination Member   HAC associated procedure   Combination Only   DRG Non-OR   Non-OR   New/Revised in GREEN

ICD-10-PCS 2020   527

Upper Bones ØP2–ØPW

Character Meanings

This Character Meaning table is provided as a guide to assist the user in the identification of character members that may be found in this section of code tables. It **SHOULD NOT** be used to build a PCS code.

Operation–Character 3	Body Part–Character 4	Approach–Character 5	Device–Character 6	Qualifier–Character 7
2 Change	Ø Sternum	Ø Open	Ø Drainage Device OR Internal Fixation Device, Rigid Plate	X Diagnostic
5 Destruction	1 Ribs, 1 to 2	3 Percutaneous	4 Internal Fixation Device	Z No Qualifier
8 Division	2 Ribs, 3 or more	4 Percutaneous Endoscopic	5 External Fixation Device	
9 Drainage	3 Cervical Vertebra	X External	6 Internal Fixation Device, Intramedullary	
B Excision	4 Thoracic Vertebra		7 Autologous Tissue Substitute OR Internal Fixation Device, Intramedullary Limb Lengthening	
C Extirpation	5 Scapula, Right		8 External Fixation Device, Limb Lengthening	
D Extraction	6 Scapula, Left		B External Fixation Device, Monoplanar	
H Insertion	7 Glenoid Cavity, Right		C External Fixation Device, Ring	
J Inspection	8 Glenoid Cavity, Left		D External Fixation Device, Hybrid	
N Release	9 Clavicle, Right		J Synthetic Substitute	
P Removal	B Clavicle, Left		K Nonautologous Tissue Substitute	
Q Repair	C Humeral Head, Right		M Bone Growth Stimulator	
R Replacement	D Humeral Head, Left		Y Other Device	
S Reposition	F Humeral Shaft, Right		Z No Device	
T Resection	G Humeral Shaft, Left			
U Supplement	H Radius, Right			
W Revision	J Radius, Left			
	K Ulna, Right			
	L Ulna, Left			
	M Carpal, Right			
	N Carpal, Left			
	P Metacarpal, Right			
	Q Metacarpal, Left			
	R Thumb Phalanx, Right			
	S Thumb Phalanx, Left			
	T Finger Phalanx, Right			
	V Finger Phalanx, Left			
	Y Upper Bone			

AHA Coding Clinic for table ØPB
2015, 3Q, 3-8   Excisional and nonexcisional debridement
2015, 2Q, 34   Decompressive laminectomy
2013, 4Q, 109   Separating conjoined twins
2013, 4Q, 116   Spinal decompression
2013, 3Q, 20   Superior labrum anterior posterior (SLAP) repair and subacromialdecompression
2012, 4Q, 101   Rib resection with reconstruction of anterior chest wall
2012, 2Q, 19   Multiple decompressive cervical laminectomies

AHA Coding Clinic for table ØPD
2017, 4Q, 41   Extraction procedures

AHA Coding Clinic for table ØPH
2018, 3Q, 26   Anterior vertebral tethering using Dynesys Tethering System
2017, 2Q, 20   Exchange of intramedullary antibiotic impregnated spacer
2016, 4Q, 117   Placement of magnetic growth rods
2014, 4Q, 28   Removal and replacement of displaced growing rods

AHA Coding Clinic for table ØPP
2017, 2Q, 20   Exchange of intramedullary antibiotic impregnated spacer
2016, 4Q, 117   Placement of magnetic growth rods
2014, 4Q, 28   Removal and replacement of displaced growing rods

AHA Coding Clinic for table ØPR
2018, 4Q, 92   Radial head arthroplasty

AHA Coding Clinic for table ØPS
2018, 3Q, 26   Anterior vertebral tethering using Dynesys Tethering System
2017, 4Q, 53   New and revised body part values - Ribs
2016, 1Q, 21   Elongation derotation flexion casting
2015, 4Q, 33   Ravitch operation
2015, 2Q, 35   Application of tongs to reduce and stabilize cervical fracture
2014, 4Q, 26   Placement of vertical expandable prosthetic titanium rib (VEPTR)
2014, 4Q, 32   Open reduction internal fixation of fracture with debridement
2014, 3Q, 33   Radial fracture treatment with open reduction internal fixation, and release of carpal ligament

AHA Coding Clinic for table ØPT
2015, 3Q, 26   Thumb arthroplasty with resection of trapezium

AHA Coding Clinic for table ØPU
2015, 2Q, 20   Cervical laminoplasty
2013, 4Q, 109   Separating conjoined twins

AHA Coding Clinic for table ØPW
2014, 4Q, 26   Adjustment of VEPTR lengthening mechanism
2014, 4Q, 27   Bilateral lengthening of growing rods

Upper Bones

Cervical vertebra **3**

Clavicle **9, B**

Sternum **Ø**

Scapula **5, 6**

Rib **1, 2**

Humerus **C, D, F, G**

Thoracic vertebra **4**

Ulna **K, L**

Radius **H, J**

Carpal **M, N**

Metacarpal **P, Q**

Thumb phalanx **R, S**

Finger phalanx **T, V**

Humerus and Scapula

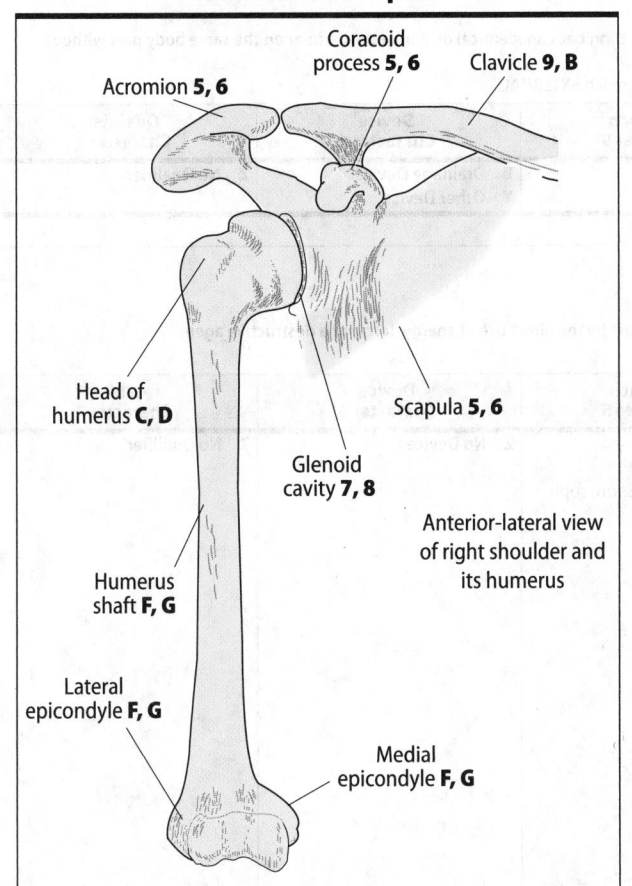

Acromion **5, 6**

Coracoid process **5, 6**

Clavicle **9, B**

Head of humerus **C, D**

Glenoid cavity **7, 8**

Scapula **5, 6**

Anterior-lateral view of right shoulder and its humerus

Humerus shaft **F, G**

Lateral epicondyle **F, G**

Medial epicondyle **F, G**

Radius and Ulna

Radius **H, J**

Olecranon process **K, L**

Coronoid process **K, L**

Ulna **K, L**

Shaft **H, J**

Shaft **K, L**

Radial styloid process **H, J**

Ulnar styloid process **K, L**

Carpal **M, N**

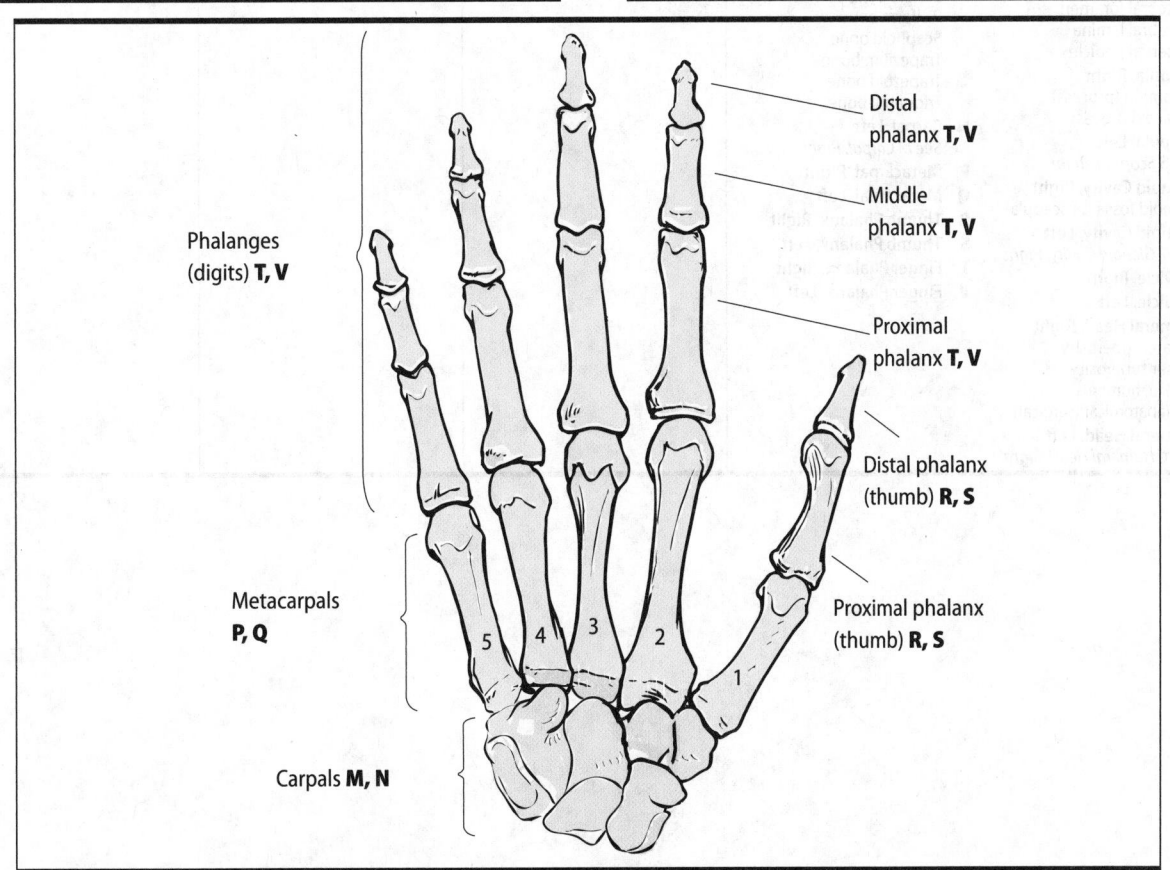

Phalanges (digits) **T, V**

Distal phalanx **T, V**

Middle phalanx **T, V**

Proximal phalanx **T, V**

Distal phalanx (thumb) **R, S**

Proximal phalanx (thumb) **R, S**

Metacarpals **P, Q**

Carpals **M, N**

Ø **Medical and Surgical**
P **Upper Bones**
2 **Change**   Definition: Taking out or off a device from a body part and putting back an identical or similar device in or on the same body part without cutting or puncturing the skin or a mucous membrane

Explanation: All CHANGE procedures are coded using the approach EXTERNAL

Body Part Character 4	Approach Character 5	Device Character 6	Qualifier Character 7
Y Upper Bone	X External	Ø Drainage Device Y Other Device	Z No Qualifier

Non-OR   All body part, approach, device, and qualifier values

Ø **Medical and Surgical**
P **Upper Bones**
5 **Destruction**   Definition: Physical eradication of all or a portion of a body part by the direct use of energy, force, or a destructive agent

Explanation: None of the body part is physically taken out

Body Part Character 4	Approach Character 5	Device Character 6	Qualifier Character 7

Ø Sternum
  Manubrium
  Suprasternal notch
  Xiphoid process
1 Ribs, 1 to 2
2 Ribs, 3 or More
3 Cervical Vertebra
  Dens
  Odontoid process
  Spinous process
  Transverse foramen
  Transverse process
  Vertebral arch
  Vertebral body
  Vertebral foramen
  Vertebral lamina
  Vertebral pedicle
4 Thoracic Vertebra
  Spinous process
  Transverse process
  Vertebral arch
  Vertebral body
  Vertebral foramen
  Vertebral lamina
  Vertebral pedicle
5 Scapula, Right
  Acromion (process)
  Coracoid process
6 Scapula, Left
  See 5 Scapula, Right
7 Glenoid Cavity, Right
  Glenoid fossa (of scapula)
8 Glenoid Cavity, Left
  See 7 Glenoid Cavity, Right
9 Clavicle, Right
B Clavicle, Left
C Humeral Head, Right
  Greater tuberosity
  Lesser tuberosity
  Neck of humerus
    (anatomical)(surgical)
D Humeral Head, Left
  See C Humeral Head, Right
	F Humeral Shaft, Right
	  Distal humerus
	  Humerus, distal
	  Lateral epicondyle of
	    humerus
	  Medial epicondyle of
	    humerus
	G Humeral Shaft, Left
	  See F Humeral Shaft, Right
	H Radius, Right
	  Ulnar notch
	J Radius, Left
	  See H Radius, Right
	K Ulna, Right
	  Olecranon process
	  Radial notch
	L Ulna, Left
	  See K Ulna, Right
	M Carpal, Right
	  Capitate bone
	  Hamate bone
	  Lunate bone
	  Pisiform bone
	  Scaphoid bone
	  Trapezium bone
	  Trapezoid bone
	  Triquetral bone
	N Carpal, Left
	  See M Carpal, Right
	P Metacarpal, Right
	Q Metacarpal, Left
	R Thumb Phalanx, Right
	S Thumb Phalanx, Left
	T Finger Phalanx, Right
	V Finger Phalanx, Left
		Ø Open
		3 Percutaneous
		4 Percutaneous Endoscopic
			Z No Device	Z No Qualifier

Ø   **Medical and Surgical**
P   **Upper Bones**
8   **Division**   Definition: Cutting into a body part, without draining fluids and/or gases from the body part, in order to separate or transect a body part
                              Explanation: All or a portion of the body part is separated into two or more portions

Body Part Character 4		Approach Character 5	Device Character 6	Qualifier Character 7

Ø   **Sternum**
    Manubrium
    Suprasternal notch
    Xiphoid process
1   **Ribs, 1 to 2**
2   **Ribs, 3 or More**
3   **Cervical Vertebra**
    Dens
    Odontoid process
    Spinous process
    Transverse foramen
    Transverse process
    Vertebral arch
    Vertebral body
    Vertebral foramen
    Vertebral lamina
    Vertebral pedicle
4   **Thoracic Vertebra**
    Spinous process
    Transverse process
    Vertebral arch
    Vertebral body
    Vertebral foramen
    Vertebral lamina
    Vertebral pedicle
5   **Scapula, Right**
    Acromion (process)
    Coracoid process
6   **Scapula, Left**
    See 5 Scapula, Right
7   **Glenoid Cavity, Right**
    Glenoid fossa (of scapula)
8   **Glenoid Cavity, Left**
    See 7 Glenoid Cavity, Right
9   **Clavicle, Right**
B   **Clavicle, Left**
C   **Humeral Head, Right**
    Greater tuberosity
    Lesser tuberosity
    Neck of humerus
      (anatomical)(surgical)
D   **Humeral Head, Left**
    See C Humeral Head, Right
	F **Humeral Shaft, Right**
	    Distal humerus
	    Humerus, distal
	    Lateral epicondyle of
	      humerus
	    Medial epicondyle of
	      humerus
	G **Humeral Shaft, Left**
	    See F Humeral Shaft, Right
	H **Radius, Right**
	    Ulnar notch
	J **Radius, Left**
	    See H Radius, Right
	K **Ulna, Right**
	    Olecranon process
	    Radial notch
	L **Ulna, Left**
	    See K Ulna, Right
	M **Carpal, Right**
	    Capitate bone
	    Hamate bone
	    Lunate bone
	    Pisiform bone
	    Scaphoid bone
	    Trapezium bone
	    Trapezoid bone
	    Triquetral bone
	N **Carpal, Left**
	    See M Carpal, Right
	P **Metacarpal, Right**
	Q **Metacarpal, Left**
	R **Thumb Phalanx, Right**
	S **Thumb Phalanx, Left**
	T **Finger Phalanx, Right**
	V **Finger Phalanx, Left**
		Ø **Open**
		3 **Percutaneous**
		4 **Percutaneous Endoscopic**
			Z **No Device**	**Z** **No Qualifier**

LC Limited Coverage   **NC** Noncovered   ⊞ Combination Member   HAC associated procedure   Combination Only   DRG Non-OR   Non-OR   New/Revised in GREEN

ICD-10-PCS 2020   533

ØP8–ØP8

Upper Bones

Ø   Medical and Surgical
P   Upper Bones
9   Drainage

Definition: Taking or letting out fluids and/or gases from a body part

Explanation: The qualifier DIAGNOSTIC is used to identify drainage procedures that are biopsies

Body Part Character 4		Approach Character 5	Device Character 6	Qualifier Character 7

Ø **Sternum**
  Manubrium
  Suprasternal notch
  Xiphoid process
1 **Ribs, 1 to 2**
2 **Ribs, 3 or More**
3 **Cervical Vertebra**
  Dens
  Odontoid process
  Spinous process
  Transverse foramen
  Transverse process
  Vertebral arch
  Vertebral body
  Vertebral foramen
  Vertebral lamina
  Vertebral pedicle
4 **Thoracic Vertebra**
  Spinous process
  Transverse process
  Vertebral arch
  Vertebral body
  Vertebral foramen
  Vertebral lamina
  Vertebral pedicle
5 **Scapula, Right**
  Acromion (process)
  Coracoid process
6 **Scapula, Left**
  See 5 Scapula, Right
7 **Glenoid Cavity, Right**
  Glenoid fossa (of scapula)
8 **Glenoid Cavity, Left**
  See 7 Glenoid Cavity, Right
9 **Clavicle, Right**
B **Clavicle, Left**
C **Humeral Head, Right**
  Greater tuberosity
  Lesser tuberosity
  Neck of humerus
    (anatomical)(surgical)
	D **Humeral Head, Left**
	  See C Humeral Head, Right
	F **Humeral Shaft, Right**
	  Distal humerus
	  Humerus, distal
	  Lateral epicondyle of
	    humerus
	  Medial epicondyle of
	    humerus
	G **Humeral Shaft, Left**
	  See F Humeral Shaft, Right
	H **Radius, Right**
	  Ulnar notch
	J **Radius, Left**
	  See H Radius, Right
	K **Ulna, Right**
	  Olecranon process
	  Radial notch
	L **Ulna, Left**
	  See K Ulna, Right
	M **Carpal, Right**
	  Capitate bone
	  Hamate bone
	  Lunate bone
	  Pisiform bone
	  Scaphoid bone
	  Trapezium bone
	  Trapezoid bone
	  Triquetral bone
	N **Carpal, Left**
	  See M Carpal, Right
	P **Metacarpal, Right**
	Q **Metacarpal, Left**
	R **Thumb Phalanx, Right**
	S **Thumb Phalanx, Left**
	T **Finger Phalanx, Right**
	V **Finger Phalanx, Left**
		Ø Open
		3 Percutaneous
		4 Percutaneous Endoscopic
			Ø Drainage Device	**Z** No Qualifier

ØP9 Continued on next page

Non-OR   ØP9[Ø,1,2,3,4,5,6,7,8,9,B,C,D,F,G,H,J,K,L,M,N,P,Q,R,S,T,V]3ØZ

0   **Medical and Surgical**   *0P9 Continued*
P   **Upper Bones**
9   **Drainage**   Definition: Taking or letting out fluids and/or gases from a body part
                       Explanation: The qualifier DIAGNOSTIC is used to identify drainage procedures that are biopsies

Body Part Character 4		Approach Character 5	Device Character 6	Qualifier Character 7

0 **Sternum**
   Manubrium
   Suprasternal notch
   Xiphoid process
1 **Ribs, 1 to 2**
2 **Ribs, 3 or More**
3 **Cervical Vertebra**
   Dens
   Odontoid process
   Spinous process
   Transverse foramen
   Transverse process
   Vertebral arch
   Vertebral body
   Vertebral foramen
   Vertebral lamina
   Vertebral pedicle
4 **Thoracic Vertebra**
   Spinous process
   Transverse process
   Vertebral arch
   Vertebral body
   Vertebral foramen
   Vertebral lamina
   Vertebral pedicle
5 **Scapula, Right**
   Acromion (process)
   Coracoid process
6 **Scapula, Left**
   See 5 Scapula, Right
7 **Glenoid Cavity, Right**
   Glenoid fossa (of scapula)
8 **Glenoid Cavity, Left**
   See 7 Glenoid Cavity, Right
9 **Clavicle, Right**
B **Clavicle, Left**
C **Humeral Head, Right**
   Greater tuberosity
   Lesser tuberosity
   Neck of humerus
     (anatomical)(surgical)
	D **Humeral Head, Left**
	   See C Humeral Head, Right
	F **Humeral Shaft, Right**
	   Distal humerus
	   Humerus, distal
	   Lateral epicondyle of
	     humerus
	   Medial epicondyle of
	     humerus
	G **Humeral Shaft, Left**
	   See F Humeral Shaft, Right
	H **Radius, Right**
	   Ulnar notch
	J **Radius, Left**
	   See H Radius, Right
	K **Ulna, Right**
	   Olecranon process
	   Radial notch
	L **Ulna, Left**
	   See K Ulna, Right
	M **Carpal, Right**
	   Capitate bone
	   Hamate bone
	   Lunate bone
	   Pisiform bone
	   Scaphoid bone
	   Trapezium bone
	   Trapezoid bone
	   Triquetral bone
	N **Carpal, Left**
	   See M Carpal, Right
	P **Metacarpal, Right**
	Q **Metacarpal, Left**
	R **Thumb Phalanx, Right**
	S **Thumb Phalanx, Left**
	T **Finger Phalanx, Right**
	V **Finger Phalanx, Left**
		0 Open
		3 Percutaneous
		4 Percutaneous Endoscopic
			Z No Device	**X** Diagnostic
				Z No Qualifier

Non-OR   0P9[0,1,2,3,4,5,6,7,8,9,B,C,D,F,G,H,J,K,L,M,N,P,Q,R,S,T,V]3ZZ

Ø   Medical and Surgical
P   Upper Bones
B   Excision   Definition: Cutting out or off, without replacement, a portion of a body part

Explanation: The qualifier DIAGNOSTIC is used to identify excision procedures that are biopsies

Body Part Character 4		Approach Character 5	Device Character 6	Qualifier Character 7

Ø   Sternum
    Manubrium
    Suprasternal notch
    Xiphoid process
1   Ribs, 1 to 2
2   Ribs, 3 or More
3   Cervical Vertebra
    Dens
    Odontoid process
    Spinous process
    Transverse foramen
    Transverse process
    Vertebral arch
    Vertebral body
    Vertebral foramen
    Vertebral lamina
    Vertebral pedicle
4   Thoracic Vertebra
    Spinous process
    Transverse process
    Vertebral arch
    Vertebral body
    Vertebral foramen
    Vertebral lamina
    Vertebral pedicle
5   Scapula, Right
    Acromion (process)
    Coracoid process
6   Scapula, Left
    See 5 Scapula, Right
7   Glenoid Cavity, Right
    Glenoid fossa (of scapula)
8   Glenoid Cavity, Left
    See 7 Glenoid Cavity, Right
9   Clavicle, Right
B   Clavicle, Left
C   Humeral Head, Right
    Greater tuberosity
    Lesser tuberosity
    Neck of humerus
      (anatomical)(surgical)
D   Humeral Head, Left
    See C Humeral Head, Right
	F Humeral Shaft, Right
	    Distal humerus
	    Humerus, distal
	    Lateral epicondyle of
	      humerus
	    Medial epicondyle of
	      humerus
	G Humeral Shaft, Left
	    See F Humeral Shaft, Right
	H Radius, Right
	    Ulnar notch
	J Radius, Left
	    See H Radius, Right
	K Ulna, Right
	    Olecranon process
	    Radial notch
	L Ulna, Left
	    See K Ulna, Right
	M Carpal, Right
	    Capitate bone
	    Hamate bone
	    Lunate bone
	    Pisiform bone
	    Scaphoid bone
	    Trapezium bone
	    Trapezoid bone
	    Triquetral bone
	N Carpal, Left
	    See M Carpal, Right
	P Metacarpal, Right
	Q Metacarpal, Left
	R Thumb Phalanx, Right
	S Thumb Phalanx, Left
	T Finger Phalanx, Right
	V Finger Phalanx, Left
		Ø Open
		3 Percutaneous
		4 Percutaneous Endoscopic
			Z No Device	**X** Diagnostic
				Z No Qualifier

LC Limited Coverage   NC Noncovered   ⊞ Combination Member   HAC associated procedure   Combination Only   DRG Non-OR   Non-OR   New/Revised in GREEN

536   ICD-10-PCS 2020

ØPB–ØPB

Ø   **Medical and Surgical**
P   **Upper Bones**
C   **Extirpation**   Definition: Taking or cutting out solid matter from a body part

Explanation: The solid matter may be an abnormal byproduct of a biological function or a foreign body; it may be imbedded in a body part or in the lumen of a tubular body part. The solid matter may or may not have been previously broken into pieces.

Body Part Character 4		Approach Character 5	Device Character 6	Qualifier Character 7

Ø **Sternum**
Manubrium
Suprasternal notch
Xiphoid process
1 **Ribs, 1 to 2**
2 **Ribs, 3 or More**
3 **Cervical Vertebra**
Dens
Odontoid process
Spinous process
Transverse foramen
Transverse process
Vertebral arch
Vertebral body
Vertebral foramen
Vertebral lamina
Vertebral pedicle
4 **Thoracic Vertebra**
Spinous process
Transverse process
Vertebral arch
Vertebral body
Vertebral foramen
Vertebral lamina
Vertebral pedicle
5 **Scapula, Right**
Acromion (process)
Coracoid process
6 **Scapula, Left**
See 5 Scapula, Right
7 **Glenoid Cavity, Right**
Glenoid fossa (of scapula)
8 **Glenoid Cavity, Left**
See 7 Glenoid Cavity, Right
9 **Clavicle, Right**
B **Clavicle, Left**
C **Humeral Head, Right**
Greater tuberosity
Lesser tuberosity
Neck of humerus
   (anatomical)(surgical)
D **Humeral Head, Left**
See C Humeral Head, Right
	F **Humeral Shaft, Right**
	Distal humerus
	Humerus, distal
	Lateral epicondyle of
	   humerus
	Medial epicondyle of
	   humerus
	G **Humeral Shaft, Left**
	See F Humeral Shaft, Right
	H **Radius, Right**
	Ulnar notch
	J **Radius, Left**
	See H Radius, Right
	K **Ulna, Right**
	Olecranon process
	Radial notch
	L **Ulna, Left**
	See K Ulna, Right
	M **Carpal, Right**
	Capitate bone
	Hamate bone
	Lunate bone
	Pisiform bone
	Scaphoid bone
	Trapezium bone
	Trapezoid bone
	Triquetral bone
	N **Carpal, Left**
	See M Carpal, Right
	P **Metacarpal, Right**
	Q **Metacarpal, Left**
	R **Thumb Phalanx, Right**
	S **Thumb Phalanx, Left**
	T **Finger Phalanx, Right**
	V **Finger Phalanx, Left**
		Ø Open
		3 Percutaneous
		4 Percutaneous Endoscopic
			Z No Device	**Z** No Qualifier

Upper Bones

Ø   **Medical and Surgical**
P   **Upper Bones**
D   **Extraction**

Definition: Pulling or stripping out or off all or a portion of a body part by the use of force
Explanation: The qualifier DIAGNOSTIC is used to identify extraction procedures that are biopsies

Body Part Character 4		Approach Character 5	Device Character 6	Qualifier Character 7
Ø **Sternum**	**F** **Humeral Shaft, Right**	**Ø** Open	**Z** No Device	**Z** No Qualifier
Manubrium	Distal humerus			
Suprasternal notch	Humerus, distal			
Xiphoid process	Lateral epicondyle of			
1 **Ribs, 1 to 2**	humerus			
2 **Ribs, 3 or More**	Medial epicondyle of			
3 **Cervical Vertebra**	humerus			
Dens	**G** **Humeral Shaft, Left**			
Odontoid process	*See F Humeral Shaft, Right*			
Spinous process	**H** **Radius, Right**			
Transverse foramen	Ulnar notch			
Transverse process	**J** **Radius, Left**			
Vertebral arch	*See H Radius, Right*			
Vertebral body	**K** **Ulna, Right**			
Vertebral foramen	Olecranon process			
Vertebral lamina	Radial notch			
Vertebral pedicle	**L** **Ulna, Left**			
4 **Thoracic Vertebra**	*See K Ulna, Right*			
Spinous process	**M** **Carpal, Right**			
Transverse process	Capitate bone			
Vertebral arch	Hamate bone			
Vertebral body	Lunate bone			
Vertebral foramen	Pisiform bone			
Vertebral lamina	Scaphoid bone			
Vertebral pedicle	Trapezium bone			
5 **Scapula, Right**	Trapezoid bone			
Acromion (process)	Triquetral bone			
Coracoid process	**N** **Carpal, Left**			
6 **Scapula, Left**	*See M Carpal, Right*			
See 5 Scapula, Right	**P** **Metacarpal, Right**			
7 **Glenoid Cavity, Right**	**Q** **Metacarpal, Left**			
Glenoid fossa (of scapula)	**R** **Thumb Phalanx, Right**			
8 **Glenoid Cavity, Left**	**S** **Thumb Phalanx, Left**			
See 7 Glenoid Cavity, Right	**T** **Finger Phalanx, Right**			
9 **Clavicle, Right**	**V** **Finger Phalanx, Left**			
B **Clavicle, Left**				
C **Humeral Head, Right**				
Greater tuberosity				
Lesser tuberosity				
Neck of humerus				
(anatomical)(surgical)				
D **Humeral Head, Left**				
See C Humeral Head, Right				

LC Limited Coverage   **NC** Noncovered   ⊞ Combination Member   HAC associated procedure   Combination Only   DRG Non-OR   Non-OR   New/Revised in GREEN

538   ICD-10-PCS 2020

ØPD–ØPD

Ø Medical and Surgical
P Upper Bones
H Insertion   Definition: Putting in a nonbiological appliance that monitors, assists, performs, or prevents a physiological function but does not physically take the place of a body part
                 Explanation: None

Body Part Character 4		Approach Character 5	Device Character 6	Qualifier Character 7
Ø Sternum Manubrium Suprasternal notch Xiphoid process		**Ø** Open **3** Percutaneous **4** Percutaneous Endoscopic	**Ø** Internal Fixation Device, Rigid Plate **4** Internal Fixation Device	**Z** No Qualifier
1 Ribs, 1 to 2 **2 Ribs, 3 or More** **3 Cervical Vertebra** Dens Odontoid process Spinous process Transverse foramen Transverse process Vertebral arch Vertebral body Vertebral foramen Vertebral lamina Vertebral pedicle **4 Thoracic Vertebra** Spinous process Transverse process Vertebral arch Vertebral body Vertebral foramen Vertebral lamina Vertebral pedicle	**5 Scapula, Right** Acromion (process) Coracoid process **6 Scapula, Left** *See 5 Scapula, Right* **7 Glenoid Cavity, Right** Glenoid fossa (of scapula) **8 Glenoid Cavity, Left** *See 7 Glenoid Cavity, Right* **9 Clavicle, Right** **B Clavicle, Left**	**Ø** Open **3** Percutaneous **4** Percutaneous Endoscopic	**4** Internal Fixation Device	**Z** No Qualifier
C Humeral Head, Right Greater tuberosity Lesser tuberosity Neck of humerus (anatomical)(surgical) **D Humeral Head, Left** *See C Humeral Head, Right*	**H Radius, Right** Ulnar notch **J Radius, Left** *See H Radius, Right* **K Ulna, Right** Olecranon process Radial notch **L Ulna, Left** *See K Ulna, Right*	**Ø** Open **3** Percutaneous **4** Percutaneous Endoscopic	**4** Internal Fixation Device **5** External Fixation Device **6** Internal Fixation Device, Intramedullary **8** External Fixation Device, Limb Lengthening **B** External Fixation Device, Monoplanar **C** External Fixation Device, Ring **D** External Fixation Device, Hybrid	**Z** No Qualifier
F Humeral Shaft, Right Distal humerus Humerus, distal Lateral epicondyle of humerus Medial epicondyle of humerus	**G Humeral Shaft, Left** *See F Humeral Shaft, Right*	**Ø** Open **3** Percutaneous **4** Percutaneous Endoscopic	**4** Internal Fixation Device **5** External Fixation Device **6** Internal Fixation Device, Intramedullary **7 Internal Fixation Device, Intramedullary Limb Lengthening** **8** External Fixation Device, Limb Lengthening **B** External Fixation Device, Monoplanar **C** External Fixation Device, Ring **D** External Fixation Device, Hybrid	**Z** No Qualifier
M Carpal, Right Capitate bone Hamate bone Lunate bone Pisiform bone Scaphoid bone Trapezium bone Trapezoid bone Triquetral bone **N Carpal, Left** *See M Carpal, Right*	**P Metacarpal, Right** **Q Metacarpal, Left** **R Thumb Phalanx, Right** **S Thumb Phalanx, Left** **T Finger Phalanx, Right** **V Finger Phalanx, Left**	**Ø** Open **3** Percutaneous **4** Percutaneous Endoscopic	**4** Internal Fixation Device **5** External Fixation Device	**Z** No Qualifier
Y Upper Bone		**Ø** Open **3** Percutaneous **4** Percutaneous Endoscopic	**M** Bone Growth Stimulator	**Z** No Qualifier

Non-OR	ØPH[C,D,H,J,K,L][Ø,3,4]8Z
Non-OR	ØPH[F,G][Ø,3,4]8Z

LC Limited Coverage   **NC** Noncovered   ⊞ Combination Member   HAC associated procedure   Combination Only   DRG Non-OR   Non-OR   New/Revised in GREEN

ICD-10-PCS 2020   539

ØPH–ØPH

Ø Medical and Surgical
P Upper Bones
J Inspection   Definition: Visually and/or manually exploring a body part

Explanation: Visual exploration may be performed with or without optical instrumentation. Manual exploration may be performed directly or through intervening body layers.

Body Part Character 4	Approach Character 5	Device Character 6	Qualifier Character 7
Y Upper Bone	Ø Open 3 Percutaneous 4 Percutaneous Endoscopic X External	Z No Device	Z No Qualifier

Non-OR   ØPJY[3,X]ZZ

Ø Medical and Surgical
P Upper Bones
N Release   Definition: Freeing a body part from an abnormal physical constraint by cutting or by the use of force

Explanation: Some of the restraining tissue may be taken out but none of the body part is taken out

Body Part Character 4	Approach Character 5	Device Character 6	Qualifier Character 7

Ø Sternum
  Manubrium
  Suprasternal notch
  Xiphoid process
1 Ribs, 1 to 2
2 Ribs, 3 or More
3 Cervical Vertebra
  Dens
  Odontoid process
  Spinous process
  Transverse foramen
  Transverse process
  Vertebral arch
  Vertebral body
  Vertebral foramen
  Vertebral lamina
  Vertebral pedicle
4 Thoracic Vertebra
  Spinous process
  Transverse process
  Vertebral arch
  Vertebral body
  Vertebral foramen
  Vertebral lamina
  Vertebral pedicle
5 Scapula, Right
  Acromion (process)
  Coracoid process
6 Scapula, Left
  See 5 Scapula, Right
7 Glenoid Cavity, Right
  Glenoid fossa (of scapula)
8 Glenoid Cavity, Left
  See 7 Glenoid Cavity, Right
9 Clavicle, Right
B Clavicle, Left
C Humeral Head, Right
  Greater tuberosity
  Lesser tuberosity
  Neck of humerus
    (anatomical) (surgical)
D Humeral Head, Left
  See C Humeral Head, Right
	F Humeral Shaft, Right
	  Distal humerus
	  Humerus, distal
	  Lateral epicondyle of
	    humerus
	  Medial epicondyle of
	    humerus
	G Humeral Shaft, Left
	  See F Humeral Shaft, Right
	H Radius, Right
	  Ulnar notch
	J Radius, Left
	  See H Radius, Right
	K Ulna, Right
	  Olecranon process
	  Radial notch
	L Ulna, Left
	  See K Ulna, Right
	M Carpal, Right
	  Capitate bone
	  Hamate bone
	  Lunate bone
	  Pisiform bone
	  Scaphoid bone
	  Trapezium bone
	  Trapezoid bone
	  Triquetral bone
	N Carpal, Left
	  See M Carpal, Right
	P Metacarpal, Right
	Q Metacarpal, Left
	R Thumb Phalanx, Right
	S Thumb Phalanx, Left
	T Finger Phalanx, Right
	V Finger Phalanx, Left
		Ø Open
		3 Percutaneous
		4 Percutaneous Endoscopic
			Z No Device	Z No Qualifier

LC Limited Coverage   **NC** Noncovered   ⊞ Combination Member   HAC associated procedure   Combination Only   DRG Non-OR   Non-OR   New/Revised in GREEN

540   ICD-10-PCS 2020

Ø   Medical and Surgical
P   Upper Bones
P   Removal   Definition: Taking out or off a device from a body part

Explanation: If a device is taken out and a similar device put in without cutting or puncturing the skin or mucous membrane, the procedure is coded to the root operation CHANGE. Otherwise, the procedure for taking out a device is coded to the root operation REMOVAL.

Body Part Character 4		Approach Character 5	Device Character 6	Qualifier Character 7
Ø Sternum Manubrium Suprasternal notch Xiphoid process **1 Ribs, 1 to 2** **2 Ribs, 3 or More** **3 Cervical Vertebra** Dens Odontoid process Spinous process Transverse foramen Transverse process Vertebral arch Vertebral body Vertebral foramen Vertebral lamina Vertebral pedicle	**4 Thoracic Vertebra** Spinous process Transverse process Vertebral arch Vertebral body Vertebral foramen Vertebral lamina Vertebral pedicle **5 Scapula, Right** Acromion (process) Coracoid process **6 Scapula, Left** *See 5 Scapula, Right* **7 Glenoid Cavity, Right** Glenoid fossa (of scapula) **8 Glenoid Cavity, Left** *See 7 Glenoid Cavity, Right* **9 Clavicle, Right** **B Clavicle, Left**	**Ø Open** **3 Percutaneous** **4 Percutaneous Endoscopic**	**4 Internal Fixation Device** **7 Autologous Tissue Substitute** **J Synthetic Substitute** **K Nonautologous Tissue Substitute**	**Z No Qualifier**
Ø Sternum Manubrium Suprasternal notch Xiphoid process **1 Ribs, 1 to 2** **2 Ribs, 3 or More** **3 Cervical Vertebra** Dens Odontoid process Spinous process Transverse foramen Transverse process Vertebral arch Vertebral body Vertebral foramen Vertebral lamina Vertebral pedicle	**4 Thoracic Vertebra** Spinous process Transverse process Vertebral arch Vertebral body Vertebral foramen Vertebral lamina Vertebral pedicle **5 Scapula, Right** Acromion (process) Coracoid process **6 Scapula, Left** *See 5 Scapula, Right* **7 Glenoid Cavity, Right** Glenoid fossa (of scapula) **8 Glenoid Cavity, Left** *See 7 Glenoid Cavity, Right* **9 Clavicle, Right** **B Clavicle, Left**	**X External**	**4 Internal Fixation Device**	**Z No Qualifier**
C Humeral Head, Right Greater tuberosity Lesser tuberosity Neck of humerus (anatomical) (surgical) **D Humeral Head, Left** *See C Humeral Head, Right* **F Humeral Shaft, Right** Distal humerus Humerus, distal Lateral epicondyle of humerus Medial epicondyle of humerus **G Humeral Shaft, Left** *See F Humeral Shaft, Right* **H Radius, Right** Ulnar notch **J Radius, Left** *See H Radius, Right* **K Ulna, Right** Olecranon process Radial notch	**L Ulna, Left** *See K Ulna, Right* **M Carpal, Right** Capitate bone Hamate bone Lunate bone Pisiform bone Scaphoid bone Trapezium bone Trapezoid bone Triquetral bone **N Carpal, Left** *See M Carpal, Right* **P Metacarpal, Right** **Q Metacarpal, Left** **R Thumb Phalanx, Right** **S Thumb Phalanx, Left** **T Finger Phalanx, Right** **V Finger Phalanx, Left**	**Ø Open** **3 Percutaneous** **4 Percutaneous Endoscopic**	**4 Internal Fixation Device** **5 External Fixation Device** **7 Autologous Tissue Substitute** **J Synthetic Substitute** **K Nonautologous Tissue Substitute**	**Z No Qualifier**

ØPP Continued on next page

Non-OR	ØPP[Ø,1,2,3,4,5,6,7,8,9,B]X4Z

LC Limited Coverage   NC Noncovered   ⊞ Combination Member   HAC associated procedure   Combination Only   DRG Non-OR   Non-OR   New/Revised in GREEN

ICD-10-PCS 2020   541

ØPP–ØPP

Upper Bones

Ø	Medical and Surgical
P	Upper Bones
P	Removal

Definition: Taking out or off a device from a body part

Explanation: If a device is taken out and a similar device put in without cutting or puncturing the skin or mucous membrane, the procedure is coded to the root operation CHANGE. Otherwise, the procedure for taking out a device is coded to the root operation REMOVAL.

Body Part Character 4		Approach Character 5	Device Character 6	Qualifier Character 7

C **Humeral Head, Right**
  Greater tuberosity
  Lesser tuberosity
  Neck of humerus
    (anatomical) (surgical)
D **Humeral Head, Left**
  See C Humeral Head, Right
F **Humeral Shaft, Right**
  Distal humerus
  Humerus, distal
  Lateral epicondyle of
    humerus
  Medial epicondyle of
    humerus
G **Humeral Shaft, Left**
  See F Humeral Shaft, Right
H **Radius, Right**
  Ulnar notch
J **Radius, Left**
  See H Radius, Right
K **Ulna, Right**
  Olecranon process
  Radial notch
	L **Ulna, Left**
	  See K Ulna, Right
	M **Carpal, Right**
	  Capitate bone
	  Hamate bone
	  Lunate bone
	  Pisiform bone
	  Scaphoid bone
	  Trapezium bone
	  Trapezoid bone
	  Triquetral bone
	N **Carpal, Left**
	  See M Carpal, Right
	P **Metacarpal, Right**
	Q **Metacarpal, Left**
	R **Thumb Phalanx, Right**
	S **Thumb Phalanx, Left**
	T **Finger Phalanx, Right**
	V **Finger Phalanx, Left**
		X **External**	4 **Internal Fixation Device**
			5 **External Fixation Device**
				Z **No Qualifier**

Y **Upper Bone**		Ø **Open** 3 **Percutaneous** 4 **Percutaneous Endoscopic** X **External**	Ø **Drainage Device** M **Bone Growth Stimulator**	Z **No Qualifier**

Non-OR	ØPP[C,D,F,G,H,J,K,L,M,N,P,Q,R,S,T,V]X[4,5]Z
Non-OR	ØPPY3ØZ
Non-OR	ØPPYX[Ø,M]Z

Ø   Medical and Surgical
P   Upper Bones
Q   Repair   Definition: Restoring, to the extent possible, a body part to its normal anatomic structure and function
                    Explanation: Used only when the method to accomplish the repair is not one of the other root operations

Body Part Character 4		Approach Character 5	Device Character 6	Qualifier Character 7

Ø   **Sternum**
     Manubrium
     Suprasternal notch
     Xiphoid process
1   **Ribs, 1 to 2**
2   **Ribs, 3 or More**
3   **Cervical Vertebra**
     Dens
     Odontoid process
     Spinous process
     Transverse foramen
     Transverse process
     Vertebral arch
     Vertebral body
     Vertebral foramen
     Vertebral lamina
     Vertebral pedicle
4   **Thoracic Vertebra**
     Spinous process
     Transverse process
     Vertebral arch
     Vertebral body
     Vertebral foramen
     Vertebral lamina
     Vertebral pedicle
5   **Scapula, Right**
     Acromion (process)
     Coracoid process
6   **Scapula, Left**
     See 5 Scapula, Right
7   **Glenoid Cavity, Right**
     Glenoid fossa (of scapula)
8   **Glenoid Cavity, Left**
     See 7 Glenoid Cavity, Right
9   **Clavicle, Right**
B   **Clavicle, Left**
C   **Humeral Head, Right**
     Greater tuberosity
     Lesser tuberosity
     Neck of humerus
        (anatomical)(surgical)
D   **Humeral Head, Left**
     See C Humeral Head, Right
	F **Humeral Shaft, Right**
	     Distal humerus
	     Humerus, distal
	     Lateral epicondyle of
	        humerus
	     Medial epicondyle of
	        humerus
	G **Humeral Shaft, Left**
	     See F Humeral Shaft, Right
	H **Radius, Right**
	     Ulnar notch
	J **Radius, Left**
	     See H Radius, Right
	K **Ulna, Right**
	     Olecranon process
	     Radial notch
	L **Ulna, Left**
	     See K Ulna, Right
	M **Carpal, Right**
	     Capitate bone
	     Hamate bone
	     Lunate bone
	     Pisiform bone
	     Scaphoid bone
	     Trapezium bone
	     Trapezoid bone
	     Triquetral bone
	N **Carpal, Left**
	     See M Carpal, Right
	P **Metacarpal, Right**
	Q **Metacarpal, Left**
	R **Thumb Phalanx, Right**
	S **Thumb Phalanx, Left**
	T **Finger Phalanx, Right**
	V **Finger Phalanx, Left**
		Ø Open
		3 Percutaneous
		4 Percutaneous Endoscopic
		X External
			Z No Device	**Z** No Qualifier

Non-OR   ØPQ[Ø,1,2,3,4,5,6,7,8,9,B,C,D,F,G,H,J,K,L,M,N,P,Q,R,S,T,V]XZZ

Ø   Medical and Surgical
P   Upper Bones
R   Replacement   Definition: Putting in or on biological or synthetic material that physically takes the place and/or function of all or a portion of a body part
Explanation: The body part may have been taken out or replaced, or may be taken out, physically eradicated, or rendered nonfunctional during the REPLACEMENT procedure. A REMOVAL procedure is coded for taking out the device used in a previous replacement procedure.

Body Part Character 4		Approach Character 5	Device Character 6	Qualifier Character 7

Ø Sternum
  Manubrium
  Suprasternal notch
  Xiphoid process
1 Ribs, 1 to 2
2 Ribs, 3 or More
3 Cervical Vertebra
  Dens
  Odontoid process
  Spinous process
  Transverse foramen
  Transverse process
  Vertebral arch
  Vertebral body
  Vertebral foramen
  Vertebral lamina
  Vertebral pedicle
4 Thoracic Vertebra
  Spinous process
  Transverse process
  Vertebral arch
  Vertebral body
  Vertebral foramen
  Vertebral lamina
  Vertebral pedicle
5 Scapula, Right
  Acromion (process)
  Coracoid process
6 Scapula, Left
  See 5 Scapula, Right
7 Glenoid Cavity, Right
  Glenoid fossa (of scapula)
8 Glenoid Cavity, Left
  See 7 Glenoid Cavity, Right
9 Clavicle, Right
B Clavicle, Left
C Humeral Head, Right
  Greater tuberosity
  Lesser tuberosity
  Neck of humerus
    (anatomical)(surgical)
D Humeral Head, Left
  See C Humeral Head, Right
	F Humeral Shaft, Right
	  Distal humerus
	  Humerus, distal
	  Lateral epicondyle of
	    humerus
	  Medial epicondyle of
	    humerus
	G Humeral Shaft, Left
	  See F Humeral Shaft, Right
	H Radius, Right
	  Ulnar notch
	J Radius, Left
	  See H Radius, Right
	K Ulna, Right
	  Olecranon process
	  Radial notch
	L Ulna, Left
	  See K Ulna, Right
	M Carpal, Right
	  Capitate bone
	  Hamate bone
	  Lunate bone
	  Pisiform bone
	  Scaphoid bone
	  Trapezium bone
	  Trapezoid bone
	  Triquetral bone
	N Carpal, Left
	  See M Carpal, Right
	P Metacarpal, Right
	Q Metacarpal, Left
	R Thumb Phalanx, Right
	S Thumb Phalanx, Left
	T Finger Phalanx, Right
	V Finger Phalanx, Left
		Ø Open
		3 Percutaneous
		4 Percutaneous Endoscopic
			**7 Autologous Tissue
			    Substitute**
			J Synthetic Substitute
			**K Nonautologous Tissue
			    Substitute**
				Z No Qualifier

Ø   Medical and Surgical
P   Upper Bones
S   Reposition   Definition: Moving to its normal location, or other suitable location, all or a portion of a body part

Explanation: The body part is moved to a new location from an abnormal location, or from a normal location where it is not functioning correctly. The body part may or may not be cut out or off to be moved to the new location.

Body Part Character 4		Approach Character 5	Device Character 6	Qualifier Character 7
Ø Sternum Manubrium Suprasternal notch Xiphoid process		**Ø** Open **3** Percutaneous **4** Percutaneous Endoscopic	**Ø** Internal Fixation Device, Rigid Plate **4** Internal Fixation Device **Z** No Device	**Z** No Qualifier
Ø Sternum Manubrium Suprasternal notch Xiphoid process		**X** External	**Z** No Device	**Z** No Qualifier

1 Ribs, 1 to 2
2 Ribs, 3 or More
3 Cervical Vertebra ⊞
  Dens
  Odontoid process
  Spinous process
  Transverse foramen
  Transverse process
  Vertebral arch
  Vertebral body
  Vertebral foramen
  Vertebral lamina
  Vertebral pedicle
4 Thoracic Vertebra ⊞
  Spinous process
  Transverse process
  Vertebral arch
  Vertebral body
  Vertebral foramen
  Vertebral lamina
  Vertebral pedicle
	5 Scapula, Right
	  Acromion (process)
	  Coracoid process
	6 Scapula, Left
	  See 5 Scapula, Right
	7 Glenoid Cavity, Right
	  Glenoid fossa (of scapula)
	8 Glenoid Cavity, Left
	  See 7 Glenoid Cavity, Right
	9 Clavicle, Right
	B Clavicle, Left
		Ø Open
		3 Percutaneous
		4 Percutaneous Endoscopic
			4 Internal Fixation Device
			Z No Device
				Z No Qualifier

1 Ribs, 1 to 2
2 Ribs, 3 or More
3 Cervical Vertebra
  Dens
  Odontoid process
  Spinous process
  Transverse foramen
  Transverse process
  Vertebral arch
  Vertebral body
  Vertebral foramen
  Vertebral lamina
  Vertebral pedicle
4 Thoracic Vertebra
  Spinous process
  Transverse process
  Vertebral arch
  Vertebral body
  Vertebral foramen
  Vertebral lamina
  Vertebral pedicle
	5 Scapula, Right
	  Acromion (process)
	  Coracoid process
	6 Scapula, Left
	  See 5 Scapula, Right
	7 Glenoid Cavity, Right
	  Glenoid fossa (of scapula)
	8 Glenoid Cavity, Left
	  See 7 Glenoid Cavity, Right
	9 Clavicle, Right
	B Clavicle, Left
		X External	**Z** No Device	**Z** No Qualifier

C Humeral Head, Right
  Greater tuberosity
  Lesser tuberosity
  Neck of humerus
    (anatomical)(surgical)
D Humeral Head, Left
  See C Humeral Head, Right
F Humeral Shaft, Right
  Distal humerus
  Humerus, distal
  Lateral epicondyle of
    humerus
  Medial epicondyle of
    humerus
	G Humeral Shaft, Left
	  See F Humeral Shaft, Right
	H Radius, Right
	  Ulnar notch
	J Radius, Left
	  See H Radius, Right
	K Ulna, Right
	  Olecranon process
	  Radial notch
	L Ulna, Left
	  See K Ulna, Right
		Ø Open
		3 Percutaneous
		4 Percutaneous Endoscopic
			4 Internal Fixation Device
			5 External Fixation Device
			6 Internal Fixation Device, Intramedullary
			B External Fixation Device, Monoplanar
			C External Fixation Device, Ring
			D External Fixation Device, Hybrid
			Z No Device
				Z No Qualifier

ØPS Continued on next page

Non-OR ØPSØ[3,4]ZZ **Non-OR** ØPSØXZZ **Non-OR** ØPS[1,2,5,6,7,8,9,B][3,4]ZZ **Non-OR** ØPS[1,2,3,4,5,6,7,8,9,B]XZZ **Non-OR** ØPS[C,D,F,G,H,J,K,L][3,4]ZZ	**See Appendix L for Procedure Combinations** ⊞ ØPS[3,4]3ZZ

🄻🄲 Limited Coverage   🄽🄲 Noncovered   ⊞ Combination Member   HAC associated procedure   Combination Only   DRG Non-OR   Non-OR   New/Revised in GREEN

ICD-10-PCS 2020   **545**

ØPS–ØPS

Ø   Medical and Surgical   *ØPS Continued*
P   Upper Bones
S   Reposition   Definition: Moving to its normal location, or other suitable location, all or a portion of a body part

Explanation: The body part is moved to a new location from an abnormal location, or from a normal location where it is not functioning correctly. The body part may or may not be cut out or off to be moved to the new location.

Body Part Character 4		Approach Character 5	Device Character 6	Qualifier Character 7
C Humeral Head, Right Greater tuberosity Lesser tuberosity Neck of humerus (anatomical)(surgical) **D** Humeral Head, Left *See C Humeral Head, Right* **F** Humeral Shaft, Right Distal humerus Humerus, distal Lateral epicondyle of humerus Medial epicondyle of humerus	**G** Humeral Shaft, Left *See F Humeral Shaft, Right* **H** Radius, Right Ulnar notch **J** Radius, Left *See H Radius, Right* **K** Ulna, Right Olecranon process Radial notch **L** Ulna, Left *See K Ulna, Right*	**X** External	**Z** No Device	**Z** No Qualifier
M Carpal, Right Capitate bone Hamate bone Lunate bone Pisiform bone Scaphoid bone Trapezium bone Trapezoid bone Triquetral bone	**N** Carpal, Left *See M Carpal, Right* **P** Metacarpal, Right **Q** Metacarpal, Left **R** Thumb Phalanx, Right **S** Thumb Phalanx, Left **T** Finger Phalanx, Right **V** Finger Phalanx, Left	**Ø** Open **3** Percutaneous **4** Percutaneous Endoscopic	**4** Internal Fixation Device **5** External Fixation Device **Z** No Device	**Z** No Qualifier
M Carpal, Right Capitate bone Hamate bone Lunate bone Pisiform bone Scaphoid bone Trapezium bone Trapezoid bone Triquetral bone	**N** Carpal, Left *See M Carpal, Right* **P** Metacarpal, Right **Q** Metacarpal, Left **R** Thumb Phalanx, Right **S** Thumb Phalanx, Left **T** Finger Phalanx, Right **V** Finger Phalanx, Left	**X** External	**Z** No Device	**Z** No Qualifier

Non-OR   ØPS[C,D,F,G,H,J,K,L]XZZ
Non-OR   ØPS[M,N,P,Q,R,S,T,V][3,4]ZZ
Non-OR   ØPS[M,N,P,Q,R,S,T,V]XZZ

Ø   Medical and Surgical
P   Upper Bones
T   Resection   Definition: Cutting out or off, without replacement, all of a body part

Explanation: None

Body Part Character 4		Approach Character 5	Device Character 6	Qualifier Character 7
Ø Sternum Manubrium Suprasternal notch Xiphoid process **1** Ribs, 1 to 2 **2** Ribs, 3 or More **5** Scapula, Right Acromion (process) Coracoid process **6** Scapula, Left *See 5 Scapula, Right* **7** Glenoid Cavity, Right Glenoid fossa (of scapula) **8** Glenoid Cavity, Left *See 7 Glenoid Cavity, Right* **9** Clavicle, Right **B** Clavicle, Left **C** Humeral Head, Right Greater tuberosity Lesser tuberosity Neck of humerus (anatomical) (surgical) **D** Humeral Head, Left *See C Humeral Head, Right* **F** Humeral Shaft, Right Distal humerus Humerus, distal Lateral epicondyle of humerus Medial epicondyle of humerus	**G** Humeral Shaft, Left *See F Humeral Shaft, Right* **H** Radius, Right Ulnar notch **J** Radius, Left *See H Radius, Right* **K** Ulna, Right Olecranon process Radial notch **L** Ulna, Left *See K Ulna, Right* **M** Carpal, Right Capitate bone Hamate bone Lunate bone Pisiform bone Scaphoid bone Trapezium bone Trapezoid bone Triquetral bone **N** Carpal, Left *See M Carpal, Right* **P** Metacarpal, Right **Q** Metacarpal, Left **R** Thumb Phalanx, Right **S** Thumb Phalanx, Left **T** Finger Phalanx, Right **V** Finger Phalanx, Left	**Ø** Open	**Z** No Device	**Z** No Qualifier

LC Limited Coverage   NC Noncovered   ⊞ Combination Member   HAC associated procedure   Combination Only   DRG Non-OR   Non-OR   New/Revised in GREEN
546   ICD-10-PCS 2020

ØPS–ØPT

Ø   **Medical and Surgical**
P   **Upper Bones**
U   **Supplement**   Definition: Putting in or on biological or synthetic material that physically reinforces and/or augments the function of a portion of a body part

                               Explanation: The biological material is non-living, or is living and from the same individual. The body part may have been previously replaced, and the SUPPLEMENT procedure is performed to physically reinforce and/or augment the function of the replaced body part.

Body Part Character 4		Approach Character 5	Device Character 6	Qualifier Character 7

Ø **Sternum**
   Manubrium
   Suprasternal notch
   Xiphoid process
1 **Ribs, 1 to 2**
2 **Ribs, 3 or More**
3 **Cervical Vertebra** ⊞
   Dens
   Odontoid process
   Spinous process
   Transverse foramen
   Transverse process
   Vertebral arch
   Vertebral body
   Vertebral foramen
   Vertebral lamina
   Vertebral pedicle
4 **Thoracic Vertebra** ⊞
   Spinous process
   Transverse process
   Vertebral arch
   Vertebral body
   Vertebral foramen
   Vertebral lamina
   Vertebral pedicle
5 **Scapula, Right**
   Acromion (process)
   Coracoid process
6 **Scapula, Left**
   See 5 Scapula, Right
7 **Glenoid Cavity, Right**
   Glenoid fossa (of scapula)
8 **Glenoid Cavity, Left**
   See 7 Glenoid Cavity, Right
9 **Clavicle, Right**
B **Clavicle, Left**
C **Humeral Head, Right**
   Greater tuberosity
   Lesser tuberosity
   Neck of humerus
     (anatomical) (surgical)
	D **Humeral Head, Left**
	   See C Humeral Head, Right
	F **Humeral Shaft, Right**
	   Distal humerus
	   Humerus, distal
	   Lateral epicondyle of
	     humerus
	   Medial epicondyle of
	     humerus
	G **Humeral Shaft, Left**
	   See F Humeral Shaft, Right
	H **Radius, Right**
	   Ulnar notch
	J **Radius, Left**
	   See H Radius, Right
	K **Ulna, Right**
	   Olecranon process
	   Radial notch
	L **Ulna, Left**
	   See K Ulna, Right
	M **Carpal, Right**
	   Capitate bone
	   Hamate bone
	   Lunate bone
	   Pisiform bone
	   Scaphoid bone
	   Trapezium bone
	   Trapezoid bone
	   Triquetral bone
	N **Carpal, Left**
	   See M Carpal, Right
	P **Metacarpal, Right**
	Q **Metacarpal, Left**
	R **Thumb Phalanx, Right**
	S **Thumb Phalanx, Left**
	T **Finger Phalanx, Right**
	V **Finger Phalanx, Left**
		Ø **Open**
		3 **Percutaneous**
		4 **Percutaneous Endoscopic**
			7 **Autologous Tissue**
			    Substitute
			J **Synthetic Substitute**
			K **Nonautologous Tissue**
			    Substitute
				Z **No Qualifier**

See Appendix L for Procedure Combinations
  ⊞   ØPU[3,4]3JZ

Upper Bones

Ø   **Medical and Surgical**
P   **Upper Bones**
W   **Revision**   Definition: Correcting, to the extent possible, a portion of a malfunctioning device or the position of a displaced device

Explanation: Revision can include correcting a malfunctioning or displaced device by taking out or putting in components of the device such as a screw or pin

Body Part Character 4		Approach Character 5	Device Character 6	Qualifier Character 7

Ø **Sternum**
   Manubrium
   Suprasternal notch
   Xiphoid process
1 **Ribs, 1 to 2**
2 **Ribs, 3 or More**
3 **Cervical Vertebra**
   Dens
   Odontoid process
   Spinous process
   Transverse foramen
   Transverse process
   Vertebral arch
   Vertebral body
   Vertebral foramen
   Vertebral lamina
   Vertebral pedicle
4 **Thoracic Vertebra**
   Spinous process
   Transverse process
   Vertebral arch
   Vertebral body
   Vertebral foramen
   Vertebral lamina
   Vertebral pedicle
	5 **Scapula, Right**
	   Acromion (process)
	   Coracoid process
	6 **Scapula, Left**
	   See 5 Scapula, Right
	7 **Glenoid Cavity, Right**
	   Glenoid fossa (of scapula)
	8 **Glenoid Cavity, Left**
	   See 7 Glenoid Cavity, Right
	9 **Clavicle, Right**
	B **Clavicle, Left**
		Ø Open
		3 Percutaneous
		4 Percutaneous Endoscopic
		X External
			4 Internal Fixation Device
			7 Autologous Tissue
			   Substitute
			J Synthetic Substitute
			K Nonautologous Tissue
			   Substitute
				Z No Qualifier

C **Humeral Head, Right**
   Greater tuberosity
   Lesser tuberosity
   Neck of humerus
     (anatomical)(surgical)
D **Humeral Head, Left**
   See C Humeral Head, Right
F **Humeral Shaft, Right**
   Distal humerus
   Humerus, distal
   Lateral epicondyle of
     humerus
   Medial epicondyle of
     humerus
G **Humeral Shaft, Left**
   See F Humeral Shaft, Right
H **Radius, Right**
   Ulnar notch
J **Radius, Left**
   See H Radius, Right
K **Ulna, Right**
   Olecranon process
   Radial notch
	L **Ulna, Left**
	   See K Ulna, Right
	M **Carpal, Right**
	   Capitate bone
	   Hamate bone
	   Lunate bone
	   Pisiform bone
	   Scaphoid bone
	   Trapezium bone
	   Trapezoid bone
	   Triquetral bone
	N **Carpal, Left**
	   See M Carpal, Right
	P **Metacarpal, Right**
	Q **Metacarpal, Left**
	R **Thumb Phalanx, Right**
	S **Thumb Phalanx, Left**
	T **Finger Phalanx, Right**
	V **Finger Phalanx, Left**
		Ø Open
		3 Percutaneous
		4 Percutaneous Endoscopic
		X External
			4 Internal Fixation Device
			5 External Fixation Device
			7 Autologous Tissue
			   Substitute
			J Synthetic Substitute
			K Nonautologous Tissue
			   Substitute
				Z No Qualifier

Y **Upper Bone**		**Ø** Open **3** Percutaneous **4** Percutaneous Endoscopic **X** External	**Ø** Drainage Device **M** Bone Growth Stimulator	**Z** No Qualifier

Non-OR   ØPW[Ø,1,2,3,4,5,6,7,8,9,B]X[4,7,J,K]Z
Non-OR   ØPW[C,D,F,G,H,J,K,L,M,N,P,Q,R,S,T,V]X[4,5,7,J,K]Z
Non-OR   ØPWYX[Ø,M]Z

LC Limited Coverage   NC Noncovered   ⊞ Combination Member   HAC associated procedure   Combination Only   DRG Non-OR   Non-OR   New/Revised in GREEN

548   ICD-10-PCS 2020

Lower Bones 0Q2–0QW

Character Meanings

This Character Meaning table is provided as a guide to assist the user in the identification of character members that may be found in this section of code tables. It **SHOULD NOT** be used to build a PCS code.

Operation–Character 3		Body Part–Character 4		Approach–Character 5		Device–Character 6		Qualifier–Character 7	
2	Change	0	Lumbar Vertebra	0	Open	0	Drainage Device	2	Sesamoid Bone(s) 1st Toe
5	Destruction	1	Sacrum	3	Percutaneous	4	Internal Fixation Device	X	Diagnostic
8	Division	2	Pelvic Bone, Right	4	Percutaneous Endoscopic	5	External Fixation Device	Z	No Qualifier
9	Drainage	3	Pelvic Bone, Left	X	External	6	Internal Fixation Device, Intramedullary		
B	Excision	4	Acetabulum, Right			7	Autologous Tissue Substitute OR Internal Fixation Device, Intramedullary Limb Lengthening		
C	Extirpation	5	Acetabulum, Left			8	External Fixation Device, Limb Lengthening		
D	Extraction	6	Upper Femur, Right			B	External Fixation Device, Monoplanar		
H	Insertion	7	Upper Femur, Left			C	External Fixation Device, Ring		
J	Inspection	8	Femoral Shaft, Right			D	External Fixation Device, Hybrid		
N	Release	9	Femoral Shaft, Left			J	Synthetic Substitute		
P	Removal	B	Lower Femur, Right			K	Nonautologous Tissue Substitute		
Q	Repair	C	Lower Femur, Left			M	Bone Growth Stimulator		
R	Replacement	D	Patella, Right			Y	Other Device		
S	Reposition	F	Patella, Left			Z	No Device		
T	Resection	G	Tibia, Right						
U	Supplement	H	Tibia, Left						
W	Revision	J	Fibula, Right						
		K	Fibula, Left						
		L	Tarsal, Right						
		M	Tarsal, Left						
		N	Metatarsal, Right						
		P	Metatarsal, Left						
		Q	Toe Phalanx, Right						
		R	Toe Phalanx, Left						
		S	Coccyx						
		Y	Lower Bone						

AHA Coding Clinic for table 0Q8
2018, 1Q, 25   Periacetabular osteotomy for repair of congenital hip dysplasia
2016, 2Q, 31   Periacetabular ostectomy for repair of congenital hip dysplasia

AHA Coding Clinic for table 0QB
2018, 3Q, 17   Excisional debridement of periosteum
2017, 1Q, 23   Reconstruction of mandible using titanium and bone
2016, 3Q, 30   Resection of femur with interposition arthroplasty
2015, 3Q, 3-8   Excisional and nonexcisional debridement
2015, 3Q, 26   Femoral head resection
2015, 2Q, 34   Decompressive laminectomy
2014, 4Q, 25   Femoroacetabular impingement and labral tear with repair
2014, 2Q, 6   Posterior lumbar fusion with discectomy
2013, 4Q, 116   Spinal decompression
2013, 2Q, 39   Ankle fusion, osteotomy, and removal of hardware
2012, 2Q, 19   Multiple decompressive cervical laminectomies

AHA Coding Clinic for table 0QD
2017, 4Q, 41   Extraction procedures

AHA Coding Clinic for table 0QH
2017, 1Q, 21   Staged scoliosis surgery with iliac fixation and spinal fusion
2016, 3Q, 34   Tibial/fibula epiphysiodesis

AHA Coding Clinic for table 0QP
2017, 4Q, 74-75   Magnetic growth rods
2015, 2Q, 6   Planned implant break

AHA Coding Clinic for table 0QQ
2018, 1Q, 15   Pubic symphysis fusion
2014, 3Q, 24   Repair of lipomyelomeningocele and tethered cord

AHA Coding Clinic for table 0QR
2017, 1Q, 22   Total knee replacement and patellar component
2016, 3Q, 30   Resection of femur with interposition arthroplasty

AHA Coding Clinic for table 0QS
2018, 1Q, 13   Bilateral cuboid osteotomy for repair of congenital talipes equinovarus
2018, 1Q, 25   Periacetabular osteotomy for repair of congenital hip dysplasia
2016, 3Q, 34   Tibial/fibula epiphysiodesis
2014, 4Q, 29   Rotational osteosynthesis
2014, 4Q, 31   Reposition of femur for correction of valgus and recurvatum deformities

AHA Coding Clinic for table 0QT
2017, 1Q, 22   Chopart amputation of foot
2016, 3Q, 30   Resection of femur with interposition arthroplasty
2015, 3Q, 26   Femoral head resection
2014, 4Q, 29   Rotational osteosynthesis

AHA Coding Clinic for table 0QU
2015, 3Q, 18   Total hip replacement with acetabular reconstruction
2014, 4Q, 31   Reposition of femur for correction of valgus and recurvatum deformities
2014, 2Q, 12   Percutaneous vertebroplasty using cement
2013, 2Q, 35   Use of bone void filler in grafting

AHA Coding Clinic for table 0QW
2017, 4Q, 74-75   Magnetic growth rods

Lower Bones

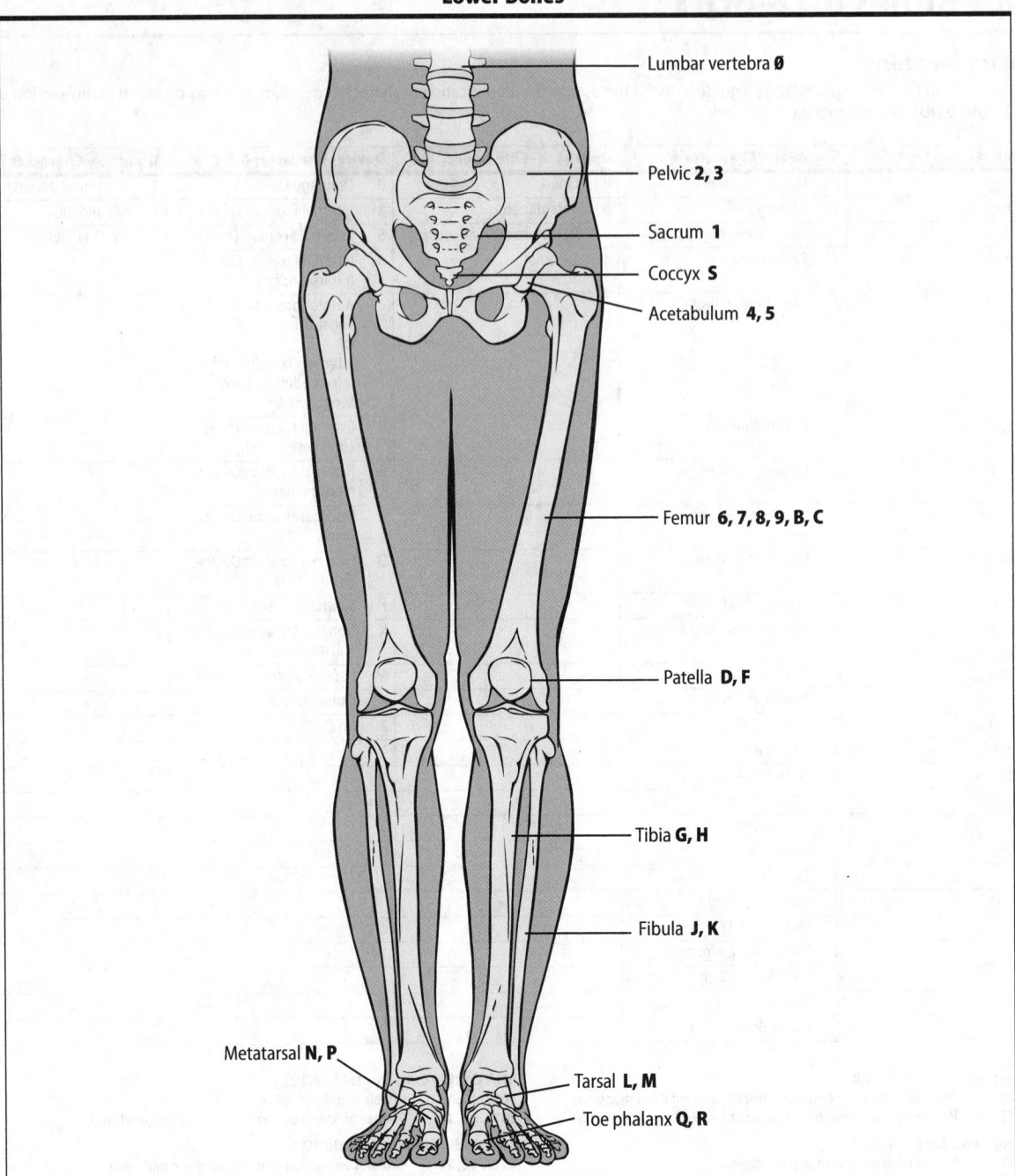

Lumbar vertebra **Ø**

Pelvic **2, 3**

Sacrum **1**

Coccyx **S**

Acetabulum **4, 5**

Femur **6, 7, 8, 9, B, C**

Patella **D, F**

Tibia **G, H**

Fibula **J, K**

Metatarsal **N, P**

Tarsal **L, M**

Toe phalanx **Q, R**

Hip Bone Anatomy

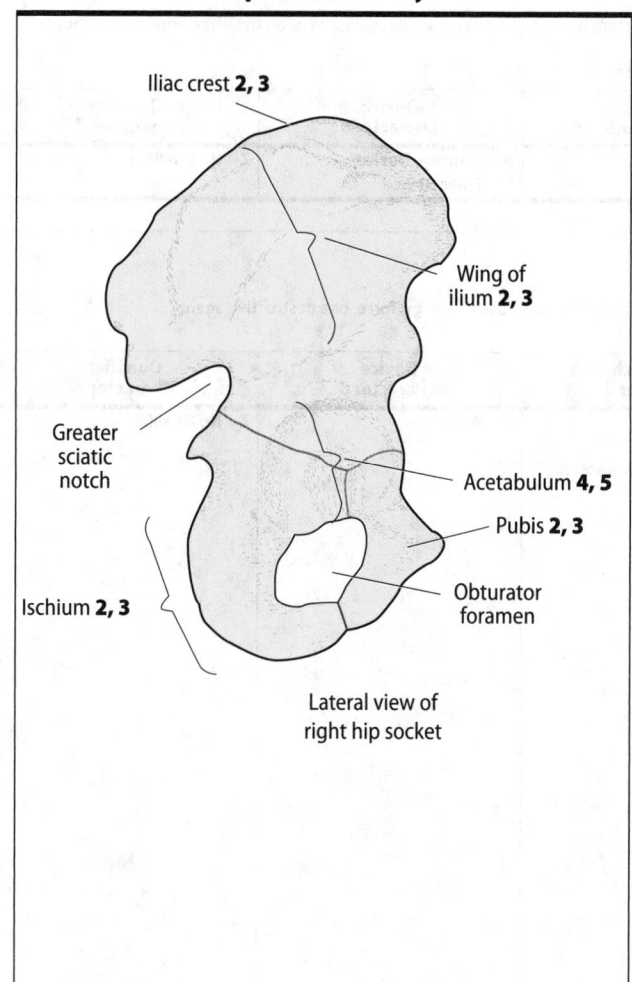

Iliac crest **2, 3**

Wing of ilium **2, 3**

Greater sciatic notch

Acetabulum **4, 5**

Pubis **2, 3**

Obturator foramen

Ischium **2, 3**

Lateral view of right hip socket

Pelvic and Lower Extremity Bones

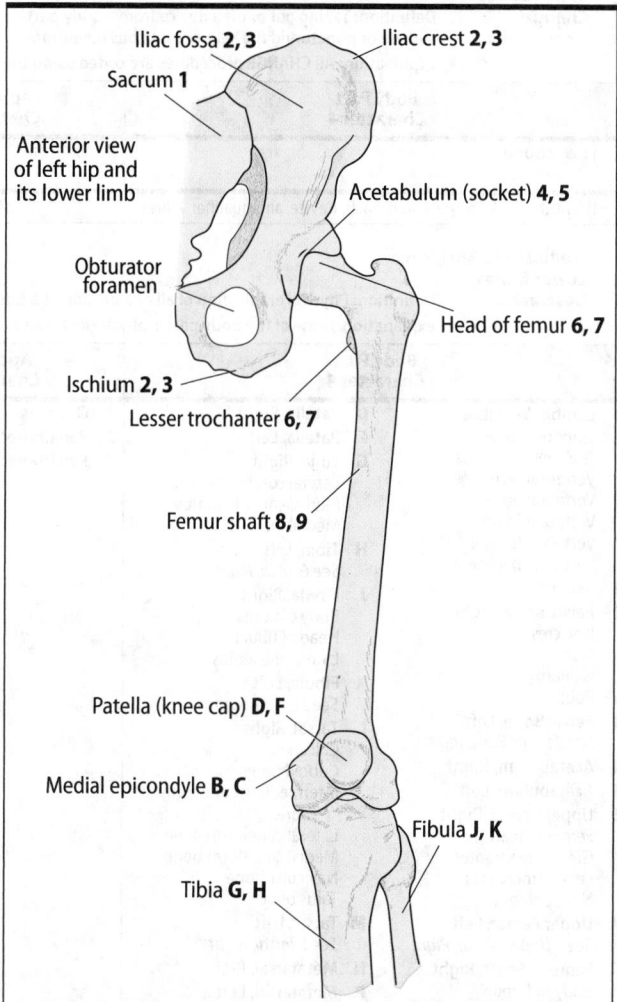

Iliac fossa **2, 3**

Iliac crest **2, 3**

Sacrum **1**

Anterior view of left hip and its lower limb

Acetabulum (socket) **4, 5**

Obturator foramen

Head of femur **6, 7**

Ischium **2, 3**

Lesser trochanter **6, 7**

Femur shaft **8, 9**

Patella (knee cap) **D, F**

Medial epicondyle **B, C**

Fibula **J, K**

Tibia **G, H**

Foot Bones

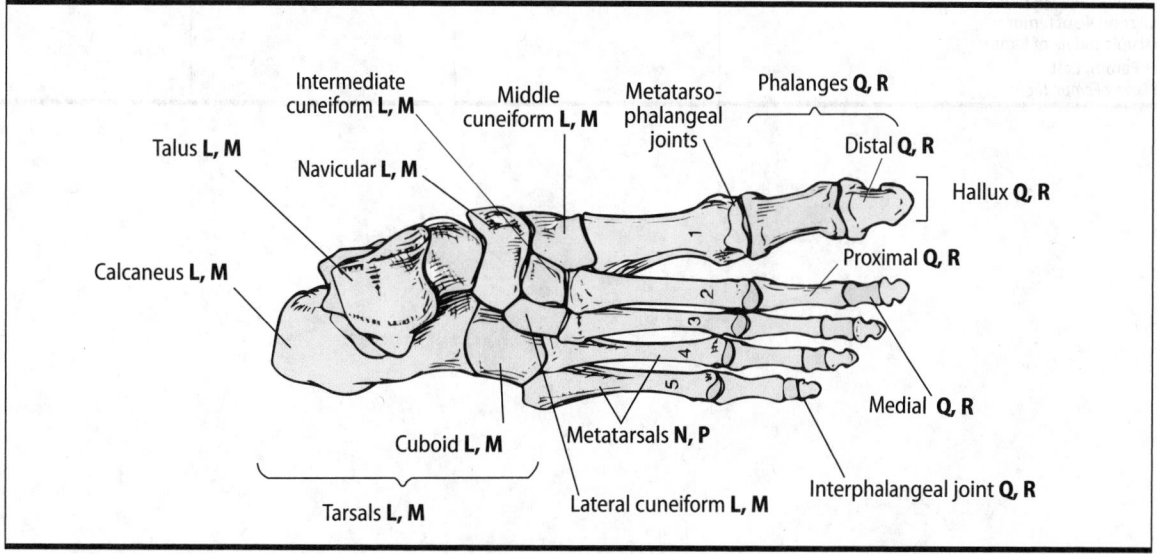

Intermediate cuneiform **L, M**

Middle cuneiform **L, M**

Metatarso-phalangeal joints

Phalanges **Q, R**

Talus **L, M**

Navicular **L, M**

Distal **Q, R**

Hallux **Q, R**

Calcaneus **L, M**

Proximal **Q, R**

Medial **Q, R**

Cuboid **L, M**

Metatarsals **N, P**

Interphalangeal joint **Q, R**

Tarsals **L, M**

Lateral cuneiform **L, M**

Lower Bones (side tab, left)

Ø **Medical and Surgical**
Q **Lower Bones**
2 **Change**   Definition: Taking out or off a device from a body part and putting back an identical or similar device in or on the same body part without cutting or puncturing the skin or a mucous membrane

         Explanation: All CHANGE procedures are coded using the approach EXTERNAL

Body Part Character 4	Approach Character 5	Device Character 6	Qualifier Character 7
Y Lower Bone	**X** External	**Ø** Drainage Device **Y** Other Device	**Z** No Qualifier

Non-OR   All body part, approach, device, and qualifier values

Ø **Medical and Surgical**
Q **Lower Bones**
5 **Destruction**   Definition: Physical eradication of all or a portion of a body part by the direct use of energy, force, or a destructive agent

         Explanation: None of the body part is physically taken out

Body Part Character 4		Approach Character 5	Device Character 6	Qualifier Character 7

Ø   Lumbar Vertebra
    Spinous process
    Transverse process
    Vertebral arch
    Vertebral body
    Vertebral foramen
    Vertebral lamina
    Vertebral pedicle
1   Sacrum
2   Pelvic Bone, Right
    Iliac crest
    Ilium
    Ischium
    Pubis
3   Pelvic Bone, Left
    See 2 Pelvic Bone, Right
4   Acetabulum, Right
5   Acetabulum, Left
6   Upper Femur, Right
    Femoral head
    Greater trochanter
    Lesser trochanter
    Neck of femur
7   Upper Femur, Left
    See 6 Upper Femur, Right
8   Femoral Shaft, Right
    Body of femur
9   Femoral Shaft, Left
    See 8 Femoral Shaft, Right
B   Lower Femur, Right
    Lateral condyle of femur
    Lateral epicondyle of femur
    Medial condyle of femur
    Medial epicondyle of femur
C   Lower Femur, Left
    See B Lower Femur, Right
	D Patella, Right
	F Patella, Left
	G Tibia, Right
	    Lateral condyle of tibia
	    Medial condyle of tibia
	    Medial malleolus
	H Tibia, Left
	    See G Tibia, Right
	J Fibula, Right
	    Body of fibula
	    Head of fibula
	    Lateral malleolus
	K Fibula, Left
	    See J Fibula, Right
	L Tarsal, Right
	    Calcaneus
	    Cuboid bone
	    Intermediate cuneiform
	      bone
	    Lateral cuneiform bone
	    Medial cuneiform bone
	    Navicular bone
	    Talus bone
	M Tarsal, Left
	    See L Tarsal, Right
	N Metatarsal, Right
	P Metatarsal, Left
	Q Toe Phalanx, Right
	R Toe Phalanx, Left
	S Coccyx
		Ø Open
		3 Percutaneous
		4 Percutaneous Endoscopic
			Z No Device	**Z** No Qualifier

LC Limited Coverage   **NC** Noncovered   ⊞ Combination Member   HAC associated procedure   Combination Only   DRG Non-OR   Non-OR   New/Revised in **GREEN**

552   ICD-10-PCS 2020

0Q2–0Q5 (side tab, left)

0   **Medical and Surgical**
Q   **Lower Bones**
8   **Division**   Definition: Cutting into a body part, without draining fluids and/or gases from the body part, in order to separate or transect a body part
                 Explanation: All or a portion of the body part is separated into two or more portions

Body Part Character 4	Approach Character 5	Device Character 6	Qualifier Character 7
0 **Lumbar Vertebra** Spinous process Transverse process Vertebral arch Vertebral body Vertebral foramen Vertebral lamina Vertebral pedicle **1** **Sacrum** **2** **Pelvic Bone, Right** Iliac crest Ilium Ischium Pubis **3** **Pelvic Bone, Left** *See 2 Pelvic Bone, Right* **4** **Acetabulum, Right** **5** **Acetabulum, Left** **6** **Upper Femur, Right** Femoral head Greater trochanter Lesser trochanter Neck of femur **7** **Upper Femur, Left** *See 6 Upper Femur, Right* **8** **Femoral Shaft, Right** Body of femur **9** **Femoral Shaft, Left** *See 8 Femoral Shaft, Right* **B** **Lower Femur, Right** Lateral condyle of femur Lateral epicondyle of femur Medial condyle of femur Medial epicondyle of femur **C** **Lower Femur, Left** *See B Lower Femur, Right* **D** **Patella, Right** **F** **Patella, Left** **G** **Tibia, Right** Lateral condyle of tibia Medial condyle of tibia Medial malleolus **H** **Tibia, Left** *See G Tibia, Right* **J** **Fibula, Right** Body of fibula Head of fibula Lateral malleolus **K** **Fibula, Left** *See J Fibula, Right* **L** **Tarsal, Right** Calcaneus Cuboid bone Intermediate cuneiform bone Lateral cuneiform bone Medial cuneiform bone Navicular bone Talus bone **M** **Tarsal, Left** *See L Tarsal, Right* **N** **Metatarsal, Right** **P** **Metatarsal, Left** **Q** **Toe Phalanx, Right** **R** **Toe Phalanx, Left** **S** **Coccyx**	**0** Open **3** Percutaneous **4** Percutaneous Endoscopic	**Z** No Device	**Z** No Qualifier

LC Limited Coverage NC Noncovered ⊞ Combination Member HAC associated procedure Combination Only DRG Non-OR Non-OR New/Revised in GREEN

ICD-10-PCS 2020

0Q8–0Q8

553

Ø Medical and Surgical
Q Lower Bones
9 Drainage   Definition: Taking or letting out fluids and/or gases from a body part

Explanation: The qualifier DIAGNOSTIC is used to identify drainage procedures that are biopsies

Body Part Character 4		Approach Character 5	Device Character 6	Qualifier Character 7
Ø **Lumbar Vertebra** Spinous process Transverse process Vertebral arch Vertebral body Vertebral foramen Vertebral lamina Vertebral pedicle **1** **Sacrum** **2** **Pelvic Bone, Right** Iliac crest Ilium Ischium Pubis **3** **Pelvic Bone, Left** *See 2 Pelvic Bone, Right* **4** **Acetabulum, Right** **5** **Acetabulum, Left** **6** **Upper Femur, Right** Femoral head Greater trochanter Lesser trochanter Neck of femur **7** **Upper Femur, Left** *See 6 Upper Femur, Right* **8** **Femoral Shaft, Right** Body of femur **9** **Femoral Shaft, Left** *See 8 Femoral Shaft, Right* **B** **Lower Femur, Right** Lateral condyle of femur Lateral epicondyle of femur Medial condyle of femur Medial epicondyle of femur	**C** **Lower Femur, Left** *See B Lower Femur, Right* **D** **Patella, Right** **F** **Patella, Left** **G** **Tibia, Right** Lateral condyle of tibia Medial condyle of tibia Medial malleolus **H** **Tibia, Left** *See G Tibia, Right* **J** **Fibula, Right** Body of fibula Head of fibula Lateral malleolus **K** **Fibula, Left** *See J Fibula, Right* **L** **Tarsal, Right** Calcaneus Cuboid bone Intermediate cuneiform bone Lateral cuneiform bone Medial cuneiform bone Navicular bone Talus bone **M** **Tarsal, Left** *See L Tarsal, Right* **N** **Metatarsal, Right** **P** **Metatarsal, Left** **Q** **Toe Phalanx, Right** **R** **Toe Phalanx, Left** **S** **Coccyx**	**Ø** Open **3** Percutaneous **4** Percutaneous Endoscopic	**Ø** Drainage Device	**Z** No Qualifier
Ø **Lumbar Vertebra** Spinous process Transverse process Vertebral arch Vertebral body Vertebral foramen Vertebral lamina Vertebral pedicle **1** **Sacrum** **2** **Pelvic Bone, Right** Iliac crest Ilium Ischium Pubis **3** **Pelvic Bone, Left** *See 2 Pelvic Bone, Right* **4** **Acetabulum, Right** **5** **Acetabulum, Left** **6** **Upper Femur, Right** Femoral head Greater trochanter Lesser trochanter Neck of femur **7** **Upper Femur, Left** *See 6 Upper Femur, Right* **8** **Femoral Shaft, Right** Body of femur **9** **Femoral Shaft, Left** *See 8 Femoral Shaft, Right* **B** **Lower Femur, Right** Lateral condyle of femur Lateral epicondyle of femur Medial condyle of femur Medial epicondyle of femur	**C** **Lower Femur, Left** *See B Lower Femur, Right* **D** **Patella, Right** **F** **Patella, Left** **G** **Tibia, Right** Lateral condyle of tibia Medial condyle of tibia Medial malleolus **H** **Tibia, Left** *See G Tibia, Right* **J** **Fibula, Right** Body of fibula Head of fibula Lateral malleolus **K** **Fibula, Left** *See J Fibula, Right* **L** **Tarsal, Right** Calcaneus Cuboid bone Intermediate cuneiform bone Lateral cuneiform bone Medial cuneiform bone Navicular bone Talus bone **M** **Tarsal, Left** *See L Tarsal, Right* **N** **Metatarsal, Right** **P** **Metatarsal, Left** **Q** **Toe Phalanx, Right** **R** **Toe Phalanx, Left** **S** **Coccyx**	**Ø** Open **3** Percutaneous **4** Percutaneous Endoscopic	**Z** No Device	**X** Diagnostic **Z** No Qualifier

Non-OR   ØQ9[Ø,1,2,3,4,5,6,7,8,9,B,C,D,F,G,H,J,K,L,M,P,Q,R,S]3ØZ
Non-OR   ØQ9[Ø,1,2,3,4,5,6,7,8,9,B,C,D,F,G,H,J,K,L,M,P,Q,R,S]3ZZ

Ø   Medical and Surgical
Q   Lower Bones
B   Excision   Definition: Cutting out or off, without replacement, a portion of a body part
                             Explanation: The qualifier DIAGNOSTIC is used to identify excision procedures that are biopsies

Body Part Character 4	Approach Character 5	Device Character 6	Qualifier Character 7

Ø   **Lumbar Vertebra**
    Spinous process
    Transverse process
    Vertebral arch
    Vertebral body
    Vertebral foramen
    Vertebral lamina
    Vertebral pedicle
1   **Sacrum**
2   **Pelvic Bone, Right**
    Iliac crest
    Ilium
    Ischium
    Pubis
3   **Pelvic Bone, Left**
    See 2 Pelvic Bone, Right
4   **Acetabulum, Right**
5   **Acetabulum, Left**
6   **Upper Femur, Right**
    Femoral head
    Greater trochanter
    Lesser trochanter
    Neck of femur
7   **Upper Femur, Left**
    See 6 Upper Femur, Right
8   **Femoral Shaft, Right**
    Body of femur
9   **Femoral Shaft, Left**
    See 8 Femoral Shaft, Right
B   **Lower Femur, Right**
    Lateral condyle of femur
    Lateral epicondyle of femur
    Medial condyle of femur
    Medial epicondyle of femur
C   **Lower Femur, Left**
    See B Lower Femur, Right
D   **Patella, Right**
F   **Patella, Left**
G   **Tibia, Right**
    Lateral condyle of tibia
    Medial condyle of tibia
    Medial malleolus
H   **Tibia, Left**
    See G Tibia, Right
J   **Fibula, Right**
    Body of fibula
    Head of fibula
    Lateral malleolus
K   **Fibula, Left**
    See J Fibula, Right
L   **Tarsal, Right**
    Calcaneus
    Cuboid bone
    Intermediate cuneiform bone
    Lateral cuneiform bone
    Medial cuneiform bone
    Navicular bone
    Talus bone
M   **Tarsal, Left**
    See L Tarsal, Right
N   **Metatarsal, Right**
P   **Metatarsal, Left**
Q   **Toe Phalanx, Right**
R   **Toe Phalanx, Left**
S   **Coccyx**
	Ø Open
	3 Percutaneous
	4 Percutaneous Endoscopic
		Z No Device	**X** Diagnostic
			Z No Qualifier

Lower Bones

Ø   **Medical and Surgical**
Q   **Lower Bones**
C   **Extirpation**   Definition: Taking or cutting out solid matter from a body part

Explanation: The solid matter may be an abnormal byproduct of a biological function or a foreign body; it may be imbedded in a body part or in the lumen of a tubular body part. The solid matter may or may not have been previously broken into pieces.

Body Part Character 4		Approach Character 5	Device Character 6	Qualifier Character 7

Ø **Lumbar Vertebra**
   Spinous process
   Transverse process
   Vertebral arch
   Vertebral body
   Vertebral foramen
   Vertebral lamina
   Vertebral pedicle
1 **Sacrum**
2 **Pelvic Bone, Right**
   Iliac crest
   Ilium
   Ischium
   Pubis
3 **Pelvic Bone, Left**
   See 2 Pelvic Bone, Right
4 **Acetabulum, Right**
5 **Acetabulum, Left**
6 **Upper Femur, Right**
   Femoral head
   Greater trochanter
   Lesser trochanter
   Neck of femur
7 **Upper Femur, Left**
   See 6 Upper Femur, Right
8 **Femoral Shaft, Right**
   Body of femur
9 **Femoral Shaft, Left**
   See 8 Femoral Shaft, Right
B **Lower Femur, Right**
   Lateral condyle of femur
   Lateral epicondyle of femur
   Medial condyle of femur
   Medial epicondyle of femur
	C **Lower Femur, Left**
	   See B Lower Femur, Right
	D **Patella, Right**
	F **Patella, Left**
	G **Tibia, Right**
	   Lateral condyle of tibia
	   Medial condyle of tibia
	   Medial malleolus
	H **Tibia, Left**
	   See G Tibia, Right
	J **Fibula, Right**
	   Body of fibula
	   Head of fibula
	   Lateral malleolus
	K **Fibula, Left**
	   See J Fibula, Right
	L **Tarsal, Right**
	   Calcaneus
	   Cuboid bone
	   Intermediate cuneiform bone
	   Lateral cuneiform bone
	   Medial cuneiform bone
	   Navicular bone
	   Talus bone
	M **Tarsal, Left**
	   See L Tarsal, Right
	N **Metatarsal, Right**
	P **Metatarsal, Left**
	Q **Toe Phalanx, Right**
	R **Toe Phalanx, Left**
	S **Coccyx**
		Ø Open
		3 Percutaneous
		4 Percutaneous Endoscopic
			Z No Device	**Z** No Qualifier

Ø   **Medical and Surgical**
Q   **Lower Bones**
D   **Extraction**   Definition: Pulling or stripping out or off all or a portion of a body part by the use of force

Explanation: The qualifier DIAGNOSTIC is used to identify extraction procedures that are biopsies

Body Part Character 4		Approach Character 5	Device Character 6	Qualifier Character 7

Ø **Lumbar Vertebra**
   Spinous process
   Transverse process
   Vertebral arch
   Vertebral body
   Vertebral foramen
   Vertebral lamina
   Vertebral pedicle
1 **Sacrum**
2 **Pelvic Bone, Right**
   Iliac crest
   Ilium
   Ischium
   Pubis
3 **Pelvic Bone, Left**
   See 2 Pelvic Bone, Right
4 **Acetabulum, Right**
5 **Acetabulum, Left**
6 **Upper Femur, Right**
   Femoral head
   Greater trochanter
   Lesser trochanter
   Neck of femur
7 **Upper Femur, Left**
   See 6 Upper Femur, Right
8 **Femoral Shaft, Right**
   Body of femur
9 **Femoral Shaft, Left**
   See 8 Femoral Shaft, Right
B **Lower Femur, Right**
   Lateral condyle of femur
   Lateral epicondyle of femur
   Medial condyle of femur
   Medial epicondyle of femur
	C **Lower Femur, Left**
	   See B Lower Femur, Right
	D **Patella, Right**
	F **Patella, Left**
	G **Tibia, Right**
	   Lateral condyle of tibia
	   Medial condyle of tibia
	   Medial malleolus
	H **Tibia, Left**
	   See G Tibia, Right
	J **Fibula, Right**
	   Body of fibula
	   Head of fibula
	   Lateral malleolus
	K **Fibula, Left**
	   See J Fibula, Right
	L **Tarsal, Right**
	   Calcaneus
	   Cuboid bone
	   Intermediate cuneiform bone
	   Lateral cuneiform bone
	   Medial cuneiform bone
	   Navicular bone
	   Talus bone
	M **Tarsal, Left**
	   See L Tarsal, Right
	N **Metatarsal, Right**
	P **Metatarsal, Left**
	Q **Toe Phalanx, Right**
	R **Toe Phalanx, Left**
	S **Coccyx**
		Ø Open	**Z** No Device	**Z** No Qualifier

LC Limited Coverage   NC Noncovered   ⊞ Combination Member   HAC associated procedure   Combination Only   DRG Non-OR   Non-OR   New/Revised in GREEN

556   ICD-10-PCS 2020

Ø   Medical and Surgical
Q   Lower Bones
H   Insertion   Definition: Putting in a nonbiological appliance that monitors, assists, performs, or prevents a physiological function but does not physically take the place of a body part

         Explanation: None

Body Part Character 4		Approach Character 5	Device Character 6	Qualifier Character 7

Ø **Lumbar Vertebra**
  Spinous process
  Transverse process
  Vertebral arch
  Vertebral body
  Vertebral foramen
  Vertebral lamina
  Vertebral pedicle
1 **Sacrum**
2 **Pelvic Bone, Right**
  Iliac crest
  Ilium
  Ischium
  Pubis
3 **Pelvic Bone, Left**
  See 2 Pelvic Bone, Right
4 **Acetabulum, Right**
5 **Acetabulum, Left**
	D **Patella, Right**
	F **Patella, Left**
	L **Tarsal, Right**
	  Calcaneus
	  Cuboid bone
	  Intermediate cuneiform bone
	  Lateral cuneiform bone
	  Medial cuneiform bone
	  Navicular bone
	  Talus bone
	M **Tarsal, Left**
	  See L Tarsal, Right
	N **Metatarsal, Right**
	P **Metatarsal, Left**
	Q **Toe Phalanx, Right**
	R **Toe Phalanx, Left**
	S **Coccyx**
		Ø **Open**
		3 **Percutaneous**
		4 **Percutaneous Endoscopic**
			4 **Internal Fixation Device**
			5 **External Fixation Device**
				Z **No Qualifier**

6 **Upper Femur, Right**
  Femoral head
  Greater trochanter
  Lesser trochanter
  Neck of femur
7 **Upper Femur, Left**
  See 6 Upper Femur, Right
B **Lower Femur, Right**
  Lateral condyle of femur
  Lateral epicondyle of femur
  Medial condyle of femur
  Medial epicondyle of femur
	C **Lower Femur, Left**
	  See B Lower Femur, Right
	J **Fibula, Right**
	  Body of fibula
	  Head of fibula
	  Lateral malleolus
	K **Fibula, Left**
	  See J Fibula, Right
		Ø **Open**
		3 **Percutaneous**
		4 **Percutaneous Endoscopic**
			4 **Internal Fixation Device**
			5 **External Fixation Device**
			6 **Internal Fixation Device,
			  Intramedullary**
			8 **External Fixation Device,
			  Limb Lengthening**
			B **External Fixation Device,
			  Monoplanar**
			C **External Fixation Device,
			  Ring**
			D **External Fixation Device,
			  Hybrid**
				Z **No Qualifier**

8 **Femoral Shaft, Right**
  Body of femur
9 **Femoral Shaft, Left**
  See 8 Femoral Shaft, Right
	G **Tibia, Right**
	  Lateral condyle of tibia
	  Medial condyle of tibia
	  Medial malleolus
	H **Tibia, Left**
	  See G Tibia, Right
		Ø **Open**
		3 **Percutaneous**
		4 **Percutaneous Endoscopic**
			4 **Internal Fixation Device**
			5 **External Fixation Device**
			6 **Internal Fixation Device,
			  Intramedullary**
			7 **Internal Fixation Device,
			  Intramedullary Limb
			  Lengthening**
			8 **External Fixation Device,
			  Limb Lengthening**
			B **External Fixation Device,
			  Monoplanar**
			C **External Fixation Device,
			  Ring**
			D **External Fixation Device,
			  Hybrid**
				Z **No Qualifier**

Y **Lower Bone**		Ø **Open** 3 **Percutaneous** 4 **Percutaneous Endoscopic**	M **Bone Growth Stimulator**	Z **No Qualifier**

    Non-OR   ØQH[6,7,B,C,J,K][Ø,3,4]8Z
    Non-OR   ØQH[8,9,G,H][Ø,3,4]8Z

Ø   Medical and Surgical
Q   Lower Bones
J   Inspection   Definition: Visually and/or manually exploring a body part

         Explanation: Visual exploration may be performed with or without optical instrumentation. Manual exploration may be performed directly or through intervening body layers.

Body Part Character 4	Approach Character 5	Device Character 6	Qualifier Character 7
Y **Lower Bone**	Ø **Open** 3 **Percutaneous** 4 **Percutaneous Endoscopic** X **External**	Z **No Device**	Z **No Qualifier**

    Non-OR   ØQJY[3,X]ZZ

LC Limited Coverage   NC Noncovered   ⊞ Combination Member   HAC associated procedure   Combination Only   DRG Non-OR   Non-OR   New/Revised in GREEN

Lower Bones

Ø Medical and Surgical
Q Lower Bones
N Release

Definition: Freeing a body part from an abnormal physical constraint by cutting or by the use of force

Explanation: Some of the restraining tissue may be taken out but none of the body part is taken out

Body Part Character 4		Approach Character 5	Device Character 6	Qualifier Character 7
Ø Lumbar Vertebra Spinous process Transverse process Vertebral arch Vertebral body Vertebral foramen Vertebral lamina Vertebral pedicle **1 Sacrum** **2 Pelvic Bone, Right** Iliac crest Ilium Ischium Pubis **3 Pelvic Bone, Left** *See 2 Pelvic Bone, Right* **4 Acetabulum, Right** **5 Acetabulum, Left** **6 Upper Femur, Right** Femoral head Greater trochanter Lesser trochanter Neck of femur **7 Upper Femur, Left** *See 6 Upper Femur, Right* **8 Femoral Shaft, Right** Body of femur **9 Femoral Shaft, Left** *See 8 Femoral Shaft, Right* **B Lower Femur, Right** Lateral condyle of femur Lateral epicondyle of femur Medial condyle of femur Medial epicondyle of femur	**C Lower Femur, Left** *See B Lower Femur, Right* **D Patella, Right** **F Patella, Left** **G Tibia, Right** Lateral condyle of tibia Medial condyle of tibia Medial malleolus **H Tibia, Left** *See G Tibia, Right* **J Fibula, Right** Body of fibula Head of fibula Lateral malleolus **K Fibula, Left** *See J Fibula, Right* **L Tarsal, Right** Calcaneus Cuboid bone Intermediate cuneiform bone Lateral cuneiform bone Medial cuneiform bone Navicular bone Talus bone **M Tarsal, Left** *See L Tarsal, Right* **N Metatarsal, Right** **P Metatarsal, Left** **Q Toe Phalanx, Right** **R Toe Phalanx, Left** **S Coccyx**	**Ø Open** **3 Percutaneous** **4 Percutaneous Endoscopic**	**Z No Device**	**Z No Qualifier**

Ø Medical and Surgical
Q Lower Bones
P Removal

Definition: Taking out or off a device from a body part

Explanation: If a device is taken out and a similar device put in without cutting or puncturing the skin or mucous membrane, the procedure is coded to the root operation CHANGE. Otherwise, the procedure for taking out a device is coded to the root operation REMOVAL.

Body Part Character 4	Approach Character 5	Device Character 6	Qualifier Character 7
Ø Lumbar Vertebra Spinous process Transverse process Vertebral arch Vertebral body Vertebral foramen Vertebral lamina Vertebral pedicle **1 Sacrum** **4 Acetabulum, Right** **5 Acetabulum, Left** **S Coccyx**	**Ø Open** **3 Percutaneous** **4 Percutaneous Endoscopic**	**4 Internal Fixation Device** **7 Autologous Tissue Substitute** **J Synthetic Substitute** **K Nonautologous Tissue Substitute**	**Z No Qualifier**
Ø Lumbar Vertebra Spinous process Transverse process Vertebral arch Vertebral body Vertebral foramen Vertebral lamina Vertebral pedicle **1 Sacrum** **4 Acetabulum, Right** **5 Acetabulum, Left** **S Coccyx**	**X External**	**4 Internal Fixation Device**	**Z No Qualifier**

ØQP Continued on next page

Non-OR   ØQP[Ø,1,4,5,S]X4Z

LC Limited Coverage   NC Noncovered   ⊞ Combination Member   HAC associated procedure   Combination Only   DRG Non-OR   Non-OR   New/Revised in **GREEN**

558   ICD-10-PCS 2020

Ø   **Medical and Surgical**   *ØQP Continued*
Q   **Lower Bones**
P   **Removal**

Definition: Taking out or off a device from a body part

Explanation: If a device is taken out and a similar device put in without cutting or puncturing the skin or mucous membrane, the procedure is coded to the root operation CHANGE. Otherwise, the procedure for taking out a device is coded to the root operation REMOVAL.

Body Part Character 4		Approach Character 5	Device Character 6	Qualifier Character 7

2 **Pelvic Bone, Right**
  Iliac crest
  Ilium
  Ischium
  Pubis
3 **Pelvic Bone, Left**
  See 2 Pelvic Bone, Right
6 **Upper Femur, Right**
  Femoral head
  Greater trochanter
  Lesser trochanter
  Neck of femur
7 **Upper Femur, Left**
  See 6 Upper Femur, Right
8 **Femoral Shaft, Right**
  Body of femur
9 **Femoral Shaft, Left**
  See 8 Femoral Shaft, Right
B **Lower Femur, Right**
  Lateral condyle of femur
  Lateral epicondyle of femur
  Medial condyle of femur
  Medial epicondyle of femur
C **Lower Femur, Left**
  See B Lower Femur, Right
D **Patella, Right**
F **Patella, Left**
	G **Tibia, Right**
	  Lateral condyle of tibia
	  Medial condyle of tibia
	  Medial malleolus
	H **Tibia, Left**
	  See G Tibia, Right
	J **Fibula, Right**
	  Body of fibula
	  Head of fibula
	  Lateral malleolus
	K **Fibula, Left**
	  See J Fibula, Right
	L **Tarsal, Right**
	  Calcaneus
	  Cuboid bone
	  Intermediate cuneiform bone
	  Lateral cuneiform bone
	  Medial cuneiform bone
	  Navicular bone
	  Talus bone
	M **Tarsal, Left**
	  See L Tarsal, Right
	N **Metatarsal, Right**
	P **Metatarsal, Left**
	Q **Toe Phalanx, Right**
	R **Toe Phalanx, Left**
		Ø **Open**
		3 **Percutaneous**
		4 **Percutaneous Endoscopic**
			4 **Internal Fixation Device**
			5 **External Fixation Device**
			7 **Autologous Tissue Substitute**
			J **Synthetic Substitute**
			K **Nonautologous Tissue Substitute**
				Z **No Qualifier**

2 **Pelvic Bone, Right**
  Iliac crest
  Ilium
  Ischium
  Pubis
3 **Pelvic Bone, Left**
  See 2 Pelvic Bone, Right
6 **Upper Femur, Right**
  Femoral head
  Greater trochanter
  Lesser trochanter
  Neck of femur
7 **Upper Femur, Left**
  See 6 Upper Femur, Right
8 **Femoral Shaft, Right**
  Body of femur
9 **Femoral Shaft, Left**
  See 8 Femoral Shaft, Right
B **Lower Femur, Right**
  Lateral condyle of femur
  Lateral epicondyle of femur
  Medial condyle of femur
  Medial epicondyle of femur
C **Lower Femur, Left**
  See B Lower Femur, Right
D **Patella, Right**
F **Patella, Left**
	G **Tibia, Right**
	  Lateral condyle of tibia
	  Medial condyle of tibia
	  Medial malleolus
	H **Tibia, Left**
	  See G Tibia, Right
	J **Fibula, Right**
	  Body of fibula
	  Head of fibula
	  Lateral malleolus
	K **Fibula, Left**
	  See J Fibula, Right
	L **Tarsal, Right**
	  Calcaneus
	  Cuboid bone
	  Intermediate cuneiform bone
	  Lateral cuneiform bone
	  Medial cuneiform bone
	  Navicular bone
	  Talus bone
	M **Tarsal, Left**
	  See L Tarsal, Right
	N **Metatarsal, Right**
	P **Metatarsal, Left**
	Q **Toe Phalanx, Right**
	R **Toe Phalanx, Left**
		X **External**	4 **Internal Fixation Device**
			5 **External Fixation Device**
				Z **No Qualifier**

Y **Lower Bone**		Ø **Open** 3 **Percutaneous** 4 **Percutaneous Endoscopic** X **External**	Ø **Drainage Device** M **Bone Growth Stimulator**	Z **No Qualifier**

Non-OR   ØQP[2,3,6,7,8,9,B,C,D,F,G,H,J,K,L,M,N,P,Q,R]X[4,5]Z
Non-OR   ØQPY3ØZ
Non-OR   ØQPYX[Ø,M]Z

Lower Bones

Ø   **Medical and Surgical**
Q   **Lower Bones**
Q   **Repair**   Definition: Restoring, to the extent possible, a body part to its normal anatomic structure and function
                Explanation: Used only when the method to accomplish the repair is not one of the other root operations

Body Part Character 4	Approach Character 5	Device Character 6	Qualifier Character 7

Ø   **Lumbar Vertebra**
     Spinous process
     Transverse process
     Vertebral arch
     Vertebral body
     Vertebral foramen
     Vertebral lamina
     Vertebral pedicle
1   **Sacrum**
2   **Pelvic Bone, Right**
     Iliac crest
     Ilium
     Ischium
     Pubis
3   **Pelvic Bone, Left**
     See 2 Pelvic Bone, Right
4   **Acetabulum, Right**
5   **Acetabulum, Left**
6   **Upper Femur, Right**
     Femoral head
     Greater trochanter
     Lesser trochanter
     Neck of femur
7   **Upper Femur, Left**
     See 6 Upper Femur, Right
8   **Femoral Shaft, Right**
     Body of femur
9   **Femoral Shaft, Left**
     See 8 Femoral Shaft, Right
B   **Lower Femur, Right**
     Lateral condyle of femur
     Lateral epicondyle of femur
     Medial condyle of femur
     Medial epicondyle of femur
C   **Lower Femur, Left**
     See B Lower Femur, Right
D   **Patella, Right**
F   **Patella, Left**
G   **Tibia, Right**
     Lateral condyle of tibia
     Medial condyle of tibia
     Medial malleolus
H   **Tibia, Left**
     See G Tibia, Right
J   **Fibula, Right**
     Body of fibula
     Head of fibula
     Lateral malleolus
K   **Fibula, Left**
     See J Fibula, Right
L   **Tarsal, Right**
     Calcaneus
     Cuboid bone
     Intermediate cuneiform bone
     Lateral cuneiform bone
     Medial cuneiform bone
     Navicular bone
     Talus bone
M   **Tarsal, Left**
     See L Tarsal, Right
N   **Metatarsal, Right**
P   **Metatarsal, Left**
Q   **Toe Phalanx, Right**
R   **Toe Phalanx, Left**
S   **Coccyx**
	Ø **Open**
	3 **Percutaneous**
	4 **Percutaneous Endoscopic**
	X **External**
		Z **No Device**	**Z** **No Qualifier**

Non-OR   ØQQ[Ø,1,2,3,4,5,6,7,8,9,B,C,D,F,G,H,J,K,L,M,N,P,Q,R,S]XZZ

LC Limited Coverage   **NC** Noncovered   ⊞ Combination Member   HAC associated procedure   Combination Only   DRG Non-OR   Non-OR   New/Revised in GREEN

560   ICD-10-PCS 2020

Ø   **Medical and Surgical**
Q   **Lower Bones**
R   **Replacement**   Definition: Putting in or on biological or synthetic material that physically takes the place and/or function of all or a portion of a body part

Explanation: The body part may have been taken out or replaced, or may be taken out, physically eradicated, or rendered nonfunctional during the REPLACEMENT procedure. A REMOVAL procedure is coded for taking out the device used in a previous replacement procedure.

Body Part Character 4	Approach Character 5	Device Character 6	Qualifier Character 7

Ø Lumbar Vertebra
   Spinous process
   Transverse process
   Vertebral arch
   Vertebral body
   Vertebral foramen
   Vertebral lamina
   Vertebral pedicle
1 Sacrum
2 Pelvic Bone, Right
   Iliac crest
   Ilium
   Ischium
   Pubis
3 Pelvic Bone, Left
   See 2 Pelvic Bone, Right
4 Acetabulum, Right
5 Acetabulum, Left
6 Upper Femur, Right
   Femoral head
   Greater trochanter
   Lesser trochanter
   Neck of femur
7 Upper Femur, Left
   See 6 Upper Femur, Right
8 Femoral Shaft, Right
   Body of femur
9 Femoral Shaft, Left
   See 8 Femoral Shaft, Right
B Lower Femur, Right
   Lateral condyle of femur
   Lateral epicondyle of femur
   Medial condyle of femur
   Medial epicondyle of femur
C Lower Femur, Left
   See B Lower Femur, Right
D Patella, Right
F Patella, Left
G Tibia, Right
   Lateral condyle of tibia
   Medial condyle of tibia
   Medial malleolus
H Tibia, Left
   See G Tibia, Right
J Fibula, Right
   Body of fibula
   Head of fibula
   Lateral malleolus
K Fibula, Left
   See J Fibula, Right
L Tarsal, Right
   Calcaneus
   Cuboid bone
   Intermediate cuneiform bone
   Lateral cuneiform bone
   Medial cuneiform bone
   Navicular bone
   Talus bone
M Tarsal, Left
   See L Tarsal, Right
N Metatarsal, Right
P Metatarsal, Left
Q Toe Phalanx, Right
R Toe Phalanx, Left
S Coccyx
	Ø Open
	3 Percutaneous
	4 Percutaneous Endoscopic
		7 Autologous Tissue Substitute
		J Synthetic Substitute
		K Nonautologous Tissue Substitute
			Z No Qualifier

LC Limited Coverage NC Noncovered ⊞ Combination Member HAC associated procedure Combination Only DRG Non-OR Non-OR New/Revised in GREEN

ICD-10-PCS 2020   561

Lower Bones

Ø   **Medical and Surgical**
Q   **Lower Bones**
S   **Reposition**   Definition: Moving to its normal location, or other suitable location, all or a portion of a body part

Explanation: The body part is moved to a new location from an abnormal location, or from a normal location where it is not functioning correctly. The body part may or may not be cut out or off to be moved to the new location.

Body Part Character 4	Approach Character 5	Device Character 6	Qualifier Character 7

Ø Lumbar Vertebra ⊞
  Spinous process
  Transverse process
  Vertebral arch
  Vertebral body
  Vertebral foramen
  Vertebral lamina
  Vertebral pedicle
1 Sacrum ⊞
4 Acetabulum, Right
5 Acetabulum, Left
S Coccyx ⊞
	Ø Open
	3 Percutaneous
	4 Percutaneous Endoscopic
		4 Internal Fixation Device
		Z No Device
			Z No Qualifier

Ø Lumbar Vertebra
  Spinous process
  Transverse process
  Vertebral arch
  Vertebral body
  Vertebral foramen
  Vertebral lamina
  Vertebral pedicle
1 Sacrum
4 Acetabulum, Right
5 Acetabulum, Left
S Coccyx
	X External	**Z** No Device	**Z** No Qualifier

2 Pelvic Bone, Right
  Iliac crest
  Ilium
  Ischium
  Pubis
3 Pelvic Bone, Left
  See 2 Pelvic Bone, Right
D Patella, Right
F Patella, Left
L Tarsal, Right
  Calcaneus
  Cuboid bone
  Intermediate cuneiform bone
  Lateral cuneiform bone
  Medial cuneiform bone
  Navicular bone
  Talus bone
M Tarsal, Left
  See L Tarsal, Right
Q Toe Phalanx, Right
R Toe Phalanx, Left
	Ø Open
	3 Percutaneous
	4 Percutaneous Endoscopic
		4 Internal Fixation Device
		5 External Fixation Device
		Z No Device
			Z No Qualifier

2 Pelvic Bone, Right
  Iliac crest
  Ilium
  Ischium
  Pubis
3 Pelvic Bone, Left
  See 2 Pelvic Bone, Right
D Patella, Right
F Patella, Left
L Tarsal, Right
  Calcaneus
  Cuboid bone
  Intermediate cuneiform bone
  Lateral cuneiform bone
  Medial cuneiform bone
  Navicular bone
  Talus bone
M Tarsal, Left
  See L Tarsal, Right
Q Toe Phalanx, Right
R Toe Phalanx, Left
	X External	**Z** No Device	**Z** No Qualifier

ØQS Continued on next page

Non-OR   ØQS[4,5][3,4]ZZ
Non-OR   ØQS[Ø,1,4,5,S]XZZ
Non-OR   ØQS[2,3,D,F,L,M,Q,R][3,4]ZZ
Non-OR   ØQS[2,3,D,F,L,M,Q,R]XZZ

See Appendix L for Procedure Combinations
⊞   ØQS[Ø,1,S]3ZZ

Ø Medical and Surgical
Q Lower Bones
S Reposition

ØQS Continued

Definition: Moving to its normal location, or other suitable location, all or a portion of a body part

Explanation: The body part is moved to a new location from an abnormal location, or from a normal location where it is not functioning correctly. The body part may or may not be cut out or off to be moved to the new location.

Body Part Character 4	Approach Character 5	Device Character 6	Qualifier Character 7
6 Upper Femur, Right Femoral head Greater trochanter Lesser trochanter Neck of femur **7 Upper Femur, Left** *See 6 Upper Femur, Right* **8 Femoral Shaft, Right** Body of femur **9 Femoral Shaft, Left** *See 8 Femoral Shaft, Right* **B Lower Femur, Right** Lateral condyle of femur Lateral epicondyle of femur Medial condyle of femur Medial epicondyle of femur **C Lower Femur, Left** *See B Lower Femur, Right* **G Tibia, Right** Lateral condyle of tibia Medial condyle of tibia Medial malleolus **H Tibia, Left** *See G Tibia, Right* **J Fibula, Right** Body of fibula Head of fibula Lateral malleolus **K Fibula, Left** *See J Fibula, Right*	**Ø Open** **3 Percutaneous** **4 Percutaneous Endoscopic**	**4 Internal Fixation Device** **5 External Fixation Device** **6 Internal Fixation Device, Intramedullary** **B External Fixation Device, Monoplanar** **C External Fixation Device, Ring** **D External Fixation Device, Hybrid** **Z No Device**	**Z No Qualifier**
6 Upper Femur, Right Femoral head Greater trochanter Lesser trochanter Neck of femur **7 Upper Femur, Left** *See 6 Upper Femur, Right* **8 Femoral Shaft, Right** Body of femur **9 Femoral Shaft, Left** *See 8 Femoral Shaft, Right* **B Lower Femur, Right** Lateral condyle of femur Lateral epicondyle of femur Medial condyle of femur Medial epicondyle of femur **C Lower Femur, Left** *See B Lower Femur, Right* **G Tibia, Right** Lateral condyle of tibia Medial condyle of tibia Medial malleolus **H Tibia, Left** *See G Tibia, Right* **J Fibula, Right** Body of fibula Head of fibula Lateral malleolus **K Fibula, Left** *See J Fibula, Right*	**X External**	**Z No Device**	**Z No Qualifier**
N Metatarsal, Right **P Metatarsal, Left**	**Ø Open** **3 Percutaneous** **4 Percutaneous Endoscopic**	**4 Internal Fixation Device** **5 External Fixation Device** **Z No Device**	**2 Sesamoid Bone(s) 1st Toe** **Z No Qualifier**
N Metatarsal, Right **P Metatarsal, Left**	**X External**	**Z No Device**	**2 Sesamoid Bone(s) 1st Toe** **Z No Qualifier**

Non-OR ØQS[6,7,8,9,B,C,G,H,J,K][3,4]ZZ
Non-OR ØQS[6,7,8,9,B,C,G,H,J,K]XZZ
Non-OR ØQS[N,P][3,4]Z[2,Z]
Non-OR ØQS[N,P]XZ[2,Z]

ØQS Continued

LC Limited Coverage   NC Noncovered   ⊞ Combination Member   HAC associated procedure   Combination Only   DRG Non-OR   Non-OR   New/Revised in GREEN

Ø   Medical and Surgical
Q   Lower Bones
T   Resection   Definition: Cutting out or off, without replacement, all of a body part
                      Explanation: None

Body Part Character 4		Approach Character 5	Device Character 6	Qualifier Character 7

2 Pelvic Bone, Right
Iliac crest
Ilium
Ischium
Pubis
	F Patella, Left
	G Tibia, Right
	    Lateral condyle of tibia
	    Medial condyle of tibia
	    Medial malleolus
		Ø Open	**Z No Device**	**Z No Qualifier**

3 Pelvic Bone, Left *See 2 Pelvic Bone, Right*	**H Tibia, Left** *See G Tibia, Right*			
4 Acetabulum, Right	**J Fibula, Right** Body of fibula			
5 Acetabulum, Left	Head of fibula			

6 Upper Femur, Right
Femoral head
Greater trochanter
Lesser trochanter
Neck of femur
	Lateral malleolus
	K Fibula, Left
	    See J Fibula, Right
	L Tarsal, Right
	    Calcaneus			

7 Upper Femur, Left *See 6 Upper Femur, Right*	Cuboid bone Intermediate cuneiform bone			
8 Femoral Shaft, Right Body of femur	Lateral cuneiform bone Medial cuneiform bone			
9 Femoral Shaft, Left *See 8 Femoral Shaft, Right*	Navicular bone Talus bone			
B Lower Femur, Right Lateral condyle of femur Lateral epicondyle of femur Medial condyle of femur Medial epicondyle of femur	**M Tarsal, Left** *See L Tarsal, Right* **N Metatarsal, Right** **P Metatarsal, Left**			
C Lower Femur, Left *See B Lower Femur, Right*	**Q Toe Phalanx, Right** **R Toe Phalanx, Left**			
D Patella, Right	**S Coccyx**			

Ø   Medical and Surgical
Q   Lower Bones
U   Supplement   Definition: Putting in or on biological or synthetic material that physically reinforces and/or augments the function of a portion of a body part
                       Explanation: The biological material is non-living, or is living and from the same individual. The body part may have been previously replaced, and the SUPPLEMENT procedure is performed to physically reinforce and/or augment the function of the replaced body part.

Body Part Character 4		Approach Character 5	Device Character 6	Qualifier Character 7

Ø Lumbar Vertebra ⊞
Spinous process
Transverse process
Vertebral arch
Vertebral body
Vertebral foramen
Vertebral lamina
Vertebral pedicle
	C Lower Femur, Left
	    See B Lower Femur, Right
	D Patella, Right
	F Patella, Left
	G Tibia, Right
	    Lateral condyle of tibia
	    Medial condyle of tibia
	    Medial malleolus
		Ø Open
		3 Percutaneous
		4 Percutaneous Endoscopic
			**7 Autologous Tissue
			    Substitute**
			J Synthetic Substitute
			**K Nonautologous Tissue
			    Substitute**
				Z No Qualifier

1 Sacrum ⊞	**H Tibia, Left** *See G Tibia, Right*			

2 Pelvic Bone, Right
Iliac crest
Ilium
Ischium
Pubis
	J Fibula, Right
	    Body of fibula
	    Head of fibula
	    Lateral malleolus			

3 Pelvic Bone, Left *See 2 Pelvic Bone, Right*	**K Fibula, Left** *See J Fibula, Right*			
4 Acetabulum, Right	**L Tarsal, Right**			
5 Acetabulum, Left	Calcaneus			
6 Upper Femur, Right Femoral head Greater trochanter Lesser trochanter Neck of femur	Cuboid bone Intermediate cuneiform bone Lateral cuneiform bone Medial cuneiform bone			
7 Upper Femur, Left *See 6 Upper Femur, Right*	Navicular bone Talus bone			
8 Femoral Shaft, Right Body of femur	**M Tarsal, Left** *See L Tarsal, Right*			
9 Femoral Shaft, Left *See 8 Femoral Shaft, Right*	**N Metatarsal, Right** **P Metatarsal, Left**			
B Lower Femur, Right Lateral condyle of femur Lateral epicondyle of femur Medial condyle of femur Medial epicondyle of femur	**Q Toe Phalanx, Right** **R Toe Phalanx, Left** **S Coccyx** ⊞			

See Appendix L for Procedure Combinations
⊞   ØQU[Ø,1,S]3JZ

LC Limited Coverage   **NC** Noncovered   ⊞ Combination Member   HAC associated procedure   Combination Only   DRG Non-OR   Non-OR   New/Revised in GREEN
564   ICD-10-PCS 2020

ØQT–ØQU

Ø   Medical and Surgical
Q   Lower Bones
W   Revision   Definition: Correcting, to the extent possible, a portion of a malfunctioning device or the position of a displaced device

            Explanation: Revision can include correcting a malfunctioning or displaced device by taking out or putting in components of the device such as a screw or pin

Body Part Character 4	Approach Character 5	Device Character 6	Qualifier Character 7

Ø   Lumbar Vertebra
   Spinous process
   Transverse process
   Vertebral arch
   Vertebral body
   Vertebral foramen
   Vertebral lamina
   Vertebral pedicle
1   Sacrum
4   Acetabulum, Right
5   Acetabulum, Left
S   Coccyx
	Ø Open
	3 Percutaneous
	4 Percutaneous Endoscopic
	X External
		4 Internal Fixation Device
		**7 Autologous Tissue
		     Substitute**
		J Synthetic Substitute
		**K Nonautologous Tissue
		     Substitute**
			Z No Qualifier

2   Pelvic Bone, Right
   Iliac crest
   Ilium
   Ischium
   Pubis
3   Pelvic Bone, Left
   See 2 Pelvic Bone, Right
6   Upper Femur, Right
   Femoral head
   Greater trochanter
   Lesser trochanter
   Neck of femur
7   Upper Femur, Left
   See 6 Upper Femur, Right
8   Femoral Shaft, Right
   Body of femur
9   Femoral Shaft, Left
   See 8 Femoral Shaft, Right
B   Lower Femur, Right
   Lateral condyle of femur
   Lateral epicondyle of femur
   Medial condyle of femur
   Medial epicondyle of femur
C   Lower Femur, Left
   See B Lower Femur, Right
D   Patella, Right
F   Patella, Left
G   Tibia, Right
   Lateral condyle of tibia
   Medial condyle of tibia
   Medial malleolus
H   Tibia, Left
   See G Tibia, Right
J   Fibula, Right
   Body of fibula
   Head of fibula
   Lateral malleolus
K   Fibula, Left
   See J Fibula, Right
L   Tarsal, Right
   Calcaneus
   Cuboid bone
   Intermediate cuneiform bone
   Lateral cuneiform bone
   Medial cuneiform bone
   Navicular bone
   Talus bone
M   Tarsal, Left
   See L Tarsal, Right
N   Metatarsal, Right
P   Metatarsal, Left
Q   Toe Phalanx, Right
R   Toe Phalanx, Left
	Ø Open
	3 Percutaneous
	4 Percutaneous Endoscopic
	X External
		4 Internal Fixation Device
		5 External Fixation Device
		**7 Autologous Tissue
		     Substitute**
		J Synthetic Substitute
		**K Nonautologous Tissue
		     Substitute**
			Z No Qualifier

Y Lower Bone	**Ø Open** **3 Percutaneous** **4 Percutaneous Endoscopic** **X External**	**Ø Drainage Device** **M Bone Growth Stimulator**	**Z No Qualifier**

Non-OR   ØQW[Ø,1,4,5,S]X[4,7,J,K]Z
Non-OR   ØQW[2,3,6,7,8,9,B,C,D,F,G,H,J,K,L,M,N,P,Q,R]X[4,5,7,J,K]Z
Non-OR   ØQWYX[Ø,M]Z

LC Limited Coverage   NC Noncovered   ⊞ Combination Member   HAC associated procedure   Combination Only   DRG Non-OR   Non-OR   New/Revised in GREEN

ICD-10-PCS 2020   565

0QW–0QW

Upper Joints ØR2–ØRW

Character Meanings*

This Character Meaning table is provided as a guide to assist the user in the identification of character members that may be found in this section of code tables. It **SHOULD NOT** be used to build a PCS code.

Operation–Character 3	Body Part–Character 4	Approach–Character 5	Device–Character 6	Qualifier–Character 7
2 Change	Ø Occipital-cervical Joint	Ø Open	Ø Drainage Device OR Synthetic Substitute, Reverse Ball and Socket	Ø Anterior Approach, Anterior Column
5 Destruction	1 Cervical Vertebral Joint	3 Percutaneous	3 Infusion Device	1 Posterior Approach, Posterior Column
9 Drainage	2 Cervical Vertebral Joint, 2 or more	4 Percutaneous Endoscopic	4 Internal Fixation Device	6 Humeral Surface
B Excision	3 Cervical Vertebral Disc	X External	5 External Fixation Device	7 Glenoid Surface
C Extirpation	4 Cervicothoracic Vertebral Joint		7 Autologous Tissue Substitute	J Posterior Approach, Anterior Column
G Fusion	5 Cervicothoracic Vertebral Disc		8 Spacer	X Diagnostic
H Insertion	6 Thoracic Vertebral Joint		A Interbody Fusion Device	Z No Qualifier
J Inspection	7 Thoracic Vertebral Joint, 2 to 7		B Spinal Stabilization Device, Interspinous Process	
N Release	8 Thoracic Vertebral Joint, 8 or more		C Spinal Stabilization Device, Pedicle-Based	
P Removal	9 Thoracic Vertebral Disc		D Spinal Stabilization Device, Facet Replacement	
Q Repair	A Thoracolumbar Vertebral Joint		J Synthetic Substitute	
R Replacement	B Thoracolumbar Vertebral Disc		K Nonautologous Tissue Substitute	
S Reposition	C Temporomandibular Joint, Right		Y Other Device	
T Resection	D Temporomandibular Joint, Left		Z No Device	
U Supplement	E Sternoclavicular Joint, Right			
W Revision	F Sternoclavicular Joint, Left			
	G Acromioclavicular Joint, Right			
	H Acromioclavicular Joint, Left			
	J Shoulder Joint, Right			
	K Shoulder Joint, Left			
	L Elbow Joint, Right			
	M Elbow Joint, Left			
	N Wrist Joint, Right			
	P Wrist Joint, Left			
	Q Carpal Joint, Right			
	R Carpal Joint, Left			
	S Carpometacarpal Joint, Right			
	T Carpometacarpal Joint, Left			
	U Metacarpophalangeal Joint, Right			
	V Metacarpophalangeal Joint, Left			
	W Finger Phalangeal Joint, Right			
	X Finger Phalangeal Joint, Left			
	Y Upper Joint			

* Includes synovial membrane.

AHA Coding Clinic for table ØRG

2019, 1Q, 30	Spinal fusion performed at same level as decompressive laminectomy
2018, 4Q, 43	Joint fusion device value
2018, 1Q, 22	Spinal fusion procedures without bone graft
2017, 4Q, 62	Added and revised device values - Nerve substitutes
2017, 4Q, 76	Radiolucent porous interbody fusion device
2017, 2Q, 23	Decompression of spinal cord and placement of instrumentation
2014, 3Q, 30	Spinal fusion and fixation instrumentation
2014, 2Q, 7	Anterior cervical thoracic fusion with total discectomy
2013, 1Q, 21-23	Spinal fusion of thoracic and lumbar vertebrae
2013, 1Q, 29	Cervical and thoracic spinal fusion

AHA Coding Clinic for table ØRH

2018, 3Q, 26	Anterior vertebral tethering using Dynesys Tethering System
2017, 2Q, 23	Decompression of spinal cord and placement of instrumentation
2016, 3Q, 32	Rotator cuff repair, tenodesis, decompression, acromioplasty and coracoplasty

AHA Coding Clinic for table ØRN

2019, 1Q, 30	Spinal fusion performed at same level as decompressive laminectomy
2016, 3Q, 32	Rotator cuff repair, tenodesis, decompression, acromioplasty and coracoplasty
2015, 2Q, 22	Arthroscopic subacromial decompression
2015, 2Q, 23	Arthroscopic release of shoulder joint

AHA Coding Clinic for table ØRP

2017, 4Q, 107	Total ankle replacement versus revision

AHA Coding Clinic for table ØRQ

2016, 1Q, 30	Thermal capsulorrhapy of shoulder

AHA Coding Clinic for table ØRR

2018, 4Q, 92	Radial head arthroplasty
2017, 4Q, 107	Total ankle replacement versus revision
2015, 3Q, 14	Endoprosthetic replacement of humerus and tendon reattachment
2015, 1Q, 27	Reverse total shoulder arthroplasty

AHA Coding Clinic for table ØRS

2018, 3Q, 26	Anterior vertebral tethering using Dynesys Tethering System
2015, 2Q, 35	Application of tongs to reduce and stabilize cervical fracture
2014, 4Q, 32	Open reduction internal fixation of fracture with debridement
2014, 3Q, 33	Radial fracture treatment with open reduction internal fixation, and release of carpal ligament
2013, 2Q, 39	Application of cervical tongs for reduction of cervical fracture

AHA Coding Clinic for table ØRT

2014, 2Q, 7	Anterior cervical thoracic fusion with total discectomy

AHA Coding Clinic for table ØRU

2015, 3Q, 26	Thumb arthroplasty with resection of trapezium

AHA Coding Clinic for table ØRW

2017, 4Q, 107	Total ankle replacement versus revision

Upper Joints

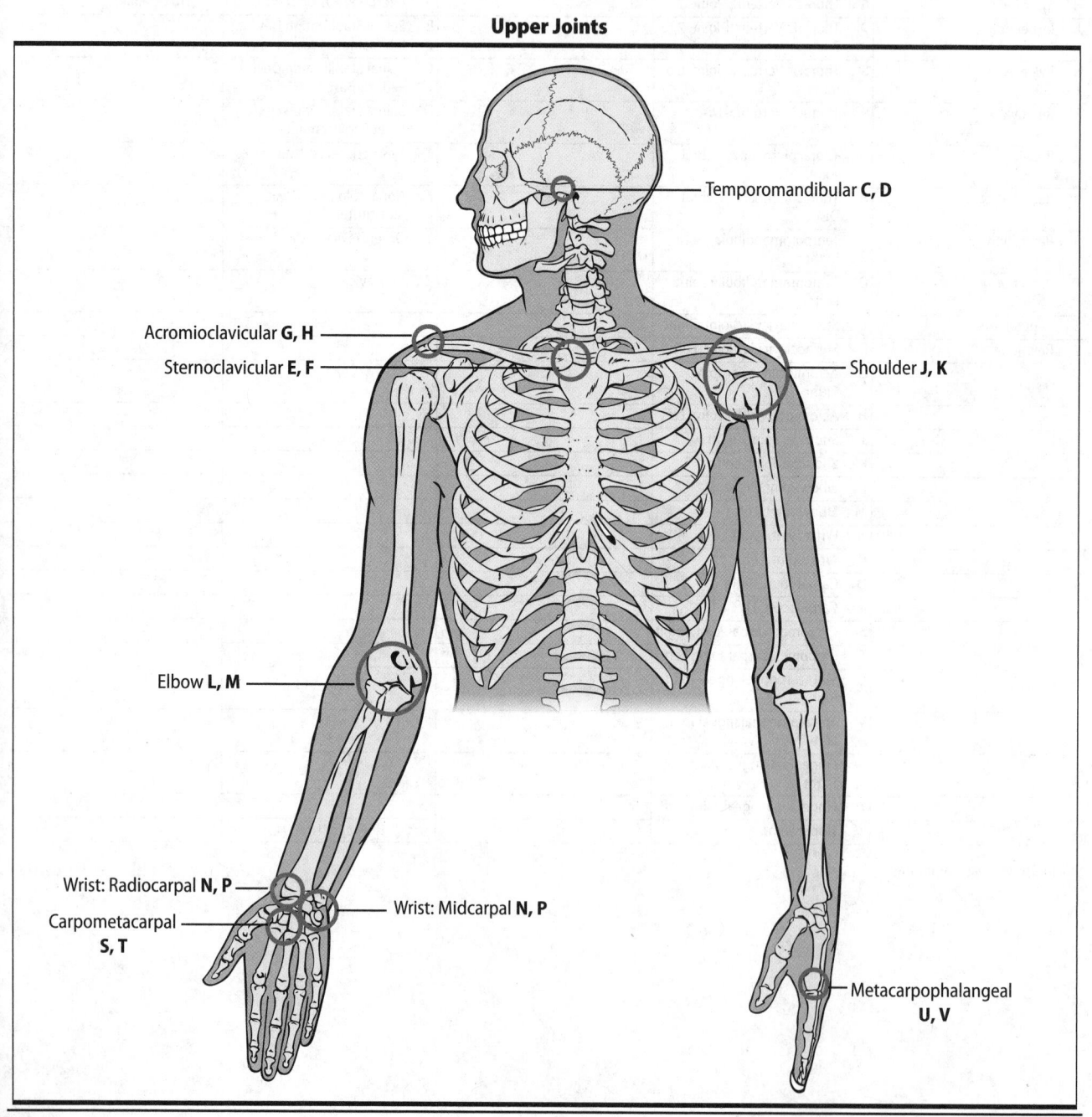

Temporomandibular **C, D**

Acromioclavicular **G, H**

Sternoclavicular **E, F**

Shoulder **J, K**

Elbow **L, M**

Wrist: Radiocarpal **N, P**

Wrist: Midcarpal **N, P**

Carpometacarpal **S, T**

Metacarpophalangeal **U, V**

Hand Joints

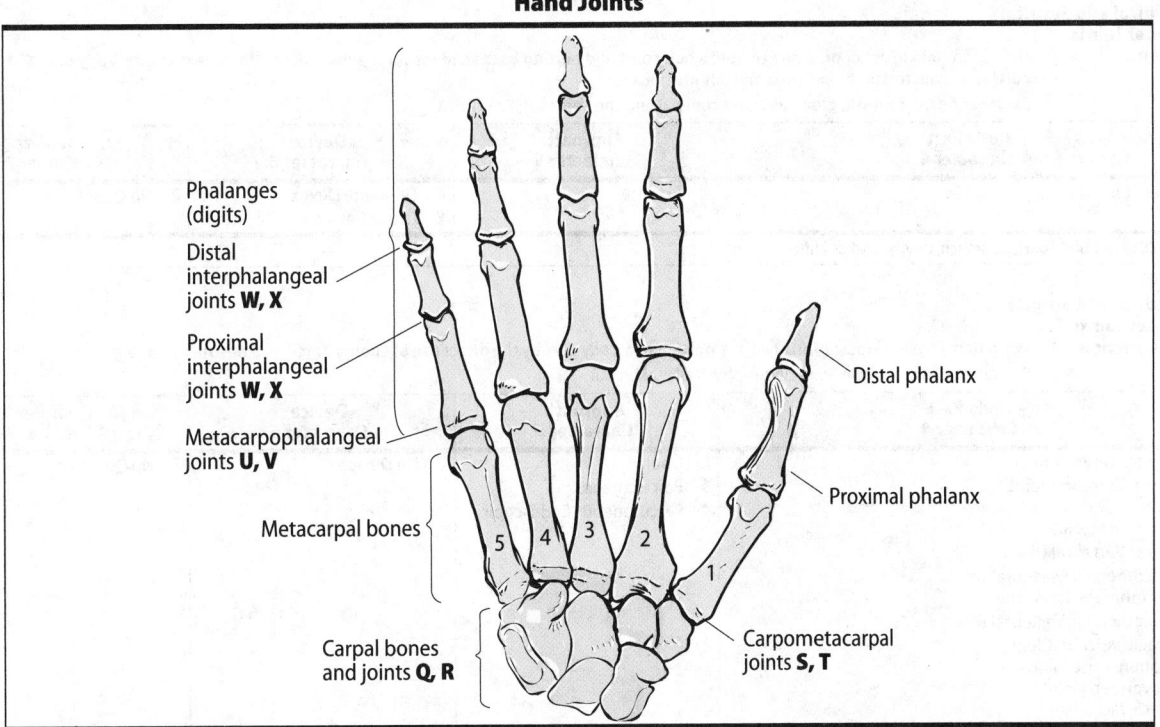

Phalanges (digits)

Distal interphalangeal joints **W, X**

Proximal interphalangeal joints **W, X**

Metacarpophalangeal joints **U, V**

Metacarpal bones

Carpal bones and joints **Q, R**

Distal phalanx

Proximal phalanx

Carpometacarpal joints **S, T**

Shoulder Joints

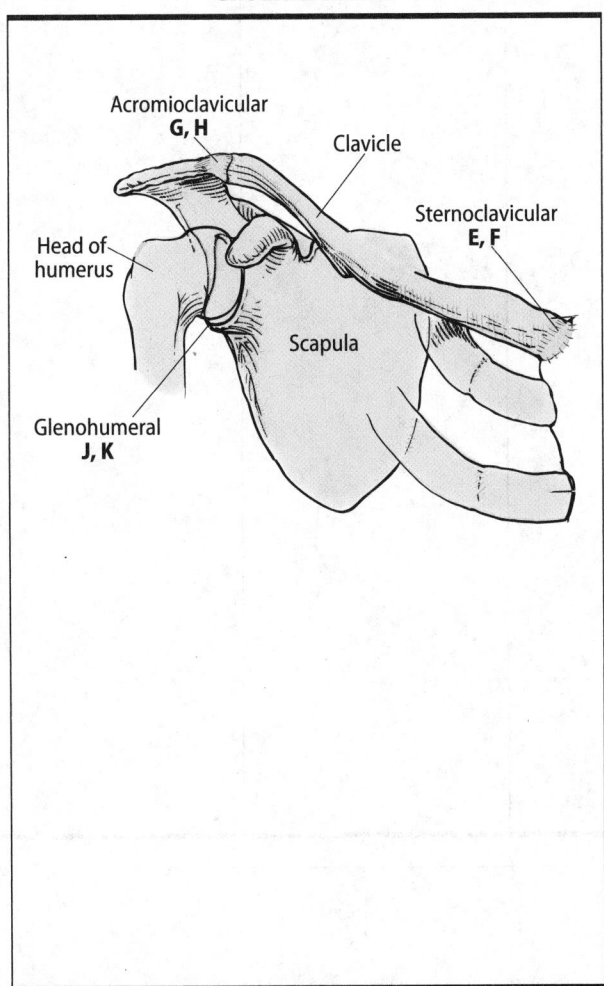

Acromioclavicular **G, H**

Clavicle

Head of humerus

Sternoclavicular **E, F**

Scapula

Glenohumeral **J, K**

Upper Vertebral Joints

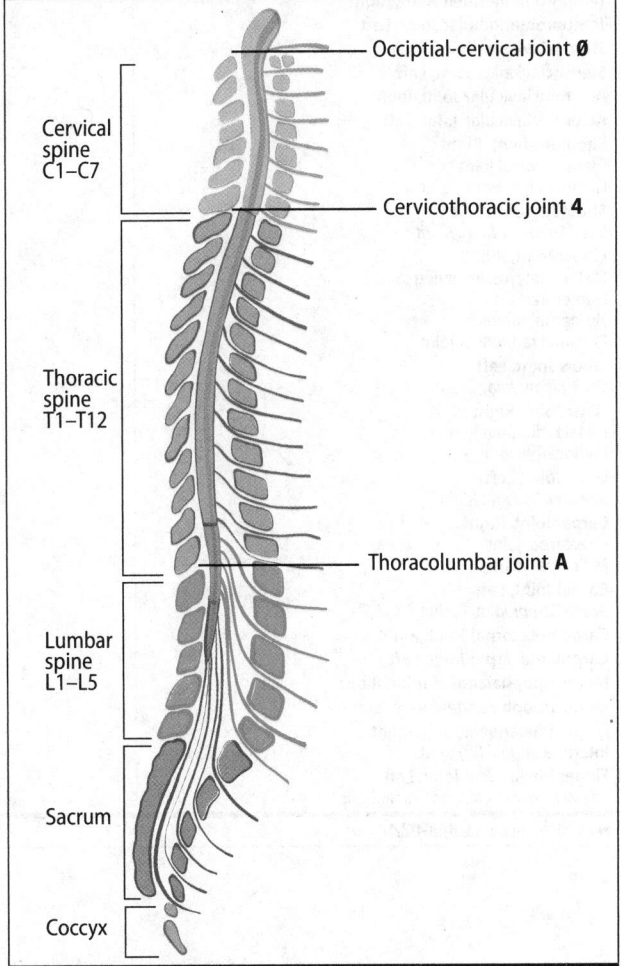

Occiptial-cervical joint **Ø**

Cervical spine C1–C7

Cervicothoracic joint **4**

Thoracic spine T1–T12

Thoracolumbar joint **A**

Lumbar spine L1–L5

Sacrum

Coccyx

Ø Medical and Surgical
R Upper Joints
2 Change   Definition: Taking out or off a device from a body part and putting back an identical or similar device in or on the same body part without cutting or puncturing the skin or a mucous membrane

Explanation: All CHANGE procedures are coded using the approach EXTERNAL

Body Part Character 4	Approach Character 5	Device Character 6	Qualifier Character 7
Y Upper Joint	X External	Ø Drainage Device Y Other Device	Z No Qualifier

Non-OR   All body part, approach, device, and qualifier values

Ø Medical and Surgical
R Upper Joints
5 Destruction   Definition: Physical eradication of all or a portion of a body part by the direct use of energy, force, or a destructive agent

Explanation: None of the body part is physically taken out

Body Part Character 4	Approach Character 5	Device Character 6	Qualifier Character 7

Ø Occipital-cervical Joint
1 Cervical Vertebral Joint
   Atlantoaxial joint
   Cervical facet joint
3 Cervical Vertebral Disc
4 Cervicothoracic Vertebral Joint
   Cervicothoracic facet joint
5 Cervicothoracic Vertebral Disc
6 Thoracic Vertebral Joint
   Costotransverse joint
   Costovertebral joint
   Thoracic facet joint
9 Thoracic Vertebral Disc
A Thoracolumbar Vertebral Joint
   Thoracolumbar facet joint
B Thoracolumbar Vertebral Disc
C Temporomandibular Joint, Right
D Temporomandibular Joint, Left
E Sternoclavicular Joint, Right
F Sternoclavicular Joint, Left
G Acromioclavicular Joint, Right
H Acromioclavicular Joint, Left
J Shoulder Joint, Right
   Glenohumeral joint
   Glenoid ligament (labrum)
K Shoulder Joint, Left
   See J Shoulder Joint, Right
L Elbow Joint, Right
   Distal humerus, involving joint
   Humeroradial joint
   Humeroulnar joint
   Proximal radioulnar joint
M Elbow Joint, Left
   See L Elbow Joint, Right
N Wrist Joint, Right
   Distal radioulnar joint
   Radiocarpal joint
P Wrist Joint, Left
   See N Wrist Joint, Right
Q Carpal Joint, Right
   Intercarpal joint
   Midcarpal joint
R Carpal Joint, Left
   See Q Carpal Joint, Right
S Carpometacarpal Joint, Right
T Carpometacarpal Joint, Left
U Metacarpophalangeal Joint, Right
V Metacarpophalangeal Joint, Left
W Finger Phalangeal Joint, Right
   Interphalangeal (IP) joint
X Finger Phalangeal Joint, Left
   See W Finger Phalangeal Joint, Right
	Ø Open
	3 Percutaneous
	4 Percutaneous Endoscopic
		Z No Device	Z No Qualifier

Non-OR   ØR5[3,5,9,B][3,4]ZZ

LC Limited Coverage   NC Noncovered   ⊞ Combination Member   HAC associated procedure   Combination Only   DRG Non-OR   Non-OR   New/Revised in GREEN

Ø   **Medical and Surgical**
R   **Upper Joints**
9   **Drainage**   Definition: Taking or letting out fluids and/or gases from a body part
                   Explanation: The qualifier DIAGNOSTIC is used to identify drainage procedures that are biopsies

Body Part Character 4		Approach Character 5	Device Character 6	Qualifier Character 7

Ø Occipital-cervical Joint
1 Cervical Vertebral Joint
  Atlantoaxial joint
  Cervical facet joint
3 Cervical Vertebral Disc
4 Cervicothoracic Vertebral Joint
  Cervicothoracic facet joint
5 Cervicothoracic Vertebral Disc
6 Thoracic Vertebral Joint
  Costotransverse joint
  Costovertebral joint
  Thoracic facet joint
9 Thoracic Vertebral Disc
A Thoracolumbar Vertebral Joint
  Thoracolumbar facet joint
B Thoracolumbar Vertebral Disc
C Temporomandibular Joint, Right
D Temporomandibular Joint, Left
E Sternoclavicular Joint, Right
F Sternoclavicular Joint, Left
G Acromioclavicular Joint, Right
H Acromioclavicular Joint, Left
J Shoulder Joint, Right
  Glenohumeral joint
  Glenoid ligament (labrum)
K Shoulder Joint, Left
  See J Shoulder Joint, Right
	L Elbow Joint, Right
	  Distal humerus, involving joint
	  Humeroradial joint
	  Humeroulnar joint
	  Proximal radioulnar joint
	M Elbow Joint, Left
	  See L Elbow Joint, Right
	N Wrist Joint, Right
	  Distal radioulnar joint
	  Radiocarpal joint
	P Wrist Joint, Left
	  See N Wrist Joint, Right
	Q Carpal Joint, Right
	  Intercarpal joint
	  Midcarpal joint
	R Carpal Joint, Left
	  See Q Carpal Joint, Right
	S Carpometacarpal Joint, Right
	T Carpometacarpal Joint, Left
	U Metacarpophalangeal Joint, Right
	V Metacarpophalangeal Joint, Left
	W Finger Phalangeal Joint, Right
	  Interphalangeal (IP) joint
	X Finger Phalangeal Joint, Left
	  See W Finger Phalangeal Joint, Right
		Ø Open
		3 Percutaneous
		4 Percutaneous Endoscopic
			Ø Drainage Device	**Z No Qualifier**

Ø Occipital-cervical Joint
1 Cervical Vertebral Joint
  Atlantoaxial joint
  Cervical facet joint
3 Cervical Vertebral Disc
4 Cervicothoracic Vertebral Joint
  Cervicothoracic facet joint
5 Cervicothoracic Vertebral Disc
6 Thoracic Vertebral Joint
  Costotransverse joint
  Costovertebral joint
  Thoracic facet joint
9 Thoracic Vertebral Disc
A Thoracolumbar Vertebral Joint
  Thoracolumbar facet joint
B Thoracolumbar Vertebral Disc
C Temporomandibular Joint, Right
D Temporomandibular Joint, Left
E Sternoclavicular Joint, Right
F Sternoclavicular Joint, Left
G Acromioclavicular Joint, Right
H Acromioclavicular Joint, Left
J Shoulder Joint, Right
  Glenohumeral joint
  Glenoid ligament (labrum)
K Shoulder Joint, Left
  See J Shoulder Joint, Right
	L Elbow Joint, Right
	  Distal humerus, involving joint
	  Humeroradial joint
	  Humeroulnar joint
	  Proximal radioulnar joint
	M Elbow Joint, Left
	  See L Elbow Joint, Right
	N Wrist Joint, Right
	  Distal radioulnar joint
	  Radiocarpal joint
	P Wrist Joint, Left
	  See N Wrist Joint, Right
	Q Carpal Joint, Right
	  Intercarpal joint
	  Midcarpal joint
	R Carpal Joint, Left
	  See Q Carpal Joint, Right
	S Carpometacarpal Joint, Right
	T Carpometacarpal Joint, Left
	U Metacarpophalangeal Joint, Right
	V Metacarpophalangeal Joint, Left
	W Finger Phalangeal Joint, Right
	  Interphalangeal (IP) joint
	X Finger Phalangeal Joint, Left
	  See W Finger Phalangeal Joint, Right
		Ø Open
		3 Percutaneous
		4 Percutaneous Endoscopic
			Z No Device	**X Diagnostic**
				Z No Qualifier

Non-OR   ØR9[Ø,1,3,4,5,6,9,A,B,E,F,G,H,J,K,L,M,N,P,Q,R,S,T,U,V,W,X][3,4]ØZ
Non-OR   ØR9[C,D]3ØZ
Non-OR   ØR9[Ø,1,3,4,5,6,9,A,B,E,F,G,H,J,K,L,M,N,P,Q,R,S,T,U,V,W,X][Ø,3,4]ZX
Non-OR   ØR9[Ø,1,3,4,5,6,9,A,B,E,F,G,H,J,K,L,M,N,P,Q,R,S,T,U,V,W,X][3,4]ZZ
Non-OR   ØR9[C,D]3ZZ

LC Limited Coverage   **NC** Noncovered   ⊞ Combination Member   HAC associated procedure   Combination Only   DRG Non-OR   Non-OR   New/Revised in GREEN

ICD-10-PCS 2020   571

ØR9–ØR9

Ø **Medical and Surgical**
R **Upper Joints**
B **Excision**

Definition: Cutting out or off, without replacement, a portion of a body part

Explanation: The qualifier DIAGNOSTIC is used to identify excision procedures that are biopsies

Body Part Character 4	Approach Character 5	Device Character 6	Qualifier Character 7
Ø **Occipital-cervical Joint**	**Ø** **Open**	**Z** **No Device**	**X** **Diagnostic**
1 **Cervical Vertebral Joint**	**3** **Percutaneous**		**Z** **No Qualifier**
Atlantoaxial joint	**4** **Percutaneous Endoscopic**		
Cervical facet joint			
3 **Cervical Vertebral Disc**			
4 **Cervicothoracic Vertebral Joint**			
Cervicothoracic facet joint			
5 **Cervicothoracic Vertebral Disc**			
6 **Thoracic Vertebral Joint**			
Costotransverse joint			
Costovertebral joint			
Thoracic facet joint			
9 **Thoracic Vertebral Disc**			
A **Thoracolumbar Vertebral Joint**			
Thoracolumbar facet joint			
B **Thoracolumbar Vertebral Disc**			
C **Temporomandibular Joint, Right**			
D **Temporomandibular Joint, Left**			
E **Sternoclavicular Joint, Right**			
F **Sternoclavicular Joint, Left**			
G **Acromioclavicular Joint, Right**			
H **Acromioclavicular Joint, Left**			
J **Shoulder Joint, Right**			
Glenohumeral joint			
Glenoid ligament (labrum)			
K **Shoulder Joint, Left**			
See J Shoulder Joint, Right			
L **Elbow Joint, Right**			
Distal humerus, involving joint			
Humeroradial joint			
Humeroulnar joint			
Proximal radioulnar joint			
M **Elbow Joint, Left**			
See L Elbow Joint, Right			
N **Wrist Joint, Right**			
Distal radioulnar joint			
Radiocarpal joint			
P **Wrist Joint, Left**			
See N Wrist Joint, Right			
Q **Carpal Joint, Right**			
Intercarpal joint			
Midcarpal joint			
R **Carpal Joint, Left**			
See Q Carpal Joint, Right			
S **Carpometacarpal Joint, Right**			
T **Carpometacarpal Joint, Left**			
U **Metacarpophalangeal Joint, Right**			
V **Metacarpophalangeal Joint, Left**			
W **Finger Phalangeal Joint, Right**			
Interphalangeal (IP) joint			
X **Finger Phalangeal Joint, Left**			
See W Finger Phalangeal Joint, Right			

Non-OR   ØRB[Ø,1,3,4,5,6,9,A,B,E,F,G,H,J,K,L,M,N,P,Q,R,S,T,U,V,W,X][Ø,3,4]ZX

Upper Joints

Ø   **Medical and Surgical**
R   **Upper Joints**
C   **Extirpation**   Definition: Taking or cutting out solid matter from a body part

Explanation: The solid matter may be an abnormal byproduct of a biological function or a foreign body; it may be imbedded in a body part or in the lumen of a tubular body part. The solid matter may or may not have been previously broken into pieces.

Body Part Character 4	Approach Character 5	Device Character 6	Qualifier Character 7
Ø **Occipital-cervical Joint**	**Ø** **Open**	**Z** **No Device**	**Z** **No Qualifier**

1 **Cervical Vertebral Joint**
    Atlantoaxial joint
    Cervical facet joint
	3 **Percutaneous**
	4 **Percutaneous Endoscopic**		

3 **Cervical Vertebral Disc**			
4 **Cervicothoracic Vertebral Joint** Cervicothoracic facet joint			
5 **Cervicothoracic Vertebral Disc**			

6 **Thoracic Vertebral Joint**
    Costotransverse joint
    Costovertebral joint
    Thoracic facet joint			

9 **Thoracic Vertebral Disc**			
A **Thoracolumbar Vertebral Joint** Thoracolumbar facet joint			
B **Thoracolumbar Vertebral Disc**			
C **Temporomandibular Joint, Right**			
D **Temporomandibular Joint, Left**			
E **Sternoclavicular Joint, Right**			
F **Sternoclavicular Joint, Left**			
G **Acromioclavicular Joint, Right**			
H **Acromioclavicular Joint, Left**			

J **Shoulder Joint, Right**
    Glenohumeral joint
    Glenoid ligament (labrum)			

K **Shoulder Joint, Left** *See J Shoulder Joint, Right*			

L **Elbow Joint, Right**
    Distal humerus, involving joint
    Humeroradial joint
    Humeroulnar joint
    Proximal radioulnar joint			

M **Elbow Joint, Left** *See L Elbow Joint, Right*			

N **Wrist Joint, Right**
    Distal radioulnar joint
    Radiocarpal joint			

P **Wrist Joint, Left** *See N Wrist Joint, Right*			

Q **Carpal Joint, Right**
    Intercarpal joint
    Midcarpal joint			

R **Carpal Joint, Left** *See Q Carpal Joint, Right*			
S **Carpometacarpal Joint, Right**			
T **Carpometacarpal Joint, Left**			
U **Metacarpophalangeal Joint, Right**			
V **Metacarpophalangeal Joint, Left**			
W **Finger Phalangeal Joint, Right** Interphalangeal (IP) joint			
X **Finger Phalangeal Joint, Left** *See W Finger Phalangeal Joint, Right*			

LC Limited Coverage   **NC** Noncovered   ⊞ Combination Member   HAC associated procedure   Combination Only   DRG Non-OR   Non-OR   New/Revised in GREEN

ICD-10-PCS 2020   573

Ø   Medical and Surgical
R   Upper Joints
G   Fusion   Definition: Joining together portions of an articular body part rendering the articular body part immobile
                  Explanation: The body part is joined together by fixation device, bone graft, or other means

Body Part Character 4	Approach Character 5	Device Character 6	Qualifier Character 7
Ø Occipital-cervical Joint **1 Cervical Vertebral Joint** Atlantoaxial joint Cervical facet joint **2 Cervical Vertebral Joints, 2 or more** Cervical facet joint **4 Cervicothoracic Vertebral Joint** Cervicothoracic facet joint **6 Thoracic Vertebral Joint** Costotransverse joint Costovertebral joint Thoracic facet joint **7 Thoracic Vertebral Joints, 2 to 7** ⊞ **8 Thoracic Vertebral Joints, 8 or more** **A Thoracolumbar Vertebral Joint** Thoracolumbar facet joint	**Ø Open** **3 Percutaneous** **4 Percutaneous Endoscopic**	**7 Autologous Tissue Substitute** **J Synthetic Substitute** **K Nonautologous Tissue Substitute**	**Ø Anterior Approach, Anterior Column** **1 Posterior Approach, Posterior Column** **J Posterior Approach, Anterior Column**
Ø Occipital-cervical Joint **1 Cervical Vertebral Joint** Atlantoaxial joint Cervical facet joint **2 Cervical Vertebral Joints, 2 or more** Cervical facet joint **4 Cervicothoracic Vertebral Joint** Cervicothoracic facet joint **6 Thoracic Vertebral Joint** Costotransverse joint Costovertebral joint Thoracic facet joint **7 Thoracic Vertebral Joints, 2 to 7** ⊞ **8 Thoracic Vertebral Joints, 8 or more** **A Thoracolumbar Vertebral Joint** Thoracolumbar facet joint	**Ø Open** **3 Percutaneous** **4 Percutaneous Endoscopic**	**A Interbody Fusion Device**	**Ø Anterior Approach, Anterior Column** **J Posterior Approach, Anterior Column**
C Temporomandibular Joint, Right **D Temporomandibular Joint, Left** **E Sternoclavicular Joint, Right** **F Sternoclavicular Joint, Left** **G Acromioclavicular Joint, Right** **H Acromioclavicular Joint, Left** **J Shoulder Joint, Right** Glenohumeral joint Glenoid ligament (labrum) **K Shoulder Joint, Left** *See J Shoulder Joint, Right*	**Ø Open** **3 Percutaneous** **4 Percutaneous Endoscopic**	**4 Internal Fixation Device** **7 Autologous Tissue Substitute** **J Synthetic Substitute** **K Nonautologous Tissue Substitute**	**Z No Qualifier**
L Elbow Joint, Right Distal humerus, involving joint Humeroradial joint Humeroulnar joint Proximal radioulnar joint **M Elbow Joint, Left** *See L Elbow Joint, Right* **N Wrist Joint, Right** Distal radioulnar joint Radiocarpal joint **P Wrist Joint, Left** *See N Wrist Joint, Right* **Q Carpal Joint, Right** Intercarpal joint Midcarpal joint **R Carpal Joint, Left** *See Q Carpal Joint, Right* **S Carpometacarpal Joint, Right** **T Carpometacarpal Joint, Left** **U Metacarpophalangeal Joint, Right** **V Metacarpophalangeal Joint, Left** **W Finger Phalangeal Joint, Right** Interphalangeal (IP) joint **X Finger Phalangeal Joint, Left** *See W Finger Phalangeal Joint, Right*	**Ø Open** **3 Percutaneous** **4 Percutaneous Endoscopic**	**4 Internal Fixation Device** **5 External Fixation Device** **7 Autologous Tissue Substitute** **J Synthetic Substitute** **K Nonautologous Tissue Substitute**	**Z No Qualifier**

HAC ØRG[Ø,1,2,4,6,7,8,A][Ø][Ø,3,4][7,J,K][Ø,1,J] when reported with SDx K68.11 or T81.4Ø–T81.49, T84.6Ø-T84.619, T84.63–T84.7 with 7th character A	
HAC ØRG[Ø,1,2,4,6,7,8,A][Ø][Ø,3,4]A[Ø,J] when reported with SDx K68.11 or T81.4Ø–T81.49, T84.6Ø-T84.619, T84.63–T84.7 with 7th character A	
HAC ØRG[E,F,G,H,J,K][Ø,3,4][4,7,J,K]Z when reported with SDx K68.11 or T81.4Ø–T81.49, T84.6Ø-T84.619, T84.63–T84.7 with 7th character A	
HAC ØRG[L,M][Ø,3,4][4,5,7,J,K]Z when reported with SDx K68.11 or T81.4Ø–T81.49, T84.6Ø-T84.619, T84.63–T84.7 with 7th character A	

See Appendix L for Procedure Combinations
⊞   ØRG7[Ø,3,4][7,J,K][Ø,1,J]
⊞   ØRG7[Ø,3,4]A[Ø,J]

LC Limited Coverage   **NC** Noncovered   ⊞ Combination Member   HAC associated procedure   Combination Only   DRG Non-OR   Non-OR   New/Revised in GREEN

574   ICD-10-PCS 2020

Ø   Medical and Surgical
R   Upper Joints
H   Insertion   Definition: Putting in a nonbiological appliance that monitors, assists, performs, or prevents a physiological function but does not physically
                                take the place of a body part
                                Explanation: None

Body Part Character 4	Approach Character 5	Device Character 6	Qualifier Character 7
Ø Occipital-cervical Joint	**Ø Open**	**3 Infusion Device**	**Z No Qualifier**
1 Cervical Vertebral Joint	**3 Percutaneous**	**4 Internal Fixation Device**	
Atlantoaxial joint	**4 Percutaneous Endoscopic**	**8 Spacer**	
Cervical facet joint		**B Spinal Stabilization Device,**	
4 Cervicothoracic Vertebral Joint		**Interspinous Process**	
Cervicothoracic facet joint		**C Spinal Stabilization Device,**	
6 Thoracic Vertebral Joint		**Pedicle-Based**	
Costotransverse joint		**D Spinal Stabilization Device,**	
Costovertebral joint		**Facet Replacement**	
Thoracic facet joint			
A Thoracolumbar Vertebral Joint			
Thoracolumbar facet joint			
3 Cervical Vertebral Disc	**Ø Open**	**3 Infusion Device**	**Z No Qualifier**
5 Cervicothoracic Vertebral Disc	**3 Percutaneous**		
9 Thoracic Vertebral Disc	**4 Percutaneous Endoscopic**		
B Thoracolumbar Vertebral Disc			
C Temporomandibular Joint, Right	**Ø Open**	**3 Infusion Device**	**Z No Qualifier**
D Temporomandibular Joint, Left	**3 Percutaneous**	**4 Internal Fixation Device**	
E Sternoclavicular Joint, Right	**4 Percutaneous Endoscopic**	**8 Spacer**	
F Sternoclavicular Joint, Left			
G Acromioclavicular Joint, Right			
H Acromioclavicular Joint, Left			
J Shoulder Joint, Right			
Glenohumeral joint			
Glenoid ligament (labrum)			
K Shoulder Joint, Left			
See J Shoulder Joint, Right			
L Elbow Joint, Right	**Ø Open**	**3 Infusion Device**	**Z No Qualifier**
Distal humerus, involving joint	**3 Percutaneous**	**4 Internal Fixation Device**	
Humeroradial joint	**4 Percutaneous Endoscopic**	**5 External Fixation Device**	
Humeroulnar joint		**8 Spacer**	
Proximal radioulnar joint			
M Elbow Joint, Left			
See L Elbow Joint, Right			
N Wrist Joint, Right			
Distal radioulnar joint			
Radiocarpal joint			
P Wrist Joint, Left			
See N Wrist Joint, Right			
Q Carpal Joint, Right			
Intercarpal joint			
Midcarpal joint			
R Carpal Joint, Left			
See Q Carpal Joint, Right			
S Carpometacarpal Joint, Right			
T Carpometacarpal Joint, Left			
U Metacarpophalangeal Joint, Right			
V Metacarpophalangeal Joint, Left			
W Finger Phalangeal Joint, Right			
Interphalangeal (IP) joint			
X Finger Phalangeal Joint, Left			
See W Finger Phalangeal Joint, Right			

Non-OR	ØRH[Ø,1,4,6,A][Ø,3,4][3,8]Z
Non-OR	ØRH[3,5,9,B][Ø,3,4]3Z
Non-OR	ØRH[C,D][Ø,4]8Z
Non-OR	ØRH[C,D]3[3,8]Z
Non-OR	ØRH[E,F,G,H,J,K][Ø,3,4][3,8]Z
Non-OR	ØRH[L,M,N,P,Q,R,S,T,U,V,W,X][Ø,3,4][3,8]Z

Ø   **Medical and Surgical**
R   **Upper Joints**
J   **Inspection**   Definition: Visually and/or manually exploring a body part

Explanation: Visual exploration may be performed with or without optical instrumentation. Manual exploration may be performed directly or through intervening body layers.

Body Part Character 4	Approach Character 5	Device Character 6	Qualifier Character 7

Ø Occipital-cervical Joint
1 Cervical Vertebral Joint
   Atlantoaxial joint
   Cervical facet joint
3 Cervical Vertebral Disc
4 Cervicothoracic Vertebral Joint
   Cervicothoracic facet joint
5 Cervicothoracic Vertebral Disc
6 Thoracic Vertebral Joint
   Costotransverse joint
   Costovertebral joint
   Thoracic facet joint
9 Thoracic Vertebral Disc
A Thoracolumbar Vertebral Joint
   Thoracolumbar facet joint
B Thoracolumbar Vertebral Disc
C Temporomandibular Joint, Right
D Temporomandibular Joint, Left
E Sternoclavicular Joint, Right
F Sternoclavicular Joint, Left
G Acromioclavicular Joint, Right
H Acromioclavicular Joint, Left
J Shoulder Joint, Right
   Glenohumeral joint
   Glenoid ligament (labrum)
K Shoulder Joint, Left
   See J Shoulder Joint, Right
L Elbow Joint, Right
   Distal humerus, involving joint
   Humeroradial joint
   Humeroulnar joint
   Proximal radioulnar joint
M Elbow Joint, Left
   See L Elbow Joint, Right
N Wrist Joint, Right
   Distal radioulnar joint
   Radiocarpal joint
P Wrist Joint, Left
   See N Wrist Joint, Right
Q Carpal Joint, Right
   Intercarpal joint
   Midcarpal joint
R Carpal Joint, Left
   See Q Carpal Joint, Right
S Carpometacarpal Joint, Right
T Carpometacarpal Joint, Left
U Metacarpophalangeal Joint, Right
V Metacarpophalangeal Joint, Left
W Finger Phalangeal Joint, Right
   Interphalangeal (IP) joint
X Finger Phalangeal Joint, Left
   See W Finger Phalangeal Joint, Right
	Ø Open
	3 Percutaneous
	4 Percutaneous Endoscopic
	X External
		Z No Device	**Z** No Qualifier

Non-OR   ØRJ[Ø,1,3,4,5,6,9,A,B,C,D,E,F,G,H,J,K,L,M,N,P,Q,R,S,T,U,V,W,X][3,X]ZZ

LC Limited Coverage   **NC** Noncovered   ⊞ Combination Member   HAC associated procedure   Combination Only   DRG Non-OR   Non-OR   New/Revised in GREEN

576   ICD-10-PCS 2020

ØRJ–ØRJ

Ø   Medical and Surgical
R   Upper Joints
N   Release   Definition: Freeing a body part from an abnormal physical constraint by cutting or by the use of force
                      Explanation: Some of the restraining tissue may be taken out but none of the body part is taken out

Body Part Character 4	Approach Character 5	Device Character 6	Qualifier Character 7
Ø Occipital-cervical Joint	**Ø Open**	**Z No Device**	**Z No Qualifier**
1 Cervical Vertebral Joint	**3 Percutaneous**		
Atlantoaxial joint	**4 Percutaneous Endoscopic**		
Cervical facet joint	**X External**		
3 Cervical Vertebral Disc			
4 Cervicothoracic Vertebral Joint			
Cervicothoracic facet joint			
5 Cervicothoracic Vertebral Disc			
6 Thoracic Vertebral Joint			
Costotransverse joint			
Costovertebral joint			
Thoracic facet joint			
9 Thoracic Vertebral Disc			
A Thoracolumbar Vertebral Joint			
Thoracolumbar facet joint			
B Thoracolumbar Vertebral Disc			
C Temporomandibular Joint, Right			
D Temporomandibular Joint, Left			
E Sternoclavicular Joint, Right			
F Sternoclavicular Joint, Left			
G Acromioclavicular Joint, Right			
H Acromioclavicular Joint, Left			
J Shoulder Joint, Right			
Glenohumeral joint			
Glenoid ligament (labrum)			
K Shoulder Joint, Left			
See J Shoulder Joint, Right			
L Elbow Joint, Right			
Distal humerus, involving joint			
Humeroradial joint			
Humeroulnar joint			
Proximal radioulnar joint			
M Elbow Joint, Left			
See L Elbow Joint, Right			
N Wrist Joint, Right			
Distal radioulnar joint			
Radiocarpal joint			
P Wrist Joint, Left			
See N Wrist Joint, Right			
Q Carpal Joint, Right			
Intercarpal joint			
Midcarpal joint			
R Carpal Joint, Left			
See Q Carpal Joint, Right			
S Carpometacarpal Joint, Right			
T Carpometacarpal Joint, Left			
U Metacarpophalangeal Joint, Right			
V Metacarpophalangeal Joint, Left			
W Finger Phalangeal Joint, Right			
Interphalangeal (IP) joint			
X Finger Phalangeal Joint, Left			
See W Finger Phalangeal Joint, Right			

Non-OR   ØRN[Ø,1,3,4,5,6,9,A,B,C,D,E,F,G,H,J,K,L,M,N,P,Q,R,S,T,U,V,W,X]XZZ

Upper Joints

Ø Medical and Surgical
R Upper Joints
P Removal   Definition: Taking out or off a device from a body part

Explanation: If a device is taken out and a similar device put in without cutting or puncturing the skin or mucous membrane, the procedure is coded to the root operation CHANGE. Otherwise, the procedure for taking out the device is coded to the root operation REMOVAL.

Body Part Character 4	Approach Character 5	Device Character 6	Qualifier Character 7

Ø Occipital-cervical Joint
1 Cervical Vertebral Joint
  Atlantoaxial joint
  Cervical facet joint
4 Cervicothoracic Vertebral Joint
  Cervicothoracic facet joint
6 Thoracic Vertebral Joint
  Costotransverse joint
  Costovertebral joint
  Thoracic facet joint
A Thoracolumbar Vertebral Joint
  Thoracolumbar facet joint
	Ø Open
	3 Percutaneous
	4 Percutaneous Endoscopic
		Ø Drainage Device
		3 Infusion Device
		4 Internal Fixation Device
		7 Autologous Tissue Substitute
		8 Spacer
		A Interbody Fusion Device
		J Synthetic Substitute
		K Nonautologous Tissue Substitute
			Z No Qualifier

Ø Occipital-cervical Joint
1 Cervical Vertebral Joint
  Atlantoaxial joint
  Cervical facet joint
4 Cervicothoracic Vertebral Joint
  Cervicothoracic facet joint
6 Thoracic Vertebral Joint
  Costotransverse joint
  Costovertebral joint
  Thoracic facet joint
A Thoracolumbar Vertebral Joint
  Thoracolumbar facet joint
	X External	**Ø** Drainage Device
		3 Infusion Device
		4 Internal Fixation Device
			Z No Qualifier

3 Cervical Vertebral Disc **5** Cervicothoracic Vertebral Disc **9** Thoracic Vertebral Disc **B** Thoracolumbar Vertebral Disc	**Ø** Open **3** Percutaneous **4** Percutaneous Endoscopic	**Ø** Drainage Device **3** Infusion Device **7** Autologous Tissue Substitute **J** Synthetic Substitute **K** Nonautologous Tissue Substitute	**Z** No Qualifier
3 Cervical Vertebral Disc **5** Cervicothoracic Vertebral Disc **9** Thoracic Vertebral Disc **B** Thoracolumbar Vertebral Disc	**X** External	**Ø** Drainage Device **3** Infusion Device	**Z** No Qualifier

C Temporomandibular Joint, Right
D Temporomandibular Joint, Left
E Sternoclavicular Joint, Right
F Sternoclavicular Joint, Left
G Acromioclavicular Joint, Right
H Acromioclavicular Joint, Left
J Shoulder Joint, Right
  Glenohumeral joint
  Glenoid ligament (labrum)
K Shoulder Joint, Left
  See J Shoulder Joint, Right
	Ø Open
	3 Percutaneous
	4 Percutaneous Endoscopic
		Ø Drainage Device
		3 Infusion Device
		4 Internal Fixation Device
		7 Autologous Tissue Substitute
		8 Spacer
		J Synthetic Substitute
		K Nonautologous Tissue Substitute
			Z No Qualifier

C Temporomandibular Joint, Right
D Temporomandibular Joint, Left
E Sternoclavicular Joint, Right
F Sternoclavicular Joint, Left
G Acromioclavicular Joint, Right
H Acromioclavicular Joint, Left
J Shoulder Joint, Right
  Glenohumeral joint
  Glenoid ligament (labrum)
K Shoulder Joint, Left
  See J Shoulder Joint, Right
	X External	**Ø** Drainage Device
		3 Infusion Device
		4 Internal Fixation Device
			Z No Qualifier

ØRP Continued on next page

Non-OR	ØRP[Ø,1,4,6,A]3[Ø,3,8]Z
Non-OR	ØRP[Ø,1,4,6,A][Ø,4]8Z
Non-OR	ØRP[Ø,1,4,6,A]X[Ø,3,4]Z
Non-OR	ØRP[3,5,9,B]3[Ø,3]Z
Non-OR	ØRP[3,5,9,B]X[Ø,3]Z
Non-OR	ØRP[C,D,E,F,G,H,J,K]3[Ø,3,8]Z
Non-OR	ØRP[C,D,E,F,G,H,J,K][Ø,4]8Z
Non-OR	ØRP[C,D]X[Ø,3]Z
Non-OR	ØRP[E,F,G,H,J,K]X[Ø,3,4]Z

Ø   **Medical and Surgical**   *ØRP Continued*
R   **Upper Joints**
P   **Removal**   Definition: Taking out or off a device from a body part

                       Explanation: If a device is taken out and a similar device put in without cutting or puncturing the skin or mucous membrane, the procedure is coded to the root operation CHANGE. Otherwise, the procedure for taking out the device is coded to the root operation REMOVAL.

Body Part Character 4	Approach Character 5	Device Character 6	Qualifier Character 7

L   **Elbow Joint, Right**
    Distal humerus, involving joint
    Humeroradial joint
    Humeroulnar joint
    Proximal radioulnar joint
M   **Elbow Joint, Left**
    See L Elbow Joint, Right
N   **Wrist Joint, Right**
    Distal radioulnar joint
    Radiocarpal joint
P   **Wrist Joint, Left**
    See N Wrist Joint, Right
Q   **Carpal Joint, Right**
    Intercarpal joint
    Midcarpal joint
R   **Carpal Joint, Left**
    See Q Carpal Joint, Right
S   **Carpometacarpal Joint, Right**
T   **Carpometacarpal Joint, Left**
U   **Metacarpophalangeal Joint, Right**
V   **Metacarpophalangeal Joint, Left**
W   **Finger Phalangeal Joint, Right**
    Interphalangeal (IP) joint
X   **Finger Phalangeal Joint, Left**
    See W Finger Phalangeal Joint, Right
	Ø Open
	3 Percutaneous
	4 Percutaneous Endoscopic
		Ø Drainage Device
		3 Infusion Device
		4 Internal Fixation Device
		5 External Fixation Device
		7 Autologous Tissue
		    Substitute
		8 Spacer
		J Synthetic Substitute
		K Nonautologous Tissue
		    Substitute
			Z No Qualifier

L   **Elbow Joint, Right**
    Distal humerus, involving joint
    Humeroradial joint
    Humeroulnar joint
    Proximal radioulnar joint
M   **Elbow Joint, Left**
    See L Elbow Joint, Right
N   **Wrist Joint, Right**
    Distal radioulnar joint
    Radiocarpal joint
P   **Wrist Joint, Left**
    See N Wrist Joint, Right
Q   **Carpal Joint, Right**
    Intercarpal joint
    Midcarpal joint
R   **Carpal Joint, Left**
    See Q Carpal Joint, Right
S   **Carpometacarpal Joint, Right**
T   **Carpometacarpal Joint, Left**
U   **Metacarpophalangeal Joint, Right**
V   **Metacarpophalangeal Joint, Left**
W   **Finger Phalangeal Joint, Right**
    Interphalangeal (IP) joint
X   **Finger Phalangeal Joint, Left**
    See W Finger Phalangeal Joint, Right
	X External	**Ø** Drainage Device
		3 Infusion Device
		4 Internal Fixation Device
		5 External Fixation Device
			Z No Qualifier

Non-OR   ØRP[L,M,N,P,Q,R,S,T,U,V,W,X]3[Ø,3,8]Z
Non-OR   ØRP[L,M,N,P,Q,R,S,T,U,V,W,X][Ø,4]8Z
Non-OR   ØRP[L,M,N,P,Q,R,S,T,U,V,W,X]X[Ø,3,4,5]Z

LC Limited Coverage   **NC** Noncovered   ⊞ Combination Member   HAC associated procedure   Combination Only   DRG Non-OR   Non-OR   New/Revised in GREEN
ICD-10-PCS 2020   **579**

ØRP–ØRP

Upper Joints

Ø Medical and Surgical
R Upper Joints
Q Repair   Definition: Restoring, to the extent possible, a body part to its normal anatomic structure and function

Explanation: Used only when the method to accomplish the repair is not one of the other root operations

Body Part Character 4	Approach Character 5	Device Character 6	Qualifier Character 7
Ø Occipital-cervical Joint	**Ø Open**	**Z No Device**	**Z No Qualifier**
1 Cervical Vertebral Joint	**3 Percutaneous**		
Atlantoaxial joint	**4 Percutaneous Endoscopic**		
Cervical facet joint	**X External**		
3 Cervical Vertebral Disc			
4 Cervicothoracic Vertebral Joint			
Cervicothoracic facet joint			
5 Cervicothoracic Vertebral Disc			
6 Thoracic Vertebral Joint			
Costotransverse joint			
Costovertebral joint			
Thoracic facet joint			
9 Thoracic Vertebral Disc			
A Thoracolumbar Vertebral Joint			
Thoracolumbar facet joint			
B Thoracolumbar Vertebral Disc			
C Temporomandibular Joint, Right			
D Temporomandibular Joint, Left			
E Sternoclavicular Joint, Right			
F Sternoclavicular Joint, Left			
G Acromioclavicular Joint, Right			
H Acromioclavicular Joint, Left			
J Shoulder Joint, Right			
Glenohumeral joint			
Glenoid ligament (labrum)			
K Shoulder Joint, Left			
See J Shoulder Joint, Right			
L Elbow Joint, Right			
Distal humerus, involving joint			
Humeroradial joint			
Humeroulnar joint			
Proximal radioulnar joint			
M Elbow Joint, Left			
See L Elbow Joint, Right			
N Wrist Joint, Right			
Distal radioulnar joint			
Radiocarpal joint			
P Wrist Joint, Left			
See N Wrist Joint, Right			
Q Carpal Joint, Right			
Intercarpal joint			
Midcarpal joint			
R Carpal Joint, Left			
See Q Carpal Joint, Right			
S Carpometacarpal Joint, Right			
T Carpometacarpal Joint, Left			
U Metacarpophalangeal Joint, Right			
V Metacarpophalangeal Joint, Left			
W Finger Phalangeal Joint, Right			
Interphalangeal (IP) joint			
X Finger Phalangeal Joint, Left			
See W Finger Phalangeal Joint, Right			

Non-OR   ØRQ[Ø,1,3,4,5,6,9,A,B,C,D,E,F,G,H,J,K,L,M,N,P,Q,R,S,T,U,V,W,X]XZZ

HAC   ØRQ[E,F,G,H,J,K,L,M][Ø,3,4,X]ZZ when reported with SDx K68.11 or T81.4Ø–T81.49, T84.6Ø-T84.619, T84.63-T84.7 with 7th character A

LC Limited Coverage   NC Noncovered   ⊞ Combination Member   HAC associated procedure   Combination Only   DRG Non-OR   Non-OR   New/Revised in GREEN

580   ICD-10-PCS 2020

Ø   Medical and Surgical
R   Upper Joints
R   Replacement   Definition: Putting in or on biological or synthetic material that physically takes the place and/or function of all or a portion of a body part

Explanation: The body part may have been taken out or replaced, or may be taken out, physically eradicated, or rendered nonfunctional during the REPLACEMENT procedure. A REMOVAL procedure is coded for taking out the device used in a previous replacement procedure.

Body Part Character 4	Approach Character 5	Device Character 6	Qualifier Character 7
Ø Occipital-cervical Joint	**Ø** Open	**7** Autologous Tissue Substitute	**Z** No Qualifier

1 Cervical Vertebral Joint
   Atlantoaxial joint
   Cervical facet joint
		J Synthetic Substitute
		K Nonautologous Tissue Substitute	

3 Cervical Vertebral Disc			
4 Cervicothoracic Vertebral Joint Cervicothoracic facet joint			
5 Cervicothoracic Vertebral Disc			

6 Thoracic Vertebral Joint
   Costotransverse joint
   Costovertebral joint
   Thoracic facet joint			

9 Thoracic Vertebral Disc			
A Thoracolumbar Vertebral Joint Thoracolumbar facet joint			
B Thoracolumbar Vertebral Disc			
C Temporomandibular Joint, Right			
D Temporomandibular Joint, Left			
E Sternoclavicular Joint, Right			
F Sternoclavicular Joint, Left			
G Acromioclavicular Joint, Right			
H Acromioclavicular Joint, Left			

L Elbow Joint, Right
   Distal humerus, involving joint
   Humeroradial joint
   Humeroulnar joint
   Proximal radioulnar joint			

M Elbow Joint, Left *See L Elbow Joint, Right*			

N Wrist Joint, Right
   Distal radioulnar joint
   Radiocarpal joint			

P Wrist Joint, Left *See N Wrist Joint, Right*			

Q Carpal Joint, Right
   Intercarpal joint
   Midcarpal joint			

R Carpal Joint, Left *See Q Carpal Joint, Right*			
S Carpometacarpal Joint, Right			
T Carpometacarpal Joint, Left			
U Metacarpophalangeal Joint, Right			
V Metacarpophalangeal Joint, Left			
W Finger Phalangeal Joint, Right Interphalangeal (IP) joint			
X Finger Phalangeal Joint, Left *See W Finger Phalangeal Joint, Right*			

J Shoulder Joint, Right
   Glenohumeral joint
   Glenoid ligament (labrum)
	Ø Open	**Ø** Synthetic Substitute, Reverse Ball and Socket
		7 Autologous Tissue Substitute
		K Nonautologous Tissue Substitute
			Z No Qualifier

K Shoulder Joint, Left *See J Shoulder Joint, Right*			

J Shoulder Joint, Right
   Glenohumeral joint
   Glenoid ligament (labrum)
	Ø Open	**J** Synthetic Substitute	**6** Humeral Surface
			7 Glenoid Surface
			Z No Qualifier

K Shoulder Joint, Left *See J Shoulder Joint, Right*			

Ø   Medical and Surgical
R   Upper Joints
S   Reposition   Definition: Moving to its normal location, or other suitable location, all or a portion of a body part

Explanation: The body part is moved to a new location from an abnormal location, or from a normal location where it is not functioning correctly. The body part may or may not be cut out or off to be moved to the new location.

Body Part Character 4	Approach Character 5	Device Character 6	Qualifier Character 7
Ø **Occipital-cervical Joint**	**Ø** Open	**4** Internal Fixation Device	**Z** No Qualifier
1 **Cervical Vertebral Joint**	**3** Percutaneous	**Z** No Device	
Atlantoaxial joint	**4** Percutaneous Endoscopic		
Cervical facet joint	**X** External		
4 **Cervicothoracic Vertebral Joint**			
Cervicothoracic facet joint			
6 **Thoracic Vertebral Joint**			
Costotransverse joint			
Costovertebral joint			
Thoracic facet joint			
A **Thoracolumbar Vertebral Joint**			
Thoracolumbar facet joint			
C **Temporomandibular Joint, Right**			
D **Temporomandibular Joint, Left**			
E **Sternoclavicular Joint, Right**			
F **Sternoclavicular Joint, Left**			
G **Acromioclavicular Joint, Right**			
H **Acromioclavicular Joint, Left**			
J **Shoulder Joint, Right**			
Glenohumeral joint			
Glenoid ligament (labrum)			
K **Shoulder Joint, Left**			
See J Shoulder Joint, Right			
L **Elbow Joint, Right**	**Ø** Open	**4** Internal Fixation Device	**Z** No Qualifier
Distal humerus, involving joint	**3** Percutaneous	**5** External Fixation Device	
Humeroradial joint	**4** Percutaneous Endoscopic	**Z** No Device	
Humeroulnar joint	**X** External		
Proximal radioulnar joint			
M **Elbow Joint, Left**			
See L Elbow Joint, Right			
N **Wrist Joint, Right**			
Distal radioulnar joint			
Radiocarpal joint			
P **Wrist Joint, Left**			
See N Wrist Joint, Right			
Q **Carpal Joint, Right**			
Intercarpal joint			
Midcarpal joint			
R **Carpal Joint, Left**			
See Q Carpal Joint, Right			
S **Carpometacarpal Joint, Right**			
T **Carpometacarpal Joint, Left**			
U **Metacarpophalangeal Joint, Right**			
V **Metacarpophalangeal Joint, Left**			
W **Finger Phalangeal Joint, Right**			
Interphalangeal (IP) joint			
X **Finger Phalangeal Joint, Left**			
See W Finger Phalangeal Joint, Right			

Non-OR   ØRS[Ø,1,4,6,A,C,D,E,F,G,H,J,K][3,4,X][4,Z]Z
Non-OR   ØRS[L,M,N,P,Q,R,S,T,U,V,W,X][3,4,X][4,5,Z]Z

LC Limited Coverage   NC Noncovered   ⊞ Combination Member   HAC associated procedure   Combination Only   DRG Non-OR   Non-OR   New/Revised in GREEN

582   ICD-10-PCS 2020

Ø   Medical and Surgical
R   Upper Joints
T   Resection   Definition: Cutting out or off, without replacement, all of a body part
                Explanation: None

Body Part Character 4		Approach Character 5	Device Character 6	Qualifier Character 7

3 Cervical Vertebral Disc
4 Cervicothoracic Vertebral Joint
   Cervicothoracic facet joint
5 Cervicothoracic Vertebral Disc
9 Thoracic Vertebral Disc
B Thoracolumbar Vertebral Disc
C Temporomandibular Joint, Right
D Temporomandibular Joint, Left
E Sternoclavicular Joint, Right
F Sternoclavicular Joint, Left
G Acromioclavicular Joint, Right
H Acromioclavicular Joint, Left
J Shoulder Joint, Right
   Glenohumeral joint
   Glenoid ligament (labrum)
K Shoulder Joint, Left
   See J Shoulder Joint, Right
L Elbow Joint, Right
   Distal humerus, involving joint
   Humeroradial joint
   Humeroulnar joint
   Proximal radioulnar joint
	M Elbow Joint, Left
	   See L Elbow Joint, Right
	N Wrist Joint, Right
	   Distal radioulnar joint
	   Radiocarpal joint
	P Wrist Joint, Left
	   See N Wrist Joint, Right
	Q Carpal Joint, Right
	   Intercarpal joint
	   Midcarpal joint
	R Carpal Joint, Left
	   See Q Carpal Joint, Right
	S Carpometacarpal Joint, Right
	T Carpometacarpal Joint, Left
	U Metacarpophalangeal Joint, Right
	V Metacarpophalangeal Joint, Left
	W Finger Phalangeal Joint, Right
	   Interphalangeal (IP) joint
	X Finger Phalangeal Joint, Left
	   See W Finger Phalangeal Joint, Right
		Ø Open	**Z** No Device	**Z** No Qualifier

Ø   Medical and Surgical
R   Upper Joints
U   Supplement   Definition: Putting in or on biological or synthetic material that physically reinforces and/or augments the function of a portion of a body part
                Explanation: The biological material is non-living, or is living and from the same individual. The body part may have been previously replaced, and the SUPPLEMENT procedure is performed to physically reinforce and/or augment the function of the replaced body part.

Body Part Character 4		Approach Character 5	Device Character 6	Qualifier Character 7

Ø Occipital-cervical Joint
1 Cervical Vertebral Joint
   Atlantoaxial joint
   Cervical facet joint
3 Cervical Vertebral Disc
4 Cervicothoracic Vertebral Joint
   Cervicothoracic facet joint
5 Cervicothoracic Vertebral Disc
6 Thoracic Vertebral Joint
   Costotransverse joint
   Costovertebral joint
   Thoracic facet joint
9 Thoracic Vertebral Disc
A Thoracolumbar Vertebral Joint
   Thoracolumbar facet joint
B Thoracolumbar Vertebral Disc
C Temporomandibular Joint, Right
D Temporomandibular Joint, Left
E Sternoclavicular Joint, Right
F Sternoclavicular Joint, Left
G Acromioclavicular Joint, Right
H Acromioclavicular Joint, Left
J Shoulder Joint, Right
   Glenohumeral joint
   Glenoid ligament (labrum)
K Shoulder Joint, Left
   See J Shoulder Joint, Right
	L Elbow Joint, Right
	   Distal humerus, involving joint
	   Humeroradial joint
	   Humeroulnar joint
	   Proximal radioulnar joint
	M Elbow Joint, Left
	   See L Elbow Joint, Right
	N Wrist Joint, Right
	   Distal radioulnar joint
	   Radiocarpal joint
	P Wrist Joint, Left
	   See N Wrist Joint, Right
	Q Carpal Joint, Right
	   Intercarpal joint
	   Midcarpal joint
	R Carpal Joint, Left
	   See Q Carpal Joint, Right
	S Carpometacarpal Joint, Right
	T Carpometacarpal Joint, Left
	U Metacarpophalangeal Joint, Right
	V Metacarpophalangeal Joint, Left
	W Finger Phalangeal Joint, Right
	   Interphalangeal (IP) joint
	X Finger Phalangeal Joint, Left
	   See W Finger Phalangeal Joint, Right
		Ø Open
		3 Percutaneous
		4 Percutaneous Endoscopic
			7 Autologous Tissue Substitute
			J Synthetic Substitute
			K Nonautologous Tissue Substitute
				Z No Qualifier

HAC   ØRU[E,F,G,H,J,K,L,M][Ø,3,4][7,J,K]Z when reported with SDx K68.11 or T81.4Ø–T81.49, T84.6Ø-T84.619, T84.63-T84.7 with 7th character A

LC Limited Coverage   **NC** Noncovered   ⊞ Combination Member   HAC associated procedure   Combination Only   DRG Non-OR   Non-OR   New/Revised in GREEN

ICD-10-PCS 2020   583

ØRT–ØRU

Upper Joints

Ø **Medical and Surgical**
R **Upper Joints**
W **Revision**

Definition: Correcting, to the extent possible, a portion of a malfunctioning device or the position of a displaced device

Explanation: Revision can include correcting a malfunctioning or displaced device by taking out or putting in components of the device such as a screw or pin

Body Part Character 4	Approach Character 5	Device Character 6	Qualifier Character 7

Ø Occipital-cervical Joint
1 Cervical Vertebral Joint
  Atlantoaxial joint
  Cervical facet joint
4 Cervicothoracic Vertebral Joint
  Cervicothoracic facet joint
6 Thoracic Vertebral Joint
  Costotransverse joint
  Costovertebral joint
  Thoracic facet joint
A Thoracolumbar Vertebral Joint
  Thoracolumbar facet joint
	Ø Open
	3 Percutaneous
	4 Percutaneous Endoscopic
	X External
		Ø Drainage Device
		3 Infusion Device
		4 Internal Fixation Device
		7 Autologous Tissue Substitute
		8 Spacer
		A Interbody Fusion Device
		J Synthetic Substitute
		K Nonautologous Tissue Substitute
			Z No Qualifier

3 Cervical Vertebral Disc 5 Cervicothoracic Vertebral Disc 9 Thoracic Vertebral Disc B Thoracolumbar Vertebral Disc	Ø Open 3 Percutaneous 4 Percutaneous Endoscopic X External	Ø Drainage Device 3 Infusion Device 7 Autologous Tissue Substitute J Synthetic Substitute K Nonautologous Tissue Substitute	Z No Qualifier

C Temporomandibular Joint, Right
D Temporomandibular Joint, Left
E Sternoclavicular Joint, Right
F Sternoclavicular Joint, Left
G Acromioclavicular Joint, Right
H Acromioclavicular Joint, Left
J Shoulder Joint, Right
  Glenohumeral joint
  Glenoid ligament (labrum)
K Shoulder Joint, Left
  See J Shoulder Joint, Right
	Ø Open
	3 Percutaneous
	4 Percutaneous Endoscopic
	X External
		Ø Drainage Device
		3 Infusion Device
		4 Internal Fixation Device
		7 Autologous Tissue Substitute
		8 Spacer
		J Synthetic Substitute
		K Nonautologous Tissue Substitute
			Z No Qualifier

L Elbow Joint, Right
  Distal humerus, involving joint
  Humeroradial joint
  Humeroulnar joint
  Proximal radioulnar joint
M Elbow Joint, Left
  See L Elbow Joint, Right
N Wrist Joint, Right
  Distal radioulnar joint
  Radiocarpal joint
P Wrist Joint, Left
  See N Wrist Joint, Right
Q Carpal Joint, Right
  Intercarpal joint
  Midcarpal joint
R Carpal Joint, Left
  See Q Carpal Joint, Right
S Carpometacarpal Joint, Right
T Carpometacarpal Joint, Left
U Metacarpophalangeal Joint, Right
V Metacarpophalangeal Joint, Left
W Finger Phalangeal Joint, Right
  Interphalangeal (IP) joint
X Finger Phalangeal Joint, Left
  See W Finger Phalangeal Joint, Right
	Ø Open
	3 Percutaneous
	4 Percutaneous Endoscopic
	X External
		Ø Drainage Device
		3 Infusion Device
		4 Internal Fixation Device
		5 External Fixation Device
		7 Autologous Tissue Substitute
		8 Spacer
		J Synthetic Substitute
		K Nonautologous Tissue Substitute
			Z No Qualifier

Non-OR   ØRW[Ø,1,4,6,A]X[Ø,3,4,7,8,A,J,K]Z
Non-OR   ØRW[3,5,9,B]X[Ø,3,7,J,K]Z
Non-OR   ØRW[C,D,E,F,G,H,J,K]X[Ø,3,4,7,8,J,K]Z
Non-OR   ØRW[L,M,N,P,Q,R,S,T,U,V,W,X]X[Ø,3,4,5,7,8,J,K]Z

LC Limited Coverage   NC Noncovered   ⊞ Combination Member   HAC associated procedure   Combination Only   DRG Non-OR   Non-OR   New/Revised in GREEN

584   ICD-10-PCS 2020

Lower Joints ØS2–ØSW

Character Meanings*

This Character Meaning table is provided as a guide to assist the user in the identification of character members that may be found in this section of code tables. It **SHOULD NOT** be used to build a PCS code.

Operation–Character 3	Body Part–Character 4	Approach–Character 5	Device–Character 6	Qualifier–Character 7
2 Change	Ø Lumbar Vertebral Joint	Ø Open	Ø Drainage Device OR Synthetic Substitute, Polyethylene	Ø Anterior Approach, Anterior Column
5 Destruction	1 Lumbar Vertebral Joint, 2 or more	3 Percutaneous	1 Synthetic Substitute, Metal	1 Posterior Approach, Posterior Column
9 Drainage	2 Lumbar Vertebral Disc	4 Percutaneous Endoscopic	2 Synthetic Substitute, Metal on Polyethylene	9 Cemented
B Excision	3 Lumbosacral Joint	X External	3 Infusion Device OR Synthetic Substitute, Ceramic	A Uncemented
C Extirpation	4 Lumbosacral Disc		4 Internal Fixation Device OR Synthetic Substitute, Ceramic on Polyethylene	C Patellar Surface
G Fusion	5 Sacrococcygeal Joint		5 External Fixation Device	J Posterior Approach, Anterior Column
H Insertion	6 Coccygeal Joint		6 Synthetic Substitute, Oxidized Zirconium on Polyethylene	X Diagnostic
J Inspection	7 Sacroiliac Joint, Right		7 Autologous Tissue Substitute	Z No Qualifier
N Release	8 Sacroiliac Joint, Left		8 Spacer	
P Removal	9 Hip Joint, Right		9 Liner	
Q Repair	A Hip Joint, Acetabular Surface, Right		A Interbody Fusion Device	
R Replacement	B Hip Joint, Left		B Resurfacing Device OR Spinal Stabilization Device, Interspinous Process	
S Reposition	C Knee Joint, Right		C Spinal Stabilization Device, Pedicle-Based	
T Resection	D Knee Joint, Left		D Spinal Stabilization Device, Facet Replacement	
U Supplement	E Hip Joint, Acetabular Surface, Left		E Articulating Spacer	
W Revision	F Ankle Joint, Right		J Synthetic Substitute	
	G Ankle Joint, Left		K Nonautologous Tissue Substitute	
	H Tarsal Joint, Right		L Synthetic Substitute, Unicondylar Medial	
	J Tarsal Joint, Left		M Synthetic Substitute, Unicondylar Lateral	
	K Tarsometatarsal Joint, Right		N Synthetic Substitute, Patellofemoral	
	L Tarsometatarsal Joint, Left		Y Other Device	
	M Metatarsal-Phalangeal Joint, Right		Z No Device	
	N Metatarsal-Phalangeal Joint, Left			
	P Toe Phalangeal Joint, Right			
	Q Toe Phalangeal Joint, Left			
	R Hip Joint, Femoral Surface, Right			
	S Hip Joint, Femoral Surface, Left			
	T Knee Joint, Femoral Surface, Right			
	U Knee Joint, Femoral Surface, Left			
	V Knee Joint, Tibial Surface, Right			
	W Knee Joint, Tibial Surface, Left			
	Y Lower Joint			

* Includes synovial membrane.

AHA Coding Clinic for table ØS9

2018, 2Q, 17	Arthroscopic drainage of knee and nonexcisional debridement
2017, 1Q, 50	Dry aspiration of ankle joint

AHA Coding Clinic for table ØSB

2017, 4Q, 76	Radiolucent porous interbody fusion device
2016, 2Q, 16	Decompressive laminectomy/foraminotomy and lumbar discectomy
2016, 1Q, 20	Metatarsophalangeal joint resection arthroplasty
2015, 1Q, 34	Arthroscopic meniscectomy with debridement and abrasion chondroplasty
2014, 2Q, 6	Posterior lumbar fusion with discectomy

AHA Coding Clinic for table ØSG

2019, 1Q, 30	Spinal fusion performed at same level as decompressive laminectomy
2018, 4Q, 43	Joint fusion device value
2018, 1Q, 22	Spinal fusion procedures without bone graft
2017, 4Q, 76	Radiolucent porous interbody fusion device
2017, 2Q, 23	Decompression of spinal cord and placement of instrumentation
2014, 3Q, 30	Spinal fusion and fixation instrumentation
2014, 3Q, 36	Lumbar interbody fusion of two vertebral levels
2014, 2Q, 6	Posterior lumbar fusion with discectomy
2013, 3Q, 25	360-degree spinal fusion
2013, 2Q, 39	Ankle fusion, osteotomy, and removal of hardware
2013, 1Q, 21-23	Spinal fusion of thoracic and lumbar vertebrae

AHA Coding Clinic for table ØSH

2017, 2Q, 23	Decompression of spinal cord and placement of instrumentation

AHA Coding Clinic for table ØSJ

2017, 1Q, 50	Dry aspiration of ankle joint

AHA Coding Clinic for table ØSN

2019, 1Q, 30	Spinal fusion performed at same level as decompressive laminectomy

AHA Coding Clinic for table ØSP

2018, 4Q, 43	Articulating spacer for hip and knee joint
2018, 2Q, 16	Exchange of tibial polyethylene component with stabilizing insert (tibial tray)
2017, 4Q, 107	Total ankle replacement versus revision
2016, 4Q, 110-112	Removal and revision of hip and knee devices
2015, 2Q, 18	Total knee revision
2015, 2Q, 19	Revision of femoral head and acetabular liner
2013, 2Q, 39	Ankle fusion, osteotomy, and removal of hardware

AHA Coding Clinic for table ØSQ

2014, 4Q, 25	Femoroacetabular impingement and labral tear with repair

AHA Coding Clinic for table ØSR

2018, 4Q, 43	Articulating spacer for hip and knee joint
2018, 2Q, 16	Exchange of tibial polyethylene component with stabilizing insert (tibial tray)
2017, 4Q, 38-39	Oxidized zirconium on polyethylene bearing surface
2017, 4Q, 107	Total ankle replacement versus revision
2017, 1Q, 22	Total knee replacement and patellar component
2016, 4Q, 110-111	Partial (unicondylar) knee replacement
2016, 4Q, 111-112	Removal and revision of hip and knee devices
2016, 3Q, 35	Use of cemented versus uncemented qualifier for joint replacement
2015, 3Q, 18	Total hip replacement with acetabular reconstruction
2015, 2Q, 18	Total knee revision
2015, 2Q, 19	Revision of femoral head and acetabular liner

AHA Coding Clinic for table ØSS

2016, 2Q, 31	Periacetabular ostectomy for repair of congenital hip dysplasia

AHA Coding Clinic for table ØST

2016, 1Q, 20	Metatarsophalangeal joint resection arthroplasty
2014, 4Q, 29	Rotational osteosynthesis

AHA Coding Clinic for table ØSU

2018, 2Q, 16	Exchange of tibial polyethylene component with stabilizing insert (tibial tray)
2016, 4Q, 111	Removal and revision of hip and knee devices
2015, 2Q, 19	Revision of femoral head and acetabular liner

AHA Coding Clinic for table ØSW

2017, 4Q, 107	Total ankle replacement versus revision
2016, 4Q, 110-112	Removal and revision of hip and knee devices
2015, 2Q, 18	Total knee revision
2015, 2Q, 19	Revision of femoral head and acetabular liner

Lower Joints

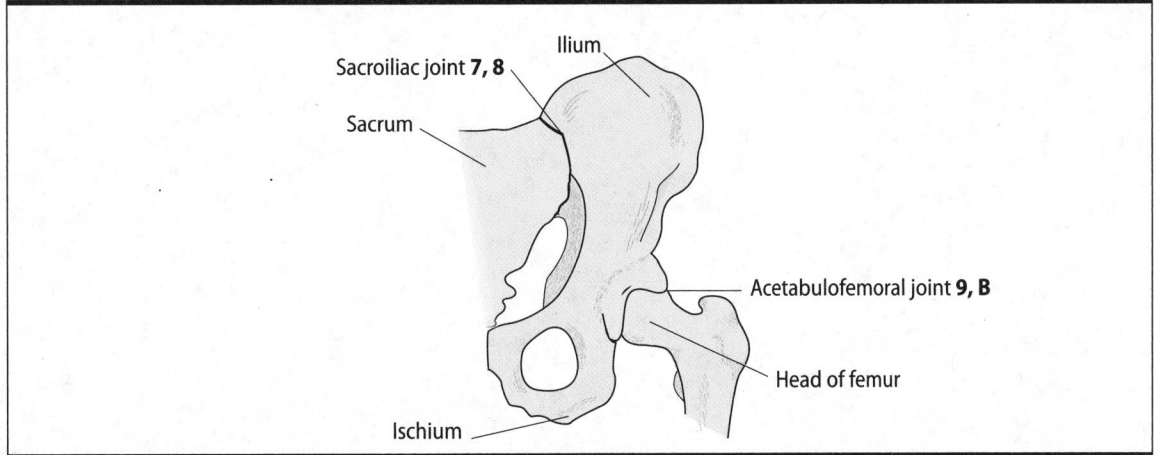

Sacroiliac **7, 8**

Lumbosacral **3**

Sacrococcygeal joint **5**

Hip **9, B**

Knee **C, D**

(Transverse) tarsal **H, J**

Metatarsal-phalangeal **M, N**

Ankle **F, G**

Hip Joint

Sacroiliac joint **7, 8**

Ilium

Sacrum

Acetabulofemoral joint **9, B**

Head of femur

Ischium

Knee Joint

Anterior view

Patella

Medial meniscus cartilage

Lateral meniscus cartilage

Lateral view

Femur

Synovial cavity

Patella

Tibia

Foot Joints

Phalanges

Metatarso-phalangeal joints **M, N**

Tarsal joints **H, J**

Tarsometatarsal joints **K, L**

Distal interphalangeal joint **P, Q**

Proximal interphalangeal joint **P, Q**

Tarsals

Metatarsals

Ø   **Medical and Surgical**
S   **Lower Joints**
2   **Change**   Definition: Taking out or off a device from a body part and putting back an identical or similar device in or on the same body part without cutting or puncturing the skin or a mucous membrane
                 Explanation: All CHANGE procedures are coded using the approach EXTERNAL

Body Part Character 4	Approach Character 5	Device Character 6	Qualifier Character 7
Y Lower Joint	**X** External	**Ø** Drainage Device **Y** Other Device	**Z** No Qualifier

Non-OR	All body part, approach, device, and qualifier values

Ø   **Medical and Surgical**
S   **Lower Joints**
5   **Destruction**   Definition: Physical eradication of all or a portion of a body part by the direct use of energy, force, or a destructive agent
                     Explanation: None of the body part is physically taken out

Body Part Character 4	Approach Character 5	Device Character 6	Qualifier Character 7

Ø   **Lumbar Vertebral Joint**
     Lumbar facet joint
2   **Lumbar Vertebral Disc**
3   **Lumbosacral Joint**
     Lumbosacral facet joint
4   **Lumbosacral Disc**
5   **Sacrococcygeal Joint**
     Sacrococcygeal symphysis
6   **Coccygeal Joint**
7   **Sacroiliac Joint, Right**
8   **Sacroiliac Joint, Left**
9   **Hip Joint, Right**
     Acetabulofemoral joint
B   **Hip Joint, Left**
     See 9 Hip Joint, Right
C   **Knee Joint, Right**
     Femoropatellar joint
     Femorotibial joint
     Lateral meniscus
     Medial meniscus
     Patellofemoral joint
     Tibiofemoral joint
D   **Knee Joint, Left**
     See C Knee Joint, Right
F   **Ankle Joint, Right**
     Inferior tibiofibular joint
     Talocrural joint
G   **Ankle Joint, Left**
     See F Ankle Joint, Right
H   **Tarsal Joint, Right**
     Calcaneocuboid joint
     Cuboideonavicular joint
     Cuneonavicular joint
     Intercuneiform joint
     Subtalar (talocalcaneal) joint
     Talocalcaneal (subtalar) joint
     Talocalcaneonavicular joint
J   **Tarsal Joint, Left**
     See H Tarsal Joint, Right
K   **Tarsometatarsal Joint, Right**
L   **Tarsometatarsal Joint, Left**
M   **Metatarsal-Phalangeal Joint, Right**
     Metatarsophalangeal (MTP) joint
N   **Metatarsal-Phalangeal Joint, Left**
     See M Metatarsal-Phalangeal Joint, Right
P   **Toe Phalangeal Joint, Right**
     Interphalangeal (IP) joint
Q   **Toe Phalangeal Joint, Left**
     See P Toe Phalangeal Joint, Right
	Ø Open
	3 Percutaneous
	4 Percutaneous Endoscopic
		Z No Device	**Z** No Qualifier

LC Limited Coverage   **NC** Noncovered   ⊞ Combination Member   HAC associated procedure   Combination Only   DRG Non-OR   Non-OR   New/Revised in GREEN

ICD-10-PCS 2020   589

ØS2–ØS5

Lower Joints

Ø **Medical and Surgical**
S **Lower Joints**
9 **Drainage**   Definition: Taking or letting out fluids and/or gases from a body part
                Explanation: The qualifier DIAGNOSTIC is used to identify drainage procedures that are biopsies

Body Part Character 4		Approach Character 5	Device Character 6	Qualifier Character 7
Ø **Lumbar Vertebral Joint** Lumbar facet joint 2 **Lumbar Vertebral Disc** 3 **Lumbosacral Joint** Lumbosacral facet joint 4 **Lumbosacral Disc** 5 **Sacrococcygeal Joint** Sacrococcygeal symphysis 6 **Coccygeal Joint** 7 **Sacroiliac Joint, Right** 8 **Sacroiliac Joint, Left** 9 **Hip Joint, Right** Acetabulofemoral joint B **Hip Joint, Left** *See 9 Hip Joint, Right* C **Knee Joint, Right** Femoropatellar joint Femorotibial joint Lateral meniscus Medial meniscus Patellofemoral joint Tibiofemoral joint D **Knee Joint, Left** *See C Knee Joint, Right* F **Ankle Joint, Right** Inferior tibiofibular joint Talocrural joint G **Ankle Joint, Left** *See F Ankle Joint, Right*	H **Tarsal Joint, Right** Calcaneocuboid joint Cuboideonavicular joint Cuneonavicular joint Intercuneiform joint Subtalar (talocalcaneal) joint Talocalcaneal (subtalar) joint Talocalcaneonavicular joint J **Tarsal Joint, Left** *See H Tarsal Joint, Right* K **Tarsometatarsal Joint, Right** L **Tarsometatarsal Joint, Left** M **Metatarsal-Phalangeal Joint, Right** Metatarsophalangeal (MTP) joint N **Metatarsal-Phalangeal Joint, Left** *See M Metatarsal-Phalangeal Joint, Right* P **Toe Phalangeal Joint, Right** Interphalangeal (IP) joint Q **Toe Phalangeal Joint, Left** *See P Toe Phalangeal Joint, Right*	Ø Open 3 Percutaneous 4 Percutaneous Endoscopic	Ø Drainage Device	Z No Qualifier
Ø **Lumbar Vertebral Joint** Lumbar facet joint 2 **Lumbar Vertebral Disc** 3 **Lumbosacral Joint** Lumbosacral facet joint 4 **Lumbosacral Disc** 5 **Sacrococcygeal Joint** Sacrococcygeal symphysis 6 **Coccygeal Joint** 7 **Sacroiliac Joint, Right** 8 **Sacroiliac Joint, Left** 9 **Hip Joint, Right** Acetabulofemoral joint B **Hip Joint, Left** *See 9 Hip Joint, Right* C **Knee Joint, Right** Femoropatellar joint Femorotibial joint Lateral meniscus Medial meniscus Patellofemoral joint Tibiofemoral joint D **Knee Joint, Left** *See C Knee Joint, Right* F **Ankle Joint, Right** Inferior tibiofibular joint Talocrural joint G **Ankle Joint, Left** *See F Ankle Joint, Right*	H **Tarsal Joint, Right** Calcaneocuboid joint Cuboideonavicular joint Cuneonavicular joint Intercuneiform joint Subtalar (talocalcaneal) joint Talocalcaneal (subtalar) joint Talocalcaneonavicular joint J **Tarsal Joint, Left** *See H Tarsal Joint, Right* K **Tarsometatarsal Joint, Right** L **Tarsometatarsal Joint, Left** M **Metatarsal-Phalangeal Joint, Right** Metatarsophalangeal (MTP) joint N **Metatarsal-Phalangeal Joint, Left** *See M Metatarsal-Phalangeal Joint, Right* P **Toe Phalangeal Joint, Right** Interphalangeal (IP) joint Q **Toe Phalangeal Joint, Left** *See P Toe Phalangeal Joint, Right*	Ø Open 3 Percutaneous 4 Percutaneous Endoscopic	Z No Device	X Diagnostic Z No Qualifier

Non-OR   ØS9[Ø,2,3,4,5,6,7,8,9,B,C,D,F,G,H,J,K,L,M,N,P,Q][3,4]ØZ
Non-OR   ØS9[Ø,2,3,4,5,6,7,8,9,B,C,D,F,G,H,J,K,L,M,N,P,Q][Ø,3,4]ZX
Non-OR   ØS9[Ø,2,3,4,5,6,7,8,9,B,C,D,F,G,H,J,K,L,M,N,P,Q][3,4]ZZ

Ø   **Medical and Surgical**
S   **Lower Joints**
B   **Excision**   Definition: Cutting out or off, without replacement, a portion of a body part

         Explanation: The qualifier DIAGNOSTIC is used to identify excision procedures that are biopsies

Body Part — Character 4		Approach — Character 5	Device — Character 6	Qualifier — Character 7
Ø **Lumbar Vertebral Joint** Lumbar facet joint **2** **Lumbar Vertebral Disc** **3** **Lumbosacral Joint** Lumbosacral facet joint **4** **Lumbosacral Disc** **5** **Sacrococcygeal Joint** Sacrococcygeal symphysis **6** **Coccygeal Joint** **7** **Sacroiliac Joint, Right** **8** **Sacroiliac Joint, Left** **9** **Hip Joint, Right** Acetabulofemoral joint **B** **Hip Joint, Left** *See 9 Hip Joint, Right* **C** **Knee Joint, Right** Femoropatellar joint Femorotibial joint Lateral meniscus Medial meniscus Patellofemoral joint Tibiofemoral joint **D** **Knee Joint, Left** *See C Knee Joint, Right* **F** **Ankle Joint, Right** Inferior tibiofibular joint Talocrural joint **G** **Ankle Joint, Left** *See F Ankle Joint, Right*	**H** **Tarsal Joint, Right** Calcaneocuboid joint Cuboideonavicular joint Cuneonavicular joint Intercuneiform joint Subtalar (talocalcaneal) joint Talocalcaneal (subtalar) joint Talocalcaneonavicular joint **J** **Tarsal Joint, Left** *See H Tarsal Joint, Right* **K** **Tarsometatarsal Joint, Right** **L** **Tarsometatarsal Joint, Left** **M** **Metatarsal-Phalangeal Joint, Right** Metatarsophalangeal (MTP) joint **N** **Metatarsal-Phalangeal Joint, Left** *See M Metatarsal-Phalangeal Joint, Right* **P** **Toe Phalangeal Joint, Right** Interphalangeal (IP) joint **Q** **Toe Phalangeal Joint, Left** *See P Toe Phalangeal Joint, Right*	**Ø** **Open** **3** **Percutaneous** **4** **Percutaneous Endoscopic**	**Z** **No Device**	**X** **Diagnostic** **Z** **No Qualifier**

Non-OR   ØSB[Ø,2,3,4,5,6,7,8,9,B,C,D,F,G,H,J,K,L,M,N,P,Q][Ø,3,4]ZX

Ø   **Medical and Surgical**
S   **Lower Joints**
C   **Extirpation**   Definition: Taking or cutting out solid matter from a body part

         Explanation: The solid matter may be an abnormal byproduct of a biological function or a foreign body; it may be imbedded in a body part or in the lumen of a tubular body part. The solid matter may or may not have been previously broken into pieces.

Body Part — Character 4		Approach — Character 5	Device — Character 6	Qualifier — Character 7
Ø **Lumbar Vertebral Joint** Lumbar facet joint **2** **Lumbar Vertebral Disc** **3** **Lumbosacral Joint** Lumbosacral facet joint **4** **Lumbosacral Disc** **5** **Sacrococcygeal Joint** Sacrococcygeal symphysis **6** **Coccygeal Joint** **7** **Sacroiliac Joint, Right** **8** **Sacroiliac Joint, Left** **9** **Hip Joint, Right** Acetabulofemoral joint **B** **Hip Joint, Left** *See 9 Hip Joint, Right* **C** **Knee Joint, Right** Femoropatellar joint Femorotibial joint Lateral meniscus Medial meniscus Patellofemoral joint Tibiofemoral joint **D** **Knee Joint, Left** *See C Knee Joint, Right* **F** **Ankle Joint, Right** Inferior tibiofibular joint Talocrural joint **G** **Ankle Joint, Left** *See F Ankle Joint, Right*	**H** **Tarsal Joint, Right** Calcaneocuboid joint Cuboideonavicular joint Cuneonavicular joint Intercuneiform joint Subtalar (talocalcaneal) joint Talocalcaneal (subtalar) joint Talocalcaneonavicular joint **J** **Tarsal Joint, Left** *See H Tarsal Joint, Right* **K** **Tarsometatarsal Joint, Right** **L** **Tarsometatarsal Joint, Left** **M** **Metatarsal-Phalangeal Joint, Right** Metatarsophalangeal (MTP) joint **N** **Metatarsal-Phalangeal Joint, Left** *See M Metatarsal-Phalangeal Joint, Right* **P** **Toe Phalangeal Joint, Right** Interphalangeal (IP) joint **Q** **Toe Phalangeal Joint, Left** *See P Toe Phalangeal Joint, Right*	**Ø** **Open** **3** **Percutaneous** **4** **Percutaneous Endoscopic**	**Z** **No Device**	**Z** **No Qualifier**

LC Limited Coverage   **NC** Noncovered   ⊞ Combination Member   HAC associated procedure   Combination Only   DRG Non-OR   Non-OR   New/Revised in GREEN

ICD-10-PCS 2020   **591**

ØSB–ØSC

Lower Joints *(side tab)*

Ø   Medical and Surgical
S   Lower Joints
G   Fusion   Definition: Joining together portions of an articular body part rendering the articular body part immobile
                 Explanation: The body part is joined together by fixation device, bone graft, or other means

Body Part Character 4	Approach Character 5	Device Character 6	Qualifier Character 7

Ø Lumbar Vertebral Joint
Lumbar facet joint
1 Lumbar Vertebral Joints, 2 or more ⊞
3 Lumbosacral Joint
Lumbosacral facet joint
	Ø Open
	3 Percutaneous
	4 Percutaneous Endoscopic
		7 Autologous Tissue
		   Substitute
		J Synthetic Substitute
		K Nonautologous Tissue
		   Substitute
			Ø Anterior Approach, Anterior
			   Column
			1 Posterior Approach,
			   Posterior Column
			J Posterior Approach,
			   Anterior Column

Ø Lumbar Vertebral Joint
Lumbar facet joint
1 Lumbar Vertebral Joints, 2 or more ⊞
3 Lumbosacral Joint
Lumbosacral facet joint
	Ø Open
	3 Percutaneous
	4 Percutaneous Endoscopic
		A Interbody Fusion Device	Ø Anterior Approach, Anterior
			   Column
			J Posterior Approach,
			   Anterior Column

5 Sacrococcygeal Joint
Sacrococcygeal symphysis
6 Coccygeal Joint
7 Sacroiliac Joint, Right
8 Sacroiliac Joint, Left
	Ø Open
	3 Percutaneous
	4 Percutaneous Endoscopic
		4 Internal Fixation Device
		7 Autologous Tissue
		   Substitute
		J Synthetic Substitute
		K Nonautologous Tissue
		   Substitute
			Z No Qualifier

9 Hip Joint, Right
Acetabulofemoral joint
B Hip Joint, Left
See 9 Hip Joint, Right
C Knee Joint, Right
Femoropatellar joint
Femorotibial joint
Lateral meniscus
Medial meniscus
Patellofemoral joint
Tibiofemoral joint
D Knee Joint, Left
See C Knee Joint, Right
F Ankle Joint, Right
Inferior tibiofibular joint
Talocrural joint
G Ankle Joint, Left
See F Ankle Joint, Right
H Tarsal Joint, Right
Calcaneocuboid joint
Cuboideonavicular joint
Cuneonavicular joint
Intercuneiform joint
Subtalar (talocalcaneal) joint
Talocalcaneal (subtalar) joint
Talocalcaneonavicular joint
J Tarsal Joint, Left
See H Tarsal Joint, Right
K Tarsometatarsal Joint, Right
L Tarsometatarsal Joint, Left
M Metatarsal-Phalangeal Joint, Right
Metatarsophalangeal (MTP) joint
N Metatarsal-Phalangeal Joint, Left
See M Metatarsal-Phalangeal Joint, Right
P Toe Phalangeal Joint, Right
Interphalangeal (IP) joint
Q Toe Phalangeal Joint, Left
See P Toe Phalangeal Joint, Right
	Ø Open
	3 Percutaneous
	4 Percutaneous Endoscopic
		4 Internal Fixation Device
		5 External Fixation Device
		7 Autologous Tissue
		   Substitute
		J Synthetic Substitute
		K Nonautologous Tissue
		   Substitute
			Z No Qualifier

HAC   ØSG[Ø,1,3][Ø,3,4][7,J,K][Ø,1,J] when reported with SDx K68.11 or T81.4Ø–T81.49, T84.6Ø-
       T84.619, T84.63-T84.7 with 7th character A
HAC   ØSG[Ø,1,3][Ø,3,4]A[Ø,J] when reported with SDx K68.11 or T81.4Ø–T81.49, T84.6Ø-T84.619,
       T84.63-T84.7 with 7th character A
HAC   ØSG[7,8][Ø,3,4][4,7,J,K]Z when reported with SDx K68.11 or T81.4Ø–T81.49, T84.6Ø-
       T84.619, T84.63-T84.7 with 7th character A
	See Appendix L for Procedure Combinations
	⊞ ØSG1[Ø,3,4][7,J,K][Ø,1,J]
	⊞ ØSG1[Ø,3,4]A[Ø,J]

Lower Joints

Ø   **Medical and Surgical**
S   **Lower Joints**
H   **Insertion**   Definition: Putting in a nonbiological appliance that monitors, assists, performs, or prevents a physiological function but does not physically take the place of a body part

                      Explanation: None

Body Part Character 4	Approach Character 5	Device Character 6	Qualifier Character 7
Ø Lumbar Vertebral Joint Lumbar facet joint **3 Lumbosacral Joint** Lumbosacral facet joint	**Ø** Open **3** Percutaneous **4** Percutaneous Endoscopic	**3** Infusion Device **4** Internal Fixation Device **8** Spacer **B** Spinal Stabilization Device, Interspinous Process **C** Spinal Stabilization Device, Pedicle-Based **D** Spinal Stabilization Device, Facet Replacement	**Z** No Qualifier
2 Lumbar Vertebral Disc **4 Lumbosacral Disc**	**Ø** Open **3** Percutaneous **4** Percutaneous Endoscopic	**3** Infusion Device **8** Spacer	**Z** No Qualifier
5 Sacrococcygeal Joint Sacrococcygeal symphysis **6 Coccygeal Joint** **7 Sacroiliac Joint, Right** **8 Sacroiliac Joint, Left**	**Ø** Open **3** Percutaneous **4** Percutaneous Endoscopic	**3** Infusion Device **4** Internal Fixation Device **8** Spacer	**Z** No Qualifier
9 Hip Joint, Right Acetabulofemoral joint **B Hip Joint, Left** *See 9 Hip Joint, Right* **C Knee Joint, Right** Femoropatellar joint Femorotibial joint Lateral meniscus Medial meniscus Patellofemoral joint Tibiofemoral joint **D Knee Joint, Left** *See C Knee Joint, Right* **F Ankle Joint, Right** Inferior tibiofibular joint Talocrural joint **G Ankle Joint, Left** *See F Ankle Joint, Right* **H Tarsal Joint, Right** Calcaneocuboid joint Cuboideonavicular joint Cuneonavicular joint Intercuneiform joint Subtalar (talocalcaneal) joint Talocalcaneal (subtalar) joint Talocalcaneonavicular joint **J Tarsal Joint, Left** *See H Tarsal Joint, Right* **K Tarsometatarsal Joint, Right** **L Tarsometatarsal Joint, Left** **M Metatarsal-Phalangeal Joint, Right** Metatarsophalangeal (MTP) joint **N Metatarsal-Phalangeal Joint, Left** *See M Metatarsal-Phalangeal Joint, Right* **P Toe Phalangeal Joint, Right** Interphalangeal (IP) joint **Q Toe Phalangeal Joint, Left** *See P Toe Phalangeal Joint, Right*	**Ø** Open **3** Percutaneous **4** Percutaneous Endoscopic	**3** Infusion Device **4** Internal Fixation Device **5** External Fixation Device **8** Spacer	**Z** No Qualifier

Non-OR   ØSH[Ø,3][Ø,3,4][3,8]Z
Non-OR   ØSH[2,4][Ø,3,4][3,8]Z
Non-OR   ØSH[5,6,7,8][Ø,3,4][3,8]Z
Non-OR   ØSH[9,B,C,D][Ø,3,4]3Z
Non-OR   ØSH[9,B,C,D][3,4]8Z
Non-OR   ØSH[F,G,H,J,K,L,M,N,P,Q][Ø,3,4][3,8]Z

LC Limited Coverage   **NC** Noncovered   ⊞ Combination Member   HAC associated procedure   Combination Only   DRG Non-OR   Non-OR   New/Revised in GREEN

Ø Medical and Surgical
S Lower Joints
J Inspection Definition: Visually and/or manually exploring a body part

Explanation: Visual exploration may be performed with or without optical instrumentation. Manual exploration may be performed directly or through intervening body layers.

Body Part Character 4		Approach Character 5	Device Character 6	Qualifier Character 7
Ø Lumbar Vertebral Joint Lumbar facet joint	**H Tarsal Joint, Right** Calcaneocuboid joint Cuboideonavicular joint Cuneonavicular joint Intercuneiform joint Subtalar (talocalcaneal) joint Talocalcaneal (subtalar) joint Talocalcaneonavicular joint	**Ø Open** **3 Percutaneous** **4 Percutaneous Endoscopic** **X External**	**Z No Device**	**Z No Qualifier**
2 Lumbar Vertebral Disc				
3 Lumbosacral Joint Lumbosacral facet joint				
4 Lumbosacral Disc				
5 Sacrococcygeal Joint Sacrococcygeal symphysis	**J Tarsal Joint, Left** *See H Tarsal Joint, Right*			
6 Coccygeal Joint	**K Tarsometatarsal Joint, Right**			
7 Sacroiliac Joint, Right				
8 Sacroiliac Joint, Left	**L Tarsometatarsal Joint, Left**			
9 Hip Joint, Right Acetabulofemoral joint	**M Metatarsal-Phalangeal Joint, Right** Metatarsophalangeal (MTP) joint			
B Hip Joint, Left *See 9 Hip Joint, Right*				
C Knee Joint, Right Femoropatellar joint Femorotibial joint Lateral meniscus Medial meniscus Patellofemoral joint Tibiofemoral joint	**N Metatarsal-Phalangeal Joint, Left** *See M Metatarsal-Phalangeal Joint, Right*			
	P Toe Phalangeal Joint, Right Interphalangeal (IP) joint			
D Knee Joint, Left *See C Knee Joint, Right*	**Q Toe Phalangeal Joint, Left** *See P Toe Phalangeal Joint, Right*			
F Ankle Joint, Right Inferior tibiofibular joint Talocrural joint				
G Ankle Joint, Left *See F Ankle Joint, Right*				

Non-OR ØSJ[Ø,2,3,4,5,6,7,8,9,B,C,D,F,G,H,J,K,L,M,N,P,Q][3,X]ZZ

Ø Medical and Surgical
S Lower Joints
N Release Definition: Freeing a body part from an abnormal physical constraint by cutting or by the use of force

Explanation: Some of the restraining tissue may be taken out but none of the body part is taken out

Body Part Character 4		Approach Character 5	Device Character 6	Qualifier Character 7
Ø Lumbar Vertebral Joint Lumbar facet joint	**H Tarsal Joint, Right** Calcaneocuboid joint Cuboideonavicular joint Cuneonavicular joint Intercuneiform joint Subtalar (talocalcaneal) joint Talocalcaneal (subtalar) joint Talocalcaneonavicular joint	**Ø Open** **3 Percutaneous** **4 Percutaneous Endoscopic** **X External**	**Z No Device**	**Z No Qualifier**
2 Lumbar Vertebral Disc				
3 Lumbosacral Joint Lumbosacral facet joint				
4 Lumbosacral Disc				
5 Sacrococcygeal Joint Sacrococcygeal symphysis	**J Tarsal Joint, Left** *See H Tarsal Joint, Right*			
6 Coccygeal Joint	**K Tarsometatarsal Joint, Right**			
7 Sacroiliac Joint, Right				
8 Sacroiliac Joint, Left	**L Tarsometatarsal Joint, Left**			
9 Hip Joint, Right Acetabulofemoral joint	**M Metatarsal-Phalangeal Joint, Right** Metatarsophalangeal (MTP) joint			
B Hip Joint, Left *See 9 Hip Joint, Right*				
C Knee Joint, Right Femoropatellar joint Femorotibial joint Lateral meniscus Medial meniscus Patellofemoral joint Tibiofemoral joint	**N Metatarsal-Phalangeal Joint, Left** *See M Metatarsal-Phalangeal Joint, Right*			
	P Toe Phalangeal Joint, Right Interphalangeal (IP) joint			
D Knee Joint, Left *See C Knee Joint, Right*	**Q Toe Phalangeal Joint, Left** *See P Toe Phalangeal Joint, Right*			
F Ankle Joint, Right Inferior tibiofibular joint Talocrural joint				
G Ankle Joint, Left *See F Ankle Joint, Right*				

Non-OR ØSN[Ø,2,3,4,5,6,7,8,9,B,C,D,F,G,H,J,K,L,M,N,P,Q]XZZ

LC Limited Coverage   NC Noncovered   ⊞ Combination Member   HAC associated procedure   Combination Only   DRG Non-OR   Non-OR   New/Revised in GREEN

594   ICD-10-PCS 2020

Ø Medical and Surgical
S Lower Joints
P Removal　　　Definition: Taking out or off a device from a body part

Explanation: If a device is taken out and a similar device put in without cutting or puncturing the skin or mucous membrane, the procedure is coded to the root operation CHANGE. Otherwise, the procedure for taking out the device is coded to the root operation REMOVAL.

Body Part Character 4	Approach Character 5	Device Character 6	Qualifier Character 7
Ø Lumbar Vertebral Joint 　Lumbar facet joint 3 Lumbosacral Joint 　Lumbosacral facet joint	Ø Open 3 Percutaneous 4 Percutaneous Endoscopic	Ø Drainage Device 3 Infusion Device 4 Internal Fixation Device 7 Autologous Tissue Substitute 8 Spacer A Interbody Fusion Device J Synthetic Substitute K Nonautologous Tissue Substitute	Z No Qualifier
Ø Lumbar Vertebral Joint 　Lumbar facet joint 3 Lumbosacral Joint 　Lumbosacral facet joint	X External	Ø Drainage Device 3 Infusion Device 4 Internal Fixation Device	Z No Qualifier
2 Lumbar Vertebral Disc 4 Lumbosacral Disc	Ø Open 3 Percutaneous 4 Percutaneous Endoscopic	Ø Drainage Device 3 Infusion Device 7 Autologous Tissue Substitute J Synthetic Substitute K Nonautologous Tissue Substitute	Z No Qualifier
2 Lumbar Vertebral Disc 4 Lumbosacral Disc	X External	Ø Drainage Device 3 Infusion Device	Z No Qualifier
5 Sacrococcygeal Joint 　Sacrococcygeal symphysis 6 Coccygeal Joint 7 Sacroiliac Joint, Right 8 Sacroiliac Joint, Left	Ø Open 3 Percutaneous 4 Percutaneous Endoscopic	Ø Drainage Device 3 Infusion Device 4 Internal Fixation Device 7 Autologous Tissue Substitute 8 Spacer J Synthetic Substitute K Nonautologous Tissue Substitute	Z No Qualifier
5 Sacrococcygeal Joint 　Sacrococcygeal symphysis 6 Coccygeal Joint 7 Sacroiliac Joint, Right 8 Sacroiliac Joint, Left	X External	Ø Drainage Device 3 Infusion Device 4 Internal Fixation Device	Z No Qualifier
9 Hip Joint, Right ⊞ 　Acetabulofemoral joint B Hip Joint, Left ⊞ 　See 9 Hip Joint, Right	Ø Open	Ø Drainage Device 3 Infusion Device 4 Internal Fixation Device 5 External Fixation Device 7 Autologous Tissue Substitute 8 Spacer 9 Liner B Resurfacing Device E Articulating Spacer J Synthetic Substitute K Nonautologous Tissue Substitute	Z No Qualifier
9 Hip Joint, Right ⊞ 　Acetabulofemoral joint B Hip Joint, Left ⊞ 　See 9 Hip Joint, Right	3 Percutaneous 4 Percutaneous Endoscopic	Ø Drainage Device 3 Infusion Device 4 Internal Fixation Device 5 External Fixation Device 7 Autologous Tissue Substitute 8 Spacer J Synthetic Substitute K Nonautologous Tissue Substitute	Z No Qualifier
9 Hip Joint, Right ⊞ 　Acetabulofemoral joint B Hip Joint, Left ⊞ 　See 9 Hip Joint, Right	X External	Ø Drainage Device 3 Infusion Device 4 Internal Fixation Device 5 External Fixation Device	Z No Qualifier

ØSP Continued on next page

Non-OR ØSP[Ø,3][Ø,3,4]8Z		
Non-OR ØSP[Ø,3]3[Ø,3]Z	**See Appendix L for Procedure Combinations**	
Non-OR ØSP[Ø,3]X[Ø,3,4]Z	**Combo-only** ØSP[9,B]48Z	
Non-OR ØSP[2,4]3[Ø,3]Z	⊞　ØSP[9,B]Ø[8,9,B,E,J]Z	
Non-OR ØSP[2,4]X[Ø,3]Z	⊞　ØSP[9,B]4JZ	
Non-OR ØSP[5,6,7,8][Ø,3,4]8Z		
Non-OR ØSP[5,6,7,8]3[Ø,3]Z		
Non-OR ØSP[5,6,7,8]X[Ø,3,4]Z		
Non-OR ØSP[9,B]3[Ø,3,8]Z		
Non-OR ØSP[9,B]X[Ø,3,4,5]Z		

LC Limited Coverage　　NC Noncovered　　⊞ Combination Member　　HAC associated procedure　　Combination Only　　DRG Non-OR　　Non-OR　　New/Revised in GREEN

Lower Joints *(side tab)*

Ø　**Medical and Surgical**
S　**Lower Joints**
P　**Removal**　　Definition: Taking out or off a device from a body part

ØSP Continued

Explanation: If a device is taken out and a similar device put in without cutting or puncturing the skin or mucous membrane, the procedure is coded to the root operation CHANGE. Otherwise, the procedure for taking out the device is coded to the root operation REMOVAL.

Body Part Character 4	Approach Character 5	Device Character 6	Qualifier Character 7
A Hip Joint, Acetabular Surface, Right ⊞ E Hip Joint, Acetabular Surface, Left ⊞ R Hip Joint, Femoral Surface, Right ⊞ S Hip Joint, Femoral Surface, Left ⊞ T Knee Joint, Femoral Surface, Right ⊞ 　Femoropatellar joint 　Patellofemoral joint U Knee Joint, Femoral Surface, Left ⊞ 　*See T Knee Joint, Femoral Surface, Right* V Knee Joint, Tibial Surface, Right ⊞ 　Femorotibial joint 　Tibiofemoral joint W Knee Joint, Tibial Surface, Left ⊞ 　*See V Knee Joint, Tibial Surface, Right*	Ø Open 3 Percutaneous 4 Percutaneous Endoscopic	J Synthetic Substitute	Z No Qualifier
C Knee Joint, Right ⊞ 　Femoropatellar joint 　Femorotibial joint 　Lateral meniscus 　Medial meniscus 　Patellofemoral joint 　Tibiofemoral joint D Knee Joint, Left ⊞ 　*See C Knee Joint, Right*	Ø Open	Ø Drainage Device 3 Infusion Device 4 Internal Fixation Device 5 External Fixation Device 7 Autologous Tissue Substitute 8 Spacer 9 Liner E Articulating Spacer K Nonautologous Tissue Substitute L Synthetic Substitute, Unicondylar Medial M Synthetic Substitute, Unicondylar Lateral N Synthetic Substitute, Patellofemoral	Z No Qualifier
C Knee Joint, Right ⊞ 　Femoropatellar joint 　Femorotibial joint 　Lateral meniscus 　Medial meniscus 　Patellofemoral joint 　Tibiofemoral joint D Knee Joint, Left ⊞ 　*See C Knee Joint, Right*	Ø Open	J Synthetic Substitute	C Patellar Surface Z No Qualifier
C Knee Joint, Right ⊞ 　Femoropatellar joint 　Femorotibial joint 　Lateral meniscus 　Medial meniscus 　Patellofemoral joint 　Tibiofemoral joint D Knee Joint, Left ⊞ 　*See C Knee Joint, Right*	3 Percutaneous 4 Percutaneous Endoscopic	Ø Drainage Device 3 Infusion Device 4 Internal Fixation Device 5 External Fixation Device 7 Autologous Tissue Substitute 8 Spacer K Nonautologous Tissue Substitute L Synthetic Substitute, Unicondylar Medial M Synthetic Substitute, Unicondylar Lateral N Synthetic Substitute, Patellofemoral	Z No Qualifier
C Knee Joint, Right ⊞ 　Femoropatellar joint 　Femorotibial joint 　Lateral meniscus 　Medial meniscus 　Patellofemoral joint 　Tibiofemoral joint D Knee Joint, Left ⊞ 　*See C Knee Joint, Right*	3 Percutaneous 4 Percutaneous Endoscopic	J Synthetic Substitute	C Patellar Surface Z No Qualifier

ØSP Continued on next page

Non-OR	ØSP[C,D]3[Ø,3]Z

See Appendix L for Procedure Combinations

Combo-only	ØSP[C,D][3,4]8Z	⊞	ØSP[C,D]ØJ[C,Z]
⊞	ØSP[A,E,R,S,T,U,V,W][Ø,4]JZ	⊞	ØSP[C,D]4[L,M,N]Z
⊞	ØSP[C,D]Ø[8,9,E,L,M,N]Z	⊞	ØSP[C,D]4J[C,Z]

ᴸᶜ Limited Coverage　ᴺᶜ Noncovered　⊞ Combination Member　HAC associated procedure　Combination Only　DRG Non-OR　Non-OR　New/Revised in GREEN

596　　　　　　　　　　　　　　　　　　　　　　　　　　　　　ICD-10-PCS 2020

Ø   Medical and Surgical
S   Lower Joints
P   Removal

ØSP Continued

Definition: Taking out or off a device from a body part

Explanation: If a device is taken out and a similar device put in without cutting or puncturing the skin or mucous membrane, the procedure is coded to the root operation CHANGE. Otherwise, the procedure for taking out the device is coded to the root operation REMOVAL.

Body Part Character 4	Approach Character 5	Device Character 6	Qualifier Character 7

C   **Knee Joint, Right**
    Femoropatellar joint
    Femorotibial joint
    Lateral meniscus
    Medial meniscus
    Patellofemoral joint
    Tibiofemoral joint
D   **Knee Joint, Left**
    See C Knee Joint, Right
	X External	**Ø** Drainage Device
		3 Infusion Device
		4 Internal Fixation Device
		5 External Fixation Device
			Z No Qualifier

F   **Ankle Joint, Right**
    Inferior tibiofibular joint
    Talocrural joint
G   **Ankle Joint, Left**
    See F Ankle Joint, Right
H   **Tarsal Joint, Right**
    Calcaneocuboid joint
    Cuboideonavicular joint
    Cuneonavicular joint
    Intercuneiform joint
    Subtalar (talocalcaneal) joint
    Talocalcaneal (subtalar) joint
    Talocalcaneonavicular joint
J   **Tarsal Joint, Left**
    See H Tarsal Joint, Right
K   **Tarsometatarsal Joint, Right**
L   **Tarsometatarsal Joint, Left**
M   **Metatarsal-Phalangeal Joint, Right**
    Metatarsophalangeal (MTP) joint
N   **Metatarsal-Phalangeal Joint, Left**
    See M Metatarsal-Phalangeal Joint,
    Right
P   **Toe Phalangeal Joint, Right**
    Interphalangeal (IP) joint
Q   **Toe Phalangeal Joint, Left**
    See P Toe Phalangeal Joint, Right
	Ø Open
	3 Percutaneous
	4 Percutaneous Endoscopic
		Ø Drainage Device
		3 Infusion Device
		4 Internal Fixation Device
		5 External Fixation Device
		7 Autologous Tissue Substitute
		8 Spacer
		J Synthetic Substitute
		K Nonautologous Tissue Substitute
			Z No Qualifier

F   **Ankle Joint, Right**
    Inferior tibiofibular joint
    Talocrural joint
G   **Ankle Joint, Left**
    See F Ankle Joint, Right
H   **Tarsal Joint, Right**
    Calcaneocuboid joint
    Cuboideonavicular joint
    Cuneonavicular joint
    Intercuneiform joint
    Subtalar (talocalcaneal) joint
    Talocalcaneal (subtalar) joint
    Talocalcaneonavicular joint
J   **Tarsal Joint, Left**
    See H Tarsal Joint, Right
K   **Tarsometatarsal Joint, Right**
L   **Tarsometatarsal Joint, Left**
M   **Metatarsal-Phalangeal Joint, Right**
    Metatarsophalangeal (MTP) joint
N   **Metatarsal-Phalangeal Joint, Left**
    See M Metatarsal-Phalangeal Joint,
    Right
P   **Toe Phalangeal Joint, Right**
    Interphalangeal (IP) joint
Q   **Toe Phalangeal Joint, Left**
    See P Toe Phalangeal Joint, Right
	X External	**Ø** Drainage Device
		3 Infusion Device
		4 Internal Fixation Device
		5 External Fixation Device
			Z No Qualifier

Non-OR   ØSP[C,D]X[Ø,3,4,5]Z
Non-OR   ØSP[F,G,H,J,K,L,M,N,P,Q]3[Ø,3,8]Z
Non-OR   ØSP[F,G,H,J,K,L,M,N,P,Q][Ø,4]8Z
Non-OR   ØSP[F,G,H,J,K,L,M,N,P,Q]X[Ø,3,4,5]Z

LC Limited Coverage   NC Noncovered   ⊞ Combination Member   HAC associated procedure   Combination Only   DRG Non-OR   Non-OR   New/Revised in GREEN

ICD-10-PCS 2020   597

ØSP–ØSP

Ø Medical and Surgical
S Lower Joints
Q Repair Definition: Restoring, to the extent possible, a body part to its normal anatomic structure and function

Explanation: Used only when the method to accomplish the repair is not one of the other root operations

Body Part Character 4	Approach Character 5	Device Character 6	Qualifier Character 7
Ø Lumbar Vertebral Joint Lumbar facet joint	Ø Open	Z No Device	Z No Qualifier
2 Lumbar Vertebral Disc	3 Percutaneous		
3 Lumbosacral Joint Lumbosacral facet joint	4 Percutaneous Endoscopic		
4 Lumbosacral Disc	X External		
5 Sacrococcygeal Joint Sacrococcygeal symphysis			
6 Coccygeal Joint			
7 Sacroiliac Joint, Right			
8 Sacroiliac Joint, Left			
9 Hip Joint, Right Acetabulofemoral joint			
B Hip Joint, Left See 9 Hip Joint, Right			

C Knee Joint, Right
  Femoropatellar joint
  Femorotibial joint
  Lateral meniscus
  Medial meniscus
  Patellofemoral joint
  Tibiofemoral joint			

D Knee Joint, Left See C Knee Joint, Right			

F Ankle Joint, Right
  Inferior tibiofibular joint
  Talocrural joint			

G Ankle Joint, Left See F Ankle Joint, Right			

H Tarsal Joint, Right
  Calcaneocuboid joint
  Cuboideonavicular joint
  Cuneonavicular joint
  Intercuneiform joint
  Subtalar (talocalcaneal) joint
  Talocalcaneal (subtalar) joint
  Talocalcaneonavicular joint			

J Tarsal Joint, Left See H Tarsal Joint, Right			
K Tarsometatarsal Joint, Right			
L Tarsometatarsal Joint, Left			
M Metatarsal-Phalangeal Joint, Right Metatarsophalangeal (MTP) joint			
N Metatarsal-Phalangeal Joint, Left See M Metatarsal-Phalangeal Joint, Right			
P Toe Phalangeal Joint, Right Interphalangeal (IP) joint			
Q Toe Phalangeal Joint, Left See P Toe Phalangeal Joint, Right			

Non-OR ØSQ[Ø,2,3,4,5,6,7,8,9,B,C,D,F,G,H,J,K,L,M,N,P,Q]XZZ

Ø   **Medical and Surgical**
S   **Lower Joints**
R   **Replacement**   Definition: Putting in or on biological or synthetic material that physically takes the place and/or function of all or a portion of a body part

                             Explanation: The body part may have been taken out or replaced, or may be taken out, physically eradicated, or rendered nonfunctional during the REPLACEMENT procedure. A REMOVAL procedure is coded for taking out the device used in a previous replacement procedure.

Body Part Character 4	Approach Character 5	Device Character 6	Qualifier Character 7

Ø Lumbar Vertebral Joint
   Lumbar facet joint
2 Lumbar Vertebral Disc NC
3 Lumbosacral Joint
   Lumbosacral facet joint
4 Lumbosacral Disc NC
5 Sacrococcygeal Joint
   Sacrococcygeal symphysis
6 Coccygeal Joint
7 Sacroiliac Joint, Right
8 Sacroiliac Joint, Left
H Tarsal Joint, Right
   Calcaneocuboid joint
   Cuboideonavicular joint
   Cuneonavicular joint
   Intercuneiform joint
   Subtalar (talocalcaneal) joint
   Talocalcaneal (subtalar) joint
   Talocalcaneonavicular joint
J Tarsal Joint, Left
   See H Tarsal Joint, Right
K Tarsometatarsal Joint, Right
L Tarsometatarsal Joint, Left
M Metatarsal-Phalangeal Joint, Right
   Metatarsophalangeal (MTP) joint
N Metatarsal-Phalangeal Joint, Left
   See M Metatarsal-Phalangeal Joint, Right
P Toe Phalangeal Joint, Right
   Interphalangeal (IP) joint
Q Toe Phalangeal Joint, Left
   See P Toe Phalangeal Joint, Right
	Ø Open	**7** Autologous Tissue Substitute
		J Synthetic Substitute
		K Nonautologous Tissue Substitute
			Z No Qualifier

9 Hip Joint, Right ⊞
   Acetabulofemoral joint
B Hip Joint, Left ⊞
   See 9 Hip Joint, Right
	Ø Open	**1** Synthetic Substitute, Metal
		2 Synthetic Substitute, Metal on Polyethylene
		3 Synthetic Substitute, Ceramic
		4 Synthetic Substitute, Ceramic on Polyethylene
		6 Synthetic Substitute, Oxidized Zirconium on Polyethylene
		J Synthetic Substitute
			9 Cemented
			A Uncemented
			Z No Qualifier

9 Hip Joint, Right ⊞
   Acetabulofemoral joint
B Hip Joint, Left ⊞
   See 9 Hip Joint, Right
	Ø Open	**7** Autologous Tissue Substitute
		E Articulating Spacer
		K Nonautologous Tissue Substitute
			Z No Qualifier

A Hip Joint, Acetabular Surface, Right ⊞ **E** Hip Joint, Acetabular Surface, Left ⊞	**Ø** Open	**Ø** Synthetic Substitute, Polyethylene **1** Synthetic Substitute, Metal **3** Synthetic Substitute, Ceramic **J** Synthetic Substitute	**9** Cemented **A** Uncemented **Z** No Qualifier
A Hip Joint, Acetabular Surface, Right **E** Hip Joint, Acetabular Surface, Left	**Ø** Open	**7** Autologous Tissue Substitute **K** Nonautologous Tissue Substitute	**Z** No Qualifier

ØSR Continued on next page

HAC ØSR[9,B]Ø[1,2,3,4,6,J][9,A,Z] when reported with SDx of I26.Ø2-I26.Ø9, I26.92-I26.99, or I82.4Ø1-I82.4Z9	**See Appendix L for Procedure Combinations** ⊞ ØSR[9,B]Ø[1,2,3,4,6,J][9,A,Z]
HAC ØSR[9,B]Ø[7,E,K]Z when reported with SDx of I26.Ø2-I26.Ø9, I26.92-I26.99, or I82.4Ø1-I82.4Z9	⊞ ØSR[9,B]ØEZ ⊞ ØSR[A,E]Ø[Ø,1,3,J][9,A,Z]
HAC ØSR[A,E]Ø[Ø,1,3,J][9,A,Z] when reported with SDx of I26.Ø2-I26.Ø9, I26.92-I26.99, or I82.4Ø1-I82.4Z9	
HAC ØSR[A,E]Ø[7,K]Z when reported with SDx of I26.Ø2-I26.Ø9, I26.92-I26.99, or I82.4Ø1-I82.4Z9	
NC ØSR[2,4]ØJZ when beneficiary age is over 6Ø	

LC Limited Coverage   **NC** Noncovered   ⊞ Combination Member   HAC associated procedure   Combination Only   DRG Non-OR   Non-OR   New/Revised in GREEN

ICD-10-PCS 2020   599

ØSR–ØSR

Lower Joints (side tab)

Ø   **Medical and Surgical**
S   **Lower Joints**
R   **Replacement**

ØSR Continued

Definition: Putting in or on biological or synthetic material that physically takes the place and/or function of all or a portion of a body part

Explanation: The body part may have been taken out or replaced, or may be taken out, physically eradicated, or rendered nonfunctional during the REPLACEMENT procedure. A REMOVAL procedure is coded for taking out the device used in a previous replacement procedure.

Body Part Character 4	Approach Character 5	Device Character 6	Qualifier Character 7
C Knee Joint, Right ⊞ Femoropatellar joint Femorotibial joint Lateral meniscus Medial meniscus Patellofemoral joint Tibiofemoral joint **D** Knee Joint, Left ⊞ *See C Knee Joint, Right*	Ø Open	6 Synthetic Substitute, Oxidized Zirconium on Polyethylene J Synthetic Substitute L Synthetic Substitute, Unicondylar Medial M Synthetic Substitute, Unicondylar Lateral N Synthetic Substitute, Patellofemoral	9 Cemented A Uncemented Z No Qualifier
C Knee Joint, Right ⊞ Femoropatellar joint Femorotibial joint Lateral meniscus Medial meniscus Patellofemoral joint Tibiofemoral joint **D** Knee Joint, Left ⊞ *See C Knee Joint, Right*	Ø Open	7 Autologous Tissue Substitute E Articulating Spacer K Nonautologous Tissue Substitute	Z No Qualifier
F Ankle Joint, Right Inferior tibiofibular joint Talocrural joint **G** Ankle Joint, Left *See F Ankle Joint, Right* **T** Knee Joint, Femoral Surface, Right Femoropatellar joint Patellofemoral joint **U** Knee Joint, Femoral Surface, Left *See T Knee Joint, Femoral Surface, Right* **V** Knee Joint, Tibial Surface, Right Femorotibial joint Tibiofemoral joint **W** Knee Joint, Tibial Surface, Left *See V Knee Joint, Tibial Surface, Right*	Ø Open	7 Autologous Tissue Substitute K Nonautologous Tissue Substitute	Z No Qualifier
F Ankle Joint, Right Inferior tibiofibular joint Talocrural joint **G** Ankle Joint, Left *See F Ankle Joint, Right* **T** Knee Joint, Femoral Surface, Right ⊞ Femoropatellar joint Patellofemoral joint **U** Knee Joint, Femoral Surface, Left ⊞ *See T Knee Joint, Femoral Surface, Right* **V** Knee Joint, Tibial Surface, Right ⊞ Femorotibial joint Tibiofemoral joint **W** Knee Joint, Tibial Surface, Left ⊞ *See V Knee Joint, Tibial Surface, Right*	Ø Open	J Synthetic Substitute	9 Cemented A Uncemented Z No Qualifier
R Hip Joint, Femoral Surface, Right ⊞ **S** Hip Joint, Femoral Surface, Left ⊞	Ø Open	1 Synthetic Substitute, Metal 3 Synthetic Substitute, Ceramic J Synthetic Substitute	9 Cemented A Uncemented Z No Qualifier
R Hip Joint, Femoral Surface, Right **S** Hip Joint, Femoral Surface, Left	Ø Open	7 Autologous Tissue Substitute K Nonautologous Tissue Substitute	Z No Qualifier

HAC   ØSR[C,D]Ø[6,J,L,M,N][9,A,Z] when reported with SDx of I26.Ø2-I26.Ø9, I26.92-I26.99 or I82.4Ø1-I82.4Z9

HAC   ØSR[C,D]Ø[7,E,K]Z when reported with SDx of I26.Ø2-I26.Ø9, I26.92-I26.99 or I82.4Ø1-I82.4Z9

HAC   ØSR[T,U,V,W]Ø[7,K]Z when reported with SDx of I26.Ø2-I26.Ø9, I26.92-I26.99 or I82.4Ø1-I82.4Z9

HAC   ØSR[T,U,V,W]ØJ[9,A,Z] when reported with SDx of I26.Ø2-I26.Ø9, I26.92-I26.99 or I82.4Ø1-I82.4Z9

HAC   ØSR[R,S]Ø[1,3,J][9,A,Z] when reported with SDx of I26.Ø2-I26.Ø9, I26.92-I26.99, or I82.4Ø1-I82.4Z9

HAC   ØSR[R,S]Ø[7,K]Z when reported with SDx of I26.Ø2-I26.Ø9, I26.92-I26.99, or I82.4Ø1-I82.4Z9

See Appendix L for Procedure Combinations
⊞   ØSR[C,D]Ø[6,J,L,M,N][9,A,Z]
⊞   ØSR[C,D]ØEZ
⊞   ØSR[T,U,V,W]ØJ[9,A,Z]
⊞   ØSR[R,S]Ø[1,3,J][9,A,Z]

Ø   **Medical and Surgical**
S   **Lower Joints**
S   **Reposition**   Definition: Moving to its normal location, or other suitable location, all or a portion of a body part

                  Explanation: The body part is moved to a new location from an abnormal location, or from a normal location where it is not functioning correctly. The body part may or may not be cut out or off to be moved to the new location.

Body Part Character 4		Approach Character 5	Device Character 6	Qualifier Character 7
Ø Lumbar Vertebral Joint Lumbar facet joint **3 Lumbosacral Joint** Lumbosacral facet joint **5 Sacrococcygeal Joint** Sacrococcygeal symphysis **6 Coccygeal Joint** **7 Sacroiliac Joint, Right** **8 Sacroiliac Joint, Left**		**Ø** Open **3** Percutaneous **4** Percutaneous Endoscopic **X** External	**4** Internal Fixation Device **Z** No Device	**Z** No Qualifier
9 Hip Joint, Right Acetabulofemoral joint **B Hip Joint, Left** *See 9 Hip Joint, Right* **C Knee Joint, Right** Femoropatellar joint Femorotibial joint Lateral meniscus Medial meniscus Patellofemoral joint Tibiofemoral joint **D Knee Joint, Left** *See C Knee Joint, Right* **F Ankle Joint, Right** Inferior tibiofibular joint Talocrural joint **G Ankle Joint, Left** *See F Ankle Joint, Right* **H Tarsal Joint, Right** Calcaneocuboid joint Cuboideonavicular joint Cuneonavicular joint Intercuneiform joint Subtalar (talocalcaneal) joint Talocalcaneal (subtalar) joint Talocalcaneonavicular joint	**J Tarsal Joint, Left** *See H Tarsal Joint, Right* **K Tarsometatarsal Joint, Right** **L Tarsometatarsal Joint, Left** **M Metatarsal-Phalangeal Joint, Right** Metatarsophalangeal (MTP) joint **N Metatarsal-Phalangeal Joint, Left** *See M Metatarsal-Phalangeal Joint, Right* **P Toe Phalangeal Joint, Right** Interphalangeal (IP) joint **Q Toe Phalangeal Joint, Left** *See P Toe Phalangeal Joint, Right*	**Ø** Open **3** Percutaneous **4** Percutaneous Endoscopic **X** External	**4** Internal Fixation Device **5** External Fixation Device **Z** No Device	**Z** No Qualifier

Non-OR   ØSS[Ø,3,5,6,7,8][3,4,X][4,Z]Z
Non-OR   ØSS[9,B,C,D,F,G,H,J,K,L,M,N,P,Q][3,4,X][4,5,Z]Z

Ø   **Medical and Surgical**
S   **Lower Joints**
T   **Resection**   Definition: Cutting out or off, without replacement, all of a body part

                  Explanation: None

Body Part Character 4		Approach Character 5	Device Character 6	Qualifier Character 7
2 Lumbar Vertebral Disc **4 Lumbosacral Disc** **5 Sacrococcygeal Joint** Sacrococcygeal symphysis **6 Coccygeal Joint** **7 Sacroiliac Joint, Right** **8 Sacroiliac Joint, Left** **9 Hip Joint, Right** Acetabulofemoral joint **B Hip Joint, Left** *See 9 Hip Joint, Right* **C Knee Joint, Right** Femoropatellar joint Femorotibial joint Lateral meniscus Medial meniscus Patellofemoral joint Tibiofemoral joint **D Knee Joint, Left** *See C Knee Joint, Right* **F Ankle Joint, Right** Inferior tibiofibular joint Talocrural joint **G Ankle Joint, Left** *See F Ankle Joint, Right*	**H Tarsal Joint, Right** Calcaneocuboid joint Cuboideonavicular joint Cuneonavicular joint Intercuneiform joint Subtalar (talocalcaneal) joint Talocalcaneal (subtalar) joint Talocalcaneonavicular joint **J Tarsal Joint, Left** *See H Tarsal Joint, Right* **K Tarsometatarsal Joint, Right** **L Tarsometatarsal Joint, Left** **M Metatarsal-Phalangeal Joint, Right** Metatarsophalangeal (MTP) joint **N Metatarsal-Phalangeal Joint, Left** *See M Metatarsal-Phalangeal Joint, Right* **P Toe Phalangeal Joint, Right** Interphalangeal (IP) joint **Q Toe Phalangeal Joint, Left** *See P Toe Phalangeal Joint, Right*	**Ø** Open	**Z** No Device	**Z** No Qualifier

LC Limited Coverage   NC Noncovered   ⊞ Combination Member   HAC associated procedure   Combination Only   DRG Non-OR   Non-OR   New/Revised in GREEN
ICD-10-PCS 2020   601

ØSS–ØST

Lower Joints (side tab)

Ø   Medical and Surgical
S   Lower Joints
U   Supplement   Definition: Putting in or on biological or synthetic material that physically reinforces and/or augments the function of a portion of a body part

                   Explanation: The biological material is non-living, or is living and from the same individual. The body part may have been previously replaced, and the SUPPLEMENT procedure is performed to physically reinforce and/or augment the function of the replaced body part.

Body Part — Character 4	Approach — Character 5	Device — Character 6	Qualifier — Character 7

Ø Lumbar Vertebral Joint
  Lumbar facet joint
2 Lumbar Vertebral Disc
3 Lumbosacral Joint
  Lumbosacral facet joint
4 Lumbosacral Disc
5 Sacrococcygeal Joint
  Sacrococcygeal symphysis
6 Coccygeal Joint
7 Sacroiliac Joint, Right
8 Sacroiliac Joint, Left
F Ankle Joint, Right
  Inferior tibiofibular joint
  Talocrural joint
G Ankle Joint, Left
  See F Ankle Joint, Right
H Tarsal Joint, Right
  Calcaneocuboid joint
  Cuboideonavicular joint
  Cuneonavicular joint
  Intercuneiform joint
  Subtalar (talocalcaneal) joint
  Talocalcaneal (subtalar) joint
  Talocalcaneonavicular joint
	J Tarsal Joint, Left
	  See H Tarsal Joint, Right
	K Tarsometatarsal Joint, Right
	L Tarsometatarsal Joint, Left
	M Metatarsal-Phalangeal Joint, Right
	  Metatarsophalangeal (MTP) joint
	N Metatarsal-Phalangeal Joint, Left
	  See M Metatarsal-Phalangeal Joint, Right
	P Toe Phalangeal Joint, Right
	  Interphalangeal (IP) joint
	Q Toe Phalangeal Joint, Left
	  See P Toe Phalangeal Joint, Right
		Ø Open
		3 Percutaneous
		4 Percutaneous Endoscopic
			7 Autologous Tissue Substitute
			J Synthetic Substitute
			K Nonautologous Tissue Substitute
				Z No Qualifier

9 Hip Joint, Right ⊞
  Acetabulofemoral joint
B Hip Joint, Left ⊞
  See 9 Hip Joint, Right
	Ø Open	7 Autologous Tissue Substitute
		9 Liner
		B Resurfacing Device
		J Synthetic Substitute
		K Nonautologous Tissue Substitute
			Z No Qualifier

9 Hip Joint, Right
  Acetabulofemoral joint
B Hip Joint, Left
  See 9 Hip Joint, Right
	3 Percutaneous
	4 Percutaneous Endoscopic
		7 Autologous Tissue Substitute
		J Synthetic Substitute
		K Nonautologous Tissue Substitute
			Z No Qualifier

A Hip Joint, Acetabular Surface, Right ⊞ E Hip Joint, Acetabular Surface, Left ⊞ R Hip Joint, Femoral Surface, Right ⊞ S Hip Joint, Femoral Surface, Left ⊞	Ø Open	9 Liner B Resurfacing Device	Z No Qualifier

C Knee Joint, Right
  Femoropatellar joint
  Femorotibial joint
  Lateral meniscus
  Medial meniscus
  Patellofemoral joint
  Tibiofemoral joint
D Knee Joint, Left
  See C Knee Joint, Right
	Ø Open	7 Autologous Tissue Substitute
		J Synthetic Substitute
		K Nonautologous Tissue Substitute
			Z No Qualifier

C Knee Joint, Right
  Femoropatellar joint
  Femorotibial joint
  Lateral meniscus
  Medial meniscus
  Patellofemoral joint
  Tibiofemoral joint
D Knee Joint, Left
  See C Knee Joint, Right
	Ø Open	9 Liner	C Patellar Surface
			Z No Qualifier

ØSU Continued on next page

HAC	ØSU[9,B]ØBZ when reported with SDx of I26.Ø2-I26.Ø9, I26.92-I26.99, or I82.4Ø1-I82.4Z9	See Appendix L for Procedure Combinations
HAC	ØSU[A,E,R,S]ØBZ when reported with SDx of I26.Ø2-I26.Ø9, I26.92-I26.99, or I82.4Ø1-I82.4Z9	⊞ ØSU[9,B]Ø9Z ⊞ ØSU[A,E,R,S]Ø9Z

LC Limited Coverage   NC Noncovered   ⊞ Combination Member   HAC associated procedure   Combination Only   DRG Non-OR   Non-OR   New/Revised in GREEN

602   ICD-10-PCS 2020

Ø   Medical and Surgical
S   Lower Joints
U   Supplement

ØSU Continued

Definition: Putting in or on biological or synthetic material that physically reinforces and/or augments the function of a portion of a body part

Explanation: The biological material is non-living, or is living and from the same individual. The body part may have been previously replaced, and the SUPPLEMENT procedure is performed to physically reinforce and/or augment the function of the replaced body part.

Body Part Character 4		Approach Character 5	Device Character 6	Qualifier Character 7

C	**Knee Joint, Right**
	Femoropatellar joint
	Femorotibial joint
	Lateral meniscus
	Medial meniscus
	Patellofemoral joint
	Tibiofemoral joint
		3 Percutaneous
		4 Percutaneous Endoscopic
			7 Autologous Tissue
			     Substitute
			J Synthetic Substitute
			K Nonautologous Tissue
			     Substitute
				Z No Qualifier

D	**Knee Joint, Left** *See C Knee Joint, Right*			
T	**Knee Joint, Femoral Surface, Right** Femoropatellar joint Patellofemoral joint	**Ø** Open	**9** Liner	**Z** No Qualifier
U	**Knee Joint, Femoral Surface, Left** *See T Knee Joint, Femoral Surface, Right*			
V	**Knee Joint, Tibial Surface, Right** ⊞ Femorotibial joint Tibiofemoral joint			
W	**Knee Joint, Tibial Surface, Left** ⊞ *See V Knee Joint, Tibial Surface, Right*			

See Appendix L for Procedure Combinations
    ⊞   ØSU[V,W]Ø9Z

⸬ Limited Coverage   ⸬ Noncovered   ⊞ Combination Member   HAC associated procedure   Combination Only   DRG Non-OR   Non-OR   New/Revised in GREEN

ICD-10-PCS 2020   603

ØSU–ØSU

Lower Joints

Ø　**Medical and Surgical**
S　**Lower Joints**
W　**Revision**　　Definition: Correcting, to the extent possible, a portion of a malfunctioning device or the position of a displaced device

Explanation: Revision can include correcting a malfunctioning or displaced device by taking out or putting in components of the device such as a screw or pin

Body Part Character 4	Approach Character 5	Device Character 6	Qualifier Character 7
Ø Lumbar Vertebral Joint Lumbar facet joint **3 Lumbosacral Joint** Lumbosacral facet joint	Ø Open 3 Percutaneous 4 Percutaneous Endoscopic X External	Ø Drainage Device 3 Infusion Device 4 Internal Fixation Device 7 Autologous Tissue Substitute 8 Spacer A Interbody Fusion Device J Synthetic Substitute K Nonautologous Tissue Substitute	Z No Qualifier
2 Lumbar Vertebral Disc **4 Lumbosacral Disc**	Ø Open 3 Percutaneous 4 Percutaneous Endoscopic X External	Ø Drainage Device 3 Infusion Device 7 Autologous Tissue Substitute J Synthetic Substitute K Nonautologous Tissue Substitute	Z No Qualifier
5 Sacrococcygeal Joint Sacrococcygeal symphysis **6 Coccygeal Joint** **7 Sacroiliac Joint, Right** **8 Sacroiliac Joint, Left**	Ø Open 3 Percutaneous 4 Percutaneous Endoscopic X External	Ø Drainage Device 3 Infusion Device 4 Internal Fixation Device 7 Autologous Tissue Substitute 8 Spacer J Synthetic Substitute K Nonautologous Tissue Substitute	Z No Qualifier
9 Hip Joint, Right Acetabulofemoral joint **B Hip Joint, Left** *See 9 Hip Joint, Right*	Ø Open	Ø Drainage Device 3 Infusion Device 4 Internal Fixation Device 5 External Fixation Device 7 Autologous Tissue Substitute 8 Spacer 9 Liner B Resurfacing Device J Synthetic Substitute K Nonautologous Tissue Substitute	Z No Qualifier
9 Hip Joint, Right Acetabulofemoral joint **B Hip Joint, Left** *See 9 Hip Joint, Right*	3 Percutaneous 4 Percutaneous Endoscopic X External	Ø Drainage Device 3 Infusion Device 4 Internal Fixation Device 5 External Fixation Device 7 Autologous Tissue Substitute 8 Spacer J Synthetic Substitute K Nonautologous Tissue Substitute	Z No Qualifier
A Hip Joint, Acetabular Surface, Right **E Hip Joint, Acetabular Surface, Left** **R Hip Joint, Femoral Surface, Right** **S Hip Joint, Femoral Surface, Left** **T Knee Joint, Femoral Surface, Right** Femoropatellar joint Patellofemoral joint **U Knee Joint, Femoral Surface, Left** *See T Knee Joint, Femoral Surface, Right* **V Knee Joint, Tibial Surface, Right** Femorotibial joint Tibiofemoral joint **W Knee Joint, Tibial Surface, Left** *See V Knee Joint, Tibial Surface, Right*	Ø Open 3 Percutaneous 4 Percutaneous Endoscopic X External	J Synthetic Substitute	Z No Qualifier
C Knee Joint, Right Femoropatellar joint Femorotibial joint Lateral meniscus Medial meniscus Patellofemoral joint Tibiofemoral joint **D Knee Joint, Left** *See C Knee Joint, Right*	Ø Open	Ø Drainage Device 3 Infusion Device 4 Internal Fixation Device 5 External Fixation Device 7 Autologous Tissue Substitute 8 Spacer 9 Liner K Nonautologous Tissue Substitute	Z No Qualifier

ØSW Continued on next page

Non-OR　ØSW[Ø,3]X[Ø,3,4,7,8,A,J,K]Z
Non-OR　ØSW[2,4]X[Ø,3,7,J,K]Z
Non-OR　ØSW[5,6,7,8]X[Ø,3,4,7,8,J,K]Z
Non-OR　ØSW[9,B]X[Ø,3,4,5,7,8,J,K]Z
Non-OR　ØSW[A,E,R,S,T,U,V,W]XJZ

LC Limited Coverage　**NC** Noncovered　⊞ Combination Member　HAC associated procedure　Combination Only　DRG Non-OR　Non-OR　New/Revised in GREEN

604　　　　　　　　　　　　　　　　　　　　　　　　　　　　　　　　　　ICD-10-PCS 2020

Ø   **Medical and Surgical**
S   **Lower Joints**
W   **Revision**

ØSW Continued

Definition: Correcting, to the extent possible, a portion of a malfunctioning device or the position of a displaced device

Explanation: Revision can include correcting or malfunctioning or displaced device by taking out or putting in components of the device such as a screw or pin

Body Part Character 4	Approach Character 5	Device Character 6	Qualifier Character 7

C   **Knee Joint, Right**
    Femoropatellar joint
    Femorotibial joint
    Lateral meniscus
    Medial meniscus
    Patellofemoral joint
    Tibiofemoral joint
D   **Knee Joint, Left**
    See C Knee Joint, Right
	Ø Open	**J** Synthetic Substitute	**C** Patellar Surface
			Z No Qualifier

C   **Knee Joint, Right**
    Femoropatellar joint
    Femorotibial joint
    Lateral meniscus
    Medial meniscus
    Patellofemoral joint
    Tibiofemoral joint
D   **Knee Joint, Left**
    See C Knee Joint, Right
	3 Percutaneous
	4 Percutaneous Endoscopic
	X External
		Ø Drainage Device
		3 Infusion Device
		4 Internal Fixation Device
		5 External Fixation Device
		7 Autologous Tissue Substitute
		8 Spacer
		K Nonautologous Tissue Substitute
			Z No Qualifier

C   **Knee Joint, Right**
    Femoropatellar joint
    Femorotibial joint
    Lateral meniscus
    Medial meniscus
    Patellofemoral joint
    Tibiofemoral joint
D   **Knee Joint, Left**
    See C Knee Joint, Right
	3 Percutaneous
	4 Percutaneous Endoscopic
	X External
		J Synthetic Substitute	**C** Patellar Surface
			Z No Qualifier

F   **Ankle Joint, Right**
    Inferior tibiofibular joint
    Talocrural joint
G   **Ankle Joint, Left**
    See F Ankle Joint, Right
H   **Tarsal Joint, Right**
    Calcaneocuboid joint
    Cuboideonavicular joint
    Cuneonavicular joint
    Intercuneiform joint
    Subtalar (talocalcaneal) joint
    Talocalcaneal (subtalar) joint
    Talocalcaneonavicular joint
J   **Tarsal Joint, Left**
    See H Tarsal Joint, Right
K   **Tarsometatarsal Joint, Right**
L   **Tarsometatarsal Joint, Left**
M   **Metatarsal-Phalangeal Joint, Right**
    Metatarsophalangeal (MTP) joint
N   **Metatarsal-Phalangeal Joint, Left**
    See M Metatarsal-Phalangeal Joint, Right
P   **Toe Phalangeal Joint, Right**
    Interphalangeal (IP) joint
Q   **Toe Phalangeal Joint, Left**
    See P Toe Phalangeal Joint, Right
	Ø Open
	3 Percutaneous
	4 Percutaneous Endoscopic
	X External
		Ø Drainage Device
		3 Infusion Device
		4 Internal Fixation Device
		5 External Fixation Device
		7 Autologous Tissue Substitute
		8 Spacer
		J Synthetic Substitute
		K Nonautologous Tissue Substitute
			Z No Qualifier

Non-OR   ØSW[C,D]X[Ø,3,4,5,7,8,K]Z
Non-OR   ØSW[C,D]XJ[C,Z]
Non-OR   ØSW[F,G,H,J,K,L,M,N,P,Q]X[Ø,3,4,5,7,8,J,K]Z

LC Limited Coverage   NC Noncovered   ⊞ Combination Member   HAC associated procedure   Combination Only   DRG Non-OR   Non-OR   New/Revised in GREEN

ICD-10-PCS 2020   605

ØSW–ØSW

Urinary System ØT1–ØTY

Character Meanings

This Character Meaning table is provided as a guide to assist the user in the identification of character members that may be found in this section of code tables. It **SHOULD NOT** be used to build a PCS code.

Operation–Character 3	Body Part–Character 4	Approach–Character 5	Device–Character 6	Qualifier–Character 7
1 Bypass	Ø Kidney, Right	Ø Open	Ø Drainage Device	Ø Allogeneic
2 Change	1 Kidney, Left	3 Percutaneous	2 Monitoring Device	1 Syngeneic
5 Destruction	2 Kidneys, Bilateral	4 Percutaneous Endoscopic	3 Infusion Device	2 Zooplastic
7 Dilation	3 Kidney Pelvis, Right	7 Via Natural or Artificial Opening	7 Autologous Tissue Substitute	3 Kidney Pelvis, Right
8 Division	4 Kidney Pelvis, Left	8 Via Natural or Artificial Opening Endoscopic	C Extraluminal Device	4 Kidney Pelvis, Left
9 Drainage	5 Kidney	X External	D Intraluminal Device	6 Ureter, Right
B Excision	6 Ureter, Right		J Synthetic Substitute	7 Ureter, Left
C Extirpation	7 Ureter, Left		K Nonautologous Tissue Substitute	8 Colon
D Extraction	8 Ureters, Bilateral		L Artificial Sphincter	9 Colocutaneous
F Fragmentation	9 Ureter		M Stimulator Lead	A Ileum
H Insertion	B Bladder		Y Other Device	B Bladder
J Inspection	C Bladder Neck		Z No Device	C Ileocutaneous
L Occlusion	D Urethra			D Cutaneous
M Reattachment				X Diagnostic
N Release				Z No Qualifier
P Removal				
Q Repair				
R Replacement				
S Reposition				
T Resection				
U Supplement				
V Restriction				
W Revision				
Y Transplantation				

AHA Coding Clinic for table ØT1
2017, 3Q, 20	Creation of Indiana pouch
2017, 3Q, 21	Augmentation cystoplasty with Indiana pouch and continent urinary diversion
2017, 1Q, 37	Perineal urethrostomy
2015, 3Q, 34	Redo urinary diversion surgery via left ureteral reimplantation

AHA Coding Clinic for table ØT7
2017, 4Q, 111	Exchange of ureteral stent
2016, 2Q, 27	Exchange of ureteral stents
2015, 2Q, 8	Urinary calculi fragmentation and evacuation
2013, 4Q, 123	Urolift® procedure

AHA Coding Clinic for table ØT9
2017, 3Q, 19	Ureteral stent placement for urinary leakage
2017, 3Q, 20	Creation of Indiana pouch
2017, 3Q, 21	Augmentation cystoplasty with Indiana pouch and continent urinary diversion

AHA Coding Clinic for table ØTB
2016, 1Q, 19	Biopsy of neobladder malignancy
2015, 3Q, 34	Excision of Mitrofanoff polyp
2014, 2Q, 8	Ileoscopy with excision of polyp of Ileal loop urinary diversion

AHA Coding Clinic for table ØTC
2016, 3Q, 23	Ureteral stone migrating into bladder
2015, 2Q, 7	Urinary calculi fragmentation and evacuation
2015, 2Q, 8	Urinary calculi fragmentation and evacuation
2013, 4Q, 122	Laser lithotripsy with removal of fragments

AHA Coding Clinic for table ØTF
2015, 2Q, 7	Urinary calculi fragmentation and evacuation
2013, 4Q, 122	Extracorporeal shock wave lithotripsy
2013, 4Q, 122	Laser lithotripsy with removal of fragments

AHA Coding Clinic for table ØTP
2017, 4Q, 111	Exchange of ureteral stent
2016, 2Q, 27	Exchange of ureteral stents

AHA Coding Clinic for table ØTQ
2018, 2Q, 27	Dismembered pyeloplasty
2017, 1Q, 37	Perineal urethrostomy

AHA Coding Clinic for table ØTR
2017, 3Q, 20	Creation of Indiana pouch

AHA Coding Clinic for table ØTS
2019, 1Q, 29	Young-Dees-Leadbetter bladder neck reconstruction
2018, 2Q, 27	Dismembered pyeloplasty
2017, 1Q, 36	Dismembered pyeloplasty
2016, 1Q, 15	Pubovaginal sling placement

AHA Coding Clinic for table ØTT
2014, 3Q, 16	Hand-assisted laparoscopy nephroureterectomy

AHA Coding Clinic for table ØTU
2019, 1Q, 29	Young-Dees-Leadbetter bladder neck reconstruction
2017, 3Q, 21	Augmentation cystoplasty with Indiana pouch and continent urinary diversion

AHA Coding Clinic for table ØTV
2015, 2Q, 11	Cystourethroscopic Deflux® injection

Urinary System

Inferior vena cava
Aorta
Right kidney Ø
Left kidney 1
Left ureter 7
Right ureter 6
Urinary bladder B
Ureteral orifice 6, 7, 8, 9
Bladder neck C
Urethra D
Urogenital diaphragm

Kidney

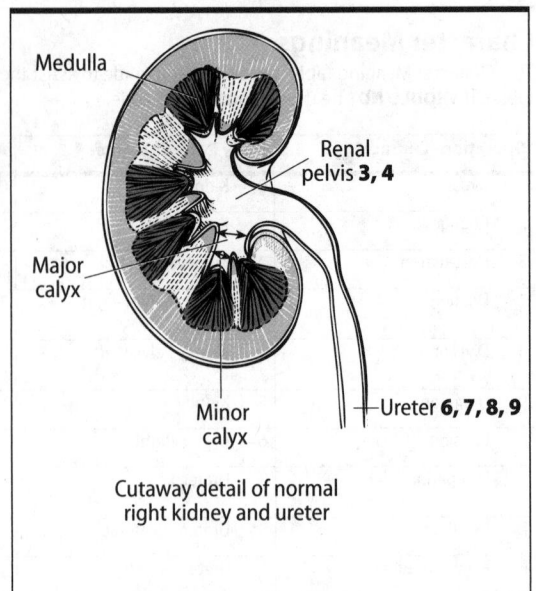

Medulla
Renal pelvis 3, 4
Major calyx
Minor calyx
Ureter 6, 7, 8, 9

Cutaway detail of normal
right kidney and ureter

Bladder

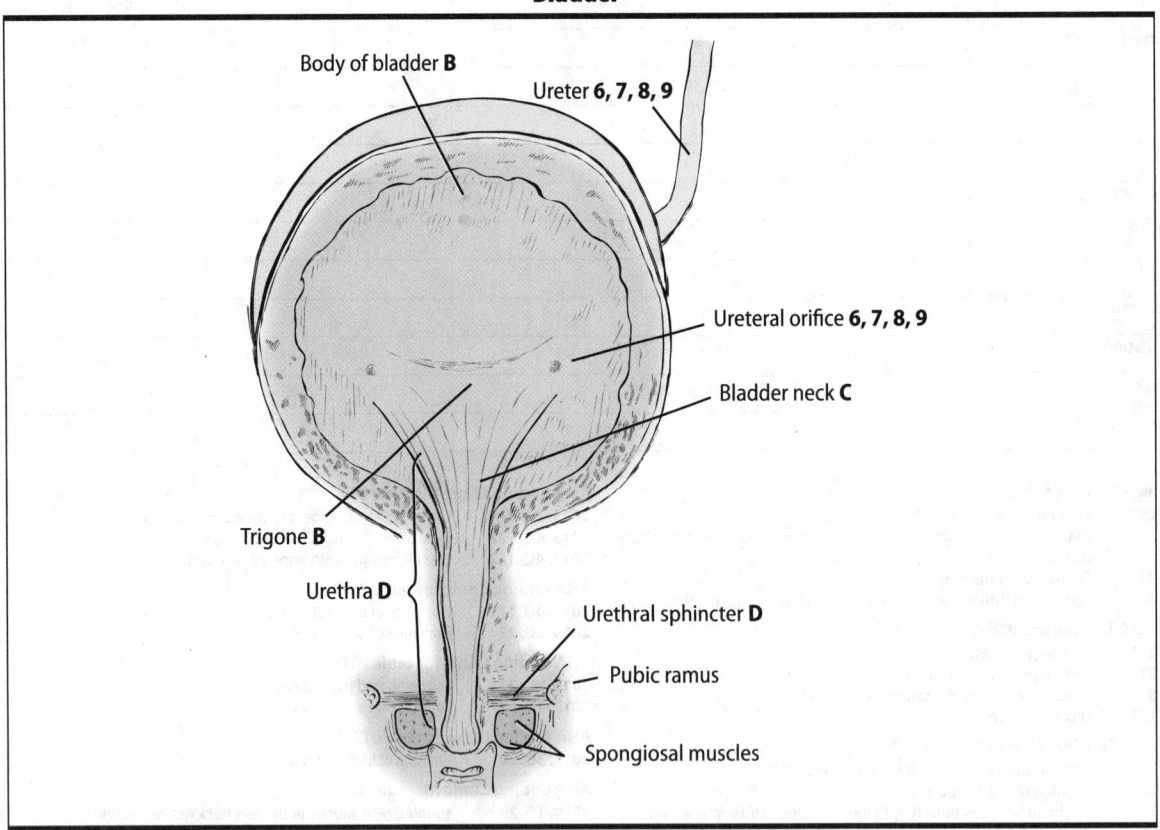

Body of bladder B
Ureter 6, 7, 8, 9
Ureteral orifice 6, 7, 8, 9
Bladder neck C
Trigone B
Urethra D
Urethral sphincter D
Pubic ramus
Spongiosal muscles

0   Medical and Surgical
T   Urinary System
1   Bypass

Definition: Altering the route of passage of the contents of a tubular body part

Explanation: Rerouting contents of a body part to a downstream area of the normal route, to a similar route and body part, or to an abnormal route and dissimilar body part. Includes one or more anastomoses, with or without the use of a device.

Body Part Character 4	Approach Character 5	Device Character 6	Qualifier Character 7
3 Kidney Pelvis, Right Ureteropelvic junction (UPJ) **4 Kidney Pelvis, Left** *See 3 Kidney Pelvis, Right*	**0 Open** **4 Percutaneous Endoscopic**	**7 Autologous Tissue Substitute** **J Synthetic Substitute** **K Nonautologous Tissue Substitute** **Z No Device**	**3 Kidney Pelvis, Right** **4 Kidney Pelvis, Left** **6 Ureter, Right** **7 Ureter, Left** **8 Colon** **9 Colocutaneous** **A Ileum** **B Bladder** **C Ileocutaneous** **D Cutaneous**
3 Kidney Pelvis, Right Ureteropelvic junction (UPJ) **4 Kidney Pelvis, Left** *See 3 Kidney Pelvis, Right*	**3 Percutaneous**	**J Synthetic Substitute**	**D Cutaneous**
6 Ureter, Right Ureteral orifice Ureterovesical orifice **7 Ureter, Left** *See 6 Ureter, Right* **8 Ureters, Bilateral** *See 6 Ureter, Right*	**0 Open** **4 Percutaneous Endoscopic**	**7 Autologous Tissue Substitute** **J Synthetic Substitute** **K Nonautologous Tissue Substitute** **Z No Device**	**6 Ureter, Right** **7 Ureter, Left** **8 Colon** **9 Colocutaneous** **A Ileum** **B Bladder** **C Ileocutaneous** **D Cutaneous**
6 Ureter, Right Ureteral orifice Ureterovesical orifice **7 Ureter, Left** *See 6 Ureter, Right* **8 Ureters, Bilateral** *See 6 Ureter, Right*	**3 Percutaneous**	**J Synthetic Substitute**	**D Cutaneous**
B Bladder Trigone of bladder	**0 Open** **4 Percutaneous Endoscopic**	**7 Autologous Tissue Substitute** **J Synthetic Substitute** **K Nonautologous Tissue Substitute** **Z No Device**	**9 Colocutaneous** **C Ileocutaneous** **D Cutaneous**
B Bladder Trigone of bladder	**3 Percutaneous**	**J Synthetic Substitute**	**D Cutaneous**

0   Medical and Surgical
T   Urinary System
2   Change

Definition: Taking out or off a device from a body part and putting back an identical or similar device in or on the same body part without cutting or puncturing the skin or a mucous membrane

Explanation: All CHANGE procedures are coded using the approach EXTERNAL

Body Part Character 4	Approach Character 5	Device Character 6	Qualifier Character 7
5 Kidney Renal calyx Renal capsule Renal cortex Renal segment **9 Ureter** Ureteral orifice Ureterovesical orifice **B Bladder** Trigone of bladder **D Urethra** Bulbourethral (Cowper's) gland Cowper's (bulbourethral) gland External urethral sphincter Internal urethral sphincter Membranous urethra Penile urethra Prostatic urethra	**X External**	**0 Drainage Device** **Y Other Device**	**Z No Qualifier**

Non-OR   All body part, approach, device, and qualifier values

---

LC Limited Coverage   **NC** Noncovered   ⊞ Combination Member   HAC associated procedure   Combination Only   DRG Non-OR   Non-OR   New/Revised in GREEN

ICD-10-PCS 2020   **609**

0T1–0T2

Urinary System

Ø   Medical and Surgical
T   Urinary System
5   Destruction   Definition: Physical eradication of all or a portion of a body part by the direct use of energy, force, or a destructive agent

Explanation: None of the body part is physically taken out

Body Part Character 4	Approach Character 5	Device Character 6	Qualifier Character 7
Ø Kidney, Right Renal calyx Renal capsule Renal cortex Renal segment **1 Kidney, Left** *See Ø Kidney, Right* **3 Kidney Pelvis, Right** Ureteropelvic junction (UPJ) **4 Kidney Pelvis, Left** *See 3 Kidney Pelvis, Right* **6 Ureter, Right** Ureteral orifice Ureterovesical orifice **7 Ureter, Left** *See 6 Ureter, Right* **B Bladder** Trigone of bladder **C Bladder Neck**	**Ø** Open **3** Percutaneous **4** Percutaneous Endoscopic **7** Via Natural or Artificial Opening **8** Via Natural or Artificial Opening Endoscopic	**Z** No Device	**Z** No Qualifier
D Urethra Bulbourethral (Cowper's) gland Cowper's (bulbourethral) gland External urethral sphincter Internal urethral sphincter Membranous urethra Penile urethra Prostatic urethra	**Ø** Open **3** Percutaneous **4** Percutaneous Endoscopic **7** Via Natural or Artificial Opening **8** Via Natural or Artificial Opening Endoscopic **X** External	**Z** No Device	**Z** No Qualifier

Non-OR   ØT5D[Ø,3,4,7,8,X]ZZ

Ø   Medical and Surgical
T   Urinary System
7   Dilation   Definition: Expanding an orifice or the lumen of a tubular body part

Explanation: The orifice can be a natural orifice or an artificially created orifice. Accomplished by stretching a tubular body part using intraluminal pressure or by cutting part of the orifice or wall of the tubular body part.

Body Part Character 4	Approach Character 5	Device Character 6	Qualifier Character 7
3 Kidney Pelvis, Right Ureteropelvic junction (UPJ) **4 Kidney Pelvis, Left** *See 3 Kidney Pelvis, Right* **6 Ureter, Right** Ureteral orifice Ureterovesical orifice **7 Ureter, Left** *See 6 Ureter, Right* **8 Ureters, Bilateral** *See 6 Ureter, Right* **B Bladder** Trigone of bladder **C Bladder Neck** **D Urethra** Bulbourethral (Cowper's) gland Cowper's (bulbourethral) gland External urethral sphincter Internal urethral sphincter Membranous urethra Penile urethra Prostatic urethra	**Ø** Open **3** Percutaneous **4** Percutaneous Endoscopic **7** Via Natural or Artificial Opening **8** Via Natural or Artificial Opening Endoscopic	**D** Intraluminal Device **Z** No Device	**Z** No Qualifier

Non-OR   ØT7[6,7,8][Ø,3,4,7]DZ   Non-OR   ØT7B7[D,Z]Z   Non-OR   ØT7[C,D][7,8][D,Z]Z
Non-OR   ØT7[6,7,8]7ZZ   Non-OR   ØT7C[Ø,3,4]ZZ
Non-OR   ØT788ZZ   Non-OR   ØT7[C,D][Ø,3,4]DZ

Ø   Medical and Surgical
T   Urinary System
8   Division   Definition: Cutting into a body part, without draining fluids and/or gases from the body part, in order to separate or transect a body part

Explanation: All or a portion of the body part is separated into two or more portions

Body Part Character 4	Approach Character 5	Device Character 6	Qualifier Character 7
2 Kidneys, Bilateral Renal calyx Renal capsule Renal cortex Renal segment **C Bladder Neck**	**Ø** Open **3** Percutaneous **4** Percutaneous Endoscopic	**Z** No Device	**Z** No Qualifier

Ø   Medical and Surgical
T   Urinary System
9   Drainage   Definition: Taking or letting out fluids and/or gases from a body part
                     Explanation: The qualifier DIAGNOSTIC is used to identify drainage procedures that are biopsies

Body Part Character 4	Approach Character 5	Device Character 6	Qualifier Character 7
Ø Kidney, Right Renal calyx Renal capsule Renal cortex Renal segment **1 Kidney, Left** *See Ø Kidney, Right* **3 Kidney Pelvis, Right** Ureteropelvic junction (UPJ) **4 Kidney Pelvis, Left** *See 3 Kidney Pelvis, Right* **6 Ureter, Right** Ureteral orifice Ureterovesical orifice **7 Ureter, Left** *See 6 Ureter, Right* **8 Ureters, Bilateral** *See 6 Ureter, Right* **B Bladder** Trigone of bladder **C Bladder Neck**	**Ø Open** **3 Percutaneous** **4 Percutaneous Endoscopic** **7 Via Natural or Artificial Opening** **8 Via Natural or Artificial Opening Endoscopic**	**Ø Drainage Device**	**Z No Qualifier**
Ø Kidney, Right Renal calyx Renal capsule Renal cortex Renal segment **1 Kidney, Left** *See Ø Kidney, Right* **3 Kidney Pelvis, Right** Ureteropelvic junction (UPJ) **4 Kidney Pelvis, Left** *See 3 Kidney Pelvis, Right* **6 Ureter, Right** Ureteral orifice Ureterovesical orifice **7 Ureter, Left** *See 6 Ureter, Right* **8 Ureters, Bilateral** *See 6 Ureter, Right* **B Bladder** Trigone of bladder **C Bladder Neck**	**Ø Open** **3 Percutaneous** **4 Percutaneous Endoscopic** **7 Via Natural or Artificial Opening** **8 Via Natural or Artificial Opening Endoscopic**	**Z No Device**	**X Diagnostic** **Z No Qualifier**
D Urethra Bulbourethral (Cowper's) gland Cowper's (bulbourethral) gland External urethral sphincter Internal urethral sphincter Membranous urethra Penile urethra Prostatic urethra	**Ø Open** **3 Percutaneous** **4 Percutaneous Endoscopic** **7 Via Natural or Artificial Opening** **8 Via Natural or Artificial Opening Endoscopic** **X External**	**Ø Drainage Device**	**Z No Qualifier**
D Urethra Bulbourethral (Cowper's) gland Cowper's (bulbourethral) gland External urethral sphincter Internal urethral sphincter Membranous urethra Penile urethra Prostatic urethra	**Ø Open** **3 Percutaneous** **4 Percutaneous Endoscopic** **7 Via Natural or Artificial Opening** **8 Via Natural or Artificial Opening Endoscopic** **X External**	**Z No Device**	**X Diagnostic** **Z No Qualifier**

Non-OR	ØT9[Ø,1,3,4]3ØZ
Non-OR	ØT9[6,7,8][Ø,3,4,7,8]ØZ
Non-OR	ØT9[B,C][3,4,7,8]ØZ
Non-OR	ØT9[Ø,1,3,4,6,7,8][3,4,7,8]ZX
Non-OR	ØT9[Ø,1,3,4][3,4]ZZ
Non-OR	ØT9[6,7,8]3ZZ
Non-OR	ØT9[B,C][3,4,7,8]ZZ
Non-OR	ØT9D3ØZ
Non-OR	ØT9D[Ø,3,4,7,8,X]ZX
Non-OR	ØT9D3ZZ

LC Limited Coverage   NC Noncovered   ⊞ Combination Member   HAC associated procedure   Combination Only   DRG Non-OR   Non-OR   New/Revised in GREEN

ICD-10-PCS 2020   611

ØT9–ØT9

Ø   **Medical and Surgical**
T   **Urinary System**
B   **Excision**   Definition: Cutting out or off, without replacement, a portion of a body part

                                Explanation: The qualifier DIAGNOSTIC is used to identify excision procedures that are biopsies

Body Part Character 4	Approach Character 5	Device Character 6	Qualifier Character 7

Ø **Kidney, Right**
    Renal calyx
    Renal capsule
    Renal cortex
    Renal segment
1 **Kidney, Left**
    See Ø Kidney, Right
3 **Kidney Pelvis, Right**
    Ureteropelvic junction (UPJ)
4 **Kidney Pelvis, Left**
    See 3 Kidney Pelvis, Right
6 **Ureter, Right**
    Ureteral orifice
    Ureterovesical orifice
7 **Ureter, Left**
    See 6 Ureter, Right
B **Bladder**
    Trigone of bladder
C **Bladder Neck**
	Ø Open
	3 Percutaneous
	4 Percutaneous Endoscopic
	7 Via Natural or Artificial Opening
	8 Via Natural or Artificial Opening
	    Endoscopic
		Z No Device	**X** Diagnostic
			Z No Qualifier

D **Urethra**
    Bulbourethral (Cowper's) gland
    Cowper's (bulbourethral) gland
    External urethral sphincter
    Internal urethral sphincter
    Membranous urethra
    Penile urethra
    Prostatic urethra
	Ø Open
	3 Percutaneous
	4 Percutaneous Endoscopic
	7 Via Natural or Artificial Opening
	8 Via Natural or Artificial Opening
	    Endoscopic
	X External
		Z No Device	**X** Diagnostic
			Z No Qualifier

Non-OR   ØTB[Ø,1,3,4,6,7][3,4,7,8]ZX
Non-OR   ØTBD[Ø,3,4,7,8,X]ZX

Ø   **Medical and Surgical**
T   **Urinary System**
C   **Extirpation**   Definition: Taking or cutting out solid matter from a body part

                                 Explanation: The solid matter may be an abnormal byproduct of a biological function or a foreign body; it may be imbedded in a body part or in the lumen of a tubular body part. The solid matter may or may not have been previously broken into pieces.

Body Part Character 4	Approach Character 5	Device Character 6	Qualifier Character 7

Ø **Kidney, Right**
    Renal calyx
    Renal capsule
    Renal cortex
    Renal segment
1 **Kidney, Left**
    See Ø Kidney, Right
3 **Kidney Pelvis, Right**
    Ureteropelvic junction (UPJ)
4 **Kidney Pelvis, Left**
    See 3 Kidney Pelvis, Right
6 **Ureter, Right**
    Ureteral orifice
    Ureterovesical orifice
7 **Ureter, Left**
    See 6 Ureter, Right
B **Bladder**
    Trigone of bladder
C **Bladder Neck**
	Ø Open
	3 Percutaneous
	4 Percutaneous Endoscopic
	7 Via Natural or Artificial Opening
	8 Via Natural or Artificial Opening
	    Endoscopic
		Z No Device	**Z** No Qualifier

D **Urethra**
    Bulbourethral (Cowper's) gland
    Cowper's (bulbourethral) gland
    External urethral sphincter
    Internal urethral sphincter
    Membranous urethra
    Penile urethra
    Prostatic urethra
	Ø Open
	3 Percutaneous
	4 Percutaneous Endoscopic
	7 Via Natural or Artificial Opening
	8 Via Natural or Artificial Opening
	    Endoscopic
	X External
		Z No Device	**Z** No Qualifier

Non-OR   ØTC[B,C][7,8]ZZ
Non-OR   ØTCD[7,8,X]ZZ

LC Limited Coverage   **NC** Noncovered   ⊞ Combination Member   HAC associated procedure   Combination Only   DRG Non-OR   Non-OR   New/Revised in GREEN

612   ICD-10-PCS 2020

Ø   **Medical and Surgical**
T   **Urinary System**
D   **Extraction**   Definition: Pulling or stripping out or off all or a portion of a body part by the use of force

                           Explanation: The qualifier DIAGNOSTIC is used to identify extraction procedures that are biopsies

Body Part Character 4	Approach Character 5	Device Character 6	Qualifier Character 7

Ø   **Kidney, Right**
    Renal calyx
    Renal capsule
    Renal cortex
    Renal segment
1   **Kidney, Left**
    See Ø Kidney, Right
	Ø Open
	3 Percutaneous
	4 Percutaneous Endoscopic
		Z No Device	**Z** No Qualifier

Ø   **Medical and Surgical**
T   **Urinary System**
F   **Fragmentation**   Definition: Breaking solid matter in a body part into pieces

                             Explanation: Physical force (e.g., manual, ultrasonic) applied directly or indirectly is used to break the solid matter into pieces. The solid matter may be an abnormal byproduct of a biological function or a foreign body. The pieces of solid matter are not taken out.

Body Part Character 4	Approach Character 5	Device Character 6	Qualifier Character 7

3   **Kidney Pelvis, Right**
    Ureteropelvic junction (UPJ)
4   **Kidney Pelvis, Left**
    See 3 Kidney Pelvis, Right
6   **Ureter, Right**
    Ureteral orifice
    Ureterovesical orifice
7   **Ureter, Left**
    See 6 Ureter, Right
B   **Bladder**
    Trigone of bladder
C   **Bladder Neck**
D   **Urethra**   `NC`
    Bulbourethral (Cowper's) gland
    Cowper's (bulbourethral) gland
    External urethral sphincter
    Internal urethral sphincter
    Membranous urethra
    Penile urethra
    Prostatic urethra
	Ø Open
	3 Percutaneous
	4 Percutaneous Endoscopic
	7 Via Natural or Artificial Opening
	8 Via Natural or Artificial Opening
	     Endoscopic
	X External
		Z No Device	**Z** No Qualifier

DRG Non-OR	ØTF[3,4,6,7,B,C]XZZ
Non-OR	ØTF[3,4][Ø,7,8]ZZ
Non-OR	ØTF[6,7,B,C][Ø,3,4,7,8]ZZ
Non-OR	ØTFD[Ø,3,4,7,8,X]ZZ
`NC`	ØTFDXZZ

`LC` Limited Coverage   `NC` Noncovered   ⊞ Combination Member   HAC associated procedure   Combination Only   DRG Non-OR   Non-OR   New/Revised in GREEN

ICD-10-PCS 2020   **613**

Urinary System

Ø   **Medical and Surgical**
T   **Urinary System**
H   **Insertion**   Definition: Putting in a nonbiological appliance that monitors, assists, performs, or prevents a physiological function but does not physically take the place of a body part
                       Explanation: None

Body Part Character 4	Approach Character 5	Device Character 6	Qualifier Character 7
5 Kidney Renal calyx Renal capsule Renal cortex Renal segment	**Ø** Open **3** Percutaneous **4** Percutaneous Endoscopic **7** Via Natural or Artificial Opening **8** Via Natural or Artificial Opening Endoscopic	**2** Monitoring Device **3** Infusion Device **Y** Other Device	**Z** No Qualifier
9 Ureter Ureteral orifice Ureterovesical orifice	**Ø** Open **3** Percutaneous **4** Percutaneous Endoscopic **7** Via Natural or Artificial Opening **8** Via Natural or Artificial Opening Endoscopic	**2** Monitoring Device **3** Infusion Device **M** Stimulator Lead **Y** Other Device	**Z** No Qualifier
B Bladder NC Trigone of bladder	**Ø** Open **3** Percutaneous **4** Percutaneous Endoscopic **7** Via Natural or Artificial Opening **8** Via Natural or Artificial Opening Endoscopic	**2** Monitoring Device **3** Infusion Device **L** Artificial Sphincter **M** Stimulator Lead **Y** Other Device	**Z** No Qualifier
C Bladder Neck	**Ø** Open **3** Percutaneous **4** Percutaneous Endoscopic **7** Via Natural or Artificial Opening **8** Via Natural or Artificial Opening Endoscopic	**L** Artificial Sphincter	**Z** No Qualifier
D Urethra Bulbourethral (Cowper's) gland Cowper's (bulbourethral) gland External urethral sphincter Internal urethral sphincter Membranous urethra Penile urethra Prostatic urethra	**Ø** Open **3** Percutaneous **4** Percutaneous Endoscopic **7** Via Natural or Artificial Opening **8** Via Natural or Artificial Opening Endoscopic	**2** Monitoring Device **3** Infusion Device **L** Artificial Sphincter **Y** Other Device	**Z** No Qualifier
D Urethra Bulbourethral (Cowper's) gland Cowper's (bulbourethral) gland External urethral sphincter Internal urethral sphincter Membranous urethra Penile urethra Prostatic urethra	**X** External	**2** Monitoring Device **3** Infusion Device **L** Artificial Sphincter	**Z** No Qualifier

Non-OR ØTH5Ø3Z		**Non-OR** ØTHB[3,4][3,Y]Z	
Non-OR ØTH5[3,4][3,Y]Z		**Non-OR** ØTHB7[2,3,Y]Z	
Non-OR ØTH57[2,3,Y]Z		**Non-OR** ØTHB8[2,3]Z	
Non-OR ØTH58[2,3]Z		**Non-OR** ØTHDØ3Z	
Non-OR ØTH9Ø3Z		**Non-OR** ØTHD[3,4][3,Y]Z	
Non-OR ØTH9[3,4][3,Y]Z		**Non-OR** ØTHD[7,8][2,3,Y]Z	
Non-OR ØTH97[2,3,Y]Z		**Non-OR** ØTHDX3Z	
Non-OR ØTH98[2,3]Z		NC ØTHB[Ø,3,4,7,8]MZ	
Non-OR ØTHBØ3Z			

Ø   **Medical and Surgical**
T   **Urinary System**
J   **Inspection**   Definition: Visually and/or manually exploring a body part

Explanation: Visual exploration may be performed with or without optical instrumentation. Manual exploration may be performed directly or through intervening body layers.

Body Part Character 4	Approach Character 5	Device Character 6	Qualifier Character 7
5 Kidney Renal calyx Renal capsule Renal cortex Renal segment **9 Ureter** Ureteral orifice Ureterovesical orifice **B Bladder** Trigone of bladder **D Urethra** Bulbourethral (Cowper's) gland Cowper's (bulbourethral) gland External urethral sphincter Internal urethral sphincter Membranous urethra Penile urethra Prostatic urethra	**Ø** Open **3** Percutaneous **4** Percutaneous Endoscopic **7** Via Natural or Artificial Opening **8** Via Natural or Artificial Opening Endoscopic **X** External	**Z** No Device	**Z** No Qualifier

Non-OR   ØTJ[5,9,D][3,4,7,8,X]ZZ
Non-OR   ØTJB[3,7,8,X]ZZ

Ø   **Medical and Surgical**
T   **Urinary System**
L   **Occlusion**   Definition: Completely closing an orifice or the lumen of a tubular body part

Explanation: The orifice can be a natural orifice or an artificially created orifice

Body Part Character 4	Approach Character 5	Device Character 6	Qualifier Character 7
3 Kidney Pelvis, Right Ureteropelvic junction (UPJ) **4 Kidney Pelvis, Left** *See 3 Kidney Pelvis, Right* **6 Ureter, Right** Ureteral orifice Ureterovesical orifice **7 Ureter, Left** *See 6 Ureter, Right* **B Bladder** Trigone of bladder **C Bladder Neck**	**Ø** Open **3** Percutaneous **4** Percutaneous Endoscopic	**C** Extraluminal Device **D** Intraluminal Device **Z** No Device	**Z** No Qualifier
3 Kidney Pelvis, Right Ureteropelvic junction (UPJ) **4 Kidney Pelvis, Left** *See 3 Kidney Pelvis, Right* **6 Ureter, Right** Ureteral orifice Ureterovesical orifice **7 Ureter, Left** *See 6 Ureter, Right* **B Bladder** Trigone of bladder **C Bladder Neck**	**7** Via Natural or Artificial Opening **8** Via Natural or Artificial Opening Endoscopic	**D** Intraluminal Device **Z** No Device	**Z** No Qualifier
D Urethra Bulbourethral (Cowper's) gland Cowper's (bulbourethral) gland External urethral sphincter Internal urethral sphincter Membranous urethra Penile urethra Prostatic urethra	**Ø** Open **3** Percutaneous **4** Percutaneous Endoscopic **X** External	**C** Extraluminal Device **D** Intraluminal Device **Z** No Device	**Z** No Qualifier
D Urethra Bulbourethral (Cowper's) gland Cowper's (bulbourethral) gland External urethral sphincter Internal urethral sphincter Membranous urethra Penile urethra Prostatic urethra	**7** Via Natural or Artificial Opening **8** Via Natural or Artificial Opening Endoscopic	**D** Intraluminal Device **Z** No Device	**Z** No Qualifier

LC Limited Coverage   NC Noncovered   ⊞ Combination Member   HAC associated procedure   Combination Only   DRG Non-OR   Non-OR   New/Revised in GREEN

ICD-10-PCS 2020   **615**

Urinary System

Ø   Medical and Surgical
T   Urinary System
M   Reattachment   Definition: Putting back in or on all or a portion of a separated body part to its normal location or other suitable location
Explanation: Vascular circulation and nervous pathways may or may not be reestablished

Body Part Character 4	Approach Character 5	Device Character 6	Qualifier Character 7

Ø Kidney, Right
  Renal calyx
  Renal capsule
  Renal cortex
  Renal segment
1 Kidney, Left
  See Ø Kidney, Right
2 Kidneys, Bilateral
  See Ø Kidney, Right
3 Kidney Pelvis, Right
  Ureteropelvic junction (UPJ)
4 Kidney Pelvis, Left
  See 3 Kidney Pelvis, Right
6 Ureter, Right
  Ureteral orifice
  Ureterovesical orifice
7 Ureter, Left
  See 6 Ureter, Right
8 Ureters, Bilateral
  See 6 Ureter, Right
B Bladder
  Trigone of bladder
C Bladder Neck
D Urethra
  Bulbourethral (Cowper's) gland
  Cowper's (bulbourethral) gland
  External urethral sphincter
  Internal urethral sphincter
  Membranous urethra
  Penile urethra
  Prostatic urethra
	Ø Open
	4 Percutaneous Endoscopic
		Z No Device	**Z No Qualifier**

Ø   Medical and Surgical
T   Urinary System
N   Release   Definition: Freeing a body part from an abnormal physical constraint by cutting or by the use of force
Explanation: Some of the restraining tissue may be taken out but none of the body part is taken out

Body Part Character 4	Approach Character 5	Device Character 6	Qualifier Character 7

Ø Kidney, Right
  Renal calyx
  Renal capsule
  Renal cortex
  Renal segment
1 Kidney, Left
  See Ø Kidney, Right
3 Kidney Pelvis, Right
  Ureteropelvic junction (UPJ)
4 Kidney Pelvis, Left
  See 3 Kidney Pelvis, Right
6 Ureter, Right
  Ureteral orifice
  Ureterovesical orifice
7 Ureter, Left
  See 6 Ureter, Right
B Bladder
  Trigone of bladder
C Bladder Neck
	Ø Open
	3 Percutaneous
	4 Percutaneous Endoscopic
	7 Via Natural or Artificial Opening
	8 Via Natural or Artificial Opening Endoscopic
		Z No Device	**Z No Qualifier**

D Urethra
  Bulbourethral (Cowper's) gland
  Cowper's (bulbourethral) gland
  External urethral sphincter
  Internal urethral sphincter
  Membranous urethra
  Penile urethra
  Prostatic urethra
	Ø Open
	3 Percutaneous
	4 Percutaneous Endoscopic
	7 Via Natural or Artificial Opening
	8 Via Natural or Artificial Opening Endoscopic
	X External
		Z No Device	**Z No Qualifier**

Ø   Medical and Surgical
T   Urinary System
P   Removal   Definition: Taking out or off a device from a body part

Explanation: If a device is taken out and a similar device put in without cutting or puncturing the skin or mucous membrane, the procedure is coded to the root operation CHANGE. Otherwise, the procedure for taking out the device is coded to the root operation REMOVAL.

Body Part Character 4	Approach Character 5	Device Character 6	Qualifier Character 7
5 Kidney Renal calyx Renal capsule Renal cortex Renal segment	Ø Open 3 Percutaneous 4 Percutaneous Endoscopic 7 Via Natural or Artificial Opening 8 Via Natural or Artificial Opening Endoscopic	Ø Drainage Device 2 Monitoring Device 3 Infusion Device 7 Autologous Tissue Substitute C Extraluminal Device D Intraluminal Device J Synthetic Substitute K Nonautologous Tissue Substitute Y Other Device	Z No Qualifier
5 Kidney Renal calyx Renal capsule Renal cortex Renal segment	X External	Ø Drainage Device 2 Monitoring Device 3 Infusion Device D Intraluminal Device	Z No Qualifier
9 Ureter Ureteral orifice Ureterovesical orifice	Ø Open 3 Percutaneous 4 Percutaneous Endoscopic 7 Via Natural or Artificial Opening 8 Via Natural or Artificial Opening Endoscopic	Ø Drainage Device 2 Monitoring Device 3 Infusion Device 7 Autologous Tissue Substitute C Extraluminal Device D Intraluminal Device J Synthetic Substitute K Nonautologous Tissue Substitute M Stimulator Lead Y Other Device	Z No Qualifier
9 Ureter Ureteral orifice Ureterovesical orifice	X External	Ø Drainage Device 2 Monitoring Device 3 Infusion Device D Intraluminal Device M Stimulator Lead	Z No Qualifier
B Bladder NC Trigone of bladder	Ø Open 3 Percutaneous 4 Percutaneous Endoscopic 7 Via Natural or Artificial Opening 8 Via Natural or Artificial Opening Endoscopic	Ø Drainage Device 2 Monitoring Device 3 Infusion Device 7 Autologous Tissue Substitute C Extraluminal Device D Intraluminal Device J Synthetic Substitute K Nonautologous Tissue Substitute L Artificial Sphincter M Stimulator Lead Y Other Device	Z No Qualifier
B Bladder Trigone of bladder	X External	Ø Drainage Device 2 Monitoring Device 3 Infusion Device D Intraluminal Device L Artificial Sphincter M Stimulator Lead	Z No Qualifier
D Urethra Bulbourethral (Cowper's) gland Cowper's (bulbourethral) gland External urethral sphincter Internal urethral sphincter Membranous urethra Penile urethra Prostatic urethra	Ø Open 3 Percutaneous 4 Percutaneous Endoscopic 7 Via Natural or Artificial Opening 8 Via Natural or Artificial Opening Endoscopic	Ø Drainage Device 2 Monitoring Device 3 Infusion Device 7 Autologous Tissue Substitute C Extraluminal Device D Intraluminal Device J Synthetic Substitute K Nonautologous Tissue Substitute L Artificial Sphincter Y Other Device	Z No Qualifier
D Urethra Bulbourethral (Cowper's) gland Cowper's (bulbourethral) gland External urethral sphincter Internal urethral sphincter Membranous urethra Penile urethra Prostatic urethra	X External	Ø Drainage Device 2 Monitoring Device 3 Infusion Device D Intraluminal Device L Artificial Sphincter	Z No Qualifier

Non-OR ØTP5[3,4,7]YZ	**Non-OR** ØTP9[7,8][Ø,2,3,D]Z	**Non-OR** ØTPB[7,8][Ø,2,3,D]Z	**Non-OR** ØTPD[7,8][Ø,2,3,D,Y]Z
Non-OR ØTP5[7,8][Ø,2,3,D]Z	**Non-OR** ØTP9X[Ø,2,3,D]Z	**Non-OR** ØTPBX[Ø,2,3,D,L]Z	**Non-OR** ØTPDX[Ø,2,3,D]Z
Non-OR ØTP5X[Ø,2,3,D]Z	**Non-OR** ØTPB[3,4,7]YZ	**Non-OR** ØTPD[3,4]YZ	**NC** ØTPB[Ø,3,4,7,8]MZ
Non-OR ØTP9[3,4,7]YZ			

LC Limited Coverage   **NC** Noncovered   ⊞ Combination Member   HAC associated procedure   Combination Only   DRG Non-OR   Non-OR   New/Revised in GREEN

ICD-10-PCS 2020   617

ØTP–ØTP

Urinary System

Ø Medical and Surgical
T Urinary System
Q Repair Definition: Restoring, to the extent possible, a body part to its normal anatomic structure and function
Explanation: Used only when the method to accomplish the repair is not one of the other root operations

Body Part Character 4	Approach Character 5	Device Character 6	Qualifier Character 7
Ø Kidney, Right Renal calyx Renal capsule Renal cortex Renal segment **1 Kidney, Left** *See Ø Kidney, Right* **3 Kidney Pelvis, Right** Ureteropelvic junction (UPJ) **4 Kidney Pelvis, Left** *See 3 Kidney Pelvis, Right* **6 Ureter, Right** Ureteral orifice Ureterovesical orifice **7 Ureter, Left** *See 6 Ureter, Right* **B Bladder** ⊞ Trigone of bladder **C Bladder Neck**	**Ø Open** **3 Percutaneous** **4 Percutaneous Endoscopic** **7 Via Natural or Artificial Opening** **8 Via Natural or Artificial Opening Endoscopic**	**Z No Device**	**Z No Qualifier**
D Urethra Bulbourethral (Cowper's) gland Cowper's (bulbourethral) gland External urethral sphincter Internal urethral sphincter Membranous urethra Penile urethra Prostatic urethra	**Ø Open** **3 Percutaneous** **4 Percutaneous Endoscopic** **7 Via Natural or Artificial Opening** **8 Via Natural or Artificial Opening Endoscopic** **X External**	**Z No Device**	**Z No Qualifier**

See Appendix L for Procedure Combinations
  ⊞ ØTQB[Ø,3,4]ZZ

Ø Medical and Surgical
T Urinary System
R Replacement Definition: Putting in or on biological or synthetic material that physically takes the place and/or function of all or a portion of a body part
Explanation: The body part may have been taken out or replaced, or may be taken out, physically eradicated, or rendered nonfunctional during the REPLACEMENT procedure. A REMOVAL procedure is coded for taking out the device used in a previous replacement procedure.

Body Part Character 4	Approach Character 5	Device Character 6	Qualifier Character 7
3 Kidney Pelvis, Right Ureteropelvic junction (UPJ) **4 Kidney Pelvis, Left** *See 3 Kidney Pelvis, Right* **6 Ureter, Right** Ureteral orifice Ureterovesical orifice **7 Ureter, Left** *See 6 Ureter, Right* **B Bladder** Trigone of bladder **C Bladder Neck**	**Ø Open** **4 Percutaneous Endoscopic** **7 Via Natural or Artificial Opening** **8 Via Natural or Artificial Opening Endoscopic**	**7 Autologous Tissue Substitute** **J Synthetic Substitute** **K Nonautologous Tissue Substitute**	**Z No Qualifier**
D Urethra Bulbourethral (Cowper's) gland Cowper's (bulbourethral) gland External urethral sphincter Internal urethral sphincter Membranous urethra Penile urethra Prostatic urethra	**Ø Open** **4 Percutaneous Endoscopic** **7 Via Natural or Artificial Opening** **8 Via Natural or Artificial Opening Endoscopic** **X External**	**7 Autologous Tissue Substitute** **J Synthetic Substitute** **K Nonautologous Tissue Substitute**	**Z No Qualifier**

Ø   **Medical and Surgical**
T   **Urinary System**
S   **Reposition**   Definition: Moving to its normal location, or other suitable location, all or a portion of a body part

         Explanation: The body part is moved to a new location from an abnormal location, or from a normal location where it is not functioning correctly. The body part may or may not be cut out or off to be moved to the new location.

Body Part Character 4	Approach Character 5	Device Character 6	Qualifier Character 7
Ø **Kidney, Right** Renal calyx Renal capsule Renal cortex Renal segment 1 **Kidney, Left** *See Ø Kidney, Right* 2 **Kidneys, Bilateral** *See Ø Kidney, Right* 3 **Kidney Pelvis, Right** Ureteropelvic junction (UPJ) 4 **Kidney Pelvis, Left** *See 3 Kidney Pelvis, Right* 6 **Ureter, Right** Ureteral orifice Ureterovesical orifice 7 **Ureter, Left** *See 6 Ureter, Right* 8 **Ureters, Bilateral** *See 6 Ureter, Right* B **Bladder** Trigone of bladder C **Bladder Neck** D **Urethra** Bulbourethral (Cowper's) gland Cowper's (bulbourethral) gland External urethral sphincter Internal urethral sphincter Membranous urethra Penile urethra Prostatic urethra	Ø **Open** 4 **Percutaneous Endoscopic**	Z **No Device**	Z **No Qualifier**

Ø   **Medical and Surgical**
T   **Urinary System**
T   **Resection**   Definition: Cutting out or off, without replacement, all of a body part

         Explanation: None

Body Part Character 4	Approach Character 5	Device Character 6	Qualifier Character 7
Ø **Kidney, Right** Renal calyx Renal capsule Renal cortex Renal segment 1 **Kidney, Left** *See Ø Kidney, Right* 2 **Kidneys, Bilateral** *See Ø Kidney, Right*	Ø **Open** 4 **Percutaneous Endoscopic**	Z **No Device**	Z **No Qualifier**
3 **Kidney Pelvis, Right** Ureteropelvic junction (UPJ) 4 **Kidney Pelvis, Left** *See 3 Kidney Pelvis, Right* 6 **Ureter, Right** Ureteral orifice Ureterovesical orifice 7 **Ureter, Left** *See 6 Ureter, Right* B **Bladder** ⊞ Trigone of bladder C **Bladder Neck** D Urethra Bulbourethral (Cowper's) gland Cowper's (bulbourethral) gland External urethral sphincter Internal urethral sphincter Membranous urethra Penile urethra Prostatic urethra	Ø **Open** 4 **Percutaneous Endoscopic** 7 **Via Natural or Artificial Opening** 8 **Via Natural or Artificial Opening Endoscopic**	Z **No Device**	Z **No Qualifier**

Non-OR   ØTTD[4,7,8]ZZ

See Appendix L for Procedure Combinations
    Combo-only   ØTTDØZZ
    ⊞   ØTTBØZZ

LC Limited Coverage   **NC** Noncovered   ⊞ Combination Member   HAC associated procedure   Combination Only   DRG Non-OR   Non-OR   New/Revised in **GREEN**

ICD-10-PCS 2020   619

Urinary System (side tab)

Ø **Medical and Surgical**
T **Urinary System**
U **Supplement**　　Definition: Putting in or on biological or synthetic material that physically reinforces and/or augments the function of a portion of a body part
　　　　　Explanation: The biological material is non-living, or is living and from the same individual. The body part may have been previously replaced, and the SUPPLEMENT procedure is performed to physically reinforce and/or augment the function of the replaced body part.

Body Part Character 4	Approach Character 5	Device Character 6	Qualifier Character 7
3 Kidney Pelvis, Right 　Ureteropelvic junction (UPJ) **4** Kidney Pelvis, Left 　*See 3 Kidney Pelvis, Right* **6** Ureter, Right 　Ureteral orifice 　Ureterovesical orifice **7** Ureter, Left 　*See 6 Ureter, Right* **B** Bladder 　Trigone of bladder **C** Bladder Neck	**Ø** Open **4** Percutaneous Endoscopic **7** Via Natural or Artificial Opening **8** Via Natural or Artificial Opening Endoscopic	**7** Autologous Tissue Substitute **J** Synthetic Substitute **K** Nonautologous Tissue Substitute	**Z** No Qualifier
D Urethra 　Bulbourethral (Cowper's) gland 　Cowper's (bulbourethral) gland 　External urethral sphincter 　Internal urethral sphincter 　Membranous urethra 　Penile urethra 　Prostatic urethra	**Ø** Open **4** Percutaneous Endoscopic **7** Via Natural or Artificial Opening **8** Via Natural or Artificial Opening Endoscopic **X** External	**7** Autologous Tissue Substitute **J** Synthetic Substitute **K** Nonautologous Tissue Substitute	**Z** No Qualifier

Ø **Medical and Surgical**
T **Urinary System**
V **Restriction**　　Definition: Partially closing an orifice or the lumen of a tubular body part
　　　　　Explanation: The orifice can be a natural orifice or an artificially created orifice

Body Part Character 4	Approach Character 5	Device Character 6	Qualifier Character 7
3 Kidney Pelvis, Right 　Ureteropelvic junction (UPJ) **4** Kidney Pelvis, Left 　*See 3 Kidney Pelvis, Right* **6** Ureter, Right 　Ureteral orifice 　Ureterovesical orifice **7** Ureter, Left 　*See 6 Ureter, Right* **B** Bladder 　Trigone of bladder **C** Bladder Neck	**Ø** Open **3** Percutaneous **4** Percutaneous Endoscopic	**C** Extraluminal Device **D** Intraluminal Device **Z** No Device	**Z** No Qualifier
3 Kidney Pelvis, Right 　Ureteropelvic junction (UPJ) **4** Kidney Pelvis, Left 　*See 3 Kidney Pelvis, Right* **6** Ureter, Right 　Ureteral orifice 　Ureterovesical orifice **7** Ureter, Left 　*See 6 Ureter, Right* **B** Bladder 　Trigone of bladder **C** Bladder Neck	**7** Via Natural or Artificial Opening **8** Via Natural or Artificial Opening Endoscopic	**D** Intraluminal Device **Z** No Device	**Z** No Qualifier
D Urethra 　Bulbourethral (Cowper's) gland 　Cowper's (bulbourethral) gland 　External urethral sphincter 　Internal urethral sphincter 　Membranous urethra 　Penile urethra 　Prostatic urethra	**Ø** Open **3** Percutaneous **4** Percutaneous Endoscopic	**C** Extraluminal Device **D** Intraluminal Device **Z** No Device	**Z** No Qualifier
D Urethra 　Bulbourethral (Cowper's) gland 　Cowper's (bulbourethral) gland 　External urethral sphincter 　Internal urethral sphincter 　Membranous urethra 　Penile urethra 　Prostatic urethra	**7** Via Natural or Artificial Opening **8** Via Natural or Artificial Opening Endoscopic	**D** Intraluminal Device **Z** No Device	**Z** No Qualifier
D Urethra 　Bulbourethral (Cowper's) gland 　Cowper's (bulbourethral) gland 　External urethral sphincter 　Internal urethral sphincter 　Membranous urethra 　Penile urethra 　Prostatic urethra	**X** External	**Z** No Device	**Z** No Qualifier

Ø   **Medical and Surgical**
T   **Urinary System**
W   **Revision**   Definition: Correcting, to the extent possible, a portion of a malfunctioning device or the position of a displaced device
                       Explanation: Revision can include correcting a malfunctioning or displaced device by taking out or putting in components of the device such as a screw or pin

Body Part Character 4	Approach Character 5	Device Character 6	Qualifier Character 7
5 **Kidney** Renal calyx Renal capsule Renal cortex Renal segment	**Ø** Open **3** Percutaneous **4** Percutaneous Endoscopic **7** Via Natural or Artificial Opening **8** Via Natural or Artificial Opening Endoscopic	**Ø** Drainage Device **2** Monitoring Device **3** Infusion Device **7** Autologous Tissue Substitute **C** Extraluminal Device **D** Intraluminal Device **J** Synthetic Substitute **K** Nonautologous Tissue Substitute **Y** Other Device	**Z** No Qualifier
5 **Kidney** Renal calyx Renal capsule Renal cortex Renal segment	**X** External	**Ø** Drainage Device **2** Monitoring Device **3** Infusion Device **7** Autologous Tissue Substitute **C** Extraluminal Device **D** Intraluminal Device **J** Synthetic Substitute **K** Nonautologous Tissue Substitute	**Z** No Qualifier
9 **Ureter** Ureteral orifice Ureterovesical orifice	**Ø** Open **3** Percutaneous **4** Percutaneous Endoscopic **7** Via Natural or Artificial Opening **8** Via Natural or Artificial Opening Endoscopic	**Ø** Drainage Device **2** Monitoring Device **3** Infusion Device **7** Autologous Tissue Substitute **C** Extraluminal Device **D** Intraluminal Device **J** Synthetic Substitute **K** Nonautologous Tissue Substitute **M** Stimulator Lead **Y** Other Device	**Z** No Qualifier
9 **Ureter** Ureteral orifice Ureterovesical orifice	**X** External	**Ø** Drainage Device **2** Monitoring Device **3** Infusion Device **7** Autologous Tissue Substitute **C** Extraluminal Device **D** Intraluminal Device **J** Synthetic Substitute **K** Nonautologous Tissue Substitute **M** Stimulator Lead	**Z** No Qualifier
B **Bladder** Trigone of bladder	**Ø** Open **3** Percutaneous **4** Percutaneous Endoscopic **7** Via Natural or Artificial Opening **8** Via Natural or Artificial Opening Endoscopic	**Ø** Drainage Device **2** Monitoring Device **3** Infusion Device **7** Autologous Tissue Substitute **C** Extraluminal Device **D** Intraluminal Device **J** Synthetic Substitute **K** Nonautologous Tissue Substitute **L** Artificial Sphincter **M** Stimulator Lead **Y** Other Device	**Z** No Qualifier
B **Bladder** Trigone of bladder	**X** External	**Ø** Drainage Device **2** Monitoring Device **3** Infusion Device **7** Autologous Tissue Substitute **C** Extraluminal Device **D** Intraluminal Device **J** Synthetic Substitute **K** Nonautologous Tissue Substitute **L** Artificial Sphincter **M** Stimulator Lead	**Z** No Qualifier

ØTW Continued on next page

Non-OR ØTW5[3,4,7]YZ	**Non-OR** ØTW9X[Ø,2,3,7,C,D,J,K,M]Z
Non-OR ØTW5X[Ø,2,3,7,C,D,J,K]Z	**Non-OR** ØTWB[3,4,7]YZ
Non-OR ØTW9[3,4,7]YZ	**Non-OR** ØTWBX[Ø,2,3,7,C,D,J,K,L,M]Z

LC Limited Coverage   **NC** Noncovered   ⊞ Combination Member   HAC associated procedure   Combination Only   DRG Non-OR   Non-OR   New/Revised in GREEN

ICD-10-PCS 2020   **621**

ØTW–ØTW

Urinary System

ØTW Continued

Ø   **Medical and Surgical**
T   **Urinary System**
W   **Revision**   Definition: Correcting, to the extent possible, a portion of a malfunctioning device or the position of a displaced device

Explanation: Revision can include correcting a malfunctioning or displaced device by taking out or putting in components of the device such as a screw or pin

Body Part Character 4	Approach Character 5	Device Character 6	Qualifier Character 7
D **Urethra** Bulbourethral (Cowper's) gland Cowper's (bulbourethral) gland External urethral sphincter Internal urethral sphincter Membranous urethra Penile urethra Prostatic urethra	**Ø** **Open** **3** **Percutaneous** **4** **Percutaneous Endoscopic** **7** **Via Natural or Artificial Opening** **8** **Via Natural or Artificial Opening** **Endoscopic**	**Ø** **Drainage Device** **2** **Monitoring Device** **3** **Infusion Device** **7** **Autologous Tissue Substitute** **C** **Extraluminal Device** **D** **Intraluminal Device** **J** **Synthetic Substitute** **K** **Nonautologous Tissue Substitute** **L** **Artificial Sphincter** **Y** **Other Device**	**Z** **No Qualifier**
D **Urethra** Bulbourethral (Cowper's) gland Cowper's (bulbourethral) gland External urethral sphincter Internal urethral sphincter Membranous urethra Penile urethra Prostatic urethra	**X** **External**	**Ø** **Drainage Device** **2** **Monitoring Device** **3** **Infusion Device** **7** **Autologous Tissue Substitute** **C** **Extraluminal Device** **D** **Intraluminal Device** **J** **Synthetic Substitute** **K** **Nonautologous Tissue Substitute** **L** **Artificial Sphincter**	**Z** **No Qualifier**

Non-OR   ØTWD[3,4,7,8]YZ
Non-OR   ØTWDX[Ø,2,3,7,C,D,J,K,L]Z

Ø   **Medical and Surgical**
T   **Urinary System**
Y   **Transplantation**   Definition: Putting in or on all or a portion of a living body part taken from another individual or animal to physically take the place and/or function of all or a portion of a similar body part

Explanation: The native body part may or may not be taken out, and the transplanted body part may take over all or a portion of its function

Body Part Character 4	Approach Character 5	Device Character 6	Qualifier Character 7
Ø **Kidney, Right** LC ⊞ Renal calyx Renal capsule Renal cortex Renal segment **1** **Kidney, Left** LC ⊞ *See Ø Kidney, Right*	**Ø** **Open**	**Z** **No Device**	**Ø** **Allogeneic** **1** **Syngeneic** **2** **Zooplastic**

LC   ØTY[Ø,1]ØZ[Ø,1,2]

See Appendix L for Procedure Combinations
⊞   ØTY[Ø,1]ØZ[Ø,1,2]

LC Limited Coverage   NC Noncovered   ⊞ Combination Member   HAC associated procedure   Combination Only   DRG Non-OR   Non-OR   New/Revised in GREEN

622   ICD-10-PCS 2020

Female Reproductive System ØU1–ØUY

Character Meanings

This Character Meaning table is provided as a guide to assist the user in the identification of character members that may be found in this section of code tables. It **SHOULD NOT** be used to build a PCS code.

Operation–Character 3		Body Part–Character 4		Approach–Character 5		Device–Character 6		Qualifier–Character 7	
1	Bypass	Ø	Ovary, Right	Ø	Open	Ø	Drainage Device	Ø	Allogeneic
2	Change	1	Ovary, Left	3	Percutaneous	1	Radioactive Element	1	Syngeneic
5	Destruction	2	Ovaries, Bilateral	4	Percutaneous Endoscopic	3	Infusion Device	2	Zooplastic
7	Dilation	3	Ovary	7	Via Natural or Artificial Opening	7	Autologous Tissue Substitute	5	Fallopian Tube, Right
8	Division	4	Uterine Supporting Structure	8	Via Natural or Artificial Opening Endoscopic	C	Extraluminal Device	6	Fallopian Tube, Left
9	Drainage	5	Fallopian Tube, Right	F	Via Natural or Artificial Opening With Percutaneous Endoscopic Assistance	D	Intraluminal Device	9	Uterus
B	Excision	6	Fallopian Tube, Left	X	External	G	Intraluminal Device, Pessary	L	Supracervical
C	Extirpation	7	Fallopian Tubes, Bilateral			H	Contraceptive Device	X	Diagnostic
D	Extraction	8	Fallopian Tube			J	Synthetic Substitute	Z	No Qualifier
F	Fragmentation	9	Uterus			K	Nonautologous Tissue Substitute		
H	Insertion	B	Endometrium			Y	Other Device		
J	Inspection	C	Cervix			Z	No Device		
L	Occlusion	D	Uterus and Cervix						
M	Reattachment	F	Cul-de-sac						
N	Release	G	Vagina						
P	Removal	H	Vagina and Cul-de-sac						
Q	Repair	J	Clitoris						
S	Reposition	K	Hymen						
T	Resection	L	Vestibular Gland						
U	Supplement	M	Vulva						
V	Restriction	N	Ova						
W	Revision								
Y	Transplantation								

Female Reproductive System

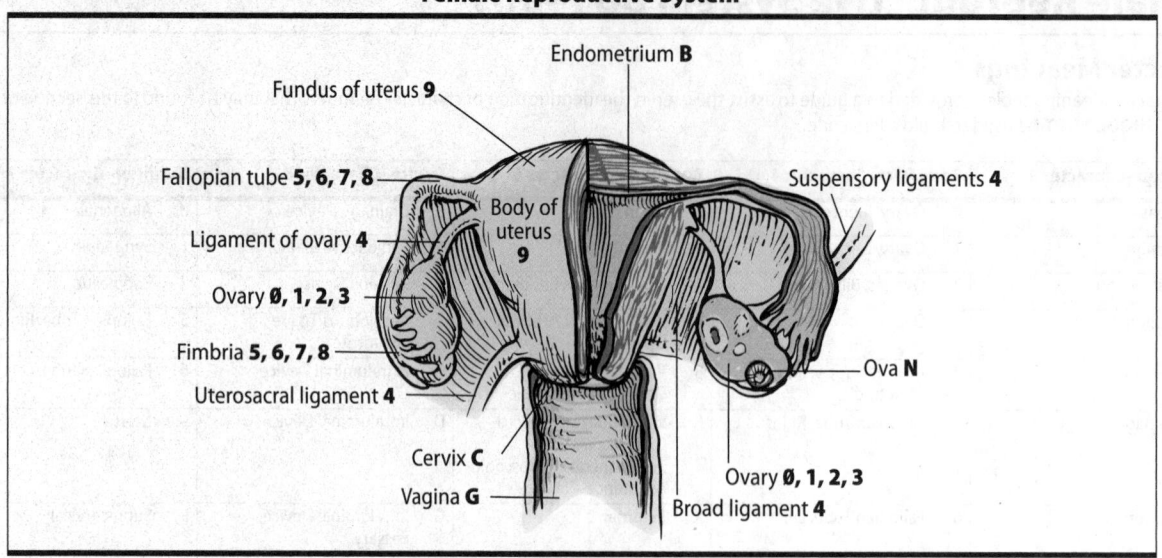

Endometrium **B**

Fundus of uterus **9**

Fallopian tube **5, 6, 7, 8**

Suspensory ligaments **4**

Body of uterus **9**

Ligament of ovary **4**

Ovary **Ø, 1, 2, 3**

Fimbria **5, 6, 7, 8**

Ova **N**

Uterosacral ligament **4**

Cervix **C**

Vagina **G**

Ovary **Ø, 1, 2, 3**

Broad ligament **4**

Female Internal/External Structures

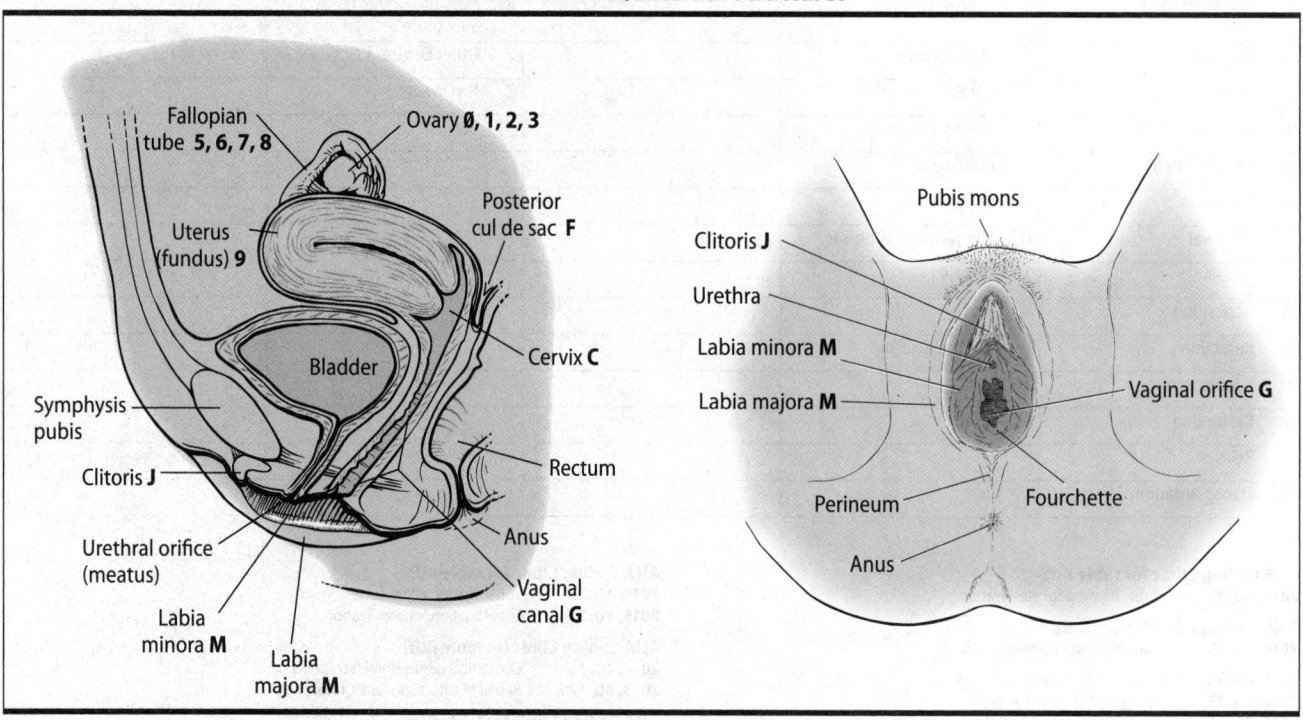

Fallopian tube **5, 6, 7, 8**

Ovary **Ø, 1, 2, 3**

Uterus (fundus) **9**

Posterior cul de sac **F**

Bladder

Cervix **C**

Symphysis pubis

Clitoris **J**

Rectum

Urethral orifice (meatus)

Anus

Labia minora **M**

Labia majora **M**

Vaginal canal **G**

Pubis mons

Clitoris **J**

Urethra

Labia minora **M**

Vaginal orifice **G**

Labia majora **M**

Perineum

Fourchette

Anus

0   **Medical and Surgical**
U   **Female Reproductive System**
1   **Bypass**   Definition: Altering the route of passage of the contents of a tubular body part

                    Explanation: Rerouting contents of a body part to a downstream area of the normal route, to a similar route and body part, or to an abnormal route and dissimilar body part. Includes one or more anastomoses, with or without the use of a device.

Body Part Character 4		Approach Character 5	Device Character 6	Qualifier Character 7

5 Fallopian Tube, Right
    Oviduct
    Salpinx
    Uterine tube
6 Fallopian Tube, Left
    See 5 Fallopian Tube, Right
	♀
	
	♀
		0 Open
		4 Percutaneous Endoscopic
			7 Autologous Tissue Substitute
			J Synthetic Substitute
			K Nonautologous Tissue Substitute
			Z No Device
				5 Fallopian Tube, Right
				6 Fallopian Tube, Left
				9 Uterus

    ♀   All body part, approach, device, and qualifier values

0   **Medical and Surgical**
U   **Female Reproductive System**
2   **Change**   Definition: Taking out or off a device from a body part and putting back an identical or similar device in or on the same body part without cutting or puncturing the skin or a mucous membrane

                    Explanation: All CHANGE procedures are coded using the approach EXTERNAL

Body Part Character 4		Approach Character 5	Device Character 6	Qualifier Character 7

3 Ovary
8 Fallopian Tube
M Vulva
    Labia majora
    Labia minora
	♀
	♀
	♀
		X External	**0** Drainage Device
			Y Other Device
				Z No Qualifier

D Uterus and Cervix	♀	**X** External	**0** Drainage Device **H** Contraceptive Device **Y** Other Device	**Z** No Qualifier
H Vagina and Cul-de-sac	♀	**X** External	**0** Drainage Device **G** Intraluminal Device, Pessary **Y** Other Device	**Z** No Qualifier

    Non-OR   All body part, approach, device, and qualifier values   ♀   All body part, approach, device, and qualifier values

Female Reproductive System

Ø   Medical and Surgical
U   Female Reproductive System
5   Destruction   Definition: Physical eradication of all or a portion of a body part by the direct use of energy, force, or a destructive agent
                     Explanation: None of the body part is physically taken out

Body Part Character 4	Approach Character 5	Device Character 6	Qualifier Character 7

Ø Ovary, Right ♀
1 Ovary, Left ♀
2 Ovaries, Bilateral ♀
4 Uterine Supporting Structure ♀
   Broad ligament
   Infundibulopelvic ligament
   Ovarian ligament
   Round ligament of uterus
	Ø Open
	3 Percutaneous
	4 Percutaneous Endoscopic
	8 Via Natural or Artificial Opening
	   Endoscopic
		Z No Device	**Z** No Qualifier

5 Fallopian Tube, Right ♀
   Oviduct
   Salpinx
   Uterine tube
6 Fallopian Tube, Left ♀
   See 5 Fallopian Tube, Right
7 Fallopian Tubes, Bilateral NC ♀
9 Uterus ♀
   Fundus uteri
   Myometrium
   Perimetrium
   Uterine cornu
B Endometrium ♀
C Cervix ♀
F Cul-de-sac ♀
	Ø Open
	3 Percutaneous
	4 Percutaneous Endoscopic
	7 Via Natural or Artificial Opening
	8 Via Natural or Artificial Opening
	   Endoscopic
		Z No Device	**Z** No Qualifier

G Vagina ♀ **K** Hymen ♀	**Ø** Open **3** Percutaneous **4** Percutaneous Endoscopic **7** Via Natural or Artificial Opening **8** Via Natural or Artificial Opening Endoscopic **X** External	**Z** No Device	**Z** No Qualifier

J Clitoris ♀
L Vestibular Gland ♀
   Bartholin's (greater vestibular) gland
   Greater vestibular (Bartholin's) gland
   Paraurethral (Skene's) gland
   Skene's (paraurethral) gland
M Vulva ♀
   Labia majora
   Labia minora
	Ø Open
	X External
		Z No Device	**Z** No Qualifier

NC   ØU57[Ø,3,4,7,8]ZZ with principal or secondary diagnosis of Z30.2   ♀   All body part, approach, device, and qualifier values

Ø Medical and Surgical
U Female Reproductive System
7 Dilation   Definition: Expanding an orifice or the lumen of a tubular body part

Explanation: The orifice can be a natural orifice or an artificially created orifice. Accomplished by stretching a tubular body part using intraluminal pressure or by cutting part of the orifice or wall of the tubular body part.

Body Part Character 4	Approach Character 5	Device Character 6	Qualifier Character 7

5 Fallopian Tube, Right ♀
  Oviduct
  Salpinx
  Uterine tube
6 Fallopian Tube, Left ♀
  See 5 Fallopian Tube, Right
7 Fallopian Tubes, Bilateral ♀
9 Uterus ♀
  Fundus uteri
  Myometrium
  Perimetrium
  Uterine cornu
C Cervix ♀
G Vagina ♀
	Ø Open
	3 Percutaneous
	4 Percutaneous Endoscopic
	7 Via Natural or Artificial Opening
	8 Via Natural or Artificial Opening Endoscopic
		D Intraluminal Device
		Z No Device
			Z No Qualifier

K Hymen ♀	Ø Open 3 Percutaneous 4 Percutaneous Endoscopic 7 Via Natural or Artificial Opening 8 Via Natural or Artificial Opening Endoscopic X External	D Intraluminal Device Z No Device	Z No Qualifier

Non-OR ØU7C[Ø,3,4,7,8][D,Z]Z
Non-OR ØU7G[7,8][D,Z]Z

♀   All body part, approach, device, and qualifier values

Ø Medical and Surgical
U Female Reproductive System
8 Division   Definition: Cutting into a body part, without draining fluids and/or gases from the body part, in order to separate or transect a body part

Explanation: All or a portion of the body part is separated into two or more portions

Body Part Character 4	Approach Character 5	Device Character 6	Qualifier Character 7

Ø Ovary, Right ♀
1 Ovary, Left ♀
2 Ovaries, Bilateral ♀
4 Uterine Supporting Structure ♀
  Broad ligament
  Infundibulopelvic ligament
  Ovarian ligament
  Round ligament of uterus
	Ø Open
	3 Percutaneous
	4 Percutaneous Endoscopic
		Z No Device	Z No Qualifier

K Hymen ♀	7 Via Natural or Artificial Opening 8 Via Natural or Artificial Opening Endoscopic X External	Z No Device	Z No Qualifier

Non-OR ØU8K[7,8,X]ZZ

♀   All body part, approach, device, and qualifier values

LC Limited Coverage   NC Noncovered   ⊞ Combination Member   HAC associated procedure   Combination Only   DRG Non-OR   Non-OR   New/Revised in GREEN

ICD-10-PCS 2020   627

ØU7–ØU8

Female Reproductive System

Ø   **Medical and Surgical**
U   **Female Reproductive System**
9   **Drainage**   Definition: Taking or letting out fluids and/or gases from a body part

                       Explanation: The qualifier DIAGNOSTIC is used to identify drainage procedures that are biopsies

Body Part Character 4	Approach Character 5	Device Character 6	Qualifier Character 7
Ø Ovary, Right ♀ **1** Ovary, Left ♀ **2** Ovaries, Bilateral ♀	**Ø** Open **3** Percutaneous **4** Percutaneous Endoscopic **8** Via Natural or Artificial Opening Endoscopic	**Ø** Drainage Device	**Z** No Qualifier
Ø Ovary, Right ♀ **1** Ovary, Left ♀ **2** Ovaries, Bilateral ♀	**Ø** Open **3** Percutaneous **4** Percutaneous Endoscopic **8** Via Natural or Artificial Opening Endoscopic	**Z** No Device	**X** Diagnostic **Z** No Qualifier
Ø Ovary, Right ♀ **1** Ovary, Left ♀ **2** Ovaries, Bilateral ♀	**X** External	**Z** No Device	**Z** No Qualifier
4 Uterine Supporting Structure ♀ Broad ligament Infundibulopelvic ligament Ovarian ligament Round ligament of uterus	**Ø** Open **3** Percutaneous **4** Percutaneous Endoscopic **8** Via Natural or Artificial Opening Endoscopic	**Ø** Drainage Device	**Z** No Qualifier
4 Uterine Supporting Structure ♀ Broad ligament Infundibulopelvic ligament Ovarian ligament Round ligament of uterus	**Ø** Open **3** Percutaneous **4** Percutaneous Endoscopic **8** Via Natural or Artificial Opening Endoscopic	**Z** No Device	**X** Diagnostic **Z** No Qualifier
5 Fallopian Tube, Right ♀ Oviduct Salpinx Uterine tube **6** Fallopian Tube, Left ♀ *See 5 Fallopian Tube, Right* **7** Fallopian Tubes, Bilateral ♀ **9** Uterus ♀ Fundus uteri Myometrium Perimetrium Uterine cornu **C** Cervix ♀ **F** Cul-de-sac ♀	**Ø** Open **3** Percutaneous **4** Percutaneous Endoscopic **7** Via Natural or Artificial Opening **8** Via Natural or Artificial Opening Endoscopic	**Ø** Drainage Device	**Z** No Qualifier
5 Fallopian Tube, Right ♀ Oviduct Salpinx Uterine tube **6** Fallopian Tube, Left ♀ *See 5 Fallopian Tube, Right* **7** Fallopian Tubes, Bilateral ♀ **9** Uterus ♀ Fundus uteri Myometrium Perimetrium Uterine cornu **C** Cervix ♀ **F** Cul-de-sac ♀	**Ø** Open **3** Percutaneous **4** Percutaneous Endoscopic **7** Via Natural or Artificial Opening **8** Via Natural or Artificial Opening Endoscopic	**Z** No Device	**X** Diagnostic **Z** No Qualifier

ØU9 Continued on next page

Non-OR ØU9[Ø,1,2][3,8]ØZ	Non-OR ØU9[5,6,7,9,C]3ØZ
Non-OR ØU9[Ø,1,2][3,8]ZZ	Non-OR ØU9F[3,4]ØZ
Non-OR ØU9[Ø,1,2]8ZX	Non-OR ØU9[5,6,7][3,4,7,8]ZZ
Non-OR ØU94[3,8]ØZ	Non-OR ØU9[9,C]3ZZ
Non-OR ØU94[3,8]ZZ	Non-OR ØU9F[3,4]ZZ
Non-OR ØU948ZX	♀ All body part, approach, device, and qualifier values

LC Limited Coverage   NC Noncovered   ⊞ Combination Member   HAC associated procedure   Combination Only   DRG Non-OR   Non-OR   New/Revised in GREEN

628   ICD-10-PCS 2020

0   **Medical and Surgical**
U   **Female Reproductive System**
9   **Drainage**   Definition: Taking or letting out fluids and/or gases from a body part
                     Explanation: The qualifier DIAGNOSTIC is used to identify drainage procedures that are biopsies

Body Part Character 4	Approach Character 5	Device Character 6	Qualifier Character 7
G Vagina ♀ **K** Hymen ♀	**0** Open **3** Percutaneous **4** Percutaneous Endoscopic **7** Via Natural or Artificial Opening **8** Via Natural or Artificial Opening Endoscopic **X** External	**0** Drainage Device	**Z** No Qualifier
G Vagina ♀ **K** Hymen ♀	**0** Open **3** Percutaneous **4** Percutaneous Endoscopic **7** Via Natural or Artificial Opening **8** Via Natural or Artificial Opening Endoscopic **X** External	**Z** No Device	**X** Diagnostic **Z** No Qualifier

J Clitoris ♀
L Vestibular Gland ♀
     Bartholin's (greater vestibular) gland
     Greater vestibular (Bartholin's) gland
     Paraurethral (Skene's) gland
     Skene's (paraurethral) gland
M Vulva ♀
     Labia majora
     Labia minora
	0 Open
	X External
		0 Drainage Device	**Z** No Qualifier

J Clitoris ♀
L Vestibular Gland ♀
     Bartholin's (greater vestibular) gland
     Greater vestibular (Bartholin's) gland
     Paraurethral (Skene's) gland
     Skene's (paraurethral) gland
M Vulva ♀
     Labia majora
     Labia minora
	0 Open
	X External
		Z No Device	**X** Diagnostic
			Z No Qualifier

Non-OR 0U9G30Z		**Non-OR** 0U9L[0,X]0Z	
Non-OR 0U9K[0,3,4,7,8,X]0Z		**Non-OR** 0U9L[0,X]ZZ	
Non-OR 0U9G3ZZ		♀ All body part, approach, device, and qualifier values	
Non-OR 0U9K[0,3,4,7,8,X]ZZ			

LC Limited Coverage   **NC** Noncovered   ⊞ Combination Member   HAC associated procedure   Combination Only   DRG Non-OR   Non-OR   New/Revised in GREEN

ICD-10-PCS 2020   629

0U9–0U9

Female Reproductive System

Ø　**Medical and Surgical**
U　**Female Reproductive System**
B　**Excision**　　　　Definition: Cutting out or off, without replacement, a portion of a body part
　　　　　　　　　　　Explanation: The qualifier DIAGNOSTIC is used to identify excision procedures that are biopsies

Body Part Character 4	Approach Character 5	Device Character 6	Qualifier Character 7
Ø　Ovary, Right　♀ 1　Ovary, Left　♀ 2　Ovaries, Bilateral　♀ 4　Uterine Supporting Structure　♀ 　　Broad ligament 　　Infundibulopelvic ligament 　　Ovarian ligament 　　Round ligament of uterus 5　Fallopian Tube, Right　♀ 　　Oviduct 　　Salpinx 　　Uterine tube 6　Fallopian Tube, Left　♀ 　　See 5 Fallopian Tube, Right 7　Fallopian Tubes, Bilateral　♀ 9　Uterus　♀ 　　Fundus uteri 　　Myometrium 　　Perimetrium 　　Uterine cornu C　Cervix　♀ F　Cul-de-sac　♀	Ø　Open 3　Percutaneous 4　Percutaneous Endoscopic 7　Via Natural or Artificial Opening 8　Via Natural or Artificial Opening 　　Endoscopic	Z　No Device	X　Diagnostic Z　No Qualifier
G　Vagina　♀ K　Hymen　♀	Ø　Open 3　Percutaneous 4　Percutaneous Endoscopic 7　Via Natural or Artificial Opening 8　Via Natural or Artificial Opening 　　Endoscopic X　External	Z　No Device	X　Diagnostic Z　No Qualifier
J　Clitoris　♀ L　Vestibular Gland　♀ 　　Bartholin's (greater vestibular) gland 　　Greater vestibular (Bartholin's) gland 　　Paraurethral (Skene's) gland 　　Skene's (paraurethral) gland M　Vulva　♀ 　　Labia majora 　　Labia minora	Ø　Open X　External	Z　No Device	X　Diagnostic Z　No Qualifier

♀　All body part, approach, device, and qualifier values

Ø   Medical and Surgical
U   Female Reproductive System
C   Extirpation   Definition: Taking or cutting out solid matter from a body part

                     Explanation: The solid matter may be an abnormal byproduct of a biological function or a foreign body; it may be imbedded in a body part or in the lumen of a tubular body part. The solid matter may or may not have been previously broken into pieces.

Body Part Character 4	Approach Character 5	Device Character 6	Qualifier Character 7

Ø Ovary, Right ♀
1 Ovary, Left ♀
2 Ovaries, Bilateral ♀
4 Uterine Supporting Structure ♀
   Broad ligament
   Infundibulopelvic ligament
   Ovarian ligament
   Round ligament of uterus
	Ø Open
	3 Percutaneous
	4 Percutaneous Endoscopic
	8 Via Natural or Artificial Opening
	   Endoscopic
		Z No Device	Z No Qualifier

5 Fallopian Tube, Right ♀
   Oviduct
   Salpinx
   Uterine tube
6 Fallopian Tube, Left ♀
   See 5 Fallopian Tube, Right
7 Fallopian Tubes, Bilateral ♀
9 **Uterus** ♀
   Fundus uteri
   Myometrium
   Perimetrium
   Uterine cornu
B Endometrium ♀
C Cervix ♀
F Cul-de-sac ♀
	Ø Open
	3 Percutaneous
	4 Percutaneous Endoscopic
	7 Via Natural or Artificial Opening
	8 Via Natural or Artificial Opening
	   Endoscopic
		Z No Device	Z No Qualifier

G Vagina ♀ K **Hymen** ♀	Ø Open 3 Percutaneous 4 Percutaneous Endoscopic 7 Via Natural or Artificial Opening 8 Via Natural or Artificial Opening Endoscopic X External	Z No Device	Z No Qualifier

J Clitoris ♀
L Vestibular Gland ♀
   Bartholin's (greater vestibular) gland
   Greater vestibular (Bartholin's) gland
   Paraurethral (Skene's) gland
   Skene's (paraurethral) gland
M **Vulva** ♀
   Labia majora
   Labia minora
	Ø Open
	X External
		Z No Device	Z No Qualifier

Non-OR ØUC9[7,8]ZZ **Non-OR** ØUCG[7,8,X]ZZ **Non-OR** ØUCK[Ø,3,4,7,8,X]ZZ	**Non-OR** ØUCMXZZ ♀ All body part, approach, device, and qualifier values

Ø   Medical and Surgical
U   Female Reproductive System
D   Extraction   Definition: Pulling or stripping out or off all or a portion of a body part by the use of force

                     Explanation: The qualifier DIAGNOSTIC is used to identify extraction procedures that are biopsies

Body Part Character 4	Approach Character 5	Device Character 6	Qualifier Character 7
B Endometrium ♀	7 Via Natural or Artificial Opening 8 Via Natural or Artificial Opening Endoscopic	Z No Device	X Diagnostic Z No Qualifier
N Ova ♀	Ø Open 3 Percutaneous 4 Percutaneous Endoscopic	Z No Device	Z No Qualifier

♀   All body part, approach, device, and qualifier values

Ø Medical and Surgical
U Female Reproductive System
F Fragmentation — Definition: Breaking solid matter in a body part into pieces

Explanation: Physical force (e.g., manual, ultrasonic) applied directly or indirectly is used to break the solid matter into pieces. The solid matter may be an abnormal byproduct of a biological function or a foreign body. The pieces of solid matter are not taken out.

Body Part Character 4	Approach Character 5	Device Character 6	Qualifier Character 7

5 Fallopian Tube, Right NC ♀
  Oviduct
  Salpinx
  Uterine tube
6 Fallopian Tube, Left NC ♀
  See 5 Fallopian Tube, Right
7 Fallopian Tubes, Bilateral NC ♀
9 Uterus NC ♀
  Fundus uteri
  Myometrium
  Perimetrium
  Uterine cornu
	Ø Open
	3 Percutaneous
	4 Percutaneous Endoscopic
	7 Via Natural or Artificial Opening
	8 Via Natural or Artificial Opening
	  Endoscopic
	X External
		Z No Device	Z No Qualifier

Non-OR	ØUF[5,6,7,9]XZZ
NC	ØUF[5,6,7,9]XZZ

♀   All body part, approach, device, and qualifier values

Ø Medical and Surgical
U Female Reproductive System
H Insertion — Definition: Putting in a nonbiological appliance that monitors, assists, performs, or prevents a physiological function but does not physically take the place of a body part

Explanation: None

Body Part Character 4	Approach Character 5	Device Character 6	Qualifier Character 7
3 Ovary ♀	Ø Open 3 Percutaneous 4 Percutaneous Endoscopic	3 Infusion Device Y Other Device	Z No Qualifier
3 Ovary ♀	7 Via Natural or Artificial Opening 8 Via Natural or Artificial Opening Endoscopic	Y Other Device	Z No Qualifier
8 Fallopian Tube ♀ D Uterus and Cervix ♀ H Vagina and Cul-de-sac ♀	Ø Open 3 Percutaneous 4 Percutaneous Endoscopic 7 Via Natural or Artificial Opening 8 Via Natural or Artificial Opening Endoscopic	3 Infusion Device Y Other Device	Z No Qualifier

9 Uterus ♀
  Fundus uteri
  Myometrium
  Perimetrium
  Uterine cornu
	Ø Open
	7 Via Natural or Artificial Opening
	8 Via Natural or Artificial Opening
	  Endoscopic
		H Contraceptive Device	Z No Qualifier

C Cervix ♀	Ø Open 3 Percutaneous 4 Percutaneous Endoscopic	1 Radioactive Element	Z No Qualifier
C Cervix ♀	7 Via Natural or Artificial Opening 8 Via Natural or Artificial Opening Endoscopic	1 Radioactive Element H Contraceptive Device	Z No Qualifier
F Cul-de-sac ♀	7 Via Natural or Artificial Opening 8 Via Natural or Artificial Opening Endoscopic	G Intraluminal Device, Pessary	Z No Qualifier
G Vagina ♀	Ø Open 3 Percutaneous 4 Percutaneous Endoscopic X External	1 Radioactive Element	Z No Qualifier
G Vagina ♀	7 Via Natural or Artificial Opening 8 Via Natural or Artificial Opening Endoscopic	1 Radioactive Element G Intraluminal Device, Pessary	Z No Qualifier

Non-OR	ØUH3[Ø,3,4][3,Y]Z
Non-OR	ØUH3[7,8]YZ
Non-OR	ØUH[8,D][Ø,3,4,7,8][3,Y]Z
Non-OR	ØUHH[3,4]YZ
Non-OR	ØUHH[7,8][3,Y]Z

Non-OR	ØUH9[Ø,7,8]HZ
Non-OR	ØUHC[7,8]HZ
Non-OR	ØUHF[7,8]GZ
Non-OR	ØUHG[7,8]GZ

♀   All body part, approach, device, and qualifier values

Ø   **Medical and Surgical**
U   **Female Reproductive System**
J   **Inspection**   Definition: Visually and/or manually exploring a body part

       Explanation: Visual exploration may be performed with or without optical instrumentation. Manual exploration may be performed directly or through intervening body layers.

Body Part Character 4	Approach Character 5	Device Character 6	Qualifier Character 7
3 Ovary ♀	**Ø** Open **3** Percutaneous **4** Percutaneous Endoscopic **8** Via Natural or Artificial Opening Endoscopic **X** External	**Z** No Device	**Z** No Qualifier
8 Fallopian Tube ♀ **D** Uterus and Cervix ♀ **H** Vagina and Cul-de-sac ♀	**Ø** Open **3** Percutaneous **4** Percutaneous Endoscopic **7** Via Natural or Artificial Opening **8** Via Natural or Artificial Opening Endoscopic **X** External	**Z** No Device	**Z** No Qualifier

M Vulva   ♀
    Labia majora
    Labia minora
	Ø Open
	X External
		Z No Device	**Z** No Qualifier

Non-OR   ØUJ3[3,8,X]ZZ
Non-OR   ØUJ[8,D,H][3,7,8,X]ZZ

Non-OR   ØUJMXZZ
♀   All body part, approach, device, and qualifier values

Ø   **Medical and Surgical**
U   **Female Reproductive System**
L   **Occlusion**   Definition: Completely closing an orifice or the lumen of a tubular body part

       Explanation: The orifice can be a natural orifice or an artificially created orifice

Body Part Character 4	Approach Character 5	Device Character 6	Qualifier Character 7

5 Fallopian Tube, Right   ♀
    Oviduct
    Salpinx
    Uterine tube
6 Fallopian Tube, Left   ♀
    See 5 Fallopian Tube, Right
7 Fallopian Tubes, Bilateral NC ♀
	Ø Open
	3 Percutaneous
	4 Percutaneous Endoscopic
		C Extraluminal Device
		D Intraluminal Device
		Z No Device
			Z No Qualifier

5 Fallopian Tube, Right   ♀
    Oviduct
    Salpinx
    Uterine tube
6 Fallopian Tube, Left   ♀
    See 5 Fallopian Tube, Right
7 Fallopian Tubes, Bilateral NC ♀
	7 Via Natural or Artificial Opening
	8 Via Natural or Artificial Opening Endoscopic
		D Intraluminal Device
		Z No Device
			Z No Qualifier

F Cul-de-sac ♀ **G** Vagina ♀	**7** Via Natural or Artificial Opening **8** Via Natural or Artificial Opening Endoscopic	**D** Intraluminal Device **Z** No Device	**Z** No Qualifier

NC   ØUL7[Ø,3,4][C,D,Z]Z with principal or secondary diagnosis of Z3Ø.2
NC   ØUL7[7,8][D,Z]Z with principal or secondary diagnosis of Z3Ø.2

♀   All body part, approach, device, and qualifier values

LC Limited Coverage   NC Noncovered   ⊞ Combination Member   HAC associated procedure   Combination Only   DRG Non-OR   Non-OR   New/Revised in GREEN
ICD-10-PCS 2020   633

ØUJ–ØUL

Female Reproductive System

Ø **Medical and Surgical**
U **Female Reproductive System**
M **Reattachment** Definition: Putting back in or on all or a portion of a separated body part to its normal location or other suitable location
Explanation: Vascular circulation and nervous pathways may or may not be reestablished

Body Part Character 4	Approach Character 5	Device Character 6	Qualifier Character 7
Ø Ovary, Right ♀ 1 Ovary, Left ♀ 2 Ovaries, Bilateral ♀ 4 Uterine Supporting Structure ♀ Broad ligament Infundibulopelvic ligament Ovarian ligament Round ligament of uterus 5 Fallopian Tube, Right ♀ Oviduct Salpinx Uterine tube 6 Fallopian Tube, Left ♀ See 5 Fallopian Tube, Right 7 Fallopian Tubes, Bilateral ♀ 9 Uterus ♀ Fundus uteri Myometrium Perimetrium Uterine cornu C Cervix ♀ F Cul-de-sac ♀ G Vagina ♀	Ø Open 4 Percutaneous Endoscopic	Z No Device	Z No Qualifier
J Clitoris ♀ M Vulva ♀ Labia majora Labia minora	X External	Z No Device	Z No Qualifier
K Hymen ♀	Ø Open 4 Percutaneous Endoscopic X External	Z No Device	Z No Qualifier

♀ All body part, approach, device, and qualifier values

Ø   **Medical and Surgical**
U   **Female Reproductive System**
N   **Release**   Definition: Freeing a body part from an abnormal physical constraint by cutting or by the use of force
                     Explanation: Some of the restraining tissue may be taken out but none of the body part is taken out

Body Part Character 4	Approach Character 5	Device Character 6	Qualifier Character 7

Ø   Ovary, Right ♀
1   Ovary, Left ♀
2   Ovaries, Bilateral ♀
4   Uterine Supporting Structure ♀
     Broad ligament
     Infundibulopelvic ligament
     Ovarian ligament
     Round ligament of uterus
	Ø Open
	3 Percutaneous
	4 Percutaneous Endoscopic
	8 Via Natural or Artificial Opening
	     Endoscopic
		Z No Device	Z No Qualifier

5   Fallopian Tube, Right ♀
     Oviduct
     Salpinx
     Uterine tube
6   Fallopian Tube, Left ♀
     See 5 Fallopian Tube, Right
7   Fallopian Tubes, Bilateral ♀
9   Uterus ♀
     Fundus uteri
     Myometrium
     Perimetrium
     Uterine cornu
C   Cervix ♀
F   Cul-de-sac ♀
	Ø Open
	3 Percutaneous
	4 Percutaneous Endoscopic
	7 Via Natural or Artificial Opening
	8 Via Natural or Artificial Opening
	     Endoscopic
		Z No Device	Z No Qualifier

G Vagina ♀ K Hymen ♀	Ø Open 3 Percutaneous 4 Percutaneous Endoscopic 7 Via Natural or Artificial Opening 8 Via Natural or Artificial Opening Endoscopic X External	Z No Device	Z No Qualifier

J   Clitoris ♀
L   Vestibular Gland ♀
     Bartholin's (greater vestibular) gland
     Greater vestibular (Bartholin's) gland
     Paraurethral (Skene's) gland
     Skene's (paraurethral) gland
M   Vulva ♀
     Labia majora
     Labia minora
	Ø Open
	X External
		Z No Device	Z No Qualifier

♀   All body part, approach, device, and qualifier values

Ø   **Medical and Surgical**
U   **Female Reproductive System**
P   **Removal**   Definition: Taking out or off a device from a body part

Explanation: If a device is taken out and a similar device put in without cutting or puncturing the skin or mucous membrane, the procedure is coded to the root operation CHANGE. Otherwise, the procedure for taking out the device is coded to the root operation REMOVAL.

Body Part Character 4	Approach Character 5	Device Character 6	Qualifier Character 7
3 Ovary ♀	**Ø** Open **3** Percutaneous **4** Percutaneous Endoscopic	**Ø** Drainage Device **3** Infusion Device **Y** Other Device	**Z** No Qualifier
3 Ovary ♀	**7** Via Natural or Artificial Opening **8** Via Natural or Artificial Opening Endoscopic	**Y** Other Device	**Z** No Qualifier
3 Ovary ♀	**X** External	**Ø** Drainage Device **3** Infusion Device	**Z** No Qualifier
8 Fallopian Tube ♀	**Ø** Open **3** Percutaneous **4** Percutaneous Endoscopic **7** Via Natural or Artificial Opening **8** Via Natural or Artificial Opening Endoscopic	**Ø** Drainage Device **3** Infusion Device **7** Autologous Tissue Substitute **C** Extraluminal Device **D** Intraluminal Device **J** Synthetic Substitute **K** Nonautologous Tissue Substitute **Y** Other Device	**Z** No Qualifier
8 Fallopian Tube ♀	**X** External	**Ø** Drainage Device **3** Infusion Device **D** Intraluminal Device	**Z** No Qualifier
D Uterus and Cervix ♀	**Ø** Open **3** Percutaneous **4** Percutaneous Endoscopic **7** Via Natural or Artificial Opening **8** Via Natural or Artificial Opening Endoscopic	**Ø** Drainage Device **1** Radioactive Element **3** Infusion Device **7** Autologous Tissue Substitute **C** Extraluminal Device **D** Intraluminal Device **H** Contraceptive Device **J** Synthetic Substitute **K** Nonautologous Tissue Substitute **Y** Other Device	**Z** No Qualifier
D Uterus and Cervix ♀	**X** External	**Ø** Drainage Device **3** Infusion Device **D** Intraluminal Device **H** Contraceptive Device	**Z** No Qualifier
H Vagina and Cul-de-sac ♀	**Ø** Open **3** Percutaneous **4** Percutaneous Endoscopic **7** Via Natural or Artificial Opening **8** Via Natural or Artificial Opening Endoscopic	**Ø** Drainage Device **1** Radioactive Element **3** Infusion Device **7** Autologous Tissue Substitute **D** Intraluminal Device **J** Synthetic Substitute **K** Nonautologous Tissue Substitute **Y** Other Device	**Z** No Qualifier
H Vagina and Cul-de-sac ♀	**X** External	**Ø** Drainage Device **1** Radioactive Element **3** Infusion Device **D** Intraluminal Device	**Z** No Qualifier
M Vulva ♀ Labia majora Labia minora	**Ø** Open	**Ø** Drainage Device **7** Autologous Tissue Substitute **J** Synthetic Substitute **K** Nonautologous Tissue Substitute	**Z** No Qualifier
M Vulva ♀ Labia majora Labia minora	**X** External	**Ø** Drainage Device	**Z** No Qualifier

Non-OR ØUP3[3,4]YZ		**Non-OR** ØUPD[7,8][Ø,3,C,D,H,Y]Z	
Non-OR ØUP3[7,8]YZ		**Non-OR** ØUPDX[Ø,3,D,H]Z	
Non-OR ØUP3X[Ø,3]Z		**Non-OR** ØUPH[3,4]YZ	
Non-OR ØUP8[3,4]YZ		**Non-OR** ØUPH[7,8][Ø,3,D,Y]Z	
Non-OR ØUP8[7,8][Ø,3,D,Y]Z		**Non-OR** ØUPHX[Ø,1,3,D]Z	
Non-OR ØUP8X[Ø,3,D]Z		**Non-OR** ØUPMXØZ	
Non-OR ØUPD[3,4][C,Y]Z		♀ All body part, approach, device, and qualifier values	

LC Limited Coverage   **NC** Noncovered   ⊞ Combination Member   HAC associated procedure   Combination Only   DRG Non-OR   Non-OR   New/Revised in GREEN

636   ICD-10-PCS 2020

ØUP–ØUP

Ø   **Medical and Surgical**
U   **Female Reproductive System**
Q   **Repair**   Definition: Restoring, to the extent possible, a body part to its normal anatomic structure and function

Explanation: Used only when the method to accomplish the repair is not one of the other root operations

Body Part Character 4	Approach Character 5	Device Character 6	Qualifier Character 7

Ø   **Ovary, Right** ♀
1   **Ovary, Left** ♀
2   **Ovaries, Bilateral** ♀
4   **Uterine Supporting Structure** ♀
    Broad ligament
    Infundibulopelvic ligament
    Ovarian ligament
    Round ligament of uterus
	Ø Open
	3 Percutaneous
	4 Percutaneous Endoscopic
	8 Via Natural or Artificial Opening
	    Endoscopic
		Z No Device	**Z** No Qualifier

5   **Fallopian Tube, Right** ♀
    Oviduct
    Salpinx
    Uterine tube
6   **Fallopian Tube, Left** ♀
    See 5 Fallopian Tube, Right
7   **Fallopian Tubes, Bilateral** ♀
9   **Uterus** ♀
    Fundus uteri
    Myometrium
    Perimetrium
    Uterine cornu
C   **Cervix** ♀
F   **Cul-de-sac** ♀
	Ø Open
	3 Percutaneous
	4 Percutaneous Endoscopic
	7 Via Natural or Artificial Opening
	8 Via Natural or Artificial Opening
	    Endoscopic
		Z No Device	**Z** No Qualifier

G **Vagina** ♀ **K** **Hymen** ♀	**Ø** Open **3** Percutaneous **4** Percutaneous Endoscopic **7** Via Natural or Artificial Opening **8** Via Natural or Artificial Opening Endoscopic **X** External	**Z** No Device	**Z** No Qualifier

J   **Clitoris** ♀
L   **Vestibular Gland** ♀
    Bartholin's (greater vestibular) gland
    Greater vestibular (Bartholin's) gland
    Paraurethral (Skene's) gland
    Skene's (paraurethral) gland
M   **Vulva** ♀
    Labia majora
    Labia minora
	Ø Open
	X External
		Z No Device	**Z** No Qualifier

Non-OR	ØUQG[7,X]ZZ
Non-OR	ØUQKXZZ

Non-OR	ØUQMXZZ
♀	All body part, approach, device, and qualifier values

Ø   **Medical and Surgical**
U   **Female Reproductive System**
S   **Reposition**   Definition: Moving to its normal location, or other suitable location, all or a portion of a body part

Explanation: The body part is moved to a new location from an abnormal location, or from a normal location where it is not functioning correctly. The body part may or may not be cut out or off to be moved to the new location.

Body Part Character 4	Approach Character 5	Device Character 6	Qualifier Character 7

Ø   **Ovary, Right** ♀
1   **Ovary, Left** ♀
2   **Ovaries, Bilateral** ♀
4   **Uterine Supporting Structure** ♀
    Broad ligament
    Infundibulopelvic ligament
    Ovarian ligament
    Round ligament of uterus
5   **Fallopian Tube, Right** ♀
    Oviduct
    Salpinx
    Uterine tube
6   **Fallopian Tube, Left** ♀
    See 5 Fallopian Tube, Right
7   **Fallopian Tubes, Bilateral** ♀
C   **Cervix** ♀
F   **Cul-de-sac** ♀
	Ø Open
	4 Percutaneous Endoscopic
	8 Via Natural or Artificial Opening
	    Endoscopic
		Z No Device	**Z** No Qualifier

9   **Uterus** ♀
    Fundus uteri
    Myometrium
    Perimetrium
    Uterine cornu
G   **Vagina** ♀
	Ø Open
	4 Percutaneous Endoscopic
	7 Via Natural or Artificial Opening
	8 Via Natural or Artificial Opening
	    Endoscopic
	X External
		Z No Device	**Z** No Qualifier

Non-OR	ØUS9XZZ		♀	All body part, approach, device, and qualifier values

LC Limited Coverage   NC Noncovered   ⊞ Combination Member   HAC associated procedure   Combination Only   DRG Non-OR   Non-OR   New/Revised in GREEN

ICD-10-PCS 2020   637

Female Reproductive System

Ø Medical and Surgical
U Female Reproductive System
T Resection　　Definition: Cutting out or off, without replacement, all of a body part
　　　　　　　　　　Explanation: None

Body Part Character 4	Approach Character 5	Device Character 6	Qualifier Character 7
Ø Ovary, Right ♀ **1** Ovary, Left ♀ **2** Ovaries, Bilateral ⊞♀ **5** Fallopian Tube, Right ♀ 　Oviduct 　Salpinx 　Uterine tube **6** Fallopian Tube, Left ♀ 　*See 5 Fallopian Tube, Right* **7** Fallopian Tubes, Bilateral ⊞♀	**Ø** Open **4** Percutaneous Endoscopic **7** Via Natural or Artificial Opening **8** Via Natural or Artificial Opening Endoscopic **F** Via Natural or Artificial Opening With Percutaneous Endoscopic Assistance	**Z** No Device	**Z** No Qualifier
4 Uterine Supporting Structure ⊞♀ 　Broad ligament 　Infundibulopelvic ligament 　Ovarian ligament 　Round ligament of uterus **C** Cervix ⊞♀ **F** Cul-de-sac ♀ **G** Vagina ⊞♀	**Ø** Open **4** Percutaneous Endoscopic **7** Via Natural or Artificial Opening **8** Via Natural or Artificial Opening Endoscopic	**Z** No Device	**Z** No Qualifier
9 Uterus ⊞♀ 　Fundus uteri 　Myometrium 　Perimetrium 　Uterine cornu	**Ø** Open **4** Percutaneous Endoscopic **7** Via Natural or Artificial Opening **8** Via Natural or Artificial Opening Endoscopic **F** Via Natural or Artificial Opening With Percutaneous Endoscopic Assistance	**Z** No Device	**L** Supracervical **Z** No Qualifier
J Clitoris ♀ **L** Vestibular Gland ♀ 　Bartholin's (greater vestibular) gland 　Greater vestibular (Bartholin's) gland 　Paraurethral (Skene's) gland 　Skene's (paraurethral) gland **M** Vulva ⊞♀ 　Labia majora 　Labia minora	**Ø** Open **X** External	**Z** No Device	**Z** No Qualifier
K Hymen ♀	**Ø** Open **4** Percutaneous Endoscopic **7** Via Natural or Artificial Opening **8** Via Natural or Artificial Opening Endoscopic **X** External	**Z** No Device	**Z** No Device

♀　All body part, approach, device, and qualifier values

See Appendix L for Procedure Combinations
⊞　ØUT[2,7]ØZZ
⊞　ØUT[4,C][Ø,4,7,8]ZZ
⊞　ØUTGØZZ
⊞　ØUT9[Ø,4,7,8,F]ZZ
⊞　ØUTM[Ø,X]ZZ

Ø Medical and Surgical
U Female Reproductive System
U Supplement Definition: Putting in or on biological or synthetic material that physically reinforces and/or augments the function of a portion of a body part

Explanation: The biological material is non-living, or is living and from the same individual. The body part may have been previously replaced, and the SUPPLEMENT procedure is performed to physically reinforce and/or augment the function of the replaced body part.

Body Part Character 4		Approach Character 5	Device Character 6	Qualifier Character 7

4 Uterine Supporting Structure ♀
  Broad ligament
  Infundibulopelvic ligament
  Ovarian ligament
  Round ligament of uterus
		Ø Open
		4 Percutaneous Endoscopic
			7 Autologous Tissue Substitute
			J Synthetic Substitute
			K Nonautologous Tissue Substitute
				Z No Qualifier

5 Fallopian Tube, Right ♀
  Oviduct
  Salpinx
  Uterine tube
6 Fallopian Tube, Left ♀
  See 5 Fallopian Tube, Right
7 Fallopian Tubes, Bilateral ♀
F Cul-de-sac ♀
		Ø Open
		4 Percutaneous Endoscopic
		7 Via Natural or Artificial Opening
		8 Via Natural or Artificial Opening Endoscopic
			7 Autologous Tissue Substitute
			J Synthetic Substitute
			K Nonautologous Tissue Substitute
				Z No Qualifier

G Vagina ♀ **K** Hymen ♀		**Ø** Open **4** Percutaneous Endoscopic **7** Via Natural or Artificial Opening **8** Via Natural or Artificial Opening Endoscopic **X** External	**7** Autologous Tissue Substitute **J** Synthetic Substitute **K** Nonautologous Tissue Substitute	**Z** No Qualifier

J Clitoris ♀
M Vulva ♀
  Labia majora
  Labia minora
		Ø Open
		X External
			7 Autologous Tissue Substitute
			J Synthetic Substitute
			K Nonautologous Tissue Substitute
				Z No Qualifier

♀ All body part, approach, device, and qualifier values

Ø Medical and Surgical
U Female Reproductive System
V Restriction Definition: Partially closing an orifice or the lumen of a tubular body part

Explanation: The orifice can be a natural orifice or an artificially created orifice

Body Part Character 4		Approach Character 5	Device Character 6	Qualifier Character 7
C Cervix ♀		**Ø** Open **3** Percutaneous **4** Percutaneous Endoscopic	**C** Extraluminal Device **D** Intraluminal Device **Z** No Device	**Z** No Qualifier
C Cervix ♀		**7** Via Natural or Artificial Opening **8** Via Natural or Artificial Opening Endoscopic	**D** Intraluminal Device **Z** No Device	**Z** No Qualifier

♀ All body part, approach, device, and qualifier values

Female Reproductive System *(side margin)*

Ø　**Medical and Surgical**
U　**Female Reproductive System**
W　**Revision**　　Definition: Correcting, to the extent possible, a portion of a malfunctioning device or the position of a displaced device

Explanation: Revision can include correcting a malfunctioning or displaced device by taking out or putting in components of the device such as a screw or pin

Body Part Character 4	Approach Character 5	Device Character 6	Qualifier Character 7
3　Ovary　♀	Ø　Open 3　Percutaneous 4　Percutaneous Endoscopic	Ø　Drainage Device 3　Infusion Device Y　Other Device	Z　No Qualifier
3　Ovary　♀	7　Via Natural or Artificial Opening 8　Via Natural or Artificial Opening Endoscopic	Y　Other Device	Z　No Qualifier
3　Ovary　♀	X　External	Ø　Drainage Device 3　Infusion Device	Z　No Qualifier
8　Fallopian Tube　♀	Ø　Open 3　Percutaneous 4　Percutaneous Endoscopic 7　Via Natural or Artificial Opening 8　Via Natural or Artificial Opening Endoscopic	Ø　Drainage Device 3　Infusion Device 7　Autologous Tissue Substitute C　Extraluminal Device D　Intraluminal Device J　Synthetic Substitute K　Nonautologous Tissue Substitute Y　Other Device	Z　No Qualifier
8　Fallopian Tube　♀	X　External	Ø　Drainage Device 3　Infusion Device 7　Autologous Tissue Substitute C　Extraluminal Device D　Intraluminal Device J　Synthetic Substitute K　Nonautologous Tissue Substitute	Z　No Qualifier
D　Uterus and Cervix　♀	Ø　Open 3　Percutaneous 4　Percutaneous Endoscopic 7　Via Natural or Artificial Opening 8　Via Natural or Artificial Opening Endoscopic	Ø　Drainage Device 1　Radioactive Element 3　Infusion Device 7　Autologous Tissue Substitute C　Extraluminal Device D　Intraluminal Device H　Contraceptive Device J　Synthetic Substitute K　Nonautologous Tissue Substitute Y　Other Device	Z　No Qualifier
D　Uterus and Cervix　♀	X　External	Ø　Drainage Device 3　Infusion Device 7　Autologous Tissue Substitute C　Extraluminal Device D　Intraluminal Device H　Contraceptive Device J　Synthetic Substitute K　Nonautologous Tissue Substitute	Z　No Qualifier
H　Vagina and Cul-de-sac　♀	Ø　Open 3　Percutaneous 4　Percutaneous Endoscopic 7　Via Natural or Artificial Opening 8　Via Natural or Artificial Opening Endoscopic	Ø　Drainage Device 1　Radioactive Element 3　Infusion Device 7　Autologous Tissue Substitute D　Intraluminal Device J　Synthetic Substitute K　Nonautologous Tissue Substitute Y　Other Device	Z　No Qualifier
H　Vagina and Cul-de-sac　♀	X　External	Ø　Drainage Device 3　Infusion Device 7　Autologous Tissue Substitute D　Intraluminal Device J　Synthetic Substitute K　Nonautologous Tissue Substitute	Z　No Qualifier
M　Vulva 　　Labia majora 　　Labia minora　♀	Ø　Open X　External	Ø　Drainage Device 7　Autologous Tissue Substitute J　Synthetic Substitute K　Nonautologous Tissue Substitute	Z　No Qualifier

Non-OR	ØUW3[3,4]YZ	Non-OR	ØUWDX[Ø,3,7,C,D,H,J,K]Z
Non-OR	ØUW3[7,8]YZ	Non-OR	ØUWH[3,4,7,8]YZ
Non-OR	ØUW3X[Ø,3]Z	Non-OR	ØUWHX[Ø,3,7,D,J,K]Z
Non-OR	ØUW8[3,4,7,8]YZ	Non-OR	ØUWMX[Ø,7,J,K]Z
Non-OR	ØUW8X[Ø,3,7,C,D,J,K]Z	♀	All body part, approach, device, and qualifier values
Non-OR	ØUWD[3,4,7,8]YZ		

LC Limited Coverage　NC Noncovered　⊞ Combination Member　HAC associated procedure　Combination Only　DRG Non-OR　Non-OR　New/Revised in GREEN

640　　ICD-10-PCS 2020

Ø   **Medical and Surgical**
U   **Female Reproductive System**
Y   **Transplantation**   Definition: Putting in or on all or a portion of a living body part taken from another individual or animal to physically take the place and/or
                            function of all or a portion of a similar body part

                            Explanation: The native body part may or may not be taken out, and the transplanted body part may take over all or a portion of its function

Body Part Character 4		Approach Character 5	Device Character 6	Qualifier Character 7
Ø Ovary, Right	♀	Ø Open	Z No Device	Ø Allogeneic
1 Ovary, Left	♀			1 Syngeneic
9 Uterus	♀			2 Zooplastic
♀	All body part, approach, device, and qualifier values			

Male Reproductive System ØV1–ØVX

Character Meanings

This Character Meaning table is provided as a guide to assist the user in the identification of character members that may be found in this section of code tables. It **SHOULD NOT** be used to build a PCS code.

Operation–Character 3		Body Part–Character 4		Approach–Character 5		Device–Character 6		Qualifier–Character 7	
1	Bypass	Ø	Prostate	Ø	Open	Ø	Drainage Device	D	Urethra
2	Change	1	Seminal Vesicle, Right	3	Percutaneous	1	Radioactive Element	J	Epididymis, Right
5	Destruction	2	Seminal Vesicle, Left	4	Percutaneous Endoscopic	3	Infusion Device	K	Epididymis, Left
7	Dilation	3	Seminal Vesicles, Bilateral	7	Via Natural or Artificial Opening	7	Autologous Tissue Substitute	N	Vas Deferens, Right
9	Drainage	4	Prostate and Seminal Vesicles	8	Via Natural or Artificial Opening Endoscopic	C	Extraluminal Device	P	Vas Deferens, Left
B	Excision	5	Scrotum	X	External	D	Intraluminal Device	S	Penis
C	Extirpation	6	Tunica Vaginalis, Right			J	Synthetic Substitute	X	Diagnostic
H	Insertion	7	Tunica Vaginalis, Left			K	Nonautologous Tissue Substitute	Z	No Qualifier
J	Inspection	8	Scrotum and Tunica Vaginalis			Y	Other Device		
L	Occlusion	9	Testis, Right			Z	No Device		
M	Reattachment	B	Testis, Left						
N	Release	C	Testes, Bilateral						
P	Removal	D	Testis						
Q	Repair	F	Spermatic Cord, Right						
R	Replacement	G	Spermatic Cord, Left						
S	Reposition	H	Spermatic Cords, Bilateral						
T	Resection	J	Epididymis, Right						
U	Supplement	K	Epididymis, Left						
W	Revision	L	Epididymis, Bilateral						
X	Transfer	M	Epididymis and Spermatic Cord						
		N	Vas Deferens, Right						
		P	Vas Deferens, Left						
		Q	Vas Deferens, Bilateral						
		R	Vas Deferens						
		S	Penis						
		T	Prepuce						

AHA Coding Clinic for table ØV1
2018, 3Q, 12   Al-Ghorab distal penile shunt surgery

AHA Coding Clinic for table ØV9
2018, 3Q, 12   Al-Ghorab distal penile shunt surgery

AHA Coding Clinic for table ØVB
2016, 1Q, 23   Transurethral resection of ejaculatory ducts
2014, 4Q, 33   Radical prostatectomy

AHA Coding Clinic for table ØVP
2016, 2Q, 28   Removal of multi-component inflatable penile prosthesis with placement of new malleable device

AHA Coding Clinic for table ØVQ
2018, 3Q, 12   Al-Ghorab distal penile shunt surgery

AHA Coding Clinic for table ØVT
2014, 4Q, 33   Radical prostatectomy

AHA Coding Clinic for table ØVU
2016, 2Q, 28   Removal of multi-component inflatable penile prosthesis with placement of new malleable device
2015, 3Q, 25   Placement of inflatable penile prosthesis

AHA Coding Clinic for table ØVX
2018, 4Q, 40   Transfer of prepuce

Male Reproductive System

Penis

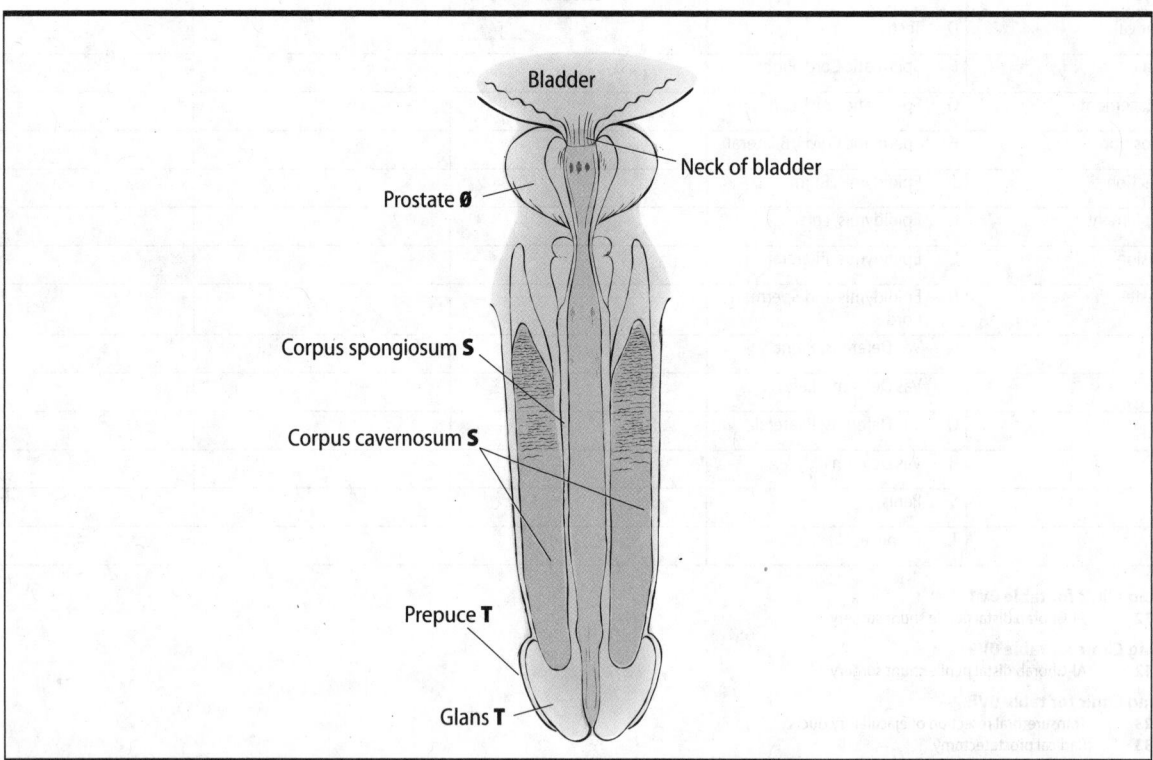

Ø   **Medical and Surgical**
V   **Male Reproductive System**
1   **Bypass**   Definition: Altering the route of passage of the contents of a tubular body part

                  Explanation: Rerouting contents of a body part to a downstream area of the normal route, to a similar route and body part, or to an abnormal route and dissimilar body part. Includes one or more anastomoses, with or without the use of a device.

Body Part Character 4	Approach Character 5	Device Character 6	Qualifier Character 7

N Vas Deferens, Right ♂
     Ductus deferens
     Ejaculatory duct
P Vas Deferens, Left ♂
     See N Vas Deferens, Right
Q Vas Deferens, Bilateral ♂
     See N Vas Deferens, Right
	Ø Open
	4 Percutaneous Endoscopic
		7 Autologous Tissue Substitute
		J Synthetic Substitute
		K Nonautologous Tissue Substitute
		Z No Device
			J Epididymis, Right
			K Epididymis, Left
			N Vas Deferens, Right
			P Vas Deferens, Left

    ♂   All body part, approach, device, and qualifier values

---

Ø   **Medical and Surgical**
V   **Male Reproductive System**
2   **Change**   Definition: Taking out or off a device from a body part and putting back an identical or similar device in or on the same body part without cutting or puncturing the skin or a mucous membrane

                  Explanation: All CHANGE procedures are coded using the approach EXTERNAL

Body Part Character 4	Approach Character 5	Device Character 6	Qualifier Character 7

4 Prostate and Seminal Vesicles ♂
8 Scrotum and Tunica Vaginalis ♂
D Testis ♂
M Epididymis and Spermatic Cord ♂
R Vas Deferens ♂
     Ductus deferens
     Ejaculatory duct
S Penis ♂
     Corpus cavernosum
     Corpus spongiosum
	X External	**Ø** Drainage Device
		Y Other Device
			Z No Qualifier

    Non-OR   All body part, approach, device, and qualifier values   ♂   All body part, approach, device, and qualifier values

---

Ø   **Medical and Surgical**
V   **Male Reproductive System**
5   **Destruction**   Definition: Physical eradication of all or a portion of a body part by the direct use of energy, force, or a destructive agent

                  Explanation: None of the body part is physically taken out

Body Part Character 4	Approach Character 5	Device Character 6	Qualifier Character 7
Ø Prostate ♂	**Ø** Open **3** Percutaneous **4** Percutaneous Endoscopic **7** Via Natural or Artificial Opening **8** Via Natural or Artificial Opening Endoscopic	**Z** No Device	**Z** No Qualifier
1 Seminal Vesicle, Right ♂ **2** Seminal Vesicle, Left ♂ **3** Seminal Vesicles, Bilateral ♂ **6** Tunica Vaginalis, Right ♂ **7** Tunica Vaginalis, Left ♂ **9** Testis, Right ♂ **B** Testis, Left ♂ **C** Testes, Bilateral ♂	**Ø** Open **3** Percutaneous **4** Percutaneous Endoscopic	**Z** No Device	**Z** No Qualifier

5 Scrotum ♂
S Penis ♂
     Corpus cavernosum
     Corpus spongiosum
T Prepuce ♂
     Foreskin
     Glans penis
	Ø Open
	3 Percutaneous
	4 Percutaneous Endoscopic
	X External
		Z No Device	**Z** No Qualifier

F Spermatic Cord, Right ♂
G Spermatic Cord, Left ♂
H Spermatic Cords, Bilateral ♂
J Epididymis, Right ♂
K Epididymis, Left ♂
L Epididymis, Bilateral ♂
N Vas Deferens, Right NC ♂
     Ductus deferens
     Ejaculatory duct
P Vas Deferens, Left NC ♂
     See N Vas Deferens, Right
Q Vas Deferens, Bilateral NC ♂
     See N Vas Deferens, Right
	Ø Open
	3 Percutaneous
	4 Percutaneous Endoscopic
	8 Via Natural or Artificial Opening
	     Endoscopic
		Z No Device	**Z** No Qualifier

    Non-OR   ØV55[Ø,3,4,X]ZZ   **NC**   ØV5[N,P,Q][Ø,3,4]ZZ with principal or secondary diagnosis of Z3Ø.2
    Non-OR   ØV5[N,P,Q][Ø,3,4,8]ZZ   ♂   All body part, approach, device, and qualifier values

---

LC Limited Coverage   **NC** Noncovered   ⊞ Combination Member   HAC associated procedure   Combination Only   DRG Non-OR   Non-OR   New/Revised in GREEN

ICD-10-PCS 2020   **645**

ØV1–ØV5

Male Reproductive System

Ø   **Medical and Surgical**
V   **Male Reproductive System**
7   **Dilation**   Definition: Expanding an orifice or the lumen of a tubular body part

          Explanation: The orifice can be a natural orifice or an artificially created orifice. Accomplished by stretching a tubular body part using intraluminal pressure or by cutting part of the orifice or wall of the tubular body part.

Body Part Character 4	Approach Character 5	Device Character 6	Qualifier Character 7

N Vas Deferens, Right ♂
    Ductus deferens
    Ejaculatory duct
P Vas Deferens, Left ♂
    See N Vas Deferens, Right
Q Vas Deferens, Bilateral ♂
    See N Vas Deferens, Right
	Ø Open
	3 Percutaneous
	4 Percutaneous Endoscopic
		D Intraluminal Device
		Z No Device
			Z No Qualifier

♂   All body part, approach, device, and qualifier values

Ø   **Medical and Surgical**
V   **Male Reproductive System**
9   **Drainage**   Definition: Taking or letting out fluids and/or gases from a body part

          Explanation: The qualifier DIAGNOSTIC is used to identify drainage procedures that are biopsies

Body Part Character 4	Approach Character 5	Device Character 6	Qualifier Character 7
Ø Prostate ♂	**Ø** Open **3** Percutaneous **4** Percutaneous Endoscopic **7** Via Natural or Artificial Opening **8** Via Natural or Artificial Opening Endoscopic	**Ø** Drainage Device	**Z** No Qualifier
Ø Prostate ♂	**Ø** Open **3** Percutaneous **4** Percutaneous Endoscopic **7** Via Natural or Artificial Opening **8** Via Natural or Artificial Opening Endoscopic	**Z** No Device	**X** Diagnostic **Z** No Qualifier

1 Seminal Vesicle, Right ♂
2 Seminal Vesicle, Left ♂
3 Seminal Vesicles, Bilateral ♂
6 Tunica Vaginalis, Right ♂
7 Tunica Vaginalis, Left ♂
9 Testis, Right ♂
B Testis, Left ♂
C Testes, Bilateral ♂
F Spermatic Cord, Right ♂
G Spermatic Cord, Left ♂
H Spermatic Cords, Bilateral ♂
J Epididymis, Right ♂
K Epididymis, Left ♂
L Epididymis, Bilateral ♂
N Vas Deferens, Right ♂
    Ductus deferens
    Ejaculatory duct
P Vas Deferens, Left ♂
    See N Vas Deferens, Right
Q Vas Deferens, Bilateral ♂
    See N Vas Deferens, Right
	Ø Open
	3 Percutaneous
	4 Percutaneous Endoscopic
		Ø Drainage Device	**Z** No Qualifier

ØV9 Continued on next page

Non-OR ØV9Ø[3,4]ØZ	**Non-OR** ØV9[6,7,F,G,H,N,P,Q][Ø,3,4]ØZ	
Non-OR ØV9Ø[3,4]Z[X,Z]	**Non-OR** ØV9[J,K,L]3ØZ	
Non-OR ØV9Ø[7,8]ZX	♂ All body part, approach, device, and qualifier values	
Non-OR ØV9[1,2,3,9,B,C][3,4]ØZ		

LC Limited Coverage   **NC** Noncovered   ⊞ Combination Member   HAC associated procedure   Combination Only   DRG Non-OR   Non-OR   New/Revised in GREEN

646   ICD-10-PCS 2020

Ø   Medical and Surgical   *ØV9 Continued*
V   Male Reproductive System
9   Drainage   Definition: Taking or letting out fluids and/or gases from a body part
                  Explanation: The qualifier DIAGNOSTIC is used to identify drainage procedures that are biopsies

Body Part Character 4	Approach Character 5	Device Character 6	Qualifier Character 7

1 Seminal Vesicle, Right ♂
2 Seminal Vesicle, Left ♂
3 Seminal Vesicles, Bilateral ♂
6 Tunica Vaginalis, Right ♂
7 Tunica Vaginalis, Left ♂
9 Testis, Right ♂
B Testis, Left ♂
C Testes, Bilateral ♂
F Spermatic Cord, Right ♂
G Spermatic Cord, Left ♂
H Spermatic Cords, Bilateral ♂
J Epididymis, Right ♂
K Epididymis, Left ♂
L Epididymis, Bilateral ♂
N Vas Deferens, Right ♂
    Ductus deferens
    Ejaculatory duct
P Vas Deferens, Left ♂
    See N Vas Deferens, Right
Q Vas Deferens, Bilateral ♂
    See N Vas Deferens, Right
	Ø Open
	3 Percutaneous
	4 Percutaneous Endoscopic
		Z No Device	**X** Diagnostic
			Z No Qualifier

5 Scrotum ♂
S Penis ♂
    Corpus cavernosum
    Corpus spongiosum
T Prepuce ♂
    Foreskin
    Glans penis
	Ø Open
	3 Percutaneous
	4 Percutaneous Endoscopic
	X External
		Ø Drainage Device	**Z** No Qualifier

5 Scrotum ♂
S Penis ♂
    Corpus cavernosum
    Corpus spongiosum
T Prepuce ♂
    Foreskin
    Glans penis
	Ø Open
	3 Percutaneous
	4 Percutaneous Endoscopic
	X External
		Z No Device	**X** Diagnostic
			Z No Qualifier

Non-OR   ØV9[1,2,3,9,B,C][3,4]Z[X,Z]   **Non-OR**   ØV9[S,T]30Z
Non-OR   ØV9[6,7,F,G,H,J,K,L,N,P,Q][Ø,3,4]ZX   **Non-OR**   ØV950ZX
Non-OR   ØV9[6,7,F,G,H,N,P,Q][Ø,3,4]ZZ   **Non-OR**   ØV95[3,4,X]Z[X,Z]
Non-OR   ØV9[J,K,L]3ZZ   **Non-OR**   ØV9[S,T]3ZZ
Non-OR   ØV95[Ø,3,4,X]ØZ   ♂   All body part, approach, device, and qualifier values

---

LC Limited Coverage   NC Noncovered   ⊞ Combination Member   HAC associated procedure   Combination Only   DRG Non-OR   Non-OR   New/Revised in GREEN

Ø   **Medical and Surgical**
V   **Male Reproductive System**
B   **Excision**   Definition: Cutting out or off, without replacement, a portion of a body part
                    Explanation: The qualifier DIAGNOSTIC is used to identify excision procedures that are biopsies

Body Part Character 4	Approach Character 5	Device Character 6	Qualifier Character 7
Ø Prostate ♂	**Ø** Open **3** Percutaneous **4** Percutaneous Endoscopic **7** Via Natural or Artificial Opening **8** Via Natural or Artificial Opening Endoscopic	**Z** No Device	**X** Diagnostic **Z** No Qualifier
1 Seminal Vesicle, Right ♂ **2** Seminal Vesicle, Left ♂ **3** Seminal Vesicles, Bilateral ♂ **6** Tunica Vaginalis, Right ♂ **7** Tunica Vaginalis, Left ♂ **9** Testis, Right ♂ **B** Testis, Left ♂ **C** Testes, Bilateral ♂	**Ø** Open **3** Percutaneous **4** Percutaneous Endoscopic	**Z** No Device	**X** Diagnostic **Z** No Qualifier

5 Scrotum ♂
S Penis ♂
    Corpus cavernosum
    Corpus spongiosum
T Prepuce ♂
    Foreskin
    Glans penis
	Ø Open
	3 Percutaneous
	4 Percutaneous Endoscopic
	X External
		Z No Device	**X** Diagnostic
			Z No Qualifier

F Spermatic Cord, Right ♂
G Spermatic Cord, Left ♂
H Spermatic Cords, Bilateral ♂
J Epididymis, Right ♂
K Epididymis, Left ♂
L Epididymis, Bilateral ♂
N Vas Deferens, Right NC ♂
    Ductus deferens
    Ejaculatory duct
P Vas Deferens, Left NC ♂
    See N Vas Deferens, Right
Q Vas Deferens, Bilateral NC ♂
    See N Vas Deferens, Right
	Ø Open
	3 Percutaneous
	4 Percutaneous Endoscopic
	8 Via Natural or Artificial Opening
	    Endoscopic
		Z No Device	**X** Diagnostic
			Z No Qualifier

Non-OR	ØVBØ[3,4,7,8]ZX	**Non-OR**	ØVB[F,G,H,J,K,L][Ø,3,4,8]ZX
Non-OR	ØVB[1,2,3,9,B,C][3,4]ZX	**Non-OR**	ØVB[N,P,Q][Ø,3,4,8]Z[X,Z]
Non-OR	ØVB[6,7][Ø,3,4]ZX	**NC**	ØVB[N,P,Q][Ø,3,4]ZZ with principal or secondary diagnosis of Z30.2
Non-OR	ØVB5ØZX	♂	All body part, approach, device, and qualifier values
Non-OR	ØVB5[3,4,X]Z[X,Z]		

LC Limited Coverage **NC** Noncovered ⊞ Combination Member HAC associated procedure Combination Only DRG Non-OR Non-OR New/Revised in **GREEN**

Ø   Medical and Surgical
V   Male Reproductive System
C   Extirpation   Definition: Taking or cutting out solid matter from a body part

                 Explanation: The solid matter may be an abnormal byproduct of a biological function or a foreign body; it may be imbedded in a body part or in the lumen of a tubular body part. The solid matter may or may not have been previously broken into pieces.

Body Part Character 4		Approach Character 5	Device Character 6	Qualifier Character 7
Ø Prostate	♂	Ø Open 3 Percutaneous 4 Percutaneous Endoscopic 7 Via Natural or Artificial Opening 8 Via Natural or Artificial Opening Endoscopic	Z No Device	Z No Qualifier

1 Seminal Vesicle, Right
2 Seminal Vesicle, Left
3 Seminal Vesicles, Bilateral
6 Tunica Vaginalis, Right
7 Tunica Vaginalis, Left
9 Testis, Right
B Testis, Left
C Testes, Bilateral
F Spermatic Cord, Right
G Spermatic Cord, Left
H Spermatic Cords, Bilateral
J Epididymis, Right
K Epididymis, Left
L Epididymis, Bilateral
N Vas Deferens, Right
     Ductus deferens
     Ejaculatory duct
P Vas Deferens, Left
     See N Vas Deferens, Right
Q Vas Deferens, Bilateral
     See N Vas Deferens, Right
	♂
	♂
	♂
	♂
	♂
	♂
	♂
	♂
	♂
	♂
	♂
	♂
	♂
	♂
	♂
	
	♂
	
	♂
		Ø Open
		3 Percutaneous
		4 Percutaneous Endoscopic
			Z No Device	Z No Qualifier

5 Scrotum
S Penis
     Corpus cavernosum
     Corpus spongiosum
T Prepuce
     Foreskin
     Glans penis
	♂
	♂
	
	♂
		Ø Open
		3 Percutaneous
		4 Percutaneous Endoscopic
		X External
			Z No Device	Z No Qualifier

Non-OR   ØVC[6,7,N,P,Q][Ø,3,4]ZZ
Non-OR   ØVC5[3,4,X]ZZ

Non-OR   ØVCSXZZ
♂   All body part, approach, device, and qualifier values

LC Limited Coverage   NC Noncovered   ⊞ Combination Member   HAC associated procedure   Combination Only   DRG Non-OR   Non-OR   New/Revised in GREEN

ICD-10-PCS 2020   649

Ø **Medical and Surgical**
V **Male Reproductive System**
H **Insertion**   Definition: Putting in a nonbiological appliance that monitors, assists, performs, or prevents a physiological function but does not physically take the place of a body part
               Explanation: None

Body Part Character 4	Approach Character 5	Device Character 6	Qualifier Character 7
Ø **Prostate** ♂	**Ø** Open **3** Percutaneous **4** Percutaneous Endoscopic **7** Via Natural or Artificial Opening **8** Via Natural or Artificial Opening Endoscopic	**1** Radioactive Element	**Z** No Qualifier

4 **Prostate and Seminal Vesicles** ♂
8 **Scrotum and Tunica Vaginalis** ♂
D **Testis** ♂
M **Epididymis and Spermatic Cord** ♂
R **Vas Deferens** ♂
    Ductus deferens
    Ejaculatory duct
	Ø Open
	3 Percutaneous
	4 Percutaneous Endoscopic
	7 Via Natural or Artificial Opening
	8 Via Natural or Artificial Opening Endoscopic
		3 Infusion Device
		Y Other Device
			Z No Qualifier

S **Penis** ♂
    Corpus cavernosum
    Corpus spongiosum
	Ø Open
	3 Percutaneous
	4 Percutaneous Endoscopic
		3 Infusion Device
		Y Other Device
			Z No Qualifier

S **Penis** ♂
    Corpus cavernosum
    Corpus spongiosum
	7 Via Natural or Artificial Opening
	8 Via Natural or Artificial Opening Endoscopic
		Y Other Device	**Z** No Qualifier

S **Penis** ♂
    Corpus cavernosum
    Corpus spongiosum
	X External	**3** Infusion Device	**Z** No Qualifier

Non-OR ØVH[4,8,D,M,R][Ø,3,4,7,8][3,Y]Z
Non-OR ØVHS[Ø,3,4][3,Y]Z
Non-OR ØVHS[7,8]YZ

Non-OR ØVHSX3Z
♂   All body part, approach, device, and qualifier values

Ø **Medical and Surgical**
V **Male Reproductive System**
J **Inspection**   Definition: Visually and/or manually exploring a body part
               Explanation: Visual exploration may be performed with or without optical instrumentation. Manual exploration may be performed directly or through intervening body layers.

Body Part Character 4	Approach Character 5	Device Character 6	Qualifier Character 7

4 **Prostate and Seminal Vesicles** ♂
8 **Scrotum and Tunica Vaginalis** ♂
D **Testis** ♂
M **Epididymis and Spermatic Cord** ♂
R **Vas Deferens** ♂
    Ductus deferens
    Ejaculatory duct
S **Penis** ♂
    Corpus cavernosum
    Corpus spongiosum
	Ø Open
	3 Percutaneous
	4 Percutaneous Endoscopic
	X External
		Z No Device	**Z** No Qualifier

Non-OR ØVJ[4,D,M,R][3,X]ZZ
Non-OR ØVJ[8,S][Ø,3,4,X]ZZ

♂   All body part, approach, device, and qualifier values

Ø **Medical and Surgical**
V **Male Reproductive System**
L **Occlusion**   Definition: Completely closing an orifice or the lumen of a tubular body part
               Explanation: The orifice can be a natural orifice or an artificially created orifice

Body Part Character 4	Approach Character 5	Device Character 6	Qualifier Character 7

F **Spermatic Cord, Right** NC ♂
G **Spermatic Cord, Left** NC ♂
H **Spermatic Cords, Bilateral** NC ♂
N **Vas Deferens, Right** NC ♂
    Ductus deferens
    Ejaculatory duct
P **Vas Deferens, Left** NC ♂
    See N Vas Deferens, Right
Q **Vas Deferens, Bilateral** NC ♂
    See N Vas Deferens, Right
	Ø Open
	3 Percutaneous
	4 Percutaneous Endoscopic
	8 Via Natural or Artificial Opening Endoscopic
		C Extraluminal Device
		D Intraluminal Device
		Z No Device
			Z No Qualifier

Non-OR ØVL[F,G,H][Ø,3,4,8][C,D,Z]Z
Non-OR ØVL[N,P,Q][Ø,3,4,8][C,Z]Z

NC ØVL[F,G,H][Ø,3,4][C,D,Z]Z with principal or secondary diagnosis of Z3Ø.2
NC ØVL[N,P,Q][Ø,3,4][C,Z]Z with principal or secondary diagnosis of Z3Ø.2
♂ All body part, approach, device, and qualifier values

LC Limited Coverage   **NC** Noncovered   ⊞ Combination Member   HAC associated procedure   Combination Only   DRG Non-OR   Non-OR   New/Revised in **GREEN**

650   ICD-10-PCS 2020

Ø   **Medical and Surgical**
V   **Male Reproductive System**
M   **Reattachment**   Definition: Putting back in or on all or a portion of a separated body part to its normal location or other suitable location
                           Explanation: Vascular circulation and nervous pathways may or may not be reestablished

Body Part Character 4	Approach Character 5	Device Character 6	Qualifier Character 7

5 Scrotum ♂
S Penis ♂
    Corpus cavernosum
    Corpus spongiosum
	X External	**Z** No Device	**Z** No Qualifier

6 Tunica Vaginalis, Right ♂ **7** Tunica Vaginalis, Left ♂ **9** Testis, Right ♂ **B** Testis, Left ♂ **C** Testes, Bilateral ♂ **F** Spermatic Cord, Right ♂ **G** Spermatic Cord, Left ♂ **H** Spermatic Cords, Bilateral ♂	**Ø** Open **4** Percutaneous Endoscopic	**Z** No Device	**Z** No Qualifier

♂   All body part, approach, device, and qualifier values

Ø   **Medical and Surgical**
V   **Male Reproductive System**
N   **Release**   Definition: Freeing a body part from an abnormal physical constraint by cutting or by the use of force
                      Explanation: Some of the restraining tissue may be taken out but none of the body part is taken out

Body Part Character 4	Approach Character 5	Device Character 6	Qualifier Character 7
Ø Prostate ♂	**Ø** Open **3** Percutaneous **4** Percutaneous Endoscopic **7** Via Natural or Artificial Opening **8** Via Natural or Artificial Opening Endoscopic	**Z** No Device	**Z** No Qualifier
1 Seminal Vesicle, Right ♂ **2** Seminal Vesicle, Left ♂ **3** Seminal Vesicles, Bilateral ♂ **6** Tunica Vaginalis, Right ♂ **7** Tunica Vaginalis, Left ♂ **9** Testis, Right ♂ **B** Testis, Left ♂ **C** Testes, Bilateral ♂	**Ø** Open **3** Percutaneous **4** Percutaneous Endoscopic	**Z** No Device	**Z** No Qualifier

5 Scrotum ♂
S Penis ♂
    Corpus cavernosum
    Corpus spongiosum
T Prepuce ♂
    Foreskin
    Glans penis
	Ø Open
	3 Percutaneous
	4 Percutaneous Endoscopic
	X External
		Z No Device	**Z** No Qualifier

F Spermatic Cord, Right ♂
G Spermatic Cord, Left ♂
H Spermatic Cords, Bilateral ♂
J Epididymis, Right ♂
K Epididymis, Left ♂
L Epididymis, Bilateral ♂
N Vas Deferens, Right ♂
    Ductus deferens
    Ejaculatory duct
P Vas Deferens, Left ♂
    See N Vas Deferens, Right
Q Vas Deferens, Bilateral ♂
    See N Vas Deferens, Right
	Ø Open
	3 Percutaneous
	4 Percutaneous Endoscopic
	8 Via Natural or Artificial Opening
	    Endoscopic
		Z No Device	**Z** No Qualifier

Non-OR   ØVN[9,B,C][Ø,3,4]ZZ
Non-OR   ØVNT[Ø,3,4,X]ZZ

♂   All body part, approach, device, and qualifier values

Male Reproductive System

Ø   **Medical and Surgical**
V   **Male Reproductive System**
P   **Removal**   Definition: Taking out or off a device from a body part

        Explanation: If a device is taken out and a similar device put in without cutting or puncturing the skin or mucous membrane, the procedure is coded to the root operation CHANGE. Otherwise, the procedure for taking out the device is coded to the root operation REMOVAL.

Body Part Character 4	Approach Character 5	Device Character 6	Qualifier Character 7
4 Prostate and Seminal Vesicles ♂	Ø Open 3 Percutaneous 4 Percutaneous Endoscopic 7 Via Natural or Artificial Opening 8 Via Natural or Artificial Opening Endoscopic	Ø Drainage Device 1 Radioactive Element 3 Infusion Device 7 Autologous Tissue Substitute J Synthetic Substitute K Nonautologous Tissue Substitute Y Other Device	Z No Qualifier
4 Prostate and Seminal Vesicles ♂	X External	Ø Drainage Device 1 Radioactive Element 3 Infusion Device	Z No Qualifier

8   Scrotum and Tunica Vaginalis ♂
D   Testis ♂
S   Penis ♂
    Corpus cavernosum
    Corpus spongiosum
	Ø Open
	3 Percutaneous
	4 Percutaneous Endoscopic
	7 Via Natural or Artificial Opening
	8 Via Natural or Artificial Opening Endoscopic
		Ø Drainage Device
		3 Infusion Device
		7 Autologous Tissue Substitute
		J Synthetic Substitute
		K Nonautologous Tissue Substitute
		Y Other Device
			Z No Qualifier

8   Scrotum and Tunica Vaginalis ♂
D   Testis ♂
S   Penis ♂
    Corpus cavernosum
    Corpus spongiosum
	X External	Ø Drainage Device
		3 Infusion Device
			Z No Qualifier

M Epididymis and Spermatic Cord ♂	Ø Open 3 Percutaneous 4 Percutaneous Endoscopic 7 Via Natural or Artificial Opening 8 Via Natural or Artificial Opening Endoscopic	Ø Drainage Device 3 Infusion Device 7 Autologous Tissue Substitute C Extraluminal Device J Synthetic Substitute K Nonautologous Tissue Substitute Y Other Device	Z No Qualifier
M Epididymis and Spermatic Cord ♂	X External	Ø Drainage Device 3 Infusion Device	Z No Qualifier

R   Vas Deferens ♂
    Ductus deferens
    Ejaculatory duct
	Ø Open
	3 Percutaneous
	4 Percutaneous Endoscopic
	7 Via Natural or Artificial Opening
	8 Via Natural or Artificial Opening Endoscopic
		Ø Drainage Device
		3 Infusion Device
		7 Autologous Tissue Substitute
		C Extraluminal Device
		D Intraluminal Device
		J Synthetic Substitute
		K Nonautologous Tissue Substitute
		Y Other Device
			Z No Qualifier

R   Vas Deferens ♂
    Ductus deferens
    Ejaculatory duct
	X External	Ø Drainage Device
		3 Infusion Device
		D Intraluminal Device
			Z No Qualifier

Non-OR	ØVP4[3,4]YZ	**Non-OR**	ØVPM[3,4]YZ
Non-OR	ØVP4[7,8][Ø,3,Y]Z	**Non-OR**	ØVPM[7,8][Ø,3,Y]Z
Non-OR	ØVP4X[Ø,1,3]Z	**Non-OR**	ØVPMX[Ø,3]Z
Non-OR	ØVP8[Ø,3,4,7,8][Ø,3,7,J,K,Y]Z	**Non-OR**	ØVPR[Ø,3,4][Ø,3,7,C,J,K,Y]Z
Non-OR	ØVP[D,S][3,4]YZ	**Non-OR**	ØVPR[7,8][Ø,3,7,C,D,J,K,Y]Z
Non-OR	ØVP[D,S][7,8][Ø,3,Y]Z	**Non-OR**	ØVPRX[Ø,3,D]Z
Non-OR	ØVP[8,D,S]X[Ø,3]Z	♂	All body part, approach, device, and qualifier values

🔟 Limited Coverage   🔟 Noncovered   ⊞ Combination Member   HAC associated procedure   Combination Only   DRG Non-OR   Non-OR   New/Revised in GREEN

652   ICD-10-PCS 2020

Ø Medical and Surgical
V Male Reproductive System
Q Repair   Definition: Restoring, to the extent possible, a body part to its normal anatomic structure and function

Explanation: Used only when the method to accomplish the repair is not one of the other root operations

Body Part Character 4		Approach Character 5	Device Character 6	Qualifier Character 7
Ø Prostate	♂	Ø Open 3 Percutaneous 4 Percutaneous Endoscopic 7 Via Natural or Artificial Opening 8 Via Natural or Artificial Opening Endoscopic	Z No Device	Z No Qualifier
1 Seminal Vesicle, Right 2 Seminal Vesicle, Left 3 Seminal Vesicles, Bilateral 6 Tunica Vaginalis, Right 7 Tunica Vaginalis, Left 9 Testis, Right B Testis, Left C Testes, Bilateral	♂ ♂ ♂ ♂ ♂ ♂ ♂ ♂	Ø Open 3 Percutaneous 4 Percutaneous Endoscopic	Z No Device	Z No Qualifier

5 Scrotum
S Penis
   Corpus cavernosum
   Corpus spongiosum
T Prepuce
   Foreskin
   Glans penis
	♂
	♂
	
	♂
		Ø Open
		3 Percutaneous
		4 Percutaneous Endoscopic
		X External
			Z No Device	Z No Qualifier

F Spermatic Cord, Right
G Spermatic Cord, Left
H Spermatic Cords, Bilateral
J Epididymis, Right
K Epididymis, Left
L Epididymis, Bilateral
N Vas Deferens, Right
   Ductus deferens
   Ejaculatory duct
P Vas Deferens, Left
   See N Vas Deferens, Right
Q Vas Deferens, Bilateral
   See N Vas Deferens, Right
	♂
	♂
	♂
	♂
	♂
	♂
	♂
	
	♂
	
	♂
		Ø Open
		3 Percutaneous
		4 Percutaneous Endoscopic
		8 Via Natural or Artificial Opening Endoscopic
			Z No Device	Z No Qualifier

Non-OR ØVQ[6,7][Ø,3,4]ZZ   ♂   All body part, approach, device, and qualifier values
Non-OR ØVQ5[Ø,3,4,X]ZZ

Ø Medical and Surgical
V Male Reproductive System
R Replacement   Definition: Putting in or on biological or synthetic material that physically takes the place and/or function of all or a portion of a body part

Explanation: The body part may have been taken out or replaced, or may be taken out, physically eradicated, or rendered nonfunctional during the REPLACEMENT procedure. A REMOVAL procedure is coded for taking out the device used in a previous replacement procedure.

Body Part Character 4		Approach Character 5	Device Character 6	Qualifier Character 7
9 Testis, Right B Testis, Left C Testes, Bilateral	♂ ♂ ♂	Ø Open	J Synthetic Substitute	Z No Qualifier

♂   All body part, approach, device, and qualifier values

Ø Medical and Surgical
V Male Reproductive System
S Reposition   Definition: Moving to its normal location, or other suitable location, all or a portion of a body part

Explanation: The body part is moved to a new location from an abnormal location, or from a normal location where it is not functioning correctly. The body part may or may not be cut out or off to be moved to the new location.

Body Part Character 4		Approach Character 5	Device Character 6	Qualifier Character 7
9 Testis, Right B Testis, Left C Testes, Bilateral F Spermatic Cord, Right G Spermatic Cord, Left H Spermatic Cords, Bilateral	♂ ♂ ♂ ♂ ♂ ♂	Ø Open 3 Percutaneous 4 Percutaneous Endoscopic 8 Via Natural or Artificial Opening Endoscopic	Z No Device	Z No Qualifier

♂   All body part, approach, device, and qualifier values

LC Limited Coverage NC Noncovered ⊞ Combination Member HAC associated procedure Combination Only DRG Non-OR Non-OR New/Revised in GREEN

Ø **Medical and Surgical**
V **Male Reproductive System**
T **Resection**   Definition: Cutting out or off, without replacement, all of a body part
    Explanation: None

Body Part Character 4		Approach Character 5	Device Character 6	Qualifier Character 7
Ø	Prostate ⊞♂	Ø Open 4 Percutaneous Endoscopic 7 Via Natural or Artificial Opening 8 Via Natural or Artificial Opening Endoscopic	Z No Device	Z No Qualifier
1 2 3 6 7 9 B C F G H J K L N P Q	Seminal Vesicle, Right ♂ Seminal Vesicle, Left ♂ Seminal Vesicles, Bilateral ⊞♂ Tunica Vaginalis, Right ♂ Tunica Vaginalis, Left ♂ Testis, Right ♂ Testis, Left ♂ Testes, Bilateral ♂ Spermatic Cord, Right ♂ Spermatic Cord, Left ♂ Spermatic Cords, Bilateral ♂ Epididymis, Right ♂ Epididymis, Left ♂ Epididymis, Bilateral ♂ Vas Deferens, Right NC♂ Ductus deferens Ejaculatory duct Vas Deferens, Left NC♂ See N Vas Deferens, Right Vas Deferens, Bilateral NC♂ See N Vas Deferens, Right	Ø Open 4 Percutaneous Endoscopic	Z No Device	Z No Qualifier
5 S T	Scrotum ♂ Penis ♂ Corpus cavernosum Corpus spongiosum Prepuce ♂ Foreskin Glans penis	Ø Open 4 Percutaneous Endoscopic X External	Z No Device	Z No Qualifier

Non-OR	ØVT[N,P,Q][Ø,4]ZZ
Non-OR	ØVT[5,T][Ø,4,X]ZZ
NC	ØVT[N,P,Q][Ø,4]ZZ with principal or secondary diagnosis of Z30.2
♂	All body part, approach, device, and qualifier values

See Appendix L for Procedure Combinations
⊞   ØVTØ[Ø,4,7,8]ZZ
⊞   ØVT3[Ø,4]ZZ

LC Limited Coverage   NC Noncovered   ⊞ Combination Member   HAC associated procedure   Combination Only   DRG Non-OR   Non-OR   New/Revised in GREEN
654   ICD-10-PCS 2020

ØVT–ØVT

Ø   Medical and Surgical
V   Male Reproductive System
U   Supplement   Definition: Putting in or on biological or synthetic material that physically reinforces and/or augments the function of a portion of a body part
                 Explanation: The biological material is non-living, or is living and from the same individual. The body part may have been previously replaced, and the SUPPLEMENT procedure is performed to physically reinforce and/or augment the function of the replaced body part.

Body Part Character 4		Approach Character 5	Device Character 6	Qualifier Character 7
1 Seminal Vesicle, Right	♂	Ø Open	7 Autologous Tissue Substitute	Z No Qualifier
2 Seminal Vesicle, Left	♂	4 Percutaneous Endoscopic	J Synthetic Substitute	
3 Seminal Vesicles, Bilateral	♂	8 Via Natural or Artificial Opening	K Nonautologous Tissue Substitute	
6 Tunica Vaginalis, Right	♂	Endoscopic		
7 Tunica Vaginalis, Left	♂			
F Spermatic Cord, Right	♂			
G Spermatic Cord, Left	♂			
H Spermatic Cords, Bilateral	♂			
J Epididymis, Right	♂			
K Epididymis, Left	♂			
L Epididymis, Bilateral	♂			

N   Vas Deferens, Right
     Ductus deferens
     Ejaculatory duct
	♂			

P Vas Deferens, Left *See* N Vas Deferens, Right	♂			
Q Vas Deferens, Bilateral *See* N Vas Deferens, Right	♂			
5 Scrotum	♂	Ø Open	7 Autologous Tissue Substitute	Z No Qualifier

S   Penis
     Corpus cavernosum
     Corpus spongiosum
	♂	4 Percutaneous Endoscopic
		X External
			J Synthetic Substitute
			K Nonautologous Tissue Substitute	

T   Prepuce
     Foreskin
     Glans penis
	♂			

9 Testis, Right	♂	Ø Open	7 Autologous Tissue Substitute	Z No Qualifier
B Testis, Left	♂		J Synthetic Substitute	
C Testes, Bilateral	♂		K Nonautologous Tissue Substitute	

Non-OR ØVUSX[7,J,K]Z	♂ All body part, approach, device, and qualifier values

Ø   **Medical and Surgical**
V   **Male Reproductive System**
W   **Revision**   Definition: Correcting, to the extent possible, a portion of a malfunctioning device or the position of a displaced device

           Explanation: Revision can include correcting a malfunctioning or displaced device by taking out or putting in components of the device such as a screw or pin

Body Part Character 4	Approach Character 5	Device Character 6	Qualifier Character 7

4   **Prostate and Seminal Vesicles** ♂
8   **Scrotum and Tunica Vaginalis** ♂
D   **Testis** ♂
S   **Penis** ♂
     Corpus cavernosum
     Corpus spongiosum
	Ø Open
	3 Percutaneous
	4 Percutaneous Endoscopic
	7 Via Natural or Artificial Opening
	8 Via Natural or Artificial Opening
	     Endoscopic
		Ø Drainage Device
		3 Infusion Device
		7 Autologous Tissue Substitute
		J Synthetic Substitute
		K Nonautologous Tissue Substitute
		Y Other Device
			Z No Qualifier

4   **Prostate and Seminal Vesicles** ♂
8   **Scrotum and Tunica Vaginalis** ♂
D   **Testis** ♂
S   **Penis** ♂
     Corpus cavernosum
     Corpus spongiosum
	X External	**Ø** Drainage Device
		3 Infusion Device
		7 Autologous Tissue Substitute
		J Synthetic Substitute
		K Nonautologous Tissue Substitute
			Z No Qualifier

M **Epididymis and Spermatic Cord** ♂	**Ø** Open **3** Percutaneous **4** Percutaneous Endoscopic **7** Via Natural or Artificial Opening **8** Via Natural or Artificial Opening Endoscopic	**Ø** Drainage Device **3** Infusion Device **7** Autologous Tissue Substitute **C** Extraluminal Device **J** Synthetic Substitute **K** Nonautologous Tissue Substitute **Y** Other Device	**Z** No Qualifier
M **Epididymis and Spermatic Cord** ♂	**X** External	**Ø** Drainage Device **3** Infusion Device **7** Autologous Tissue Substitute **C** Extraluminal Device **J** Synthetic Substitute **K** Nonautologous Tissue Substitute	**Z** No Qualifier

R   **Vas Deferens** ♂
     Ductus deferens
     Ejaculatory duct
	Ø Open
	3 Percutaneous
	4 Percutaneous Endoscopic
	7 Via Natural or Artificial Opening
	8 Via Natural or Artificial Opening
	     Endoscopic
		Ø Drainage Device
		3 Infusion Device
		7 Autologous Tissue Substitute
		C Extraluminal Device
		D Intraluminal Device
		J Synthetic Substitute
		K Nonautologous Tissue Substitute
		Y Other Device
			Z No Qualifier

R   **Vas Deferens** ♂
     Ductus deferens
     Ejaculatory duct
	X External	**Ø** Drainage Device
		3 Infusion Device
		7 Autologous Tissue Substitute
		C Extraluminal Device
		D Intraluminal Device
		J Synthetic Substitute
		K Nonautologous Tissue Substitute
			Z No Qualifier

Non-OR	ØVW[4,D,S][3,4,7,8]YZ	Non-OR	ØVWMX[Ø,3,7,C,J,K]Z
Non-OR	ØVW8[Ø,3,4,7,8][Ø,3,7,J,K,Y]Z	Non-OR	ØVWR[Ø,3,4,7,8][Ø,3,7,C,D,J,K,Y]Z
Non-OR	ØVW[4,8,D,S]X[Ø,3,7,J,K]Z	Non-OR	ØVWRX[Ø,3,7,C,D,J,K]Z
Non-OR	ØVWM[3,4,7,8]YZ	♂	All body part, approach, device, and qualifier values

Ø   **Medical and Surgical**
V   **Male Reproductive System**
X   **Transfer**   Definition: Moving, without taking out, all or a portion of a body part to another location to take over the function of all or a portion of a body part

           Explanation: The body part transferred remains connected to its vascular and nervous supply

Body Part Character 4	Approach Character 5	Device Character 6	Qualifier Character 7

T   Prepuce
     Foreskin
     Glans penis
	Ø Open
	X External
		Z No Device	**D** Urethra
			S Penis

🄻🄲 Limited Coverage   🄽🄲 Noncovered   ⊞ Combination Member   HAC associated procedure   Combination Only   DRG Non-OR   Non-OR   New/Revised in GREEN

656   ICD-10-PCS 2020

Anatomical Regions, General ØWØ–ØWY

Character Meanings

This Character Meaning table is provided as a guide to assist the user in the identification of character members that may be found in this section of code tables. It **SHOULD NOT** be used to build a PCS code.

Operation–Character 3	Body Region–Character 4	Approach–Character 5	Device–Character 6	Qualifier–Character 7
Ø Alteration	Ø Head	Ø Open	Ø Drainage Device	Ø Vagina OR Allogeneic
1 Bypass	1 Cranial Cavity	3 Percutaneous	1 Radioactive Element	1 Penis OR Syngeneic
2 Change	2 Face	4 Percutaneous Endoscopic	3 Infusion Device	2 Stoma
3 Control	3 Oral Cavity and Throat	7 Via Natural or Artificial Opening	7 Autologous Tissue Substitute	4 Cutaneous
4 Creation	4 Upper Jaw	8 Via Natural or Artificial Opening Endoscopic	J Synthetic Substitute	9 Pleural Cavity, Right
8 Division	5 Lower Jaw	X External	K Nonautologous Tissue Substitute	B Pleural Cavity, Left
9 Drainage	6 Neck		Y Other Device	G Peritoneal Cavity
B Excision	8 Chest Wall		Z No Device	J Pelvic Cavity
C Extirpation	9 Pleural Cavity, Right			W Upper Vein
F Fragmentation	B Pleural Cavity, Left			X Diagnostic
H Insertion	C Mediastinum			Y Lower Vein
J Inspection	D Pericardial Cavity			Z No Qualifier
M Reattachment	F Abdominal Wall			
P Removal	G Peritoneal Cavity			
Q Repair	H Retroperitoneum			
U Supplement	J Pelvic Cavity			
W Revision	K Upper Back			
Y Transplantation	L Lower Back			
	M Perineum, Male			
	N Perineum, Female			
	P Gastrointestinal Tract			
	Q Respiratory Tract			
	R Genitourinary Tract			

AHA Coding Clinic for table ØWØ
2015, 1Q, 31   Bilateral browpexy

AHA Coding Clinic for table ØW1
2018, 4Q, 41-42   Anatomical regions bypass qualifiers
2015, 2Q, 36   Insertion of infusion device into peritoneal cavity
2013, 4Q, 126-127 Creation of percutaneous cutaneoperitoneal fistula

AHA Coding Clinic for table ØW3
2018, 4Q, 38   Control of epistaxis
2018, 1Q, 19   Argon plasma coagulation of duodenal arteriovenous malformation
2018, 1Q, 19   Control of epistaxis via silver nitrate cauterization
2017, 4Q, 57-58   Added approach values - Transorifice esophageal vein banding
2017, 4Q, 105   Control of gastrointestinal bleeding
2017, 4Q, 106   Control of bleeding of external naris using suture
2017, 4Q, 106   Nasal packing for epistaxis
2016, 4Q, 99-100   Root operation Control
2014, 4Q, 44   Bakri balloon for control of postpartum hemorrhage
2013, 3Q, 23   Control of intraoperative bleeding

AHA Coding Clinic for table ØW4
2016, 4Q, 101   Root operation Creation

AHA Coding Clinic for table ØW9
2017, 3Q, 12   Therapeutic and diagnostic paracentesis
2017, 2Q, 16   Incision and drainage of floor of mouth

AHA Coding Clinic for table ØWB
2019, 1Q, 27   Excision of pelvic sidewall mass
2017, 2Q, 16   Excision of floor of mouth
2016, 1Q, 21   Excision of urachal mass
2013, 4Q, 119   Excision of inclusion cyst of perineum

AHA Coding Clinic for table ØWC
2017, 2Q, 16   Excision of floor of mouth

AHA Coding Clinic for table ØWH
2018, 1Q, 25   Intrauterine brachytherapy & placement of tandems & ovoids
2017, 4Q, 104   Intrauterine brachytherapy & placement of tandems & ovoids
2016, 2Q, 14   Insertion of peritoneal totally implantable venous access device
2015, 2Q, 36   Insertion of infusion device into peritoneal cavity

AHA Coding Clinic for table ØWJ
2019, 1Q, 3-8   Whipple procedure
2019, 1Q, 25   Laparoscopic appendectomy converted to open procedure
2018, 3Q, 29   Decommissioning of left ventricular assist device with exploration of mediastinum
2016, 4Q, 58   Longitudinal vaginal septum
2013, 2Q, 36   Insertion of ventriculoperitoneal shunt with laparoscopic assistance

AHA Coding Clinic for table ØWQ
2017, 4Q, 106   Control of bleeding of external naris using suture
2017, 3Q, 8   Removal of silo and closure of gastroschisis
2016, 3Q, 3-7   Stoma creation & takedown procedures
2014, 4Q, 38   Abdominoplasty and abdominal wall plication for hernia repair
2014, 3Q, 28   Ileostomy takedown and parastomal hernia repair

AHA Coding Clinic for table ØWU
2017, 3Q, 8   First stage of gastroschisis repair with silo placement
2016, 3Q, 40   Omentoplasty
2015, 2Q, 29   Placement of Ioban™ antimicrobial drape over surgical wound
2014, 4Q, 39   Abdominal component release with placement of mesh for hernia repair
2012, 4Q, 101   Rib resection with reconstruction of anterior chest wall

AHA Coding Clinic for table ØWW
2015, 2Q, 9   Revision of ventriculoperitoneal (VP) shunt

AHA Coding Clinic for table ØWY
2016, 4Q, 112-113 Transplantation

Ø Medical and Surgical
W Anatomical Regions, General
Ø Alteration   Definition: Modifying the anatomic structure of a body part without affecting the function of the body part

         Explanation: Principal purpose is to improve appearance

Body Part Character 4	Approach Character 5	Device Character 6	Qualifier Character 7
Ø Head 2 Face 4 Upper Jaw 5 Lower Jaw 6 Neck 8 Chest Wall F Abdominal Wall K Upper Back L Lower Back M Perineum, Male ♂ N Perineum, Female ♀	Ø Open 3 Percutaneous 4 Percutaneous Endoscopic	7 Autologous Tissue Substitute J Synthetic Substitute K Nonautologous Tissue Substitute Z No Device	Z No Qualifier

    ♂   ØWØM[Ø,3,4][7,J,K,Z]Z
    ♀   ØWØN[Ø,3,4][7,J,K,Z]Z

Ø Medical and Surgical
W Anatomical Regions, General
1 Bypass   Definition: Altering the route of passage of the contents of a tubular body part

         Explanation: Rerouting contents of a body part to a downstream area of the normal route, to a similar route and body part, or to an abnormal route and dissimilar body part. Includes one or more anastomoses, with or without the use of a device.

Body Part Character 4	Approach Character 5	Device Character 6	Qualifier Character 7
1 Cranial Cavity	Ø Open	J Synthetic Substitute	9 Pleural Cavity, Right B Pleural Cavity, Left G Peritoneal Cavity J Pelvic Cavity
9 Pleural Cavity, Right B Pleural Cavity, Left G Peritoneal Cavity J Pelvic Cavity Retropubic space	Ø Open 3 Percutaneous 4 Percutaneous Endoscopic	J Synthetic Substitute	4 Cutaneous 9 Pleural Cavity, Right B Pleural Cavity, Left G Peritoneal Cavity J Pelvic Cavity W Upper Vein Y Lower Vein

    Non-OR   ØW1[9,B][Ø,3,4]J[4,G,W,Y]
    Non-OR   ØW1G[Ø,3,4]J[9,B,G,J]
    Non-OR   ØW1J[Ø,3,4]J[4,W,Y]

Ø Medical and Surgical
W Anatomical Regions, General
2 Change   Definition: Taking out or off a device from a body part and putting back an identical or similar device in or on the same body part without cutting or puncturing the skin or a mucous membrane

         Explanation: All CHANGE procedures are coded using the approach EXTERNAL

Body Part Character 4	Approach Character 5	Device Character 6	Qualifier Character 7

Ø Head
1 Cranial Cavity
2 Face
4 Upper Jaw
5 Lower Jaw
6 Neck
8 Chest Wall
9 Pleural Cavity, Right
B Pleural Cavity, Left
C Mediastinum
  Mediastinal cavity
  Mediastinal space
D Pericardial Cavity
F Abdominal Wall
G Peritoneal Cavity
H Retroperitoneum
  Retroperitoneal cavity
  Retroperitoneal space
J Pelvic Cavity
  Retropubic space
K Upper Back
L Lower Back
M Perineum, Male   ♂
N Perineum, Female   ♀
	X External	Ø Drainage Device
		Y Other Device
			Z No Qualifier

    Non-OR   All body part, approach, device, and qualifier values   ♂   ØW2MX[Ø,Y]Z
                                                      ♀   ØW2NX[Ø,Y]Z

LC Limited Coverage   NC Noncovered   ⊞ Combination Member   HAC associated procedure   Combination Only   DRG Non-OR   Non-OR   New/Revised in GREEN

658   ICD-10-PCS 2020

Ø   **Medical and Surgical**
W   **Anatomical Regions, General**
3   **Control**   Definition: Stopping, or attempting to stop, postprocedural or other acute bleeding
                       Explanation: None

Body Part Character 4	Approach Character 5	Device Character 6	Qualifier Character 7

Ø Head
1 Cranial Cavity
2 Face
4 Upper Jaw
5 Lower Jaw
6 Neck
8 Chest Wall
9 Pleural Cavity, Right
B Pleural Cavity, Left
C Mediastinum
    Mediastinal cavity
    Mediastinal space
D Pericardial Cavity
F Abdominal Wall
G Peritoneal Cavity
H Retroperitoneum
    Retroperitoneal cavity
    Retroperitoneal space
J Pelvic Cavity
    Retropubic space
K Upper Back
L Lower Back
M Perineum, Male   ♂
N Perineum, Female   ♀
	Ø Open
	3 Percutaneous
	4 Percutaneous Endoscopic
		Z No Device	Z No Qualifier

3 Oral Cavity and Throat	Ø Open 3 Percutaneous 4 Percutaneous Endoscopic 7 Via Natural or Artificial Opening 8 Via Natural or Artificial Opening Endoscopic X External	Z No Device	Z No Qualifier
P Gastrointestinal Tract Q Respiratory Tract R Genitourinary Tract	Ø Open 3 Percutaneous 4 Percutaneous Endoscopic 7 Via Natural or Artificial Opening 8 Via Natural or Artificial Opening Endoscopic	Z No Device	Z No Qualifier

Non-OR   ØW3GØZZ
Non-OR   ØW3P8ZZ
                                               ♂   ØW3M[Ø,3,4]ZZ
                                               ♀   ØW3N[Ø,3,4]ZZ

Ø   **Medical and Surgical**
W   **Anatomical Regions, General**
4   **Creation**   Definition: Putting in or on biological or synthetic material to form a new body part that to the extent possible replicates the anatomic structure or function of an absent body part
                       Explanation: Used for gender reassignment surgery and corrective procedures in individuals with congenital anomalies

Body Part Character 4	Approach Character 5	Device Character 6	Qualifier Character 7
M Perineum, Male ♂	Ø Open	7 Autologous Tissue Substitute J Synthetic Substitute K Nonautologous Tissue Substitute	Ø Vagina
N Perineum, Female ♀	Ø Open	7 Autologous Tissue Substitute J Synthetic Substitute K Nonautologous Tissue Substitute	1 Penis

♂   ØW4MØ[7,J,K]Ø
♀   ØW4NØ[7,J,K]1

Ø   **Medical and Surgical**
W   **Anatomical Regions, General**
8   **Division**   Definition: Cutting into a body part, without draining fluids and/or gases from the body part, in order to separate or transect a body part
                       Explanation: All or a portion of the body part is separated into two or more portions

Body Part Character 4	Approach Character 5	Device Character 6	Qualifier Character 7
N Perineum, Female ♀	X External	Z No Device	Z No Qualifier

Non-OR   ØW8NXZZ   ♀   ØW8NXZZ

Anatomical Regions, General (left margin)

Ø   **Medical and Surgical**
W   **Anatomical Regions, General**
9   **Drainage**   Definition: Taking or letting out fluids and/or gases from a body part
      Explanation: The qualifier DIAGNOSTIC is used to identify drainage procedures that are biopsies

Body Part Character 4	Approach Character 5	Device Character 6	Qualifier Character 7

Ø Head
1 Cranial Cavity
2 Face
3 Oral Cavity and Throat
4 Upper Jaw
5 Lower Jaw
6 Neck
8 Chest Wall
9 Pleural Cavity, Right
B Pleural Cavity, Left
C Mediastinum
  Mediastinal cavity
  Mediastinal space
D Pericardial Cavity
F Abdominal Wall
G Peritoneal Cavity
H Retroperitoneum
  Retroperitoneal cavity
  Retroperitoneal space
J Pelvic Cavity
  Retropubic space
K Upper Back
L Lower Back
M Perineum, Male ♂
N Perineum, Female ♀
	Ø Open
	3 Percutaneous
	4 Percutaneous Endoscopic
		Ø Drainage Device	Z No Qualifier

Ø Head
1 Cranial Cavity
2 Face
3 Oral Cavity and Throat
4 Upper Jaw
5 Lower Jaw
6 Neck
8 Chest Wall
9 Pleural Cavity, Right
B Pleural Cavity, Left
C Mediastinum
  Mediastinal cavity
  Mediastinal space
D Pericardial Cavity
F Abdominal Wall
G Peritoneal Cavity
H Retroperitoneum
  Retroperitoneal cavity
  Retroperitoneal space
J Pelvic Cavity
  Retropubic space
K Upper Back
L Lower Back
M Perineum, Male ♂
N Perineum, Female ♀
	Ø Open
	3 Percutaneous
	4 Percutaneous Endoscopic
		Z No Device	X Diagnostic
			Z No Qualifier

Non-OR   ØW9[Ø,8,9,B,K,L,M]ØØZ
Non-OR   ØW9[Ø,1,2,3,4,5,6,8,9,B,C,D,F,G,H,J,K,L,M,N]3ØZ
Non-OR   ØW9[Ø,1,8,F,G,K,L,M]4ØZ
Non-OR   ØW9[Ø,2,3,4,5,6,8,9,B,K,L,M,N]ØZX
Non-OR   ØW9[Ø,1,2,3,4,5,6,8,9,B,C,D,G,K,L,M,N]3ZX
Non-OR   ØW9[Ø,1,2,3,4,5,6,8,C,K,L,M,N]4ZX
Non-OR   ØW9[Ø,8,9,B,K,L,M]ØZZ
Non-OR   ØW9[Ø,1,2,3,4,5,6,8,9,B,C,D,F,G,H,J,K,L,M,N]3ZZ
Non-OR   ØW9[Ø,1,8,F,G,K,L,M]4ZZ

♂ ØW9M[Ø,3,4]ØZ
♂ ØW9M[Ø,3,4]Z[X,Z]
♀ ØW9N[Ø,3,4]ØZ
♀ ØW9N[Ø,3]Z[X,Z]
♀ ØW9N4ZZ

Ø   **Medical and Surgical**
W   **Anatomical Regions, General**
B   **Excision**   Definition: Cutting out or off, without replacement, a portion of a body part
                       Explanation: The qualifier DIAGNOSTIC is used to identify excision procedures that are biopsies

Body Part Character 4	Approach Character 5	Device Character 6	Qualifier Character 7
Ø Head **2** Face **3** Oral Cavity and Throat **4** Upper Jaw **5** Lower Jaw **8** Chest Wall **K** Upper Back **L** Lower Back **M** Perineum, Male ♂ **N** Perineum, Female ♀	**Ø** Open **3** Percutaneous **4** Percutaneous Endoscopic **X** External	**Z** No Device	**X** Diagnostic **Z** No Qualifier
6 Neck **F** Abdominal Wall	**Ø** Open **3** Percutaneous **4** Percutaneous Endoscopic	**Z** No Device	**X** Diagnostic **Z** No Qualifier
6 Neck **F** Abdominal Wall	**X** External	**Z** No Device	**2** Stoma **X** Diagnostic **Z** No Qualifier

C Mediastinum
    Mediastinal cavity
    Mediastinal space
H Retroperitoneum
    Retroperitoneal cavity
    Retroperitoneal space
	Ø Open
	3 Percutaneous
	4 Percutaneous Endoscopic
		Z No Device	**X** Diagnostic
			Z No Qualifier

Non-OR ØWB[Ø,2,4,5,8,K,L,M][Ø,3,4,X]ZX		♂	ØWBM[Ø,3,4,X]Z[X,Z]
Non-OR ØWB6[Ø,3,4]ZX		♀	ØWBN[Ø,3,4,X]Z[X,Z]
Non-OR ØWB6XZX			
Non-OR ØWB[C,H][3,4]ZX			

Ø   **Medical and Surgical**
W   **Anatomical Regions, General**
C   **Extirpation**   Definition: Taking or cutting out solid matter from a body part
                       Explanation: The solid matter may be an abnormal byproduct of a biological function or a foreign body; it may be imbedded in a body part or in
                       the lumen of a tubular body part. The solid matter may or may not have been previously broken into pieces.

Body Part Character 4	Approach Character 5	Device Character 6	Qualifier Character 7

1 Cranial Cavity
3 Oral Cavity and Throat
9 Pleural Cavity, Right
B Pleural Cavity, Left
C Mediastinum
    Mediastinal cavity
    Mediastinal space
D Pericardial Cavity
G Peritoneal Cavity
H Retroperitoneum
    Retroperitoneal cavity
    Retroperitoneal space
J Pelvic Cavity
    Retropubic space
	Ø Open
	3 Percutaneous
	4 Percutaneous Endoscopic
	X External
		Z No Device	**Z** No Qualifier

4 Upper Jaw **5** Lower Jaw	**Ø** Open **3** Percutaneous **4** Percutaneous Endoscopic	**Z** No Device	**Z** No Qualifier
P Gastrointestinal Tract **Q** Respiratory Tract **R** Genitourinary Tract	**Ø** Open **3** Percutaneous **4** Percutaneous Endoscopic **7** Via Natural or Artificial Opening **8** Via Natural or Artificial Opening Endoscopic **X** External	**Z** No Device	**Z** No Qualifier

Non-OR   ØWC[1,3]XZZ
Non-OR   ØWC[9,B][Ø,3,4,X]ZZ
Non-OR   ØWC[C,D,G,H,J]XZZ
Non-OR   ØWC[P,R][7,8,X]ZZ
Non-OR   ØWCQ[Ø,3,4,X]ZZ

LC Limited Coverage   **NC** Noncovered   ⊞ Combination Member   HAC associated procedure   Combination Only   DRG Non-OR   Non-OR   New/Revised in GREEN

ICD-10-PCS 2020   **661**

Ø Medical and Surgical
W Anatomical Regions, General
F Fragmentation   Definition: Breaking solid matter in a body part into pieces

     Explanation: Physical force (e.g., manual, ultrasonic) applied directly or indirectly is used to break the solid matter into pieces. The solid matter may be an abnormal byproduct of a biological function or a foreign body. The pieces of solid matter are not taken out.

Body Part Character 4	Approach Character 5	Device Character 6	Qualifier Character 7

1 Cranial Cavity   NC
3 Oral Cavity and Throat   NC
9 Pleural Cavity, Right   NC
B Pleural Cavity, Left   NC
C Mediastinum   NC
    Mediastinal cavity
    Mediastinal space
D Pericardial Cavity
G Peritoneal Cavity   NC
J Pelvic Cavity   NC
    Retropubic space
	Ø Open
	3 Percutaneous
	4 Percutaneous Endoscopic
	X External
		Z No Device	Z No Qualifier

P Gastrointestinal Tract NC Q Respiratory Tract NC R Genitourinary Tract	Ø Open 3 Percutaneous 4 Percutaneous Endoscopic 7 Via Natural or Artificial Opening 8 Via Natural or Artificial Opening Endoscopic X External	Z No Device	Z No Qualifier

DRG Non-OR	ØWFRXZZ	NC	ØWF[1,3,9,B,C,G,J]XZZ
Non-OR	ØWF[1,3,9,B,C,G]XZZ	NC	ØWF[P,Q]XZZ
Non-OR	ØWFJ[Ø,3,4,X]ZZ		
Non-OR	ØWFP[Ø,3,4,7,8,X]ZZ		
Non-OR	ØWFQXZZ		
Non-OR	ØWFR[Ø,3,4,7,8]ZZ		

Ø Medical and Surgical
W Anatomical Regions, General
H Insertion   Definition: Putting in a nonbiological appliance that monitors, assists, performs, or prevents a physiological function but does not physically take the place of a body part

     Explanation: None

Body Part Character 4	Approach Character 5	Device Character 6	Qualifier Character 7

Ø Head
1 Cranial Cavity
2 Face
3 Oral Cavity and Throat
4 Upper Jaw
5 Lower Jaw
6 Neck
8 Chest Wall
9 Pleural Cavity, Right
B Pleural Cavity, Left
C Mediastinum
    Mediastinal cavity
    Mediastinal space
D Pericardial Cavity
F Abdominal Wall
G Peritoneal Cavity
H Retroperitoneum
    Retroperitoneal cavity
    Retroperitoneal space
J Pelvic Cavity
    Retropubic space
K Upper Back
L Lower Back
M Perineum, Male
N Perineum, Female   ♀
	Ø Open
	3 Percutaneous
	4 Percutaneous Endoscopic
		1 Radioactive Element
		3 Infusion Device
		Y Other Device
			Z No Qualifier

P Gastrointestinal Tract Q Respiratory Tract R Genitourinary Tract	Ø Open 3 Percutaneous 4 Percutaneous Endoscopic 7 Via Natural or Artificial Opening 8 Via Natural or Artificial Opening Endoscopic	1 Radioactive Element 3 Infusion Device Y Other Device	Z No Qualifier

DRG Non-OR	ØWH[Ø,2,4,5,6,K,L,M][Ø,3,4][3,Y]Z	Non-OR	ØWHP[3,4,7,8][3,Y]Z
Non-OR	ØWH1[Ø,3,4]3Z	Non-OR	ØWHQ[Ø,7,8][3,Y]Z
Non-OR	ØWH[8,9,B][Ø,3,4][3,Y]Z	Non-OR	ØWHR[Ø,3,4,7,8][3,Y]Z
Non-OR	ØWHPØYZ	♀	ØWHN[Ø,3,4][3,Y]Z

Ø   Medical and Surgical
W   Anatomical Regions, General
J   Inspection   Definition: Visually and/or manually exploring a body part

Explanation: Visual exploration may be performed with or without optical instrumentation. Manual exploration may be performed directly or through intervening body layers.

Body Part Character 4	Approach Character 5	Device Character 6	Qualifier Character 7
Ø Head 2 Face 3 Oral Cavity and Throat 4 Upper Jaw 5 Lower Jaw 6 Neck 8 Chest Wall F Abdominal Wall K Upper Back L Lower Back M Perineum, Male ♂ N Perineum, Female ♀	Ø Open 3 Percutaneous 4 Percutaneous Endoscopic X External	Z No Device	Z No Qualifier

1 Cranial Cavity
9 Pleural Cavity, Right
B Pleural Cavity, Left
C Mediastinum
   Mediastinal cavity
   Mediastinal space
D Pericardial Cavity
G Peritoneal Cavity
H Retroperitoneum
   Retroperitoneal cavity
   Retroperitoneal space
J Pelvic Cavity
   Retropubic space
	Ø Open
	3 Percutaneous
	4 Percutaneous Endoscopic
		Z No Device	Z No Qualifier

P Gastrointestinal Tract Q Respiratory Tract R Genitourinary Tract	Ø Open 3 Percutaneous 4 Percutaneous Endoscopic 7 Via Natural or Artificial Opening 8 Via Natural or Artificial Opening Endoscopic	Z No Device	Z No Qualifier

DRG Non-OR ØWJ[Ø,2,4,5,K,L]ØZZ	♂ ØWJM[Ø,3,4,X]ZZ
DRG Non-OR ØWJM[Ø,4]ZZ	♀ ØWJN[Ø,3,4,X]ZZ
Non-OR ØWJ3ØZZ	
Non-OR ØWJ[Ø,2,3,4,5,6,8,F,K,L,M,N][3,X]ZZ	
Non-OR ØWJ[Ø,2,3,4,5,K,L]4ZZ	
Non-OR ØWJDØZZ	
Non-OR ØWJ[1,9,B,C,D,G,H,J]3ZZ	
Non-OR ØWJ[P,Q,R][3,7,8]ZZ	

Ø   Medical and Surgical
W   Anatomical Regions, General
M   Reattachment   Definition: Putting back in or on all or a portion of a separated body part to its normal location or other suitable location

Explanation: Vascular circulation and nervous pathways may or may not be reestablished

Body Part Character 4	Approach Character 5	Device Character 6	Qualifier Character 7
2 Face 4 Upper Jaw 5 Lower Jaw 6 Neck 8 Chest Wall F Abdominal Wall K Upper Back L Lower Back M Perineum, Male ♂ N Perineum, Female ♀	Ø Open	Z No Device	Z No Qualifier

♂ ØWMMØZZ	
♀ ØWMNØZZ	

LC Limited Coverage   **NC** Noncovered   ⊞ Combination Member   HAC associated procedure   Combination Only   DRG Non-OR   Non-OR   New/Revised in GREEN

ICD-10-PCS 2020   **663**

Anatomical Regions, General

ØWJ–ØWM

Anatomical Regions, General

Ø Medical and Surgical
W Anatomical Regions, General
P Removal   Definition: Taking out or off a device from a body part

Explanation: If a device is taken out and a similar device put in without cutting or puncturing the skin or mucous membrane, the procedure is coded to the root operation CHANGE. Otherwise, the procedure for taking out the device is coded to the root operation REMOVAL.

Body Part Character 4	Approach Character 5	Device Character 6	Qualifier Character 7

Ø Head
2 Face
4 Upper Jaw
5 Lower Jaw
6 Neck
8 Chest Wall
C Mediastinum
   Mediastinal cavity
   Mediastinal space
F Abdominal Wall
K Upper Back
L Lower Back
M Perineum, Male ♂
N Perineum, Female ♀
	Ø Open
	3 Percutaneous
	4 Percutaneous Endoscopic
	X External
		Ø Drainage Device
		1 Radioactive Element
		3 Infusion Device
		7 Autologous Tissue Substitute
		J Synthetic Substitute
		K Nonautologous Tissue Substitute
		Y Other Device
			Z No Qualifier

1 Cranial Cavity 9 Pleural Cavity, Right B Pleural Cavity, Left G Peritoneal Cavity J Pelvic Cavity Retropubic space	Ø Open 3 Percutaneous 4 Percutaneous Endoscopic	Ø Drainage Device 1 Radioactive Element 3 Infusion Device J Synthetic Substitute Y Other Device	Z No Qualifier
1 Cranial Cavity 9 Pleural Cavity, Right B Pleural Cavity, Left G Peritoneal Cavity J Pelvic Cavity Retropubic space	X External	Ø Drainage Device 1 Radioactive Element 3 Infusion Device	Z No Qualifier

D Pericardial Cavity
H Retroperitoneum
   Retroperitoneal cavity
   Retroperitoneal space
	Ø Open
	3 Percutaneous
	4 Percutaneous Endoscopic
		Ø Drainage Device
		1 Radioactive Element
		3 Infusion Device
		Y Other Device
			Z No Qualifier

D Pericardial Cavity
H Retroperitoneum
   Retroperitoneal cavity
   Retroperitoneal space
	X External	Ø Drainage Device
		1 Radioactive Element
		3 Infusion Device
			Z No Qualifier

P Gastrointestinal Tract Q Respiratory Tract R Genitourinary Tract	Ø Open 3 Percutaneous 4 Percutaneous Endoscopic 7 Via Natural or Artificial Opening 8 Via Natural or Artificial Opening Endoscopic X External	1 Radioactive Element 3 Infusion Device Y Other Device	Z No Qualifier

Non-OR	ØWP[Ø,2,4,5,6,8][Ø,3,4,X][Ø,1,3,7,J,K,Y]Z	♂	ØWPM[Ø,3,4,X][Ø,1,3,7,J,K,Y]Z
Non-OR	ØWP[C,F]X[Ø,1,3,7,J,K,Y]Z	♀	ØWPN[Ø,3,4,X][Ø,1,3,7,J,K,Y]Z
Non-OR	ØWP[K,L][Ø,3,4,X][Ø,1,3,7,J,K,Y]Z		
Non-OR	ØWPM[Ø,3,4][Ø,1,3,J,Y]Z		
Non-OR	ØWPMX[Ø,1,3,Y]Z		
Non-OR	ØWPNX[Ø,1,3,7,J,K,Y]Z		
Non-OR	ØWP1[Ø,3,4]3Z		
Non-OR	ØWP[9,B,J][Ø,3,4][Ø,1,3,J,Y]Z		
Non-OR	ØWP[1,9,B,G,J]X[Ø,1,3]Z		
Non-OR	ØWP[D,H]X[Ø,1,3]Z		
Non-OR	ØWPP[3,4,7,8,X][1,3,Y]Z		
Non-OR	ØWPQ73Z		
Non-OR	ØWPQ8[3,Y]Z		
Non-OR	ØWPQ[Ø,X][1,3,Y]Z		
Non-OR	ØWPR[Ø,3,4,7,8,X][1,3,Y]Z		

LC Limited Coverage   NC Noncovered   ⊞ Combination Member   HAC associated procedure   Combination Only   DRG Non-OR   Non-OR   New/Revised in GREEN

664   ICD-10-PCS 2020

Ø   **Medical and Surgical**
W   **Anatomical Regions, General**
Q   **Repair**   Definition: Restoring, to the extent possible, a body part to its normal anatomic structure and function

                         Explanation: Used only when the method to accomplish the repair is not one of the other root operations

Body Part Character 4	Approach Character 5	Device Character 6	Qualifier Character 7
Ø Head **2** Face **3** Oral Cavity and Throat **4** Upper Jaw **5** Lower Jaw **8** Chest Wall **K** Upper Back **L** Lower Back **M** Perineum, Male ♂ **N** Perineum, Female ♀	**Ø** Open **3** Percutaneous **4** Percutaneous Endoscopic **X** External	**Z** No Device	**Z** No Qualifier
6 Neck **F** Abdominal Wall	**Ø** Open **3** Percutaneous **4** Percutaneous Endoscopic	**Z** No Device	**Z** No Qualifier
6 Neck **F** Abdominal Wall ⊞	**X** External	**Z** No Device	**2** Stoma **Z** No Qualifier

C Mediastinum
     Mediastinal cavity
     Mediastinal space
	Ø Open
	3 Percutaneous
	4 Percutaneous Endoscopic
		Z No Device	**Z** No Qualifier

Non-OR   ØWQNXZZ
♂   ØWQM[Ø,3,4,X]ZZ
♀   ØWQN[Ø,3,4,X]ZZ

See Appendix L for Procedure Combinations
⊞   ØWQFXZ[2,Z]

Ø   **Medical and Surgical**
W   **Anatomical Regions, General**
U   **Supplement**   Definition: Putting in or on biological or synthetic material that physically reinforces and/or augments the function of a portion of a body part

                       Explanation: The biological material is non-living, or is living and from the same individual. The body part may have been previously replaced, and the SUPPLEMENT procedure is performed to physically reinforce and/or augment the function of the replaced body part.

Body Part Character 4	Approach Character 5	Device Character 6	Qualifier Character 7

Ø Head
2 Face
4 Upper Jaw
5 Lower Jaw
6 Neck
8 Chest Wall
C Mediastinum
     Mediastinal cavity
     Mediastinal space
F Abdominal Wall
K Upper Back
L Lower Back
M Perineum, Male   ♂
N Perineum, Female   ♀
	Ø Open
	4 Percutaneous Endoscopic
		7 Autologous Tissue Substitute
		J Synthetic Substitute
		K Nonautologous Tissue Substitute
			Z No Qualifier

♂   ØWUM[Ø,4][7,J,K]Z
♀   ØWUN[Ø,4][7,J,K]Z

LC Limited Coverage   **NC** Noncovered   ⊞ Combination Member   HAC associated procedure   Combination Only   DRG Non-OR   Non-OR   New/Revised in GREEN

ICD-10-PCS 2020   665

ØWQ–ØWU

Ø　Medical and Surgical
W　Anatomical Regions, General
W　Revision　　Definition: Correcting, to the extent possible, a portion of a malfunctioning device or the position of a displaced device

Explanation: Revision can include correcting a malfunctioning or displaced device by taking out or putting in components of the device such as a screw or pin

Body Part Character 4	Approach Character 5	Device Character 6	Qualifier Character 7
Ø　Head 2　Face 4　Upper Jaw 5　Lower Jaw 6　Neck 8　Chest Wall C　Mediastinum 　　Mediastinal cavity 　　Mediastinal space F　Abdominal Wall K　Upper Back L　Lower Back M　Perineum, Male　　♂ N　Perineum, Female　　♀	Ø　Open 3　Percutaneous 4　Percutaneous Endoscopic X　External	Ø　Drainage Device 1　Radioactive Element 3　Infusion Device 7　Autologous Tissue Substitute J　Synthetic Substitute K　Nonautologous Tissue Substitute Y　Other Device	Z　No Qualifier
1　Cranial Cavity 9　Pleural Cavity, Right B　Pleural Cavity, Left G　Peritoneal Cavity J　Pelvic Cavity 　　Retropubic space	Ø　Open 3　Percutaneous 4　Percutaneous Endoscopic X　External	Ø　Drainage Device 1　Radioactive Element 3　Infusion Device J　Synthetic Substitute Y　Other Device	Z　No Qualifier
D　Pericardial Cavity H　Retroperitoneum 　　Retroperitoneal cavity 　　Retroperitoneal space	Ø　Open 3　Percutaneous 4　Percutaneous Endoscopic X　External	Ø　Drainage Device 1　Radioactive Element 3　Infusion Device Y　Other Device	Z　No Qualifier
P　Gastrointestinal Tract Q　Respiratory Tract R　Genitourinary Tract	Ø　Open 3　Percutaneous 4　Percutaneous Endoscopic 7　Via Natural or Artificial Opening 8　Via Natural or Artificial Opening 　　Endoscopic X　External	1　Radioactive Element 3　Infusion Device Y　Other Device	Z　No Qualifier

DRG Non-OR	ØWW[Ø,2,4,5,6,K,L][Ø,3,4][Ø,1,3,7,J,K,Y]Z	♂	ØWWM[Ø,3,4,X][Ø,1,3,7,K,Y]Z
DRG Non-OR	ØWWM[Ø,3,4][Ø,1,3,J,Y]Z	♀	ØWWN[Ø,3,4,X][Ø,1,3,7,K,Y]Z
Non-OR	ØWW[Ø,2,4,5,6,C,F,K,L,M,N]X[Ø,1,3,7,J,K,Y]Z		
Non-OR	ØWW8[Ø,3,4,X][Ø,1,3,7,J,K,Y]Z		
Non-OR	ØWW[1,G,J]X[Ø,1,3,J,Y]Z		
Non-OR	ØWW[9,B][Ø,3,4,X][Ø,1,3,J,Y]Z		
Non-OR	ØWW[D,H]X[Ø,1,3,Y]Z		
Non-OR	ØWWP[3,4,7,8,X][1,3,Y]Z		
Non-OR	ØWWQ[Ø,X][1,3,Y]Z		
Non-OR	ØWWR[Ø,3,4,7,8,X][1,3,Y]Z		

Ø　Medical and Surgical
W　Anatomical Regions, General
Y　Transplantation　　Definition: Putting in or on all or a portion of a living body part taken from another individual or animal to physically take the place and/or function of all or a portion of a similar body part

Explanation: The native body part may or may not be taken out, and the transplanted body part may take over all or a portion of its function

Body Part Character 4	Approach Character 5	Device Character 6	Qualifier Character 7
2　Face	Ø　Open	Z　No Device	Ø　Allogeneic 1　Syngeneic

LC Limited Coverage　NC Noncovered　⊞ Combination Member　HAC associated procedure　Combination Only　DRG Non-OR　Non-OR　New/Revised in GREEN
666　　ICD-10-PCS 2020

ØWW–ØWY

Anatomical Regions, Upper Extremities ØXØ–ØXY

Character Meanings

This Character Meaning table is provided as a guide to assist the user in the identification of character members that may be found in this section of code tables. It **SHOULD NOT** be used to build a PCS code.

Operation–Character 3	Body Part–Character 4	Approach–Character 5	Device–Character 6	Qualifier–Character 7
Ø Alteration	Ø Forequarter, Right	Ø Open	Ø Drainage Device	Ø Complete OR Allogeneic
2 Change	1 Forequarter, Left	3 Percutaneous	1 Radioactive Element	1 High OR Syngeneic
3 Control	2 Shoulder Region, Right	4 Percutaneous Endoscopic	3 Infusion Device	2 Mid
6 Detachment	3 Shoulder Region, Left	X External	7 Autologous Tissue Substitute	3 Low
9 Drainage	4 Axilla, Right		J Synthetic Substitute	4 Complete 1st Ray
B Excision	5 Axilla, Left		K Nonautologous Tissue Substitute	5 Complete 2nd Ray
H Insertion	6 Upper Extremity, Right		Y Other Device	6 Complete 3rd Ray
J Inspection	7 Upper Extremity, Left		Z No Device	7 Complete 4th Ray
M Reattachment	8 Upper Arm, Right			8 Complete 5th Ray
P Removal	9 Upper Arm, Left			9 Partial 1st Ray
Q Repair	B Elbow Region, Right			B Partial 2nd Ray
R Replacement	C Elbow Region, Left			C Partial 3rd Ray
U Supplement	D Lower Arm, Right			D Partial 4th Ray
W Revision	F Lower Arm, Left			F Partial 5th Ray
X Transfer	G Wrist Region, Right			L Thumb, Right
Y Transplantation	H Wrist Region, Left			M Thumb, Left
	J Hand, Right			N Toe, Right
	K Hand, Left			P Toe, Left
	L Thumb, Right			X Diagnostic
	M Thumb, Left			Z No Qualifier
	N Index Finger, Right			
	P Index Finger, Left			
	Q Middle Finger, Right			
	R Middle Finger, Left			
	S Ring Finger, Right			
	T Ring Finger, Left			
	V Little Finger, Right			
	W Little Finger, Left			

AHA Coding Clinic for table ØX3

2016, 4Q, 99	Root operation Control
2015, 1Q, 35	Evacuation of hematoma for control of postprocedural bleeding
2013, 3Q, 23	Control of intraoperative bleeding

AHA Coding Clinic for table ØX6

2017, 2Q, 3-4	Qualifiers for the root operation detachment
2017, 2Q, 18	Removal of polydactyl digits
2017, 1Q, 52	Further distal phalangeal amputation
2016, 3Q, 33	Traumatic amputation of fingers with further revision amputation

AHA Coding Clinic for table ØXH

2017, 2Q, 20	Exchange of intramedullary antibiotic impregnated spacer

AHA Coding Clinic for table ØXP

2017, 2Q, 20	Exchange of intramedullary antibiotic impregnated spacer

AHA Coding Clinic for table ØXY

2016, 4Q, 112-113	Transplantation

Detachment Qualifier Descriptions

Qualifier Definition	Upper Arm	Lower Arm
1 **High:** Amputation at the proximal portion of the shaft of the:	Humerus	Radius/Ulna
2 **Mid:** Amputation at the middle portion of the shaft of the:	Humerus	Radius/Ulna
3 **Low:** Amputation at the distal portion of the shaft of the:	Humerus	Radius/Ulna

Qualifier Definition	Hand
Ø Complete 1st through 5th Rays Ray: digit of hand or foot with corresponding metacarpus or metatarsus	Through carpo-metacarpal joint, **Wrist**
4 Complete 1st Ray	Through carpo-metacarpal joint, **Thumb**
5 Complete 2nd Ray	Through carpo-metacarpal joint, **Index Finger**
6 Complete 3rd Ray	Through carpo-metacarpal joint, **Middle Finger**
7 Complete 4th Ray	Through carpo-metacarpal joint, **Ring Finger**
8 Complete 5th Ray	Through carpo-metacarpal joint, **Little Finger**
9 Partial 1st Ray	Anywhere along shaft or head of metacarpal bone, **Thumb**
B Partial 2nd Ray	Anywhere along shaft or head of metacarpal bone, **Index Finger**
C Partial 3rd Ray	Anywhere along shaft or head of metacarpal bone, **Middle Finger**
D Partial 4th Ray	Anywhere along shaft or head of metacarpal bone, **Ring Finger**
F Partial 5th Ray	Anywhere along shaft or head of metacarpal bone, **Little Finger**

Qualifier Definition	Thumb/Finger
Ø Complete	At the metacarpophalangeal joint
1 High	Anywhere along the proximal phalanx
2 Mid	Through the proximal interphalangeal joint or anywhere along the middle phalanx
3 Low	Through the distal interphalangeal joint or anywhere along the distal phalanx

Ø   Medical and Surgical
X   Anatomical Regions, Upper Extremities
Ø   Alteration   Definition: Modifying the anatomic structure of a body part without affecting the function of the body part
                    Explanation: Principal purpose is to improve appearance

Body Part Character 4	Approach Character 5	Device Character 6	Qualifier Character 7
2 Shoulder Region, Right 3 Shoulder Region, Left 4 Axilla, Right 5 Axilla, Left 6 Upper Extremity, Right 7 Upper Extremity, Left 8 Upper Arm, Right 9 Upper Arm, Left B Elbow Region, Right C Elbow Region, Left D Lower Arm, Right F Lower Arm, Left G Wrist Region, Right H Wrist Region, Left	Ø Open 3 Percutaneous 4 Percutaneous Endoscopic	7 Autologous Tissue Substitute J Synthetic Substitute K Nonautologous Tissue Substitute Z No Device	Z No Qualifier

Ø   Medical and Surgical
X   Anatomical Regions, Upper Extremities
2   Change   Definition: Taking out or off a device from a body part and putting back an identical or similar device in or on the same body part without cutting or puncturing the skin or a mucous membrane
                    Explanation: All CHANGE procedures are coded using the approach EXTERNAL

Body Part Character 4	Approach Character 5	Device Character 6	Qualifier Character 7
6 Upper Extremity, Right 7 Upper Extremity, Left	X External	Ø Drainage Device Y Other Device	Z No Qualifier

Non-OR   All body part, approach, device, and qualifier values

Ø   Medical and Surgical
X   Anatomical Regions, Upper Extremities
3   Control   Definition: Stopping, or attempting to stop, postprocedural or other acute bleeding
                    Explanation: None

Body Part Character 4	Approach Character 5	Device Character 6	Qualifier Character 7
2 Shoulder Region, Right 3 Shoulder Region, Left 4 Axilla, Right 5 Axilla, Left 6 Upper Extremity, Right 7 Upper Extremity, Left 8 Upper Arm, Right 9 Upper Arm, Left B Elbow Region, Right C Elbow Region, Left D Lower Arm, Right F Lower Arm, Left G Wrist Region, Right H Wrist Region, Left J Hand, Right K Hand, Left	Ø Open 3 Percutaneous 4 Percutaneous Endoscopic	Z No Device	Z No Qualifier

Anatomical Regions, Upper Extremities (side margin)

Ø **Medical and Surgical**
X **Anatomical Regions, Upper Extremities**
6 **Detachment**　　Definition: Cutting off all or a portion of the upper or lower extremities

Explanation: The body part value is the site of the detachment, with a qualifier if applicable to further specify the level where the extremity was detached

Body Part Character 4	Approach Character 5	Device Character 6	Qualifier Character 7
Ø Forequarter, Right 1 Forequarter, Left 2 Shoulder Region, Right 3 Shoulder Region, Left B Elbow Region, Right C Elbow Region, Left	Ø Open	Z No Device	Z No Qualifier
8 Upper Arm, Right 9 Upper Arm, Left D Lower Arm, Right F Lower Arm, Left	Ø Open	Z No Device	1 High 2 Mid 3 Low
J Hand, Right K Hand, Left	Ø Open	Z No Device	Ø Complete 4 Complete 1st Ray 5 Complete 2nd Ray 6 Complete 3rd Ray 7 Complete 4th Ray 8 Complete 5th Ray 9 Partial 1st Ray B Partial 2nd Ray C Partial 3rd Ray D Partial 4th Ray F Partial 5th Ray
L Thumb, Right M Thumb, Left N Index Finger, Right P Index Finger, Left Q Middle Finger, Right R Middle Finger, Left S Ring Finger, Right T Ring Finger, Left V Little Finger, Right W Little Finger, Left	Ø Open	Z No Device	Ø Complete 1 High 2 Mid 3 Low

ØX6–ØX6 (side margin, bottom)

Ø **Medical and Surgical**
X **Anatomical Regions, Upper Extremities**
9 **Drainage** Definition: Taking or letting out fluids and/or gases from a body part
    Explanation: The qualifier DIAGNOSTIC is used to identify drainage procedures that are biopsies

Body Part Character 4	Approach Character 5	Device Character 6	Qualifier Character 7
2 Shoulder Region, Right	Ø Open	Ø Drainage Device	Z No Qualifier
3 Shoulder Region, Left	3 Percutaneous		
4 Axilla, Right	4 Percutaneous Endoscopic		
5 Axilla, Left			
6 Upper Extremity, Right			
7 Upper Extremity, Left			
8 Upper Arm, Right			
9 Upper Arm, Left			
B Elbow Region, Right			
C Elbow Region, Left			
D Lower Arm, Right			
F Lower Arm, Left			
G Wrist Region, Right			
H Wrist Region, Left			
J Hand, Right			
K Hand, Left			
2 Shoulder Region, Right	Ø Open	Z No Device	X Diagnostic
3 Shoulder Region, Left	3 Percutaneous		Z No Qualifier
4 Axilla, Right	4 Percutaneous Endoscopic		
5 Axilla, Left			
6 Upper Extremity, Right			
7 Upper Extremity, Left			
8 Upper Arm, Right			
9 Upper Arm, Left			
B Elbow Region, Right			
C Elbow Region, Left			
D Lower Arm, Right			
F Lower Arm, Left			
G Wrist Region, Right			
H Wrist Region, Left			
J Hand, Right			
K Hand, Left			

Non-OR All body part, approach, device, and qualifier values

Ø **Medical and Surgical**
X **Anatomical Regions, Upper Extremities**
B **Excision** Definition: Cutting out or off, without replacement, a portion of a body part
    Explanation: The qualifier DIAGNOSTIC is used to identify excision procedures that are biopsies

Body Part Character 4	Approach Character 5	Device Character 6	Qualifier Character 7
2 Shoulder Region, Right	Ø Open	Z No Device	X Diagnostic
3 Shoulder Region, Left	3 Percutaneous		Z No Qualifier
4 Axilla, Right	4 Percutaneous Endoscopic		
5 Axilla, Left			
6 Upper Extremity, Right			
7 Upper Extremity, Left			
8 Upper Arm, Right			
9 Upper Arm, Left			
B Elbow Region, Right			
C Elbow Region, Left			
D Lower Arm, Right			
F Lower Arm, Left			
G Wrist Region, Right			
H Wrist Region, Left			
J Hand, Right			
K Hand, Left			

Non-OR ØXB[2,3,4,5,6,7,8,9,B,C,D,F,G,H,J,K][Ø,3,4]ZX

Ø   **Medical and Surgical**
X   **Anatomical Regions, Upper Extremities**
H   **Insertion**   Definition: Putting in a nonbiological appliance that monitors, assists, performs, or prevents a physiological function but does not physically take the place of a body part

                   Explanation: None

Body Part Character 4	Approach Character 5	Device Character 6	Qualifier Character 7
2 Shoulder Region, Right	Ø Open	1 Radioactive Element	Z No Qualifier
3 Shoulder Region, Left	3 Percutaneous	3 Infusion Device	
4 Axilla, Right	4 Percutaneous Endoscopic	Y Other Device	
5 Axilla, Left			
6 Upper Extremity, Right			
7 Upper Extremity, Left			
8 Upper Arm, Right			
9 Upper Arm, Left			
B Elbow Region, Right			
C Elbow Region, Left			
D Lower Arm, Right			
F Lower Arm, Left			
G Wrist Region, Right			
H Wrist Region, Left			
J Hand, Right			
K Hand, Left			

DRG Non-OR   ØXH[2,3,4,5,6,7,8,9,B,C,D,F,G,H,J,K][Ø,3,4][3,Y]Z

Ø   **Medical and Surgical**
X   **Anatomical Regions, Upper Extremities**
J   **Inspection**   Definition: Visually and/or manually exploring a body part

                   Explanation: Visual exploration may be performed with or without optical instrumentation. Manual exploration may be performed directly or through intervening body layers.

Body Part Character 4	Approach Character 5	Device Character 6	Qualifier Character 7
2 Shoulder Region, Right	Ø Open	Z No Device	Z No Qualifier
3 Shoulder Region, Left	3 Percutaneous		
4 Axilla, Right	4 Percutaneous Endoscopic		
5 Axilla, Left	X External		
6 Upper Extremity, Right			
7 Upper Extremity, Left			
8 Upper Arm, Right			
9 Upper Arm, Left			
B Elbow Region, Right			
C Elbow Region, Left			
D Lower Arm, Right			
F Lower Arm, Left			
G Wrist Region, Right			
H Wrist Region, Left			
J Hand, Right			
K Hand, Left			

DRG Non-OR   ØXJ[2,3,4,5,6,7,8,9,B,C,D,F,G,H,J,K]ØZZ
Non-OR   ØXJ[2,3,4,5,6,7,8,9,B,C,D,F,G,H][3,4,X]ZZ
Non-OR   ØXJ[J,K][3,X]ZZ

Ø   Medical and Surgical
X   Anatomical Regions, Upper Extremities
M   Reattachment   Definition: Putting back in or on all or a portion of a separated body part to its normal location or other suitable location

                 Explanation: Vascular circulation and nervous pathways may or may not be reestablished

Body Part Character 4	Approach Character 5	Device Character 6	Qualifier Character 7
Ø Forequarter, Right	Ø Open	Z No Device	Z No Qualifier
1 Forequarter, Left			
2 Shoulder Region, Right			
3 Shoulder Region, Left			
4 Axilla, Right			
5 Axilla, Left			
6 Upper Extremity, Right			
7 Upper Extremity, Left			
8 Upper Arm, Right			
9 Upper Arm, Left			
B Elbow Region, Right			
C Elbow Region, Left			
D Lower Arm, Right			
F Lower Arm, Left			
G Wrist Region, Right			
H Wrist Region, Left			
J Hand, Right			
K Hand, Left			
L Thumb, Right			
M Thumb, Left			
N Index Finger, Right			
P Index Finger, Left			
Q Middle Finger, Right			
R Middle Finger, Left			
S Ring Finger, Right			
T Ring Finger, Left			
V Little Finger, Right			
W Little Finger, Left			

Ø   Medical and Surgical
X   Anatomical Regions, Upper Extremities
P   Removal   Definition: Taking out or off a device from a body part

                Explanation: If a device is taken out and a similar device put in without cutting or puncturing the skin or mucous membrane, the procedure is coded to the root operation CHANGE. Otherwise, the procedure for taking out the device is coded to the root operation REMOVAL.

Body Part Character 4	Approach Character 5	Device Character 6	Qualifier Character 7
6 Upper Extremity, Right	Ø Open	Ø Drainage Device	Z No Qualifier
7 Upper Extremity, Left	3 Percutaneous	1 Radioactive Element	
	4 Percutaneous Endoscopic	3 Infusion Device	
	X External	7 Autologous Tissue Substitute	
		J Synthetic Substitute	
		K Nonautologous Tissue Substitute	
		Y Other Device	

Non-OR   All body part, approach, device, and qualifier values

LC Limited Coverage   NC Noncovered   ⊞ Combination Member   HAC associated procedure   Combination Only   DRG Non-OR   Non-OR   New/Revised in GREEN

ICD-10-PCS 2020   **673**

Ø   Medical and Surgical
X   Anatomical Regions, Upper Extremities
Q   Repair   Definition: Restoring, to the extent possible, a body part to its normal anatomic structure and function

                       Explanation: Used only when the method to accomplish the repair is not one of the other root operations

Body Part Character 4	Approach Character 5	Device Character 6	Qualifier Character 7
2 Shoulder Region, Right	Ø Open	Z No Device	Z No Qualifier
3 Shoulder Region, Left	3 Percutaneous		
4 Axilla, Right	4 Percutaneous Endoscopic		
5 Axilla, Left	X External		
6 Upper Extremity, Right			
7 Upper Extremity, Left			
8 Upper Arm, Right			
9 Upper Arm, Left			
B Elbow Region, Right			
C Elbow Region, Left			
D Lower Arm, Right			
F Lower Arm, Left			
G Wrist Region, Right			
H Wrist Region, Left			
J Hand, Right			
K Hand, Left			
L Thumb, Right			
M Thumb, Left			
N Index Finger, Right			
P Index Finger, Left			
Q Middle Finger, Right			
R Middle Finger, Left			
S Ring Finger, Right			
T Ring Finger, Left			
V Little Finger, Right			
W Little Finger, Left			

Ø   Medical and Surgical
X   Anatomical Regions, Upper Extremities
R   Replacement   Definition: Putting in or on biological or synthetic material that physically takes the place and/or function of all or a portion of a body part

                       Explanation: The body part may have been taken out or replaced, or may be taken out, physically eradicated, or rendered nonfunctional during the REPLACEMENT procedure. A REMOVAL procedure is coded for taking out the device used in a previous replacement procedure.

Body Part Character 4	Approach Character 5	Device Character 6	Qualifier Character 7
L Thumb, Right	Ø Open	7 Autologous Tissue Substitute	N Toe, Right
M Thumb, Left	4 Percutaneous Endoscopic		P Toe, Left

Ø Medical and Surgical
X Anatomical Regions, Upper Extremities
U Supplement   Definition: Putting in or on biological or synthetic material that physically reinforces and/or augments the function of a portion of a body part

Explanation: The biological material is non-living, or is living and from the same individual. The body part may have been previously replaced, and the SUPPLEMENT procedure is performed to physically reinforce and/or augment the function of the replaced body part.

Body Part Character 4	Approach Character 5	Device Character 6	Qualifier Character 7
2 Shoulder Region, Right	Ø Open	7 Autologous Tissue Substitute	Z No Qualifier
3 Shoulder Region, Left	4 Percutaneous Endoscopic	J Synthetic Substitute	
4 Axilla, Right		K Nonautologous Tissue Substitute	
5 Axilla, Left			
6 Upper Extremity, Right			
7 Upper Extremity, Left			
8 Upper Arm, Right			
9 Upper Arm, Left			
B Elbow Region, Right			
C Elbow Region, Left			
D Lower Arm, Right			
F Lower Arm, Left			
G Wrist Region, Right			
H Wrist Region, Left			
J Hand, Right			
K Hand, Left			
L Thumb, Right			
M Thumb, Left			
N Index Finger, Right			
P Index Finger, Left			
Q Middle Finger, Right			
R Middle Finger, Left			
S Ring Finger, Right			
T Ring Finger, Left			
V Little Finger, Right			
W Little Finger, Left			

Ø Medical and Surgical
X Anatomical Regions, Upper Extremities
W Revision   Definition: Correcting, to the extent possible, a portion of a malfunctioning device or the position of a displaced device

Explanation: Revision can include correcting a malfunctioning or displaced device by taking out or putting in components of the device such as a screw or pin

Body Part Character 4	Approach Character 5	Device Character 6	Qualifier Character 7
6 Upper Extremity, Right	Ø Open	Ø Drainage Device	Z No Qualifier
7 Upper Extremity, Left	3 Percutaneous	3 Infusion Device	
	4 Percutaneous Endoscopic	7 Autologous Tissue Substitute	
	X External	J Synthetic Substitute	
		K Nonautologous Tissue Substitute	
		Y Other Device	

DRG Non-OR   ØXW[6,7][Ø,3,4][Ø,3,7,J,K,Y]Z
Non-OR   ØXW[6,7]X[Ø,3,7,J,K,Y]Z

Ø Medical and Surgical
X Anatomical Regions, Upper Extremities
X Transfer   Definition: Moving, without taking out, all or a portion of a body part to another location to take over the function of all or a portion of a body part

Explanation: The body part transferred remains connected to its vascular and nervous supply

Body Part Character 4	Approach Character 5	Device Character 6	Qualifier Character 7
N Index Finger, Right	Ø Open	Z No Device	L Thumb, Right
P Index Finger, Left	Ø Open	Z No Device	M Thumb, Left

Ø Medical and Surgical
X Anatomical Regions, Upper Extremities
Y Transplantation   Definition: Putting in or on all or a portion of a living body part taken from another individual or animal to physically take the place and/or function of all or a portion of a similar body part

Explanation: The native body part may or may not be taken out, and the transplanted body part may take over all or a portion of its function

Body Part Character 4	Approach Character 5	Device Character 6	Qualifier Character 7
J Hand, Right	Ø Open	Z No Device	Ø Allogeneic
K Hand, Left			1 Syngeneic

Anatomical Regions, Lower Extremities ØYØ–ØYW

Character Meanings

This Character Meaning table is provided as a guide to assist the user in the identification of character members that may be found in this section of code tables. It **SHOULD NOT** be used to build a PCS code.

Operation–Character 3	Body Part–Character 4	Approach–Character 5	Device–Character 6	Qualifier–Character 7
Ø Alteration	Ø Buttock, Right	Ø Open	Ø Drainage Device	Ø Complete
2 Change	1 Buttock, Left	3 Percutaneous	1 Radioactive Element	1 High
3 Control	2 Hindquarter, Right	4 Percutaneous Endoscopic	3 Infusion Device	2 Mid
6 Detachment	3 Hindquarter, Left	X External	7 Autologous Tissue Substitute	3 Low
9 Drainage	4 Hindquarter, Bilateral		J Synthetic Substitute	4 Complete 1st Ray
B Excision	5 Inguinal Region, Right		K Nonautologous Tissue Substitute	5 Complete 2nd Ray
H Insertion	6 Inguinal Region, Left		Y Other Device	6 Complete 3rd Ray
J Inspection	7 Femoral Region, Right		Z No Device	7 Complete 4th Ray
M Reattachment	8 Femoral Region, Left			8 Complete 5th Ray
P Removal	9 Lower Extremity, Right			9 Partial 1st Ray
Q Repair	A Inguinal Region, Bilateral			B Partial 2nd Ray
U Supplement	B Lower Extremity, Left			C Partial 3rd Ray
W Revision	C Upper Leg, Right			D Partial 4th Ray
	D Upper Leg, Left			F Partial 5th Ray
	E Femoral Region, Bilateral			X Diagnostic
	F Knee Region, Right			Z No Qualifier
	G Knee Region, Left			
	H Lower Leg, Right			
	J Lower Leg, Left			
	K Ankle Region, Right			
	L Ankle Region, Left			
	M Foot, Right			
	N Foot, Left			
	P 1st Toe, Right			
	Q 1st Toe, Left			
	R 2nd Toe, Right			
	S 2nd Toe, Left			
	T 3rd Toe, Right			
	U 3rd Toe, Left			
	V 4th Toe, Right			
	W 4th Toe, Left			
	X 5th Toe, Right			
	Y 5th Toe, Left			

AHA Coding Clinic for table ØY3

2016, 4Q, 99	Root operation Control
2013, 3Q, 23	Control of intraoperative bleeding

AHA Coding Clinic for table ØY6

2017, 2Q, 3-4	Qualifiers for the root operation detachment
2017, 1Q, 22	Chopart amputation of foot
2015, 2Q, 28	Partial amputation of hallux at interphalangeal Joint
2015, 1Q, 28	Mid-foot amputation

AHA Coding Clinic for table ØY9

2015, 1Q, 22	Incision and drainage of abscess of femoropopliteal bypass site
2015, 1Q, 22	Incision and drainage of groin abscess

Detachment Qualifier Descriptions

Qualifier Definition	Upper Leg	Lower Leg
1 **High:** Amputation at the proximal portion of the shaft of the:	Femur	Tibia/Fibula
2 **Mid:** Amputation at the middle portion of the shaft of the:	Femur	Tibia/Fibula
3 **Low:** Amputation at the distal portion of the shaft of the:	Femur	Tibia/Fibula

Qualifier Definition	Foot
Ø Complete 1st through 5th Rays Ray: digit of hand or foot with corresponding metacarpus or metatarsus	Through tarso-metatarsal Joint, **Ankle**
4 Complete 1st Ray	Through tarso-metatarsal joint, **Great Toe**
5 Complete 2nd Ray	Through tarso-metatarsal joint, **2nd Toe**
6 Complete 3rd Ray	Through tarso-metatarsal joint, **3rd Toe**
7 Complete 4th Ray	Through tarso-metatarsal joint, **4th Toe**
8 Complete 5th Ray	Through tarso-metatarsal joint, **Little Toe**
9 Partial 1st Ray	Anywhere along shaft or head of metatarsal bone, **Great Toe**
B Partial 2nd Ray	Anywhere along shaft or head of metatarsal bone, **2nd Toe**
C Partial 3rd Ray	Anywhere along shaft or head of metatarsal bone, **3rd Toe**
D Partial 4th Ray	Anywhere along shaft or head of metatarsal bone, **4th Toe**
F Partial 5th Ray	Anywhere along shaft or head of metatarsal bone, **Little Toe**

Qualifier Definition	Toe
Ø Complete	At the metatarsal-phalangeal joint
1 High	Anywhere along the proximal phalanx
2 Mid	Through the proximal interphalangeal joint or anywhere along the middle phalanx
3 Low	Through the distal interphalangeal joint or anywhere along the distal phalanx

Ø Medical and Surgical
Y Anatomical Regions, Lower Extremities
Ø Alteration   Definition: Modifying the anatomic structure of a body part without affecting the function of the body part

           Explanation: Principal purpose is to improve appearance

Body Part Character 4	Approach Character 5	Device Character 6	Qualifier Character 7
Ø Buttock, Right 1 Buttock, Left 9 Lower Extremity, Right B Lower Extremity, Left C Upper Leg, Right D Upper Leg, Left F Knee Region, Right G Knee Region, Left H Lower Leg, Right J Lower Leg, Left K Ankle Region, Right L Ankle Region, Left	Ø Open 3 Percutaneous 4 Percutaneous Endoscopic	7 Autologous Tissue Substitute J Synthetic Substitute K Nonautologous Tissue Substitute Z No Device	Z No Qualifier

Ø Medical and Surgical
Y Anatomical Regions, Lower Extremities
2 Change   Definition: Taking out or off a device from a body part and putting back an identical or similar device in or on the same body part without cutting or puncturing the skin or a mucous membrane

           Explanation: All CHANGE procedures are coded using the approach EXTERNAL

Body Part Character 4	Approach Character 5	Device Character 6	Qualifier Character 7
9 Lower Extremity, Right B Lower Extremity, Left	X External	Ø Drainage Device Y Other Device	Z No Qualifier

Non-OR   All body part, approach, device, and qualifier values

Ø Medical and Surgical
Y Anatomical Regions, Lower Extremities
3 Control   Definition: Stopping, or attempting to stop, postprocedural or other acute bleeding

           Explanation: None

Body Part Character 4	Approach Character 5	Device Character 6	Qualifier Character 7

Ø Buttock, Right
1 Buttock, Left
5 Inguinal Region, Right
     Inguinal canal
     Inguinal triangle
6 Inguinal Region, Left
     See 5 Inguinal Region, Right
7 Femoral Region, Right
8 Femoral Region, Left
9 Lower Extremity, Right
B Lower Extremity, Left
C Upper Leg, Right
D Upper Leg, Left
F Knee Region, Right
G Knee Region, Left
H Lower Leg, Right
J Lower Leg, Left
K Ankle Region, Right
L Ankle Region, Left
M Foot, Right
N Foot, Left
	Ø Open
	3 Percutaneous
	4 Percutaneous Endoscopic
		Z No Device	Z No Qualifier

LC Limited Coverage   NC Noncovered   ⊞ Combination Member   HAC associated procedure   Combination Only   DRG Non-OR   Non-OR   New/Revised in GREEN

ICD-10-PCS 2020   679

Anatomical Regions, Lower Extremities

Ø   **Medical and Surgical**
Y   **Anatomical Regions, Lower Extremities**
6   **Detachment**   Definition: Cutting off all or a portion of the upper or lower extremities

                       Explanation: The body part value is the site of the detachment, with a qualifier if applicable to further specify the level where the extremity was detached

Body Part Character 4	Approach Character 5	Device Character 6	Qualifier Character 7
2 Hindquarter, Right **3** Hindquarter, Left **4** Hindquarter, Bilateral **7** Femoral Region, Right **8** Femoral Region, Left **F** Knee Region, Right **G** Knee Region, Left	**Ø** Open	**Z** No Device	**Z** No Qualifier
C Upper Leg, Right **D** Upper Leg, Left **H** Lower Leg, Right **J** Lower Leg, Left	**Ø** Open	**Z** No Device	**1** High **2** Mid **3** Low
M Foot, Right **N** Foot, Left	**Ø** Open	**Z** No Device	**Ø** Complete **4** Complete 1st Ray **5** Complete 2nd Ray **6** Complete 3rd Ray **7** Complete 4th Ray **8** Complete 5th Ray **9** Partial 1st Ray **B** Partial 2nd Ray **C** Partial 3rd Ray **D** Partial 4th Ray **F** Partial 5th Ray

P   1st Toe, Right
      Hallux
Q   1st Toe, Left
      See 1st Toe, Right
R   2nd Toe, Right
S   2nd Toe, Left
T   3rd Toe, Right
U   3rd Toe, Left
V   4th Toe, Right
W   4th Toe, Left
X   5th Toe, Right
Y   5th Toe, Left
	Ø Open	**Z** No Device	**Ø** Complete
			1 High
			2 Mid
			3 Low

LC Limited Coverage   **NC** Noncovered   ⊞ Combination Member   HAC associated procedure   Combination Only   DRG Non-OR   Non-OR   New/Revised in GREEN

680   ICD-10-PCS 2020

Ø   Medical and Surgical
Y   Anatomical Regions, Lower Extremities
9   Drainage   Definition: Taking or letting out fluids and/or gases from a body part

                        Explanation: The qualifier DIAGNOSTIC is used to identify drainage procedures that are biopsies

Body Part Character 4	Approach Character 5	Device Character 6	Qualifier Character 7

Ø   Buttock, Right
1   Buttock, Left
5   Inguinal Region, Right
     Inguinal canal
     Inguinal triangle
6   Inguinal Region, Left
     See 5 Inguinal Region, Right
7   Femoral Region, Right
8   Femoral Region, Left
9   Lower Extremity, Right
B   Lower Extremity, Left
C   Upper Leg, Right
D   Upper Leg, Left
F   Knee Region, Right
G   Knee Region, Left
H   Lower Leg, Right
J   Lower Leg, Left
K   Ankle Region, Right
L   Ankle Region, Left
M   Foot, Right
N   Foot, Left
	Ø Open
	3 Percutaneous
	4 Percutaneous Endoscopic
		Ø Drainage Device	Z No Qualifier

Ø   Buttock, Right
1   Buttock, Left
5   Inguinal Region, Right
     Inguinal canal
     Inguinal triangle
6   Inguinal Region, Left
     See 5 Inguinal Region, Right
7   Femoral Region, Right
8   Femoral Region, Left
9   Lower Extremity, Right
B   Lower Extremity, Left
C   Upper Leg, Right
D   Upper Leg, Left
F   Knee Region, Right
G   Knee Region, Left
H   Lower Leg, Right
J   Lower Leg, Left
K   Ankle Region, Right
L   Ankle Region, Left
M   Foot, Right
N   Foot, Left
	Ø Open
	3 Percutaneous
	4 Percutaneous Endoscopic
		Z No Device	X Diagnostic
			Z No Qualifier

Non-OR   ØY9[Ø,1,7,8,9,B,C,D,F,G,H,J,K,L,M,N][Ø,3,4]ØZ
Non-OR   ØY9[5,6]3ØZ
Non-OR   ØY9[Ø,1,7,8,9,B,C,D,F,G,H,J,K,L,M,N][Ø,3,4]Z[X,Z]
Non-OR   ØY9[5,6]3ZZ

Ø Medical and Surgical
Y Anatomical Regions, Lower Extremities
B Excision   Definition: Cutting out or off, without replacement, a portion of a body part

                     Explanation: The qualifier DIAGNOSTIC is used to identify excision procedures that are biopsies

Body Part Character 4	Approach Character 5	Device Character 6	Qualifier Character 7

Ø Buttock, Right
1 Buttock, Left
5 Inguinal Region, Right
   Inguinal canal
   Inguinal triangle
6 Inguinal Region, Left
   See 5 Inguinal Region, Right
7 Femoral Region, Right
8 Femoral Region, Left
9 Lower Extremity, Right
B Lower Extremity, Left
C Upper Leg, Right
D Upper Leg, Left
F Knee Region, Right
G Knee Region, Left
H Lower Leg, Right
J Lower Leg, Left
K Ankle Region, Right
L Ankle Region, Left
M Foot, Right
N Foot, Left
	Ø Open
	3 Percutaneous
	4 Percutaneous Endoscopic
		Z No Device	X Diagnostic
			Z No Qualifier

Non-OR   ØYB[Ø,1,9,B,C,D,F,G,H,J,K,L,M,N][Ø,3,4]ZX

Ø Medical and Surgical
Y Anatomical Regions, Lower Extremities
H Insertion   Definition: Putting in a nonbiological appliance that monitors, assists, performs, or prevents a physiological function but does not physically
                     take the place of a body part

                     Explanation: None

Body Part Character 4	Approach Character 5	Device Character 6	Qualifier Character 7

Ø Buttock, Right
1 Buttock, Left
5 Inguinal Region, Right
   Inguinal canal
   Inguinal triangle
6 Inguinal Region, Left
   See 5 Inguinal Region, Right
7 Femoral Region, Right
8 Femoral Region, Left
9 Lower Extremity, Right
B Lower Extremity, Left
C Upper Leg, Right
D Upper Leg, Left
F Knee Region, Right
G Knee Region, Left
H Lower Leg, Right
J Lower Leg, Left
K Ankle Region, Right
L Ankle Region, Left
M Foot, Right
N Foot, Left
	Ø Open
	3 Percutaneous
	4 Percutaneous Endoscopic
		1 Radioactive Element
		3 Infusion Device
		Y Other Device
			Z No Qualifier

DRG Non-OR   ØYH[Ø,1,5,6,7,8,9,B,C,D,F,G,H,J,K,L,M,N][Ø,3,4][3,Y]Z

LC Limited Coverage   NC Noncovered   ⊞ Combination Member   HAC associated procedure   Combination Only   DRG Non-OR   Non-OR   New/Revised in GREEN

682   ICD-10-PCS 2020

Ø   Medical and Surgical
Y   Anatomical Regions, Lower Extremities
J   Inspection   Definition: Visually and/or manually exploring a body part

Explanation: Visual exploration may be performed with or without optical instrumentation. Manual exploration may be performed directly or through intervening body layers.

Body Part Character 4	Approach Character 5	Device Character 6	Qualifier Character 7
Ø Buttock, Right	**Ø** Open	**Z** No Device	**Z** No Qualifier
1 Buttock, Left	**3** Percutaneous		
5 Inguinal Region, Right	**4** Percutaneous Endoscopic		
Inguinal canal	**X** External		
Inguinal triangle			
6 Inguinal Region, Left			
See 5 Inguinal Region, Right			
7 Femoral Region, Right			
8 Femoral Region, Left			
9 Lower Extremity, Right			
A Inguinal Region, Bilateral			
See 5 Inguinal Region, Right			
B Lower Extremity, Left			
C Upper Leg, Right			
D Upper Leg, Left			
E Femoral Region, Bilateral			
F Knee Region, Right			
G Knee Region, Left			
H Lower Leg, Right			
J Lower Leg, Left			
K Ankle Region, Right			
L Ankle Region, Left			
M Foot, Right			
N Foot, Left			

DRG Non-OR   ØYJ[Ø,1,8,9,B,C,D,E,F,G,H,J,K,L,M,N]ØZZ
Non-OR   ØYJ[Ø,1,9,B,C,D,F,G,H,J,K,L,M,N][3,4,X]ZZ
Non-OR   ØYJ[5,6,7,8,A,E][3,X]ZZ

⬛ Limited Coverage   ⬛ Noncovered   ⊞ Combination Member   HAC associated procedure   Combination Only   DRG Non-OR   Non-OR   New/Revised in GREEN

ICD-10-PCS 2020   **683**

Ø   **Medical and Surgical**
Y   **Anatomical Regions, Lower Extremities**
M   **Reattachment**   Definition: Putting back in or on all or a portion of a separated body part to its normal location or other suitable location

                        Explanation: Vascular circulation and nervous pathways may or may not be reestablished

Body Part Character 4	Approach Character 5	Device Character 6	Qualifier Character 7
Ø Buttock, Right	**Ø** Open	**Z** No Device	**Z** No Qualifier
1 Buttock, Left			
2 Hindquarter, Right			
3 Hindquarter, Left			
4 Hindquarter, Bilateral			

5 Inguinal Region, Right
    Inguinal canal
    Inguinal triangle			

6 Inguinal Region, Left *See 5 Inguinal Region, Right*			
7 Femoral Region, Right			
8 Femoral Region, Left			
9 Lower Extremity, Right			
B Lower Extremity, Left			
C Upper Leg, Right			
D Upper Leg, Left			
F Knee Region, Right			
G Knee Region, Left			
H Lower Leg, Right			
J Lower Leg, Left			
K Ankle Region, Right			
L Ankle Region, Left			
M Foot, Right			
N Foot, Left			
P 1st Toe, Right Hallux			
Q 1st Toe, Left *See 1st Toe, Right*			
R 2nd Toe, Right			
S 2nd Toe, Left			
T 3rd Toe, Right			
U 3rd Toe, Left			
V 4th Toe, Right			
W 4th Toe, Left			
X 5th Toe, Right			
Y 5th Toe, Left			

Ø   **Medical and Surgical**
Y   **Anatomical Regions, Lower Extremities**
P   **Removal**   Definition: Taking out or off a device from a body part

                  Explanation: If a device is taken out and a similar device put in without cutting or puncturing the skin or mucous membrane, the procedure is coded to the root operation CHANGE. Otherwise, the procedure for taking out the device is coded to the root operation REMOVAL.

Body Part Character 4	Approach Character 5	Device Character 6	Qualifier Character 7
9 Lower Extremity, Right	**Ø** Open	**Ø** Drainage Device	**Z** No Qualifier
B Lower Extremity, Left	**3** Percutaneous	**1** Radioactive Element	
	4 Percutaneous Endoscopic	**3** Infusion Device	
	X External	**7** Autologous Tissue Substitute	
		J Synthetic Substitute	
		K Nonautologous Tissue Substitute	
		Y Other Device	

    Non-OR   All body part, approach, device, and qualifier values

🅛🅒 Limited Coverage   🅝🅒 Noncovered   ⊞ Combination Member   HAC associated procedure   Combination Only   DRG Non-OR   Non-OR   New/Revised in GREEN

684   ICD-10-PCS 2020

Ø   **Medical and Surgical**
Y   **Anatomical Regions, Lower Extremities**
Q   **Repair**   Definition: Restoring, to the extent possible, a body part to its normal anatomic structure and function
                    Explanation: Used only when the method to accomplish the repair is not one of the other root operations

Body Part Character 4	Approach Character 5	Device Character 6	Qualifier Character 7
Ø Buttock, Right	Ø Open	Z No Device	Z No Qualifier
1 Buttock, Left	3 Percutaneous		
5 Inguinal Region, Right	4 Percutaneous Endoscopic		
Inguinal canal	X External		
Inguinal triangle			
6 Inguinal Region, Left			
See 5 Inguinal Region, Right			
7 Femoral Region, Right			
8 Femoral Region, Left			
9 Lower Extremity, Right			
A Inguinal Region, Bilateral			
See 5 Inguinal Region, Right			
B Lower Extremity, Left			
C Upper Leg, Right			
D Upper Leg, Left			
E Femoral Region, Bilateral			
F Knee Region, Right			
G Knee Region, Left			
H Lower Leg, Right			
J Lower Leg, Left			
K Ankle Region, Right			
L Ankle Region, Left			
M Foot, Right			
N Foot, Left			
P 1st Toe, Right			
Hallux			
Q 1st Toe, Left			
See 1st Toe, Right			
R 2nd Toe, Right			
S 2nd Toe, Left			
T 3rd Toe, Right			
U 3rd Toe, Left			
V 4th Toe, Right			
W 4th Toe, Left			
X 5th Toe, Right			
Y 5th Toe, Left			

Non-OR   ØYQ[5,6,7,8,A,E]XZZ

Ø Medical and Surgical
Y Anatomical Regions, Lower Extremities
U Supplement   Definition: Putting in or on biological or synthetic material that physically reinforces and/or augments the function of a portion of a body part

Explanation: The biological material is non-living, or is living and from the same individual. The body part may have been previously replaced, and the SUPPLEMENT procedure is performed to physically reinforce and/or augment the function of the replaced body part.

Body Part Character 4	Approach Character 5	Device Character 6	Qualifier Character 7
Ø Buttock, Right	Ø Open	7 Autologous Tissue Substitute	Z No Qualifier
1 Buttock, Left	4 Percutaneous Endoscopic	J Synthetic Substitute	

5 Inguinal Region, Right
   Inguinal canal
   Inguinal triangle
		K Nonautologous Tissue Substitute	

6 Inguinal Region, Left *See 5 Inguinal Region, Right*			
7 Femoral Region, Right			
8 Femoral Region, Left			
9 Lower Extremity, Right			
A Inguinal Region, Bilateral *See 5 Inguinal Region, Right*			
B Lower Extremity, Left			
C Upper Leg, Right			
D Upper Leg, Left			
E Femoral Region, Bilateral			
F Knee Region, Right			
G Knee Region, Left			
H Lower Leg, Right			
J Lower Leg, Left			
K Ankle Region, Right			
L Ankle Region, Left			
M Foot, Right			
N Foot, Left			
P 1st Toe, Right Hallux			
Q 1st Toe, Left *See 1st Toe, Right*			
R 2nd Toe, Right			
S 2nd Toe, Left			
T 3rd Toe, Right			
U 3rd Toe, Left			
V 4th Toe, Right			
W 4th Toe, Left			
X 5th Toe, Right			
Y 5th Toe, Left			

Ø Medical and Surgical
Y Anatomical Regions, Lower Extremities
W Revision   Definition: Correcting, to the extent possible, a portion of a malfunctioning device or the position of a displaced device

Explanation: Revision can include correcting a malfunctioning or displaced device by taking out or putting in components of the device such as a screw or pin

Body Part Character 4	Approach Character 5	Device Character 6	Qualifier Character 7
9 Lower Extremity, Right	Ø Open	Ø Drainage Device	Z No Qualifier
B Lower Extremity, Left	3 Percutaneous	3 Infusion Device	
	4 Percutaneous Endoscopic	7 Autologous Tissue Substitute	
	X External	J Synthetic Substitute	
		K Nonautologous Tissue Substitute	
		Y Other Device	

DRG Non-OR   ØYW[9,B][Ø,3,4][Ø,3,7,J,K,Y]Z
Non-OR   ØYW[9,B]X[Ø,3,7,J,K,Y]Z

LC Limited Coverage   NC Noncovered   ⊞ Combination Member   HAC associated procedure   Combination Only   DRG Non-OR   Non-OR   New/Revised in GREEN

Obstetrics 1Ø2–1ØY

Character Meanings

This Character Meaning table is provided as a guide to assist the user in the identification of character members that may be found in this section of code tables. It **SHOULD NOT** be used to build a PCS code.

Ø: Pregnancy

Operation–Character 3		Body Part–Character 4		Approach–Character 5		Device–Character 6		Qualifier–Character 7	
2	Change	Ø	Products of Conception	Ø	Open	3	Monitoring Electrode	Ø	High
9	Drainage	1	Products of Conception, Retained	3	Percutaneous	Y	Other Device	1	Low
A	Abortion	2	Products of Conception, Ectopic	4	Percutaneous Endoscopic	Z	No Device	2	Extraperitoneal
D	Extraction			7	Via Natural or Artificial Opening			3	Low Forceps
E	Delivery			8	Via Natural or Artificial Opening Endoscopic			4	Mid Forceps
H	Insertion			X	External			5	High Forceps
J	Inspection							6	Vacuum
P	Removal							7	Internal Version
Q	Repair							8	Other
S	Reposition							9	Fetal Blood OR Manual
T	Resection							A	Fetal Cerebrospinal Fluid
Y	Transplantation							B	Fetal Fluid, Other
								C	Amniotic Fluid, Therapeutic
								D	Fluid, Other
								E	Nervous System
								F	Cardiovascular System
								G	Lymphatics & Hemic
								H	Eye
								J	Ear, Nose & Sinus
								K	Respiratory System
								L	Mouth & Throat
								M	Gastrointestinal System
								N	Hepatobiliary & Pancreas
								P	Endocrine System
								Q	Skin
								R	Musculoskeletal System
								S	Urinary System
								T	Female Reproductive System
								U	Amniotic Fluid, Diagnostic
								V	Male Reproductive System
								W	Laminaria
								X	Abortifacient
								Y	Other Body System
								Z	No Qualifier

AHA Coding Clinic for table 1Ø9

| 2014, 3Q, 12 | Fetoscopic laser photocoagulation and laser microseptostomy for twin-twin transfusion syndrome |
| 2014, 2Q, 9 | Pitocin administration to augment labor |

AHA Coding Clinic for table 1ØD

2018, 4Q, 49-51	Revised qualifier values for root operation "extraction" (cesarean delivery)
2018, 2Q, 17	High transverse cesarean section
2016, 1Q, 9	Vaginal delivery assisted by vacuum and low forceps extraction
2014, 4Q, 43	Cesarean delivery assisted by vacuum extraction
2014, 4Q, 43	Vacuum dilation and curettage for blighted ovum

AHA Coding Clinic for table 1ØE

2017, 3Q, 5	Delivery of placenta
2016, 2Q, 34	Assisted vaginal delivery
2014, 4Q, 17	RH (D) alloimmunization (sensitization)
2014, 2Q, 9	Pitocin administration to augment labor

AHA Coding Clinic for table 1ØH

| 2013, 2Q, 36 | Intrauterine pressure monitor |

AHA Coding Clinic for table 1ØQ

| 2014, 3Q, 12 | Fetoscopic laser photocoagulation and laser microseptostomy for twin-twin transfusion syndrome |

AHA Coding Clinic for table 1ØT

| 2015, 3Q, 31 | Laparoscopic partial salpingectomy for ectopic pregnancy |

1 Obstetrics
Ø Pregnancy
2 Change   Definition: Taking out or off a device from a body part and putting back an identical or similar device in or on the same body part without cutting or puncturing the skin or a mucous membrane
Explanation: None

Body Part Character 4	Approach Character 5	Device Character 6	Qualifier Character 7
Ø Products of Conception ♀	7 Via Natural or Artificial Opening	3 Monitoring Electrode Y Other Device	Z No Qualifier

Non-OR   All body part, approach, device, and qualifier values   ♀   All body part, approach, device, and qualifier values

1 Obstetrics
Ø Pregnancy
9 Drainage   Definition: Taking or letting out fluids and/or gases from a body part
Explanation: None

Body Part Character 4	Approach Character 5	Device Character 6	Qualifier Character 7
Ø Products of Conception ♀	Ø Open 3 Percutaneous 4 Percutaneous Endoscopic 7 Via Natural or Artificial Opening 8 Via Natural or Artificial Opening Endoscopic	Z No Device	9 Fetal Blood A Fetal Cerebrospinal Fluid B Fetal Fluid, Other C Amniotic Fluid, Therapeutic D Fluid, Other U Amniotic Fluid, Diagnostic

Non-OR   All body part, approach, device, and qualifier values   ♀   All body part, approach, device, and qualifier values

1 Obstetrics
Ø Pregnancy
A Abortion   Definition: Artificially terminating a pregnancy
Explanation: None

Body Part Character 4	Approach Character 5	Device Character 6	Qualifier Character 7
Ø Products of Conception ♀	Ø Open 3 Percutaneous 4 Percutaneous Endoscopic 8 Via Natural or Artificial Opening Endoscopic	Z No Device	Z No Qualifier
Ø Products of Conception ♀	7 Via Natural or Artificial Opening	Z No Device	6 Vacuum W Laminaria X Abortifacient Z No Qualifier

Non-OR   10A07Z[6,W,X]   ♀   All body part, approach, device, and qualifier values

1 Obstetrics
Ø Pregnancy
D Extraction   Definition: Pulling or stripping out or off all or a portion of a body part by the use of force
Explanation: None

Body Part Character 4	Approach Character 5	Device Character 6	Qualifier Character 7
Ø Products of Conception ⒰Ⓐ♀	Ø Open	Z No Device	Ø High 1 Low 2 Extraperitoneal
Ø Products of Conception ⒰Ⓐ♀	7 Via Natural or Artificial Opening	Z No Device	3 Low Forceps 4 Mid Forceps 5 High Forceps 6 Vacuum 7 Internal Version 8 Other
1 Products of Conception, Retained ♀	7 Via Natural or Artificial Opening 8 Via Natural or Artificial Opening Endoscopic	Z No Device	9 Manual Z No Qualifier
2 Products of Conception, Ectopic ♀	7 Via Natural or Artificial Opening 8 Via Natural or Artificial Opening Endoscopic	Z No Device	Z No Qualifier

DRG Non-OR   10D07Z[3,4,5,6,7,8]   ♀   All body part, approach, device, and qualifier values
⒰Ⓐ   10D00Z[Ø,1,2] except when a corresponding SDX of Z37.Ø-Z37.9 is also reported
⒰Ⓐ   10D07Z[3,4,5,7] except when a corresponding SDX of Z37.Ø-Z37.9 is also reported

1   **Obstetrics**
Ø   **Pregnancy**
E   **Delivery**   Definition: Assisting the passage of the products of conception from the genital canal

                   Explanation: None

Body Part Character 4	Approach Character 5	Device Character 6	Qualifier Character 7
Ø Products of Conception QA ♀	**X** External	**Z** No Device	**Z** No Qualifier

DRG Non-OR	1ØEØXZZ	♀	All body part, approach, device, and qualifier values
QA	1ØEØXZZ except when a corresponding SDX of Z37.Ø-Z37.9 is also reported		

1   **Obstetrics**
Ø   **Pregnancy**
H   **Insertion**   Definition: Putting in a nonbiological appliance that monitors, assists, performs, or prevents a physiological function but does not physically take the place of a body part

                   Explanation: None

Body Part Character 4	Approach Character 5	Device Character 6	Qualifier Character 7
Ø Products of Conception ♀	**Ø** Open **7** Via Natural or Artificial Opening	**3** Monitoring Electrode **Y** Other Device	**Z** No Qualifier

Non-OR	All body part, approach, device, and qualifier values	♀	All body part, approach, device, and qualifier values

1   **Obstetrics**
Ø   **Pregnancy**
J   **Inspection**   Definition: Visually and/or manually exploring a body part

                   Explanation: Visual exploration may be performed with or without optical instrumentation. Manual exploration may be performed directly or through intervening body layers.

Body Part Character 4	Approach Character 5	Device Character 6	Qualifier Character 7
Ø Products of Conception ♀ **1** Products of Conception, Retained ♀ **2** Products of Conception, Ectopic ♀	**Ø** Open **3** Percutaneous **4** Percutaneous Endoscopic **7** Via Natural or Artificial Opening **8** Via Natural or Artificial Opening Endoscopic **X** External	**Z** No Device	**Z** No Qualifier

Non-OR	All body part, approach, device, and qualifier values	♀	All body part, approach, device, and qualifier values

1   **Obstetrics**
Ø   **Pregnancy**
P   **Removal**   Definition: Taking out or off a device from a body part, region or orifice

                   Explanation: If a device is taken out and a similar device put in without cutting or puncturing the skin or mucous membrane, the procedure is coded to the root operation CHANGE. Otherwise, the procedure for taking out a device is coded to the root operation REMOVAL.

Body Part Character 4	Approach Character 5	Device Character 6	Qualifier Character 7
Ø Products of Conception ♀	**Ø** Open **7** Via Natural or Artificial Opening	**3** Monitoring Electrode **Y** Other Device	**Z** No Qualifier

Non-OR	All body part, approach, device, and qualifier values	♀	All body part, approach, device, and qualifier values

1   **Obstetrics**
Ø   **Pregnancy**
Q   **Repair**   Definition: Restoring, to the extent possible, a body part to its normal anatomic structure and function

                   Explanation: Used only when the method to accomplish the repair is not one of the other root operations

Body Part Character 4	Approach Character 5	Device Character 6	Qualifier Character 7
Ø Products of Conception ♀	**Ø** Open **3** Percutaneous **4** Percutaneous Endoscopic **7** Via Natural or Artificial Opening **8** Via Natural or Artificial Opening Endoscopic	**Y** Other Device **Z** No Device	**E** Nervous System **F** Cardiovascular System **G** Lymphatics and Hemic **H** Eye **J** Ear, Nose and Sinus **K** Respiratory System **L** Mouth and Throat **M** Gastrointestinal System **N** Hepatobiliary and Pancreas **P** Endocrine System **Q** Skin **R** Musculoskeletal System **S** Urinary System **T** Female Reproductive System **V** Male Reproductive System **Y** Other Body System

Non-OR	All body part, approach, device, and qualifier values	♀	All body part, approach, device, and qualifier values

LC Limited Coverage   **NC** Noncovered   **QA** Questionable Admit   ⊞ Combination Member   HAC   Combination Only   DRG Non-OR   Non-OR   New/Revised in GREEN

ICD-10-PCS 2020   689

10E–10Q

1 Obstetrics
Ø Pregnancy
S Reposition Definition: Moving to its normal location, or other suitable location, all or a portion of a body part
Explanation: The body part is moved to a new location from an abnormal location, or from a normal location where it is not functioning correctly. The body part may or may not be cut out or off to be moved to the new location.

Body Part Character 4	Approach Character 5	Device Character 6	Qualifier Character 7
Ø Products of Conception ♀	7 Via Natural or Artificial Opening X External	Z No Device	Z No Qualifier
2 Products of Conception, Ectopic ♀	Ø Open 3 Percutaneous 4 Percutaneous Endoscopic 7 Via Natural or Artificial Opening 8 Via Natural or Artificial Opening Endoscopic	Z No Device	Z No Qualifier

Non-OR 10SØ[7,X]ZZ		♀ All body part, approach, device, and qualifier values	

1 Obstetrics
Ø Pregnancy
T Resection Definition: Cutting out or off, without replacement, all of a body part
Explanation: None

Body Part Character 4	Approach Character 5	Device Character 6	Qualifier Character 7
2 Products of Conception, Ectopic ♀	Ø Open 3 Percutaneous 4 Percutaneous Endoscopic 7 Via Natural or Artificial Opening 8 Via Natural or Artificial Opening Endoscopic	Z No Device	Z No Qualifier

♀ All body part, approach, device, and qualifier values

1 Obstetrics
Ø Pregnancy
Y Transplantation Definition: Putting in or on all or a portion of a living body part taken from another individual or animal to physically take the place and/or function of all or a portion of a similar body part
Explanation: The native body part may or may not be taken out, and the transplanted body part may take over all or a portion of its function

Body Part Character 4	Approach Character 5	Device Character 6	Qualifier Character 7
Ø Products of Conception ♀	3 Percutaneous 4 Percutaneous Endoscopic 7 Via Natural or Artificial Opening	Z No Device	E Nervous System F Cardiovascular System G Lymphatics and Hemic H Eye J Ear, Nose and Sinus K Respiratory System L Mouth and Throat M Gastrointestinal System N Hepatobiliary and Pancreas P Endocrine System Q Skin R Musculoskeletal System S Urinary System T Female Reproductive System V Male Reproductive System Y Other Body System

Non-OR All body part, approach, device, and qualifier values		♀ All body part, approach, device, and qualifier values	

Placement 2WØ–2Y5

AHA Coding Clinic for table 2W6

2015, 2Q, 35	Application of tongs to reduce and stabilize cervical fracture
2013, 2Q, 39	Application of cervical tongs for reduction of cervical fracture

AHA Coding Clinic for table 2Y4

2018, 4Q, 38	Control of epistaxis
2017, 4Q, 106	Nasal packing for epistaxis

2   Placement
W   Anatomical Regions
Ø   Change   Definition: Taking out or off a device from a body part and putting back an identical or similar device in or on the same body part without cutting or puncturing the skin or a mucous membrane

Body Region Character 4	Approach Character 5	Device Character 6	Qualifier Character 7
Ø Head	X External	Ø Traction Apparatus	Z No Qualifier
2 Neck		1 Splint	
3 Abdominal Wall		2 Cast	
4 Chest Wall		3 Brace	
5 Back		4 Bandage	
6 Inguinal Region, Right		5 Packing Material	
7 Inguinal Region, Left		6 Pressure Dressing	
8 Upper Extremity, Right		7 Intermittent Pressure Device	
9 Upper Extremity, Left		Y Other Device	
A Upper Arm, Right			
B Upper Arm, Left			
C Lower Arm, Right			
D Lower Arm, Left			
E Hand, Right			
F Hand, Left			
G Thumb, Right			
H Thumb, Left			
J Finger, Right			
K Finger, Left			
L Lower Extremity, Right			
M Lower Extremity, Left			
N Upper Leg, Right			
P Upper Leg, Left			
Q Lower Leg, Right			
R Lower Leg, Left			
S Foot, Right			
T Foot, Left			
U Toe, Right			
V Toe, Left			
1 Face	X External	Ø Traction Apparatus	Z No Qualifier
		1 Splint	
		2 Cast	
		3 Brace	
		4 Bandage	
		5 Packing Material	
		6 Pressure Dressing	
		7 Intermittent Pressure Device	
		9 Wire	
		Y Other Device	

Placement

2   **Placement**
W   **Anatomical Regions**
1   **Compression**   Definition: Putting pressure on a body region

Body Region Character 4	Approach Character 5	Device Character 6	Qualifier Character 7
Ø Head 1 Face 2 Neck 3 Abdominal Wall 4 Chest Wall 5 Back 6 Inguinal Region, Right 7 Inguinal Region, Left 8 Upper Extremity, Right 9 Upper Extremity, Left A Upper Arm, Right B Upper Arm, Left C Lower Arm, Right D Lower Arm, Left E Hand, Right F Hand, Left G Thumb, Right H Thumb, Left J Finger, Right K Finger, Left L Lower Extremity, Right M Lower Extremity, Left N Upper Leg, Right P Upper Leg, Left Q Lower Leg, Right R Lower Leg, Left S Foot, Right T Foot, Left U Toe, Right V Toe, Left	X External	6 Pressure Dressing 7 Intermittent Pressure Device	Z No Qualifier

2   **Placement**
W   **Anatomical Regions**
2   **Dressing**   Definition: Putting material on a body region for protection

Body Region Character 4	Approach Character 5	Device Character 6	Qualifier Character 7
Ø Head 1 Face 2 Neck 3 Abdominal Wall 4 Chest Wall 5 Back 6 Inguinal Region, Right 7 Inguinal Region, Left 8 Upper Extremity, Right 9 Upper Extremity, Left A Upper Arm, Right B Upper Arm, Left C Lower Arm, Right D Lower Arm, Left E Hand, Right F Hand, Left G Thumb, Right H Thumb, Left J Finger, Right K Finger, Left L Lower Extremity, Right M Lower Extremity, Left N Upper Leg, Right P Upper Leg, Left Q Lower Leg, Right R Lower Leg, Left S Foot, Right T Foot, Left U Toe, Right V Toe, Left	X External	4 Bandage	Z No Qualifier

2 Placement
W Anatomical Regions
3 Immobilization   Definition: Limiting or preventing motion of a body region

Body Region Character 4	Approach Character 5	Device Character 6	Qualifier Character 7
Ø Head 2 Neck 3 Abdominal Wall 4 Chest Wall 5 Back 6 Inguinal Region, Right 7 Inguinal Region, Left 8 Upper Extremity, Right 9 Upper Extremity, Left A Upper Arm, Right B Upper Arm, Left C Lower Arm, Right D Lower Arm, Left E Hand, Right F Hand, Left G Thumb, Right H Thumb, Left J Finger, Right K Finger, Left L Lower Extremity, Right M Lower Extremity, Left N Upper Leg, Right P Upper Leg, Left Q Lower Leg, Right R Lower Leg, Left S Foot, Right T Foot, Left U Toe, Right V Toe, Left	X External	1 Splint 2 Cast 3 Brace Y Other Device	Z No Qualifier
1 Face	X External	1 Splint 2 Cast 3 Brace 9 Wire Y Other Device	Z No Qualifier

2 Placement
W Anatomical Regions
4 Packing   Definition: Putting material in a body region or orifice

Body Region Character 4	Approach Character 5	Device Character 6	Qualifier Character 7
Ø Head 1 Face 2 Neck 3 Abdominal Wall 4 Chest Wall 5 Back 6 Inguinal Region, Right 7 Inguinal Region, Left 8 Upper Extremity, Right 9 Upper Extremity, Left A Upper Arm, Right B Upper Arm, Left C Lower Arm, Right D Lower Arm, Left E Hand, Right F Hand, Left G Thumb, Right H Thumb, Left J Finger, Right K Finger, Left L Lower Extremity, Right M Lower Extremity, Left N Upper Leg, Right P Upper Leg, Left Q Lower Leg, Right R Lower Leg, Left S Foot, Right T Foot, Left U Toe, Right V Toe, Left	X External	5 Packing Material	Z No Qualifier

LC Limited Coverage   **NC** Noncovered   ⊞ Combination Member   **HAC**   Valid OR   Combination Only   DRG Non-OR   New/Revised in GREEN

ICD-10-PCS 2020   **693**

2W3–2W4

Placement

2   Placement
W   Anatomical Regions
5   Removal   Definition: Taking out or off a device from a body part

Body Region Character 4	Approach Character 5	Device Character 6	Qualifier Character 7
Ø Head 2 Neck 3 Abdominal Wall 4 Chest Wall 5 Back 6 Inguinal Region, Right 7 Inguinal Region, Left 8 Upper Extremity, Right 9 Upper Extremity, Left A Upper Arm, Right B Upper Arm, Left C Lower Arm, Right D Lower Arm, Left E Hand, Right F Hand, Left G Thumb, Right H Thumb, Left J Finger, Right K Finger, Left L Lower Extremity, Right M Lower Extremity, Left N Upper Leg, Right P Upper Leg, Left Q Lower Leg, Right R Lower Leg, Left S Foot, Right T Foot, Left U Toe, Right V Toe, Left	X External	Ø Traction Apparatus 1 Splint 2 Cast 3 Brace 4 Bandage 5 Packing Material 6 Pressure Dressing 7 Intermittent Pressure Device Y Other Device	Z No Qualifier
1 Face	X External	Ø Traction Apparatus 1 Splint 2 Cast 3 Brace 4 Bandage 5 Packing Material 6 Pressure Dressing 7 Intermittent Pressure Device 9 Wire Y Other Device	Z No Qualifier

2 **Placement**
W **Anatomical Regions**
6 **Traction**　　　Definition: Exerting a pulling force on a body region in a distal direction

Body Region Character 4	Approach Character 5	Device Character 6	Qualifier Character 7
Ø Head **1** Face **2** Neck **3** Abdominal Wall **4** Chest Wall **5** Back **6** Inguinal Region, Right **7** Inguinal Region, Left **8** Upper Extremity, Right **9** Upper Extremity, Left **A** Upper Arm, Right **B** Upper Arm, Left **C** Lower Arm, Right **D** Lower Arm, Left **E** Hand, Right **F** Hand, Left **G** Thumb, Right **H** Thumb, Left **J** Finger, Right **K** Finger, Left **L** Lower Extremity, Right **M** Lower Extremity, Left **N** Upper Leg, Right **P** Upper Leg, Left **Q** Lower Leg, Right **R** Lower Leg, Left **S** Foot, Right **T** Foot, Left **U** Toe, Right **V** Toe, Left	**X** External	**Ø** Traction Apparatus **Z** No Device	**Z** No Qualifier

2 **Placement**
Y **Anatomical Orifices**
Ø **Change**　　　Definition: Taking out or off a device from a body part and putting back an identical or similar device in or on the same body part without cutting or puncturing the skin or a mucous membrane

Body Region Character 4	Approach Character 5	Device Character 6	Qualifier Character 7
Ø Mouth and Pharynx **1** Nasal **2** Ear **3** Anorectal **4** Female Genital Tract　♀ **5** Urethra	**X** External	**5** Packing Material	**Z** No Qualifier

　　♀　2YØ4X5Z

2 **Placement**
Y **Anatomical Orifices**
4 **Packing**　　　Definition: Putting material in a body region or orifice

Body Region Character 4	Approach Character 5	Device Character 6	Qualifier Character 7
Ø Mouth and Pharynx **1** Nasal **2** Ear **3** Anorectal **4** Female Genital Tract　♀ **5** Urethra	**X** External	**5** Packing Material	**Z** No Qualifier

　　♀　2Y44X5Z

2 **Placement**
Y **Anatomical Orifices**
5 **Removal**　　　Definition: Taking out or off a device from a body part

Body Region Character 4	Approach Character 5	Device Character 6	Qualifier Character 7
Ø Mouth and Pharynx **1** Nasal **2** Ear **3** Anorectal **4** Female Genital Tract　♀ **5** Urethra	**X** External	**5** Packing Material	**Z** No Qualifier

　　♀　2Y54X5Z

LC Limited Coverage　　NC Noncovered　　⊞ Combination Member　　HAC　　Valid OR　　Combination Only　　DRG Non-OR　　New/Revised in GREEN

Administration 3Ø2–3E1

AHA Coding Clinic for table 3Ø2

2016, 4Q, 113	Bone marrow and stem cell transfusion (Transplantation)

AHA Coding Clinic for table 3EØ

2018, 3Q, 7	Coronary brachytherapy with angioplasty
2018, 1Q, 8	Placement of bone morphogenetic protein & spinal fusion surgery
2017, 2Q, 14	Infusion of tPA into pleural cavity
2017, 1Q, 37	Injection of glue into enteric fistula tract
2016, 4Q, 113-114	Substances applied to cranial cavity and brain
2016, 3Q, 29	Closure of bilateral alveolar clefts
2016, 1Q, 20	Metatarsophalangeal joint resection arthroplasty
2015, 3Q, 24	Esophagogastroduodenoscopy with epinephrine injection for control of bleeding
2015, 3Q, 29	Placement of adhesion barrier
2015, 2Q, 29	Insertion of nasogastric tube for drainage and feeding
2015, 2Q, 31	Thoracoscopic talc pleurodesis
2015, 1Q, 31	Intrathecal chemotherapy

AHA Coding Clinic for table 3EØ (Continued)

2015, 1Q, 38	Chemoembolization of the hepatic artery
2014, 4Q, 16	Administration of RH (D) immunoglobulin
2014, 4Q, 17	RH (D) alloimmunization (sensitization)
2014, 4Q, 19	Ultrasound accelerated thrombolysis
2014, 4Q, 34	Resection of brain malignancy with implantation of chemotherapeutic wafer
2014, 4Q, 38	Placement of saline and seprafilm solution into abdominal cavity
2014, 3Q, 26	Coil embolization of gastroduodenal artery with chemoembolization of hepatic artery
2014, 2Q, 8	Medical induction of labor with Cervidil tampon insertion
2014, 2Q, 10	Prophylactic Neulasta injection for infection prevention
2013, 4Q, 124	Administration of tPA for stroke treatment prior to transfer
2013, 1Q, 27	Injection of sclerosing agent into an esophageal varix

AHA Coding Clinic for table 3E1

2017, 3Q, 14	Bronchoscopy with suctioning and washings for removal of mucus plug

3 Administration
Ø Circulatory
2 Transfusion　　Definition: Putting in blood or blood products

Body System/Region Character 4		Approach Character 5		Substance Character 6		Qualifier Character 7	
3 Peripheral Vein	NC	**Ø** Open		**A** Stem Cells, Embryonic		**Z** No Qualifier	
4 Central Vein	NC	**3** Percutaneous					
3 Peripheral Vein	NC	**Ø** Open		**G** Bone Marrow		**Ø** Autologous	
4 Central Vein	NC	**3** Percutaneous		**X** Stem Cells, Cord Blood		**2** Allogeneic, Related	
				Y Stem Cells, Hematopoietic		**3** Allogeneic, Unrelated	
						4 Allogeneic, Unspecified	
3 Peripheral Vein		**Ø** Open		**H** Whole Blood		**Ø** Autologous	
4 Central Vein		**3** Percutaneous		**J** Serum Albumin		**1** Nonautologous	
				K Frozen Plasma			
				L Fresh Plasma			
				M Plasma Cryoprecipitate			
				N Red Blood Cells			
				P Frozen Red Cells			
				Q White Cells			
				R Platelets			
				S Globulin			
				T Fibrinogen			
				V Antihemophilic Factors			
				W Factor IX			
3 Peripheral Vein		**Ø** Open		**U** Stem Cells, T-cell Depleted Hematopoietic		**2** Allogeneic, Related	
4 Central Vein		**3** Percutaneous				**3** Allogeneic, Unrelated	
						4 Allogeneic, Unspecified	
7 Products of Conception, Circulatory	♀	**3** Percutaneous		**H** Whole Blood		**1** Nonautologous	
		7 Via Natural or Artificial Opening		**J** Serum Albumin			
				K Frozen Plasma			
				L Fresh Plasma			
				M Plasma Cryoprecipitate			
				N Red Blood Cells			
				P Frozen Red Cells			
				Q White Cells			
				R Platelets			
				S Globulin			
				T Fibrinogen			
				V Antihemophilic Factors			
				W Factor IX			
8 Vein		**Ø** Open		**B** 4-Factor Prothrombin Complex Concentrate		**1** Nonautologous	
		3 Percutaneous					

Valid OR	3Ø2[3,4]ØAZ
Valid OR	3Ø2[3,4]Ø[G,X,Y][Ø,2,3,4]
Valid OR	3Ø2[3,4]3[G,X,Y][2,3,4]
Valid OR	3Ø2[3,4]ØU[2,3,4]
DRG-Non-OR	3Ø2[3,4]3AZ
DRG-Non-OR	3Ø2[3,4]3[G,X,Y]Ø
DRG-Non-OR	3Ø2[3,4]3U[2,3,4]

NC	3Ø2[3,4][Ø,3]AZ Only when reported with PDx or SDx of C91.ØØ, C92.ØØ, C92.1Ø, C92.11, C92.4Ø, C92.5Ø, C92.6Ø, C92.AØ, C93.ØØ, C94.ØØ, C95.ØØ
NC	3Ø2[3,4][Ø,3][G,Y]Ø Only when reported with PDx or SDx of C91.ØØ, C92.ØØ, C92.1Ø, C92.11, C92.4Ø, C92.5Ø, C92.6Ø, C92.AØ, C93.ØØ, C94.ØØ, C95.ØØ
NC	3Ø2[3,4][Ø,3][G,Y][2,3,4]
♀	3Ø27[3,7][H,J,K,L,M,N,P,Q,R,S,T,V,W]1

3 Administration
C Indwelling Device
1 Irrigation　　Definition: Putting in or on a cleansing substance

Body System/Region Character 4	Approach Character 5	Substance Character 6	Qualifier Character 7
Z None	**X** External	**8** Irrigating Substance	**Z** No Qualifier

Administration

3   **Administration**
E   **Physiological Systems and Anatomical Regions**
Ø   **Introduction**   Definition: Putting in or on a therapeutic, diagnostic, nutritional, physiological, or prophylactic substance except blood or blood products

Body System/Region Character 4	Approach Character 5	Substance Character 6	Qualifier Character 7
Ø Skin and Mucous Membranes	X External	Ø Antineoplastic	5 Other Antineoplastic M Monoclonal Antibody
Ø Skin and Mucous Membranes	X External	2 Anti-infective	8 Oxazolidinones 9 Other Anti-infective
Ø Skin and Mucous Membranes	X External	3 Anti-inflammatory 4 Serum, Toxoid and Vaccine B Anesthetic Agent K Other Diagnostic Substance M Pigment N Analgesics, Hypnotics, Sedatives T Destructive Agent	Z No Qualifier
Ø Skin and Mucous Membranes	X External	G Other Therapeutic Substance	C Other Substance
1 Subcutaneous Tissue	Ø Open	2 Anti-infective	A Anti-Infective Envelope
1 Subcutaneous Tissue	3 Percutaneous	Ø Antineoplastic	5 Other Antineoplastic M Monoclonal Antibody
1 Subcutaneous Tissue	3 Percutaneous	2 Anti-infective	8 Oxazolidinones 9 Other Anti-infective A Anti-Infective Envelope
1 Subcutaneous Tissue	3 Percutaneous	3 Anti-inflammatory 6 Nutritional Substance 7 Electrolytic and Water Balance Substance B Anesthetic Agent H Radioactive Substance K Other Diagnostic Substance N Analgesics, Hypnotics, Sedatives T Destructive Agent	Z No Qualifier
1 Subcutaneous Tissue	3 Percutaneous	4 Serum, Toxoid and Vaccine	Ø Influenza Vaccine Z No Qualifier
1 Subcutaneous Tissue	3 Percutaneous	G Other Therapeutic Substance	C Other Substance
1 Subcutaneous Tissue	3 Percutaneous	V Hormone	G Insulin J Other Hormone
2 Muscle	3 Percutaneous	Ø Antineoplastic	5 Other Antineoplastic M Monoclonal Antibody
2 Muscle	3 Percutaneous	2 Anti-infective	8 Oxazolidinones 9 Other Anti-infective
2 Muscle	3 Percutaneous	3 Anti-inflammatory 6 Nutritional Substance 7 Electrolytic and Water Balance Substance B Anesthetic Agent H Radioactive Substance K Other Diagnostic Substance N Analgesics, Hypnotics, Sedatives T Destructive Agent	Z No Qualifier
2 Muscle	3 Percutaneous	4 Serum, Toxoid and Vaccine	Ø Influenza Vaccine Z No Qualifier
2 Muscle	3 Percutaneous	G Other Therapeutic Substance	C Other Substance
3 Peripheral Vein	Ø Open	Ø Antineoplastic	2 High-dose Interleukin-2 3 Low-dose Interleukin-2 5 Other Antineoplastic M Monoclonal Antibody P Clofarabine
3 Peripheral Vein	Ø Open	1 Thrombolytic	6 Recombinant Human- activated Protein C 7 Other Thrombolytic
3 Peripheral Vein	Ø Open	2 Anti-infective	8 Oxazolidinones 9 Other Anti-infective

3EØ Continued on next page

DRG Non-OR   3EØ3ØØ2
DRG Non-OR   3EØ3Ø17

3   **Administration**
E   **Physiological Systems and Anatomical Regions**   *3E0 Continued*
Ø   **Introduction**   Definition: Putting in or on a therapeutic, diagnostic, nutritional, physiological, or prophylactic substance except blood or blood products

Body System/Region Character 4	Approach Character 5	Substance Character 6	Qualifier Character 7
3 Peripheral Vein	**Ø** Open	**3** Anti-inflammatory **4** Serum, Toxoid and Vaccine **6** Nutritional Substance **7** Electrolytic and Water Balance Substance **F** Intracirculatory Anesthetic **H** Radioactive Substance **K** Other Diagnostic Substance **N** Analgesics, Hypnotics, Sedatives **P** Platelet Inhibitor **R** Antiarrhythmic **T** Destructive Agent **X** Vasopressor	**Z** No Qualifier
3 Peripheral Vein	**Ø** Open	**G** Other Therapeutic Substance	**C** Other Substance **N** Blood Brain Barrier Disruption
3 Peripheral Vein	**Ø** Open	**U** Pancreatic Islet Cells	**Ø** Autologous **1** Nonautologous
3 Peripheral Vein	**Ø** Open	**V** Hormone	**G** Insulin **H** Human B-type Natriuretic Peptide **J** Other Hormone
3 Peripheral Vein	**Ø** Open	**W** Immunotherapeutic	**K** Immunostimulator **L** Immunosuppressive
3 Peripheral Vein	**3** Percutaneous	**Ø** Antineoplastic	**2** High-dose Interleukin-2 **3** Low-dose Interleukin-2 **5** Other Antineoplastic **M** Monoclonal Antibody **P** Clofarabine
3 Peripheral Vein	**3** Percutaneous	**1** Thrombolytic	**6** Recombinant Human- activated Protein C **7** Other Thrombolytic
3 Peripheral Vein	**3** Percutaneous	**2** Anti-infective	**8** Oxazolidinones **9** Other Anti-infective
3 Peripheral Vein	**3** Percutaneous	**3** Anti-inflammatory **4** Serum, Toxoid and Vaccine **6** Nutritional Substance **7** Electrolytic and Water Balance Substance **F** Intracirculatory Anesthetic **H** Radioactive Substance **K** Other Diagnostic Substance **N** Analgesics, Hypnotics, Sedatives **P** Platelet Inhibitor **R** Antiarrhythmic **T** Destructive Agent **X** Vasopressor	**Z** No Qualifier
3 Peripheral Vein	**3** Percutaneous	**G** Other Therapeutic Substance	**C** Other Substance **N** Blood Brain Barrier Disruption **Q** Glucarpidase
3 Peripheral Vein	**3** Percutaneous	**U** Pancreatic Islet Cells	**Ø** Autologous **1** Nonautologous
3 Peripheral Vein	**3** Percutaneous	**V** Hormone	**G** Insulin **H** Human B-type Natriuretic Peptide **J** Other Hormone
3 Peripheral Vein	**3** Percutaneous	**W** Immunotherapeutic	**K** Immunostimulator **L** Immunosuppressive
4 Central Vein	**Ø** Open	**Ø** Antineoplastic	**2** High-dose Interleukin-2 **3** Low-dose Interleukin-2 **5** Other Antineoplastic **M** Monoclonal Antibody **P** Clofarabine
4 Central Vein	**Ø** Open	**1** Thrombolytic	**6** Recombinant Human- activated Protein C **7** Other Thrombolytic

3E0 Continued on next page

Valid OR 3E03ØTZ		**DRG Non-OR** 3E033U[Ø,1]	
DRG Non-OR 3E03ØU[Ø,1]		**DRG Non-OR** 3E04ØØ2	
DRG Non-OR 3E033Ø2		**DRG Non-OR** 3E04Ø17	
DRG Non-OR 3E03317			

LC Limited Coverage   **NC** Noncovered   ⊞ Combination Member   HAC   Valid OR   Combination Only   DRG Non-OR   New/Revised in GREEN

Administration

3E0 Continued

3   **Administration**
E   **Physiological Systems and Anatomical Regions**
0   **Introduction**   Definition: Putting in or on a therapeutic, diagnostic, nutritional, physiological, or prophylactic substance except blood or blood products

Body System/Region Character 4	Approach Character 5	Substance Character 6	Qualifier Character 7
4 Central Vein	Ø Open	2 Anti-infective	8 Oxazolidinones 9 Other Anti-infective
4 Central Vein	Ø Open	3 Anti-inflammatory 4 Serum, Toxoid and Vaccine 6 Nutritional Substance 7 Electrolytic and Water Balance Substance F Intracirculatory Anesthetic H Radioactive Substance K Other Diagnostic Substance N Analgesics, Hypnotics, Sedatives P Platelet Inhibitor R Antiarrhythmic T Destructive Agent X Vasopressor	Z No Qualifier
4 Central Vein	Ø Open	G Other Therapeutic Substance	C Other Substance N Blood Brain Barrier Disruption
4 Central Vein	Ø Open	V Hormone	G Insulin H Human B-type Natriuretic Peptide J Other Hormone
4 Central Vein	Ø Open	W Immunotherapeutic	K Immunostimulator L Immunosuppressive
4 Central Vein	3 Percutaneous	Ø Antineoplastic	2 High-dose Interleukin-2 3 Low-dose Interleukin-2 5 Other Antineoplastic M Monoclonal Antibody P Clofarabine
4 Central Vein	3 Percutaneous	1 Thrombolytic	6 Recombinant Human- activated Protein C 7 Other Thrombolytic
4 Central Vein	3 Percutaneous	2 Anti-infective	8 Oxazolidinones 9 Other Anti-infective
4 Central Vein	3 Percutaneous	3 Anti-inflammatory 4 Serum, Toxoid and Vaccine 6 Nutritional Substance 7 Electrolytic and Water Balance Substance F Intracirculatory Anesthetic H Radioactive Substance K Other Diagnostic Substance N Analgesics, Hypnotics, Sedatives P Platelet Inhibitor R Antiarrhythmic T Destructive Agent X Vasopressor	Z No Qualifier
4 Central Vein	3 Percutaneous	G Other Therapeutic Substance	C Other Substance N Blood Brain Barrier Disruption Q Glucarpidase
4 Central Vein	3 Percutaneous	V Hormone	G Insulin H Human B-type Natriuretic Peptide J Other Hormone
4 Central Vein	3 Percutaneous	W Immunotherapeutic	K Immunostimulator L Immunosuppressive
5 Peripheral Artery 6 Central Artery	Ø Open 3 Percutaneous	Ø Antineoplastic	2 High-dose Interleukin-2 3 Low-dose Interleukin-2 5 Other Antineoplastic M Monoclonal Antibody P Clofarabine
5 Peripheral Artery 6 Central Artery	Ø Open 3 Percutaneous	1 Thrombolytic	6 Recombinant Human- activated Protein C 7 Other Thrombolytic
5 Peripheral Artery 6 Central Artery	Ø Open 3 Percutaneous	2 Anti-infective	8 Oxazolidinones 9 Other Anti-infective

3E0 Continued on next page

Valid OR	3E04ØTZ	**DRG Non-OR**	3E0[5,6][Ø,3]Ø2
DRG Non-OR	3E043Ø2	**DRG Non-OR**	3E0[5,6][Ø,3]17
DRG Non-OR	3E04317		

3   Administration
E   Physiological Systems and Anatomical Regions
0   Introduction   Definition: Putting in or on a therapeutic, diagnostic, nutritional, physiological, or prophylactic substance except blood or blood products

3E0 Continued

Body System/Region Character 4	Approach Character 5	Substance Character 6	Qualifier Character 7
5 Peripheral Artery 6 Central Artery	0 Open 3 Percutaneous	3 Anti-inflammatory 4 Serum, Toxoid and Vaccine 6 Nutritional Substance 7 Electrolytic and Water Balance Substance F Intracirculatory Anesthetic H Radioactive Substance K Other Diagnostic Substance N Analgesics, Hypnotics, Sedatives P Platelet Inhibitor R Antiarrhythmic T Destructive Agent X Vasopressor	Z No Qualifier
5 Peripheral Artery 6 Central Artery	0 Open 3 Percutaneous	G Other Therapeutic Substance	C Other Substance N Blood Brain Barrier Disruption
5 Peripheral Artery 6 Central Artery	0 Open 3 Percutaneous	V Hormone	G Insulin H Human B-type Natriuretic Peptide J Other Hormone
5 Peripheral Artery 6 Central Artery	0 Open 3 Percutaneous	W Immunotherapeutic	K Immunostimulator L Immunosuppressive
7 Coronary Artery 8 Heart	0 Open 3 Percutaneous	1 Thrombolytic	6 Recombinant Human- activated Protein C 7 Other Thrombolytic
7 Coronary Artery 8 Heart	0 Open 3 Percutaneous	G Other Therapeutic Substance	C Other Substance
7 Coronary Artery 8 Heart	0 Open 3 Percutaneous	K Other Diagnostic Substance P Platelet Inhibitor	Z No Qualifier
7 Coronary Artery 8 Heart	4 Percutaneous Endoscopic	G Other Therapeutic Substance	C Other Substance
9 Nose	3 Percutaneous 7 Via Natural or Artificial Opening X External	0 Antineoplastic	5 Other Antineoplastic M Monoclonal Antibody
9 Nose	3 Percutaneous 7 Via Natural or Artificial Opening X External	2 Anti-infective	8 Oxazolidinones 9 Other Anti-infective
9 Nose	3 Percutaneous 7 Via Natural or Artificial Opening X External	3 Anti-inflammatory 4 Serum, Toxoid and Vaccine B Anesthetic Agent H Radioactive Substance K Other Diagnostic Substance N Analgesics, Hypnotics, Sedatives T Destructive Agent	Z No Qualifier
9 Nose	3 Percutaneous 7 Via Natural or Artificial Opening X External	G Other Therapeutic Substance	C Other Substance
A Bone Marrow	3 Percutaneous	0 Antineoplastic	5 Other Antineoplastic M Monoclonal Antibody
A Bone Marrow	3 Percutaneous	G Other Therapeutic Substance	C Other Substance
B Ear	3 Percutaneous 7 Via Natural or Artificial Opening X External	0 Antineoplastic	4 Liquid Brachytherapy Radioisotope 5 Other Antineoplastic M Monoclonal Antibody
B Ear	3 Percutaneous 7 Via Natural or Artificial Opening X External	2 Anti-infective	8 Oxazolidinones 9 Other Anti-infective
B Ear	3 Percutaneous 7 Via Natural or Artificial Opening X External	3 Anti-inflammatory B Anesthetic Agent H Radioactive Substance K Other Diagnostic Substance N Analgesics, Hypnotics, Sedatives T Destructive Agent	Z No Qualifier
B Ear	3 Percutaneous 7 Via Natural or Artificial Opening X External	G Other Therapeutic Substance	C Other Substance

3E0 Continued on next page

DRG Non-OR   3E08[0,3]17

LC Limited Coverage   NC Noncovered   ⊞ Combination Member   HAC   Valid OR   Combination Only   DRG Non-OR   New/Revised in GREEN
ICD-10-PCS 2020   701

3E0–3E0

Administration

3E0 Continued

3   **Administration**
E   **Physiological Systems and Anatomical Regions**
0   **Introduction**   Definition: Putting in or on a therapeutic, diagnostic, nutritional, physiological, or prophylactic substance except blood or blood products

Body System/Region Character 4	Approach Character 5	Substance Character 6	Qualifier Character 7
C Eye	**3** Percutaneous **7** Via Natural or Artificial Opening **X** External	**0** Antineoplastic	**4** Liquid Brachytherapy Radioisotope **5** Other Antineoplastic **M** Monoclonal Antibody
C Eye	**3** Percutaneous **7** Via Natural or Artificial Opening **X** External	**2** Anti-infective	**8** Oxazolidinones **9** Other Anti-infective
C Eye	**3** Percutaneous **7** Via Natural or Artificial Opening **X** External	**3** Anti-inflammatory **B** Anesthetic Agent **H** Radioactive Substance **K** Other Diagnostic Substance **M** Pigment **N** Analgesics, Hypnotics, Sedatives **T** Destructive Agent	**Z** No Qualifier
C Eye	**3** Percutaneous **7** Via Natural or Artificial Opening **X** External	**G** Other Therapeutic Substance	**C** Other Substance
C Eye	**3** Percutaneous **7** Via Natural or Artificial Opening **X** External	**S** Gas	**F** Other Gas
D Mouth and Pharynx	**3** Percutaneous **7** Via Natural or Artificial Opening **X** External	**0** Antineoplastic	**4** Liquid Brachytherapy Radioisotope **5** Other Antineoplastic **M** Monoclonal Antibody
D Mouth and Pharynx	**3** Percutaneous **7** Via Natural or Artificial Opening **X** External	**2** Anti-infective	**8** Oxazolidinones **9** Other Anti-infective
D Mouth and Pharynx	**3** Percutaneous **7** Via Natural or Artificial Opening **X** External	**3** Anti-inflammatory **4** Serum, Toxoid and Vaccine **6** Nutritional Substance **7** Electrolytic and Water Balance Substance **B** Anesthetic Agent **H** Radioactive Substance **K** Other Diagnostic Substance **N** Analgesics, Hypnotics, Sedatives **R** Antiarrhythmic **T** Destructive Agent	**Z** No Qualifier
D Mouth and Pharynx	**3** Percutaneous **7** Via Natural or Artificial Opening **X** External	**G** Other Therapeutic Substance	**C** Other Substance
E Products of Conception ♀ **G** Upper GI **H** Lower GI **K** Genitourinary Tract **N** Male Reproductive ♂	**3** Percutaneous **7** Via Natural or Artificial Opening **8** Via Natural or Artificial Opening Endoscopic	**0** Antineoplastic	**4** Liquid Brachytherapy Radioisotope **5** Other Antineoplastic **M** Monoclonal Antibody
E Products of Conception ♀ **G** Upper GI **H** Lower GI **K** Genitourinary Tract **N** Male Reproductive ♂	**3** Percutaneous **7** Via Natural or Artificial Opening **8** Via Natural or Artificial Opening Endoscopic	**2** Anti-infective	**8** Oxazolidinones **9** Other Anti-infective
E Products of Conception ♀ **G** Upper GI **H** Lower GI **K** Genitourinary Tract **N** Male Reproductive ♂	**3** Percutaneous **7** Via Natural or Artificial Opening **8** Via Natural or Artificial Opening Endoscopic	**3** Anti-inflammatory **6** Nutritional Substance **7** Electrolytic and Water Balance Substance **B** Anesthetic Agent **H** Radioactive Substance **K** Other Diagnostic Substance **N** Analgesics, Hypnotics, Sedatives **T** Destructive Agent	**Z** No Qualifier
E Products of Conception ♀ **G** Upper GI **H** Lower GI **K** Genitourinary Tract **N** Male Reproductive ♂	**3** Percutaneous **7** Via Natural or Artificial Opening **8** Via Natural or Artificial Opening Endoscopic	**G** Other Therapeutic Substance	**C** Other Substance

3E0 Continued on next page

♂   All approach, substance, and qualifier values for body system/region (character 4) with this icon
♀   All approach, substance, and qualifier values for body system/region (character 4) with this icon

LC Limited Coverage   **NC** Noncovered   ⊞ Combination Member   **HAC**   Valid OR   Combination Only   DRG Non-OR   New/Revised in **GREEN**

702   ICD-10-PCS 2020

3   Administration
E   Physiological Systems and Anatomical Regions
0   Introduction   Definition: Putting in or on a therapeutic, diagnostic, nutritional, physiological, or prophylactic substance except blood or blood products

Body System/Region Character 4	Approach Character 5	Substance Character 6	Qualifier Character 7
E Products of Conception ♀ G Upper GI H Lower GI K Genitourinary Tract N Male Reproductive ♂	3 Percutaneous 7 Via Natural or Artificial Opening 8 Via Natural or Artificial Opening Endoscopic	S Gas	F Other Gas
E Products of Conception ♀ G Upper GI H Lower GI K Genitourinary Tract N Male Reproductive ♂	4 Percutaneous Endoscopic	G Other Therapeutic Substance	C Other Substance
F Respiratory Tract	3 Percutaneous 7 Via Natural or Artificial Opening 8 Via Natural or Artificial Opening Endoscopic	0 Antineoplastic	4 Liquid Brachytherapy Radioisotope 5 Other Antineoplastic M Monoclonal Antibody
F Respiratory Tract	3 Percutaneous 7 Via Natural or Artificial Opening 8 Via Natural or Artificial Opening Endoscopic	2 Anti-infective	8 Oxazolidinones 9 Other Anti-infective
F Respiratory Tract	3 Percutaneous 7 Via Natural or Artificial Opening 8 Via Natural or Artificial Opening Endoscopic	3 Anti-inflammatory 6 Nutritional Substance 7 Electrolytic and Water Balance Substance B Anesthetic Agent H Radioactive Substance K Other Diagnostic Substance N Analgesics, Hypnotics, Sedatives T Destructive Agent	Z No Qualifier
F Respiratory Tract	3 Percutaneous 7 Via Natural or Artificial Opening 8 Via Natural or Artificial Opening Endoscopic	G Other Therapeutic Substance	C Other Substance
F Respiratory Tract	3 Percutaneous 7 Via Natural or Artificial Opening 8 Via Natural or Artificial Opening Endoscopic	S Gas	D Nitric Oxide F Other Gas
F Respiratory Tract	4 Percutaneous Endoscopic	G Other Therapeutic Substance	C Other Substance
J Biliary and Pancreatic Tract	3 Percutaneous 7 Via Natural or Artificial Opening 8 Via Natural or Artificial Opening Endoscopic	0 Antineoplastic	4 Liquid Brachytherapy Radioisotope 5 Other Antineoplastic M Monoclonal Antibody
J Biliary and Pancreatic Tract	3 Percutaneous 7 Via Natural or Artificial Opening 8 Via Natural or Artificial Opening Endoscopic	2 Anti-infective	8 Oxazolidinones 9 Other Anti-infective
J Biliary and Pancreatic Tract	3 Percutaneous 7 Via Natural or Artificial Opening 8 Via Natural or Artificial Opening Endoscopic	3 Anti-inflammatory 6 Nutritional Substance 7 Electrolytic and Water Balance Substance B Anesthetic Agent H Radioactive Substance K Other Diagnostic Substance N Analgesics, Hypnotics, Sedatives T Destructive Agent	Z No Qualifier
J Biliary and Pancreatic Tract	3 Percutaneous 7 Via Natural or Artificial Opening 8 Via Natural or Artificial Opening Endoscopic	G Other Therapeutic Substance	C Other Substance
J Biliary and Pancreatic Tract	3 Percutaneous 7 Via Natural or Artificial Opening 8 Via Natural or Artificial Opening Endoscopic	S Gas	F Other Gas

3E0 Continued on next page

♂   All approach, substance, and qualifier values for body system/region (character 4) with this icon
♀   All approach, substance, and qualifier values for body system/region (character 4) with this icon

Administration

3E0 Continued

3   **Administration**
E   **Physiological Systems and Anatomical Regions**
0   **Introduction**   Definition: Putting in or on a therapeutic, diagnostic, nutritional, physiological, or prophylactic substance except blood or blood products

Body System/Region Character 4		Approach Character 5	Substance Character 6	Qualifier Character 7
J	Biliary and Pancreatic Tract	3 Percutaneous 7 Via Natural or Artificial Opening 8 Via Natural or Artificial Opening Endoscopic	U Pancreatic Islet Cells	0 Autologous 1 Nonautologous
J	Biliary and Pancreatic Tract	4 Percutaneous Endoscopic	G Other Therapeutic Substance	C Other Substance
L	Pleural Cavity	0 Open	5 Adhesion Barrier	Z No Qualifier
L	Pleural Cavity	3 Percutaneous	0 Antineoplastic	4 Liquid Brachytherapy Radioisotope 5 Other Antineoplastic M Monoclonal Antibody
L	Pleural Cavity	3 Percutaneous	2 Anti-infective	8 Oxazolidinones 9 Other Anti-infective
L	Pleural Cavity	3 Percutaneous	3 Anti-inflammatory 5 Adhesion Barrier 6 Nutritional Substance 7 Electrolytic and Water Balance Substance B Anesthetic Agent H Radioactive Substance K Other Diagnostic Substance N Analgesics, Hypnotics, Sedatives T Destructive Agent	Z No Qualifier
L	Pleural Cavity	3 Percutaneous	G Other Therapeutic Substance	C Other Substance
L	Pleural Cavity	3 Percutaneous	S Gas	F Other Gas
L	Pleural Cavity	4 Percutaneous Endoscopic	5 Adhesion Barrier	Z No Qualifier
L	Pleural Cavity	4 Percutaneous Endoscopic	G Other Therapeutic Substance	C Other Substance
L	Pleural Cavity	7 Via Natural or Artificial Opening	0 Antineoplastic	4 Liquid Brachytherapy Radioisotope 5 Other Antineoplastic M Monoclonal Antibody
L	Pleural Cavity	7 Via Natural or Artificial Opening	S Gas	F Other Gas
M	Peritoneal Cavity	0 Open	5 Adhesion Barrier	Z No Qualifier
M	Peritoneal Cavity	3 Percutaneous	0 Antineoplastic	4 Liquid Brachytherapy Radioisotope 5 Other Antineoplastic M Monoclonal Antibody Y Hyperthermic
M	Peritoneal Cavity	3 Percutaneous	2 Anti-infective	8 Oxazolidinones 9 Other Anti-infective
M	Peritoneal Cavity	3 Percutaneous	3 Anti-inflammatory 5 Adhesion Barrier 6 Nutritional Substance 7 Electrolytic and Water Balance Substance B Anesthetic Agent H Radioactive Substance K Other Diagnostic Substance N Analgesics, Hypnotics, Sedatives T Destructive Agent	Z No Qualifier
M	Peritoneal Cavity	3 Percutaneous	G Other Therapeutic Substance	C Other Substance
M	Peritoneal Cavity	3 Percutaneous	S Gas	F Other Gas
M	Peritoneal Cavity	4 Percutaneous Endoscopic	5 Adhesion Barrier	Z No Qualifier
M	Peritoneal Cavity	4 Percutaneous Endoscopic	G Other Therapeutic Substance	C Other Substance
M	Peritoneal Cavity	7 Via Natural or Artificial Opening	0 Antineoplastic	4 Liquid Brachytherapy Radioisotope 5 Other Antineoplastic M Monoclonal Antibody
M	Peritoneal Cavity	7 Via Natural or Artificial Opening	S Gas	F Other Gas
P	Female Reproductive ♀	0 Open	5 Adhesion Barrier	Z No Qualifier
P	Female Reproductive ♀	3 Percutaneous	0 Antineoplastic	4 Liquid Brachytherapy Radioisotope 5 Other Antineoplastic M Monoclonal Antibody
P	Female Reproductive ♀	3 Percutaneous	2 Anti-infective	8 Oxazolidinones 9 Other Anti-infective

3E0 Continued on next page

LC Limited Coverage   **NC** Noncovered   ⊞ Combination Member   **HAC**   Valid OR   Combination Only   DRG Non-OR   New/Revised in GREEN

704   ICD-10-PCS 2020

3   **Administration**
E   **Physiological Systems and Anatomical Regions**
0   **Introduction**   Definition: Putting in or on a therapeutic, diagnostic, nutritional, physiological, or prophylactic substance except blood or blood products

Body System/Region Character 4			Approach Character 5	Substance Character 6	Qualifier Character 7
P	Female Reproductive	♀	3 Percutaneous	3 Anti-inflammatory 5 Adhesion Barrier 6 Nutritional Substance 7 Electrolytic and Water Balance Substance B Anesthetic Agent H Radioactive Substance K Other Diagnostic Substance L Sperm N Analgesics, Hypnotics, Sedatives T Destructive Agent V Hormone	Z No Qualifier
P	Female Reproductive	♀	3 Percutaneous	G Other Therapeutic Substance	C Other Substance
P	Female Reproductive	♀	3 Percutaneous	Q Fertilized Ovum	0 Autologous 1 Nonautologous
P	Female Reproductive	♀	3 Percutaneous	S Gas	F Other Gas
P	Female Reproductive	♀	4 Percutaneous Endoscopic	5 Adhesion Barrier	Z No Qualifier
P	Female Reproductive	♀	4 Percutaneous Endoscopic	G Other Therapeutic Substance	C Other Substance
P	Female Reproductive	♀	7 Via Natural or Artificial Opening	0 Antineoplastic	4 Liquid Brachytherapy Radioisotope 5 Other Antineoplastic M Monoclonal Antibody
P	Female Reproductive	♀	7 Via Natural or Artificial Opening	2 Anti-infective	8 Oxazolidinones 9 Other Anti-infective
P	Female Reproductive	♀	7 Via Natural or Artificial Opening	3 Anti-inflammatory 6 Nutritional Substance 7 Electrolytic and Water Balance Substance B Anesthetic Agent H Radioactive Substance K Other Diagnostic Substance L Sperm N Analgesics, Hypnotics, Sedatives T Destructive Agent V Hormone	Z No Qualifier
P	Female Reproductive	♀	7 Via Natural or Artificial Opening	G Other Therapeutic Substance	C Other Substance
P	Female Reproductive	♀	7 Via Natural or Artificial Opening	Q Fertilized Ovum	0 Autologous 1 Nonautologous
P	Female Reproductive	♀	7 Via Natural or Artificial Opening	S Gas	F Other Gas
P	Female Reproductive	♀	8 Via Natural or Artificial Opening Endoscopic	0 Antineoplastic	4 Liquid Brachytherapy Radioisotope 5 Other Antineoplastic M Monoclonal Antibody
P	Female Reproductive	♀	8 Via Natural or Artificial Opening Endoscopic	2 Anti-infective	8 Oxazolidinones 9 Other Anit-infection
P	Female Reproductive	♀	8 Via Natural or Artificial Opening Endoscopic	3 Anti-inflammatory 6 Nutritional Substance 7 Electrolytic and Water Balance Substance B Anesthetic Agent H Radioactive Substance K Other Diagnostic Substance N Analgesics, Hypnotics, Sedative T Destructive Agent	Z No Qualifier
P	Female Reproductive	♀	8 Via Natural or Artificial Opening Endoscopic	G Other Therapeutic Substance	C Other Substance
P	Female Reproductive	♀	8 Via Natural or Artificial Opening Endoscopic	S Gas	F Other Gas
Q	Cranial Cavity and Brain		0 Open 3 Percutaneous	0 Antineoplastic	4 Liquid Brachytherapy Radioisotope 5 Other Antineoplastic M Monoclonal Antibody
Q	Cranial Cavity and Brain		0 Open 3 Percutaneous	2 Anti-infective	8 Oxazolidinones 9 Other Anti-infective

3E0 Continued on next page

Valid OR	3E0P3Q[0,1]	
Valid OR	3E0P7Q[0,1]	
DRG Non-OR	3E0Q[0,3]05	
♀	All approach, substance, and qualifier values for body system/region (character 4) with this icon	

3 Administration
E Physiological Systems and Anatomical Regions
0 Introduction Definition: Putting in or on a therapeutic, diagnostic, nutritional, physiological, or prophylactic substance except blood or blood products

3E0 Continued

Body System/Region Character 4	Approach Character 5	Substance Character 6	Qualifier Character 7
Q Cranial Cavity and Brain	0 Open 3 Percutaneous	3 Anti-inflammatory 6 Nutritional Substance 7 Electrolytic and Water Balance Substance A Stem Cells, Embryonic B Anesthetic Agent H Radioactive Substance K Other Diagnostic Substance N Analgesics, Hypnotics, Sedatives T Destructive Agent	Z No Qualifier
Q Cranial Cavity and Brain	0 Open 3 Percutaneous	E Stem Cells, Somatic	0 Autologous 1 Nonautologous
Q Cranial Cavity and Brain	0 Open 3 Percutaneous	G Other Therapeutic Substance	C Other Substance
Q Cranial Cavity and Brain	0 Open 3 Percutaneous	S Gas	F Other Gas
Q Cranial Cavity and Brain	7 Via Natural or Artificial Opening	0 Antineoplastic	4 Liquid Brachytherapy Radioisotope 5 Other Antineoplastic M Monoclonal Antibody
Q Cranial Cavity and Brain	7 Via Natural or Artificial Opening	S Gas	F Other Gas
R Spinal Canal	0 Open	A Stem Cells, Embryonic	Z No Qualifier
R Spinal Canal	0 Open	E Stem Cells, Somatic	0 Autologous 1 Nonautologous
R Spinal Canal	3 Percutaneous	0 Antineoplastic	2 High-dose Interleukin-2 3 Low-dose Interleukin-2 4 Liquid Brachytherapy Radioisotope 5 Other Antineoplastic M Monoclonal Antibody
R Spinal Canal	3 Percutaneous	2 Anti-infective	8 Oxazolidinones 9 Other Anti-infective
R Spinal Canal	3 Percutaneous	3 Anti-inflammatory 6 Nutritional Substance 7 Electrolytic and Water Balance Substance A Stem Cells, Embryonic B Anesthetic Agent H Radioactive Substance K Other Diagnostic Substance N Analgesics, Hypnotics, Sedatives T Destructive Agent	Z No Qualifier
R Spinal Canal	3 Percutaneous	E Stem Cells, Somatic	0 Autologous 1 Nonautologous
R Spinal Canal	3 Percutaneous	G Other Therapeutic Substance	C Other Substance
R Spinal Canal	3 Percutaneous	S Gas	F Other Gas
R Spinal Canal	7 Via Natural or Artificial Opening	S Gas	F Other Gas
S Epidural Space	3 Percutaneous	0 Antineoplastic	2 High-dose Interleukin-2 3 Low-dose Interleukin-2 4 Liquid Brachytherapy Radioisotope 5 Other Antineoplastic M Monoclonal Antibody
S Epidural Space	3 Percutaneous	2 Anti-infective	8 Oxazolidinones 9 Other Anti-infective
S Epidural Space	3 Percutaneous	3 Anti-inflammatory 6 Nutritional Substance 7 Electrolytic and Water Balance Substance B Anesthetic Agent H Radioactive Substance K Other Diagnostic Substance N Analgesics, Hypnotics, Sedatives T Destructive Agent	Z No Qualifier

3E0 Continued on next page

DRG Non-OR	3E0Q705
DRG Non-OR	3E0R302
DRG Non-OR	3E0S302

3EØ Continued

3   **Administration**
E   **Physiological Systems and Anatomical Regions**
Ø   **Introduction**   Definition: Putting in or on a therapeutic, diagnostic, nutritional, physiological, or prophylactic substance except blood or blood products

Body System/Region Character 4	Approach Character 5	Substance Character 6	Qualifier Character 7
S Epidural Space	**3** Percutaneous	**G** Other Therapeutic Substance	**C** Other Substance
S Epidural Space	**3** Percutaneous	**S** Gas	**F** Other Gas
S Epidural Space	**7** Via Natural or Artificial Opening	**S** Gas	**F** Other Gas
T Peripheral Nerves and Plexi **X** Cranial Nerves	**3** Percutaneous	**3** Anti-inflammatory **B** Anesthetic Agent **T** Destructive Agent	**Z** No Qualifier
T Peripheral Nerves and Plexi **X** Cranial Nerves	**3** Percutaneous	**G** Other Therapeutic Substance	**C** Other Substance
U Joints	**Ø** Open	**2** Anti-infective	**8** Oxazolidinones **9** Other Anti-infective
U Joints	**Ø** Open	**G** Other Therapeutic Substance	**B** Recombinant Bone Morphogenetic Protein
U Joints	**3** Percutaneous	**Ø** Antineoplastic	**4** Liquid Brachytherapy Radioisotope **5** Other Antineoplastic **M** Monoclonal Antibody
U Joints	**3** Percutaneous	**2** Anti-infective	**8** Oxazolidinones **9** Other Anti-infective
U Joints	**3** Percutaneous	**3** Anti-inflammatory **6** Nutritional Substance **7** Electrolytic and Water Balance Substance **B** Anesthetic Agent **H** Radioactive Substance **K** Other Diagnostic Substance **N** Analgesics, Hypnotics, Sedatives **T** Destructive Agent	**Z** No Qualifier
U Joints	**3** Percutaneous	**G** Other Therapeutic Substance	**B** Recombinant Bone Morphogenetic Protein **C** Other Substance
U Joints	**3** Percutaneous	**S** Gas	**F** Other Gas
U Joints	**4** Percutaneous Endoscopic	**G** Other Therapeutic Substance	**C** Other Substance
V Bones	**Ø** Open	**G** Other Therapeutic Substance	**B** Recombinant Bone Morphogenetic Protein
V Bones	**3** Percutaneous	**Ø** Antineoplastic	**5** Other Antineoplastic **M** Monoclonal Antibody
V Bones	**3** Percutaneous	**2** Anti-infective	**8** Oxazolidinones **9** Other Anti-infective
V Bones	**3** Percutaneous	**3** Anti-inflammatory **6** Nutritional Substance **7** Electrolytic and Water Balance Substance **B** Anesthetic Agent **H** Radioactive Substance **K** Other Diagnostic Substance **N** Analgesics, Hypnotics, Sedatives **T** Destructive Agent	**Z** No Qualifier
V Bones	**3** Percutaneous	**G** Other Therapeutic Substance	**B** Recombinant Bone Morphogenetic Protein **C** Other Substance
W Lymphatics	**3** Percutaneous	**Ø** Antineoplastic	**5** Other Antineoplastic **M** Monoclonal Antibody
W Lymphatics	**3** Percutaneous	**2** Anti-infective	**8** Oxazolidinones **9** Other Anti-infective
W Lymphatics	**3** Percutaneous	**3** Anti-inflammatory **6** Nutritional Substance **7** Electrolytic and Water Balance Substance **B** Anesthetic Agent **H** Radioactive Substance **K** Other Diagnostic Substance **N** Analgesics, Hypnotics, Sedatives **T** Destructive Agent	**Z** No Qualifier
W Lymphatics	**3** Percutaneous	**G** Other Therapeutic Substance	**C** Other Substance

3EØ Continued on next page

LC Limited Coverage   **NC** Noncovered   ⊞ Combination Member   HAC   Valid OR   Combination Only   DRG Non-OR   New/Revised in GREEN

ICD-10-PCS 2020   **707**

3   **Administration**
E   **Physiological Systems and Anatomical Regions**
Ø   **Introduction**   Definition: Putting in or on a therapeutic, diagnostic, nutritional, physiological, or prophylactic substance except blood or blood products

3EØ Continued

Body System/Region Character 4	Approach Character 5	Substance Character 6	Qualifier Character 7
Y Pericardial Cavity	3 Percutaneous	Ø Antineoplastic	4 Liquid Brachytherapy Radioisotope 5 Other Antineoplastic M Monoclonal Antibody
Y Pericardial Cavity	3 Percutaneous	2 Anti-infective	8 Oxazolidinones 9 Other Anti-infective
Y Pericardial Cavity	3 Percutaneous	3 Anti-inflammatory 6 Nutritional Substance 7 Electrolytic and Water Balance Substance B Anesthetic Agent H Radioactive Substance K Other Diagnostic Substance N Analgesics, Hypnotics, Sedatives T Destructive Agent	Z No Qualifier
Y Pericardial Cavity	3 Percutaneous	G Other Therapeutic Substance	C Other Substance
Y Pericardial Cavity	3 Percutaneous	S Gas	F Other Gas
Y Pericardial Cavity	4 Percutaneous Endoscopic	G Other Therapeutic Substance	C Other Substance
Y Pericardial Cavity	7 Via Natural or Artificial Opening	Ø Antineoplastic	4 Liquid Brachytherapy Radioisotope 5 Other Antineoplastic M Monoclonal Antibody
Y Pericardial Cavity	7 Via Natural or Artificial Opening	S Gas	F Other Gas

3   **Administration**
E   **Physiological Systems and Anatomical Regions**
1   **Irrigation**   Definition: Putting in or on a cleansing substance

Body System/Region Character 4	Approach Character 5	Substance Character 6	Qualifier Character 7
Ø Skin and Mucous Membranes C Eye	3 Percutaneous X External	8 Irrigating Substance	X Diagnostic Z No Qualifier
9 Nose B Ear F Respiratory Tract G Upper GI H Lower GI J Biliary and Pancreatic Tract K Genitourinary Tract N Male Reproductive ♂ P Female Reproductive ♀	3 Percutaneous 7 Via Natural or Artificial Opening 8 Via Natural or Artificial Opening Endoscopic	8 Irrigating Substance	X Diagnostic Z No Qualifier
L Pleural Cavity Q Cranial Cavity and Brain R Spinal Canal S Epidural Space Y Pericardial Cavity	3 Percutaneous	8 Irrigating Substance	X Diagnostic Z No Qualifier
M Peritoneal Cavity	3 Percutaneous	8 Irrigating Substance	X Diagnostic Z No Qualifier
M Peritoneal Cavity	3 Percutaneous	9 Dialysate	Z No Qualifier
U Joints	3 Percutaneous 4 Percutaneous Endoscopic	8 Irrigating Substance	X Diagnostic Z No Qualifier

♂   3E1N[3,7,8]8[X,Z]
♀   3E1P[3,7,8]8[X,Z]

LC Limited Coverage   **NC** Noncovered   ⊞ Combination Member   **HAC**   Valid OR   Combination Only   DRG Non-OR   New/Revised in GREEN

708   ICD-10-PCS 2020

Measurement and Monitoring 4A0–4B0

AHA Coding Clinic for table 4A0

2018, 1Q, 12	Percutaneous balloon valvuloplasty & cardiac catheterization with ventriculogram
2016, 3Q, 37	Fractional flow reserve
2015, 3Q, 29	Approach value for esophageal electrophysiology study

AHA Coding Clinic for table 4A1

2016, 4Q, 114	Fluorescence vascular angiography
2016, 2Q, 29	Decompressive craniectomy with cryopreservation and storage of bone flap
2016, 2Q, 33	Monitoring of arterial pressure & pulse
2015, 3Q, 35	Swan Ganz catheterization
2015, 2Q, 14	Intraoperative EMG monitoring via endotracheal tube
2015, 1Q, 26	Intraoperative monitoring using Sentio MMG®
2014, 4Q, 28	Removal and replacement of displaced growing rods

4   **Measurement and Monitoring**
A   **Physiological Systems**
0   **Measurement**   Definition: Determining the level of a physiological or physical function at a point in time

Body System Character 4	Approach Character 5	Function/Device Character 6	Qualifier Character 7
0 Central Nervous	0 Open	2 Conductivity 4 Electrical Activity B Pressure	Z No Qualifier
0 Central Nervous	3 Percutaneous 7 Via Natural or Artificial Opening 8 Via Natural or Artificial Opening Endoscopic	4 Electrical Activity	Z No Qualifier
0 Central Nervous	3 Percutaneous 7 Via Natural or Artificial Opening 8 Via Natural or Artificial Opening Endoscopic	B Pressure K Temperature R Saturation	D Intracranial
0 Central Nervous	X External	2 Conductivity 4 Electrical Activity	Z No Qualifier
1 Peripheral Nervous	0 Open 3 Percutaneous 7 Via Natural or Artificial Opening 8 Via Natural or Artificial Opening Endoscopic X External	2 Conductivity	9 Sensory B Motor
1 Peripheral Nervous	0 Open 3 Percutaneous 7 Via Natural or Artificial Opening 8 Via Natural or Artificial Opening Endoscopic X External	4 Electrical Activity	Z No Qualifier
2 Cardiac	0 Open 3 Percutaneous 7 Via Natural or Artificial Opening 8 Via Natural or Artificial Opening Endoscopic	4 Electrical Activity 9 Output C Rate F Rhythm H Sound P Action Currents	Z No Qualifier
2 Cardiac	0 Open 3 Percutaneous 7 Via Natural or Artificial Opening 8 Via Natural or Artificial Opening Endoscopic	N Sampling and Pressure	6 Right Heart 7 Left Heart 8 Bilateral
2 Cardiac	X External	4 Electrical Activity	A Guidance Z No Qualifier
2 Cardiac	X External	9 Output C Rate F Rhythm H Sound P Action Currents	Z No Qualifier
2 Cardiac	X External	M Total Activity	4 Stress
3 Arterial	0 Open 3 Percutaneous	5 Flow J Pulse	1 Peripheral 3 Pulmonary C Coronary
3 Arterial	0 Open 3 Percutaneous	B Pressure	1 Peripheral 3 Pulmonary C Coronary F Other Thoracic

4A0 Continued on next page

DRG Non-OR	4A02[3,7,8]FZ
DRG Non-OR	4A02[0,3,7,8]N[6,7,8]

4   **Measurement and Monitoring**   *4A0 Continued*
A   **Physiological Systems**
0   **Measurement**   Definition: Determining the level of a physiological or physical function at a point in time

Body System Character 4	Approach Character 5	Function/Device Character 6	Qualifier Character 7
3 Arterial	**0** Open **3** Percutaneous	**H** Sound **R** Saturation	**1** Peripheral
3 Arterial	**X** External	**5** Flow **B** Pressure **H** Sound **J** Pulse **R** Saturation	**1** Peripheral
4 Venous	**0** Open **3** Percutaneous	**5** Flow **B** Pressure **J** Pulse	**0** Central **1** Peripheral **2** Portal **3** Pulmonary
4 Venous	**0** Open **3** Percutaneous	**R** Saturation	**1** Peripheral
4 Venous	**X** External	**5** Flow **B** Pressure **J** Pulse **R** Saturation	**1** Peripheral
5 Circulatory	**X** External	**L** Volume	**Z** No Qualifier
6 Lymphatic	**0** Open **3** Percutaneous **7** Via Natural or Artificial Opening **8** Via Natural or Artificial Opening Endoscopic	**5** Flow **B** Pressure	**Z** No Qualifier
7 Visual	**X** External	**0** Acuity **7** Mobility **B** Pressure	**Z** No Qualifier
8 Olfactory	**X** External	**0** Acuity	**Z** No Qualifier
9 Respiratory	**7** Via Natural or Artificial Opening **8** Via Natural or Artificial Opening Endoscopic **X** External	**1** Capacity **5** Flow **C** Rate **D** Resistance **L** Volume **M** Total Activity	**Z** No Qualifier
B Gastrointestinal	**7** Via Natural or Artificial Opening **8** Via Natural or Artificial Opening Endoscopic	**8** Motility **B** Pressure **G** Secretion	**Z** No Qualifier
C Biliary	**3** Percutaneous **4** Percutaneous Endoscopic **7** Via Natural or Artificial Opening **8** Via Natural or Artificial Opening Endoscopic	**5** Flow **B** Pressure	**Z** No Qualifier
D Urinary	**7** Via Natural or Artificial Opening **8** Via Natural or Artificial Opening Endoscopic	**3** Contractility **5** Flow **B** Pressure **D** Resistance **L** Volume	**Z** No Qualifier
F Musculoskeletal	**3** Percutaneous **X** External	**3** Contractility	**Z** No Qualifier
H Products of Conception, ♀ Cardiac	**7** Via Natural or Artificial Opening **8** Via Natural or Artificial Opening Endoscopic **X** External	**4** Electrical Activity **C** Rate **F** Rhythm **H** Sound	**Z** No Qualifier
J Products of Conception, ♀ Nervous	**7** Via Natural or Artificial Opening **8** Via Natural or Artificial Opening Endoscopic **X** External	**2** Conductivity **4** Electrical Activity **B** Pressure	**Z** No Qualifier
Z None	**7** Via Natural or Artificial Opening	**6** Metabolism **K** Temperature	**Z** No Qualifier
Z None	**X** External	**6** Metabolism **K** Temperature **Q** Sleep	**Z** No Qualifier

Valid OR	4A060[5,B]Z		
Valid OR	4A0C4[5,B]Z	♀	4A0H[7,8,X][4,C,F,H]Z
		♀	4A0J[7,8,X][2,4,B]Z

[LC] Limited Coverage   [NC] Noncovered   ⊞ Combination Member   HAC   Valid OR   Combination Only   DRG Non-OR   New/Revised in GREEN

710   ICD-10-PCS 2020

4 Measurement and Monitoring
A Physiological Systems
1 Monitoring Definition: Determining the level of a physiological or physical function repetitively over a period of time

Body System Character 4	Approach Character 5	Function/Device Character 6	Qualifier Character 7
Ø Central Nervous	Ø Open	2 Conductivity B Pressure	Z No Qualifier
Ø Central Nervous	Ø Open	4 Electrical Activity	G Intraoperative Z No Qualifier
Ø Central Nervous	3 Percutaneous 7 Via Natural or Artificial Opening 8 Via Natural or Artificial Opening Endoscopic	4 Electrical Activity	G Intraoperative Z No Qualifier
Ø Central Nervous	3 Percutaneous 7 Via Natural or Artificial Opening 8 Via Natural or Artificial Opening Endoscopic	B Pressure K Temperature R Saturation	D Intracranial
Ø Central Nervous	X External	2 Conductivity	Z No Qualifier
Ø Central Nervous	X External	4 Electrical Activity	G Intraoperative Z No Qualifier
1 Peripheral Nervous	Ø Open 3 Percutaneous 7 Via Natural or Artificial Opening 8 Via Natural or Artificial Opening Endoscopic X External	2 Conductivity	9 Sensory B Motor
1 Peripheral Nervous	Ø Open 3 Percutaneous 7 Via Natural or Artificial Opening 8 Via Natural or Artificial Opening Endoscopic X External	4 Electrical Activity	G Intraoperative Z No Qualifier
2 Cardiac	Ø Open 3 Percutaneous 7 Via Natural or Artificial Opening 8 Via Natural or Artificial Opening Endoscopic	4 Electrical Activity 9 Output C Rate F Rhythm H Sound	Z No Qualifier
2 Cardiac	X External	4 Electrical Activity	5 Ambulatory Z No Qualifier
2 Cardiac	X External	9 Output C Rate F Rhythm H Sound	Z No Qualifier
2 Cardiac	X External	M Total Activity	4 Stress
2 Cardiac	X External	S Vascular Perfusion	H Indocyanine Green Dye
3 Arterial	Ø Open 3 Percutaneous	5 Flow B Pressure J Pulse	1 Peripheral 3 Pulmonary C Coronary
3 Arterial	Ø Open 3 Percutaneous	H Sound R Saturation	1 Peripheral
3 Arterial	X External	5 Flow B Pressure H Sound J Pulse R Saturation	1 Peripheral
4 Venous	Ø Open 3 Percutaneous	5 Flow B Pressure J Pulse	Ø Central 1 Peripheral 2 Portal 3 Pulmonary
4 Venous	Ø Open 3 Percutaneous	R Saturation	Ø Central 2 Portal 3 Pulmonary
4 Venous	X External	5 Flow B Pressure J Pulse	1 Peripheral
6 Lymphatic	Ø Open 3 Percutaneous 7 Via Natural or Artificial Opening 8 Via Natural or Artificial Opening Endoscopic	5 Flow	H Indocyanine Green Dye Z No Qualifier

4A1 Continued on next page

Valid OR 4A16Ø5Z

4   **Measurement and Monitoring**
A   **Physiological Systems**   *4A1 Continued*
1   **Monitoring**   Definition: Determining the level of a physiological or physical function repetitively over a period of time

Body System Character 4	Approach Character 5	Function/Device Character 6	Qualifier Character 7
6 Lymphatic	Ø Open 3 Percutaneous 7 Via Natural or Artificial Opening 8 Via Natural or Artificial Opening Endoscopic	B Pressure	Z No Qualifier
9 Respiratory	7 Via Natural or Artificial Opening X External	1 Capacity 5 Flow C Rate D Resistance L Volume	Z No Qualifier
B Gastrointestinal	7 Via Natural or Artificial Opening 8 Via Natural or Artificial Opening Endoscopic	8 Motility B Pressure G Secretion	Z No Qualifier
B Gastrointestinal	X External	S Vascular Perfusion	H Indocyanine Green Dye
D Urinary	7 Via Natural or Artificial Opening 8 Via Natural or Artificial Opening Endoscopic	3 Contractility 5 Flow B Pressure D Resistance L Volume	Z No Qualifier
G Skin and Breast	X External	S Vascular Perfusion	H Indocyanine Green Dye
H Products of Conception, ♀ Cardiac	7 Via Natural or Artificial Opening 8 Via Natural or Artificial Opening Endoscopic X External	4 Electrical Activity C Rate F Rhythm H Sound	Z No Qualifier
J Products of Conception, ♀ Nervous	7 Via Natural or Artificial Opening 8 Via Natural or Artificial Opening Endoscopic X External	2 Conductivity 4 Electrical Activity B Pressure	Z No Qualifier
Z None	7 Via Natural or Artificial Opening	K Temperature	Z No Qualifier
Z None	X External	K Temperature Q Sleep	Z No Qualifier

Valid OR   4A16ØBZ
♀   4A1H[7,8,X][4,C,F,H]Z
♀   4A1J[7,8,X][2,4,B]Z

4   **Measurement and Monitoring**
B   **Physiological Devices**
Ø   **Measurement**   Definition: Determining the level of a physiological or physical function at a point in time

Body System Character 4	Approach Character 5	Function/Device Character 6	Qualifier Character 7
Ø Central Nervous 1 Peripheral Nervous F Musculoskeletal	X External	V Stimulator	Z No Qualifier
2 Cardiac	X External	S Pacemaker T Defibrillator	Z No Qualifier
9 Respiratory	X External	S Pacemaker	Z No Qualifier

Extracorporeal or Systemic Assistance and Performance 5A0–5A2

AHA Coding Clinic for table 5A0

2018, 2Q, 3-5	Intra-aortic balloon pump
2017, 4Q, 43-44	Insertion of external heart assist devices
2017, 3Q, 18	Intra-aortic balloon pump removal
2017, 1Q, 10-11	External heart assist device
2017, 1Q, 29	Newborn resuscitation using positive pressure ventilation
2017, 1Q, 29	Newborn noninvasive ventilation
2016, 4Q, 137-139	Heart assist device systems
2014, 4Q, 9	Mechanical ventilation
2014, 3Q, 19	Ablation of ventricular tachycardia with Impella® support
2013, 3Q, 18	Heart transplant surgery

AHA Coding Clinic for table 5A1

2018, 4Q, 52-54	Percutaneous extracorporeal membrane oxygenation
2018, 1Q, 13	Mechanical ventilation using patient's equipment
2017, 4Q, 71-73	Hemodialysis and renal replacement therapy
2017, 3Q, 7	Senning procedure (arterial switch)
2017, 1Q, 19	Norwood Sano procedure
2016, 1Q, 27	Aortocoronary bypass graft utilizing Y-graft
2016, 1Q, 28	Extracorporeal liver assist device
2016, 1Q, 29	Duration of hemodialysis
2015, 4Q, 22-24	Congenital heart corrective procedures
2014, 4Q, 3-10	Mechanical ventilation
2014, 4Q, 11-15	Sequencing of mechanical ventilation with other procedures
2014, 3Q, 16	Repair of Tetralogy of Fallot
2014, 3Q, 20	MAZE procedure performed with coronary artery bypass graft
2014, 1Q, 10	Repair of thoracic aortic aneurysm & coronary artery bypass graft
2013, 3Q, 18	Heart transplant surgery

5   Extracorporeal or Systemic Assistance and Performance
A   Physiological Systems
0   Assistance   Definition: Taking over a portion of a physiological function by extracorporeal means

Body System Character 4	Duration Character 5	Function Character 6	Qualifier Character 7
2 Cardiac	1 Intermittent 2 Continuous	1 Output	0 Balloon Pump 5 Pulsatile Compression 6 Other Pump D Impeller Pump
5 Circulatory	1 Intermittent 2 Continuous	2 Oxygenation	1 Hyperbaric C Supersaturated
9 Respiratory	2 Continuous	0 Filtration	Z No Qualifier
9 Respiratory	3 Less than 24 Consecutive Hours 4 24-96 Consecutive Hours 5 Greater than 96 Consecutive Hours	5 Ventilation	7 Continuous Positive Airway Pressure 8 Intermittent Positive Airway Pressure 9 Continuous Negative Airway Pressure B Intermittent Negative Airway Pressure Z No Qualifier

Valid OR   5A02[1,2]1[0,6,D]

5   Extracorporeal or Systemic Assistance and Performance
A   Physiological Systems
1   Performance   Definition: Completely taking over a physiological function by extracorporeal means

Body System Character 4	Duration Character 5	Function Character 6	Qualifier Character 7
2 Cardiac	0 Single	1 Output	2 Manual
2 Cardiac	1 Intermittent	3 Pacing	Z No Qualifier
2 Cardiac	2 Continuous	1 Output 3 Pacing	Z No Qualifier
5 Circulatory	2 Continuous A Intraoperative	2 Oxygenation	F Membrane, Central G Membrane, Peripheral Veno-arterial H Membrane, Peripheral Veno-venous
9 Respiratory	0 Single	5 Ventilation	4 Nonmechanical
9 Respiratory	3 Less than 24 Consecutive Hours 4 24-96 Consecutive Hours 5 Greater than 96 Consecutive Hours	5 Ventilation	Z No Qualifier
C Biliary	0 Single 6 Multiple	0 Filtration	Z No Qualifier
D Urinary	7 Intermittent, Less than 6 Hours per day 8 Prolonged Intermittent, 6-18 Hours per day 9 Continuous, Greater than 18 Hours per day	0 Filtration	Z No Qualifier

Valid OR   5A1522F
DRG Non-OR   5A1522[G,H]

DRG Non-OR   5A19[3,4,5]5Z
Note: For code 5A1955Z, length of stay must be > 4 consecutive days.

5   Extracorporeal or Systemic Assistance and Performance
A   Physiological Systems
2   Restoration   Definition: Returning, or attempting to return, a physiological function to its original state by extracorporeal means.

Body System Character 4	Duration Character 5	Function Character 6	Qualifier Character 7
2 Cardiac	0 Single	4 Rhythm	Z No Qualifier

Extracorporeal or Systemic Therapies 6A0–6AB

AHA Coding Clinic for table 6A7
2014, 4Q, 19   Ultrasound accelerated thrombolysis

AHA Coding Clinic for table 6AB
2016, 4Q, 115   Donor organ perfusion

6   Extracorporeal or Systemic Therapies
A   Physiological Systems
0   Atmospheric Control   Definition: Extracorporeal control of atmospheric pressure and composition

Body System Character 4	Duration Character 5	Qualifier Character 6	Qualifier Character 7
Z None	0 Single 1 Multiple	Z No Qualifier	Z No Qualifier

6   Extracorporeal or Systemic Therapies
A   Physiological Systems
1   Decompression   Definition: Extracorporeal elimination of undissolved gas from body fluids

Body System Character 4	Duration Character 5	Qualifier Character 6	Qualifier Character 7
5 Circulatory	0 Single 1 Multiple	Z No Qualifier	Z No Qualifier

6   Extracorporeal or Systemic Therapies
A   Physiological Systems
2   Electromagnetic Therapy   Definition: Extracorporeal treatment by electromagnetic rays

Body System Character 4	Duration Character 5	Qualifier Character 6	Qualifier Character 7
1 Urinary 2 Central Nervous	0 Single 1 Multiple	Z No Qualifier	Z No Qualifier

6   Extracorporeal or Systemic Therapies
A   Physiological Systems
3   Hyperthermia   Definition: Extracorporeal raising of body temperature

Body System Character 4	Duration Character 5	Qualifier Character 6	Qualifier Character 7
Z None	0 Single 1 Multiple	Z No Qualifier	Z No Qualifier

6   Extracorporeal or Systemic Therapies
A   Physiological Systems
4   Hypothermia   Definition: Extracorporeal lowering of body temperature

Body System Character 4	Duration Character 5	Qualifier Character 6	Qualifier Character 7
Z None	0 Single 1 Multiple	Z No Qualifier	Z No Qualifier

6   Extracorporeal or Systemic Therapies
A   Physiological Systems
5   Pheresis   Definition: Extracorporeal separation of blood products

Body System Character 4	Duration Character 5	Qualifier Character 6	Qualifier Character 7
5 Circulatory	0 Single 1 Multiple	Z No Qualifier	0 Erythrocytes 1 Leukocytes 2 Platelets 3 Plasma T Stem Cells, Cord Blood V Stem Cells, Hematopoietic

6   Extracorporeal or Systemic Therapies
A   Physiological Systems
6   Phototherapy   Definition: Extracorporeal treatment by light rays

Body System Character 4	Duration Character 5	Qualifier Character 6	Qualifier Character 7
0 Skin 5 Circulatory	0 Single 1 Multiple	Z No Qualifier	Z No Qualifier

6　**Extracorporeal or Systemic Therapies**
A　**Physiological Systems**
7　**Ultrasound Therapy**　　　Definition: Extracorporeal treatment by ultrasound

Body System Character 4	Duration Character 5	Qualifier Character 6	Qualifier Character 7
5　Circulatory	Ø　Single 1　Multiple	Z　No Qualifier	4　Head and Neck Vessels 5　Heart 6　Peripheral Vessels 7　Other Vessels Z　No Qualifier

6　**Extracorporeal or Systemic Therapies**
A　**Physiological Systems**
8　**Ultraviolet Light Therapy**　　　Definition: Extracorporeal treatment by ultraviolet light

Body System Character 4	Duration Character 5	Qualifier Character 6	Qualifier Character 7
Ø　Skin	Ø　Single 1　Multiple	Z　No Qualifier	Z　No Qualifier

6　**Extracorporeal or Systemic Therapies**
A　**Physiological Systems**
9　**Shock Wave Therapy**　　　Definition: Extracorporeal treatment by shock waves

Body System Character 4	Duration Character 5	Qualifier Character 6	Qualifier Character 7
3　Musculoskeletal	Ø　Single 1　Multiple	Z　No Qualifier	Z　No Qualifier

6　**Extracorporeal or Systemic Therapies**
A　**Physiological Systems**
B　**Perfusion**　　　Definition: Extracorporeal treatment by diffusion of therapeutic fluid

Body System Character 4	Duration Character 5	Qualifier Character 6	Qualifier Character 7
5　Circulatory B　Respiratory System F　Hepatobiliary System and Pancreas T　Urinary System	Ø　Single	B　Donor Organ	Z　No Qualifier

LC Limited Coverage　　**NC** Noncovered　　⊞ Combination Member　　HAC　　Valid OR　　Combination Only　　DRG Non-OR　　New/Revised in GREEN

716　　　　　　　　　　　　　　　　　　　　　　　　　　　　　　　　　　ICD-10-PCS 2020

Osteopathic 7WØ

7   Osteopathic
W   Anatomical Regions
Ø   Treatment   Definition: Manual treatment to eliminate or alleviate somatic dysfunction and related disorders

Body Region Character 4	Approach Character 5	Method Character 6	Qualifier Character 7
Ø Head	X External	Ø Articulatory-Raising	Z None
1 Cervical		1 Fascial Release	
2 Thoracic		2 General Mobilization	
3 Lumbar		3 High Velocity-Low Amplitude	
4 Sacrum		4 Indirect	
5 Pelvis		5 Low Velocity-High Amplitude	
6 Lower Extremities		6 Lymphatic Pump	
7 Upper Extremities		7 Muscle Energy-Isometric	
8 Rib Cage		8 Muscle Energy-Isotonic	
9 Abdomen		9 Other Method	

Other Procedures 8CØ–8EØ

AHA Coding Clinic for table 8EØ

2019, 1Q, 30	Laparoscopic-assisted rectopexy with manual reduction of prolapse
2015, 1Q, 33	Robotic-assisted laparoscopic hysterectomy converted to open procedure
2014, 4Q, 33	Radical prostatectomy

8   Other Procedures
C   Indwelling Device
Ø   Other Procedures   Definition: Methodologies which attempt to remediate or cure a disorder or disease

Body Region Character 4	Approach Character 5	Method Character 6	Qualifier Character 7
1 Nervous System	X External	6 Collection	J Cerebrospinal Fluid L Other Fluid
2 Circulatory System	X External	6 Collection	K Blood L Other Fluid

8   Other Procedures
E   Physiological Systems and Anatomical Regions
Ø   Other Procedures   Definition: Methodologies which attempt to remediate or cure a disorder or disease

Body Region Character 4	Approach Character 5	Method Character 6	Qualifier Character 7
1 Nervous System U Female Reproductive System ♀	X External	Y Other Method	7 Examination
2 Circulatory System	3 Percutaneous	D Near Infrared Spectroscopy	Z No Qualifier
9 Head and Neck Region	Ø Open	C Robotic Assisted Procedure	Z No Qualifier
9 Head and Neck Region	Ø Open	E Fluorescence Guided Procedure	M Aminolevulinic Acid Z No Qualifier
9 Head and Neck Region	3 Percutaneous 4 Percutaneous Endoscopic 7 Via Natural or Artificial Opening 8 Via Natural or Artificial Opening Endoscopic	C Robotic Assisted Procedure E Fluorescence Guided Procedure	Z No Qualifier
9 Head and Neck Region	X External	B Computer Assisted Procedure	F With Fluoroscopy G With Computerized Tomography H With Magnetic Resonance Imaging Z No Qualifier
9 Head and Neck Region	X External	C Robotic Assisted Procedure	Z No Qualifier
9 Head and Neck Region	X External	Y Other Method	8 Suture Removal
H Integumentary System and Breast	3 Percutaneous	Ø Acupuncture	Ø Anesthesia Z No Qualifier
H Integumentary System and Breast ♀	X External	6 Collection	2 Breast Milk
H Integumentary System and Breast	X External	Y Other Method	9 Piercing
K Musculoskeletal System	X External	1 Therapeutic Massage	Z No Qualifier
K Musculoskeletal System	X External	Y Other Method	7 Examination
V Male Reproductive System ♂	X External	1 Therapeutic Massage	C Prostate D Rectum
V Male Reproductive System ♂	X External	6 Collection	3 Sperm
W Trunk Region	Ø Open 3 Percutaneous 4 Percutaneous Endoscopic 7 Via Natural or Artificial Opening 8 Via Natural or Artificial Opening Endoscopic	C Robotic Assisted Procedure E Fluorescence Guided Procedure	Z No Qualifier
W Trunk Region	X External	B Computer Assisted Procedure	F With Fluoroscopy G With Computerized Tomography H With Magnetic Resonance Imaging Z No Qualifier
W Trunk Region	X External	C Robotic Assisted Procedure	Z No Qualifier
W Trunk Region	X External	Y Other Method	8 Suture Removal
X Upper Extremity Y Lower Extremity	Ø Open 3 Percutaneous 4 Percutaneous Endoscopic	C Robotic Assisted Procedure E Fluorescence Guided Procedure	Z No Qualifier
X Upper Extremity Y Lower Extremity	X External	B Computer Assisted Procedure	F With Fluoroscopy G With Computerized Tomography H With Magnetic Resonance Imaging Z No Qualifier

8EØ Continued on next page

♂	8EØVX1C
♂	8EØVX63
♀	8EØUXY7
♀	8EØHX62

8   Other Procedures
E   Physiological Systems and Anatomical Regions
0   Other Procedures   Definition: Methodologies which attempt to remediate or cure a disorder or disease

Body Region Character 4	Approach Character 5	Method Character 6	Qualifier Character 7
X Upper Extremity **Y** Lower Extremity	**X** External	**C** Robotic Assisted Procedure	**Z** No Qualifier
X Upper Extremity **Y** Lower Extremity	**X** External	**Y** Other Method	**8** Suture Removal
Z None	**X** External	**Y** Other Method	**1** In Vitro Fertilization **4** Yoga Therapy **5** Meditation **6** Isolation

Chiropractic 9WB

9   **Chiropractic**
W   **Anatomical Regions**
B   **Manipulation**   Definition: Manual procedure that involves a directed thrust to move a joint past the physiological range of motion, without exceeding the anatomical limit

Body Region Character 4	Approach Character 5	Method Character 6	Qualifier Character 7
Ø Head 1 Cervical 2 Thoracic 3 Lumbar 4 Sacrum 5 Pelvis 6 Lower Extremities 7 Upper Extremities 8 Rib Cage 9 Abdomen	X External	B Non-Manual C Indirect Visceral D Extra-Articular F Direct Visceral G Long Lever Specific Contact H Short Lever Specific Contact J Long and Short Lever Specific Contact K Mechanically Assisted L Other Method	Z None

Imaging B00–BY4

AHA Coding Clinic for table B21

2018, 1Q, 12   Percutaneous balloon valvuloplasty & cardiac catheterization with ventriculogram
2016, 3Q, 36   Type of contrast medium for angiography (high osmolar, low osmolar, and other)

AHA Coding Clinic for table B41

2015, 3Q, 9   Aborted endovascular stenting of superficial femoral artery

AHA Coding Clinic for table B51

2015, 4Q, 30   Vascular access devices

AHA Coding Clinic for table BF4

2014, 3Q, 15   Drainage of pancreatic pseudocyst

B   **Imaging**
0   **Central Nervous System**
0   **Plain Radiography**   Definition: Planar display of an image developed from the capture of external ionizing radiation on photographic or photoconductive plate

Body Part Character 4	Contrast Character 5	Qualifier Character 6	Qualifier Character 7
B Spinal Cord	0 High Osmolar 1 Low Osmolar Y Other Contrast Z None	Z None	Z None

B   **Imaging**
0   **Central Nervous System**
1   **Fluoroscopy**   Definition: Single plane or bi-plane real time display of an image developed from the capture of external ionizing radiation on a fluorescent screen. The image may also be stored by either digital or analog means.

Body Part Character 4	Contrast Character 5	Qualifier Character 6	Qualifier Character 7
B Spinal Cord	0 High Osmolar 1 Low Osmolar Y Other Contrast Z None	Z None	Z None

B   **Imaging**
0   **Central Nervous System**
2   **Computerized Tomography (CT Scan)**   Definition: Computer reformatted digital display of multiplanar images developed from the capture of multiple exposures of external ionizing radiation

Body Part Character 4	Contrast Character 5	Qualifier Character 6	Qualifier Character 7
0 Brain 7 Cisterna 8 Cerebral Ventricle(s) 9 Sella Turcica/Pituitary Gland B Spinal Cord	0 High Osmolar 1 Low Osmolar Y Other Contrast	0 Unenhanced and Enhanced Z None	Z None
0 Brain 7 Cisterna 8 Cerebral Ventricle(s) 9 Sella Turcica/Pituitary Gland B Spinal Cord	Z None	Z None	Z None

B   **Imaging**
0   **Central Nervous System**
3   **Magnetic Resonance Imaging (MRI)**   Definition: Computer reformatted digital display of multiplanar images developed from the capture of radio-frequency signals emitted by nuclei in a body site excited within a magnetic field

Body Part Character 4	Contrast Character 5	Qualifier Character 6	Qualifier Character 7
0 Brain 9 Sella Turcica/Pituitary Gland B Spinal Cord C Acoustic Nerves	Y Other Contrast	0 Unenhanced and Enhanced Z None	Z None
0 Brain 9 Sella Turcica/Pituitary Gland B Spinal Cord C Acoustic Nerves	Z None	Z None	Z None

B   **Imaging**
0   **Central Nervous System**
4   **Ultrasonography**   Definition: Real time display of images of anatomy or flow information developed from the capture of relected and attenuated high frequency sound waves

Body Part Character 4	Contrast Character 5	Qualifier Character 6	Qualifier Character 7
0 Brain B Spinal Cord	Z None	Z None	Z None

B   **Imaging**
2   **Heart**
0   **Plain Radiography**   Definition: Planar display of an image developed from the capture of external ionizing radiation on photographic or photoconductive plate

Body Part Character 4	Contrast Character 5	Qualifier Character 6	Qualifier Character 7
0 Coronary Artery, Single 1 Coronary Arteries, Multiple 2 Coronary Artery Bypass Graft, Single 3 Coronary Artery Bypass Grafts, Multiple 4 Heart, Right 5 Heart, Left 6 Heart, Right and Left 7 Internal Mammary Bypass Graft, Right 8 Internal Mammary Bypass Graft, Left F Bypass Graft, Other	0 High Osmolar 1 Low Osmolar Y Other Contrast	Z None	Z None

DRG Non-OR   All body part, contrast, and qualifier values

B   **Imaging**
2   **Heart**
1   **Fluoroscopy**   Definition: Single plane or bi-plane real time display of an image developed from the capture of external ionizing radioation on a fluorescent screen. The image may also be stored by either digital or analog means.

Body Part Character 4	Contrast Character 5	Qualifier Character 6	Qualifier Character 7
0 Coronary Artery, Single 1 Coronary Arteries, Multiple 2 Coronary Artery Bypass Graft, Single 3 Coronary Artery Bypass Grafts, Multiple	0 High Osmolar 1 Low Osmolar Y Other Contrast	1 Laser	0 Intraoperative
0 Coronary Artery, Single 1 Coronary Arteries, Multiple 2 Coronary Artery Bypass Graft, Single 3 Coronary Artery Bypass Grafts, Multiple	0 High Osmolar 1 Low Osmolar Y Other Contrast	Z None	Z None
4 Heart, Right 5 Heart, Left 6 Heart, Right and Left 7 Internal Mammary Bypass Graft, Right 8 Internal Mammary Bypass Graft, Left F Bypass Graft, Other	0 High Osmolar 1 Low Osmolar Y Other Contrast	Z None	Z None

DRG Non-OR   All body part, contrast, and qualifier values

B   **Imaging**
2   **Heart**
2   **Computerized Tomography (CT Scan)**   Definition: Computer reformatted digital display of multiplanar images developed from the capture of multiple exposures of external ionizing radiation

Body Part Character 4	Contrast Character 5	Qualifier Character 6	Qualifier Character 7
1 Coronary Arteries, Multiple 3 Coronary Artery Bypass Grafts, Multiple 6 Heart, Right and Left	0 High Osmolar 1 Low Osmolar Y Other Contrast	0 Unenhanced and Enhanced Z None	Z None
1 Coronary Arteries, Multiple 3 Coronary Artery Bypass Grafts, Multiple 6 Heart, Right and Left	Z None	2 Intravascular Optical Coherence Z None	Z None

B   Imaging
2   Heart
3   Magnetic Resonance Imaging (MRI)   Definition: Computer reformatted digital display of multiplanar images developed from the capture of radio-frequency signals emitted by nuclei in a body site excited within a magnetic field

Body Part Character 4	Contrast Character 5	Qualifier Character 6	Qualifier Character 7
1 Coronary Arteries, Multiple 3 Coronary Artery Bypass Grafts, Multiple 6 Heart, Right and Left	Y Other Contrast	Ø Unenhanced and Enhanced Z None	Z None
1 Coronary Arteries, Multiple 3 Coronary Artery Bypass Grafts, Multiple 6 Heart, Right and Left	Z None	Z None	Z None

B   Imaging
2   Heart
4   Ultrasonography   Definition: Real time display of images of anatomy or flow information developed from the capture of relected and attenuated high frequency sound waves

Body Part Character 4	Contrast Character 5	Qualifier Character 6	Qualifier Character 7
Ø Coronary Artery, Single 1 Coronary Arteries, Multiple 4 Heart, Right 5 Heart, Left 6 Heart, Right and Left B Heart with Aorta C Pericardium D Pediatric Heart	Y Other Contrast	Z None	Z None
Ø Coronary Artery, Single 1 Coronary Arteries, Multiple 4 Heart, Right 5 Heart, Left 6 Heart, Right and Left B Heart with Aorta C Pericardium D Pediatric Heart	Z None	Z None	3 Intravascular 4 Transesophageal Z None

B   Imaging
3   Upper Arteries
Ø   Plain Radiography   Definition: Planar display of an image developed from the capture of external ionizing radiation on photographic or photoconductive plate

Body Part Character 4	Contrast Character 5	Qualifier Character 6	Qualifier Character 7
Ø Thoracic Aorta 1 Brachiocephalic-Subclavian Artery, Right 2 Subclavian Artery, Left 3 Common Carotid Artery, Right 4 Common Carotid Artery, Left 5 Common Carotid Arteries, Bilateral 6 Internal Carotid Artery, Right 7 Internal Carotid Artery, Left 8 Internal Carotid Arteries, Bilateral 9 External Carotid Artery, Right B External Carotid Artery, Left C External Carotid Arteries, Bilateral D Vertebral Artery, Right F Vertebral Artery, Left G Vertebral Arteries, Bilateral H Upper Extremity Arteries, Right J Upper Extremity Arteries, Left K Upper Extremity Arteries, Bilateral L Intercostal and Bronchial Arteries M Spinal Arteries N Upper Arteries, Other P Thoraco-Abdominal Aorta Q Cervico-Cerebral Arch R Intracranial Arteries S Pulmonary Artery, Right T Pulmonary Artery, Left	Ø High Osmolar 1 Low Osmolar Y Other Contrast Z None	Z None	Z None

B   **Imaging**
3   **Upper Arteries**
1   **Fluoroscopy**   Definition: Single plane or bi-plane real time display of an image developed from the capture of external ionizing radiation on a fluorescent screen. The image may also be stored by either digital or analog means.

Body Part Character 4	Contrast Character 5	Qualifier Character 6	Qualifier Character 7
0 Thoracic Aorta 1 Brachiocephalic-Subclavian Artery, Right 2 Subclavian Artery, Left 3 Common Carotid Artery, Right 4 Common Carotid Artery, Left 5 Common Carotid Arteries, Bilateral 6 Internal Carotid Artery, Right 7 Internal Carotid Artery, Left 8 Internal Carotid Arteries, Bilateral 9 External Carotid Artery, Right B External Carotid Artery, Left C External Carotid Arteries, Bilateral D Vertebral Artery, Right F Vertebral Artery, Left G Vertebral Arteries, Bilateral H Upper Extremity Arteries, Right J Upper Extremity Arteries, Left K Upper Extremity Arteries, Bilateral L Intercostal and Bronchial Arteries M Spinal Arteries N Upper Arteries, Other P Thoraco-Abdominal Aorta Q Cervico-Cerebral Arch R Intracranial Arteries S Pulmonary Artery, Right T Pulmonary Artery, Left U Pulmonary Trunk	0 High Osmolar 1 Low Osmolar Y Other Contrast	1 Laser	0 Intraoperative
0 Thoracic Aorta 1 Brachiocephalic-Subclavian Artery, Right 2 Subclavian Artery, Left 3 Common Carotid Artery, Right 4 Common Carotid Artery, Left 5 Common Carotid Arteries, Bilateral 6 Internal Carotid Artery, Right 7 Internal Carotid Artery, Left 8 Internal Carotid Arteries, Bilateral 9 External Carotid Artery, Right B External Carotid Artery, Left C External Carotid Arteries, Bilateral D Vertebral Artery, Right F Vertebral Artery, Left G Vertebral Arteries, Bilateral H Upper Extremity Arteries, Right J Upper Extremity Arteries, Left K Upper Extremity Arteries, Bilateral L Intercostal and Bronchial Arteries M Spinal Arteries N Upper Arteries, Other P Thoraco-Abdominal Aorta Q Cervico-Cerebral Arch R Intracranial Arteries S Pulmonary Artery, Right T Pulmonary Artery, Left U Pulmonary Trunk	0 High Osmolar 1 Low Osmolar Y Other Contrast	Z None	Z None

B31 Continued on next page

B31 Continued

B   **Imaging**
3   **Upper Arteries**
1   **Fluoroscopy**   Definition: Single plane or bi-plane real time display of an image developed from the capture of external ionizing radiation on a fluorescent screen. The image may also be stored by either digital or analog means.

Body Part Character 4	Contrast Character 5	Qualifier Character 6	Qualifier Character 7
Ø Thoracic Aorta	Z None	Z None	Z None
1 Brachiocephalic-Subclavian Artery, Right			
2 Subclavian Artery, Left			
3 Common Carotid Artery, Right			
4 Common Carotid Artery, Left			
5 Common Carotid Arteries, Bilateral			
6 Internal Carotid Artery, Right			
7 Internal Carotid Artery, Left			
8 Internal Carotid Arteries, Bilateral			
9 External Carotid Artery, Right			
B External Carotid Artery, Left			
C External Carotid Arteries, Bilateral			
D Vertebral Artery, Right			
F Vertebral Artery, Left			
G Vertebral Arteries, Bilateral			
H Upper Extremity Arteries, Right			
J Upper Extremity Arteries, Left			
K Upper Extremity Arteries, Bilateral			
L Intercostal and Bronchial Arteries			
M Spinal Arteries			
N Upper Arteries, Other			
P Thoraco-Abdominal Aorta			
Q Cervico-Cerebral Arch			
R Intracranial Arteries			
S Pulmonary Artery, Right			
T Pulmonary Artery, Left			
U Pulmonary Trunk			

B   **Imaging**
3   **Upper Arteries**
2   **Computerized Tomography (CT Scan)**   Definition: Computer reformatted digital display of multiplanar images developed from the capture of multiple exposures of external ionizing radiation

Body Part Character 4	Contrast Character 5	Qualifier Character 6	Qualifier Character 7
Ø Thoracic Aorta	Ø High Osmolar	Z None	Z None
5 Common Carotid Arteries, Bilateral	1 Low Osmolar		
8 Internal Carotid Arteries, Bilateral	Y Other Contrast		
G Vertebral Arteries, Bilateral			
R Intracranial Arteries			
S Pulmonary Artery, Right			
T Pulmonary Artery, Left			
Ø Thoracic Aorta	Z None	2 Intravascular Optical Coherence	Z None
5 Common Carotid Arteries, Bilateral		Z None	
8 Internal Carotid Arteries, Bilateral			
G Vertebral Arteries, Bilateral			
R Intracranial Arteries			
S Pulmonary Artery, Right			
T Pulmonary Artery, Left			

LC Limited Coverage   NC Noncovered   ⊞ Combination Member   HAC   Valid OR   Combination Only   DRG Non-OR   New/Revised in GREEN
ICD-10-PCS 2020   727

B31–B32

B   **Imaging**
3   **Upper Arteries**
3   **Magnetic Resonance Imaging (MRI)**   Definition: Computer reformatted digital display of multiplanar images developed from the capture of radio-frequency signals emitted by nuclei in a body site excited within a magnetic field

Body Part Character 4	Contrast Character 5	Qualifier Character 6	Qualifier Character 7
Ø Thoracic Aorta 5 Common Carotid Arteries, Bilateral 8 Internal Carotid Arteries, Bilateral G Vertebral Arteries, Bilateral H Upper Extremity Arteries, Right J Upper Extremity Arteries, Left K Upper Extremity Arteries, Bilateral M Spinal Arteries Q Cervico-Cerebral Arch R Intracranial Arteries	Y Other Contrast	Ø Unenhanced and Enhanced Z None	Z None
Ø Thoracic Aorta 5 Common Carotid Arteries, Bilateral 8 Internal Carotid Arteries, Bilateral G Vertebral Arteries, Bilateral H Upper Extremity Arteries, Right J Upper Extremity Arteries, Left K Upper Extremity Arteries, Bilateral M Spinal Arteries Q Cervico-Cerebral Arch R Intracranial Arteries	Z None	Z None	Z None

B   **Imaging**
3   **Upper Arteries**
4   **Ultrasonography**   Definition: Real time display of images of anatomy or flow information developed from the capture of reflected and attenuated high frequency sound waves

Body Part Character 4	Contrast Character 5	Qualifier Character 6	Qualifier Character 7
Ø Thoracic Aorta 1 Brachiocephalic-Subclavian Artery, Right 2 Subclavian Artery, Left 3 Common Carotid Artery, Right 4 Common Carotid Artery, Left 5 Common Carotid Arteries, Bilateral 6 Internal Carotid Artery, Right 7 Internal Carotid Artery, Left 8 Internal Carotid Arteries, Bilateral H Upper Extremity Arteries, Right J Upper Extremity Arteries, Left K Upper Extremity Arteries, Bilateral R Intracranial Arteries S Pulmonary Artery, Right T Pulmonary Artery, Left V Ophthalmic Arteries	Z None	Z None	3 Intravascular Z None

B   **Imaging**
4   **Lower Arteries**
Ø   **Plain Radiography**   Definition: Planar display of an image developed from the capture of external ionizing radiation on photographic or photoconductive plate

Body Part Character 4	Contrast Character 5	Qualifier Character 6	Qualifier Character 7
Ø Abdominal Aorta 2 Hepatic Artery 3 Splenic Arteries 4 Superior Mesenteric Artery 5 Inferior Mesenteric Artery 6 Renal Artery, Right 7 Renal Artery, Left 8 Renal Arteries, Bilateral 9 Lumbar Arteries B Intra-Abdominal Arteries, Other C Pelvic Arteries D Aorta and Bilateral Lower Extremity Arteries F Lower Extremity Arteries, Right G Lower Extremity Arteries, Left J Lower Arteries, Other M Renal Artery Transplant	Ø High Osmolar 1 Low Osmolar Y Other Contrast	Z None	Z None

B   **Imaging**
4   **Lower Arteries**
1   **Fluoroscopy**   Definition: Single plane or bi-plane real time display of an image developed from the capture of external ionizing radiation on a fluorescent screen. The image may also be stored by either digital or analog means.

Body Part Character 4	Contrast Character 5	Qualifier Character 6	Qualifier Character 7
Ø Abdominal Aorta **2** Hepatic Artery **3** Splenic Arteries **4** Superior Mesenteric Artery **5** Inferior Mesenteric Artery **6** Renal Artery, Right **7** Renal Artery, Left **8** Renal Arteries, Bilateral **9** Lumbar Arteries **B** Intra-Abdominal Arteries, Other **C** Pelvic Arteries **D** Aorta and Bilateral Lower Extremity Arteries **F** Lower Extremity Arteries, Right **G** Lower Extremity Arteries, Left **J** Lower Arteries, Other	**Ø** High Osmolar **1** Low Osmolar **Y** Other Contrast	**1** Laser	**Ø** Intraoperative
Ø Abdominal Aorta **2** Hepatic Artery **3** Splenic Arteries **4** Superior Mesenteric Artery **5** Inferior Mesenteric Artery **6** Renal Artery, Right **7** Renal Artery, Left **8** Renal Arteries, Bilateral **9** Lumbar Arteries **B** Intra-Abdominal Arteries, Other **C** Pelvic Arteries **D** Aorta and Bilateral Lower Extremity Arteries **F** Lower Extremity Arteries, Right **G** Lower Extremity Arteries, Left **J** Lower Arteries, Other	**Ø** High Osmolar **1** Low Osmolar **Y** Other Contrast	**Z** None	**Z** None
Ø Abdominal Aorta **2** Hepatic Artery **3** Splenic Arteries **4** Superior Mesenteric Artery **5** Inferior Mesenteric Artery **6** Renal Artery, Right **7** Renal Artery, Left **8** Renal Arteries, Bilateral **9** Lumbar Arteries **B** Intra-Abdominal Arteries, Other **C** Pelvic Arteries **D** Aorta and Bilateral Lower Extremity Arteries **F** Lower Extremity Arteries, Right **G** Lower Extremity Arteries, Left **J** Lower Arteries, Other	**Z** None	**Z** None	**Z** None

B **Imaging**
4 **Lower Arteries**
2 **Computerized Tomography (CT Scan)** Definition: Computer reformatted digital display of multiplanar images developed from the capture of multiple exposures of external ionizing radiation

Body Part Character 4	Contrast Character 5	Qualifier Character 6	Qualifier Character 7
Ø Abdominal Aorta **1** Celiac Artery **4** Superior Mesenteric Artery **8** Renal Arteries, Bilateral **C** Pelvic Arteries **F** Lower Extremity Arteries, Right **G** Lower Extremity Arteries, Left **H** Lower Extremity Arteries, Bilateral **M** Renal Artery Transplant	**Ø** High Osmolar **1** Low Osmolar **Y** Other Contrast	**Z** None	**Z** None
Ø Abdominal Aorta **1** Celiac Artery **4** Superior Mesenteric Artery **8** Renal Arteries, Bilateral **C** Pelvic Arteries **F** Lower Extremity Arteries, Right **G** Lower Extremity Arteries, Left **H** Lower Extremity Arteries, Bilateral **M** Renal Artery Transplant	**Z** None	**2** Intravascular Optical Coherence **Z** None	**Z** None

B **Imaging**
4 **Lower Arteries**
3 **Magnetic Resonance Imaging (MRI)** Definition: Computer reformatted digital display of multiplanar images developed from the capture of radio-frequency signals emitted by nuclei in a body site excited within a magnetic field

Body Part Character 4	Contrast Character 5	Qualifier Character 6	Qualifier Character 7
Ø Abdominal Aorta **1** Celiac Artery **4** Superior Mesenteric Artery **8** Renal Arteries, Bilateral **C** Pelvic Arteries **F** Lower Extremity Arteries, Right **G** Lower Extremity Arteries, Left **H** Lower Extremity Arteries, Bilateral	**Y** Other Contrast	**Ø** Unenhanced and Enhanced **Z** None	**Z** None
Ø Abdominal Aorta **1** Celiac Artery **4** Superior Mesenteric Artery **8** Renal Arteries, Bilateral **C** Pelvic Arteries **F** Lower Extremity Arteries, Right **G** Lower Extremity Arteries, Left **H** Lower Extremity Arteries, Bilateral	**Z** None	**Z** None	**Z** None

B **Imaging**
4 **Lower Arteries**
4 **Ultrasonography** Definition: Real time display of images of anatomy or flow information developed from the capture of reflected and attenuated high frequency sound waves

Body Part Character 4	Contrast Character 5	Qualifier Character 6	Qualifier Character 7
Ø Abdominal Aorta **4** Superior Mesenteric Artery **5** Inferior Mesenteric Artery **6** Renal Artery, Right **7** Renal Artery, Left **8** Renal Arteries, Bilateral **B** Intra-Abdominal Arteries, Other **F** Lower Extremity Arteries, Right **G** Lower Extremity Arteries, Left **H** Lower Extremity Arteries, Bilateral **K** Celiac and Mesenteric Arteries **L** Femoral Artery **N** Penile Arteries	**Z** None	**Z** None	**3** Intravascular **Z** None

LC Limited Coverage   **NC** Noncovered   ⊞ Combination Member   HAC   Valid OR   Combination Only   DRG Non-OR   New/Revised in GREEN

730

ICD-10-PCS 2020

B42–B44

B   **Imaging**
5   **Veins**
Ø   **Plain Radiography**   Definition: Planar display of an image developed from the capture of external ionizing radiation on photographic or photoconductive plate

Body Part Character 4	Contrast Character 5	Qualifier Character 6	Qualifier Character 7
Ø Epidural Veins	Ø High Osmolar	Z None	Z None
1 Cerebral and Cerebellar Veins	1 Low Osmolar		
2 Intracranial Sinuses	Y Other Contrast		
3 Jugular Veins, Right			
4 Jugular Veins, Left			
5 Jugular Veins, Bilateral			
6 Subclavian Vein, Right			
7 Subclavian Vein, Left			
8 Superior Vena Cava			
9 Inferior Vena Cava			
B Lower Extremity Veins, Right			
C Lower Extremity Veins, Left			
D Lower Extremity Veins, Bilateral			
F Pelvic (Iliac) Veins, Right			
G Pelvic (Iliac) Veins, Left			
H Pelvic (Iliac) Veins, Bilateral			
J Renal Vein, Right			
K Renal Vein, Left			
L Renal Veins, Bilateral			
M Upper Extremity Veins, Right			
N Upper Extremity Veins, Left			
P Upper Extremity Veins, Bilateral			
Q Pulmonary Vein, Right			
R Pulmonary Vein, Left			
S Pulmonary Veins, Bilateral			
T Portal and Splanchnic Veins			
V Veins, Other			
W Dialysis Shunt/Fistula			

B   **Imaging**
5   **Veins**
1   **Fluoroscopy**   Definition: Single plane or bi-plane real time display of an image developed from the capture of external ionizing radioation on a fluorescent screen. The image may also be stored by either digital or analog means.

Body Part Character 4	Contrast Character 5	Qualifier Character 6	Qualifier Character 7
Ø Epidural Veins	Ø High Osmolar	Z None	A Guidance
1 Cerebral and Cerebellar Veins	1 Low Osmolar		Z None
2 Intracranial Sinuses	Y Other Contrast		
3 Jugular Veins, Right	Z None		
4 Jugular Veins, Left			
5 Jugular Veins, Bilateral			
6 Subclavian Vein, Right			
7 Subclavian Vein, Left			
8 Superior Vena Cava			
9 Inferior Vena Cava			
B Lower Extremity Veins, Right			
C Lower Extremity Veins, Left			
D Lower Extremity Veins, Bilateral			
F Pelvic (Iliac) Veins, Right			
G Pelvic (Iliac) Veins, Left			
H Pelvic (Iliac) Veins, Bilateral			
J Renal Vein, Right			
K Renal Vein, Left			
L Renal Veins, Bilateral			
M Upper Extremity Veins, Right			
N Upper Extremity Veins, Left			
P Upper Extremity Veins, Bilateral			
Q Pulmonary Vein, Right			
R Pulmonary Vein, Left			
S Pulmonary Veins, Bilateral			
T Portal and Splanchnic Veins			
V Veins, Other			
W Dialysis Shunt/Fistula			

LC Limited Coverage   NC Noncovered   ⊞ Combination Member   HAC   Valid OR   Combination Only   DRG Non-OR   New/Revised in GREEN
ICD-10-PCS 2020

B5Ø–B51

731

B   Imaging
5   Veins
2   Computerized Tomography (CT Scan) Definition: Computer reformatted digital display of multiplanar images developed from the capture of multiple exposures of external ionizing radiation

Body Part Character 4	Contrast Character 5	Qualifier Character 6	Qualifier Character 7
2 Intracranial Sinuses 8 Superior Vena Cava 9 Inferior Vena Cava F Pelvic (Iliac) Veins, Right G Pelvic (Iliac) Veins, Left H Pelvic (Iliac) Veins, Bilateral J Renal Vein, Right K Renal Vein, Left L Renal Veins, Bilateral Q Pulmonary Vein, Right R Pulmonary Vein, Left S Pulmonary Veins, Bilateral T Portal and Splanchnic Veins	Ø High Osmolar 1 Low Osmolar Y Other Contrast	Ø Unenhanced and Enhanced Z None	Z None
2 Intracranial Sinuses 8 Superior Vena Cava 9 Inferior Vena Cava F Pelvic (Iliac) Veins, Right G Pelvic (Iliac) Veins, Left H Pelvic (Iliac) Veins, Bilateral J Renal Vein, Right K Renal Vein, Left L Renal Veins, Bilateral Q Pulmonary Vein, Right R Pulmonary Vein, Left S Pulmonary Veins, Bilateral T Portal and Splanchnic Veins	Z None	2 Intravascular Optical Coherence Z None	Z None

B   Imaging
5   Veins
3   Magnetic Resonance Imaging (MRI) Definition: Computer reformatted digital display of multiplanar images developed from the capture of radio-frequency signals emitted by nuclei in a body site excited within a magnetic field

Body Part Character 4	Contrast Character 5	Qualifier Character 6	Qualifier Character 7
1 Cerebral and Cerebellar Veins 2 Intracranial Sinuses 5 Jugular Veins, Bilateral 8 Superior Vena Cava 9 Inferior Vena Cava B Lower Extremity Veins, Right C Lower Extremity Veins, Left D Lower Extremity Veins, Bilateral H Pelvic (Iliac) Veins, Bilateral L Renal Veins, Bilateral M Upper Extremity Veins, Right N Upper Extremity Veins, Left P Upper Extremity Veins, Bilateral S Pulmonary Veins, Bilateral T Portal and Splanchnic Veins V Veins, Other	Y Other Contrast	Ø Unenhanced and Enhanced Z None	Z None
1 Cerebral and Cerebellar Veins 2 Intracranial Sinuses 5 Jugular Veins, Bilateral 8 Superior Vena Cava 9 Inferior Vena Cava B Lower Extremity Veins, Right C Lower Extremity Veins, Left D Lower Extremity Veins, Bilateral H Pelvic (Iliac) Veins, Bilateral L Renal Veins, Bilateral M Upper Extremity Veins, Right N Upper Extremity Veins, Left P Upper Extremity Veins, Bilateral S Pulmonary Veins, Bilateral T Portal and Splanchnic Veins V Veins, Other	Z None	Z None	Z None

B   **Imaging**
5   **Veins**
4   **Ultrasonography**   Definition: Real time display of images of anatomy or flow information developed from the capture of relected and attenuated high frequency sound waves

Body Part Character 4	Contrast Character 5	Qualifier Character 6	Qualifier Character 7
3 Jugular Veins, Right **4** Jugular Veins, Left **6** Subclavian Vein, Right **7** Subclavian Vein, Left **8** Superior Vena Cava **9** Inferior Vena Cava **B** Lower Extremity Veins, Right **C** Lower Extremity Veins, Left **D** Lower Extremity Veins, Bilateral **J** Renal Vein, Right **K** Renal Vein, Left **L** Renal Veins, Bilateral **M** Upper Extremity Veins, Right **N** Upper Extremity Veins, Left **P** Upper Extremity Veins, Bilateral **T** Portal and Splanchnic Veins	**Z** None	**Z** None	**3** Intravascular **A** Guidance **Z** None

B   **Imaging**
7   **Lymphatic System**
Ø   **Plain Radiography**   Definition: Planar display of an image developed from the capture of external ionizing radiation on photographic or photoconductive plate

Body Part Character 4	Contrast Character 5	Qualifier Character 6	Qualifier Character 7

Ø Abdominal/Retroperitoneal
   Lymphatics, Unilateral
1 Abdominal/Retroperitoneal
   Lymphatics, Bilateral
4 Lymphatics, Head and Neck
5 Upper Extremity Lymphatics, Right
6 Upper Extremity Lymphatics, Left
7 Upper Extremity Lymphatics,
   Bilateral
8 Lower Extremity Lymphatics, Right
9 Lower Extremity Lymphatics, Left
B Lower Extremity Lymphatics,
   Bilateral
C Lymphatics, Pelvic
	Ø High Osmolar
	1 Low Osmolar
	Y Other Contrast
		Z None	**Z** None

B   **Imaging**
8   **Eye**
Ø   **Plain Radiography**   Definition: Planar display of an image developed from the capture of external ionizing radiation on photographic or photoconductive plate

Body Part Character 4	Contrast Character 5	Qualifier Character 6	Qualifier Character 7
Ø Lacrimal Duct, Right **1** Lacrimal Duct, Left **2** Lacrimal Ducts, Bilateral	**Ø** High Osmolar **1** Low Osmolar **Y** Other Contrast	**Z** None	**Z** None
3 Optic Foramina, Right **4** Optic Foramina, Left **5** Eye, Right **6** Eye, Left **7** Eyes, Bilateral	**Z** None	**Z** None	**Z** None

B   **Imaging**
8   **Eye**
2   **Computerized Tomography (CT Scan)**   Definition: Computer reformatted digital display of multiplanar images developed from the capture of multiple exposures of external ionizing radiation

Body Part Character 4	Contrast Character 5	Qualifier Character 6	Qualifier Character 7
5 Eye, Right **6** Eye, Left **7** Eyes, Bilateral	**Ø** High Osmolar **1** Low Osmolar **Y** Other Contrast	**Ø** Unenhanced and Enhanced **Z** None	**Z** None
5 Eye, Right **6** Eye, Left **7** Eyes, Bilateral	**Z** None	**Z** None	**Z** None

[LC] Limited Coverage   [NC] Noncovered   ⊞ Combination Member   HAC   Valid OR   Combination Only   DRG Non-OR   New/Revised in GREEN

ICD-10-PCS 2020   733

B54–B82

B   Imaging
8   Eye
3   Magnetic Resonance Imaging (MRI)   Definition: Computer reformatted digital display of multiplanar images developed from the capture of radio-frequency signals emitted by nuclei in a body site excited within a magnetic field

Body Part Character 4	Contrast Character 5	Qualifier Character 6	Qualifier Character 7
5 Eye, Right 6 Eye, Left 7 Eyes, Bilateral	Y Other Contrast	Ø Unenhanced and Enhanced Z None	Z None
5 Eye, Right 6 Eye, Left 7 Eyes, Bilateral	Z None	Z None	Z None

B   Imaging
8   Eye
4   Ultrasonography   Definition: Real time display of images of anatomy or flow information developed from the capture of relected and attenuated high frequency sound waves

Body Part Character 4	Contrast Character 5	Qualifier Character 6	Qualifier Character 7
5 Eye, Right 6 Eye, Left 7 Eyes, Bilateral	Z None	Z None	Z None

B   Imaging
9   Ear, Nose, Mouth and Throat
Ø   Plain Radiography   Definition: Planar display of an image developed from the capture of external ionizing radiation on photographic or photoconductive plate

Body Part Character 4	Contrast Character 5	Qualifier Character 6	Qualifier Character 7
2 Paranasal Sinuses F Nasopharynx/Oropharynx H Mastoids	Z None	Z None	Z None
4 Parotid Gland, Right 5 Parotid Gland, Left 6 Parotid Glands, Bilateral 7 Submandibular Gland, Right 8 Submandibular Gland, Left 9 Submandibular Glands, Bilateral B Salivary Gland, Right C Salivary Gland, Left D Salivary Glands, Bilateral	Ø High Osmolar 1 Low Osmolar Y Other Contrast	Z None	Z None

B   Imaging
9   Ear, Nose, Mouth and Throat
1   Fluoroscopy   Definition: Single plane or bi-plane real time display of an image developed from the capture of external ionizing radioation on a fluorescent screen. The image may also be stored by either digital or analog means.

Body Part Character 4	Contrast Character 5	Qualifier Character 6	Qualifier Character 7
G Pharynx and Epiglottis J Larynx	Y Other Contrast Z None	Z None	Z None

B   Imaging
9   Ear, Nose, Mouth and Throat
2   Computerized Tomography (CT Scan)   Definition: Computer reformatted digital display of multiplanar images developed from the capture of multiple exposures of external ionizing radiation

Body Part Character 4	Contrast Character 5	Qualifier Character 6	Qualifier Character 7
Ø Ear 2 Paranasal Sinuses 6 Parotid Glands, Bilateral 9 Submandibular Glands, Bilateral D Salivary Glands, Bilateral F Nasopharynx/Oropharynx J Larynx	Ø High Osmolar 1 Low Osmolar Y Other Contrast	Ø Unenhanced and Enhanced Z None	Z None
Ø Ear 2 Paranasal Sinuses 6 Parotid Glands, Bilateral 9 Submandibular Glands, Bilateral D Salivary Glands, Bilateral F Nasopharynx/Oropharynx J Larynx	Z None	Z None	Z None

LC Limited Coverage   NC Noncovered   ⊞ Combination Member   HAC   Valid OR   Combination Only   DRG Non-OR   New/Revised in GREEN
734   ICD-10-PCS 2020

B83–B92

B   Imaging
9   Ear, Nose, Mouth and Throat
3   Magnetic Resonance Imaging (MRI)   Definition: Computer reformatted digital display of multiplanar images developed from the capture of radio-frequency signals emitted by nuclei in a body site excited within a magnetic field

Body Part Character 4	Contrast Character 5	Qualifier Character 6	Qualifier Character 7
Ø Ear 2 Paranasal Sinuses 6 Parotid Glands, Bilateral 9 Submandibular Glands, Bilateral D Salivary Glands, Bilateral F Nasopharynx/Oropharynx J Larynx	Y Other Contrast	Ø Unenhanced and Enhanced Z None	Z None
Ø Ear 2 Paranasal Sinuses 6 Parotid Glands, Bilateral 9 Submandibular Glands, Bilateral D Salivary Glands, Bilateral F Nasopharynx/Oropharynx J Larynx	Z None	Z None	Z None

B   Imaging
B   Respiratory System
Ø   Plain Radiography   Definition: Planar display of an image developed from the capture of external ionizing radiation on photographic or photoconductive plate

Body Part Character 4	Contrast Character 5	Qualifier Character 6	Qualifier Character 7
7 Tracheobronchial Tree, Right 8 Tracheobronchial Tree, Left 9 Tracheobronchial Trees, Bilateral	Y Other Contrast	Z None	Z None
D Upper Airways	Z None	Z None	Z None

B   Imaging
B   Respiratory System
1   Fluoroscopy   Definition: Single plane or bi-plane real time display of an image developed from the capture of external ionizing radioation on a fluorescent screen. The image may also be stored by either digital or analog means.

Body Part Character 4	Contrast Character 5	Qualifier Character 6	Qualifier Character 7
2 Lung, Right 3 Lung, Left 4 Lungs, Bilateral 6 Diaphragm C Mediastinum D Upper Airways	Z None	Z None	Z None
7 Tracheobronchial Tree, Right 8 Tracheobronchial Tree, Left 9 Tracheobronchial Trees, Bilateral	Y Other Contrast	Z None	Z None

B   Imaging
B   Respiratory System
2   Computerized Tomography (CT Scan)   Definition: Computer reformatted digital display of multiplanar images developed from the capture of multiple exposures of external ionizing radiation

Body Part Character 4	Contrast Character 5	Qualifier Character 6	Qualifier Character 7
4 Lungs, Bilateral 7 Tracheobronchial Tree, Right 8 Tracheobronchial Tree, Left 9 Tracheobronchial Trees, Bilateral F Trachea/Airways	Ø High Osmolar 1 Low Osmolar Y Other Contrast	Ø Unenhanced and Enhanced Z None	Z None
4 Lungs, Bilateral 7 Tracheobronchial Tree, Right 8 Tracheobronchial Tree, Left 9 Tracheobronchial Trees, Bilateral F Trachea/Airways	Z None	Z None	Z None

B   **Imaging**
B   **Respiratory System**
3   **Magnetic Resonance Imaging (MRI)**   Definition: Computer reformatted digital display of multiplanar images developed from the capture of radio-frequency signals emitted by nuclei in a body site excited within a magnetic field

Body Part Character 4	Contrast Character 5	Qualifier Character 6	Qualifier Character 7
G Lung Apices	Y Other Contrast	Ø Unenhanced and Enhanced Z None	Z None
G Lung Apices	Z None	Z None	Z None

B   **Imaging**
B   **Respiratory System**
4   **Ultrasonography**   Definition: Real time display of images of anatomy or flow information developed from the capture of relected and attenuated high frequency sound waves

Body Part Character 4	Contrast Character 5	Qualifier Character 6	Qualifier Character 7
B Pleura C Mediastinum	Z None	Z None	Z None

B   **Imaging**
D   **Gastrointestinal System**
1   **Fluoroscopy**   Definition: Single plane or bi-plane real time display of an image developed from the capture of external ionizing radioation on a fluorescent screen. The image may also be stored by either digital or analog means.

Body Part Character 4	Contrast Character 5	Qualifier Character 6	Qualifier Character 7
1 Esophagus 2 Stomach 3 Small Bowel 4 Colon 5 Upper GI 6 Upper GI and Small Bowel 9 Duodenum B Mouth/Oropharynx	Y Other Contrast Z None	Z None	Z None

B   **Imaging**
D   **Gastrointestinal System**
2   **Computerized Tomography (CT Scan)**   Definition: Computer reformatted digital display of multiplanar images developed from the capture of multiple exposures of external ionizing radiation

Body Part Character 4	Contrast Character 5	Qualifier Character 6	Qualifier Character 7
4 Colon	Ø High Osmolar 1 Low Osmolar Y Other Contrast	Ø Unenhanced and Enhanced Z None	Z None
4 Colon	Z None	Z None	Z None

B   **Imaging**
D   **Gastrointestinal System**
4   **Ultrasonography**   Definition: Real time display of images of anatomy or flow information developed from the capture of relected and attenuated high frequency sound waves

Body Part Character 4	Contrast Character 5	Qualifier Character 6	Qualifier Character 7
1 Esophagus 2 Stomach 7 Gastrointestinal Tract 8 Appendix 9 Duodenum C Rectum	Z None	Z None	Z None

B   **Imaging**
F   **Hepatobiliary System and Pancreas**
Ø   **Plain Radiography**   Definition: Planar display of an image developed from the capture of external ionizing radiation on photographic or photoconductive plate

Body Part Character 4	Contrast Character 5	Qualifier Character 6	Qualifier Character 7
Ø Bile Ducts 3 Gallbladder and Bile Ducts C Hepatobiliary System, All	Ø High Osmolar 1 Low Osmolar Y Other Contrast	Z None	Z None

LC Limited Coverage   **NC** Noncovered   ⊞ Combination Member   HAC   Valid OR   Combination Only   DRG Non-OR   New/Revised in GREEN

736   ICD-10-PCS 2020

BB3–BF0

B   **Imaging**
F   **Hepatobiliary System and Pancreas**
1   **Fluoroscopy**   Definition: Single plane or bi-plane real time display of an image developed from the capture of external ionizing radioation on a fluorescent screen. The image may also be stored by either digital or analog means.

Body Part Character 4	Contrast Character 5	Qualifier Character 6	Qualifier Character 7
Ø Bile Ducts 1 Biliary and Pancreatic Ducts 2 Gallbladder 3 Gallbladder and Bile Ducts 4 Gallbladder, Bile Ducts and Pancreatic Ducts 8 Pancreatic Ducts	Ø High Osmolar 1 Low Osmolar Y Other Contrast	Z None	Z None

B   **Imaging**
F   **Hepatobiliary System and Pancreas**
2   **Computerized Tomography (CT Scan)**   Definition: Computer reformatted digital display of multiplanar images developed from the capture of multiple exposures of external ionizing radiation

Body Part Character 4	Contrast Character 5	Qualifier Character 6	Qualifier Character 7
5 Liver 6 Liver and Spleen 7 Pancreas C Hepatobiliary System, All	Ø High Osmolar 1 Low Osmolar Y Other Contrast	Ø Unenhanced and Enhanced Z None	Z None
5 Liver 6 Liver and Spleen 7 Pancreas C Hepatobiliary System, All	Z None	Z None	Z None

B   **Imaging**
F   **Hepatobiliary System and Pancreas**
3   **Magnetic Resonance Imaging (MRI)**   Definition: Computer reformatted digital display of multiplanar images developed from the capture of radio-frequency signals emitted by nuclei in a body site excited within a magnetic field

Body Part Character 4	Contrast Character 5	Qualifier Character 6	Qualifier Character 7
5 Liver 6 Liver and Spleen 7 Pancreas	Y Other Contrast	Ø Unenhanced and Enhanced Z None	Z None
5 Liver 6 Liver and Spleen 7 Pancreas	Z None	Z None	Z None

B   **Imaging**
F   **Hepatobiliary System and Pancreas**
4   **Ultrasonography**   Definition: Real time display of images of anatomy or flow information developed from the capture of relected and attenuated high frequency sound waves

Body Part Character 4	Contrast Character 5	Qualifier Character 6	Qualifier Character 7
Ø Bile Ducts 2 Gallbladder 3 Gallbladder and Bile Ducts 5 Liver 6 Liver and Spleen 7 Pancreas C Hepatobiliary System, All	Z None	Z None	Z None

B   **Imaging**
G   **Endocrine System**
2   **Computerized Tomography (CT Scan)**   Definition: Computer reformatted digital display of multiplanar images developed from the capture of multiple exposures of external ionizing radiation

Body Part Character 4	Contrast Character 5	Qualifier Character 6	Qualifier Character 7
2 Adrenal Glands, Bilateral 3 Parathyroid Glands 4 Thyroid Gland	Ø High Osmolar 1 Low Osmolar Y Other Contrast	Ø Unenhanced and Enhanced Z None	Z None
2 Adrenal Glands, Bilateral 3 Parathyroid Glands 4 Thyroid Gland	Z None	Z None	Z None

B   Imaging
G   Endocrine System
3   Magnetic Resonance Imaging (MRI)   Definition: Computer reformatted digital display of multiplanar images developed from the capture of radio-frequency signals emitted by nuclei in a body site excited within a magnetic field

Body Part Character 4	Contrast Character 5	Qualifier Character 6	Qualifier Character 7
2 Adrenal Glands, Bilateral 3 Parathyroid Glands 4 Thyroid Gland	Y Other Contrast	0 Unenhanced and Enhanced Z None	Z None
2 Adrenal Glands, Bilateral 3 Parathyroid Glands 4 Thyroid Gland	Z None	Z None	Z None

B   Imaging
G   Endocrine System
4   Ultrasonography   Definition: Real time display of images of anatomy or flow information developed from the capture of relected and attenuated high frequency sound waves

Body Part Character 4	Contrast Character 5	Qualifier Character 6	Qualifier Character 7
0 Adrenal Gland, Right 1 Adrenal Gland, Left 2 Adrenal Glands, Bilateral 3 Parathyroid Glands 4 Thyroid Gland	Z None	Z None	Z None

B   Imaging
H   Skin, Subcutaneous Tissue and Breast
0   Plain Radiography   Definition: Planar display of an image developed from the capture of external ionizing radiation on photographic or photoconductive plate

Body Part Character 4	Contrast Character 5	Qualifier Character 6	Qualifier Character 7
0 Breast, Right 1 Breast, Left 2 Breasts, Bilateral	Z None	Z None	Z None
3 Single Mammary Duct, Right 4 Single Mammary Duct, Left 5 Multiple Mammary Ducts, Right 6 Multiple Mammary Ducts, Left	0 High Osmolar 1 Low Osmolar Y Other Contrast Z None	Z None	Z None

B   Imaging
H   Skin, Subcutaneous Tissue and Breast
3   Magnetic Resonance Imaging (MRI)   Definition: Computer reformatted digital display of multiplanar images developed from the capture of radio-frequency signals emitted by nuclei in a body site excited within a magnetic field

Body Part Character 4	Contrast Character 5	Qualifier Character 6	Qualifier Character 7
0 Breast, Right 1 Breast, Left 2 Breasts, Bilateral D Subcutaneous Tissue, Head/Neck F Subcutaneous Tissue, Upper Extremity G Subcutaneous Tissue, Thorax H Subcutaneous Tissue, Abdomen and Pelvis J Subcutaneous Tissue, Lower Extremity	Y Other Contrast	0 Unenhanced and Enhanced Z None	Z None
0 Breast, Right 1 Breast, Left 2 Breasts, Bilateral D Subcutaneous Tissue, Head/Neck F Subcutaneous Tissue, Upper Extremity G Subcutaneous Tissue, Thorax H Subcutaneous Tissue, Abdomen and Pelvis J Subcutaneous Tissue, Lower Extremity	Z None	Z None	Z None

B   Imaging
H   Skin, Subcutaneous Tissue and Breast
4   Ultrasonography   Definition: Real time display of images of anatomy or flow information developed from the capture of relected and attenuated high frequency sound waves

Body Part Character 4	Contrast Character 5	Qualifier Character 6	Qualifier Character 7
Ø Breast, Right 1 Breast, Left 2 Breasts, Bilateral 7 Extremity, Upper 8 Extremity, Lower 9 Abdominal Wall B Chest Wall C Head and Neck	Z None	Z None	Z None

B   Imaging
L   Connective Tissue
3   Magnetic Resonance Imaging (MRI)   Definition: Computer reformatted digital display of multiplanar images developed from the capture of radio-frequency signals emitted by nuclei in a body site excited within a magnetic field

Body Part Character 4	Contrast Character 5	Qualifier Character 6	Qualifier Character 7
Ø Connective Tissue, Upper Extremity 1 Connective Tissue, Lower Extremity 2 Tendons, Upper Extremity 3 Tendons, Lower Extremity	Y Other Contrast	Ø Unenhanced and Enhanced Z None	Z None
Ø Connective Tissue, Upper Extremity 1 Connective Tissue, Lower Extremity 2 Tendons, Upper Extremity 3 Tendons, Lower Extremity	Z None	Z None	Z None

B   Imaging
L   Connective Tissue
4   Ultrasonography   Definition: Real time display of images of anatomy or flow information developed from the capture of relected and attenuated high frequency sound waves

Body Part Character 4	Contrast Character 5	Qualifier Character 6	Qualifier Character 7
Ø Connective Tissue, Upper Extremity 1 Connective Tissue, Lower Extremity 2 Tendons, Upper Extremity 3 Tendons, Lower Extremity	Z None	Z None	Z None

B   Imaging
N   Skull and Facial Bones
Ø   Plain Radiography   Definition: Planar display of an image developed from the capture of external ionizing radiation on photographic or photoconductive plate

Body Part Character 4	Contrast Character 5	Qualifier Character 6	Qualifier Character 7
Ø Skull 1 Orbit, Right 2 Orbit, Left 3 Orbits, Bilateral 4 Nasal Bones 5 Facial Bones 6 Mandible B Zygomatic Arch, Right C Zygomatic Arch, Left D Zygomatic Arches, Bilateral G Tooth, Single H Teeth, Multiple J Teeth, All	Z None	Z None	Z None
7 Temporomandibular Joint, Right 8 Temporomandibular Joint, Left 9 Temporomandibular Joints, Bilateral	Ø High Osmolar 1 Low Osmolar Y Other Contrast Z None	Z None	Z None

B   Imaging
N   Skull and Facial Bones
1   Fluoroscopy   Definition: Single plane or bi-plane real time display of an image developed from the capture of external ionizing radioation on a fluorescent screen. The image may also be stored by either digital or analog means.

Body Part Character 4	Contrast Character 5	Qualifier Character 6	Qualifier Character 7
7 Temporomandibular Joint, Right 8 Temporomandibular Joint, Left 9 Temporomandibular Joints, Bilateral	Ø High Osmolar 1 Low Osmolar Y Other Contrast Z None	Z None	Z None

B   Imaging
N   Skull and Facial Bones
2   Computerized Tomography (CT Scan)   Definition: Computer reformatted digital display of multiplanar images developed from the capture of multiple exposures of external ionizing radiation

Body Part Character 4	Contrast Character 5	Qualifier Character 6	Qualifier Character 7
Ø Skull 3 Orbits, Bilateral 5 Facial Bones 6 Mandible 9 Temporomandibular Joints, Bilateral F Temporal Bones	Ø High Osmolar 1 Low Osmolar Y Other Contrast Z None	Z None	Z None

B   Imaging
N   Skull and Facial Bones
3   Magnetic Resonance Imaging (MRI)   Definition: Computer reformatted digital display of multiplanar images developed from the capture of radio-frequency signals emitted by nuclei in a body site excited within a magnetic field

Body Part Character 4	Contrast Character 5	Qualifier Character 6	Qualifier Character 7
9 Temporomandibular Joints, Bilateral	Y Other Contrast Z None	Z None	Z None

B   Imaging
P   Non-Axial Upper Bones
Ø   Plain Radiography   Definition: Planar display of an image developed from the capture of external ionizing radiation on photographic or photoconductive plate

Body Part Character 4	Contrast Character 5	Qualifier Character 6	Qualifier Character 7
Ø Sternoclavicular Joint, Right 1 Sternoclavicular Joint, Left 2 Sternoclavicular Joints, Bilateral 3 Acromioclavicular Joints, Bilateral 4 Clavicle, Right 5 Clavicle, Left 6 Scapula, Right 7 Scapula, Left A Humerus, Right B Humerus, Left E Upper Arm, Right F Upper Arm, Left J Forearm, Right K Forearm, Left N Hand, Right P Hand, Left R Finger(s), Right S Finger(s), Left X Ribs, Right Y Ribs, Left	Z None	Z None	Z None
8 Shoulder, Right 9 Shoulder, Left C Hand/Finger Joint, Right D Hand/Finger Joint, Left G Elbow, Right H Elbow, Left L Wrist, Right M Wrist, Left	Ø High Osmolar 1 Low Osmolar Y Other Contrast Z None	Z None	Z None

B   Imaging
P   Non-Axial Upper Bones
1   Fluoroscopy   Definition: Single plane or bi-plane real time display of an image developed from the capture of external ionizing radioation on a fluorescent screen. The image may also be stored by either digital or analog means.

Body Part Character 4	Contrast Character 5	Qualifier Character 6	Qualifier Character 7
Ø Sternoclavicular Joint, Right 1 Sternoclavicular Joint, Left 2 Sternoclavicular Joints, Bilateral 3 Acromioclavicular Joints, Bilateral 4 Clavicle, Right 5 Clavicle, Left 6 Scapula, Right 7 Scapula, Left A Humerus, Right B Humerus, Left E Upper Arm, Right F Upper Arm, Left J Forearm, Right K Forearm, Left N Hand, Right P Hand, Left R Finger(s), Right S Finger(s), Left X Ribs, Right Y Ribs, Left	Z None	Z None	Z None
8 Shoulder, Right 9 Shoulder, Left L Wrist, Right M Wrist, Left	Ø High Osmolar 1 Low Osmolar Y Other Contrast Z None	Z None	Z None
C Hand/Finger Joint, Right D Hand/Finger Joint, Left G Elbow, Right H Elbow, Left	Ø High Osmolar 1 Low Osmolar Y Other Contrast	Z None	Z None

B   Imaging
P   Non-Axial Upper Bones
2   Computerized Tomography (CT Scan)   Definition: Computer reformatted digital display of multiplanar images developed from the capture of multiple exposures of external ionizing radiation

Body Part Character 4	Contrast Character 5	Qualifier Character 6	Qualifier Character 7
Ø Sternoclavicular Joint, Right 1 Sternoclavicular Joint, Left W Thorax	Ø High Osmolar 1 Low Osmolar Y Other Contrast	Z None	Z None
2 Sternoclavicular Joints, Bilateral 3 Acromioclavicular Joints, Bilateral 4 Clavicle, Right 5 Clavicle, Left 6 Scapula, Right 7 Scapula, Left 8 Shoulder, Right 9 Shoulder, Left A Humerus, Right B Humerus, Left E Upper Arm, Right F Upper Arm, Left G Elbow, Right H Elbow, Left J Forearm, Right K Forearm, Left L Wrist, Right M Wrist, Left N Hand, Right P Hand, Left Q Hands and Wrists, Bilateral R Finger(s), Right S Finger(s), Left T Upper Extremity, Right U Upper Extremity, Left V Upper Extremities, Bilateral X Ribs, Right Y Ribs, Left	Ø High Osmolar 1 Low Osmolar Y Other Contrast Z None	Z None	Z None
C Hand/Finger Joint, Right D Hand/Finger Joint, Left	Z None	Z None	Z None

LC Limited Coverage   NC Noncovered   ⊞ Combination Member   HAC   Valid OR   Combination Only   DRG Non-OR   New/Revised in GREEN

Imaging

B   Imaging
P   Non-Axial Upper Bones
3   Magnetic Resonance Imaging (MRI)   Definition: Computer reformatted digital display of multiplanar images developed from the capture of radio-frequency signals emitted by nuclei in a body site excited within a magnetic field

Body Part Character 4	Contrast Character 5	Qualifier Character 6	Qualifier Character 7
8 Shoulder, Right 9 Shoulder, Left C Hand/Finger Joint, Right D Hand/Finger Joint, Left E Upper Arm, Right F Upper Arm, Left G Elbow, Right H Elbow, Left J Forearm, Right K Forearm, Left L Wrist, Right M Wrist, Left	Y Other Contrast	Ø Unenhanced and Enhanced Z None	Z None
8 Shoulder, Right 9 Shoulder, Left C Hand/Finger Joint, Right D Hand/Finger Joint, Left E Upper Arm, Right F Upper Arm, Left G Elbow, Right H Elbow, Left J Forearm, Right K Forearm, Left L Wrist, Right M Wrist, Left	Z None	Z None	Z None

B   Imaging
P   Non-Axial Upper Bones
4   Ultrasonography   Definition: Real time display of images of anatomy or flow information developed from the capture of relected and attenuated high frequency sound waves

Body Part Character 4	Contrast Character 5	Qualifier Character 6	Qualifier Character 7
8 Shoulder, Right 9 Shoulder, Left G Elbow, Right H Elbow, Left L Wrist, Right M Wrist, Left N Hand, Right P Hand, Left	Z None	Z None	1 Densitometry Z None

B   Imaging
Q   Non-Axial Lower Bones
Ø   Plain Radiography   Definition: Planar display of an image developed from the capture of external ionizing radiation on photographic or photoconductive plate

Body Part Character 4	Contrast Character 5	Qualifier Character 6	Qualifier Character 7
Ø Hip, Right 1 Hip, Left	Ø High Osmolar 1 Low Osmolar Y Other Contrast	Z None	Z None
Ø Hip, Right 1 Hip, Left	Z None	Z None	1 Densitometry Z None
3 Femur, Right 4 Femur, Left	Z None	Z None	1 Densitometry Z None
7 Knee, Right 8 Knee, Left G Ankle, Right H Ankle, Left	Ø High Osmolar 1 Low Osmolar Y Other Contrast Z None	Z None	Z None
D Lower Leg, Right F Lower Leg, Left J Calcaneus, Right K Calcaneus, Left L Foot, Right M Foot, Left P Toe(s), Right Q Toe(s), Left V Patella, Right W Patella, Left	Z None	Z None	Z None
X Foot/Toe Joint, Right Y Foot/Toe Joint, Left	Ø High Osmolar 1 Low Osmolar Y Other Contrast	Z None	Z None

B   **Imaging**
Q   **Non-Axial Lower Bones**
1   **Fluoroscopy**   Definition: Single plane or bi-plane real time display of an image developed from the capture of external ionizing radioation on a fluorescent screen. The image may also be stored by either digital or analog means.

Body Part Character 4	Contrast Character 5	Qualifier Character 6	Qualifier Character 7
Ø Hip, Right 1 Hip, Left 7 Knee, Right 8 Knee, Left G Ankle, Right H Ankle, Left X Foot/Toe Joint, Right Y Foot/Toe Joint, Left	Ø High Osmolar 1 Low Osmolar Y Other Contrast Z None	Z None	Z None
3 Femur, Right 4 Femur, Left D Lower Leg, Right F Lower Leg, Left J Calcaneus, Right K Calcaneus, Left L Foot, Right M Foot, Left P Toe(s), Right Q Toe(s), Left V Patella, Right W Patella, Left	Z None	Z None	Z None

B   **Imaging**
Q   **Non-Axial Lower Bones**
2   **Computerized Tomography (CT Scan)**   Definition: Computer reformatted digital display of multiplanar images developed from the capture of multiple exposures of external ionizing radiation

Body Part Character 4	Contrast Character 5	Qualifier Character 6	Qualifier Character 7
Ø Hip, Right 1 Hip, Left 3 Femur, Right 4 Femur, Left 7 Knee, Right 8 Knee, Left D Lower Leg, Right F Lower Leg, Left G Ankle, Right H Ankle, Left J Calcaneus, Right K Calcaneus, Left L Foot, Right M Foot, Left P Toe(s), Right Q Toe(s), Left R Lower Extremity, Right S Lower Extremity, Left V Patella, Right W Patella, Left X Foot/Toe Joint, Right Y Foot/Toe Joint, Left	Ø High Osmolar 1 Low Osmolar Y Other Contrast Z None	Z None	Z None
B Tibia/Fibula, Right C Tibia/Fibula, Left	Ø High Osmolar 1 Low Osmolar Y Other Contrast	Z None	Z None

B Imaging
Q Non-Axial Lower Bones
3 Magnetic Resonance Imaging (MRI) Definition: Computer reformatted digital display of multiplanar images developed from the capture of radio-frequency signals emitted by nuclei in a body site excited within a magnetic field

Body Part Character 4	Contrast Character 5	Qualifier Character 6	Qualifier Character 7
Ø Hip, Right 1 Hip, Left 3 Femur, Right 4 Femur, Left 7 Knee, Right 8 Knee, Left D Lower Leg, Right F Lower Leg, Left G Ankle, Right H Ankle, Left J Calcaneus, Right K Calcaneus, Left L Foot, Right M Foot, Left P Toe(s), Right Q Toe(s), Left V Patella, Right W Patella, Left	Y Other Contrast	Ø Unenhanced and Enhanced Z None	Z None
Ø Hip, Right 1 Hip, Left 3 Femur, Right 4 Femur, Left 7 Knee, Right 8 Knee, Left D Lower Leg, Right F Lower Leg, Left G Ankle, Right H Ankle, Left J Calcaneus, Right K Calcaneus, Left L Foot, Right M Foot, Left P Toe(s), Right Q Toe(s), Left V Patella, Right W Patella, Left	Z None	Z None	Z None

B Imaging
Q Non-Axial Lower Bones
4 Ultrasonography Definition: Real time display of images of anatomy or flow information developed from the capture of relected and attenuated high frequency sound waves

Body Part Character 4	Contrast Character 5	Qualifier Character 6	Qualifier Character 7
Ø Hip, Right 1 Hip, Left 2 Hips, Bilateral 7 Knee, Right 8 Knee, Left 9 Knees, Bilateral	Z None	Z None	Z None

B   Imaging
R   Axial Skeleton, Except Skull and Facial Bones
Ø   Plain Radiography   Definition: Planar display of an image developed from the capture of external ionizing radiation on photographic or photoconductive plate

Body Part Character 4	Contrast Character 5	Qualifier Character 6	Qualifier Character 7
Ø Cervical Spine 7 Thoracic Spine 9 Lumbar Spine G Whole Spine	Z None	Z None	1 Densitometry Z None
1 Cervical Disc(s) 2 Thoracic Disc(s) 3 Lumbar Disc(s) 4 Cervical Facet Joint(s) 5 Thoracic Facet Joint(s) 6 Lumbar Facet Joint(s) D Sacroiliac Joints	Ø High Osmolar 1 Low Osmolar Y Other Contrast Z None	Z None	Z None
8 Thoracolumbar Joint B Lumbosacral Joint C Pelvis F Sacrum and Coccyx H Sternum	Z None	Z None	Z None

B   Imaging
R   Axial Skeleton, Except Skull and Facial Bones
1   Fluoroscopy   Definition: Single plane or bi-plane real time display of an image developed from the capture of external ionizing radioation on a fluorescent screen. The image may also be stored by either digital or analog means.

Body Part Character 4	Contrast Character 5	Qualifier Character 6	Qualifier Character 7
Ø Cervical Spine 1 Cervical Disc(s) 2 Thoracic Disc(s) 3 Lumbar Disc(s) 4 Cervical Facet Joint(s) 5 Thoracic Facet Joint(s) 6 Lumbar Facet Joint(s) 7 Thoracic Spine 8 Thoracolumbar Joint 9 Lumbar Spine B Lumbosacral Joint C Pelvis D Sacroiliac Joints F Sacrum and Coccyx G Whole Spine H Sternum	Ø High Osmolar 1 Low Osmolar Y Other Contrast Z None	Z None	Z None

B   Imaging
R   Axial Skeleton, Except Skull and Facial Bones
2   Computerized Tomography (CT Scan)   Definition: Computer reformatted digital display of multiplanar images developed from the capture of multiple exposures of external ionizing radiation

Body Part Character 4	Contrast Character 5	Qualifier Character 6	Qualifier Character 7
Ø Cervical Spine 7 Thoracic Spine 9 Lumbar Spine C Pelvis D Sacroiliac Joints F Sacrum and Coccyx	Ø High Osmolar 1 Low Osmolar Y Other Contrast Z None	Z None	Z None

B   Imaging
R   Axial Skeleton, Except Skull and Facial Bones
3   Magnetic Resonance Imaging (MRI)   Definition: Computer reformatted digital display of multiplanar images developed from the capture of radio-frequency signals emitted by nuclei in a body site excited within a magnetic field

Body Part Character 4	Contrast Character 5	Qualifier Character 6	Qualifier Character 7
Ø Cervical Spine 1 Cervical Disc(s) 2 Thoracic Disc(s) 3 Lumbar Disc(s) 7 Thoracic Spine 9 Lumbar Spine C Pelvis F Sacrum and Coccyx	Y Other Contrast	Ø Unenhanced and Enhanced Z None	Z None
Ø Cervical Spine 1 Cervical Disc(s) 2 Thoracic Disc(s) 3 Lumbar Disc(s) 7 Thoracic Spine 9 Lumbar Spine C Pelvis F Sacrum and Coccyx	Z None	Z None	Z None

B   Imaging
R   Axial Skeleton, Except Skull and Facial Bones
4   Ultrasonography   Definition: Real time display of images of anatomy or flow information developed from the capture of relected and attenuated high frequency sound waves

Body Part Character 4	Contrast Character 5	Qualifier Character 6	Qualifier Character 7
Ø Cervical Spine 7 Thoracic Spine 9 Lumbar Spine F Sacrum and Coccyx	Z None	Z None	Z None

B   Imaging
T   Urinary System
Ø   Plain Radiography   Definition: Planar display of an image developed from the capture of external ionizing radiation on photographic or photoconductive plate

Body Part Character 4	Contrast Character 5	Qualifier Character 6	Qualifier Character 7
Ø Bladder 1 Kidney, Right 2 Kidney, Left 3 Kidneys, Bilateral 4 Kidneys, Ureters and Bladder 5 Urethra 6 Ureter, Right 7 Ureter, Left 8 Ureters, Bilateral B Bladder and Urethra C Ileal Diversion Loop	Ø High Osmolar 1 Low Osmolar Y Other Contrast Z None	Z None	Z None

B   Imaging
T   Urinary System
1   Fluoroscopy   Definition: Single plane or bi-plane real time display of an image developed from the capture of external ionizing radioation on a fluorescent screen. The image may also be stored by either digital or analog means.

Body Part Character 4	Contrast Character 5	Qualifier Character 6	Qualifier Character 7
Ø Bladder 1 Kidney, Right 2 Kidney, Left 3 Kidneys, Bilateral 4 Kidneys, Ureters and Bladder 5 Urethra 6 Ureter, Right 7 Ureter, Left B Bladder and Urethra C Ileal Diversion Loop D Kidney, Ureter and Bladder, Right F Kidney, Ureter and Bladder, Left G Ileal Loop, Ureters and Kidneys	Ø High Osmolar 1 Low Osmolar Y Other Contrast Z None	Z None	Z None

B   Imaging
T   Urinary System
2   Computerized Tomography (CT Scan)   Definition: Computer reformatted digital display of multiplanar images developed from the capture of multiple exposures of external ionizing radiation

Body Part Character 4	Contrast Character 5	Qualifier Character 6	Qualifier Character 7
Ø Bladder 1 Kidney, Right 2 Kidney, Left 3 Kidneys, Bilateral 9 Kidney Transplant	Ø High Osmolar 1 Low Osmolar Y Other Contrast	Ø Unenhanced and Enhanced Z None	Z None
Ø Bladder 1 Kidney, Right 2 Kidney, Left 3 Kidneys, Bilateral 9 Kidney Transplant	Z None	Z None	Z None

B   Imaging
T   Urinary System
3   Magnetic Resonance Imaging (MRI)   Definition: Computer reformatted digital display of multiplanar images developed from the capture of radio-frequency signals emitted by nuclei in a body site excited within a magnetic field

Body Part Character 4	Contrast Character 5	Qualifier Character 6	Qualifier Character 7
Ø Bladder 1 Kidney, Right 2 Kidney, Left 3 Kidneys, Bilateral 9 Kidney Transplant	Y Other Contrast	Ø Unenhanced and Enhanced Z None	Z None
Ø Bladder 1 Kidney, Right 2 Kidney, Left 3 Kidneys, Bilateral 9 Kidney Transplant	Z None	Z None	Z None

B   Imaging
T   Urinary System
4   Ultrasonography   Definition: Real time display of images of anatomy or flow information developed from the capture of relected and attenuated high frequency sound waves

Body Part Character 4	Contrast Character 5	Qualifier Character 6	Qualifier Character 7
Ø Bladder 1 Kidney, Right 2 Kidney, Left 3 Kidneys, Bilateral 5 Urethra 6 Ureter, Right 7 Ureter, Left 8 Ureters, Bilateral 9 Kidney Transplant J Kidneys and Bladder	Z None	Z None	Z None

B   Imaging
U   Female Reproductive System
Ø   Plain Radiography   Definition: Planar display of an image developed from the capture of external ionizing radiation on photographic or photoconductive plate

Body Part Character 4		Contrast Character 5	Qualifier Character 6	Qualifier Character 7
Ø Fallopian Tube, Right 1 Fallopian Tube, Left 2 Fallopian Tubes, Bilateral 6 Uterus 8 Uterus and Fallopian Tubes 9 Vagina	♀ ♀ ♀ ♀ ♀ ♀	Ø High Osmolar 1 Low Osmolar Y Other Contrast	Z None	Z None
♀	All body part, contrast, and qualifier values			

B   Imaging
U   Female Reproductive System
1   Fluoroscopy   Definition: Single plane or bi-plane real time display of an image developed from the capture of external ionizing radioation on a fluorescent screen. The image may also be stored by either digital or analog means.

Body Part Character 4		Contrast Character 5	Qualifier Character 6	Qualifier Character 7
Ø Fallopian Tube, Right	♀	Ø High Osmolar	Z None	Z None
1 Fallopian Tube, Left	♀	1 Low Osmolar		
2 Fallopian Tubes, Bilateral	♀	Y Other Contrast		
6 Uterus	♀	Z None		
8 Uterus and Fallopian Tubes	♀			
9 Vagina	♀			

♀   All body part, contrast, and qualifier values

B   Imaging
U   Female Reproductive System
3   Magnetic Resonance Imaging (MRI)   Definition: Computer reformatted digital display of multiplanar images developed from the capture of radio-frequency signals emitted by nuclei in a body site excited within a magnetic field

Body Part Character 4		Contrast Character 5	Qualifier Character 6	Qualifier Character 7
3 Ovary, Right	♀	Y Other Contrast	Ø Unenhanced and Enhanced	Z None
4 Ovary, Left	♀		Z None	
5 Ovaries, Bilateral	♀			
6 Uterus	♀			
9 Vagina	♀			
B Pregnant Uterus	♀			
C Uterus and Ovaries	♀			
3 Ovary, Right	♀	Z None	Z None	Z None
4 Ovary, Left	♀			
5 Ovaries, Bilateral	♀			
6 Uterus	♀			
9 Vagina	♀			
B Pregnant Uterus	♀			
C Uterus and Ovaries	♀			

♀   All body part, contrast, and qualifier values

B   Imaging
U   Female Reproductive System
4   Ultrasonography   Definition: Real time display of images of anatomy or flow information developed from the capture of relected and attenuated high frequency sound waves

Body Part Character 4		Contrast Character 5	Qualifier Character 6	Qualifier Character 7
Ø Fallopian Tube, Right	♀	Y Other Contrast	Z None	Z None
1 Fallopian Tube, Left	♀	Z None		
2 Fallopian Tubes, Bilateral	♀			
3 Ovary, Right	♀			
4 Ovary, Left	♀			
5 Ovaries, Bilateral	♀			
6 Uterus	♀			
C Uterus and Ovaries	♀			

♀   All body part, contrast, and qualifier values

B   Imaging
V   Male Reproductive System
Ø   Plain Radiography   Definition: Planar display of an image developed from the capture of external ionizing radiation on photographic or photoconductive plate

Body Part Character 4		Contrast Character 5	Qualifier Character 6	Qualifier Character 7
Ø Corpora Cavernosa	♂	Ø High Osmolar	Z None	Z None
1 Epididymis, Right	♂	1 Low Osmolar		
2 Epididymis, Left	♂	Y Other Contrast		
3 Prostate	♂			
5 Testicle, Right	♂			
6 Testicle, Left	♂			
8 Vasa Vasorum	♂			

♂   All body part, contrast, and qualifier values

B **Imaging**
V **Male Reproductive System**
1 **Fluoroscopy** Definition: Single plane or bi-plane real time display of an image developed from the capture of external ionizing radiation on a fluorescent screen. The image may also be stored by either digital or analog means.

Body Part Character 4	Contrast Character 5	Qualifier Character 6	Qualifier Character 7
0 Corpora Cavernosa ♂ 8 Vasa Vasorum ♂	0 High Osmolar 1 Low Osmolar Y Other Contrast Z None	Z None	Z None

♂ All body part, contrast, and qualifier values

B **Imaging**
V **Male Reproductive System**
2 **Computerized Tomography (CT Scan)** Definition: Computer reformatted digital display of multiplanar images developed from the capture of multiple exposures of external ionizing radiation

Body Part Character 4	Contrast Character 5	Qualifier Character 6	Qualifier Character 7
3 Prostate ♂	0 High Osmolar 1 Low Osmolar Y Other Contrast	0 Unenhanced and Enhanced Z None	Z None
3 Prostate ♂	Z None	Z None	Z None

♂ BV23[0,Y][0,Z]Z   ♂ BV23ZZZ
♂ BV2310Z

B **Imaging**
V **Male Reproductive System**
3 **Magnetic Resonance Imaging (MRI)** Definition: Computer reformatted digital display of multiplanar images developed from the capture of radio-frequency signals emitted by nuclei in a body site excited within a magnetic field

Body Part Character 4	Contrast Character 5	Qualifier Character 6	Qualifier Character 7
0 Corpora Cavernosa ♂ 3 Prostate ♂ 4 Scrotum ♂ 5 Testicle, Right ♂ 6 Testicle, Left ♂ 7 Testicles, Bilateral ♂	Y Other Contrast	0 Unenhanced and Enhanced Z None	Z None
0 Corpora Cavernosa ♂ 3 Prostate ♂ 4 Scrotum ♂ 5 Testicle, Right ♂ 6 Testicle, Left ♂ 7 Testicles, Bilateral ♂	Z None	Z None	Z None

♂ All body part, contrast, and qualifier values

B **Imaging**
V **Male Reproductive System**
4 **Ultrasonography** Definition: Real time display of images of anatomy or flow information developed from the capture of reflected and attenuated high frequency sound waves

Body Part Character 4	Contrast Character 5	Qualifier Character 6	Qualifier Character 7
4 Scrotum ♂ 9 Prostate and Seminal Vesicles ♂ B Penis ♂	Z None	Z None	Z None

♂ All body part, contrast, and qualifier values

B **Imaging**
W **Anatomical Regions**
0 **Plain Radiography** Definition: Planar display of an image developed from the capture of external ionizing radiation on photographic or photoconductive plate

Body Part Character 4	Contrast Character 5	Qualifier Character 6	Qualifier Character 7
0 Abdomen 1 Abdomen and Pelvis 3 Chest B Long Bones, All C Lower Extremity J Upper Extremity K Whole Body L Whole Skeleton M Whole Body, Infant	Z None	Z None	Z None

B　Imaging
W　Anatomical Regions
1　Fluoroscopy　Definition: Single plane or bi-plane real time display of an image developed from the capture of external ionizing radioation on a fluorescent screen. The image may also be stored by either digital or analog means.

Body Part Character 4	Contrast Character 5	Qualifier Character 6	Qualifier Character 7
1 Abdomen and Pelvis 9 Head and Neck C Lower Extremity J Upper Extremity	Ø High Osmolar 1 Low Osmolar Y Other Contrast Z None	Z None	Z None

B　Imaging
W　Anatomical Regions
2　Computerized Tomography (CT Scan)　Definition: Computer reformatted digital display of multiplanar images developed from the capture of multiple exposures of external ionizing radiation

Body Part Character 4	Contrast Character 5	Qualifier Character 6	Qualifier Character 7
Ø Abdomen 1 Abdomen and Pelvis 4 Chest and Abdomen 5 Chest, Abdomen and Pelvis 8 Head 9 Head and Neck F Neck G Pelvic Region	Ø High Osmolar 1 Low Osmolar Y Other Contrast	Ø Unenhanced and Enhanced Z None	Z None
Ø Abdomen 1 Abdomen and Pelvis 4 Chest and Abdomen 5 Chest, Abdomen and Pelvis 8 Head 9 Head and Neck F Neck G Pelvic Region	Z None	Z None	Z None

B　Imaging
W　Anatomical Regions
3　Magnetic Resonance Imaging (MRI)　Definition: Computer reformatted digital display of multiplanar images developed from the capture of radio-frequency signals emitted by nuclei in a body site excited within a magnetic field

Body Part Character 4	Contrast Character 5	Qualifier Character 6	Qualifier Character 7
Ø Abdomen 8 Head F Neck G Pelvic Region H Retroperitoneum P Brachial Plexus	Y Other Contrast	Ø Unenhanced and Enhanced Z None	Z None
Ø Abdomen 8 Head F Neck G Pelvic Region H Retroperitoneum P Brachial Plexus	Z None	Z None	Z None
3 Chest	Y Other Contrast	Ø Unenhanced and Enhanced Z None	Z None

B　Imaging
W　Anatomical Regions
4　Ultrasonography　Definition: Real time display of images of anatomy or flow information developed from the capture of relected and attenuated high frequency sound waves

Body Part Character 4	Contrast Character 5	Qualifier Character 6	Qualifier Character 7
Ø Abdomen 1 Abdomen and Pelvis F Neck G Pelvic Region	Z None	Z None	Z None

B   **Imaging**
Y   **Fetus and Obstetrical**
3   **Magnetic Resonance Imaging (MRI)**   Definition: Computer reformatted digital display of multiplanar images developed from the capture of radio-frequency signals emitted by nuclei in a body site excited within a magnetic field

Body Part Character 4		Contrast Character 5	Qualifier Character 6	Qualifier Character 7
Ø Fetal Head	♀	**Y** Other Contrast	**Ø** Unenhanced and Enhanced	**Z** None
1 Fetal Heart	♀		**Z** None	
2 Fetal Thorax	♀			
3 Fetal Abdomen	♀			
4 Fetal Spine	♀			
5 Fetal Extremities	♀			
6 Whole Fetus	♀			
Ø Fetal Head	♀	**Z** None	**Z** None	**Z** None
1 Fetal Heart	♀			
2 Fetal Thorax	♀			
3 Fetal Abdomen	♀			
4 Fetal Spine	♀			
5 Fetal Extremities	♀			
6 Whole Fetus	♀			

   ♀ BY3[Ø,1,2,3,5,6]Y[Ø,Z]Z
   ♀ BY34YZZ
   ♀ BY3[Ø,1,2,3,4,5,6]ZZZ

B   **Imaging**
Y   **Fetus and Obstetrical**
4   **Ultrasonography**   Definition: Real time display of images of anatomy or flow information developed from the capture of relected and attenuated high frequency sound waves

Body Part Character 4		Contrast Character 5	Qualifier Character 6	Qualifier Character 7
7 Fetal Umbilical Cord	♀	**Z** None	**Z** None	**Z** None
8 Placenta	♀			
9 First Trimester, Single Fetus	♀			
B First Trimester, Multiple Gestation	♀			
C Second Trimester, Single Fetus	♀			
D Second Trimester, Multiple Gestation	♀			
F Third Trimester, Single Fetus	♀			
G Third Trimester, Multiple Gestation	♀			

   ♀   All body part, contrast, and qualifier values

LC Limited Coverage   **NC** Noncovered   ⊞ Combination Member   HAC   Valid OR   Combination Only   DRG Non-OR   New/Revised in GREEN

ICD-10-PCS 2020   751

BY3–BY4

Nuclear Medicine CØ1–CW7

C Nuclear Medicine
Ø Central Nervous System
1 Planar Nuclear Medicine Imaging   Definition: Introduction of radioactive materials into the body for single plane display of images developed from the capture of radioactive emissions

Body Part Character 4	Radionuclide Character 5	Qualifier Character 6	Qualifier Character 7
Ø Brain	1 Technetium 99m (Tc-99m) Y Other Radionuclide	Z None	Z None
5 Cerebrospinal Fluid	D Indium 111 (In-111) Y Other Radionuclide	Z None	Z None
Y Central Nervous System	Y Other Radionuclide	Z None	Z None

C Nuclear Medicine
Ø Central Nervous System
2 Tomographic (Tomo) Nuclear Medicine Imaging   Definition: Introduction of radioactive materials into the body for three dimensional display of images developed from the capture of radioactive emissions

Body Part Character 4	Radionuclide Character 5	Qualifier Character 6	Qualifier Character 7
Ø Brain	1 Technetium 99m (Tc-99m) F Iodine 123 (I-123) S Thallium 201 (Tl-201) Y Other Radionuclide	Z None	Z None
5 Cerebrospinal Fluid	D Indium 111 (In-111) Y Other Radionuclide	Z None	Z None
Y Central Nervous System	Y Other Radionuclide	Z None	Z None

C Nuclear Medicine
Ø Central Nervous System
3 Positron Emission Tomographic (PET) Imaging   Definition: Introduction of radioactive materials into the body for three dimensional display of images developed from the simultaneous capture, 180 degrees apart, of radioactive emissions

Body Part Character 4	Radionuclide Character 5	Qualifier Character 6	Qualifier Character 7
Ø Brain	B Carbon 11 (C-11) K Fluorine 18 (F-18) M Oxygen 15 (O-15) Y Other Radionuclide	Z None	Z None
Y Central Nervous System	Y Other Radionuclide	Z None	Z None

C Nuclear Medicine
Ø Central Nervous System
5 Nonimaging Nuclear Medicine Probe   Definition: Introduction of radioactive materials into the body for the study of distribution and fate of certain substances by the detection of radioactive emissions; or, alternatively, measurement of absorption of radioactive emissions from an external source

Body Part Character 4	Radionuclide Character 5	Qualifier Character 6	Qualifier Character 7
Ø Brain	V Xenon 133 (Xe-133) Y Other Radionuclide	Z None	Z None
Y Central Nervous System	Y Other Radionuclide	Z None	Z None

C Nuclear Medicine
2 Heart
1 Planar Nuclear Medicine Imaging   Definition: Introduction of radioactive materials into the body for single plane display of images developed from the capture of radioactive emissions

Body Part Character 4	Radionuclide Character 5	Qualifier Character 6	Qualifier Character 7
6 Heart, Right and Left	1 Technetium 99m (Tc-99m) Y Other Radionuclide	Z None	Z None
G Myocardium	1 Technetium 99m (Tc-99m) D Indium 111 (In-111) S Thallium 201 (Tl-201) Y Other Radionuclide Z None	Z None	Z None
Y Heart	Y Other Radionuclide	Z None	Z None

C   **Nuclear Medicine**
2   **Heart**
2   **Tomographic (Tomo) Nuclear Medicine Imaging**   Definition: Introduction of radioactive materials into the body for three dimensional display of images developed from the capture of radioactive emissions

Body Part Character 4	Radionuclide Character 5	Qualifier Character 6	Qualifier Character 7
6 Heart, Right and Left	**1** Technetium 99m (Tc-99m) **Y** Other Radionuclide	**Z** None	**Z** None
G Myocardium	**1** Technetium 99m (Tc-99m) **D** Indium 111 (In-111) **K** Fluorine 18 (F-18) **S** Thallium 201 (Tl-201) **Y** Other Radionuclide **Z** None	**Z** None	**Z** None
Y Heart	**Y** Other Radionuclide	**Z** None	**Z** None

C   **Nuclear Medicine**
2   **Heart**
3   **Positron Emission Tomographic (PET) Imaging**   Definition: Introduction of radioactive materials into the body for three dimensional display of images developed from the simultaneous capture, 180 degrees apart, of radioactive emissions

Body Part Character 4	Radionuclide Character 5	Qualifier Character 6	Qualifier Character 7
G Myocardium	**K** Fluorine 18 (F-18) **M** Oxygen 15 (O-15) **Q** Rubidium 82 (Rb-82) **R** Nitrogen 13 (N-13) **Y** Other Radionuclide	**Z** None	**Z** None
Y Heart	**Y** Other Radionuclide	**Z** None	**Z** None

C   **Nuclear Medicine**
2   **Heart**
5   **Nonimaging Nuclear Medicine Probe**   Definition: Introduction of radioactive materials into the body for the study of distribution and fate of certain substances by the detection of radioactive emissions; or, alternatively, measurement of absorption of radioactive emissions from an external source

Body Part Character 4	Radionuclide Character 5	Qualifier Character 6	Qualifier Character 7
6 Heart, Right and Left	**1** Technetium 99m (Tc-99m) **Y** Other Radionuclide	**Z** None	**Z** None
Y Heart	**Y** Other Radionuclide	**Z** None	**Z** None

C   **Nuclear Medicine**
5   **Veins**
1   **Planar Nuclear Medicine Imaging**   Definition: Introduction of radioactive materials into the body for single plane display of images developed from the capture of radioactive emissions

Body Part Character 4	Radionuclide Character 5	Qualifier Character 6	Qualifier Character 7
B Lower Extremity Veins, Right **C** Lower Extremity Veins, Left **D** Lower Extremity Veins, Bilateral **N** Upper Extremity Veins, Right **P** Upper Extremity Veins, Left **Q** Upper Extremity Veins, Bilateral **R** Central Veins	**1** Technetium 99m (Tc-99m) **Y** Other Radionuclide	**Z** None	**Z** None
Y Veins	**Y** Other Radionuclide	**Z** None	**Z** None

C   **Nuclear Medicine**
7   **Lymphatic and Hematologic System**
1   **Planar Nuclear Medicine Imaging**   Definition: Introduction of radioactive materials into the body for single plane display of images developed from the capture of radioactive emissions

Body Part Character 4	Radionuclide Character 5	Qualifier Character 6	Qualifier Character 7
Ø Bone Marrow	1 Technetium 99m (Tc-99m) D Indium 111 (In-111) Y Other Radionuclide	Z None	Z None
2 Spleen 5 Lymphatics, Head and Neck D Lymphatics, Pelvic J Lymphatics, Head K Lymphatics, Neck L Lymphatics, Upper Chest M Lymphatics, Trunk N Lymphatics, Upper Extremity P Lymphatics, Lower Extremity	1 Technetium 99m (Tc-99m) Y Other Radionuclide	Z None	Z None
3 Blood	D Indium 111 (In-111) Y Other Radionuclide	Z None	Z None
Y Lymphatic and Hematologic System	Y Other Radionuclide	Z None	Z None

C   **Nuclear Medicine**
7   **Lymphatic and Hematologic System**
2   **Tomographic (Tomo) Nuclear Medicine Imaging**   Definition: Introduction of radioactive materials into the body for three dimensional display of images developed from the capture of radioactive emissions

Body Part Character 4	Radionuclide Character 5	Qualifier Character 6	Qualifier Character 7
2 Spleen	1 Technetium 99m (Tc-99m) Y Other Radionuclide	Z None	Z None
Y Lymphatic and Hematologic System	Y Other Radionuclide	Z None	Z None

C   **Nuclear Medicine**
7   **Lymphatic and Hematologic System**
5   **Nonimaging Nuclear Medicine Probe**   Definition: Introduction of radioactive materials into the body for the study of distribution and fate of certain substances by the detection of radioactive emissions; or, alternatively, measurement of absorption of radioactive emissions from an external source

Body Part Character 4	Radionuclide Character 5	Qualifier Character 6	Qualifier Character 7
5 Lymphatics, Head and Neck D Lymphatics, Pelvic J Lymphatics, Head K Lymphatics, Neck L Lymphatics, Upper Chest M Lymphatics, Trunk N Lymphatics, Upper Extremity P Lymphatics, Lower Extremity	1 Technetium 99m (Tc-99m) Y Other Radionuclide	Z None	Z None
Y Lymphatic and Hematologic System	Y Other Radionuclide	Z None	Z None

C   **Nuclear Medicine**
7   **Lymphatic and Hematologic System**
6   **Nonimaging Nuclear Medicine Assay**   Definition: Introduction of radioactive materials into the body for the study of body fluids and blood elements, by the detection of radioactive emissions

Body Part Character 4	Radionuclide Character 5	Qualifier Character 6	Qualifier Character 7
3 Blood	1 Technetium 99m (Tc-99m) 7 Cobalt 58 (Co-58) C Cobalt 57 (Co-57) D Indium 111 (In-111) H Iodine 125 (I-125) W Chromium (Cr-51) Y Other Radionuclide	Z None	Z None
Y Lymphatic and Hematologic System	Y Other Radionuclide	Z None	Z None

C **Nuclear Medicine**
8 **Eye**
1 **Planar Nuclear Medicine Imaging** Definition: Introduction of radioactive materials into the body for single plane display of images developed from the capture of radioactive emissions

Body Part Character 4	Radionuclide Character 5	Qualifier Character 6	Qualifier Character 7
9 Lacrimal Ducts, Bilateral	1 Technetium 99m (Tc-99m) Y Other Radionuclide	Z None	Z None
Y Eye	Y Other Radionuclide	Z None	Z None

C **Nuclear Medicine**
9 **Ear, Nose, Mouth and Throat**
1 **Planar Nuclear Medicine Imaging** Definition: Introduction of radioactive materials into the body for single plane display of images developed from the capture of radioactive emissions

Body Part Character 4	Radionuclide Character 5	Qualifier Character 6	Qualifier Character 7
B Salivary Glands, Bilateral	1 Technetium 99m (Tc-99m) Y Other Radionuclide	Z None	Z None
Y Ear, Nose, Mouth and Throat	Y Other Radionuclide	Z None	Z None

C **Nuclear Medicine**
B **Respiratory System**
1 **Planar Nuclear Medicine Imaging** Definition: Introduction of radioactive materials into the body for single plane display of images developed from the capture of radioactive emissions

Body Part Character 4	Radionuclide Character 5	Qualifier Character 6	Qualifier Character 7
2 Lungs and Bronchi	1 Technetium 99m (Tc-99m) 9 Krypton (Kr-81m) T Xenon 127 (Xe-127) V Xenon 133 (Xe-133) Y Other Radionuclide	Z None	Z None
Y Respiratory System	Y Other Radionuclide	Z None	Z None

C **Nuclear Medicine**
B **Respiratory System**
2 **Tomographic (Tomo) Nuclear Medicine Imaging** Definition: Introduction of radioactive materials into the body for three dimensional display of images developed from the capture of radioactive emissions

Body Part Character 4	Radionuclide Character 5	Qualifier Character 6	Qualifier Character 7
2 Lungs and Bronchi	1 Technetium 99m (Tc-99m) 9 Krypton (Kr-81m) Y Other Radionuclide	Z None	Z None
Y Respiratory System	Y Other Radionuclide	Z None	Z None

C **Nuclear Medicine**
B **Respiratory System**
3 **Positron Emission Tomographic (PET) Imaging** Definition: Introduction of radioactive materials into the body for three dimensional display of images developed from the simultaneous capture, 180 degrees apart, of radioactive emissions

Body Part Character 4	Radionuclide Character 5	Qualifier Character 6	Qualifier Character 7
2 Lungs and Bronchi	K Fluorine 18 (F-18) Y Other Radionuclide	Z None	Z None
Y Respiratory System	Y Other Radionuclide	Z None	Z None

C **Nuclear Medicine**
D **Gastrointestinal System**
1 **Planar Nuclear Medicine Imaging** Definition: Introduction of radioactive materials into the body for single plane display of images developed from the capture of radioactive emissions

Body Part Character 4	Radionuclide Character 5	Qualifier Character 6	Qualifier Character 7
5 Upper Gastrointestinal Tract 7 Gastrointestinal Tract	1 Technetium 99m (Tc-99m) D Indium 111 (In-111) Y Other Radionuclide	Z None	Z None
Y Digestive System	Y Other Radionuclide	Z None	Z None

C   Nuclear Medicine
D   Gastrointestinal System
2   Tomographic (Tomo) Nuclear Medicine Imaging   Definition: Introduction of radioactive materials into the body for three dimensional display of images developed from the capture of radioactive emissions

Body Part Character 4	Radionuclide Character 5	Qualifier Character 6	Qualifier Character 7
7 Gastrointestinal Tract	**1** Technetium 99m (Tc-99m) **D** Indium 111 (In-111) **Y** Other Radionuclide	**Z** None	**Z** None
Y Digestive System	**Y** Other Radionuclide	**Z** None	**Z** None

C   Nuclear Medicine
F   Hepatobiliary System and Pancreas
1   Planar Nuclear Medicine Imaging   Definition: Introduction of radioactive materials into the body for single plane display of images developed from the capture of radioactive emissions

Body Part Character 4	Radionuclide Character 5	Qualifier Character 6	Qualifier Character 7
4 Gallbladder **5** Liver **6** Liver and Spleen **C** Hepatobiliary System, All	**1** Technetium 99m (Tc-99m) **Y** Other Radionuclide	**Z** None	**Z** None
Y Hepatobiliary System and Pancreas	**Y** Other Radionuclide	**Z** None	**Z** None

C   Nuclear Medicine
F   Hepatobiliary System and Pancreas
2   Tomographic (Tomo) Nuclear Medicine Imaging   Definition: Introduction of radioactive materials into the body for three dimensional display of images developed from the capture of radioactive emissions

Body Part Character 4	Radionuclide Character 5	Qualifier Character 6	Qualifier Character 7
4 Gallbladder **5** Liver **6** Liver and Spleen	**1** Technetium 99m (Tc-99m) **Y** Other Radionuclide	**Z** None	**Z** None
Y Hepatobiliary System and Pancreas	**Y** Other Radionuclide	**Z** None	**Z** None

C   Nuclear Medicine
G   Endocrine System
1   Planar Nuclear Medicine Imaging   Definition: Introduction of radioactive materials into the body for single plane display of images developed from the capture of radioactive emissions

Body Part Character 4	Radionuclide Character 5	Qualifier Character 6	Qualifier Character 7
1 Parathyroid Glands	**1** Technetium 99m (Tc-99m) **S** Thallium 201 (Tl-201) **Y** Other Radionuclide	**Z** None	**Z** None
2 Thyroid Gland	**1** Technetium 99m (Tc-99m) **F** Iodine 123 (I-123) **G** Iodine 131 (I-131) **Y** Other Radionuclide	**Z** None	**Z** None
4 Adrenal Glands, Bilateral	**G** Iodine 131 (I-131) **Y** Other Radionuclide	**Z** None	**Z** None
Y Endocrine System	**Y** Other Radionuclide	**Z** None	**Z** None

C   Nuclear Medicine
G   Endocrine System
2   Tomographic (Tomo) Nuclear Medicine Imaging   Definition: Introduction of radioactive materials into the body for three dimensional display of images developed from the capture of radioactive emissions

Body Part Character 4	Radionuclide Character 5	Qualifier Character 6	Qualifier Character 7
1 Parathyroid Glands	**1** Technetium 99m (Tc-99m) **S** Thallium 201 (Tl-201) **Y** Other Radionuclide	**Z** None	**Z** None
Y Endocrine System	**Y** Other Radionuclide	**Z** None	**Z** None

C Nuclear Medicine
G Endocrine System
4 Nonimaging Nuclear Medicine Uptake　　Definition: Introduction of radioactive materials into the body for measurements of organ function, from the detection of radioactive emmissions

Body Part Character 4	Radionuclide Character 5	Qualifier Character 6	Qualifier Character 7
2 Thyroid Gland	**1** Technetium 99m (Tc-99m) **F** Iodine 123 (I-123) **G** Iodine 131 (I-131) **Y** Other Radionuclide	**Z** None	**Z** None
Y Endocrine System	**Y** Other Radionuclide	**Z** None	**Z** None

C Nuclear Medicine
H Skin, Subcutaneous Tissue and Breast
1 Planar Nuclear Medicine Imaging　　Definition: Introduction of radioactive materials into the body for single plane display of images developed from the capture of radioactive emissions

Body Part Character 4	Radionuclide Character 5	Qualifier Character 6	Qualifier Character 7
Ø Breast, Right **1** Breast, Left **2** Breasts, Bilateral	**1** Technetium 99m (Tc-99m) **S** Thallium 201 (Tl-201) **Y** Other Radionuclide	**Z** None	**Z** None
Y Skin, Subcutaneous Tissue and Breast	**Y** Other Radionuclide	**Z** None	**Z** None

C Nuclear Medicine
H Skin, Subcutaneous Tissue and Breast
2 Tomographic (Tomo) Nuclear Medicine Imaging　　Definition: Introduction of radioactive materials into the body for three dimensional display of images developed from the capture of radioactive emissions

Body Part Character 4	Radionuclide Character 5	Qualifier Character 6	Qualifier Character 7
Ø Breast, Right **1** Breast, Left **2** Breasts, Bilateral	**1** Technetium 99m (Tc-99m) **S** Thallium 201 (Tl-201) **Y** Other Radionuclide	**Z** None	**Z** None
Y Skin, Subcutaneous Tissue and Breast	**Y** Other Radionuclide	**Z** None	**Z** None

C Nuclear Medicine
P Musculoskeletal System
1 Planar Nuclear Medicine Imaging　　Definition: Introduction of radioactive materials into the body for single plane display of images developed from the capture of radioactive emissions

Body Part Character 4	Radionuclide Character 5	Qualifier Character 6	Qualifier Character 7
1 Skull **4** Thorax **5** Spine **6** Pelvis **7** Spine and Pelvis **8** Upper Extremity, Right **9** Upper Extremity, Left **B** Upper Extremities, Bilateral **C** Lower Extremity, Right **D** Lower Extremity, Left **F** Lower Extremities, Bilateral **Z** Musculoskeletal System, All	**1** Technetium 99m (Tc-99m) **Y** Other Radionuclide	**Z** None	**Z** None
Y Musculoskeletal System, Other	**Y** Other Radionuclide	**Z** None	**Z** None

C   **Nuclear Medicine**
P   **Musculoskeletal System**
2   **Tomographic (Tomo) Nuclear Medicine Imaging**   Definition: Introduction of radioactive materials into the body for three dimensional display of images developed from the capture of radioactive emissions

Body Part Character 4	Radionuclide Character 5	Qualifier Character 6	Qualifier Character 7
1 Skull **2** Cervical Spine **3** Skull and Cervical Spine **4** Thorax **6** Pelvis **7** Spine and Pelvis **8** Upper Extremity, Right **9** Upper Extremity, Left **B** Upper Extremities, Bilateral **C** Lower Extremity, Right **D** Lower Extremity, Left **F** Lower Extremities, Bilateral **G** Thoracic Spine **H** Lumbar Spine **J** Thoracolumbar Spine	**1** Technetium 99m (Tc-99m) **Y** Other Radionuclide	**Z** None	**Z** None
Y Musculoskeletal System, Other	**Y** Other Radionuclide	**Z** None	**Z** None

C   **Nuclear Medicine**
P   **Musculoskeletal System**
5   **Nonimaging Nuclear Medicine Probe**   Definition: Introduction of radioactive materials into the body for the study of distribution and fate of certain substances by the detection of radioactive emissions; or, alternatively, measurement of absorption of radioactive emissions from an external source

Body Part Character 4	Radionuclide Character 5	Qualifier Character 6	Qualifier Character 7
5 Spine **N** Upper Extremities **P** Lower Extremities	**Z** None	**Z** None	**Z** None
Y Musculoskeletal System, Other	**Y** Other Radionuclide	**Z** None	**Z** None

C   **Nuclear Medicine**
T   **Urinary System**
1   **Planar Nuclear Medicine Imaging**   Definition: Introduction of radioactive materials into the body for single plane display of images developed from the capture of radioactive emissions

Body Part Character 4	Radionuclide Character 5	Qualifier Character 6	Qualifier Character 7
3 Kidneys, Ureters and Bladder	**1** Technetium 99m (Tc-99m) **F** Iodine 123 (I-123) **G** Iodine 131 (I-131) **Y** Other Radionuclide	**Z** None	**Z** None
H Bladder and Ureters	**1** Technetium 99m (Tc-99m) **Y** Other Radionuclide	**Z** None	**Z** None
Y Urinary System	**Y** Other Radionuclide	**Z** None	**Z** None

C   **Nuclear Medicine**
T   **Urinary System**
2   **Tomographic (Tomo) Nuclear Medicine Imaging**   Definition: Introduction of radioactive materials into the body for three dimensional display of images developed from the capture of radioactive emissions

Body Part Character 4	Radionuclide Character 5	Qualifier Character 6	Qualifier Character 7
3 Kidneys, Ureters and Bladder	**1** Technetium 99m (Tc-99m) **Y** Other Radionuclide	**Z** None	**Z** None
Y Urinary System	**Y** Other Radionuclide	**Z** None	**Z** None

C   **Nuclear Medicine**
T   **Urinary System**
6   **Nonimaging Nuclear Medicine Assay**   Definition: Introduction of radioactive materials into the body for the study of body fluids and blood elements, by the detection of radioactive emissions

Body Part Character 4	Radionuclide Character 5	Qualifier Character 6	Qualifier Character 7
3 Kidneys, Ureters and Bladder	**1** Technetium 99m (Tc-99m) **F** Iodine 123 (I-123) **G** Iodine 131 (I-131) **H** Iodine 125 (I-125) **Y** Other Radionuclide	**Z** None	**Z** None
Y Urinary System	**Y** Other Radionuclide	**Z** None	**Z** None

Nuclear Medicine

C   Nuclear Medicine
V   Male Reproductive System
1   Planar Nuclear Medicine Imaging   Definition: Introduction of radioactive materials into the body for single plane display of images developed from the capture of radioactive emissions

Body Part Character 4	Radionuclide Character 5	Qualifier Character 6	Qualifier Character 7
9 Testicles, Bilateral ♂	1 Technetium 99m (Tc-99m) Y Other Radionuclide	Z None	Z None
Y Male Reproductive System ♂	Y Other Radionuclide	Z None	Z None

♂   All body part, radionuclide, and qualifier values

C   Nuclear Medicine
W   Anatomical Regions
1   Planar Nuclear Medicine Imaging   Definition: Introduction of radioactive materials into the body for single plane display of images developed from the capture of radioactive emissions

Body Part Character 4	Radionuclide Character 5	Qualifier Character 6	Qualifier Character 7
Ø Abdomen 1 Abdomen and Pelvis 4 Chest and Abdomen 6 Chest and Neck B Head and Neck D Lower Extremity J Pelvic Region M Upper Extremity N Whole Body	1 Technetium 99m (Tc-99m) D Indium 111 (In-111) F Iodine 123 (I-123) G Iodine 131 (I-131) L Gallium 67 (Ga-67) S Thallium 201 (Tl-201) Y Other Radionuclide	Z None	Z None
3 Chest	1 Technetium 99m (Tc-99m) D Indium 111 (In-111) F Iodine 123 (I-123) G Iodine 131 (I-131) K Fluorine 18 (F-18) L Gallium 67 (Ga-67) S Thallium 201 (Tl-201) Y Other Radionuclide	Z None	Z None
Y Anatomical Regions, Multiple	Y Other Radionuclide	Z None	Z None
Z Anatomical Region, Other	Z None	Z None	Z None

C   Nuclear Medicine
W   Anatomical Regions
2   Tomographic (Tomo) Nuclear Medicine Imaging   Definition: Introduction of radioactive materials into the body for three dimensional display of images developed from the capture of radioactive emissions

Body Part Character 4	Radionuclide Character 5	Qualifier Character 6	Qualifier Character 7
Ø Abdomen 1 Abdomen and Pelvis 3 Chest 4 Chest and Abdomen 6 Chest and Neck B Head and Neck D Lower Extremity J Pelvic Region M Upper Extremity	1 Technetium 99m (Tc-99m) D Indium 111 (In-111) F Iodine 123 (I-123) G Iodine 131 (I-131) K Fluorine 18 (F-18) L Gallium 67 (Ga-67) S Thallium 201 (Tl-201) Y Other Radionuclide	Z None	Z None
Y Anatomical Regions, Multiple	Y Other Radionuclide	Z None	Z None

C   Nuclear Medicine
W   Anatomical Regions
3   Positron Emission Tomographic (PET) Imaging   Definition: Introduction of radioactive materials into the body for three dimensional display of images developed from the simultaneous capture, 180 degrees apart, of radioactive emissions

Body Part Character 4	Radionuclide Character 5	Qualifier Character 6	Qualifier Character 7
N Whole Body	Y Other Radionuclide	Z None	Z None

C   **Nuclear Medicine**
W   **Anatomical Regions**
5   **Nonimaging Nuclear Medicine Probe**   Definition: Introduction of radioactive materials into the body for the study of distribution and fate of certain substances by the detection of radioactive emissions; or, alternatively, measurement of absorption of radioactive emissions from an external source

Body Part Character 4	Radionuclide Character 5	Qualifier Character 6	Qualifier Character 7
0 Abdomen **1** Abdomen and Pelvis **3** Chest **4** Chest and Abdomen **6** Chest and Neck **B** Head and Neck **D** Lower Extremity **J** Pelvic Region **M** Upper Extremity	**1** Technetium 99m (Tc-99m) **D** Indium 111 (In-111) **Y** Other Radionuclide	**Z** None	**Z** None

C   **Nuclear Medicine**
W   **Anatomical Regions**
7   **Systemic Nuclear Medicine Therapy**   Definition: Introduction of unsealed radioactive materials into the body for treatment

Body Part Character 4	Radionuclide Character 5	Qualifier Character 6	Qualifier Character 7
0 Abdomen **3** Chest	**N** Phosphorus 32 (P-32) **Y** Other Radionuclide	**Z** None	**Z** None
G Thyroid	**G** Iodine 131 (I-131) **Y** Other Radionuclide	**Z** None	**Z** None
N Whole Body	**8** Samarium 153 (Sm-153) **G** Iodine 131 (I-131) **N** Phosphorus 32 (P-32) **P** Strontium 89 (Sr-89) **Y** Other Radionuclide	**Z** None	**Z** None
Y Anatomical Regions, Multiple	**Y** Other Radionuclide	**Z** None	**Z** None

LC Limited Coverage   **NC** Noncovered   ⊞ Combination Member   HAC   Valid OR   Combination Only   DRG Non-OR   New/Revised in GREEN

ICD-10-PCS 2020   **761**

Radiation Therapy D00–DWY

AHA Coding Clinic for table DU1

2017, 4Q, 104   Intrauterine brachytherapy & placement of tandems & ovoids

D   **Radiation Therapy**
0   **Central and Peripheral Nervous System**
0   **Beam Radiation**

Treatment Site Character 4	Modality Qualifier Character 5	Isotope Character 6	Qualifier Character 7
0 Brain 1 Brain Stem 6 Spinal Cord 7 Peripheral Nerve	0 Photons <1 MeV 1 Photons 1- 10 MeV 2 Photons >10 MeV 4 Heavy Particles (Protons, Ions) 5 Neutrons 6 Neutron Capture	Z None	Z None
0 Brain 1 Brain Stem 6 Spinal Cord 7 Peripheral Nerve	3 Electrons	Z None	0 Intraoperative Z None

D   **Radiation Therapy**
0   **Central and Peripheral Nervous System**
1   **Brachytherapy**

Treatment Site Character 4	Modality Qualifier Character 5	Isotope Character 6	Qualifier Character 7
0 Brain 1 Brain Stem 6 Spinal Cord 7 Peripheral Nerve	9 High Dose Rate (HDR)	7 Cesium 137 (Cs-137) 8 Iridium 192 (Ir-192) 9 Iodine 125 (I-125) B Palladium 103 (Pd-103) C Californium 252 (Cf-252) Y Other Isotope	Z None
0 Brain 1 Brain Stem 6 Spinal Cord 7 Peripheral Nerve	B Low Dose Rate (LDR)	7 Cesium 137 (Cs-137) 8 Iridium 192 (Ir-192) 9 Iodine 125 (I-125) C Californium 252 (Cf-252) Y Other Isotope	Z None
0 Brain 1 Brain Stem 6 Spinal Cord 7 Peripheral Nerve	B Low Dose Rate (LDR)	B Palladium 103 (Pd-103)	1 Unidirectional Source Z None

D   **Radiation Therapy**
0   **Central and Peripheral Nervous System**
2   **Stereotactic Radiosurgery**

Treatment Site Character 4	Modality Qualifier Character 5	Isotope Character 6	Qualifier Character 7

0 Brain
1 Brain Stem
6 Spinal Cord
7 Peripheral Nerve
	D Stereotactic Other Photon
	    Radiosurgery
	H Stereotactic Particulate
	    Radiosurgery
	J Stereotactic Gamma Beam
	    Radiosurgery
		Z None	Z None

DRG Non-OR All treatment site, modality, isotope, and qualifier values

D   **Radiation Therapy**
0   **Central and Peripheral Nervous System**
Y   **Other Radiation**

Treatment Site Character 4	Modality Qualifier Character 5	Isotope Character 6	Qualifier Character 7
0 Brain 1 Brain Stem 6 Spinal Cord 7 Peripheral Nerve	7 Contact Radiation 8 Hyperthermia F Plaque Radiation K Laser Interstitial Thermal Therapy	Z None	Z None

Valid OR   D0Y[0,1,6,7]KZZ

LC Limited Coverage   **NC** Noncovered   ⊞ Combination Member   **HAC**   Valid OR   Combination Only   DRG Non-OR   New/Revised in GREEN

D Radiation Therapy
7 Lymphatic and Hematologic System
Ø Beam Radiation

Treatment Site Character 4	Modality Qualifier Character 5	Isotope Character 6	Qualifier Character 7
Ø Bone Marrow 1 Thymus 2 Spleen 3 Lymphatics, Neck 4 Lymphatics, Axillary 5 Lymphatics, Thorax 6 Lymphatics, Abdomen 7 Lymphatics, Pelvis 8 Lymphatics, Inguinal	Ø Photons <1 MeV 1 Photons 1- 10 MeV 2 Photons >10 MeV 4 Heavy Particles (Protons, Ions) 5 Neutrons 6 Neutron Capture	Z None	Z None
Ø Bone Marrow 1 Thymus 2 Spleen 3 Lymphatics, Neck 4 Lymphatics, Axillary 5 Lymphatics, Thorax 6 Lymphatics, Abdomen 7 Lymphatics, Pelvis 8 Lymphatics, Inguinal	3 Electrons	Z None	Ø Intraoperative Z None

D Radiation Therapy
7 Lymphatic and Hematologic System
1 Brachytherapy

Treatment Site Character 4	Modality Qualifier Character 5	Isotope Character 6	Qualifier Character 7
Ø Bone Marrow 1 Thymus 2 Spleen 3 Lymphatics, Neck 4 Lymphatics, Axillary 5 Lymphatics, Thorax 6 Lymphatics, Abdomen 7 Lymphatics, Pelvis 8 Lymphatics, Inguinal	9 High Dose Rate (HDR)	7 Cesium 137 (Cs-137) 8 Iridium 192 (Ir-192) 9 Iodine 125 (I-125) B Palladium 103 (Pd-103) C Californium 252 (Cf-252) Y Other Isotope	Z None
Ø Bone Marrow 1 Thymus 2 Spleen 3 Lymphatics, Neck 4 Lymphatics, Axillary 5 Lymphatics, Thorax 6 Lymphatics, Abdomen 7 Lymphatics, Pelvis 8 Lymphatics, Inguinal	B Low Dose Rate (LDR)	7 Cesium 137 (Cs-137) 8 Iridium 192 (Ir-192) 9 Iodine 125 (I-125) C Californium 252 (Cf-252) Y Other Isotope	Z None
Ø Bone Marrow 1 Thymus 2 Spleen 3 Lymphatics, Neck 4 Lymphatics, Axillary 5 Lymphatics, Thorax 6 Lymphatics, Abdomen 7 Lymphatics, Pelvis 8 Lymphatics, Inguinal	B Low Dose Rate (LDR)	B Palladium 103 (Pd-103)	1 Unidirectional Source Z None

D Radiation Therapy
7 Lymphatic and Hematologic System
2 Stereotactic Radiosurgery

Treatment Site Character 4	Modality Qualifier Character 5	Isotope Character 6	Qualifier Character 7
Ø Bone Marrow 1 Thymus 2 Spleen 3 Lymphatics, Neck 4 Lymphatics, Axillary 5 Lymphatics, Thorax 6 Lymphatics, Abdomen 7 Lymphatics, Pelvis 8 Lymphatics, Inguinal	D Stereotactic Other Photon Radiosurgery H Stereotactic Particulate Radiosurgery J Stereotactic Gamma Beam Radiosurgery	Z None	Z None

DRG Non-OR All treatment site, modality, isotope, and qualifier values

D   **Radiation Therapy**
7   **Lymphatic and Hematologic System**
Y   **Other Radiation**

Treatment Site Character 4	Modality Qualifier Character 5	Isotope Character 6	Qualifier Character 7
Ø Bone Marrow **1** Thymus **2** Spleen **3** Lymphatics, Neck **4** Lymphatics, Axillary **5** Lymphatics, Thorax **6** Lymphatics, Abdomen **7** Lymphatics, Pelvis **8** Lymphatics, Inguinal	**8** Hyperthermia **F** Plaque Radiation	**Z** None	**Z** None

D   **Radiation Therapy**
8   **Eye**
Ø   **Beam Radiation**

Treatment Site Character 4	Modality Qualifier Character 5	Isotope Character 6	Qualifier Character 7
Ø Eye	**Ø** Photons <1 MeV **1** Photons 1- 10 MeV **2** Photons >10 MeV **4** Heavy Particles (Protons, Ions) **5** Neutrons **6** Neutron Capture	**Z** None	**Z** None
Ø Eye	**3** Electrons	**Z** None	**Ø** Intraoperative **Z** None

D   **Radiation Therapy**
8   **Eye**
1   **Brachytherapy**

Treatment Site Character 4	Modality Qualifier Character 5	Isotope Character 6	Qualifier Character 7
Ø Eye	**9** High Dose Rate (HDR)	**7** Cesium 137 (Cs-137) **8** Iridium 192 (Ir-192) **9** Iodine 125 (I-125) **B** Palladium 103 (Pd-103) **C** Californium 252 (Cf-252) **Y** Other Isotope	**Z** None
Ø Eye	**B** Low Dose Rate (LDR)	**7** Cesium 137 (Cs-137) **8** Iridium 192 (Ir-192) **9** Iodine 125 (I-125) **C** Californium 252 (Cf-252) **Y** Other Isotope	**Z** None
Ø Eye	**B** Low Dose Rate (LDR)	**B** Palladium 103 (Pd-103)	**1** Unidirectional Source **Z** None

D   **Radiation Therapy**
8   **Eye**
2   **Stereotactic Radiosurgery**

Treatment Site Character 4	Modality Qualifier Character 5	Isotope Character 6	Qualifier Character 7
Ø Eye	**D** Stereotactic Other Photon Radiosurgery **H** Stereotactic Particulate Radiosurgery **J** Stereotactic Gamma Beam Radiosurgery	**Z** None	**Z** None

DRG Non-OR   All treatment site, modality, isotope, and qualifier values

D   **Radiation Therapy**
8   **Eye**
Y   **Other Radiation**

Treatment Site Character 4	Modality Qualifier Character 5	Isotope Character 6	Qualifier Character 7
Ø Eye	**7** Contact Radiation **8** Hyperthermia **F** Plaque Radiation	**Z** None	**Z** None

LC Limited Coverage   **NC** Noncovered   ⊞ Combination Member   **HAC**   Valid OR   Combination Only   DRG Non-OR   New/Revised in **GREEN**

D   Radiation Therapy
9   Ear, Nose, Mouth and Throat
Ø   Beam Radiation

Treatment Site Character 4	Modality Qualifier Character 5	Isotope Character 6	Qualifier Character 7
Ø Ear 1 Nose 3 Hypopharynx 4 Mouth 5 Tongue 6 Salivary Glands 7 Sinuses 8 Hard Palate 9 Soft Palate B Larynx D Nasopharynx F Oropharynx	Ø Photons <1 MeV 1 Photons 1- 10 MeV 2 Photons >10 MeV 4 Heavy Particles (Protons, Ions) 5 Neutrons 6 Neutron Capture	Z None	Z None
Ø Ear 1 Nose 3 Hypopharynx 4 Mouth 5 Tongue 6 Salivary Glands 7 Sinuses 8 Hard Palate 9 Soft Palate B Larynx D Nasopharynx F Oropharynx	3 Electrons	Z None	Ø Intraoperative Z None

D   Radiation Therapy
9   Ear, Nose, Mouth and Throat
1   Brachytherapy

Treatment Site Character 4	Modality Qualifier Character 5	Isotope Character 6	Qualifier Character 7
Ø Ear 1 Nose 3 Hypopharynx 4 Mouth 5 Tongue 6 Salivary Glands 7 Sinuses 8 Hard Palate 9 Soft Palate B Larynx D Nasopharynx F Oropharynx	9 High Dose Rate (HDR)	7 Cesium 137 (Cs-137) 8 Iridium 192 (Ir-192) 9 Iodine 125 (I-125) B Palladium 103 (Pd-103) C Californium 252 (Cf-252) Y Other Isotope	Z None
Ø Ear 1 Nose 3 Hypopharynx 4 Mouth 5 Tongue 6 Salivary Glands 7 Sinuses 8 Hard Palate 9 Soft Palate B Larynx D Nasopharynx F Oropharynx	B Low Dose Rate (LDR)	7 Cesium 137 (Cs-137) 8 Iridium 192 (Ir-192) 9 Iodine 125 (I-125) C Californium 252 (Cf-252) Y Other Isotope	Z None
Ø Ear 1 Nose 3 Hypopharynx 4 Mouth 5 Tongue 6 Salivary Glands 7 Sinuses 8 Hard Palate 9 Soft Palate B Larynx D Nasopharynx F Oropharynx	B Low Dose Rate (LDR)	B Palladium 103 (Pd-103)	1 Unidirectional Source Z None

D   Radiation Therapy
9   Ear, Nose, Mouth and Throat
2   Stereotactic Radiosurgery

Treatment Site Character 4	Modality Qualifier Character 5	Isotope Character 6	Qualifier Character 7

0 Ear
1 Nose
4 Mouth
5 Tongue
6 Salivary Glands
7 Sinuses
8 Hard Palate
9 Soft Palate
B Larynx
C Pharynx
D Nasopharynx
	D Stereotactic Other Photon
	    Radiosurgery
	H Stereotactic Particulate
	    Radiosurgery
	J Stereotactic Gamma Beam
	    Radiosurgery
		Z None	Z None

DRG Non-OR All treatment site, modality, isotope, and qualifier values

D   Radiation Therapy
9   Ear, Nose, Mouth and Throat
Y   Other Radiation

Treatment Site Character 4	Modality Qualifier Character 5	Isotope Character 6	Qualifier Character 7
0 Ear 1 Nose 5 Tongue 6 Salivary Glands 7 Sinuses 8 Hard Palate 9 Soft Palate	7 Contact Radiation 8 Hyperthermia F Plaque Radiation	Z None	Z None
3 Hypopharynx F Oropharynx	7 Contact Radiation 8 Hyperthermia	Z None	Z None
4 Mouth B Larynx D Nasopharynx	7 Contact Radiation 8 Hyperthermia C Intraoperative Radiation Therapy (IORT) F Plaque Radiation	Z None	Z None
C Pharynx	C Intraoperative Radiation Therapy (IORT) F Plaque Radiation	Z None	Z None

D   Radiation Therapy
B   Respiratory System
0   Beam Radiation

Treatment Site Character 4	Modality Qualifier Character 5	Isotope Character 6	Qualifier Character 7
0 Trachea 1 Bronchus 2 Lung 5 Pleura 6 Mediastinum 7 Chest Wall 8 Diaphragm	0 Photons <1 MeV 1 Photons 1- 10 MeV 2 Photons >10 MeV 4 Heavy Particles (Protons, Ions) 5 Neutrons 6 Neutron Capture	Z None	Z None
0 Trachea 1 Bronchus 2 Lung 5 Pleura 6 Mediastinum 7 Chest Wall 8 Diaphragm	3 Electrons	Z None	0 Intraoperative Z None

D Radiation Therapy
B Respiratory System
1 Brachytherapy

Treatment Site Character 4	Modality Qualifier Character 5	Isotope Character 6	Qualifier Character 7
Ø Trachea 1 Bronchus 2 Lung 5 Pleura 6 Mediastinum 7 Chest Wall 8 Diaphragm	9 High Dose Rate (HDR)	7 Cesium 137 (Cs-137) 8 Iridium 192 (Ir-192) 9 Iodine 125 (I-125) B Palladium 103 (Pd-103) C Californium 252 (Cf-252) Y Other Isotope	Z None
Ø Trachea 1 Bronchus 2 Lung 5 Pleura 6 Mediastinum 7 Chest Wall 8 Diaphragm	B Low Dose Rate (LDR)	7 Cesium 137 (Cs-137) 8 Iridium 192 (Ir-192) 9 Iodine 125 (I-125) C Californium 252 (Cf-252) Y Other Isotope	Z None
Ø Trachea 1 Bronchus 2 Lung 5 Pleura 6 Mediastinum 7 Chest Wall 8 Diaphragm	B Low Dose Rate (LDR)	B Palladium 103 (Pd-103)	1 Unidirectional Source Z None

D Radiation Therapy
B Respiratory System
2 Stereotactic Radiosurgery

Treatment Site Character 4	Modality Qualifier Character 5	Isotope Character 6	Qualifier Character 7
Ø Trachea 1 Bronchus 2 Lung 5 Pleura 6 Mediastinum 7 Chest Wall 8 Diaphragm	D Stereotactic Other Photon Radiosurgery H Stereotactic Particulate Radiosurgery J Stereotactic Gamma Beam Radiosurgery	Z None	Z None

DRG Non-OR All treatment site, modality, isotope, and qualifier values

D Radiation Therapy
B Respiratory System
Y Other Radiation

Treatment Site Character 4	Modality Qualifier Character 5	Isotope Character 6	Qualifier Character 7
Ø Trachea 1 Bronchus 2 Lung 5 Pleura 6 Mediastinum 7 Chest Wall 8 Diaphragm	7 Contact Radiation 8 Hyperthermia F Plaque Radiation K Laser Interstitial Thermal Therapy	Z None	Z None

Valid OR DBY[Ø,1,2,5,6,7,8]KZZ

D Radiation Therapy
D Gastrointestinal System
Ø Beam Radiation

Treatment Site Character 4	Modality Qualifier Character 5	Isotope Character 6	Qualifier Character 7
Ø Esophagus 1 Stomach 2 Duodenum 3 Jejunum 4 Ileum 5 Colon 7 Rectum	Ø Photons <1 MeV 1 Photons 1- 10 MeV 2 Photons >10 MeV 4 Heavy Particles (Protons, Ions) 5 Neutrons 6 Neutron Capture	Z None	Z None
Ø Esophagus 1 Stomach 2 Duodenum 3 Jejunum 4 Ileum 5 Colon 7 Rectum	3 Electrons	Z None	Ø Intraoperative Z None

D Radiation Therapy
D Gastrointestinal System
1 Brachytherapy

Treatment Site Character 4	Modality Qualifier Character 5	Isotope Character 6	Qualifier Character 7
Ø Esophagus 1 Stomach 2 Duodenum 3 Jejunum 4 Ileum 5 Colon 7 Rectum	9 High Dose Rate (HDR)	7 Cesium 137 (Cs-137) 8 Iridium 192 (Ir-192) 9 Iodine 125 (I-125) B Palladium 103 (Pd-103) C Californium 252 (Cf-252) Y Other Isotope	Z None
Ø Esophagus 1 Stomach 2 Duodenum 3 Jejunum 4 Ileum 5 Colon 7 Rectum	B Low Dose Rate (LDR)	7 Cesium 137 (Cs-137) 8 Iridium 192 (Ir-192) 9 Iodine 125 (I-125) C Californium 252 (Cf-252) Y Other Isotope	Z None
Ø Esophagus 1 Stomach 2 Duodenum 3 Jejunum 4 Ileum 5 Colon 7 Rectum	B Low Dose Rate (LDR)	B Palladium 103 (Pd-103)	1 Unidirectional Source Z None

D Radiation Therapy
D Gastrointestinal System
2 Stereotactic Radiosurgery

Treatment Site Character 4	Modality Qualifier Character 5	Isotope Character 6	Qualifier Character 7

Ø Esophagus
1 Stomach
2 Duodenum
3 Jejunum
4 Ileum
5 Colon
7 Rectum
	D Stereotactic Other Photon
	   Radiosurgery
	H Stereotactic Particulate
	   Radiosurgery
	J Stereotactic Gamma Beam
	   Radiosurgery
		Z None	Z None

DRG Non-OR All treatment site, modality, isotope, and qualifier values

Radiation Therapy

D   **Radiation therapy**
D   **Gastrointestinal System**
Y   **Other Radiation**

Treatment Site Character 4	Modality Qualifier Character 5	Isotope Character 6	Qualifier Character 7
Ø Esophagus	7 Contact Radiation 8 Hyperthermia F Plaque Radiation K Laser Interstitial Thermal Therapy	Z None	Z None
1 Stomach 2 Duodenum 3 Jejunum 4 Ileum 5 Colon 7 Rectum	7 Contact Radiation 8 Hyperthermia C Intraoperative Radiation Therapy (IORT) F Plaque Radiation K Laser Interstitial Thermal Therapy	Z None	Z None
8 Anus	C Intraoperative Radiation Therapy (IORT) F Plaque Radiation K Laser Interstitial Thermal Therapy	Z None	Z None

Valid OR   DDYØKZZ
Valid OR   DDY[1,2,3,4,5,7]KZZ
Valid OR   DDY8KZZ

D   **Radiation Therapy**
F   **Hepatobiliary System and Pancreas**
Ø   **Beam Radiation**

Treatment Site Character 4	Modality Qualifier Character 5	Isotope Character 6	Qualifier Character 7
Ø Liver 1 Gallbladder 2 Bile Ducts 3 Pancreas	Ø Photons <1 MeV 1 Photons 1- 10 MeV 2 Photons >10 MeV 4 Heavy Particles (Protons, Ions) 5 Neutrons 6 Neutron Capture	Z None	Z None
Ø Liver 1 Gallbladder 2 Bile Ducts 3 Pancreas	3 Electrons	Z None	Ø Intraoperative Z None

D   **Radiation Therapy**
F   **Hepatobiliary System and Pancreas**
1   **Brachytherapy**

Treatment Site Character 4	Modality Qualifier Character 5	Isotope Character 6	Qualifier Character 7
Ø Liver 1 Gallbladder 2 Bile Ducts 3 Pancreas	9 High Dose Rate (HDR)	7 Cesium 137 (Cs-137) 8 Iridium 192 (Ir-192) 9 Iodine 125 (I-125) B Palladium 103 (Pd-103) C Californium 252 (Cf-252) Y Other Isotope	Z None
Ø Liver 1 Gallbladder 2 Bile Ducts 3 Pancreas	B Low Dose Rate (LDR)	7 Cesium 137 (Cs-137) 8 Iridium 192 (Ir-192) 9 Iodine 125 (I-125) C Californium 252 (Cf-252) Y Other Isotope	Z None
Ø Liver 1 Gallbladder 2 Bile Ducts 3 Pancreas	B Low Dose Rate (LDR)	B Palladium 103 (Pd-103)	1 Unidirectional Source Z None

D   **Radiation Therapy**
F   **Hepatobiliary System and Pancreas**
2   **Stereotactic Radiosurgery**

Treatment Site Character 4	Modality Qualifier Character 5	Isotope Character 6	Qualifier Character 7
Ø Liver 1 Gallbladder 2 Bile Ducts 3 Pancreas	D Stereotactic Other Photon Radiosurgery H Stereotactic Particulate Radiosurgery J Stereotactic Gamma Beam Radiosurgery	Z None	Z None

DRG Non-OR   All treatment site, modality, isotope, and qualifier values

D   **Radiation Therapy**
F   **Hepatobiliary System and Pancreas**
Y   **Other Radiation**

Treatment Site Character 4	Modality Qualifier Character 5	Isotope Character 6	Qualifier Character 7
Ø Liver 1 Gallbladder 2 Bile Ducts 3 Pancreas	7 Contact Radiation 8 Hyperthermia C Intraoperative Radiation Therapy (IORT) F Plaque Radiation K Laser Interstitial Thermal Therapy	Z None	Z None

Valid OR   DFY[Ø,1,2,3]KZZ

D   **Radiation Therapy**
G   **Endocrine System**
Ø   **Beam Radiation**

Treatment Site Character 4	Modality Qualifier Character 5	Isotope Character 6	Qualifier Character 7
Ø Pituitary Gland 1 Pineal Body 2 Adrenal Glands 4 Parathyroid Glands 5 Thyroid	Ø Photons <1 MeV 1 Photons 1- 10 MeV 2 Photons >10 MeV 5 Neutrons 6 Neutron Capture	Z None	Z None
Ø Pituitary Gland 1 Pineal Body 2 Adrenal Glands 4 Parathyroid Glands 5 Thyroid	3 Electrons	Z None	Ø Intraoperative Z None

D   **Radiation Therapy**
G   **Endocrine System**
1   **Brachytherapy**

Treatment Site Character 4	Modality Qualifier Character 5	Isotope Character 6	Qualifier Character 7
Ø Pituitary Gland 1 Pineal Body 2 Adrenal Glands 4 Parathyroid Glands 5 Thyroid	9 High Dose Rate (HDR)	7 Cesium 137 (Cs-137) 8 Iridium 192 (Ir-192) 9 Iodine 125 (I-125) B Palladium 103 (Pd-103) C Californium 252 (Cf-252) Y Other Isotope	Z None
Ø Pituitary Gland 1 Pineal Body 2 Adrenal Glands 4 Parathyroid Glands 5 Thyroid	B Low Dose Rate (LDR)	7 Cesium 137 (Cs-137) 8 Iridium 192 (Ir-192) 9 Iodine 125 (I-125) C Californium 252 (Cf-252) Y Other Isotope	Z None
Ø Pituitary Gland 1 Pineal Body 2 Adrenal Glands 4 Parathyroid Glands 5 Thyroid	B Low Dose Rate (LDR)	B Palladium 103 (Pd-103)	1 Unidirectional Source Z None

D   **Radiation Therapy**
G   **Endocrine System**
2   **Stereotactic Radiosurgery**

Treatment Site Character 4	Modality Qualifier Character 5	Isotope Character 6	Qualifier Character 7

Ø Pituitary Gland
1 Pineal Body
2 Adrenal Glands
4 Parathyroid Glands
5 Thyroid
	D Stereotactic Other Photon
	    Radiosurgery
	H Stereotactic Particulate
	    Radiosurgery
	J Stereotactic Gamma Beam
	    Radiosurgery
		Z None	Z None

DRG Non-OR All treatment site, modality, isotope, and qualifier values

D　**Radiation therapy**
G　**Endocrine System**
Y　**Other Radiation**

Treatment Site Character 4	Modality Qualifier Character 5	Isotope Character 6	Qualifier Character 7
0　Pituitary Gland 1　Pineal Body 2　Adrenal Glands 4　Parathyroid Glands 5　Thyroid	7　Contact Radiation 8　Hyperthermia F　Plaque Radiation K　Laser Interstitial Thermal Therapy	Z　None	Z　None

Valid OR　　DGY[0,1,2,4,5]KZZ

D　**Radiation Therapy**
H　**Skin**
0　**Beam Radiation**

Treatment Site Character 4	Modality Qualifier Character 5	Isotope Character 6	Qualifier Character 7
2　Skin, Face 3　Skin, Neck 4　Skin, Arm 6　Skin, Chest 7　Skin, Back 8　Skin, Abdomen 9　Skin, Buttock B　Skin, Leg	0　Photons <1 MeV 1　Photons 1- 10 MeV 2　Photons >10 MeV 4　Heavy Particles (Protons, Ions) 5　Neutrons 6　Neutron Capture	Z　None	Z　None
2　Skin, Face 3　Skin, Neck 4　Skin, Arm 6　Skin, Chest 7　Skin, Back 8　Skin, Abdomen 9　Skin, Buttock B　Skin, Leg	3　Electrons	Z　None	0　Intraoperative Z　None

---

D　**Radiation Therapy**
H　**Skin**
Y　**Other Radiation**

Treatment Site Character 4	Modality Qualifier Character 5	Isotope Character 6	Qualifier Character 7
2　Skin, Face 3　Skin, Neck 4　Skin, Arm 6　Skin, Chest 7　Skin, Back 8　Skin, Abdomen 9　Skin, Buttock B　Skin, Leg	7　Contact Radiation 8　Hyperthermia F　Plaque Radiation	Z　None	Z　None
5　Skin, Hand C　Skin, Foot	F　Plaque Radiation	Z　None	Z　None

D　**Radiation Therapy**
M　**Breast**
0　**Beam Radiation**

Treatment Site Character 4	Modality Qualifier Character 5	Isotope Character 6	Qualifier Character 7
0　Breast, Left 1　Breast, Right	0　Photons <1 MeV 1　Photons 1- 10 MeV 2　Photons >10 MeV 4　Heavy Particles (Protons, Ions) 5　Neutrons 6　Neutron Capture	Z　None	Z　None
0　Breast, Left 1　Breast, Right	3　Electrons	Z　None	0　Intraoperative Z　None

D Radiation Therapy
M Breast
1 Brachytherapy

Treatment Site Character 4	Modality Qualifier Character 5	Isotope Character 6	Qualifier Character 7
0 Breast, Left 1 Breast, Right	9 High Dose Rate (HDR)	7 Cesium 137 (Cs-137) 8 Iridium 192 (Ir-192) 9 Iodine 125 (I-125) B Palladium 103 (Pd-103) C Californium 252 (Cf-252) Y Other Isotope	Z None
0 Breast, Left 1 Breast, Right	B Low Dose Rate (LDR)	7 Cesium 137 (Cs-137) 8 Iridium 192 (Ir-192) 9 Iodine 125 (I-125) C Californium 252 (Cf-252) Y Other Isotope	Z None
0 Breast, Left 1 Breast, Right	B Low Dose Rate (LDR)	B Palladium 103 (Pd-103)	1 Unidirectional Source Z None

D Radiation Therapy
M Breast
2 Stereotactic Radiosurgery

Treatment Site Character 4	Modality Qualifier Character 5	Isotope Character 6	Qualifier Character 7

0 Breast, Left
1 Breast, Right
	D Stereotactic Other Photon
	    Radiosurgery
	H Stereotactic Particulate
	    Radiosurgery
	J Stereotactic Gamma Beam
	    Radiosurgery
		Z None	Z None

DRG Non-OR All treatment site, modality, isotope, and qualifier values

D Radiation Therapy
M Breast
Y Other Radiation

Treatment Site Character 4	Modality Qualifier Character 5	Isotope Character 6	Qualifier Character 7
0 Breast, Left 1 Breast, Right	7 Contact Radiation 8 Hyperthermia F Plaque Radiation K Laser Interstitial Thermal Therapy	Z None	Z None

Valid OR   DMY[0,1]KZZ

D Radiation Therapy
P Musculoskeletal System
0 Beam Radiation

Treatment Site Character 4	Modality Qualifier Character 5	Isotope Character 6	Qualifier Character 7
0 Skull 2 Maxilla 3 Mandible 4 Sternum 5 Rib(s) 6 Humerus 7 Radius/Ulna 8 Pelvic Bones 9 Femur B Tibia/Fibula C Other Bone	0 Photons <1 MeV 1 Photons 1- 10 MeV 2 Photons >10 MeV 4 Heavy Particles (Protons, Ions) 5 Neutrons 6 Neutron Capture	Z None	Z None
0 Skull 2 Maxilla 3 Mandible 4 Sternum 5 Rib(s) 6 Humerus 7 Radius/Ulna 8 Pelvic Bones 9 Femur B Tibia/Fibula C Other Bone	3 Electrons	Z None	0 Intraoperative Z None

D   Radiation Therapy
P   Musculoskeletal System
Y   Other Radiation

Treatment Site Character 4	Modality Qualifier Character 5	Isotope Character 6	Qualifier Character 7
Ø Skull 2 Maxilla 3 Mandible 4 Sternum 5 Rib(s) 6 Humerus 7 Radius/Ulna 8 Pelvic Bones 9 Femur B Tibia/Fibula C Other Bone	7 Contact Radiation 8 Hyperthermia F Plaque Radiation	Z None	Z None

D   Radiation Therapy
T   Urinary System
Ø   Beam Radiation

Treatment Site Character 4	Modality Qualifier Character 5	Isotope Character 6	Qualifier Character 7
Ø Kidney 1 Ureter 2 Bladder 3 Urethra	Ø Photons <1 MeV 1 Photons 1- 10 MeV 2 Photons >10 MeV 4 Heavy Particles (Protons, Ions) 5 Neutrons 6 Neutron Capture	Z None	Z None
Ø Kidney 1 Ureter 2 Bladder 3 Urethra	3 Electrons	Z None	Ø Intraoperative Z None

D   Radiation Therapy
T   Urinary System
1   Brachytherapy

Treatment Site Character 4	Modality Qualifier Character 5	Isotope Character 6	Qualifier Character 7
Ø Kidney 1 Ureter 2 Bladder 3 Urethra	9 High Dose Rate (HDR)	7 Cesium 137 (Cs-137) 8 Iridium 192 (Ir-192) 9 Iodine 125 (I-125) B Palladium 103 (Pd-103) C Californium 252 (Cf-252) Y Other Isotope	Z None
Ø Kidney 1 Ureter 2 Bladder 3 Urethra	B Low Dose Rate (LDR)	7 Cesium 137 (Cs-137) 8 Iridium 192 (Ir-192) 9 Iodine 125 (I-125) C Californium 252 (Cf-252) Y Other Isotope	Z None
Ø Kidney 1 Ureter 2 Bladder 3 Urethra	B Low Dose Rate (LDR)	B Palladium 103 (Pd-103)	1 Unidirectional Source Z None

D   Radiation Therapy
T   Urinary System
2   Stereotactic Radiosurgery

Treatment Site Character 4	Modality Qualifier Character 5	Isotope Character 6	Qualifier Character 7
Ø Kidney 1 Ureter 2 Bladder 3 Urethra	D Stereotactic Other Photon Radiosurgery H Stereotactic Particulate Radiosurgery J Stereotactic Gamma Beam Radiosurgery	Z None	Z None

DRG Non-OR   All treatment site, modality, isotope, and qualifier values

D   **Radiation Therapy**
T   **Urinary System**
Y   **Other Radiation**

Treatment Site Character 4	Modality Qualifier Character 5	Isotope Character 6	Qualifier Character 7
Ø Kidney 1 Ureter 2 Bladder 3 Urethra	7 Contact Radiation 8 Hyperthermia C Intraoperative Radiation Therapy (IORT) F Plaque Radiation	Z None	Z None

D   **Radiation Therapy**
U   **Female Reproductive System**
Ø   **Beam Radiation**

Treatment Site Character 4	Modality Qualifier Character 5	Isotope Character 6	Qualifier Character 7
Ø Ovary ♀ 1 Cervix ♀ 2 Uterus ♀	Ø Photons <1 MeV 1 Photons 1- 10 MeV 2 Photons >10 MeV 4 Heavy Particles (Protons, Ions) 5 Neutrons 6 Neutron Capture	Z None	Z None
Ø Ovary ♀ 1 Cervix ♀ 2 Uterus ♀	3 Electrons	Z None	Ø Intraoperative Z None

♀   All treatment site, modality, isotope, and qualifier values

D   **Radiation Therapy**
U   **Female Reproductive System**
1   **Brachytherapy**

Treatment Site Character 4	Modality Qualifier Character 5	Isotope Character 6	Qualifier Character 7
Ø Ovary ♀ 1 Cervix ♀ 2 Uterus ♀	9 High Dose Rate (HDR)	7 Cesium 137 (Cs-137) 8 Iridium 192 (Ir-192) 9 Iodine 125 (I-125) B Palladium 103 (Pd-103) C Californium 252 (Cf-252) Y Other Isotope	Z None
Ø Ovary ♀ 1 Cervix ♀ 2 Uterus ♀	B Low Dose Rate (LDR)	7 Cesium 137 (Cs-137) 8 Iridium 192 (Ir-192) 9 Iodine 125 (I-125) C Californium 252 (Cf-252) Y Other Isotope	Z None
Ø Ovary ♀ 1 Cervix ♀ 2 Uterus ♀	B Low Dose Rate (LDR)	B Palladium 103 (Pd-103)	1 Unidirectional Source Z None

♀   All treatment site, modality, isotope, and qualifier values

D   **Radiation Therapy**
U   **Female Reproductive System**
2   **Stereotactic Radiosurgery**

Treatment Site Character 4	Modality Qualifier Character 5	Isotope Character 6	Qualifier Character 7
Ø Ovary ♀ 1 Cervix ♀ 2 Uterus ♀	D Stereotactic Other Photon Radiosurgery H Stereotactic Particulate Radiosurgery J Stereotactic Gamma Beam Radiosurgery	Z None	Z None

DRG Non-OR   All treatment site, modality, isotope, and qualifier values
♀   All treatment site, modality, isotope, and qualifier values

D Radiation Therapy
U Female Reproductive System
Y Other Radiation

Treatment Site Character 4		Modality Qualifier Character 5	Isotope Character 6	Qualifier Character 7
0 Ovary ♀ 1 Cervix ♀ 2 Uterus ♀		7 Contact Radiation 8 Hyperthermia C Intraoperative Radiation Therapy (IORT) F Plaque Radiation	Z None	Z None

♀	All treatment site, modality, isotope, and qualifier values

D Radiation Therapy
V Male Reproductive System
0 Beam Radiation

Treatment Site Character 4		Modality Qualifier Character 5	Isotope Character 6	Qualifier Character 7
0 Prostate ♂ 1 Testis ♂		0 Photons <1 MeV 1 Photons 1- 10 MeV 2 Photons >10 MeV 4 Heavy Particles (Protons, Ions) 5 Neutrons 6 Neutron Capture	Z None	Z None
0 Prostate ♂ 1 Testis ♂		3 Electrons	Z None	0 Intraoperative Z None

♂	All treatment site, modality, isotope, and qualifier values

D Radiation Therapy
V Male Reproductive System
1 Brachytherapy

Treatment Site Character 4		Modality Qualifier Character 5	Isotope Character 6	Qualifier Character 7
0 Prostate ♂ 1 Testis ♂		9 High Dose Rate (HDR)	7 Cesium 137 (Cs-137) 8 Iridium 192 (Ir-192) 9 Iodine 125 (I-125) B Palladium 103 (Pd-103) C Californium 252 (Cf-252) Y Other Isotope	Z None
0 Prostate ♂ 1 Testis ♂		B Low Dose Rate (LDR)	7 Cesium 137 (Cs-137) 8 Iridium 192 (Ir-192) 9 Iodine 125 (I-125) C Californium 252 (Cf-252) Y Other Isotope	Z None
0 Prostate ♂ 1 Testis ♂		B Low Dose Rate (LDR)	B Palladium 103 (Pd-103)	1 Unidirectional Source Z None

♂	All treatment site, modality, isotope, and qualifier values

D Radiation Therapy
V Male Reproductive System
2 Stereotactic Radiosurgery

Treatment Site Character 4		Modality Qualifier Character 5	Isotope Character 6	Qualifier Character 7
0 Prostate ♂ 1 Testis ♂		D Stereotactic Other Photon Radiosurgery H Stereotactic Particulate Radiosurgery J Stereotactic Gamma Beam Radiosurgery	Z None	Z None

DRG Non-OR	All treatment site, modality, isotope, and qualifier values
♂	All treatment site, modality, isotope, and qualifier values

LC Limited Coverage **NC** Noncovered ⊞ Combination Member HAC Valid OR Combination Only DRG Non-OR New/Revised in GREEN

776

ICD-10-PCS 2020

D   **Radiation Therapy**
V   **Male Reproductive System**
Y   **Other Radiation**

Treatment Site Character 4	Modality Qualifier Character 5	Isotope Character 6	Qualifier Character 7
Ø Prostate ♂	7 Contact Radiation 8 Hyperthermia C Intraoperative Radiation Therapy (IORT) F Plaque Radiation K Laser Interstitial Thermal Therapy	Z None	Z None
1 Testis ♂	7 Contact Radiation 8 Hyperthermia F Plaque Radiation	Z None	Z None

Valid OR	DVYØKZZ
♂	All treatment site, modality, isotope, and qualifier values

D   **Radiation Therapy**
W **Anatomical Regions**
Ø   **Beam Radiation**

Treatment Site Character 4	Modality Qualifier Character 5	Isotope Character 6	Qualifier Character 7
1 Head and Neck 2 Chest 3 Abdomen 4 Hemibody 5 Whole Body 6 Pelvic Region	Ø Photons <1 MeV 1 Photons 1- 10 MeV 2 Photons >10 MeV 4 Heavy Particles (Protons, Ions) 5 Neutrons 6 Neutron Capture	Z None	Z None
1 Head and Neck 2 Chest 3 Abdomen 4 Hemibody 5 Whole Body 6 Pelvic Region	3 Electrons	Z None	Ø Intraoperative Z None

D   **Radiation Therapy**
W **Anatomical Regions**
1   **Brachytherapy**

Treatment Site Character 4	Modality Qualifier Character 5	Isotope Character 6	Qualifier Character 7
Ø Cranial Cavity K Upper Back L Lower Back P Gastrointestinal Tract Q Respiratory Tract R Genitourinary Tract X Upper Extremity Y Lower Extremity	B Low Dose Rate (LDR)	B Palladium 103 (Pd-103)	1 Unidirectional Source Z None
1 Head and Neck 2 Chest 3 Abdomen 6 Pelvic Region	9 High Dose Rate (HDR)	7 Cesium 137 (Cs-137) 8 Iridium 192 (Ir-192) 9 Iodine 125 (I-125) B Palladium 103 (Pd-103) C Californium 252 (Cf-252) Y Other Isotope	Z None
1 Head and Neck 2 Chest 3 Abdomen 6 Pelvic Region	B Low Dose Rate (LDR)	7 Cesium 137 (Cs-137) 8 Iridium 192 (Ir-192) 9 Iodine 125 (I-125) C Californium 252 (Cf-252) Y Other Isotope	Z None
1 Head and Neck 2 Chest 3 Abdomen 6 Pelvic Region	B Low Dose Rate (LDR)	B Palladium 103 (Pd-103)	1 Unidirectional Source Z None

LC Limited Coverage   **NC** Noncovered   ⊞ Combination Member   HAC   Valid OR   Combination Only   DRG Non-OR   New/Revised in GREEN

ICD-10-PCS 2020   777

DVY–DW1

D Radiation Therapy
W Anatomical Regions
2 Stereotactic Radiosurgery

Treatment Site Character 4	Modality Qualifier Character 5	Isotope Character 6	Qualifier Character 7

1 Head and Neck
2 Chest
3 Abdomen
6 Pelvic Region
	D Stereotactic Other Photon
	    Radiosurgery
	H Stereotactic Particulate
	    Radiosurgery
	J Stereotactic Gamma Beam
	    Radiosurgery
		Z None	Z None

DRG Non-OR All treatment site, modality, isotope, and qualifier values

D Radiation Therapy
W Anatomical Regions
Y Other Radiation

Treatment Site Character 4	Modality Qualifier Character 5	Isotope Character 6	Qualifier Character 7
1 Head and Neck 2 Chest 3 Abdomen 4 Hemibody 6 Pelvic Region	7 Contact Radiation 8 Hyperthermia F Plaque Radiation	Z None	Z None
5 Whole Body	7 Contact Radiation 8 Hyperthermia F Plaque Radiation	Z None	Z None
5 Whole Body	G Isotope Administration	D Iodine 131 (I-131) F Phosphorus 32 (P-32) G Strontium 89 (Sr-89) H Strontium 90 (Sr-90) Y Other Isotope	Z None

Physical Rehabilitation and Diagnostic Audiology F00–F15

F   **Physical Rehabilitation and Diagnostic Audiology**
Ø   **Rehabilitation**
Ø   **Speech Assessment**   Definition: Measurement of speech and related functions

Body System/Region Character 4	Type Qualifier Character 5	Equipment Character 6	Qualifier Character 7
3 Neurological System - Whole Body	G Communicative/Cognitive Integration Skills	K Audiovisual M Augmentative / Alternative Communication P Computer Y Other Equipment Z None	Z None
Z None	Ø Filtered Speech 3 Staggered Spondaic Word Q Performance Intensity Phonetically Balanced Speech Discrimination R Brief Tone Stimuli S Distorted Speech T Dichotic Stimuli V Temporal Ordering of Stimuli W Masking Patterns	1 Audiometer 2 Sound Field / Booth K Audiovisual Z None	Z None
Z None	1 Speech Threshold 2 Speech/Word Recognition	1 Audiometer 2 Sound Field / Booth 9 Cochlear Implant K Audiovisual Z None	Z None
Z None	4 Sensorineural Acuity Level	1 Audiometer 2 Sound Field / Booth Z None	Z None
Z None	5 Synthetic Sentence Identification	1 Audiometer 2 Sound Field / Booth 9 Cochlear Implant K Audiovisual	Z None
Z None	6 Speech and/or Language Screening 7 Nonspoken Language 8 Receptive/Expressive Language C Aphasia G Communicative/Cognitive Integration Skills L Augmentative/Alternative Communication System	K Audiovisual M Augmentative / Alternative Communication P Computer Y Other Equipment Z None	Z None
Z None	9 Articulation/Phonology	K Audiovisual P Computer Q Speech Analysis Y Other Equipment Z None	Z None
Z None	B Motor Speech	K Audiovisual N Biosensory Feedback P Computer Q Speech Analysis T Aerodynamic Function Y Other Equipment Z None	Z None
Z None	D Fluency	K Audiovisual N Biosensory Feedback P Computer Q Speech Analysis S Voice Analysis T Aerodynamic Function Y Other Equipment Z None	Z None
Z None	F Voice	K Audiovisual N Biosensory Feedback P Computer S Voice Analysis T Aerodynamic Function Y Other Equipment Z None	Z None

F00 Continued on next page

DRG Non-OR	All body system/region, type qualifier, equipment, and qualifier values

LC Limited Coverage   **NC** Noncovered   ⊞ Combination Member   HAC   Valid OR   Combination Only   DRG Non-OR   New/Revised in GREEN

ICD-10-PCS 2020   779

F00–F00

F   Physical Rehabilitation and Diagnostic Audiology
0   Rehabilitation
0   Speech Assessment   Definition: Measurement of speech and related functions

Body System/Region Character 4	Type Qualifier Character 5	Equipment Character 6	Qualifier Character 7
Z None	H Bedside Swallowing and Oral Function P Oral Peripheral Mechanism	Y Other Equipment Z None	Z None
Z None	J Instrumental Swallowing and Oral Function	T Aerodynamic Function W Swallowing Y Other Equipment	Z None
Z None	K Orofacial Myofunctional	K Audiovisual P Computer Y Other Equipment Z None	Z None
Z None	M Voice Prosthetic	K Audiovisual P Computer S Voice Analysis V Speech Prosthesis Y Other Equipment Z None	Z None
Z None	N Non-invasive Instrumental Status	N Biosensory Feedback P Computer Q Speech Analysis S Voice Analysis T Aerodynamic Function Y Other Equipment	Z None
Z None	X Other Specified Central Auditory Processing	Z None	Z None

DRG Non-OR   All body system/region, type qualifier, equipment, and qualifier values

F   Physical Rehabilitation and Diagnostic Audiology
0   Rehabilitation
1   Motor and/or Nerve Function Assessment   Definition: Measurement of motor, nerve, and related functions

Body System/Region Character 4	Type Qualifier Character 5	Equipment Character 6	Qualifier Character 7
0 Neurological System - Head and Neck 1 Neurological System - Upper Back/ Upper Extremity 2 Neurological System - Lower Back/ Lower Extremity 3 Neurological System - Whole Body	0 Muscle Performance	E Orthosis F Assistive, Adaptive, Supportive or Protective U Prosthesis Y Other Equipment Z None	Z None
0 Neurological System - Head and Neck 1 Neurological System - Upper Back/ Upper Extremity 2 Neurological System - Lower Back/ Lower Extremity 3 Neurological System - Whole Body	1 Integumentary Integrity 3 Coordination/Dexterity 4 Motor Function G Reflex Integrity	Z None	Z None
0 Neurological System - Head and Neck 1 Neurological System - Upper Back/ Upper Extremity 2 Neurological System - Lower Back/ Lower Extremity 3 Neurological System - Whole Body	5 Range of Motion and Joint Integrity 6 Sensory Awareness/Processing/ Integrity	Y Other Equipment Z None	Z None
D Integumentary System - Head and Neck F Integumentary System - Upper Back/ Upper Extremity G Integumentary System - Lower Back/ Lower Extremity H Integumentary System - Whole Body J Musculoskeletal System - Head and Neck K Musculoskeletal System - Upper Back/ Upper Extremity L Musculoskeletal System - Lower Back/ Lower Extremity M Musculoskeletal System - Whole Body	0 Muscle Performance	E Orthosis F Assistive, Adaptive, Supportive or Protective U Prosthesis Y Other Equipment Z None	Z None

F01 Continued on next page

DRG Non-OR   All body system/region, type qualifier, equipment, and qualifier values

F   **Physical Rehabilitation and Diagnostic Audiology**
Ø   **Rehabilitation**
1   **Motor and/or Nerve Function Assessment**   Definition: Measurement of motor, nerve, and related functions

Body System/Region Character 4	Type Qualifier Character 5	Equipment Character 6	Qualifier Character 7
D Integumentary System - Head and Neck **F** Integumentary System - Upper Back/ Upper Extremity **G** Integumentary System - Lower Back/ Lower Extremity **H** Integumentary System - Whole Body **J** Musculoskeletal System - Head and Neck **K** Musculoskeletal System - Upper Back/ Upper Extremity **L** Musculoskeletal System - Lower Back/ Lower Extremity **M** Musculoskeletal System - Whole Body	**1** Integumentary Integrity	**Z** None	**Z** None
D Integumentary System - Head and Neck **F** Integumentary System - Upper Back/ Upper Extremity **G** Integumentary System - Lower Back/ Lower Extremity **H** Integumentary System - Whole Body **J** Musculoskeletal System - Head and Neck **K** Musculoskeletal System - Upper Back/ Upper Extremity **L** Musculoskeletal System - Lower Back/ Lower Extremity **M** Musculoskeletal System - Whole Body	**5** Range of Motion and Joint Integrity **6** Sensory Awareness/Processing/ Integrity	**Y** Other Equipment **Z** None	**Z** None
N Genitourinary System	**Ø** Muscle Performance	**E** Orthosis **F** Assistive, Adaptive, Supportive or Protective **U** Prosthesis **Y** Other Equipment **Z** None	**Z** None
Z None	**2** Visual Motor Integration	**K** Audiovisual **M** Augmentative / Alternative Communication **N** Biosensory Feedback **P** Computer **Q** Speech Analysis **S** Voice Analysis **Y** Other Equipment **Z** None	**Z** None
Z None	**7** Facial Nerve Function	**7** Electrophysiologic	**Z** None
Z None	**9** Somatosensory Evoked Potentials	**J** Somatosensory	**Z** None
Z None	**B** Bed Mobility **C** Transfer **F** Wheelchair Mobility	**E** Orthosis **F** Assistive, Adaptive, Supportive or Protective **U** Prosthesis **Z** None	**Z** None
Z None	**D** Gait and/or Balance	**E** Orthosis **F** Assistive, Adaptive, Supportive or Protective **U** Prosthesis **Y** Other Equipment **Z** None	**Z** None

DRG Non-OR   All body system/region, type qualifier, equipment, and qualifier values

F   **Physical Rehabilitation and Diagnostic Audiology**
Ø   **Rehabilitation**
2   **Activities of Daily Living Assessment**   Definition: Measurement of functional level for activities of daily living

Body System/Region Character 4	Type Qualifier Character 5	Equipment Character 6	Qualifier Character 7
Ø Neurological System - Head and Neck	**9** Cranial Nerve Integrity **D** Neuromotor Development	**Y** Other Equipment **Z** None	**Z** None
1 Neurological System - Upper Back/Upper Extremity **2** Neurological System - Lower Back/Lower Extremity **3** Neurological System - Whole Body	**D** Neuromotor Development	**Y** Other Equipment **Z** None	**Z** None
4 Circulatory System - Head and Neck **5** Circulatory System - Upper Back/Upper Extremity **6** Circulatory System - Lower Back/Lower Extremity **8** Respiratory System - Head and Neck **9** Respiratory System - Upper Back/Upper Extremity **B** Respiratory System - Lower Back/Lower Extremity	**G** Ventilation, Respiration and Circulation	**C** Mechanical **G** Aerobic Endurance and Conditioning **Y** Other Equipment **Z** None	**Z** None
7 Circulatory System - Whole Body **C** Respiratory System - Whole Body	**7** Aerobic Capacity and Endurance	**E** Orthosis **G** Aerobic Endurance and Conditioning **U** Prosthesis **Y** Other Equipment **Z** None	**Z** None
7 Circulatory System - Whole Body **C** Respiratory System - Whole Body	**G** Ventilation, Respiration and Circulation	**C** Mechanical **G** Aerobic Endurance and Conditioning **Y** Other Equipment **Z** None	**Z** None
Z None	**Ø** Bathing/Showering **1** Dressing **3** Grooming/Personal Hygiene **4** Home Management	**E** Orthosis **F** Assistive, Adaptive, Supportive or Protective **U** Prosthesis **Z** None	**Z** None
Z None	**2** Feeding/Eating **8** Anthropometric Characteristics **F** Pain	**Y** Other Equipment **Z** None	**Z** None
Z None	**5** Perceptual Processing	**K** Audiovisual **M** Augmentative / Alternative Communication **N** Biosensory Feedback **P** Computer **Q** Speech Analysis **S** Voice Analysis **Y** Other Equipment **Z** None	**Z** None
Z None	**6** Psychosocial Skills	**Z** None	**Z** None
Z None	**B** Environmental, Home and Work Barriers **C** Ergonomics and Body Mechanics	**E** Orthosis **F** Assistive, Adaptive, Supportive or Protective **U** Prosthesis **Y** Other Equipment **Z** None	**Z** None
Z None	**H** Vocational Activities and Functional Community or Work Reintegration Skills	**E** Orthosis **F** Assistive, Adaptive, Supportive or Protective **G** Aerobic Endurance and Conditioning **U** Prosthesis **Y** Other Equipment **Z** None	**Z** None

DRG Non-OR   All body system/region, type qualifier, equipment, and qualifier values

F   **Physical Rehabilitation and Diagnostic Audiology**
0   **Rehabilitation**
6   **Speech Treatment**   Definition: Application of techniques to improve, augment, or compensate for speech and related functional impairment

Body System/Region Character 4		Type Qualifier Character 5		Equipment Character 6		Qualifier Character 7
3 Neurological System - Whole Body	**6**	Communicative/Cognitive Integration Skills	**K** Audiovisual **M** Augmentative / Alternative Communication **P** Computer **Y** Other Equipment **Z** None		**Z** None	
Z None	**0** **3** **6**	Nonspoken Language Aphasia Communicative/Cognitive Integration Skills	**K** Audiovisual **M** Augmentative / Alternative Communication **P** Computer **Y** Other Equipment **Z** None		**Z** None	
Z None	**1** **2**	Speech-Language Pathology and Related Disorders Counseling Speech-Language Pathology and Related Disorders Prevention	**K** Audiovisual **Z** None		**Z** None	
Z None	**4**	Articulation/Phonology	**K** Audiovisual **P** Computer **Q** Speech Analysis **T** Aerodynamic Function **Y** Other Equipment **Z** None		**Z** None	
Z None	**5**	Aural Rehabilitation	**K** Audiovisual **L** Assistive Listening **M** Augmentative / Alternative Communication **N** Biosensory Feedback **P** Computer **Q** Speech Analysis **S** Voice Analysis **Y** Other Equipment **Z** None		**Z** None	
Z None	**7**	Fluency	**4** Electroacoustic Immitance / Acoustic Reflex **K** Audiovisual **N** Biosensory Feedback **Q** Speech Analysis **S** Voice Analysis **T** Aerodynamic Function **Y** Other Equipment **Z** None		**Z** None	
Z None	**8**	Motor Speech	**K** Audiovisual **N** Biosensory Feedback **P** Computer **Q** Speech Analysis **S** Voice Analysis **T** Aerodynamic Function **Y** Other Equipment **Z** None		**Z** None	
Z None	**9**	Orofacial Myofunctional	**K** Audiovisual **P** Computer **Y** Other Equipment **Z** None		**Z** None	
Z None	**B**	Receptive/Expressive Language	**K** Audiovisual **L** Assistive Listening **M** Augmentative / Alternative Communication **P** Computer **Y** Other Equipment **Z** None		**Z** None	

F06 Continued on next page

DRG Non-OR   All body system/region, type qualifier, equipment, and qualifier values

LC Limited Coverage   **NC** Noncovered   ⊞ Combination Member   **HAC**   Valid OR   Combination Only   DRG Non-OR   New/Revised in GREEN

ICD-10-PCS 2020   **783**

Physical Rehabilitation and Diagnostic Audiology

F06 Continued

F   **Physical Rehabilitation and Diagnostic Audiology**
Ø   **Rehabilitation**
6   **Speech Treatment**   Definition: Application of techniques to improve, augment, or compensate for speech and related functional impairment

Body System/Region Character 4	Type Qualifier Character 5	Equipment Character 6	Qualifier Character 7
Z None	C Voice	K Audiovisual N Biosensory Feedback P Computer S Voice Analysis T Aerodynamic Function V Speech Prosthesis Y Other Equipment Z None	Z None
Z None	D Swallowing Dysfunction	M Augmentative / Alternative Communication T Aerodynamic Function V Speech Prosthesis Y Other Equipment Z None	Z None

DRG Non-OR   All body system/region, type qualifier, equipment, and qualifier values

F   **Physical Rehabilitation and Diagnostic Audiology**
Ø   **Rehabilitation**
7   **Motor Treatment**   Definition: Exercise or activities to increase or facilitate motor function

Body System/Region Character 4	Type Qualifier Character 5	Equipment Character 6	Qualifier Character 7
Ø Neurological System - Head and Neck 1 Neurological System - Upper Back/Upper Extremity 2 Neurological System - Lower Back/Lower Extremity 3 Neurological System - Whole Body D Integumentary System - Head and Neck F Integumentary System - Upper Back/Upper Extremity G Integumentary System - Lower Back/Lower Extremity H Integumentary System - Whole Body J Musculoskeletal System - Head and Neck K Musculoskeletal System - Upper Back/Upper Extremity L Musculoskeletal System - Lower Back/Lower Extremity M Musculoskeletal System - Whole Body	Ø Range of Motion and Joint Mobility 1 Muscle Performance 2 Coordination/Dexterity 3 Motor Function	E Orthosis F Assistive, Adaptive, Supportive or Protective U Prosthesis Y Other Equipment Z None	Z None
Ø Neurological System - Head and Neck 1 Neurological System - Upper Back/Upper Extremity 2 Neurological System - Lower Back/Lower Extremity 3 Neurological System - Whole Body D Integumentary System - Head and Neck F Integumentary System - Upper Back/Upper Extremity G Integumentary System - Lower Back/Lower Extremity H Integumentary System - Whole Body J Musculoskeletal System - Head and Neck K Musculoskeletal System - Upper Back/Upper Extremity L Musculoskeletal System - Lower Back/Lower Extremity M Musculoskeletal System - Whole Body	6 Therapeutic Exercise	B Physical Agents C Mechanical D Electrotherapeutic E Orthosis F Assistive, Adaptive, Supportive or Protective G Aerobic Endurance and Conditioning H Mechanical or Electromechanical U Prosthesis Y Other Equipment Z None	Z None

F07 Continued on next page

DRG Non-OR   All body system/region, type qualifier, equipment, and qualifier values

F   **Physical Rehabilitation and Diagnostic Audiology**
Ø   **Rehabilitation**
7   **Motor Treatment**   Definition: Exercise or activities to increase or facilitate motor function

F07 Continued

Body System/Region Character 4	Type Qualifier Character 5	Equipment Character 6	Qualifier Character 7
Ø Neurological System - Head and Neck 1 Neurological System - Upper Back/ Upper Extremity 2 Neurological System - Lower Back/ Lower Extremity 3 Neurological System - Whole Body D Integumentary System - Head and Neck F Integumentary System - Upper Back/Upper Extremity G Integumentary System - Lower Back/Lower Extremity H Integumentary System - Whole Body J Musculoskeletal System - Head and Neck K Musculoskeletal System - Upper Back/Upper Extremity L Musculoskeletal System - Lower Back/Lower Extremity M Musculoskeletal System - Whole Body	7 Manual Therapy Techniques	Z None	Z None
4 Circulatory System - Head and Neck 5 Circulatory System - Upper Back / Upper Extremity 6 Circulatory System - Lower Back / Lower Extremity 7 Circulatory System - Whole Body 8 Respiratory System - Head and Neck 9 Respiratory System - Upper Back / Upper Extremity B Respiratory System -Lower Back / Lower Extremity C Respiratory System -Whole Body	6 Therapeutic Exercise	B Physical Agents C Mechanical D Electrotherapeutic E Orthosis F Assistive, Adaptive, Supportive or Protective G Aerobic Endurance and Conditioning H Mechanical or Electromechanical U Prosthesis Y Other Equipment Z None	Z None
N Genitourinary System	1 Muscle Performance	E Orthosis F Assistive, Adaptive, Supportive or Protective U Prosthesis Y Other Equipment Z None	Z None
N Genitourinary System	6 Therapeutic Exercise	B Physical Agents C Mechanical D Electrotherapeutic E Orthosis F Assistive, Adaptive, Supportive or Protective G Aerobic Endurance and Conditioning H Mechanical or Electromechanical U Prosthesis Y Other Equipment Z None	Z None
Z None	4 Wheelchair Mobility	D Electrotherapeutic E Orthosis F Assistive, Adaptive, Supportive or Protective U Prosthesis Y Other Equipment Z None	Z None
Z None	5 Bed Mobility	C Mechanical E Orthosis F Assistive, Adaptive, Supportive or Protective U Prosthesis Y Other Equipment Z None	Z None

DRG Non-OR   All body system/region, type qualifier, equipment, and qualifier values

Physical Rehabilitation and Diagnostic Audiology

F07–F07

F Physical Rehabilitation and Diagnostic Audiology
Ø Rehabilitation
8 Activities of Daily Living Treatment   Definition: Exercise or activities to facilitate functional competence for activities of daily living

Body System/Region Character 4	Type Qualifier Character 5	Equipment Character 6	Qualifier Character 7
Z None	8 Transfer Training	C Mechanical D Electrotherapeutic E Orthosis F Assistive, Adaptive, Supportive or Protective U Prosthesis Y Other Equipment Z None	Z None
Z None	9 Gait Training/Functional Ambulation	C Mechanical D Electrotherapeutic E Orthosis F Assistive, Adaptive, Supportive or Protective G Aerobic Endurance and Conditioning U Prosthesis Y Other Equipment Z None	Z None
D Integumentary System - Head and Neck F Integumentary System - Upper Back/Upper Extremity G Integumentary System - Lower Back/Lower Extremity H Integumentary System - Whole Body J Musculoskeletal System - Head and Neck K Musculoskeletal System - Upper Back/Upper Extremity L Musculoskeletal System - Lower Back/Lower Extremity M Musculoskeletal System - Whole Body	5 Wound Management	B Physical Agents C Mechanical D Electrotherapeutic E Orthosis F Assistive, Adaptive, Supportive or Protective U Prosthesis Y Other Equipment Z None	Z None
Z None	Ø Bathing/Showering Techniques 1 Dressing Techniques 2 Grooming/Personal Hygiene	E Orthosis F Assistive, Adaptive, Supportive or Protective U Prosthesis Y Other Equipment Z None	Z None
Z None	3 Feeding/Eating	C Mechanical D Electrotherapeutic E Orthosis F Assistive, Adaptive, Supportive or Protective U Prosthesis Y Other Equipment Z None	Z None
Z None	4 Home Management	D Electrotherapeutic E Orthosis F Assistive, Adaptive, Supportive or Protective U Prosthesis Y Other Equipment Z None	Z None
Z None	6 Psychosocial Skills	Z None	Z None
Z None	7 Vocational Activities and Functional Community or Work Reintegration Skills	B Physical Agents C Mechanical D Electrotherapeutic E Orthosis F Assistive, Adaptive, Supportive or Protective G Aerobic Endurance and Conditioning U Prosthesis Y Other Equipment Z None	Z None

DRG Non-OR All body system/region, type qualifier, equipment, and qualifier values

F **Physical Rehabilitation and Diagnostic Audiology**
Ø **Rehabilitation**
9 **Hearing Treatment** Definition: Application of techniques to improve, augment, or compensate for hearing and related functional impairment

Body System/Region Character 4	Type Qualifier Character 5	Equipment Character 6	Qualifier Character 7
Z None	**Ø** Hearing and Related Disorders Counseling **1** Hearing and Related Disorders Prevention	**K** Audiovisual **Z** None	**Z** None
Z None	**2** Auditory Processing	**K** Audiovisual **L** Assistive Listening **P** Computer **Y** Other Equipment **Z** None	**Z** None
Z None	**3** Cerumen Management	**X** Cerumen Management **Z** None	**Z** None

DRG Non-OR All body system/region, type qualifier, equipment, and qualifier values

F **Physical Rehabilitation and Diagnostic Audiology**
Ø **Rehabilitation**
B **Cochlear Implant Treatment** Definition: Application of techniques to improve the communication abilities of individuals with cochlear implant

Body System/Region Character 4	Type Qualifier Character 5	Equipment Character 6	Qualifier Character 7
Z None	**Ø** Cochlear Implant Rehabilitation	**1** Audiometer **2** Sound Field / Booth **9** Cochlear Implant **K** Audiovisual **P** Computer **Y** Other Equipment	**Z** None

DRG Non-OR All body system/region, type qualifier, equipment, and qualifier values

F **Physical Rehabilitation and Diagnostic Audiology**
Ø **Rehabilitation**
C **Vestibular Treatment** Definition: Application of techniques to improve, augment, or compensate for vestibular and related functional impairment

Body System/Region Character 4	Type Qualifier Character 5	Equipment Character 6	Qualifier Character 7
3 Neurological System - Whole Body **H** Integumentary System - Whole Body **M** Musculoskeletal System - Whole Body	**3** Postural Control	**E** Orthosis **F** Assistive, Adaptive, Supportive or Protective **U** Prosthesis **Y** Other Equipment **Z** None	**Z** None
Z None	**Ø** Vestibular	**8** Vestibular / Balance **Z** None	**Z** None
Z None	**1** Perceptual Processing **2** Visual Motor Integration	**K** Audiovisual **L** Assistive Listening **N** Biosensory Feedback **P** Computer **Q** Speech Analysis **S** Voice Analysis **T** Aerodynamic Function **Y** Other Equipment **Z** None	**Z** None

DRG Non-OR All body system/region, type qualifier, equipment, and qualifier values

F   **Physical Rehabilitation and Diagnostic Audiology**
Ø   **Rehabilitation**
D   **Device Fitting**   Definition: Fitting of a device designed to facilitate or support achievement of a higher level of function

Body System/Region Character 4	Type Qualifier Character 5	Equipment Character 6	Qualifier Character 7
Z None	Ø Tinnitus Masker	5 Hearing Aid Selection / Fitting / Test Z None	Z None
Z None	1 Monaural Hearing Aid 2 Binaural Hearing Aid 5 Assistive Listening Device	1 Audiometer 2 Sound Field / Booth 5 Hearing Aid Selection / Fitting / Test K Audiovisual L Assistive Listening Z None	Z None
Z None	3 Augmentative/Alternative Communication System	M Augmentative / Alternative Communication	Z None
Z None	4 Voice Prosthetic	S Voice Analysis V Speech Prosthesis	Z None
Z None	6 Dynamic Orthosis 7 Static Orthosis 8 Prosthesis 9 Assistive, Adaptive, Supportive or Protective Devices	E Orthosis F Assistive, Adaptive, Supportive or Protective U Prosthesis Z None	Z None

DRG Non-OR	FØDZØ[5,Z]Z
DRG Non-OR	FØDZ[1, 2,5][1,2,5, K,L,Z]Z
DRG Non-OR	FØDZ3MZ
DRG Non-OR	FØDZ4[S,V]Z
DRG Non-OR	FØDZ[6,7][E,F,U,Z]Z
DRG Non-OR	FØDZ8[E,F,U]Z

F   **Physical Rehabilitation and Diagnostic Audiology**
Ø   **Rehabilitation**
F   **Caregiver Training**   Definition: Training in activities to support patient's optimal level of function

Body System/Region Character 4	Type Qualifier Character 5	Equipment Character 6	Qualifier Character 7
Z None	Ø Bathing/Showering Technique 1 Dressing 2 Feeding and Eating 3 Grooming/Personal Hygiene 4 Bed Mobility 5 Transfer 6 Wheelchair Mobility 7 Therapeutic Exercise 8 Airway Clearance Techniques 9 Wound Management B Vocational Activities and Functional Community or Work Reintegration Skills C Gait Training/Functional Ambulation D Application, Proper Use and Care of Devices F Application, Proper Use and Care of Orthoses G Application, Proper Use and Care of Prosthesis H Home Management	E Orthosis F Assistive, Adaptive, Supportive or Protective U Prosthesis Z None	Z None
Z None	J Communication Skills	K Audiovisual L Assistive Listening M Augmentative / Alternative Communication P Computer Z None	Z None

DRG Non-OR	All body system/region, type qualifier, equipment, and qualifier values

F   Physical Rehabilitation and Diagnostic Audiology
1   Diagnostic Audiology
3   Hearing Assessment   Definition: Measurement of hearing and related functions

Body System/Region Character 4	Type Qualifier Character 5	Equipment Character 6	Qualifier Character 7
Z None	Ø Hearing Screening	Ø Occupational Hearing 1 Audiometer 2 Sound Field / Booth 3 Tympanometer 8 Vestibular / Balance 9 Cochlear Implant Z None	Z None
Z None	1 Pure Tone Audiometry, Air 2 Pure Tone Audiometry, Air and Bone	Ø Occupational Hearing 1 Audiometer 2 Sound Field / Booth Z None	Z None
Z None	3 Bekesy Audiometry 6 Visual Reinforcement Audiometry 9 Short Increment Sensitivity Index B Stenger C Pure Tone Stenger	1 Audiometer 2 Sound Field / Booth Z None	Z None
Z None	4 Conditioned Play Audiometry 5 Select Picture Audiometry	1 Audiometer 2 Sound Field / Booth K Audiovisual Z None	Z None
Z None	7 Alternate Binaural or Monaural Loudness Balance	1 Audiometer K Audiovisual Z None	Z None
Z None	8 Tone Decay D Tympanometry F Eustachian Tube Function G Acoustic Reflex Patterns H Acoustic Reflex Threshold J Acoustic Reflex Decay	3 Tympanometer 4 Electroacoustic Immitance / Acoustic Reflex Z None	Z None
Z None	K Electrocochleography L Auditory Evoked Potentials	7 Electrophysiologic Z None	Z None
Z None	M Evoked Otoacoustic Emissions, Screening N Evoked Otoacoustic Emissions, Diagnostic	6 Otoacoustic Emission (OAE) Z None	Z None
Z None	P Aural Rehabilitation Status	1 Audiometer 2 Sound Field / Booth 4 Electroacoustic Immitance / Acoustic Reflex 9 Cochlear Implant K Audiovisual L Assistive Listening P Computer Z None	Z None
Z None	Q Auditory Processing	K Audiovisual P Computer Y Other Equipment Z None	Z None

F   **Physical Rehabilitation and Diagnostic Audiology**
1   **Diagnostic Audiology**
4   **Hearing Aid Assessment**   Definition: Measurement of the appropriateness and/or effectiveness of a hearing device

Body System/Region Character 4	Type Qualifier Character 5	Equipment Character 6	Qualifier Character 7
Z None	**Ø** Cochlear Implant	**1** Audiometer **2** Sound Field / Booth **3** Tympanometer **4** Electroacoustic Immitance / Acoustic Reflex **5** Hearing Aid Selection / Fitting / Test **7** Electrophysiologic **9** Cochlear Implant **K** Audiovisual **L** Assistive Listening **P** Computer **Y** Other Equipment **Z** None	**Z** None

Z None	**1** Ear Canal Probe Microphone
	6 Binaural Electroacoustic Hearing
	    Aid Check
	8 Monaural Electroacoustic Hearing
	    Aid Check
		5 Hearing Aid Selection / Fitting / Test
		Z None
			Z None

Z None	**2** Monaural Hearing Aid **3** Binaural Hearing Aid	**1** Audiometer **2** Sound Field / Booth **3** Tympanometer **4** Electroacoustic Immitance / Acoustic Reflex **5** Hearing Aid Selection / Fitting / Test **K** Audiovisual **L** Assistive Listening **P** Computer **Z** None	**Z** None

Z None	**4** Assistive Listening System/Device
	    Selection
		1 Audiometer
		2 Sound Field / Booth
		3 Tympanometer
		4 Electroacoustic Immitance /
		    Acoustic Reflex
		K Audiovisual
		L Assistive Listening
		Z None
			Z None

Z None	**5** Sensory Aids	**1** Audiometer **2** Sound Field / Booth **3** Tympanometer **4** Electroacoustic Immitance / Acoustic Reflex **5** Hearing Aid Selection / Fitting / Test **K** Audiovisual **L** Assistive Listening **Z** None	**Z** None
Z None	**7** Ear Protector Attentuation	**Ø** Occupational Hearing **Z** None	**Z** None

F   **Physical Rehabilitation and Diagnostic Audiology**
1   **Diagnostic Audiology**
5   **Vestibular Assessment**   Definition: Measurement of the vestibular system and related functions

Body System/Region Character 4	Type Qualifier Character 5	Equipment Character 6	Qualifier Character 7

Z None	**Ø** Bithermal, Binaural Caloric
	    Irrigation
	1 Bithermal, Monaural Caloric
	    Irrigation
	2 Unithermal Binaural Screen
	3 Oscillating Tracking
	4 Sinusoidal Vertical Axis Rotational
	5 Dix-Hallpike Dynamic
	6 Computerized Dynamic
	    Posturography
		8 Vestibular / Balance
		Z None
			Z None

Z None	**7** Tinnitus Masker	**5** Hearing Aid Selection / Fitting / Test **Z** None	**Z** None

Mental Health GZ1–GZJ

G Mental Health
Z None
1 Psychological Tests   Definition: The administration and interpretation of standardized psychological tests and measurement instruments for the assessment of psychological function

Qualifier Character 4	Qualifier Character 5	Qualifier Character 6	Qualifier Character 7
Ø Developmental 1 Personality and Behavioral 2 Intellectual and Psychoeducational 3 Neuropsychological 4 Neurobehavioral and Cognitive Status	Z None	Z None	Z None

G Mental Health
Z None
2 Crisis Intervention   Definition: Treatment of a traumatized, acutely disturbed or distressed individual for the purpose of short-term stabilization

Qualifier Character 4	Qualifier Character 5	Qualifier Character 6	Qualifier Character 7
Z None	Z None	Z None	Z None

G Mental Health
Z None
3 Medication Management   Definition: Monitoring and adjusting the use of medications for the treatment of a mental health disorder

Qualifier Character 4	Qualifier Character 5	Qualifier Character 6	Qualifier Character 7
Z None	Z None	Z None	Z None

G Mental Health
Z None
5 Individual Psychotherapy   Definition: Treatment of an individual with a mental health disorder by behavioral, cognitive, psychoanalytic, psychodynamic or psychophysiological means to improve functioning or well-being

Qualifier Character 4	Qualifier Character 5	Qualifier Character 6	Qualifier Character 7
Ø Interactive 1 Behavioral 2 Cognitive 3 Interpersonal 4 Psychoanalysis 5 Psychodynamic 6 Supportive 8 Cognitive-Behavioral 9 Psychophysiological	Z None	Z None	Z None

G Mental Health
Z None
6 Counseling   Definition: The application of psychological methods to treat an individual with normal developmental issues and psychological problems in order to increase function, improve well-being, alleviate distress, maladjustment or resolve crises

Qualifier Character 4	Qualifier Character 5	Qualifier Character 6	Qualifier Character 7
Ø Educational 1 Vocational 3 Other Counseling	Z None	Z None	Z None

G Mental Health
Z None
7 Family Psychotherapy Definition: Treatment that includes one or more family members of an individual with a mental health disorder by behavioral, cognitive, psychoanalytic, psychodynamic or psychophysiological means to improve functioning or well-being

Explanation: Remediation of emotional or behavioral problems presented by one or more family members in cases where psychotherapy with more than one family member is indicated

Qualifier Character 4	Qualifier Character 5	Qualifier Character 6	Qualifier Character 7
2 Other Family Psychotherapy	Z None	Z None	Z None

Mental Health

G   **Mental Health**
Z   **None**
B   **Electroconvulsive Therapy**   Definition: The application of controlled electrical voltages to treat a mental health disorder

Qualifier Character 4	Qualifier Character 5	Qualifier Character 6	Qualifier Character 7
Ø Unilateral-Single Seizure 1 Unilateral-Multiple Seizure 2 Bilateral-Single Seizure 3 Bilateral-Multiple Seizure 4 Other Electroconvulsive Therapy	Z None	Z None	Z None

G   **Mental Health**
Z   **None**
C   **Biofeedback**   Definition: Provision of information from the monitoring and regulating of physiological processes in conjunction with cognitive-behavioral techniques to improve patient functioning or well-being

Qualifier Character 4	Qualifier Character 5	Qualifier Character 6	Qualifier Character 7
9 Other Biofeedback	Z None	Z None	Z None

G   **Mental Health**
Z   **None**
F   **Hypnosis**   Definition: Induction of a state of heightened suggestibility by auditory, visual and tactile techniques to elicit an emotional or behavioral response

Qualifier Character 4	Qualifier Character 5	Qualifier Character 6	Qualifier Character 7
Z None	Z None	Z None	Z None

G   **Mental Health**
Z   **None**
G   **Narcosynthesis**   Definition: Administration of intravenous barbiturates in order to release suppressed or repressed thoughts

Qualifier Character 4	Qualifier Character 5	Qualifier Character 6	Qualifier Character 7
Z None	Z None	Z None	Z None

G   **Mental Health**
Z   **None**
H   **Group Psychotherapy**   Definition: Treatment of two or more individuals with a mental health disorder by behavioral, cognitive, psychoanalytic, psychodynamic or psychophysiological means to improve functioning or well-being

Qualifier Character 4	Qualifier Character 5	Qualifier Character 6	Qualifier Character 7
Z None	Z None	Z None	Z None

G   **Mental Health**
Z   **None**
J   **Light Therapy**   Definition: Application of specialized light treatments to improve functioning or well-being

Qualifier Character 4	Qualifier Character 5	Qualifier Character 6	Qualifier Character 7
Z None	Z None	Z None	Z None

Substance Abuse Treatment HZ2–HZ9

H   **Substance Abuse Treatment**
Z   **None**
2   **Detoxification Services**   Definition: Detoxification from alcohol and/or drugs

Explanation: Not a treatment modality, but helps the patient stabilize physically and psychologically until the body becomes free of drugs and the effects of alcohol

Qualifier Character 4	Qualifier Character 5	Qualifier Character 6	Qualifier Character 7
Z None	Z None	Z None	Z None

H   **Substance Abuse Treatment**
Z   **None**
3   **Individual Counseling**   Definition: The application of psychological methods to treat an individual with addictive behavior

Explanation: Comprised of several different techniques, which apply various strategies to address drug addiction

Qualifier Character 4	Qualifier Character 5	Qualifier Character 6	Qualifier Character 7
Ø Cognitive 1 Behavioral 2 Cognitive-Behavioral 3 12-Step 4 Interpersonal 5 Vocational 6 Psychoeducation 7 Motivational Enhancement 8 Confrontational 9 Continuing Care B Spiritual C Pre/Post-Test Infectious Disease	Z None	Z None	Z None

DRG Non-OR   HZ3[Ø,1,2,3,4,5,6,7,8,9,B]ZZZ

H   **Substance Abuse Treatment**
Z   **None**
4   **Group Counseling**   Definition: The application of psychological methods to treat two or more individuals with addictive behavior

Explanation: Provides structured group counseling sessions and healing power through the connection with others

Qualifier Character 4	Qualifier Character 5	Qualifier Character 6	Qualifier Character 7
Ø Cognitive 1 Behavioral 2 Cognitive-Behavioral 3 12-Step 4 Interpersonal 5 Vocational 6 Psychoeducation 7 Motivational Enhancement 8 Confrontational 9 Continuing Care B Spiritual C Pre/Post-Test Infectious Disease	Z None	Z None	Z None

DRG Non-OR   HZ4[Ø,1,2,3,4,5,6,7,8,9,B]ZZZ

H   **Substance Abuse Treatment**
Z   **None**
5   **Individual Psychotherapy**   Definition: Treatment of an individual with addictive behavior by behavioral, cognitive, psychoanalytic, psychodynamic or psychophysiological means

Qualifier Character 4	Qualifier Character 5	Qualifier Character 6	Qualifier Character 7
Ø Cognitive 1 Behavioral 2 Cognitive-Behavioral 3 12-Step 4 Interpersonal 5 Interactive 6 Psychoeducation 7 Motivational Enhancement 8 Confrontational 9 Supportive B Psychoanalysis C Psychodynamic D Psychophysiological	Z None	Z None	Z None

DRG Non-OR   For all qualifier values

LC Limited Coverage   **NC** Noncovered   ⊞ Combination Member   **HAC**   Valid OR   Combination Only   DRG Non-OR   New/Revised in GREEN

ICD-10-PCS 2020   **793**

H   **Substance Abuse Treatment**
Z   **None**
6   **Family Counseling**   Definition: The application of psychological methods that includes one or more family members to treat an individual with addictive behavior

Explanation: Provides support and education for family members of addicted individuals. Family member participation is seen as a critical area of substance abuse treatment

Qualifier Character 4	Qualifier Character 5	Qualifier Character 6	Qualifier Character 7
3 Other Family Counseling	**Z** None	**Z** None	**Z** None

H   **Substance Abuse Treatment**
Z   **None**
8   **Medication Management**   Definition: Monitoring or adjusting the use of replacement medications for the treatment of addiction

Qualifier Character 4	Qualifier Character 5	Qualifier Character 6	Qualifier Character 7
0 Nicotine Replacement **1** Methadone Maintenance **2** Levo-alpha-acetyl-methadol (LAAM) **3** Antabuse **4** Naltrexone **5** Naloxone **6** Clonidine **7** Bupropion **8** Psychiatric Medication **9** Other Replacement Medication	**Z** None	**Z** None	**Z** None

H   **Substance Abuse Treatment**
Z   **None**
9   **Pharmacotherapy**   Definition: The use of replacement medications for the treatment of addiction

Qualifier Character 4	Qualifier Character 5	Qualifier Character 6	Qualifier Character 7
0 Nicotine Replacement **1** Methadone Maintenance **2** Levo-alpha-acetyl-methadol (LAAM) **3** Antabuse **4** Naltrexone **5** Naloxone **6** Clonidine **7** Bupropion **8** Psychiatric Medication **9** Other Replacement Medication	**Z** None	**Z** None	**Z** None

New Technology X27–XYØ

AHA Coding Clinic for all tables in the New Technology Section
2015, 4Q, 8-11

AHA Coding Clinic for table X2A
2016, 4Q, 115-116   Cerebral embolic filtration

AHA Coding Clinic for table X2C
2016, 4Q, 82-83   Coronary artery, number of arteries
2015, 4Q, 8-14   New Section X codes—New Technology procedures

AHA Coding Clinic for table X2R
2016, 4Q, 116   Aortic valve rapid deployment
2015, 4Q, 8-12   New Section X codes—New Technology procedures

AHA Coding Clinic for table XHR
2016, 4Q, 116   Application of wound matrix

AHA Coding Clinic for table XKØ
2017, 4Q, 74   Intramuscular autologous bone marrow cell therapy

AHA Coding Clinic for table XNS
2017, 4Q, 74-75   Magnetic growth rods
2016, 4Q, 117   Placement of magnetic growth rods

AHA Coding Clinic for table XRG
2017, 4Q, 76   Radiolucent porous interbody fusion device

AHA Coding Clinic for table XV5
2018, 4Q, 55   Robotic waterjet ablation

AHA Coding Clinic for table XWØ
2018, 4Q, 56   New therapeutic substances
2015, 4Q, 8-15   New Section X codes—New Technology procedures

AHA Coding Clinic for table XYØ
2017, 4Q, 78   Intraoperative treatment of vascular grafts

X   **New Technology**
2   **Cardiovascular System**
7   **Dilation**   Definition: Expanding an orifice or the lumen of a tubular body part

Explanation: The orifice can be a natural orifice or an artificially created orifice. Accomplished by stretching a tubular body part using intraluminal pressure or by cutting part of the orifice or wall of the tubular body part.

Body Part Character 4	Approach Character 5	Device/Substance/Technology Character 6	Qualifier Character 7
H Femoral Artery, Right J Femoral Artery, Left K Popliteal Artery, Proximal Right L Popliteal Artery, Proximal Left M Popliteal Artery, Distal Right N Popliteal Artery, Distal Left P Anterior Tibial Artery, Right Q Anterior Tibial Artery, Left R Posterior Tibial Artery, Right S Posterior Tibial Artery, Left T Peroneal Artery, Right U Peroneal Artery, Left	3 Percutaneous	8 Intraluminal Device, Sustained Release Drug-eluting 9 Intraluminal Device, Sustained Release Drug-eluting, Two B Intraluminal Device, Sustained Release Drug-eluting, Three C Intraluminal Device, Sustained Release Drug-eluting, Four or More	5 New Technology Group 5

X   **New Technology**
2   **Cardiovascular System**
A   **Assistance**   Definition: Taking over a portion of a physiological function by extracorporeal means

Explanation: None

Body Part Character 4	Approach Character 5	Device/Substance/Technology Character 6	Qualifier Character 7
5 Innominate Artery and Left Common Carotid Artery	3 Percutaneous	1 Cerebral Embolic Filtration, Dual Filter	2 New Technology Group 2
6 Aortic Arch	3 Percutaneous	2 Cerebral Embolic Filtration, Single Deflection Filter	5 New Technology Group 5

X   **New Technology**
2   **Cardiovascular System**
C   **Extirpation**   Definition: Taking or cutting out solid matter from a body part

Explanation: The solid matter may be an abnormal byproduct of a biological function or a foreign body; it may be imbedded in a body part or in the lumen of a tubular body part. The solid matter may or may not have been previously broken into pieces.

Body Part Character 4	Approach Character 5	Device/Substance/Technology Character 6	Qualifier Character 7
Ø Coronary Artery, One Artery 1 Coronary Artery, Two Arteries 2 Coronary Artery, Three Arteries 3 Coronary Artery, Four or More Arteries	3 Percutaneous	6 Orbital Atherectomy Technology	1 New Technology Group 1

Valid OR   All body part, approach, device/substance/technology, and qualifier values

[LC] Limited Coverage   [NC] Noncovered   ⊞ Combination Member   HAC   Valid OR   Combination Only   DRG Non-OR   New/Revised in GREEN
ICD-10-PCS 2020   795

X27–X2C

X **New Technology**
2 **Cardiovascular System**
R **Replacement** Definition: Putting in or on biological or synthetic material that physically takes the place and/or function of all or a portion of a body part

Explanation: The body part may have been taken out or replaced, or may be taken out, physically eradicated, or rendered nonfunctional during the REPLACEMENT procedure. A REMOVAL procedure is coded for taking out the device used in a previous replacement procedure

Body Part Character 4	Approach Character 5	Device/Substance/Technology Character 6	Qualifier Character 7
F Aortic Valve	**Ø** Open **3** Percutaneous **4** Percutaneous Endoscopic	**3** Zooplastic Tissue, Rapid Deployment Technique	**2** New Technology Group 2

Valid OR All body part, approach, device/substance/technology, and qualifier values

---

X **New Technology**
H **Skin, Subcutaneous Tissue, Fascia and Breast**
R **Replacement** Definition: Putting in or on biological or synthetic material that physically takes the place and/or function of all or a portion of a body part

Explanation: The body part may have been taken out or replaced, or may be taken out, physically eradicated, or rendered nonfunctional during the REPLACEMENT procedure. A REMOVAL procedure is coded for taking out the device used in a previous replacement procedure

Body Part Character 4	Approach Character 5	Device/Substance/Technology Character 6	Qualifier Character 7
P Skin	**X** External	**L** Skin Substitute, Porcine Liver Derived	**2** New Technology Group 2

Valid OR All body part, approach, device/substance/technology, and qualifier values

---

X **New Technology**
K **Muscles, Tendons, Bursae and Ligaments**
Ø **Introduction** Definition: Putting in or on a therapeutic, diagnostic, nutritional, physiological, or prophylactic substance except blood or blood products

Explanation: None

Body Part Character 4	Approach Character 5	Device/Substance/Technology Character 6	Qualifier Character 7
2 Muscle	**3** Percutaneous	**Ø** Concentrated Bone Marrow Aspirate	**3** New Technology Group 3

X **New Technology**
N **Bones**
S **Reposition** Definition: Moving to its normal location, or other suitable location, all or a portion of a body part

Explanation: The body part is moved to a new location from an abnormal location, or from a normal location where it is not functioning correctly. The body part may or may not be cut out or off to be moved to the new location.

Body Part Character 4	Approach Character 5	Device/Substance/Technology Character 6	Qualifier Character 7
Ø Lumbar Vertebra **3** Cervical Vertebra **4** Thoracic Vertebra	**Ø** Open **3** Percutaneous	**3** Magnetically Controlled Growth Rod(s)	**2** New Technology Group 2

Valid OR All body part, approach, device/substance/technology, and qualifier values

---

X **New Technology**
R **Joints**
2 **Monitoring** Definition: Determining the level of a physiological or physical function repetitively over a period of time

Explanation: None

Body Part Character 4	Approach Character 5	Device/Substance/Technology Character 6	Qualifier Character 7
G Knee Joint, Right **H** Knee Joint, Left	**Ø** Open	**2** Intraoperative Knee Replacement Sensor	**1** New Technology Group 1

Valid OR All body part, approach, device/substance/technology, and qualifier values

LC Limited Coverage   **NC** Noncovered   ⊞ Combination Member   HAC   Valid OR   Combination Only   DRG Non-OR   New/Revised in GREEN

796   ICD-10-PCS 2020

X   **New Technology**
R   **Joints**
G   **Fusion**   Definition: Joining together portions of an articular body part rendering the articular body part immobile
               Explanation: The body part is joined together by fixation device, bone graft, or other means

Body Part Character 4	Approach Character 5	Device/Substance/Technology Character 6	Qualifier Character 7
Ø Occipital-cervical Joint	**Ø** Open	**9** Interbody Fusion Device, Nanotextured Surface	**2** New Technology Group 2
Ø Occipital-cervical Joint	**Ø** Open	**F** Interbody Fusion Device, Radiolucent Porous	**3** New Technology Group 3
1 Cervical Vertebral Joint	**Ø** Open	**9** Interbody Fusion Device, Nanotextured Surface	**2** New Technology Group 2
1 Cervical Vertebral Joint	**Ø** Open	**F** Interbody Fusion Device, Radiolucent Porous	**3** New Technology Group 3
2 Cervical Vertebral Joints, 2 or more	**Ø** Open	**9** Interbody Fusion Device, Nanotextured Surface	**2** New Technology Group 2
2 Cervical Vertebral Joints, 2 or more	**Ø** Open	**F** Interbody Fusion Device, Radiolucent Porous	**3** New Technology Group 3
4 Cervicothoracic Vertebral Joint	**Ø** Open	**9** Interbody Fusion Device, Nanotextured Surface	**2** New Technology Group 2
4 Cervicothoracic Vertebral Joint	**Ø** Open	**F** Interbody Fusion Device, Radiolucent Porous	**3** New Technology Group 3
6 Thoracic Vertebral Joint	**Ø** Open	**9** Interbody Fusion Device, Nanotextured Surface	**2** New Technology Group 2
6 Thoracic Vertebral Joint	**Ø** Open	**F** Interbody Fusion Device, Radiolucent Porous	**3** New Technology Group 3
7 Thoracic Vertebral Joints, 2 to 7 ⊞	**Ø** Open	**9** Interbody Fusion Device, Nanotextured Surface	**2** New Technology Group 2
7 Thoracic Vertebral Joints, 2 to 7 ⊞	**Ø** Open	**F** Interbody Fusion Device, Radiolucent Porous	**3** New Technology Group 3
8 Thoracic Vertebral Joints, 8 or more	**Ø** Open	**9** Interbody Fusion Device, Nanotextured Surface	**2** New Technology Group 2
8 Thoracic Vertebral Joints, 8 or more	**Ø** Open	**F** Interbody Fusion Device, Radiolucent Porous	**3** New Technology Group 3
A Thoracolumbar Vertebral Joint	**Ø** Open	**9** Interbody Fusion Device, Nanotextured Surface	**2** New Technology Group 2
A Thoracolumbar Vertebral Joint	**Ø** Open	**F** Interbody Fusion Device, Radiolucent Porous	**3** New Technology Group 3
B Lumbar Vertebral Joint	**Ø** Open	**9** Interbody Fusion Device, Nanotextured Surface	**2** New Technology Group 2
B Lumbar Vertebral Joint	**Ø** Open	**F** Interbody Fusion Device, Radiolucent Porous	**3** New Technology Group 3
C Lumbar Vertebral Joints, 2 or more ⊞	**Ø** Open	**9** Interbody Fusion Device, Nanotextured Surface	**2** New Technology Group 2
C Lumbar Vertebral Joints, 2 or more ⊞	**Ø** Open	**F** Interbody Fusion Device, Radiolucent Porous	**3** New Technology Group 3
D Lumbosacral Joint	**Ø** Open	**9** Interbody Fusion Device, Nanotextured Surface	**2** New Technology Group 2
D Lumbosacral Joint	**Ø** Open	**F** Interbody Fusion Device, Radiolucent Porous	**3** New Technology Group 3

Valid OR   All body part, approach, device/substance/technology, and qualifier values
HAC   XRG[Ø,1,2,4,6,7,8,A,B,C,D]Ø92 when reported with SDx K68.11 or
          T81.4Ø–T81.49, T84.6Ø-T84.619, T84.63-T84.7 with 7th character A
HAC   XRG[Ø,1,2,4,6,7,8,A,B,C,D]ØF3 when reported with SDx K68.11 or
          T81.4Ø–T81.49, T84.6Ø-T84.619, T84.63-T84.7 with 7th character A

See Appendix L for Procedure Combinations
⊞   XRG7Ø92
⊞   XRG7ØF3
⊞   XRGCØ92
⊞   XRGCØF3

X   **New Technology**
T   **Urinary System**
2   **Monitoring**   Definition: Determining the level of a physiological or physical function repetitively over a period of time
               Explanation: None

Body Part Character 4	Approach Character 5	Device/Substance/Technology Character 6	Qualifier Character 7
5 Kidney	**X** External	**E** Fluorescent Pyrazine	**5** New Technology Group 5

X   **New Technology**
V   **Male Reproductive System**
5   **Destruction**   Definition: Physical eradication of all or a portion of a body part by the direct use of energy, force, or a destructive agent
               Explanation: None of the body part is physically taken out

Body Part Character 4	Approach Character 5	Device/Substance/Technology Character 6	Qualifier Character 7
Ø Prostate	**8** Via Natural or Artificial Opening Endoscopic	**A** Robotic Waterjet Ablation	**4** New Technology Group 4

Valid OR   XV5Ø8A4

🄛🄖 Limited Coverage   🄝🄒 Noncovered   ⊞ Combination Member   HAC   Valid OR   Combination Only   DRG Non-OR   New/Revised in GREEN
ICD-10-PCS 2020   797

XRG–XV5

New Technology

X	**New Technology**
W	**Anatomical Regions**
Ø	**Introduction**

Definition: Putting in or on a therapeutic, diagnostic, nutritional, physiological, or prophylactic substance except blood or blood products

Explanation: None

Body Part Character 4	Approach Character 5	Device/Substance/Technology Character 6	Qualifier Character 7
1 Subcutaneous Tissue	**3** Percutaneous	**W** Caplacizumab	**5** New Technology Group 5
3 Peripheral Vein	**3** Percutaneous	**2** Ceftazidime-Avibactam Anti-infective **3** Idarucizumab, Dabigatran Reversal Agent **4** Isavuconazole Anti- infective **5** Blinatumomab Antineoplastic Immunotherapy	**1** New Technology Group 1
3 Peripheral Vein	**3** Percutaneous	**7** Coagulation Factor Xa, Inactivated **9** Defibrotide Sodium Anticoagulant	**2** New Technology Group 2
3 Peripheral Vein	**3** Percutaneous	**A** Bezlotoxumab Monoclonal Antibody **B** Cytarabine and Daunorubicin Liposome Antineoplastic **C** Engineered Autologous Chimeric Antigen Receptor T-cell Immunotherapy **F** Other New Technology Therapeutic Substance	**3** New Technology Group 3
3 Peripheral Vein	**3** Percutaneous	**G** Plazomicin Anti-infective **H** Synthetic Human Angiotensin II	**4** New Technology Group 4
3 Peripheral Vein	**3** Percutaneous	**K** Fosfomycin Anti-infective **N** Meropenem-vaborbactam Anti-infective **Q** Tagraxofusp-erzs Antineoplastic **S** Iobenguane I-131 Antineoplastic **U** Imipenem-cilastatin-relebactam Anti-infective **W** Caplacizumab	**5** New Technology Group 5
4 Central Vein	**3** Percutaneous	**2** Ceftazidime-Avibactam Anti-infective **3** Idarucizumab, Dabigatran Reversal Agent **4** Isavuconazole Anti- infective **5** Blinatumomab Antineoplastic Immunotherapy	**1** New Technology Group 1
4 Central Vein	**3** Percutaneous	**7** Coagulation Factor Xa, Inactivated **9** Defibrotide Sodium Anticoagulant	**2** New Technology Group 2
4 Central Vein	**3** Percutaneous	**A** Bezlotoxumab Monoclonal Antibody **B** Cytarabine and Daunorubicin Liposome Antineoplastic **C** Engineered Autologous Chimeric Antigen Receptor T-cell Immunotherapy **F** Other New Technology Therapeutic Substance	**3** New Technology Group 3
4 Central Vein	**3** Percutaneous	**G** Plazomicin Anti-infective **H** Synthetic Human Angiotensin II	**4** New Technology Group 4
4 Central Vein	**3** Percutaneous	**K** Fosfomycin Anti-infective **N** Meropenem-vaborbactam Anti-infective **Q** Tagraxofusp-erzs Antineoplastic **S** Iobenguane I-131 Antineoplastic **U** Imipenem-cilastatin-relebactam Anti-infective **W** Caplacizumab	**5** New Technology Group 5
D Mouth and Pharynx	**X** External	**8** Uridine Triacetate	**2** New Technology Group 2
D Mouth and Pharynx	**X** External	**J** Apalutamide Antineoplastic **L** Erdafitinib Antineoplastic **R** Venetoclax Antineoplastic **T** Ruxolitinib **V** Gilteritinib Antineoplastic	**5** New Technology Group 5

DRG Non-OR XWØ33C3
DRG Non-OR XWØ43C3

LC Limited Coverage   NC Noncovered   ⊞ Combination Member   HAC   Valid OR   Combination Only   DRG Non-OR   New/Revised in GREEN

X   **New Technology**
X   **Physiological Systems**
E   **Measurement**   Definition: Determining the level of a physiological or physical function at a point in time
                         Explanation: None

Body Part Character 4	Approach Character 5	Device/Substance/Technology Character 6	Qualifier Character 7
5 Circulatory	X External	M Infection, Whole Blood Nucleic Acid-base Microbial Detection	5 New Technology Group 5

X   **New Technology**
Y   **Extracorporeal**
Ø   **Introduction**   Definition: Putting in or on a therapeutic, diagnostic, nutritional, physiological, or prophylactic substance except blood or blood products
                      Explanation: None

Body Part Character 4	Approach Character 5	Device/Substance/Technology Character 6	Qualifier Character 7
V Vein Graft	X External	8 Endothelial Damage Inhibitor	3 New Technology Group 3

Appendixes

Appendix A: Components of the Medical and Surgical Approach Definitions

ICD-10-PCS Value	Definition	Access Location	Method	Type of Instrumentation	Example
Open (Ø)	Cutting through the skin or mucous membrane and any other body layers necessary to expose the site of the procedure	Skin or mucous membrane, any other body layers	Cutting	None	Abdominal hysterectomy
Percutaneous (3)	Entry, by puncture or minor incision, of instrumentation through the skin or mucous membrane and any other body layers necessary to reach the site of the procedure	Skin or mucous membrane, any other body layers	Puncture or minor incision	Without visualization	Needle biopsy of liver, Liposuction
Percutaneous endoscopic (4)	Entry, by puncture or minor incision, of instrumentation through the skin or mucous membrane and any other body layers necessary to reach and visualize the site of the procedure	Skin or mucous membrane, any other body layers	Puncture or minor incision	With visualization	Arthroscopy, Laparoscopic cholecystectomy
Via natural or artificial opening (7)	Entry of instrumentation through a natural or artificial external opening to reach the site of the procedure	Natural or artificial external opening	Direct entry	Without visualization	Endotracheal tube insertion, Foley catheter placement
Via natural or artificial opening endoscopic (8)	Entry of instrumentation through a natural or artificial external opening to reach and visualize the site of the procedure	Natural or artificial external opening	Direct entry	With visualization	Sigmoidoscopy, EGD, ERCP
Via natural or artificial opening with percutaneous endoscopic assistance (F)	Entry of instrumentation through a natural or artificial external opening and entry, by puncture or minor incision, of instrumentation through the skin or mucous membrane and any other body layers necessary to aid in the performance of the procedure	Skin or mucous membrane, any other body layers	Direct entry with puncture or minor incision for instrumentation only	With visualization	Laparoscopic-assisted vaginal hysterectomy
External (X)	Procedures performed directly on the skin or mucous membrane and procedures performed indirectly by the application of external force through the skin or mucous membrane	Skin or mucous membrane	Direct or indirect application	None	Closed fracture reduction, Resection of tonsils

Open (Ø)

Percutaneous (3)

Percutaneous Endoscopic (4)

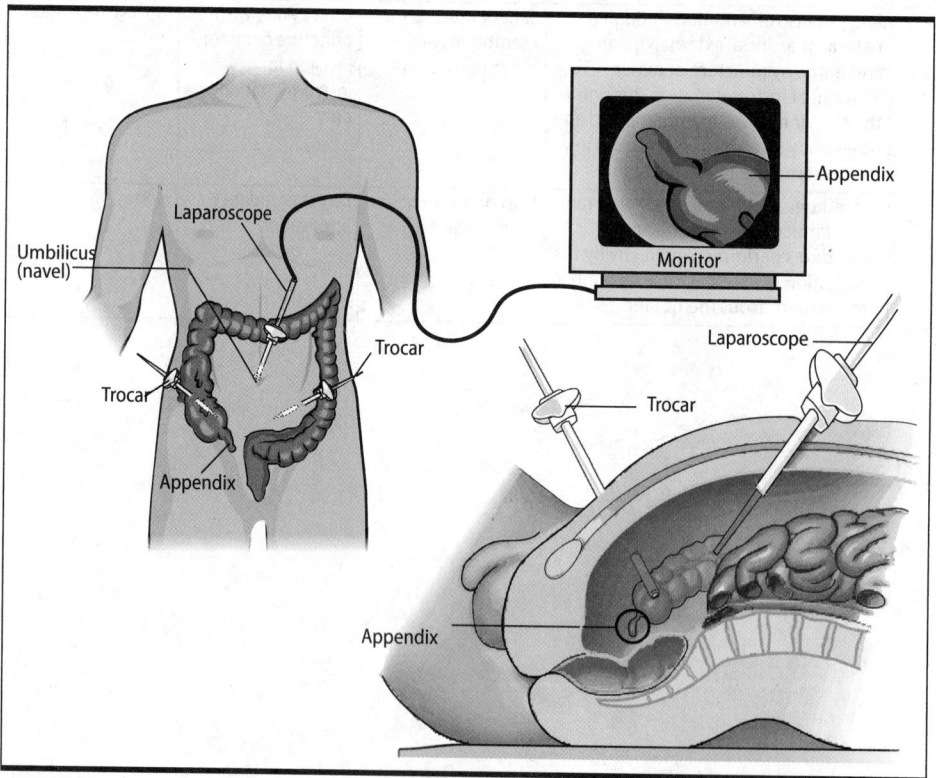

Via Natural or Artificial Opening (7)

Via Natural or Artificial Opening, Endoscopic (8)

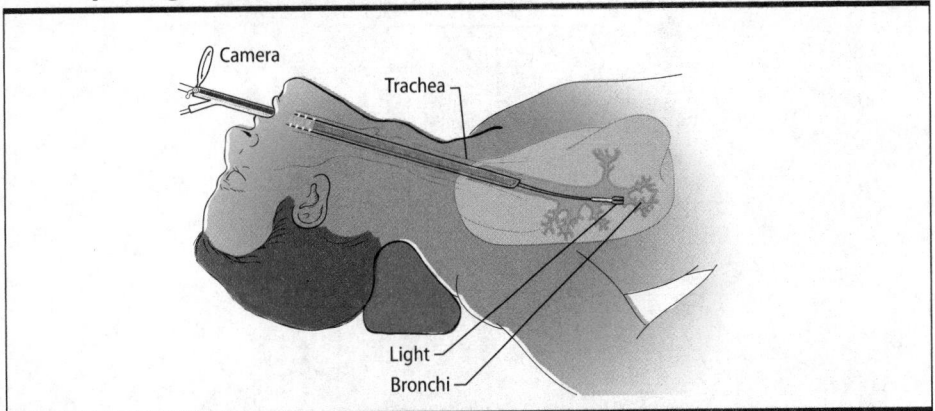

Via Natural or Artificial Opening with Percutaneous Endoscopic Assistance (F)

External (X)

Via Natural or Artificial Opening (7)

Via Natural or Artificial Opening Endoscopic (8)

Via Natural or Artificial Opening with Percutaneous Endoscopic Assistance (F)

Appendix B: Root Operation Definitions

The character 3 value in the Medical and Surgical section (Ø) and the Medical and Surgical-related sections (1-9) represents the root operation. This resource provides each root operation (character 3) value, found in sections Ø-9, as well as their associated definition, explanation, and examples, where applicable. The Ancillary sections (B-H) do not include root operations; instead the character 3 value represents the type of procedure performed with additional detail provided by the character 4 or 5 value, when applicable. For the character 3, character 4, and character 5 values used in the Ancillary sections of B-H, along with their definitions, see appendix I.

Ø	Medical and Surgical		
ICD-10-PCS Value		**Definition**	
Ø	Alteration	Definition:	Modifying the anatomic structure of a body part without affecting the function of the body part
		Explanation:	Principal purpose is to improve appearance
		Examples:	Face lift, breast augmentation
1	Bypass	Definition:	Altering the route of passage of the contents of a tubular body part
		Explanation:	Rerouting contents of a body part to a downstream area of the normal route, to a similar route and body part, or to an abnormal route and dissimilar body part. Includes one or more anastomoses, with or without the use of a device.
		Examples:	Coronary artery bypass, colostomy formation
2	Change	Definition:	Taking out or off a device from a body part and putting back an identical or similar device in or on the same body part without cutting or puncturing the skin or a mucous membrane
		Explanation:	All CHANGE procedures are coded using the approach EXTERNAL
		Example:	Urinary catheter change, gastrostomy tube change
3	Control	Definition:	Stopping, or attempting to stop, postprocedural or other acute bleeding
		Explanation:	None
		Examples:	Control of post-prostatectomy hemorrhage, control of intracranial subdural hemorrhage, control of bleeding duodenal ulcer, control of retroperitoneal hemorrhage
4	Creation	Definition:	Putting in or on biological or synthetic material to form a new body part that to the extent possible replicates the anatomic structure or function of an absent body part
		Explanation:	Used for gender reassignment surgery and corrective procedures in individuals with congenital anomalies
		Examples:	Creation of vagina in a male, creation of right and left atrioventricular valve from common atrioventricular valve
5	Destruction	Definition:	Physical eradication of all or a portion of a body part by the direct use of energy, force, or a destructive agent
		Explanation:	None of the body part is physically taken out
		Examples:	Fulguration of rectal polyp, cautery of skin lesion
6	Detachment	Definition:	Cutting off all or a portion of the upper or lower extremities
		Explanation:	The body part value is the site of the detachment, with a qualifier if applicable to further specify the level where the extremity was detached
		Examples:	Below knee amputation, disarticulation of shoulder
7	Dilation	Definition:	Expanding an orifice or the lumen of a tubular body part
		Explanation:	The orifice can be a natural orifice or an artificially created orifice. Accomplished by stretching a tubular body part using intraluminal pressure or by cutting part of the orifice or wall of the tubular body part.
		Examples:	Percutaneous transluminal angioplasty, internal urethrotomy
8	Division	Definition:	Cutting into a body part, without draining fluids and/or gases from the body part, in order to separate or transect a body part
		Explanation:	All or a portion of the body part is separated into two or more portions
		Examples:	Spinal cordotomy, osteotomy
9	Drainage	Definition:	Taking or letting out fluids and/or gases from a body part
		Explanation:	The qualifier DIAGNOSTIC is used to identify drainage procedures that are biopsies
		Examples:	Thoracentesis, incision and drainage
B	Excision	Definition:	Cutting out or off, without replacement, a portion of a body part
		Explanation:	The qualifier DIAGNOSTIC is used to identify excision procedures that are biopsies
		Examples:	Partial nephrectomy, liver biopsy

Continued on next page

Ø	**Medical and Surgical**		*Continued from previous page*
ICD-10-PCS Value			**Definition**
C	Extirpation	Definition:	Taking or cutting out solid matter from a body part
		Explanation:	The solid matter may be an abnormal byproduct of a biological function or a foreign body; it may be imbedded in a body part or in the lumen of a tubular body part. The solid matter may or may not have been previously broken into pieces.
		Examples:	Thrombectomy, choledocholithotomy
D	Extraction	Definition:	Pulling or stripping out or off all or a portion of a body part by the use of force
		Explanation:	The qualifier DIAGNOSTIC is used to identify extractions that are biopsies
		Examples:	Dilation and curettage, vein stripping
F	Fragmentation	Definition:	Breaking solid matter in a body part into pieces
		Explanation:	Physical force (e.g., manual, ultrasonic) applied directly or indirectly is used to break the solid matter into pieces. The solid matter may be an abnormal byproduct of a biological function or a foreign body. The pieces of solid matter are not taken out.
		Examples:	Extracorporeal shockwave lithotripsy, transurethral lithotripsy
G	Fusion	Definition:	Joining together portions of an articular body part rendering the articular body part immobile
		Explanation:	The body part is joined together by fixation device, bone graft, or other means
		Examples:	Spinal fusion, ankle arthrodesis
H	Insertion	Definition:	Putting in a nonbiological appliance that monitors, assists, performs, or prevents a physiological function but does not physically take the place of a body part
		Explanation:	None
		Examples:	Insertion of radioactive implant, insertion of central venous catheter
J	Inspection	Definition:	Visually and/or manually exploring a body part
		Explanation:	Visual exploration may be performed with or without optical instrumentation. Manual exploration may be performed directly or through intervening body layers.
		Examples:	Diagnostic arthroscopy, exploratory laparotomy
K	Map	Definition:	Locating the route of passage of electrical impulses and/or locating functional areas in a body part
		Explanation:	Applicable only to the cardiac conduction mechanism and the central nervous system
		Examples:	Cardiac mapping, cortical mapping
L	Occlusion	Definition:	Completely closing an orifice or lumen of a tubular body part
		Explanation:	The orifice can be a natural orifice or an artificially created orifice
		Examples:	Fallopian tube ligation, ligation of inferior vena cava
M	Reattachment	Definition:	Putting back in or on all or a portion of a separated body part to its normal location or other suitable location
		Explanation:	Vascular circulation and nervous pathways may or may not be reestablished
		Examples:	Reattachment of hand, reattachment of avulsed kidney
N	Release	Definition:	Freeing a body part from an abnormal physical constraint by cutting or by use of force
		Explanation:	Some of the restraining tissue may be taken out but none of the body part is taken out
		Examples:	Adhesiolysis, carpal tunnel release
P	Removal	Definition:	Taking out or off a device from a body part
		Explanation:	If a device is taken out and a similar device put in without cutting or puncturing the skin or mucous membrane, the procedure is coded to the root operation CHANGE. Otherwise, the procedure for taking out a device is coded to the root operation REMOVAL.
		Examples:	Drainage tube removal, cardiac pacemaker removal
Q	Repair	Definition:	Restoring, to the extent possible, a body part to its normal anatomic structure and function
		Explanation:	Used only when the method to accomplish the repair is not one of the other root operations
		Examples:	Colostomy takedown, suture of laceration
R	Replacement	Definition:	Putting in or on biological or synthetic material that physically takes the place and/or function of all or a portion of a body part
		Explanation:	The body part may have been taken out or replaced, or may be taken out, physically eradicated, or rendered nonfunctional during the REPLACEMENT procedure. A REMOVAL procedure is coded for taking out the device used in a previous replacement procedure.
		Examples:	Total hip replacement, bone graft, free skin graft

Continued on next page

Ø	**Medical and Surgical**		*Continued from previous page*
ICD-10-PCS Value		**Definition**	
S	Reposition	Definition:	Moving to its normal location, or other suitable location, all or a portion of a body part
		Explanation:	The body part is moved to a new location from an abnormal location, or from a normal location where it is not functioning correctly. The body part may or may not be cut out or off to be moved to the new location.
		Examples:	Reposition of undescended testicle, fracture reduction
T	Resection	Definition:	Cutting out or off, without replacement, all of a body part
		Explanation:	None
		Examples:	Total nephrectomy, total lobectomy of lung
V	Restriction	Definition:	Partially closing an orifice or the lumen of a tubular body part
		Explanation:	The orifice can be a natural orifice or an artificially created orifice
		Examples:	Esophagogastric fundoplication, cervical cerclage
W	Revision	Definition:	Correcting, to the extent possible, a portion of a malfunctioning device or the position of a displaced device
		Explanation:	Revision can include correcting a malfunctioning or displaced device by taking out or putting in components of the device such as a screw or pin
		Examples:	Adjustment of position of pacemaker lead, recementing of hip prosthesis
U	Supplement	Definition:	Putting in or on biological or synthetic material that physically reinforces and/or augments the function of a portion of a body part
		Explanation:	The biological material is non-living, or is living and from the same individual. The body part may have been previously replaced, and the SUPPLEMENT procedure is performed to physically reinforce and/or augment the function of the replaced body part.
		Examples:	Herniorrhaphy using mesh, free nerve graft, mitral valve ring annuloplasty, put a new acetabular liner in a previous hip replacement
X	Transfer	Definition:	Moving, without taking out, all or a portion of a body part to another location to take over the function of all or a portion of a body part
		Explanation:	The body part transferred remains connected to its vascular and nervous supply
		Examples:	Tendon transfer, skin pedicle flap transfer
Y	Transplantation	Definition:	Putting in or on all or a portion of a living body part taken from another individual or animal to physically take the place and/or function of all or a portion of a similar body part
		Explanation:	The native body part may or may not be taken out, and the transplanted body part may take over all or a portion of its function
		Examples:	Kidney transplant, heart transplant

Root Operation Definitions for Other Sections

1	**Obstetrics**		
ICD-10-PCS Value		**Definition**	
2	Change	Definition:	Taking out or off a device from a body part and putting back an identical or similar device in or on the same body part without cutting or puncturing the skin or a mucous membrane
		Explanation:	None
		Examples:	Replacement of fetal scalp electrode
9	Drainage	Definition:	Taking or letting out fluids and/or gases from a body part
		Explanation:	None
		Examples:	Biopsy of amniotic fluid
A	Abortion	Definition:	Artificially terminating a pregnancy
		Explanation:	None
		Examples:	Transvaginal abortion using vacuum aspiration technique
D	Extraction	Definition:	Pulling or stripping out or off all or a portion of a body part by the use of force
		Explanation:	None
		Examples:	Low-transverse C-section
E	Delivery	Definition:	Assisting the passage of the products of conception from the genital canal
		Explanation:	None
		Examples:	Manually-assisted delivery

Continued on next page

1   Obstetrics

Continued from previous page

ICD-10-PCS Value			Definition
H	Insertion	Definition:	Putting in a nonbiological appliance that monitors, assists, performs, or prevents a physiological function but does not physically take the place of a body part
		Explanation:	None
		Examples:	Placement of fetal scalp electrode
J	Inspection	Definition:	Visually and/or manually exploring a body part
		Explanation:	Visual exploration may be performed with or without optical instrumentation. Manual exploration may be performed directly or through intervening body layers.
		Examples:	Bimanual pregnancy exam
P	Removal	Definition:	Taking out or off a device from a body part, region or orifice
		Explanation:	If a device is taken out and a similar device put in without cutting or puncturing the skin or mucous membrane, the procedure is coded to the root operation CHANGE. Otherwise, the procedure for taking out a device is coded to the root operation REMOVAL.
		Examples:	Removal of fetal monitoring electrode
Q	Repair	Definition:	Restoring, to the extent possible, a body part to its normal anatomic structure and function
		Explanation:	Used only when the method to accomplish the repair is not one of the other root operations
		Examples:	In utero repair of congenital diaphragmatic hernia
S	Reposition	Definition:	Moving to its normal location, or other suitable location, all or a portion of a body part
		Explanation:	The body part is moved to a new location from an abnormal location, or from a normal location where it is not functioning correctly. The body part may or may not be cut out or off to be moved to the new location.
		Examples:	External version of fetus
T	Resection	Definition:	Cutting out or off, without replacement, all of a body part
		Explanation:	None
		Examples:	Total excision of tubal pregnancy
Y	Transplantation	Definition:	Putting in or on all or a portion of a living body part taken from another individual or animal to physically take the place and/or function of all or a portion of a similar body part
		Explanation:	The native body part may or may not be taken out, and the transplanted body part may take over all or a portion of its function
		Examples:	In utero fetal kidney transplant

2   Placement

ICD-10-PCS Value			Definition
Ø	Change	Definition:	Taking out or off a device from a body part and putting back an identical or similar device in or on the same body part without cutting or puncturing the skin or a mucous membrane
		Examples:	Change of vaginal packing
1	Compression	Definition:	Putting pressure on a body region
		Examples:	Placement of pressure dressing on abdominal wall
2	Dressing	Definition:	Putting material on a body region for protection
		Examples:	Application of sterile dressing to head wound
3	Immobilization	Definition:	Limiting or preventing motion of a body region
		Examples:	Placement of splint on left finger
4	Packing	Definition:	Putting material in a body region or orifice
		Examples:	Placement of nasal packing
5	Removal	Definition:	Taking out or off a device from a body part
		Examples:	Removal of stereotactic head frame
6	Traction	Definition:	Exerting a pulling force on a body region in a distal direction
		Examples:	Lumbar traction using motorized split-traction table

3   Administration

ICD-10-PCS Value			Definition
Ø	Introduction	Definition:	Putting in or on a therapeutic, diagnostic, nutritional, physiological, or prophylactic substance except blood or blood products
		Examples:	Nerve block injection to median nerve
1	Irrigation	Definition:	Putting in or on a cleansing substance
		Examples:	Flushing of eye
2	Transfusion	Definition:	Putting in blood or blood products
		Examples:	Transfusion of cell saver red cells into central venous line

4   Measurement and Monitoring

ICD-10-PCS Value			Definition
Ø	Measurement	Definition:	Determining the level of a physiological or physical function at a point in time
		Examples:	External electrocardiogram(EKG), single reading
1	Monitoring	Definition:	Determining the level of a physiological or physical function repetitively over a period of time
		Examples:	Urinary pressure monitoring

5   Extracorporeal or Systemic Assistance and Performance

ICD-10-PCS Value			Definition
Ø	Assistance	Definition:	Taking over a portion of a physiological function by extracorporeal means
		Examples:	Hyperbaric oxygenation of wound
1	Performance	Definition:	Completely taking over a physiological function by extracorporeal means
		Examples:	Cardiopulmonary bypass in conjunction with CABG
2	Restoration	Definition:	Returning, or attempting to return, a physiological function to its original state by extracorporeal means
		Examples:	Attempted cardiac defibrillation, unsuccessful

6   Extracorporeal or Systemic Therapies

ICD-10-PCS Value			Definition
Ø	Atmospheric Control	Definition:	Extracorporeal control of atmospheric pressure and composition
		Examples:	Antigen-free air conditioning, series treatment
1	Decompression	Definition:	Extracorporeal elimination of undissolved gas from body fluids
		Examples:	Hyperbaric decompression treatment, single
2	Electromagnetic Therapy	Definition:	Extracorporeal treatment by electromagnetic rays
		Examples:	TMS (transcranial magnetic stimulation), series treatment
3	Hyperthermia	Definition:	Extracorporeal raising of body temperature
		Examples:	None
4	Hypothermia	Definition:	Extracorporeal lowering of body temperature
		Examples:	Whole body hypothermia treatment for temperature imbalances, series
5	Pheresis	Definition:	Extracorporeal separation of blood products
		Examples:	Therapeutic leukopheresis, single treatment
6	Phototherapy	Definition:	Extracorporeal treatment by light rays
		Examples:	Phototherapy of circulatory system, series treatment
7	Ultrasound Therapy	Definition:	Extracorporeal treatment by ultrasound
		Examples:	Therapeutic ultrasound of peripheral vessels, single treatment
8	Ultraviolet Light Therapy	Definition:	Extracorporeal treatment by ultraviolet light
		Examples:	Ultraviolet light phototherapy, series treatment
9	Shock Wave Therapy	Definition:	Extracorporeal treatment by shock waves
		Examples:	Shockwave therapy of plantar fascia, single treatment
B	Perfusion	Definition:	Extracorporeal treatment by diffusion of therapeutic fluid
		Examples:	Perfusion of donor liver while preparing transplant patient

7   Osteopathic

ICD-10-PCS Value			Definition
Ø	Treatment	Definition:	Manual treatment to eliminate or alleviate somatic dysfunction and related disorders
		Examples:	Fascial release of abdomen, osteopathic treatment

8   Other Procedures

ICD-10-PCS Value			Definition
Ø	Other Procedures	Definition:	Methodologies which attempt to remediate or cure a disorder or disease
		Examples:	Acupuncture, yoga therapy

9   Chiropractic

ICD-10-PCS Value			Definition
B	Manipulation	Definition:	Manual procedure that involves a directed thrust to move a joint past the physiological range of motion, without exceeding the anatomical limit
		Examples:	Chiropractic treatment of cervical spine, short lever specific contact

Appendix C: Comparison of Medical and Surgical Root Operations

Note: the character associated with each operation appears in parentheses after its title.

Procedures That Take Out Some or All of a Body Part

Root Operation	Objective of Procedure	Site of Procedure	Example
Destruction (5)	Eradicating without taking out or replacement	Some/all of a body part	Fulguration of endometrium
Detachment (6)	Cutting out/off without replacement	Extremity only, any level	Amputation above elbow
Excision (B)	Cutting out/off without replacement	Some of a body part	Breast lumpectomy
Extraction (D)	Pulling out or off without replacement	Some/all of a body part	Suction D&C
Resection (T)	Cutting out/off without replacement	All of a body part	Total mastectomy

Procedures That Put in/Put Back or Move Some/All of a Body Part

Root Operation	Objective of Procedure	Site of Procedure	Example
Reattachment (M)	Putting back a detached body part	Some/all of a body part	Reattach finger
Reposition (S)	Moving a body part to normal or other suitable location	Some/all of a body part	Move undescended testicle
Transfer (X)	Moving a body part to function for a similar body part	Some/all of a body part	Skin pedicle transfer flap
Transplantation (Y)	Putting in a living body part from a person/animal	Some/all of a body part	Kidney transplant

Procedures That Take Out or Eliminate Solid Matter, Fluids, or Gases From a Body Part

Root Operation	Objective of Procedure	Site of Procedure	Example
Drainage (9)	Taking or letting out	Fluids and/or gases from a body part	Incision and drainage
Extirpation (C)	Taking or cutting out	Solid matter in a body part	Thrombectomy
Fragmentation (F)	Breaking into pieces	Solid matter within a body part	Lithotripsy

Procedures That Involve Only Examination of Body Parts and Regions

Root Operation	Objective of Procedure	Site of Procedure	Example
Inspection (J)	Visual/manual exploration	Some/all of a body part	Diagnostic cystoscopy Exploratory laparoscopy
Map (K)	Locating electrical impulse route/functional areas	Brain/cardiac conduction mechanism	Cardiac mapping

Procedures That Alter the Diameter/Route of a Tubular Body Part

Root Operation	Objective of Procedure	Site of Procedure	Example
Bypass (1)	Altering route of passage of contents	Tubular body part	Coronary artery bypass graft (CABG)
Dilation (7)	Expanding natural or artificially created orifice/lumen	Tubular body part	Percutaneous transluminal coronary angioplasty (PTCA)
Occlusion (L)	Completely closing natural or artificially created orifice/lumen	Tubular body part	Fallopian tube ligation
Restriction (V)	Partially closing natural or artificially created orifice/lumen	Tubular body part	Gastroesophageal fundoplication

Procedures That Always Involve Devices

Root Operation		Objective of Procedure	Site of Procedure	Example
Change (2)	DVC	Exchanging device w/out cutting/puncturing	In/on a body part	Gastrostomy tube change
Insertion (H)	DVC	Putting in nonbiological device	In/on a body part	Central line insertion
Removal (P)	DVC	Taking out device	In/on a body part	Central line removal
Replacement (R)	DVC	Putting in device that replaces a body part	Some/all of a body part	Total hip replacement
Revision (W)	DVC	Correcting a malfunctioning/displaced device	In/on a body part	Revision of pacemaker
Supplement (U)	DVC	Putting in device that reinforces or augments a body part	In/on a body part	Abdominal wall herniorrhaphy using mesh

DVC = Device involved in root operation

Procedures Involving Cutting or Separation Only

Root Operation	Objective of Procedure	Site of Procedure	Example
Division (8)	Cutting into/separating	A body part	Neurotomy
Release (N)	Freeing a body part from constraint	Around a body part	Adhesiolysis

Procedures That Define Other Repairs

Root Operation	Objective of Procedure	Site of Procedure	Example
Control (3)	Stopping/attempting to stop postprocedural or other acute bleeding	Anatomical region or nasal mucosa/soft tissue	Post-prostatectomy bleeding control, control subdural hemorrhage, bleeding ulcer, retroperitoneal hemorrhage
Repair (Q)	Restoring body part to its normal structure/function	Some/all of a body part	Suture laceration

Procedures That Define Other Objectives

Root Operation	Objective of Procedure	Site of Procedure	Example
Alteration (Ø)	Modifying body part for cosmetic purposes without affecting function	Some/all of a body part	Face lift
Creation (4)	Using biological or synthetic material to form a new body part that replicates the anatomic structure or function of a missing body part	Perineum, valve	Sex change/artificial vagina/penis, atrioventricular valve creation
Fusion (G)	Unification or immobilization	Joint or articular body part	Spinal fusion

Appendix D: Body Part Key

Term	ICD-10-PCS Value
Abdominal aortic plexus	Abdominal Sympathetic Nerve
Abdominal esophagus	Esophagus, Lower
Abductor hallucis muscle	Foot Muscle, Right
	Foot Muscle, Left
Accessory cephalic vein	Cephalic Vein, Right
	Cephalic Vein, Left
Accessory obturator nerve	Lumbar Plexus
Accessory phrenic nerve	Phrenic nerve
Accessory spleen	Spleen
Acetabulofemoral joint	Hip Joint, Right
	Hip Joint, Left
Achilles tendon	Lower Leg Tendon, Right
	Lower Leg Tendon, Left
Acromioclavicular ligament	Shoulder Bursa and Ligament, Right
	Shoulder Bursa and Ligament, Left
Acromion (process)	Scapula, Right
	Scapula, Left
Adductor brevis muscle	Upper Leg Muscle, Right
	Upper Leg Muscle, Left
Adductor hallucis muscle	Foot Muscle, Right
	Foot Muscle, Left
Adductor longus muscle	Upper Leg Muscle, Right
	Upper Leg Muscle, Left
Adductor magnus muscle	Upper Leg Muscle, Right
	Upper Leg Muscle, Left
Adenohypophysis	Pituitary Gland
Alar ligament of axis	Head and Neck Bursa and Ligament
Alveolar process of mandible	Mandible, Right
	Mandible, Left
Alveolar process of maxilla	Maxilla
Anal orifice	Anus
Anatomical snuffbox	Lower Arm and Wrist Muscle, Right
	Lower Arm and Wrist Muscle, Left
Angular artery	Face Artery
Angular vein	Face Vein, Right
	Face Vein, Left
Annular ligament	Elbow Bursa and Ligament, Right
	Elbow Bursa and Ligament, Left
Anorectal junction	Rectum
Ansa cervicalis	Cervical Plexus
Antebrachial fascia	Subcutaneous Tissue and Fascia, Right Lower Arm
	Subcutaneous Tissue and Fascia, Left Lower Arm
Anterior (pectoral) lymph node	Lymphatic, Right Axillary
	Lymphatic, Left Axillary
Anterior cerebral artery	Intracranial Artery
Anterior cerebral vein	Intracranial Vein
Anterior choroidal artery	Intracranial Artery
Anterior circumflex humeral artery	Axillary Artery, Right
	Axillary Artery, Left
Anterior communicating artery	Intracranial Artery

Term	ICD-10-PCS Value
Anterior cruciate ligament (ACL)	Knee Bursa and Ligament, Right
	Knee Bursa and Ligament, Left
Anterior crural nerve	Femoral Nerve
Anterior facial vein	Face Vein, Right
	Face Vein, Left
Anterior intercostal artery	Internal Mammary Artery, Right
	Internal Mammary Artery, Left
Anterior interosseous nerve	Median Nerve
Anterior lateral malleolar artery	Anterior Tibial Artery, Right
	Anterior Tibial Artery, Left
Anterior lingual gland	Minor Salivary Gland
Anterior medial malleolar artery	Anterior Tibial Artery, Right
	Anterior Tibial Artery, Left
Anterior spinal artery	Vertebral Artery, Right
	Vertebral Artery, Left
Anterior tibial recurrent artery	Anterior Tibial Artery, Right
	Anterior Tibial Artery, Left
Anterior ulnar recurrent artery	Ulnar Artery, Right
	Ulnar Artery, Left
Anterior vagal trunk	Vagus Nerve
Anterior vertebral muscle	Neck Muscle, Right
	Neck Muscle, Left
Antihelix	External Ear, Right
	External Ear, Left
	External Ear, Bilateral
Antitragus	External Ear, Right
	External Ear, Left
	External Ear, Bilateral
Antrum of Highmore	Maxillary Sinus, Right
	Maxillary Sinus, Left
Aortic annulus	Aortic Valve
Aortic arch	Thoracic Aorta, Ascending/Arch
Aortic intercostal artery	Upper Artery
Apical (subclavicular) lymph node	Lymphatic, Right Axillary
	Lymphatic, Left Axillary
Apneustic center	Pons
Aqueduct of Sylvius	Cerebral Ventricle
Aqueous humour	Anterior Chamber, Right
	Anterior Chamber, Left
Arachnoid mater, intracranial	Cerebral Meninges
Arachnoid mater, spinal	Spinal Meninges
Arcuate artery	Foot Artery, Right
	Foot Artery, Left
Areola	Nipple, Right
	Nipple, Left
Arterial canal (duct)	Pulmonary Artery, Left
Aryepiglottic fold	Larynx
Arytenoid cartilage	Larynx
Arytenoid muscle	Neck Muscle, Right
	Neck Muscle, Left
Ascending aorta	Thoracic Aorta, Ascending/Arch

Term	ICD-10-PCS Value
Ascending palatine artery	Face Artery
Ascending pharyngeal artery	External Carotid Artery, Right
	External Carotid Artery, Left
Atlantoaxial joint	Cervical Vertebral Joint
Atrioventricular node	Conduction Mechanism
Atrium dextrum cordis	Atrium, Right
Atrium pulmonale	Atrium, Left
Auditory tube	Eustachian Tube, Right
	Eustachian Tube, Left
Auerbach's (myenteric)plexus	Abdominal Sympathetic Nerve
Auricle	External Ear, Right
	External Ear, Left
	External Ear, Bilateral
Auricularis muscle	Head Muscle
Axillary fascia	Subcutaneous Tissue and Fascia, Right Upper Arm
	Subcutaneous Tissue and Fascia, Left Upper Arm
Axillary nerve	Brachial Plexus
Bartholin's (greater vestibular) gland	Vestibular Gland
Basal (internal) cerebral vein	Intracranial Vein
Basal nuclei	Basal Ganglia
Base of tongue	Pharynx
Basilar artery	Intracranial Artery
Basis pontis	Pons
Biceps brachii muscle	Upper Arm Muscle, Right
	Upper Arm Muscle, Left
Biceps femoris muscle	Upper Leg Muscle, Right
	Upper Leg Muscle, Left
Bicipital aponeurosis	Subcutaneous Tissue and Fascia, Right Lower Arm
	Subcutaneous Tissue and Fascia, Left Lower Arm
Bicuspid valve	Mitral Valve
Body of femur	Femoral Shaft, Right
	Femoral Shaft, Left
Body of fibula	Fibula, Right
	Fibula, Left
Bony labyrinth	Inner Ear, Right
	Inner Ear, Left
Bony orbit	Orbit, Right
	Orbit, Left
Bony vestibule	Inner Ear, Right
	Inner Ear, Left
Botallo's duct	Pulmonary Artery, Left
Brachial (lateral) lymph node	Lymphatic, Right Axillary
	Lymphatic, Left Axillary
Brachialis muscle	Upper Arm Muscle, Right
	Upper Arm Muscle, Left
Brachiocephalic artery	Innominate Artery
Brachiocephalic trunk	Innominate Artery
Brachiocephalic vein	Innominate Vein, Right
	Innominate Vein, Left

Term	ICD-10-PCS Value
Brachioradialis muscle	Lower Arm and Wrist Muscle, Right
	Lower Arm and Wrist Muscle, Left
Breast procedures, skin only	Skin, Chest
Broad ligament	Uterine Supporting Structure
Bronchial artery	Upper Artery
Bronchus intermedius	Main Bronchus, Right
Buccal gland	Buccal Mucosa
Buccinator lymph node	Lymphatic, Head
Buccinator muscle	Facial Muscle
Bulbospongiosus muscle	Perineum Muscle
Bulbourethral (Cowper's) gland	Urethra
Bundle of His	Conduction Mechanism
Bundle of Kent	Conduction Mechanism
Calcaneocuboid joint	Tarsal Joint, Right
	Tarsal Joint, Left
Calcaneocuboid ligament	Foot Bursa and Ligament, Right
	Foot Bursa and Ligament, Left
Calcaneofibular ligament	Ankle Bursa and Ligament, Right
	Ankle Bursa and Ligament, Left
Calcaneus	Tarsal, Right
	Tarsal, Left
Capitate bone	Carpal, Right
	Carpal, Left
Cardia	Esophagogastric Junction
Cardiac plexus	Thoracic Sympathetic Nerve
Cardioesophageal junction	Esophagogastric Junction
Caroticotympanic artery	Internal Carotid Artery, Right
	Internal Carotid Artery, Left
Carotid glomus	Carotid Body, Right
	Carotid Body, Left
	Carotid Bodies, Bilateral
Carotid sinus	Internal Carotid Artery, Right
	Internal Carotid Artery, Left
Carotid sinus nerve	Glossopharyngeal Nerve
Carpometacarpal ligament	Hand Bursa and Ligament, Right
	Hand Bursa and Ligament, Left
Cauda equina	Lumbar Spinal Cord
Cavernous plexus	Head and Neck Sympathetic Nerve
Celiac ganglion	Abdominal Sympathetic Nerve
Celiac (solar) plexus	Abdominal Sympathetic Nerve
Celiac lymph node	Lymphatic, Aortic
Celiac trunk	Celiac Artery
Central axillary lymph node	Lymphatic, Right Axillary
	Lymphatic, Left Axillary
Cerebral aqueduct (Sylvius)	Cerebral Ventricle
Cerebrum	Brain
Cervical esophagus	Esophagus, Upper
Cervical facet joint	Cervical Vertebral Joint
	Cervical Vertebral Joints, 2 or more
Cervical ganglion	Head and Neck Sympathetic Nerve
Cervical interspinous ligament	Head and Neck Bursa and Ligament

Term	ICD-10-PCS Value
Cervical intertransverse ligament	Head and Neck Bursa and Ligament
Cervical ligamentum flavum	Head and Neck Bursa and Ligament
Cervical lymph node	Lymphatic, Right Neck
	Lymphatic, Left Neck
Cervicothoracic facet joint	Cervicothoracic Vertebral Joint
Choana	Nasopharynx
Chondroglossus muscle	Tongue, Palate, Pharynx Muscle
Chorda tympani	Facial Nerve
Choroid plexus	Cerebral Ventricle
Ciliary body	Eye, Right
	Eye, Left
Ciliary ganglion	Head and Neck Sympathetic Nerve
Circle of Willis	Intracranial Artery
Circumflex illiac artery	Femoral Artery, Right
	Femoral Artery, Left
Claustrum	Basal Ganglia
Coccygeal body	Coccygeal Glomus
Coccygeus muscle	Trunk Muscle, Right
	Trunk Muscle, Left
Cochlea	Inner Ear, Right
	Inner Ear, Left
Cochlear nerve	Acoustic Nerve
Columella	Nasal Mucosa and Soft Tissue
Common digital vein	Foot Vein, Right
	Foot Vein, Left
Common facial vein	Face Vein, Right
	Face Vein, Left
Common fibular nerve	Peroneal Nerve
Common hepatic artery	Hepatic Artery
Common iliac (subaortic) lymph node	Lymphatic, Pelvis
Common interosseous artery	Ulnar Artery, Right
	Ulnar Artery, Left
Common peroneal nerve	Peroneal Nerve
Condyloid process	Mandible, Right
	Mandible, Left
Conus arteriosus	Ventricle, Right
Conus medullaris	Lumbar Spinal Cord
Coracoacromial ligament	Shoulder Bursa and Ligament, Right
	Shoulder Bursa and Ligament, Left
Coracobrachialis muscle	Upper Arm Muscle, Right
	Upper Arm Muscle, Left
Coracoclavicular ligament	Shoulder Bursa and Ligament, Right
	Shoulder Bursa and Ligament, Left
Coracohumeral ligament	Shoulder Bursa and Ligament, Right
	Shoulder Bursa and Ligament, Left
Coracoid process	Scapula, Right
	Scapula, Left
Corniculate cartilage	Larynx
Corpus callosum	Brain
Corpus cavernosum	Penis
Corpus spongiosum	Penis
Corpus striatum	Basal Ganglia

Term	ICD-10-PCS Value
Corrugator supercilii muscle	Facial Muscle
Costocervical trunk	Subclavian Artery, Right
	Subclavian Artery, Left
Costoclavicular ligament	Shoulder Bursa and Ligament, Right
	Shoulder Bursa and Ligament, Left
Costotransverse joint	Thoracic Vertebral Joint
Costotransverse ligament	Rib(s) Bursa and Ligament
Costovertebral joint	Thoracic Vertebral Joint
Costoxiphoid ligament	Sternum Bursa and Ligament
Cowper's (bulbourethral) gland	Urethra
Cremaster muscle	Perineum Muscle
Cribriform plate	Ethmoid Bone, Right
	Ethmoid Bone, Left
Cricoid cartilage	Trachea
Cricothyroid artery	Thyroid Artery, Right
	Thyroid Artery, Left
Cricothyroid muscle	Neck Muscle, Right
	Neck Muscle, Left
Crural fascia	Subcutaneous Tissue and Fascia, Right Upper Leg
	Subcutaneous Tissue and Fascia, Left Upper Leg
Cubital lymph node	Lymphatic, Right Upper Extremity
	Lymphatic, Left Upper Extremity
Cubital nerve	Ulnar Nerve
Cuboid bone	Tarsal, Right
	Tarsal, Left
Cuboideonavicular joint	Tarsal Joint, Right
	Tarsal Joint, Left
Culmen	Cerebellum
Cuneiform cartilage	Larynx
Cuneonavicular joint	Tarsal Joint, Right
	Tarsal Joint, Left
Cuneonavicular ligament	Foot Bursa and Ligament, Right
	Foot Bursa and Ligament, Left
Cutaneous (transverse) cervical nerve	Cervical Plexus
Deep cervical fascia	Subcutaneous Tissue and Fascia, Right Neck
	Subcutaneous Tissue and Fascia, Left Neck
Deep cervical vein	Vertebral Vein, Right
	Vertebral Vein, Left
Deep circumflex iliac artery	External Iliac Artery, Right
	External Iliac Artery, Left
Deep facial vein	Face Vein, Right
	Face Vein, Left
Deep femoral artery	Femoral Artery, Right
	Femoral Artery, Left
Deep femoral (profunda femoris) vein	Femoral Vein, Right
	Femoral Vein, Left
Deep palmar arch	Hand Artery, Right
	Hand Artery, Left
Deep transverse perineal muscle	Perineum Muscle

Term	ICD-10-PCS Value
Deferential artery	Internal Iliac Artery, Right
	Internal Iliac Artery, Left
Deltoid fascia	Subcutaneous Tissue and Fascia, Right Upper Arm
	Subcutaneous Tissue and Fascia, Left Upper Arm
Deltoid ligament	Ankle Bursa and Ligament, Right
	Ankle Bursa and Ligament, Left
Deltoid muscle	Shoulder Muscle, Right
	Shoulder Muscle, Left
Deltopectoral (infraclavicular) lymph node	Lymphatic, Right Upper Extremity
	Lymphatic, Left Upper Extremity
Dens	Cervical Vertebra
Denticulate (dentate) ligament	Spinal Meninges
Depressor anguli oris muscle	Facial Muscle
Depressor labii inferioris muscle	Facial Muscle
Depressor septi nasi muscle	Facial Muscle
Depressor supercilii muscle	Facial Muscle
Dermis	Skin
Descending genicular artery	Femoral Artery, Right
	Femoral Artery, Left
Diaphragma sellae	Dura Mater
Distal humerus	Humeral Shaft, Right
	Humeral Shaft, Left
Distal humerus, involving joint	Elbow Joint, Right
	Elbow Joint, Left
Distal radioulnar joint	Wrist Joint, Right
	Wrist Joint, Left
Dorsal digital nerve	Radial Nerve
Dorsal metacarpal vein	Hand Vein, Right
	Hand Vein, Left
Dorsal metatarsal artery	Foot Artery, Right
	Foot Artery, Left
Dorsal metatarsal vein	Foot Vein, Right
	Foot Vein, Left
Dorsal scapular artery	Subclavian Artery, Right
	Subclavian Artery, Left
Dorsal scapular nerve	Brachial Plexus
Dorsal venous arch	Foot Vein, Right
	Foot Vein, Left
Dorsalis pedis artery	Anterior Tibial Artery, Right
	Anterior Tibial Artery, Left
Duct of Santorini	Pancreatic Duct, Accessory
Duct of Wirsung	Pancreatic Duct
Ductus deferens	Vas Deferens, Right
	Vas Deferens, Left
	Vas Deferens, Bilateral
	Vas Deferens
Duodenal ampulla	Ampulla of Vater
Duodenojejunal flexure	Jejunum
Dura mater, intracranial	Dura Mater

Term	ICD-10-PCS Value
Dura mater, spinal	Spinal Meninges
Dural venous sinus	Intracranial Vein
Earlobe	External Ear, Right
	External Ear, Left
	External Ear, Bilateral
Eighth cranial nerve	Acoustic Nerve
Ejaculatory duct	Vas Deferens, Right
	Vas Deferens, Left
	Vas Deferens, Bilateral
	Vas Deferens
Eleventh cranial nerve	Accessory Nerve
Encephalon	Brain
Ependyma	Cerebral Ventricle
Epidermis	Skin
Epidural space, spinal	Spinal Canal
Epiploic foramen	Peritoneum
Epithalamus	Thalamus
Epitroclear lymph node	Lymphatic, Right Upper Extremity
	Lymphatic, Left Upper Extremity
Erector spinae muscle	Trunk Muscle, Right
	Trunk Muscle, Left
Esophageal artery	Upper Artery
Esophageal plexus	Thoracic Sympathetic Nerve
Ethmoidal air cell	Ethmoid Sinus, Right
	Ethmoid Sinus, Left
Extensor carpi radialis muscle	Lower Arm and Wrist Muscle, Right
	Lower Arm and Wrist Muscle, Left
Extensor carpi ulnaris muscle	Lower Arm and Wrist Muscle, Right
	Lower Arm and Wrist Muscle, Left
Extensor digitorum brevis muscle	Foot Muscle, Right
	Foot Muscle, Left
Extensor digitorum longus muscle	Lower Leg Muscle, Right
	Lower Leg Muscle, Left
Extensor hallucis brevis muscle	Foot Muscle, Right
	Foot Muscle, Left
Extensor hallucis longus muscle	Lower Leg Muscle, Right
	Lower Leg Muscle, Left
External anal sphincter	Anal Sphincter
External auditory meatus	External Auditory Canal, Right
	External Auditory Canal, Left
External maxillary artery	Face Artery
External naris	Nasal Mucosa and Soft Tissue
External oblique aponeurosis	Subcutaneous Tissue and Fascia, Trunk
External oblique muscle	Abdomen Muscle, Right
	Abdomen Muscle, Left
External popliteal nerve	Peroneal Nerve
External pudendal artery	Femoral Artery, Right
	Femoral Artery, Left
External pudenal vein	Saphenous Vein, Right
	Saphenous Vein, Left
External urethral sphincter	Urethra
Extradural space, intracranial	Epidural Space, Intracranial
Extradural space, spinal	Spinal Canal

Term	ICD-10-PCS Value
Facial artery	Face Artery
False vocal cord	Larynx
Falx cerebri	Dura Mater
Fascia lata	Subcutaneous Tissue and Fascia, Right Upper Leg
	Subcutaneous Tissue and Fascia, Left Upper Leg
Femoral head	Upper Femur, Right
	Upper Femur, Left
Femoral lymph node	Lymphatic, Right Lower Extremity
	Lymphatic, Left Lower Extremity
Femoropatellar joint	Knee Joint, Right
	Knee Joint, Left
	Knee Joint, Femoral Surface, Right
	Knee Joint, Femoral Surface, Left
Femorotibial joint	Knee Joint, Right
	Knee Joint, Left
	Knee Joint, Tibial Surface, Right
	Knee Joint, Tibial Surface, Left
Fibular artery	Peroneal Artery, Right
	Peroneal Artery, Left
Fibularis brevis muscle	Lower Leg Muscle, Right
	Lower Leg Muscle, Left
Fibularis longus muscle	Lower Leg Muscle, Right
	Lower Leg Muscle, Left
Fifth cranial nerve	Trigeminal Nerve
Filum terminale	Spinal Meninges
First cranial nerve	Olfactory Nerve
First intercostal nerve	Brachial Plexus
Flexor carpi radialis muscle	Lower Arm and Wrist Muscle, Right
	Lower Arm and Wrist Muscle, Left
Flexor carpi ulnaris muscle	Lower Arm and Wrist Muscle, Right
	Lower Arm and Wrist Muscle, Left
Flexor digitorum brevis muscle	Foot Muscle, Right
	Foot Muscle, Left
Flexor digitorum longus muscle	Lower Leg Muscle, Right
	Lower Leg Muscle, Left
Flexor hallucis brevis muscle	Foot Muscle, Right
	Foot Muscle, Left
Flexor hallucis longus muscle	Lower Leg Muscle, Right
	Lower Leg Muscle, Left
Flexor pollicis longus muscle	Lower Arm and Wrist Muscle, Right
	Lower Arm and Wrist Muscle, Left
Foramen magnum	Occipital Bone
Foramen of Monro (intraventricular)	Cerebral Ventricle
Foreskin	Prepuce
Fossa of Rosenmuller	Nasopharynx
Fourth cranial nerve	Trochlear Nerve
Fourth ventricle	Cerebral Ventricle
Fovea	Retina, Right
	Retina, Left
Frenulum labii inferioris	Lower Lip
Frenulum labii superioris	Upper Lip
Frenulum linguae	Tongue

Term	ICD-10-PCS Value
Frontal lobe	Cerebral Hemisphere
Frontal vein	Face Vein, Right
	Face Vein, Left
Fundus uteri	Uterus
Galea aponeurotica	Subcutaneous Tissue and Fascia, Scalp
Ganglion impar (ganglion of Walther)	Sacral Sympathetic Nerve
Gasserian ganglion	Trigeminal Nerve
Gastric lymph node	Lymphatic, Aortic
Gastric plexus	Abdominal Sympathetic Nerve
Gastrocnemius muscle	Lower Leg Muscle, Right
	Lower Leg Muscle, Left
Gastrocolic ligament	Omentum
Gastrocolic omentum	Omentum
Gastroduodenal artery	Hepatic Artery
Gastroesophageal (GE) junction	Esophagogastric Junction
Gastrohepatic omentum	Omentum
Gastrophrenic ligament	Omentum
Gastrosplenic ligament	Omentum
Gemellus muscle	Hip Muscle, Right
	Hip Muscle, Left
Geniculate ganglion	Facial Nerve
Geniculate nucleus	Thalamus
Genioglossus muscle	Tongue, Palate, Pharynx Muscle
Genitofemoral nerve	Lumbar Plexus
Glans penis	Prepuce
Glenohumeral joint	Shoulder Joint, Right
	Shoulder Joint, Left
Glenohumeral ligament	Shoulder Bursa and Ligament, Right
	Shoulder Bursa and Ligament, Left
Glenoid fossa (of scapula)	Glenoid Cavity, Right
	Glenoid Cavity, Left
Glenoid ligament (labrum)	Shoulder Joint, Right
	Shoulder Joint, Left
Globus pallidus	Basal Ganglia
Glossoepiglottic fold	Epiglottis
Glottis	Larynx
Gluteal lymph node	Lymphatic, Pelvis
Gluteal vein	Hypogastric Vein, Right
	Hypogastric Vein, Left
Gluteus maximus muscle	Hip Muscle, Right
	Hip Muscle, Left
Gluteus medius muscle	Hip Muscle, Right
	Hip Muscle, Left
Gluteus minimus muscle	Hip Muscle, Right
	Hip Muscle, Left
Gracilis muscle	Upper Leg Muscle, Right
	Upper Leg Muscle, Left
Great auricular nerve	Cervical Plexus
Great cerebral vein	Intracranial Vein
Great(er) saphenous vein	Saphenous Vein, Right
	Saphenous Vein, Left
Greater alar cartilage	Nasal Mucosa and Soft Tissue
Greater occipital nerve	Cervical Nerve

Term	ICD-10-PCS Value
Greater omentum	Omentum
Greater splanchnic nerve	Thoracic Sympathetic Nerve
Greater superficial petrosal nerve	Facial Nerve
Greater trochanter	Upper Femur, Right
	Upper Femur, Left
Greater tuberosity	Humeral Head, Right
	Humeral Head, Left
Greater vestibular (Bartholin's) gland	Vestibular Gland
Greater wing	Sphenoid Bone
Hallux	1st Toe, Right
	1st Toe, Left
Hamate bone	Carpal, Right
	Carpal, Left
Head of fibula	Fibula, Right
	Fibula, Left
Helix	External Ear, Right
	External Ear, Left
	External Ear, Bilateral
Hepatic artery proper	Hepatic Artery
Hepatic flexure	Transverse Colon
Hepatic lymph node	Lymphatic, Aortic
Hepatic plexus	Abdominal Sympathetic Nerve
Hepatic portal vein	Portal Vein
Hepatogastric ligament	Omentum
Hepatopancreatic ampulla	Ampulla of Vater
Humeroradial joint	Elbow Joint, Right
	Elbow Joint, Left
Humeroulnar joint	Elbow Joint, Right
	Elbow Joint, Left
Humerus, distal	Humeral Shaft, Right
	Humeral Shaft, Left
Hyoglossus muscle	Tongue, Palate, Pharynx Muscle
Hyoid artery	Thyroid Artery, Right
	Thyroid Artery, Left
Hypogastric artery	Internal Iliac Artery, Right
	Internal Iliac Artery, Left
Hypopharynx	Pharynx
Hypophysis	Pituitary Gland
Hypothenar muscle	Hand Muscle, Right
	Hand Muscle, Left
Ileal artery	Superior Mesenteric Artery
Ileocolic artery	Superior Mesenteric Artery
Ileocolic vein	Colic Vein
Iliac crest	Pelvic Bone, Right
	Pelvic Bone, Left
Iliac fascia	Subcutaneous Tissue and Fascia, Right Upper Leg
	Subcutaneous Tissue and Fascia, Left Upper Leg
Iliac lymph node	Lymphatic, Pelvis
Iliacus muscle	Hip Muscle, Right
	Hip Muscle, Left
Iliofemoral ligament	Hip Bursa and Ligament, Right
	Hip Bursa and Ligament, Left

Term	ICD-10-PCS Value
Iliohypogastric nerve	Lumbar Plexus
Ilioinguinal nerve	Lumbar Plexus
Iliolumbar artery	Internal Iliac Artery, Right
	Internal Iliac Artery, Left
Iliolumbar ligament	Lower Spine Bursa and Ligament
Iliotibial tract (band)	Subcutaneous Tissue and Fascia, Right Upper Leg
	Subcutaneous Tissue and Fascia, Left Upper Leg
Ilium	Pelvic Bone, Right
	Pelvic Bone, Left
Incus	Auditory Ossicle, Right
	Auditory Ossicle, Left
Inferior cardiac nerve	Thoracic Sympathetic Nerve
Inferior cerebellar vein	Intracranial Vein
Inferior cerebral vein	Intracranial Vein
Inferior epigastric artery	External Iliac Artery, Right
	External Iliac Artery, Left
Inferior epigastric lymph node	Lymphatic, Pelvis
Inferior genicular artery	Popliteal Artery, Right
	Popliteal Artery, Left
Inferior gluteal artery	Internal Iliac Artery, Right
	Internal Iliac Artery, Left
Inferior gluteal nerve	Sacral Plexus
Inferior hypogastric plexus	Abdominal Sympathetic Nerve
Inferior labial artery	Face Artery
Inferior longitudinal muscle	Tongue, Palate, Pharynx Muscle
Inferior mesenteric ganglion	Abdominal Sympathetic Nerve
Inferior mesenteric lymph node	Lymphatic, Mesenteric
Inferior mesenteric plexus	Abdominal Sympathetic Nerve
Inferior oblique muscle	Extraocular Muscle, Right
	Extraocular Muscle, Left
Inferior pancreaticoduo-denal artery	Superior Mesenteric Artery
Inferior phrenic artery	Abdominal Aorta
Inferior rectus muscle	Extraocular Muscle, Right
	Extraocular Muscle, Left
Inferior suprarenal artery	Renal Artery, Right
	Renal Artery, Left
Inferior tarsal plate	Lower Eyelid, Right
	Lower Eyelid, Left
Inferior thyroid vein	Innominate Vein, Right
	Innominate Vein, Left
Inferior tibiofibular joint	Ankle Joint, Right
	Ankle Joint, Left
Inferior turbinate	Nasal Turbinate
Inferior ulnar collateral artery	Brachial Artery, Right
	Brachial Artery, Left
Inferior vesical artery	Internal Iliac Artery, Right
	Internal Iliac Artery, Left
Infraauricular lymph node	Lymphatic, Head

Term	ICD-10-PCS Value
Infraclavicular (deltopectoral) lymph node	Lymphatic, Right Upper Extremity
	Lymphatic, Left Upper Extremity
Infrahyoid muscle	Neck Muscle, Right
	Neck Muscle, Left
Infraparotid lymph node	Lymphatic, Head
Infraspinatus fascia	Subcutaneous Tissue and Fascia, Right Upper Arm
	Subcutaneous Tissue and Fascia, Left Upper Arm
Infraspinatus muscle	Shoulder Muscle, Right
	Shoulder Muscle, Left
Infundibulopelvic ligament	Uterine Supporting Structure
Inguinal canal	Inguinal Region, Right
	Inguinal Region, Left
	Inguinal Region, Bilateral
Inguinal triangle	Inguinal Region, Right
	Inguinal Region, Left
	Inguinal Region, Bilateral
Interatrial septum	Atrial Septum
Intercarpal joint	Carpal Joint, Right
	Carpal Joint, Left
Intercarpal ligament	Hand Bursa and Ligament, Right
	Hand Bursa and Ligament, Left
Interclavicular ligament	Shoulder Bursa and Ligament, Right
	Shoulder Bursa and Ligament, Left
Intercostal lymph node	Lymphatic, Thorax
Intercostal muscle	Thorax Muscle, Right
	Thorax Muscle, Left
Intercostal nerve	Thoracic Nerve
Intercostobrachial nerve	Thoracic Nerve
Intercuneiform joint	Tarsal Joint, Right
	Tarsal Joint, Left
Intercuneiform ligament	Foot Bursa and Ligament, Right
	Foot Bursa and Ligament, Left
Intermediate bronchus	Main Bronchus, Right
Intermediate cuneiform bone	Tarsal, Right
	Tarsal, Left
Internal anal sphincter	Anal Sphincter
Internal (basal) cerebral vein	Intracranial Vein
Internal carotid artery, intracranial portion	Intracranial Artery
Internal carotid plexus	Head and Neck Sympathetic Nerve
Internal iliac vein	Hypogastric Vein, Right
	Hypogastric Vein, Left
Internal maxillary artery	External Carotid Artery, Right
	External Carotid Artery, Left
Internal naris	Nasal Mucosa and Soft Tissue
Internal oblique muscle	Abdomen Muscle, Right
	Abdomen Muscle, Left
Internal pudendal artery	Internal Iliac Artery, Right
	Internal Iliac Artery, Left
Internal pudendal vein	Hypogastric Vein, Right
	Hypogastric Vein, Left

Term	ICD-10-PCS Value
Internal thoracic artery	Internal Mammary Artery, Right
	Internal Mammary Artery, Left
	Subclavian Artery, Right
	Subclavian Artery, Left
Internal urethral sphincter	Urethra
Interphalangeal (IP) joint	Finger Phalangeal Joint, Right
	Finger Phalangeal Joint, Left
	Toe Phalangeal Joint, Right
	Toe Phalangeal Joint, Left
Interphalangeal ligament	Foot Bursa and Ligament, Right
	Foot Bursa and Ligament, Left
	Hand Bursa and Ligament, Right
	Hand Bursa and Ligament, Left
Interspinalis muscle	Trunk Muscle, Right
	Trunk Muscle, Left
Interspinous ligament, cervical	Head and Neck Bursa and Ligament
Interspinous ligament, lumbar	Lower Spine Bursa and Ligament
Interspinous ligament, thoracic	Upper Spine Bursa and Ligament
Intertransversarius muscle	Trunk Muscle, Right
	Trunk Muscle, Left
Intertransverse ligament, cervical	Head and Neck Bursa and Ligament
Intertransverse ligament, lumbar	Lower Spine Bursa and Ligament
Intertransverse ligament, thoracic	Upper Spine Bursa and Ligament
Interventricular foramen (Monro)	Cerebral Ventricle
Interventricular septum	Ventricular Septum
Intestinal lymphatic trunk	Cisterna Chyli
Ischiatic nerve	Sciatic Nerve
Ischiocavernosus muscle	Perineum Muscle
Ischiofemoral ligament	Hip Bursa and Ligament, Right
	Hip Bursa and Ligament, Left
Ischium	Pelvic Bone, Right
	Pelvic Bone, Left
Jejunal artery	Superior Mesenteric Artery
Jugular body	Glomus Jugulare
Jugular lymph node	Lymphatic, Right Neck
	Lymphatic, Left Neck
Labia majora	Vulva
Labia minora	Vulva
Labial gland	Upper Lip
	Lower Lip
Lacrimal canaliculus	Lacrimal Duct, Right
	Lacrimal Duct, Left
Lacrimal punctum	Lacrimal Duct, Right
	Lacrimal Duct, Left
Lacrimal sac	Lacrimal Duct, Right
	Lacrimal Duct, Left
Laryngopharynx	Pharynx
Lateral (brachial) lymph node	Lymphatic, Right Axillary
	Lymphatic, Left Axillary

Term	ICD-10-PCS Value
Lateral canthus	Upper Eyelid, Right
	Upper Eyelid, Left
Lateral collateral ligament (LCL)	Knee Bursa and Ligament, Right
	Knee Bursa and Ligament, Left
Lateral condyle of femur	Lower Femur, Right
	Lower Femur, Left
Lateral condyle of tibia	Tibia, Right
	Tibia, Left
Lateral cuneiform bone	Tarsal, Right
	Tarsal, Left
Lateral epicondyle of femur	Lower Femur, Right
	Lower Femur, Left
Lateral epicondyle of humerus	Humeral Shaft, Right
	Humeral Shaft, Left
Lateral femoral cutaneous nerve	Lumbar Plexus
Lateral malleolus	Fibula, Right
	Fibula, Left
Lateral meniscus	Knee Joint, Right
	Knee Joint, Left
Lateral nasal cartilage	Nasal Mucosa and Soft Tissue
Lateral plantar artery	Foot Artery, Right
	Foot Artery, Left
Lateral plantar nerve	Tibial Nerve
Lateral rectus muscle	Extraocular Muscle, Right
	Extraocular Muscle, Left
Lateral sacral artery	Internal Iliac Artery, Right
	Internal Iliac Artery, Left
Lateral sacral vein	Hypogastric Vein, Right
	Hypogastric Vein, Left
Lateral sural cutaneous nerve	Peroneal Nerve
Lateral tarsal artery	Foot Artery, Right
	Foot Artery, Left
Lateral temporo-mandibular ligament	Head and Neck Bursa and Ligament
Lateral thoracic artery	Axillary Artery, Right
	Axillary Artery, Left
Latissimus dorsi muscle	Trunk Muscle, Right
	Trunk Muscle, Left
Least splanchnic nerve	Thoracic Sympathetic Nerve
Left ascending lumbar vein	Hemiazygos Vein
Left atrioventricular valve	Mitral Valve
Left auricular appendix	Atrium, Left
Left colic vein	Colic Vein
Left coronary sulcus	Heart, Left
Left gastric artery	Gastric Artery
Left gastroepiploic artery	Splenic Artery
Left gastroepiploic vein	Splenic Vein
Left inferior phrenic vein	Renal Vein, Left
Left inferior pulmonary vein	Pulmonary Vein, Left
Left jugular trunk	Thoracic Duct
Left lateral ventricle	Cerebral Ventricle
Left ovarian vein	Renal Vein, Left
Left second lumbar vein	Renal Vein, Left

Term	ICD-10-PCS Value
Left subclavian trunk	Thoracic Duct
Left subcostal vein	Hemiazygos Vein
Left superior pulmonary vein	Pulmonary Vein, Left
Left suprarenal vein	Renal Vein, Left
Left testicular vein	Renal Vein, Left
Leptomeninges, intracranial	Cerebral Meninges
Leptomeninges, spinal	Spinal Meninges
Lesser alar cartilage	Nasal Mucosa and Soft Tissue
Lesser occipital nerve	Cervical Plexus
Lesser omentum	Omentum
Lesser saphenous vein	Saphenous Vein, Right
	Saphenous Vein, Left
Lesser splanchnic nerve	Thoracic Sympathetic Nerve
Lesser trochanter	Upper Femur, Right
	Upper Femur, Left
Lesser tuberosity	Humeral Head, Right
	Humeral Head, Left
Lesser wing	Sphenoid Bone
Levator anguli oris muscle	Facial Muscle
Levator ani muscle	Perineum Muscle
Levator labii superioris alaeque nasi muscle	Facial Muscle
Levator labii superioris muscle	Facial Muscle
Levator palpebrae superioris muscle	Upper Eyelid, Right
	Upper Eyelid, Left
Levator scapulae muscle	Neck Muscle, Right
	Neck Muscle, Left
Levator veli palatini muscle	Tongue, Palate, Pharynx Muscle
Levatores costarum muscle	Thorax Muscle, Right
	Thorax Muscle, Left
Ligament of head of fibula	Knee Bursa and Ligament, Right
	Knee Bursa and Ligament, Left
Ligament of the lateral malleolus	Ankle Bursa and Ligament, Right
	Ankle Bursa and Ligament, Left
Ligamentum flavum, cervical	Head and Neck Bursa and Ligament
Ligamentum flavum, lumbar	Lower Spine Bursa and Ligament
Ligamentum flavum, thoracic	Upper Spine Bursa and Ligament
Lingual artery	External Carotid Artery, Right
	External Carotid Artery, Left
Lingual tonsil	Pharynx
Locus ceruleus	Pons
Long thoracic nerve	Brachial Plexus
Lumbar artery	Abdominal Aorta
Lumbar facet joint	Lumbar Vertebral Joint
Lumbar ganglion	Lumbar Sympathetic Nerve
Lumbar lymph node	Lymphatic, Aortic
Lumbar lymphatic trunk	Cisterna Chyli
Lumbar splanchnic nerve	Lumbar Sympathetic Nerve
Lumbosacral facet joint	Lumbosacral Joint
Lumbosacral trunk	Lumbar Nerve

Term	ICD-10-PCS Value
Lunate bone	Carpal, Right
	Carpal, Left
Lunotriquetral ligament	Hand Bursa and Ligament, Right
	Hand Bursa and Ligament, Left
Macula	Retina, Right
	Retina, Left
Malleus	Auditory Ossicle, Right
	Auditory Ossicle, Left
Mammary duct	Breast, Right
	Breast, Left
	Breast, Bilateral
Mammary gland	Breast, Right
	Breast, Left
	Breast, Bilateral
Mammillary body	Hypothalamus
Mandibular nerve	Trigeminal Nerve
Mandibular notch	Mandible, Right
	Mandible, Left
Manubrium	Sternum
Masseter muscle	Head Muscle
Masseteric fascia	Subcutaneous Tissue and Fascia, Face
Mastoid (postauricular) lymph node	Lymphatic, Right Neck
	Lymphatic, Left Neck
Mastoid air cells	Mastoid Sinus, Right
	Mastoid Sinus, Left
Mastoid process	Temporal Bone, Right
	Temporal Bone, Left
Maxillary artery	External Carotid Artery, Right
	External Carotid Artery, Left
Maxillary nerve	Trigeminal Nerve
Medial canthus	Lower Eyelid, Right
	Lower Eyelid, Left
Medial collateral ligament (MCL)	Knee Bursa and Ligament, Right
	Knee Bursa and Ligament, Left
Medial condyle of femur	Lower Femur, Right
	Lower Femur, Left
Medial condyle of tibia	Tibia, Right
	Tibia, Left
Medial cuneiform bone	Tarsal, Right
	Tarsal, Left
Medial epicondyle of femur	Lower Femur, Right
	Lower Femur, Left
Medial epicondyle of humerus	Humeral Shaft, Right
	Humeral Shaft, Left
Medial malleolus	Tibia, Right
	Tibia, Left
Medial meniscus	Knee Joint, Right
	Knee Joint, Left
Medial plantar artery	Foot Artery, Right
	Foot Artery, Left
Medial plantar nerve	Tibial Nerve
Medial popliteal nerve	Tibial Nerve
Medial rectus muscle	Extraocular Muscle, Right
	Extraocular Muscle, Left

Term	ICD-10-PCS Value
Medial sural cutaneous nerve	Tibial Nerve
Median antebrachial vein	Basilic Vein, Right
	Basilic Vein, Left
Median cubital vein	Basilic Vein, Right
	Basilic Vein, Left
Median sacral artery	Abdominal Aorta
Mediastinal cavity	Mediastinum
Mediastinal lymph node	Lymphatic, Thorax
Mediastinal space	Mediastinum
Meissner's (submucous) plexus	Abdominal Sympathetic Nerve
Membranous urethra	Urethra
Mental foramen	Mandible, Right
	Mandible, Left
Mentalis muscle	Facial Muscle
Mesoappendix	Mesentery
Mesocolon	Mesentery
Metacarpal ligament	Hand Bursa and Ligament, Right
	Hand Bursa and Ligament, Left
Metacarpophalangeal ligament	Hand Bursa and Ligament, Right
	Hand Bursa and Ligament, Left
Metatarsal ligament	Foot Bursa and Ligament, Right
	Foot Bursa and Ligament, Left
Metatarsophalangeal ligament	Foot Bursa and Ligament, Right
	Foot Bursa and Ligament, Left
Metatarsophalangeal (MTP) joint	Metatarsal-Phalangeal Joint, Right
	Metatarsal-Phalangeal Joint, Left
Metathalamus	Thalamus
Midcarpal joint	Carpal Joint, Right
	Carpal Joint, Left
Middle cardiac nerve	Thoracic Sympathetic Nerve
Middle cerebral artery	Intracranial Artery
Middle cerebral vein	Intracranial Vein
Middle colic vein	Colic Vein
Middle genicular artery	Popliteal Artery, Right
	Popliteal Artery, Left
Middle hemorrhoidal vein	Hypogastric Vein, Right
	Hypogastric Vein, Left
Middle rectal artery	Internal Iliac Artery, Right
	Internal Iliac Artery, Left
Middle suprarenal artery	Abdominal Aorta
Middle temporal artery	Temporal Artery, Right
	Temporal Artery, Left
Middle turbinate	Nasal Turbinate
Mitral annulus	Mitral Valve
Molar gland	Buccal Mucosa
Musculocutaneous nerve	Brachial Plexus
Musculophrenic artery	Internal Mammary Artery, Right
	Internal Mammary Artery, Left
Musculospiral nerve	Radial Nerve
Myelencephalon	Medulla Oblongata
Myenteric (Auerbach's) plexus	Abdominal Sympathetic Nerve
Myometrium	Uterus

Term	ICD-10-PCS Value
Nail bed	Finger Nail
	Toe Nail
Nail plate	Finger Nail
	Toe Nail
Nasal cavity	Nasal Mucosa and Soft Tissue
Nasal concha	Nasal Turbinate
Nasalis muscle	Facial Muscle
Nasolacrimal duct	Lacrimal Duct, Right
	Lacrimal Duct, Left
Navicular bone	Tarsal, Right
	Tarsal, Left
Neck of femur	Upper Femur, Right
	Upper Femur, Left
Neck of humerus (anatomical) (surgical)	Humeral Head, Right
	Humeral Head, Left
Nerve to the stapedius	Facial Nerve
Neurohypophysis	Pituitary Gland
Ninth cranial nerve	Glossopharyngeal Nerve
Nostril	Nasal Mucosa and Soft Tissue
Obturator artery	Internal Iliac Artery, Right
	Internal Iliac Artery, Left
Obturator lymph node	Lymphatic, Pelvis
Obturator muscle	Hip Muscle, Right
	Hip Muscle, Left
Obturator nerve	Lumbar Plexus
Obturator vein	Hypogastric Vein, Right
	Hypogastric Vein, Left
Obtuse margin	Heart, Left
Occipital artery	External Carotid Artery, Right
	External Carotid Artery, Left
Occipital lobe	Cerebral Hemisphere
Occipital lymph node	Lymphatic, Right Neck
	Lymphatic, Left Neck
Occipitofrontalis muscle	Facial Muscle
Odontoid process	Cervical Vertebra
Olecranon bursa	Elbow Bursa and Ligament, Right
	Elbow Bursa and Ligament, Left
Olecranon process	Ulna, Right
	Ulna, Left
Olfactory bulb	Olfactory Nerve
Ophthalmic artery	Intracranial Artery
Ophthalmic nerve	Trigeminal Nerve
Ophthalmic vein	Intracranial Vein
Optic chiasma	Optic Nerve
Optic disc	Retina, Right
	Retina, Left
Optic foramen	Sphenoid Bone
Orbicularis oculi muscle	Upper Eyelid, Right
	Upper Eyelid, Left
Orbicularis oris muscle	Facial Muscle
Orbital fascia	Subcutaneous Tissue and Fascia, Face
Orbital portion of ethmoid bone	Orbit, Right
	Orbit, Left

Term	ICD-10-PCS Value
Orbital portion of frontal bone	Orbit, Right
	Orbit, Left
Orbital portion of lacrimal bone	Orbit, Right
	Orbit, Left
Orbital portion of maxilla	Orbit, Right
	Orbit, Left
Orbital portion of palatine bone	Orbit, Right
	Orbit, Left
Orbital portion of sphenoid bone	Orbit, Right
	Orbit, Left
Orbital portion of zygomatic bone	Orbit, Right
	Orbit, Left
Oropharynx	Pharynx
Otic ganglion	Head and Neck Sympathetic Nerve
Oval window	Middle Ear, Right
	Middle Ear, Left
Ovarian artery	Abdominal Aorta
Ovarian ligament	Uterine Supporting Structure
Oviduct	Fallopian Tube, Right
	Fallopian Tube, Left
Palatine gland	Buccal Mucosa
Palatine tonsil	Tonsils
Palatine uvula	Uvula
Palatoglossal muscle	Tongue, Palate, Pharynx Muscle
Palatopharyngeal muscle	Tongue, Palate, Pharynx Muscle
Palmar (volar) digital vein	Hand Vein, Right
	Hand Vein, Left
Palmar (volar) metacarpal vein	Hand Vein, Right
	Hand Vein, Left
Palmar cutaneous nerve	Median Nerve
	Radial Nerve
Palmar fascia (aponeurosis)	Subcutaneous Tissue and Fascia, Right Hand
	Subcutaneous Tissue and Fascia, Left Hand
Palmar interosseous muscle	Hand Muscle, Right
	Hand Muscle, Left
Palmar ulnocarpal ligament	Wrist Bursa and Ligament, Right
	Wrist Bursa and Ligament, Left
Palmaris longus muscle	Lower Arm and Wrist Muscle, Right
	Lower Arm and Wrist Muscle, Left
Pancreatic artery	Splenic Artery
Pancreatic plexus	Abdominal Sympathetic Nerve
Pancreatic vein	Splenic Vein
Pancreaticosplenic lymph node	Lymphatic, Aortic
Paraaortic lymph node	Lymphatic, Aortic
Pararectal lymph node	Lymphatic, Mesenteric
Parasternal lymph node	Lymphatic, Thorax
Paratracheal lymph node	Lymphatic, Thorax
Paraurethral (Skene's) gland	Vestibular Gland
Parietal lobe	Cerebral Hemisphere
Parotid lymph node	Lymphatic, Head
Parotid plexus	Facial Nerve

Term	ICD-10-PCS Value
Pars flaccida	Tympanic Membrane, Right
	Tympanic Membrane, Left
Patellar ligament	Knee Bursa and Ligament, Right
	Knee Bursa and Ligament, Left
Patellar tendon	Knee Tendon, Right
	Knee Tendon, Left
Patellofemoral joint	Knee Joint, Right
	Knee Joint, Left
	Knee Joint, Femoral Surface, Right
	Knee Joint, Femoral Surface, Left
Pectineus muscle	Upper Leg Muscle, Right
	Upper Leg Muscle, Left
Pectoral (anterior) lymph node	Lymphatic, Right Axillary
	Lymphatic, Left Axillary
Pectoral fascia	Subcutaneous Tissue and Fascia, Chest
Pectoralis major muscle	Thorax Muscle, Right
	Thorax Muscle, Left
Pectoralis minor muscle	Thorax Muscle, Right
	Thorax Muscle, Left
Pelvic splanchnic nerve	Abdominal Sympathetic Nerve
	Sacral Sympathetic Nerve
Penile urethra	Urethra
Pericardiophrenic artery	Internal Mammary Artery, Right
	Internal Mammary Artery, Left
Perimetrium	Uterus
Peroneus brevis muscle	Lower Leg Muscle, Right
	Lower Leg Muscle, Left
Peroneus longus muscle	Lower Leg Muscle, Right
	Lower Leg Muscle, Left
Petrous part of temporal bone	Temporal Bone, Right
	Temporal Bone, Left
Pharyngeal constrictor muscle	Tongue, Palate, Pharynx Muscle
Pharyngeal plexus	Vagus Nerve
Pharyngeal recess	Nasopharynx
Pharyngeal tonsil	Adenoids
Pharyngotympanic tube	Eustachian Tube, Right
	Eustachian Tube, Left
Pia mater, intracranial	Cerebral Meninges
Pia mater, spinal	Spinal Meninges
Pinna	External Ear, Right
	External Ear, Left
	External Ear, Bilateral
Piriform recess (sinus)	Pharynx
Piriformis muscle	Hip Muscle, Right
	Hip Muscle, Left
Pisiform bone	Carpal, Right
	Carpal, Left
Pisohamate ligament	Hand Bursa and Ligament, Right
	Hand Bursa and Ligament, Left
Pisometacarpal ligament	Hand Bursa and Ligament, Right
	Hand Bursa and Ligament, Left
Plantar digital vein	Foot Vein, Right
	Foot Vein, Left

Term	ICD-10-PCS Value
Plantar fascia (aponeurosis)	Subcutaneous Tissue and Fascia, Right Foot
	Subcutaneous Tissue and Fascia, Left Foot
Plantar metatarsal vein	Foot Vein, Right
	Foot Vein, Left
Plantar venous arch	Foot Vein, Right
	Foot Vein, Left
Platysma muscle	Neck Muscle, Right
	Neck Muscle, Left
Plica semilunaris	Conjunctiva, Right
	Conjunctiva, Left
Pneumogastric nerve	Vagus Nerve
Pneumotaxic center	Pons
Pontine tegmentum	Pons
Popliteal ligament	Knee Bursa and Ligament, Right
	Knee Bursa and Ligament, Left
Popliteal lymph node	Lymphatic, Left Lower Extremity
	Lymphatic, Right Lower Extremity
Popliteal vein	Femoral Vein, Right
	Femoral Vein, Left
Popliteus muscle	Lower Leg Muscle, Right
	Lower Leg Muscle, Left
Postauricular (mastoid) lymph node	Lymphatic, Right Neck
	Lymphatic, Left Neck
Postcava	Inferior Vena Cava
Posterior (subscapular) lymph node	Lymphatic, Right Axillary
	Lymphatic, Left Axillary
Posterior auricular artery	External Carotid Artery, Right
	External Carotid Artery, Left
Posterior auricular nerve	Facial Nerve
Posterior auricular vein	External Jugular Vein, Right
	External Jugular Vein, Left
Posterior cerebral artery	Intracranial Artery
Posterior chamber	Eye, Right
	Eye, Left
Posterior circumflex humeral artery	Axillary Artery, Right
	Axillary Artery, Left
Posterior communicating artery	Intracranial Artery
Posterior cruciate ligament (PCL)	Knee Bursa and Ligament, Right
	Knee Bursa and Ligament, Left
Posterior facial (retromandibular) vein	Face Vein, Right
	Face Vein, Left
Posterior femoral cutaneous nerve	Sacral Plexus
Posterior inferior cerebellar artery (PICA)	Intracranial Artery
Posterior interosseous nerve	Radial Nerve
Posterior labial nerve	Pudendal Nerve
Posterior scrotal nerve	Pudendal Nerve
Posterior spinal artery	Vertebral Artery, Right
	Vertebral Artery, Left
Posterior tibial recurrent artery	Anterior Tibial Artery, Right
	Anterior Tibial Artery, Left
Posterior ulnar recurrent artery	Ulnar Artery, Right
	Ulnar Artery, Left

Term	ICD-10-PCS Value
Posterior vagal trunk	Vagus Nerve
Preauricular lymph node	Lymphatic, Head
Precava	Superior Vena Cava
Prepatellar bursa	Knee Bursa and Ligament, Right
	Knee Bursa and Ligament, Left
Pretracheal fascia	Subcutaneous Tissue and Fascia, Right Neck
	Subcutaneous Tissue and Fascia, Left Neck
Prevertebral fascia	Subcutaneous Tissue and Fascia, Right Neck
	Subcutaneous Tissue and Fascia, Left Neck
Princeps pollicis artery	Hand Artery, Right
	Hand Artery, Left
Procerus muscle	Facial Muscle
Profunda brachii	Brachial Artery, Right
	Brachial Artery, Left
Profunda femoris (deep femoral) vein	Femoral Vein, Right
	Femoral Vein, Left
Pronator quadratus muscle	Lower Arm and Wrist Muscle, Right
	Lower Arm and Wrist Muscle, Left
Pronator teres muscle	Lower Arm and Wrist Muscle, Right
	Lower Arm and Wrist Muscle, Left
Prostatic urethra	Urethra
Proximal radioulnar joint	Elbow Joint, Right
	Elbow Joint, Left
Psoas muscle	Hip Muscle, Right
	Hip Muscle, Left
Pterygoid muscle	Head Muscle
Pterygoid process	Sphenoid Bone
Pterygopalatine (sphenopalatine) ganglion	Head and Neck Sympathetic Nerve
Pubis	Pelvic Bone, Right
	Pelvic Bone, Left
Pubofemoral ligament	Hip Bursa and Ligament, Right
	Hip Bursa and Ligament, Left
Pudendal nerve	Sacral Plexus
Pulmoaortic canal	Pulmonary Artery, Left
Pulmonary annulus	Pulmonary Valve
Pulmonary plexus	Thoracic Sympathetic Nerve
	Vagus Nerve
Pulmonic valve	Pulmonary Valve
Pulvinar	Thalamus
Pyloric antrum	Stomach, Pylorus
Pyloric canal	Stomach, Pylorus
Pyloric sphincter	Stomach, Pylorus
Pyramidalis muscle	Abdomen Muscle, Right
	Abdomen Muscle, Left
Quadrangular cartilage	Nasal Septum
Quadrate lobe	Liver
Quadratus femoris muscle	Hip Muscle, Right
	Hip Muscle, Left
Quadratus lumborum muscle	Trunk Muscle, Right
	Trunk Muscle, Left
Quadratus plantae muscle	Foot Muscle, Right
	Foot Muscle, Left

Term	ICD-10-PCS Value
Quadriceps (femoris)	Upper Leg Muscle, Right
	Upper Leg Muscle, Left
Radial collateral carpal ligament	Wrist Bursa and Ligament, Right
	Wrist Bursa and Ligament, Left
Radial collateral ligament	Elbow Bursa and Ligament, Right
	Elbow Bursa and Ligament, Left
Radial notch	Ulna, Right
	Ulna, Left
Radial recurrent artery	Radial Artery, Right
	Radial Artery, Left
Radial vein	Brachial Vein, Right
	Brachial Vein, Left
Radialis indicis	Hand Artery, Right
	Hand Artery, Left
Radiocarpal joint	Wrist Joint, Right
	Wrist Joint, Left
Radiocarpal ligament	Wrist Bursa and Ligament, Right
	Wrist Bursa and Ligament, Left
Radioulnar ligament	Wrist Bursa and Ligament, Right
	Wrist Bursa and Ligament, Left
Rectosigmoid junction	Sigmoid Colon
Rectus abdominis muscle	Abdomen Muscle, Right
	Abdomen Muscle, Left
Rectus femoris muscle	Upper Leg Muscle, Right
	Upper Leg Muscle, Left
Recurrent laryngeal nerve	Vagus Nerve
Renal calyx	Kidney, Right
	Kidney, Left
	Kidneys, Bilateral
	Kidney
Renal capsule	Kidney, Right
	Kidney, Left
	Kidneys, Bilateral
	Kidney
Renal cortex	Kidney, Right
	Kidney, Left
	Kidneys, Bilateral
	Kidney
Renal plexus	Abdominal Sympathetic Nerve
Renal segment	Kidney, Right
	Kidney, Left
	Kidneys, Bilateral
	Kidney
Renal segmental artery	Renal Artery, Right
	Renal Artery, Left
Retroperitoneal cavity	Retroperitoneum
Retroperitoneal lymph node	Lymphatic, Aortic
Retroperitoneal space	Retroperitoneum
Retropharyngeal lymph node	Lymphatic, Right Neck
	Lymphatic, Left Neck
Retropubic space	Pelvic Cavity
Rhinopharynx	Nasopharynx
Rhomboid major muscle	Trunk Muscle, Right
	Trunk Muscle, Left

Term	ICD-10-PCS Value
Rhomboid minor muscle	Trunk Muscle, Right
	Trunk Muscle, Left
Right ascending lumbar vein	Azygos Vein
Right atrioventricular valve	Tricuspid Valve
Right auricular appendix	Atrium, Right
Right colic vein	Colic Vein
Right coronary sulcus	Heart, Right
Right gastric artery	Gastric Artery
Right gastroepiploic vein	Superior Mesenteric Vein
Right inferior phrenic vein	Inferior Vena Cava
Right inferior pulmonary vein	Pulmonary Vein, Right
Right jugular trunk	Lymphatic, Right Neck
Right lateral ventricle	Cerebral Ventricle
Right lymphatic duct	Lymphatic, Right Neck
Right ovarian vein	Inferior Vena Cava
Right second lumbar vein	Inferior Vena Cava
Right subclavian trunk	Lymphatic, Right Neck
Right subcostal vein	Azygos Vein
Right superior pulmonary vein	Pulmonary Vein, Right
Right suprarenal vein	Inferior Vena Cava
Right testicular vein	Inferior Vena Cava
Rima glottidis	Larynx
Risorius muscle	Facial Muscle
Round ligament of uterus	Uterine Supporting Structure
Round window	Inner Ear, Right
	Inner Ear, Left
Sacral ganglion	Sacral Sympathetic Nerve
Sacral lymph node	Lymphatic, Pelvis
Sacral splanchnic nerve	Sacral Sympathetic Nerve
Sacrococcygeal ligament	Lower Spine Bursa and Ligament
Sacrococcygeal symphysis	Sacrococcygeal Joint
Sacroiliac ligament	Lower Spine Bursa and Ligament
Sacrospinous ligament	Lower Spine Bursa and Ligament
Sacrotuberous ligament	Lower Spine Bursa and Ligament
Salpingopharyngeus muscle	Tongue, Palate, Pharynx Muscle
Salpinx	Fallopian Tube, Right
	Fallopian Tube, Left
Saphenous nerve	Femoral Nerve
Sartorius muscle	Upper Leg Muscle, Right
	Upper Leg Muscle, Left
Scalene muscle	Neck Muscle, Right
	Neck Muscle, Left
Scaphoid bone	Carpal, Right
	Carpal, Left
Scapholunate ligament	Hand Bursa and Ligament, Right
	Hand Bursa and Ligament, Left
Scaphotrapezium ligament	Hand Bursa and Ligament, Right
	Hand Bursa and Ligament, Left
Scarpa's (vestibular) ganglion	Acoustic Nerve
Sebaceous gland	Skin

Term	ICD-10-PCS Value
Second cranial nerve	Optic Nerve
Sella turcica	Sphenoid Bone
Semicircular canal	Inner Ear, Right
	Inner Ear, Left
Semimembranosus muscle	Upper Leg Muscle, Right
	Upper Leg Muscle, Left
Semitendinosus muscle	Upper Leg Muscle, Right
	Upper Leg Muscle, Left
Septal cartilage	Nasal Septum
Serratus anterior muscle	Thorax Muscle, Right
	Thorax Muscle, Left
Serratus posterior muscle	Trunk Muscle, Right
	Trunk Muscle, Left
Seventh cranial nerve	Facial Nerve
Short gastric artery	Splenic Artery
Sigmoid artery	Inferior Mesenteric Artery
Sigmoid flexure	Sigmoid Colon
Sigmoid vein	Inferior Mesenteric Vein
Sinoatrial node	Conduction Mechanism
Sinus venosus	Atrium, Right
Sixth cranial nerve	Abducens Nerve
Skene's (paraurethral) gland	Vestibular Gland
Small saphenous vein	Saphenous Vein, Right
	Saphenous Vein, Left
Solar (celiac) plexus	Abdominal Sympathetic Nerve
Soleus muscle	Lower Leg Muscle, Right
	Lower Leg Muscle, Left
Sphenomandibular ligament	Head and Neck Bursa and Ligament
Sphenopalatine (pterygopalatine) ganglion	Head and Neck Sympathetic Nerve
Spinal nerve, cervical	Cervical Nerve
Spinal nerve, lumbar	Lumbar Nerve
Spinal nerve, sacral	Sacral Nerve
Spinal nerve, thoracic	Thoracic Nerve
Spinous process	Cervical Vertebra
	Lumbar Vertebra
	Thoracic Vertebra
Spiral ganglion	Acoustic Nerve
Splenic flexure	Transverse Colon
Splenic plexus	Abdominal Sympathetic Nerve
Splenius capitis muscle	Head Muscle
Splenius cervicis muscle	Neck Muscle, Right
	Neck Muscle, Left
Stapes	Auditory Ossicle, Right
	Auditory Ossicle, Left
Stellate ganglion	Head and Neck Sympathetic Nerve
Stensen's duct	Parotid Duct, Right
	Parotid Duct, Left
Sternoclavicular ligament	Shoulder Bursa and Ligament, Right
	Shoulder Bursa and Ligament, Left
Sternocleidomastoid artery	Thyroid Artery, Right
	Thyroid Artery, Left

Term	ICD-10-PCS Value
Sternocleidomastoid muscle	Neck Muscle, Right
	Neck Muscle, Left
Sternocostal ligament	Sternum Bursa and Ligament
Styloglossus muscle	Tongue, Palate, Pharynx Muscle
Stylomandibular ligament	Head and Neck Bursa and Ligament
Stylopharyngeus muscle	Tongue, Palate, Pharynx Muscle
Subacromial bursa	Shoulder Bursa and Ligament, Right
	Shoulder Bursa and Ligament, Left
Subaortic (common iliac) lymph node	Lymphatic, Pelvis
Subarachnoid space, spinal	Spinal Canal
Subclavicular (apical) lymph node	Lymphatic, Right Axillary
	Lymphatic, Left Axillary
Subclavius muscle	Thorax Muscle, Right
	Thorax Muscle, Left
Subclavius nerve	Brachial Plexus
Subcostal artery	Upper Artery
Subcostal muscle	Thorax Muscle, Right
	Thorax Muscle, Left
Subcostal nerve	Thoracic Nerve
Subdural space, spinal	Spinal Canal
Submandibular ganglion	Facial Nerve
	Head and Neck Sympathetic Nerve
Submandibular gland	Submaxillary Gland, Right
	Submaxillary Gland, Left
Submandibular lymph node	Lymphatic, Head
Submandibular space	Subcutaneous Tissue and Fascia, Face
Submaxillary ganglion	Head and Neck Sympathetic Nerve
Submaxillary lymph node	Lymphatic, Head
Submental artery	Face Artery
Submental lymph node	Lymphatic, Head
Submucous (Meissner's) plexus	Abdominal Sympathetic Nerve
Suboccipital nerve	Cervical Nerve
Suboccipital venous plexus	Vertebral Vein, Right
	Vertebral Vein, Left
Subparotid lymph node	Lymphatic, Head
Subscapular aponeurosis	Subcutaneous Tissue and Fascia, Right Upper Arm
	Subcutaneous Tissue and Fascia, Left Upper Arm
Subscapular artery	Axillary Artery, Right
	Axillary Artery, Left
Subscapular (posterior) lymph node	Lymphatic, Right Axillary
	Lymphatic, Left Axillary
Subscapularis muscle	Shoulder Muscle, Right
	Shoulder Muscle, Left
Substantia nigra	Basal Ganglia
Subtalar (talocalcaneal) joint	Tarsal Joint, Right
	Tarsal Joint, Left
Subtalar ligament	Foot Bursa and Ligament, Right
	Foot Bursa and Ligament, Left
Subthalamic nucleus	Basal Ganglia
Superficial circumflex iliac vein	Saphenous Vein, Right
	Saphenous Vein, Left

Term	ICD-10-PCS Value
Superficial epigastric artery	Femoral Artery, Right
	Femoral Artery, Left
Superficial epigastric vein	Saphenous Vein, Right
	Saphenous Vein, Left
Superficial palmar arch	Hand Artery, Right
	Hand Artery, Left
Superficial palmar venous arch	Hand Vein, Right
	Hand Vein, Left
Superficial temporal artery	Temporal Artery, Right
	Temporal Artery, Left
Superficial transverse perineal muscle	Perineum Muscle
Superior cardiac nerve	Thoracic Sympathetic Nerve
Superior cerebellar vein	Intracranial Vein
Superior cerebral vein	Intracranial Vein
Superior clunic (cluneal) nerve	Lumbar Nerve
Superior epigastric artery	Internal Mammary Artery, Right
	Internal Mammary Artery, Left
Superior genicular artery	Popliteal Artery, Right
	Popliteal Artery, Left
Superior gluteal artery	Internal Iliac Artery, Right
	Internal Iliac Artery, Left
Superior gluteal nerve	Lumbar Plexus
Superior hypogastric plexus	Abdominal Sympathetic Nerve
Superior labial artery	Face Artery
Superior laryngeal artery	Thyroid Artery, Right
	Thyroid Artery, Left
Superior laryngeal nerve	Vagus Nerve
Superior longitudinal muscle	Tongue, Palate, Pharynx Muscle
Superior mesenteric ganglion	Abdominal Sympathetic Nerve
Superior mesenteric lymph node	Lymphatic, Mesenteric
Superior mesenteric plexus	Abdominal Sympathetic Nerve
Superior oblique muscle	Extraocular Muscle, Right
	Extraocular Muscle, Left
Superior olivary nucleus	Pons
Superior rectal artery	Inferior Mesenteric Artery
Superior rectal vein	Inferior Mesenteric Vein
Superior rectus muscle	Extraocular Muscle, Right
	Extraocular Muscle, Left
Superior tarsal plate	Upper Eyelid, Right
	Upper Eyelid, Left
Superior thoracic artery	Axillary Artery, Right
	Axillary Artery, Left
Superior thyroid artery	External Carotid Artery, Right
	External Carotid Artery, Left
	Thyroid Artery, Right
	Thyroid Artery, Left
Superior turbinate	Nasal Turbinate
Superior ulnar collateral artery	Brachial Artery, Right
	Brachial Artery, Left
Supraclavicular nerve	Cervical Plexus

Term	ICD-10-PCS Value
Supraclavicular (Virchow's) lymph node	Lymphatic, Right Neck
	Lymphatic, Left Neck
Suprahyoid lymph node	Lymphatic, Head
Suprahyoid muscle	Neck Muscle, Right
	Neck Muscle, Left
Suprainguinal lymph node	Lymphatic, Pelvis
Supraorbital vein	Face Vein, Right
	Face Vein, Left
Suprarenal gland	Adrenal Gland, Right
	Adrenal Gland, Left
	Adrenal Glands, Bilateral
	Adrenal Gland
Suprarenal plexus	Abdominal Sympathetic Nerve
Suprascapular nerve	Brachial Plexus
Supraspinatus fascia	Subcutaneous Tissue and Fascia, Right Upper Arm
	Subcutaneous Tissue and Fascia, Left Upper Arm
Supraspinatus muscle	Shoulder Muscle, Right
	Shoulder Muscle, Left
Supraspinous ligament	Upper Spine Bursa and Ligament
	Lower Spine Bursa and Ligament
Suprasternal notch	Sternum
Supratrochlear lymph node	Lymphatic, Right Upper Extremity
	Lymphatic, Left Upper Extremity
Sural artery	Popliteal Artery, Right
	Popliteal Artery, Left
Sweat gland	Skin
Talocalcaneal ligament	Foot Bursa and Ligament, Right
	Foot Bursa and Ligament, Left
Talocalcaneal (subtalar) joint	Tarsal Joint, Right
	Tarsal Joint, Left
Talocalcaneonavicular joint	Tarsal Joint, Right
	Tarsal Joint, Left
Talocalcaneonavicular ligament	Foot Bursa and Ligament, Right
	Foot Bursa and Ligament, Left
Talocrural joint	Ankle Joint, Right
	Ankle Joint, Left
Talofibular ligament	Ankle Bursa and Ligament, Right
	Ankle Bursa and Ligament, Left
Talus bone	Tarsal, Right
	Tarsal, Left
Tarsometatarsal ligament	Foot Bursa and Ligament, Right
	Foot Bursa and Ligament, Left
Temporal lobe	Cerebral Hemisphere
Temporalis muscle	Head Muscle
Temporoparietalis muscle	Head Muscle
Tensor fasciae latae muscle	Hip Muscle, Right
	Hip Muscle, Left
Tensor veli palatini muscle	Tongue, Palate, Pharynx Muscle
Tenth cranial nerve	Vagus Nerve
Tentorium cerebelli	Dura Mater
Teres major muscle	Shoulder Muscle, Right
	Shoulder Muscle, Left

Term	ICD-10-PCS Value
Teres minor muscle	Shoulder Muscle, Right
	Shoulder Muscle, Left
Testicular artery	Abdominal Aorta
Thenar muscle	Hand Muscle, Right
	Hand Muscle, Left
Third cranial nerve	Oculomotor Nerve
Third occipital nerve	Cervical Nerve
Third ventricle	Cerebral Ventricle
Thoracic aortic plexus	Thoracic Sympathetic Nerve
Thoracic esophagus	Esophagus, Middle
Thoracic facet joint	Thoracic Vertebral Joint
Thoracic ganglion	Thoracic Sympathetic Nerve
Thoracoacromial artery	Axillary Artery, Right
	Axillary Artery, Left
Thoracolumbar facet joint	Thoracolumbar Vertebral Joint
Thymus gland	Thymus
Thyroarytenoid muscle	Neck Muscle, Right
	Neck Muscle, Left
Thyrocervical trunk	Thyroid Artery, Right
	Thyroid Artery, Left
Thyroid cartilage	Larynx
Tibialis anterior muscle	Lower Leg Muscle, Right
	Lower Leg Muscle, Left
Tibialis posterior muscle	Lower Leg Muscle, Right
	Lower Leg Muscle, Left
Tibiofemoral joint	Knee Joint, Right
	Knee Joint, Left
	Knee Joint, Tibial Surface, Right
	Knee Joint, Tibial Surface, Left
Tibioperoneal trunk	Popliteal Artery, Right
	Popliteal Artery, Left
Tongue, base of	Pharynx
Tracheobronchial lymph node	Lymphatic, Thorax
Tragus	External Ear, Right
	External Ear, Left
	External Ear, Bilateral
Transversalis fascia	Subcutaneous Tissue and Fascia, Trunk
Transverse acetabular ligament	Hip Bursa and Ligament, Right
	Hip Bursa and Ligament, Left
Transverse (cutaneous) cervical nerve	Cervical Plexus
Transverse facial artery	Temporal Artery, Right
	Temporal Artery, Left
Transverse foramen	Cervical Vertebra
Transverse humeral ligament	Shoulder Bursa and Ligament, Right
	Shoulder Bursa and Ligament, Left
Transverse ligament of atlas	Head and Neck Bursa and Ligament
Transverse process	Cervical Vertebra
	Thoracic Vertebra
	Lumbar Vertebra
Transverse scapular ligament	Shoulder Bursa and Ligament, Right
	Shoulder Bursa and Ligament, Left

Term	ICD-10-PCS Value
Transverse thoracis muscle	Thorax Muscle, Right
	Thorax Muscle, Left
Transversospinalis muscle	Trunk Muscle, Right
	Trunk Muscle, Left
Transversus abdominis muscle	Abdomen Muscle, Right
	Abdomen Muscle, Left
Trapezium bone	Carpal, Right
	Carpal, Left
Trapezius muscle	Trunk Muscle, Right
	Trunk Muscle, Left
Trapezoid bone	Carpal, Right
	Carpal, Left
Triceps brachii muscle	Upper Arm Muscle, Right
	Upper Arm Muscle, Left
Tricuspid annulus	Tricuspid Valve
Trifacial nerve	Trigeminal Nerve
Trigone of bladder	Bladder
Triquetral bone	Carpal, Right
	Carpal, Left
Trochantericbursa	Hip Bursa and Ligament, Right
	Hip Bursa and Ligament, Left
Twelfth cranial nerve	Hypoglossal Nerve
Tympanic cavity	Middle Ear, Right
	Middle Ear, Left
Tympanic nerve	Glossopharyngeal Nerve
Tympanic part of temporal bone	Temporal Bone, Right
	Temporal Bone, Left
Ulnar collateral carpal ligament	Wrist Bursa and Ligament, Right
	Wrist Bursa and Ligament, Left
Ulnar collateral ligament	Elbow Bursa and Ligament, Right
	Elbow Bursa and Ligament, Left
Ulnar notch	Radius, Right
	Radius, Left
Ulnar vein	Brachial Vein, Right
	Brachial Vein, Left
Umbilical artery	Internal Iliac Artery, Right
	Internal Iliac Artery, Left
	Lower Artery
Ureteral orifice	Ureter, Right
	Ureter, Left
	Ureters, Bilateral
	Ureter
Ureteropelvic junction (UPJ)	Kidney Pelvis, Right
	Kidney Pelvis, Left
Ureterovesical orifice	Ureter, Right
	Ureter, Left
	Ureters, Bilateral
	Ureter
Uterine artery	Internal Iliac Artery, Right
	Internal Iliac Artery, Left
Uterine cornu	Uterus
Uterine tube	Fallopian Tube, Right
	Fallopian Tube, Left
Uterine vein	Hypogastric Vein, Right
	Hypogastric Vein, Left

Term	ICD-10-PCS Value
Vaginal artery	Internal Iliac Artery, Right
	Internal Iliac Artery, Left
Vaginal vein	Hypogastric Vein, Right
	Hypogastric Vein, Left
Vastus intermedius muscle	Upper Leg Muscle, Right
	Upper Leg Muscle, Left
Vastus lateralis muscle	Upper Leg Muscle, Right
	Upper Leg Muscle, Left
Vastus medialis muscle	Upper Leg Muscle, Right
	Upper Leg Muscle, Left
Ventricular fold	Larynx
Vermiform appendix	Appendix
Vermilion border	Upper Lip
	Lower Lip
Vertebral arch	Cervical Vertebra
	Lumbar Vertebra
	Thoracic Vertebra
Vertebral body	Cervical Vertebra
	Lumbar Vertebra
	Thoracic Vertebra
Vertebral canal	Spinal Canal
Vertebral foramen	Cervical Vertebra
	Lumbar Vertebra
	Thoracic Vertebra
Vertebral lamina	Cervical Vertebra
	Lumbar Vertebra
	Thoracic Vertebra
Vertebral pedicle	Cervical Vertebra
	Lumbar Vertebra
	Thoracic Vertebra
Vesical vein	Hypogastric Vein, Right
	Hypogastric Vein, Left
Vestibular (Scarpa's) ganglion	Acoustic Nerve
Vestibular nerve	Acoustic Nerve
Vestibulocochlear nerve	Acoustic Nerve
Virchow's (supraclavicular) lymph node	Lymphatic, Right Neck
	Lymphatic, Left Neck
Vitreous body	Vitreous, Right
	Vitreous, Left
Vocal fold	Vocal Cord, Right
	Vocal Cord, Left
Volar (palmar) digital vein	Hand Vein, Right
	Hand Vein, Left
Volar (palmar) metacarpal vein	Hand Vein, Right
	Hand Vein, Left
Vomer bone	Nasal Septum
Vomer of nasal septum	Nasal Bone
Xiphoid process	Sternum
Zonule of Zinn	Lens, Right
	Lens, Left
Zygomatic process of frontal bone	Frontal Bone

Term	ICD-10-PCS Value
Zygomatic process of temporal bone	Temporal Bone, Right
	Temporal Bone, Left
Zygomaticus muscle	Facial Muscle

Appendix E: Body Part Definitions

ICD-10-PCS Value	Definition
1st Toe, Left 1st Toe, Right	**Includes:** Hallux
Abdomen Muscle, Left Abdomen Muscle, Right	**Includes:** External oblique muscle Internal oblique muscle Pyramidalis muscle Rectus abdominis muscle Transversus abdominis muscle
Abdominal Aorta	**Includes:** Inferior phrenic artery Lumbar artery Median sacral artery Middle suprarenal artery Ovarian artery Testicular artery
Abdominal Sympathetic Nerve	**Includes:** Abdominal aortic plexus Auerbach's (myenteric) plexus Celiac (solar) plexus Celiac ganglion Gastric plexus Hepatic plexus Inferior hypogastric plexus Inferior mesenteric ganglion Inferior mesenteric plexus Meissner's (submucous) plexus Myenteric (Auerbach's) plexus Pancreatic plexus Pelvic splanchnic nerve Renal plexus Solar (celiac) plexus Splenic plexus Submucous (Meissner's) plexus Superior hypogastric plexus Superior mesenteric ganglion Superior mesenteric plexus Suprarenal plexus
Abducens Nerve	**Includes:** Sixth cranial nerve
Accessory Nerve	**Includes:** Eleventh cranial nerve
Acoustic Nerve	**Includes:** Cochlear nerve Eighth cranial nerve Scarpa's (vestibular) ganglion Spiral ganglion Vestibular (Scarpa's) ganglion Vestibular nerve Vestibulocochlear nerve
Adenoids	**Includes:** Pharyngeal tonsil
Adrenal Gland Adrenal Gland, Left Adrenal Gland, Right Adrenal Glands, Bilateral	**Includes:** Suprarenal gland
Ampulla of Vater	**Includes:** Duodenal ampulla Hepatopancreatic ampulla
Anal Sphincter	**Includes:** External anal sphincter Internal anal sphincter

ICD-10-PCS Value	Definition
Ankle Bursa and Ligament, Left Ankle Bursa and Ligament, Right	**Includes:** Calcaneofibular ligament Deltoid ligament Ligament of the lateral malleolus Talofibular ligament
Ankle Joint, Left Ankle Joint, Right	**Includes:** Inferior tibiofibular joint Talocrural joint
Anterior Chamber, Left Anterior Chamber, Right	**Includes:** Aqueous humour
Anterior Tibial Artery, Left Anterior Tibial Artery, Right	**Includes:** Anterior lateral malleolar artery Anterior medial malleolar artery Anterior tibial recurrent artery Dorsalis pedis artery Posterior tibial recurrent artery
Anus	**Includes:** Anal orifice
Aortic Valve	**Includes:** Aortic annulus
Appendix	**Includes:** Vermiform appendix
Atrial Septum	**Includes:** Interatrial septum
Atrium, Left	**Includes:** Atrium pulmonale Left auricular appendix
Atrium, Right	**Includes:** Atrium dextrum cordis Right auricular appendix Sinus venosus
Auditory Ossicle, Left Auditory Ossicle, Right	**Includes:** Incus Malleus Stapes
Axillary Artery, Left Axillary Artery, Right	**Includes:** Anterior circumflex humeral artery Lateral thoracic artery Posterior circumflex humeral artery Subscapular artery Superior thoracic artery Thoracoacromial artery
Azygos Vein	**Includes:** Right ascending lumbar vein Right subcostal vein
Basal Ganglia	**Includes:** Basal nuclei Claustrum Corpus striatum Globus pallidus Substantia nigra Subthalamic nucleus
Basilic Vein, Left Basilic Vein, Right	**Includes:** Median antebrachial vein Median cubital vein
Bladder	**Includes:** Trigone of bladder
Brachial Artery, Left Brachial Artery, Right	**Includes:** Inferior ulnar collateral artery Profunda brachii Superior ulnar collateral artery

ICD-10-PCS Value	Definition
Brachial Plexus	**Includes:** Axillary nerve Dorsal scapular nerve First intercostal nerve Long thoracic nerve Musculocutaneous nerve Subclavius nerve Suprascapular nerve
Brachial Vein, Left **Brachial Vein, Right**	**Includes:** Radial vein Ulnar vein
Brain	**Includes:** Cerebrum Corpus callosum Encephalon
Breast, Bilateral **Breast, Left** **Breast, Right**	**Includes:** Mammary duct Mammary gland
Buccal Mucosa	**Includes:** Buccal gland Molar gland Palatine gland
Carotid Bodies, Bilateral **Carotid Body, Left** **Carotid Body, Right**	**Includes:** Carotid glomus
Carpal Joint, Left **Carpal Joint, Right**	**Includes:** Intercarpal joint Midcarpal joint
Carpal, Left **Carpal, Right**	**Includes:** Capitate bone Hamate bone Lunate bone Pisiform bone Scaphoid bone Trapezium bone Trapezoid bone Triquetral bone
Celiac Artery	**Includes:** Celiac trunk
Cephalic Vein, Left **Cephalic Vein, Right**	**Includes:** Accessory cephalic vein
Cerebellum	**Includes:** Culmen
Cerebral Hemisphere	**Includes:** Frontal lobe Occipital lobe Parietal lobe Temporal lobe
Cerebral Meninges	**Includes:** Arachnoid mater, intracranial Leptomeninges, intracranial Pia mater, intracranial
Cerebral Ventricle	**Includes:** Aqueduct of Sylvius Cerebral aqueduct (Sylvius) Choroid plexus Ependyma Foramen of Monro (intraventricular) Fourth ventricle Interventricular foramen (Monro) Left lateral ventricle Right lateral ventricle Third ventricle

ICD-10-PCS Value	Definition
Cervical Nerve	**Includes:** Greater occipital nerve Spinal nerve, cervical Suboccipital nerve Third occipital nerve
Cervical Plexus	**Includes:** Ansa cervicalis Cutaneous (transverse) cervical nerve Great auricular nerve Lesser occipital nerve Supraclavicular nerve Transverse (cutaneous) cervical nerve
Cervical Vertebra	**Includes:** Dens Odontoid process Spinous process Transverse foramen Transverse process Vertebral arch Vertebral body Vertebral foramen Vertebral lamina Vertebral pedicle
Cervical Vertebral Joint	**Includes:** Atlantoaxial joint Cervical facet joint
Cervical Vertebral Joints, 2 or more	**Includes:** Cervical facet joint
Cervicothoracic Vertebral Joint	**Includes:** Cervicothoracic facet joint
Cisterna Chyli	**Includes:** Intestinal lymphatic trunk Lumbar lymphatic trunk
Coccygeal Glomus	**Includes:** Coccygeal body
Colic Vein	**Includes:** Ileocolic vein Left colic vein Middle colic vein Right colic vein
Conduction Mechanism	**Includes:** Atrioventricular node Bundle of His Bundle of Kent Sinoatrial node
Conjunctiva, Left **Conjunctiva, Right**	**Includes:** Plica semilunaris
Dura Mater	**Includes:** Diaphragma sellae Dura mater, intracranial Falx cerebri Tentorium cerebelli
Elbow Bursa and Ligament, Left **Elbow Bursa and Ligament, Right**	**Includes:** Annular ligament Olecranon bursa Radial collateral ligament Ulnar collateral ligament
Elbow Joint, Left **Elbow Joint, Right**	**Includes:** Distal humerus, involving joint Humeroradial joint Humeroulnar joint Proximal radioulnar joint
Epidural Space, Intracranial	**Includes:** Extradural space, intracranial

ICD-10-PCS Value	Definition
Epiglottis	**Includes:** Glossoepiglottic fold
Esophagogastric Junction	**Includes:** Cardia Cardioesophageal junction Gastroesophageal (GE) junction
Esophagus, Lower	**Includes:** Abdominal esophagus
Esophagus, Middle	**Includes:** Thoracic esophagus
Esophagus, Upper	**Includes:** Cervical esophagus
Ethmoid Bone, Left Ethmoid Bone, Right	**Includes:** Cribriform plate
Ethmoid Sinus, Left Ethmoid Sinus, Right	**Includes:** Ethmoidal air cell
Eustachian Tube, Left Eustachian Tube, Right	**Includes:** Auditory tube Pharyngotympanic tube
External Auditory Canal, Left External Auditory Canal, Right	**Includes:** External auditory meatus
External Carotid Artery, Left External Carotid Artery, Right	**Includes:** Ascending pharyngeal artery Internal maxillary artery Lingual artery Maxillary artery Occipital artery Posterior auricular artery Superior thyroid artery
External Ear, Bilateral External Ear, Left External Ear, Right	**Includes:** Antihelix Antitragus Auricle Earlobe Helix Pinna Tragus
External Iliac Artery, Left External Iliac Artery, Right	**Includes:** Deep circumflex iliac artery Inferior epigastric artery
External Jugular Vein, Left External Jugular Vein, Right	**Includes:** Posterior auricular vein
Extraocular Muscle, Left Extraocular Muscle, Right	**Includes:** Inferior oblique muscle Inferior rectus muscle Lateral rectus muscle Medial rectus muscle Superior oblique muscle Superior rectus muscle
Eye, Left Eye, Right	**Includes:** Ciliary body Posterior chamber
Face Artery	**Includes:** Angular artery Ascending palatine artery External maxillary artery Facial artery Inferior labial artery Submental artery Superior labial artery

ICD-10-PCS Value	Definition
Face Vein, Left Face Vein, Right	**Includes:** Angular vein Anterior facial vein Common facial vein Deep facial vein Frontal vein Posterior facial (retromandibular) vein Supraorbital vein
Facial Muscle	**Includes:** Buccinator muscle Corrugator supercilii muscle Depressor anguli oris muscle Depressor labii inferioris muscle Depressor septi nasi muscle Depressor supercilii muscle Levator anguli oris muscle Levator labii superioris alaeque nasi muscle Levator labii superioris muscle Mentalis muscle Nasalis muscle Occipitofrontalis muscle Orbicularis oris muscle Procerus muscle Risorius muscle Zygomaticus muscle
Facial Nerve	**Includes:** Chorda tympani Geniculate ganglion Greater superficial petrosal nerve Nerve to the stapedius Parotid plexus Posterior auricular nerve Seventh cranial nerve Submandibular ganglion
Fallopian Tube, Left Fallopian Tube, Right	**Includes:** Oviduct Salpinx Uterine tube
Femoral Artery, Left Femoral Artery, Right	**Includes:** Circumflex iliac artery Deep femoral artery Descending genicular artery External pudendal artery Superficial epigastric artery
Femoral Nerve	**Includes:** Anterior crural nerve Saphenous nerve
Femoral Shaft, Left Femoral Shaft, Right	**Includes:** Body of femur
Femoral Vein, Left Femoral Vein, Right	**Includes:** Deep femoral (profunda femoris) vein Popliteal vein Profunda femoris (deep femoral) vein
Fibula, Left Fibula, Right	**Includes:** Body of fibula Head of fibula Lateral malleolus
Finger Nail	**Includes:** Nail bed Nail plate

ICD-10-PCS Value	Definition
Finger Phalangeal Joint, Left **Finger Phalangeal Joint, Right**	**Includes:** Interphalangeal (IP) joint
Foot Artery, Left **Foot Artery, Right**	**Includes:** Arcuate artery Dorsal metatarsal artery Lateral plantar artery Lateral tarsal artery Medial plantar artery
Foot Bursa and Ligament, Left **Foot Bursa and Ligament, Right**	**Includes:** Calcaneocuboid ligament Cuneonavicular ligament Intercuneiform ligament Interphalangeal ligament Metatarsal ligament Metatarsophalangeal ligament Subtalar ligament Talocalcaneal ligament Talocalcaneonavicular ligament Tarsometatarsal ligament
Foot Muscle, Left **Foot Muscle, Right**	**Includes:** Abductor hallucis muscle Adductor hallucis muscle Extensor digitorum brevis muscle Extensor hallucis brevis muscle Flexor digitorum brevis muscle Flexor hallucis brevis muscle Quadratus plantae muscle
Foot Vein, Left **Foot Vein, Right**	**Includes:** Common digital vein Dorsal metatarsal vein Dorsal venous arch Plantar digital vein Plantar metatarsal vein Plantar venous arch
Frontal Bone	**Includes:** Zygomatic process of frontal bone
Gastric Artery	**Includes:** Left gastric artery Right gastric artery
Glenoid Cavity, Left **Glenoid Cavity, Right**	**Includes:** Glenoid fossa (of scapula)
Glomus Jugulare	**Includes:** Jugular body
Glossopharyngeal Nerve	**Includes:** Carotid sinus nerve Ninth cranial nerve Tympanic nerve
Hand Artery, Left **Hand Artery, Right**	**Includes:** Deep palmar arch Princeps pollicis artery Radialis indicis Superficial palmar arch
Hand Bursa and Ligament, Left **Hand Bursa and Ligament, Right**	**Includes:** Carpometacarpal ligament Intercarpal ligament Interphalangeal ligament Lunotriquetral ligament Metacarpal ligament Metacarpophalangeal ligament Pisohamate ligament Pisometacarpal ligament Scapholunate ligament Scaphotrapezium ligament

ICD-10-PCS Value	Definition
Hand Muscle, Left **Hand Muscle, Right**	**Includes:** Hypothenar muscle Palmar interosseous muscle Thenar muscle
Hand Vein, Left **Hand Vein, Right**	**Includes:** Dorsal metacarpal vein Palmar (volar) digital vein Palmar (volar) metacarpal vein Superficial palmar venous arch Volar (palmar) digital vein Volar (palmar) metacarpal vein
Head and Neck Bursa and Ligament	**Includes:** Alar ligament of axis Cervical interspinous ligament Cervical intertransverse ligament Cervical ligamentum flavum Interspinous ligament, cervical Intertransverse ligament, cervical Lateral temporomandibular ligament Ligamentum flavum, cervical Sphenomandibular ligament Stylomandibular ligament Transverse ligament of atlas
Head and Neck Sympathetic Nerve	**Includes:** Cavernous plexus Cervical ganglion Ciliary ganglion Internal carotid plexus Otic ganglion Pterygopalatine (sphenopalatine) ganglion Sphenopalatine (pterygopalatine) ganglion Stellate ganglion Submandibular ganglion Submaxillary ganglion
Head Muscle	**Includes:** Auricularis muscle Masseter muscle Pterygoid muscle Splenius capitis muscle Temporalis muscle Temporoparietalis muscle
Heart, Left	**Includes:** Left coronary sulcus Obtuse margin
Heart, Right	**Includes:** Right coronary sulcus
Hemiazygos Vein	**Includes:** Left ascending lumbar vein Left subcostal vein
Hepatic Artery	**Includes:** Common hepatic artery Gastroduodenal artery Hepatic artery proper
Hip Bursa and Ligament, Left **Hip Bursa and Ligament, Right**	**Includes:** Iliofemoral ligament Ischiofemoral ligament Pubofemoral ligament Transverse acetabular ligament Trochanteric bursa
Hip Joint, Left **Hip Joint, Right**	**Includes:** Acetabulofemoral joint

ICD-10-PCS Value	Definition
Hip Muscle, Left **Hip Muscle, Right**	**Includes:** Gemellus muscle Gluteus maximus muscle Gluteus medius muscle Gluteus minimus muscle Iliacus muscle Obturator muscle Piriformis muscle Psoas muscle Quadratus femoris muscle Tensor fasciae latae muscle
Humeral Head, Left **Humeral Head, Right**	**Includes:** Greater tuberosity Lesser tuberosity Neck of humerus (anatomical)(surgical)
Humeral Shaft, Left **Humeral Shaft, Right**	**Includes:** Distal humerus Humerus, distal Lateral epicondyle of humerus Medial epicondyle of humerus
Hypogastric Vein, Left **Hypogastric Vein, Right**	**Includes:** Gluteal vein Internal iliac vein Internal pudendal vein Lateral sacral vein Middle hemorrhoidal vein Obturator vein Uterine vein Vaginal vein Vesical vein
Hypoglossal Nerve	**Includes:** Twelfth cranial nerve
Hypothalamus	**Includes:** Mammillary body
Inferior Mesenteric Artery	**Includes:** Sigmoid artery Superior rectal artery
Inferior Mesenteric Vein	**Includes:** Sigmoid vein Superior rectal vein
Inferior Vena Cava	**Includes:** Postcava Right inferior phrenic vein Right ovarian vein Right second lumbar vein Right suprarenal vein Right testicular vein
Inguinal Region, Bilateral **Inguinal Region, Left** **Inguinal Region, Right**	**Includes:** Inguinal canal Inguinal triangle
Inner Ear, Left **Inner Ear, Right**	**Includes:** Bony labyrinth Bony vestibule Cochlea Round window Semicircular canal
Innominate Artery	**Includes:** Brachiocephalic artery Brachiocephalic trunk
Innominate Vein, Left **Innominate Vein, Right**	**Includes:** Brachiocephalic vein Inferior thyroid vein
Internal Carotid Artery, Left **Internal Carotid Artery, Right**	**Includes:** Caroticotympanic artery Carotid sinus

ICD-10-PCS Value	Definition
Internal Iliac Artery, Left **Internal Iliac Artery, Right**	**Includes:** Deferential artery Hypogastric artery Iliolumbar artery Inferior gluteal artery Inferior vesical artery Internal pudendal artery Lateral sacral artery Middle rectal artery Obturator artery Superior gluteal artery Umbilical artery Uterine artery Vaginal artery
Internal Mammary Artery, Left **Internal Mammary Artery, Right**	**Includes:** Anterior intercostal artery Internal thoracic artery Musculophrenic artery Pericardiophrenic artery Superior epigastric artery
Intracranial Artery	**Includes:** Anterior cerebral artery Anterior choroidal artery Anterior communicating artery Basilar artery Circle of Willis Internal carotid artery, intracranial portion Middle cerebral artery Ophthalmic artery Posterior cerebral artery Posterior communicating artery Posterior inferior cerebellar artery (PICA)
Intracranial Vein	**Includes:** Anterior cerebral vein Basal (internal) cerebral vein Dural venous sinus Great cerebral vein Inferior cerebellar vein Inferior cerebral vein Internal (basal) cerebral vein Middle cerebral vein Ophthalmic vein Superior cerebellar vein Superior cerebral vein
Jejunum	**Includes:** Duodenojejunal flexure
Kidney	**Includes:** Renal calyx Renal capsule Renal cortex Renal segment
Kidney Pelvis, Left **Kidney Pelvis, Right**	**Includes:** Ureteropelvic junction (UPJ)
Kidney, Left **Kidney, Right** **Kidneys, Bilateral**	**Includes:** Renal calyx Renal capsule Renal cortex Renal segment

ICD-10-PCS Value	Definition
Knee Bursa and Ligament, Left Knee Bursa and Ligament, Right	**Includes:** Anterior cruciate ligament (ACL) Lateral collateral ligament (LCL) Ligament of head of fibula Medial collateral ligament (MCL) Patellar ligament Popliteal ligament Posterior cruciate ligament (PCL) Prepatellar bursa
Knee Joint, Femoral Surface, Left Knee Joint, Femoral Surface, Right	**Includes:** Femoropatellar joint Patellofemoral joint
Knee Joint, Left Knee Joint, Right	**Includes:** Femoropatellar joint Femorotibial joint Lateral meniscus Medial meniscus Patellofemoral joint Tibiofemoral joint
Knee Joint, Tibial Surface, Left Knee Joint, Tibial Surface, Right	**Includes:** Femorotibial joint Tibiofemoral joint
Knee Tendon, Left Knee Tendon, Right	**Includes:** Patellar tendon
Lacrimal Duct, Left Lacrimal Duct, Right	**Includes:** Lacrimal canaliculus Lacrimal punctum Lacrimal sac Nasolacrimal duct
Larynx	**Includes:** Aryepiglottic fold Arytenoid cartilage Corniculate cartilage Cuneiform cartilage False vocal cord Glottis Rima glottidis Thyroid cartilage Ventricular fold
Lens, Left Lens, Right	**Includes:** Zonule of Zinn
Liver	**Includes:** Quadrate lobe
Lower Arm and Wrist Muscle, Left Lower Arm and Wrist Muscle, Right	**Includes:** Anatomical snuffbox Brachioradialis muscle Extensor carpi radialis muscle Extensor carpi ulnaris muscle Flexor carpi radialis muscle Flexor carpi ulnaris muscle Flexor pollicis longus muscle Palmaris longus muscle Pronator quadratus muscle Pronator teres muscle
Lower Artery	**Includes:** Umbilical artery
Lower Eyelid, Left Lower Eyelid, Right	**Includes:** Inferior tarsal plate Medial canthus
Lower Femur, Left Lower Femur, Right	**Includes:** Lateral condyle of femur Lateral epicondyle of femur Medial condyle of femur Medial epicondyle of femur

ICD-10-PCS Value	Definition
Lower Leg Muscle, Left Lower Leg Muscle, Right	**Includes:** Extensor digitorum longus muscle Extensor hallucis longus muscle Fibularis brevis muscle Fibularis longus muscle Flexor digitorum longus muscle Flexor hallucis longus muscle Gastrocnemius muscle Peroneus brevis muscle Peroneus longus muscle Popliteus muscle Soleus muscle Tibialis anterior muscle Tibialis posterior muscle
Lower Leg Tendon, Left Lower Leg Tendon, Right	**Includes:** Achilles tendon
Lower Lip	**Includes:** Frenulum labii inferioris Labial gland Vermilion border
Lower Spine Bursa and Ligament	**Includes:** Iliolumbar ligament Interspinous ligament, lumbar Intertransverse ligament, lumbar Ligamentum flavum, lumbar Sacrococcygeal ligament Sacroiliac ligament Sacrospinous ligament Sacrotuberous ligament Supraspinous ligament
Lumbar Nerve	**Includes:** Lumbosacral trunk Spinal nerve, lumbar Superior clunic (cluneal) nerve
Lumbar Plexus	**Includes:** Accessory obturator nerve Genitofemoral nerve Iliohypogastric nerve Ilioinguinal nerve Lateral femoral cutaneous nerve Obturator nerve Superior gluteal nerve
Lumbar Spinal Cord	**Includes:** Cauda equina Conus medullaris
Lumbar Sympathetic Nerve	**Includes:** Lumbar ganglion Lumbar splanchnic nerve
Lumbar Vertebra	**Includes:** Spinous process Transverse process Vertebral arch Vertebral body Vertebral foramen Vertebral lamina Vertebral pedicle
Lumbar Vertebral Joint	**Includes:** Lumbar facet joint
Lumbosacral Joint	**Includes:** Lumbosacral facet joint

ICD-10-PCS Value	Definition
Lymphatic, Aortic	**Includes:** Celiac lymph node Gastric lymph node Hepatic lymph node Lumbar lymph node Pancreaticosplenic lymph node Paraaortic lymph node Retroperitoneal lymph node
Lymphatic, Head	**Includes:** Buccinator lymph node Infraauricular lymph node Infraparotid lymph node Parotid lymph node Preauricular lymph node Submandibular lymph node Submaxillary lymph node Submental lymph node Subparotid lymph node Suprahyoid lymph node
Lymphatic, Left Axillary	**Includes:** Anterior (pectoral) lymph node Apical (subclavicular) lymph node Brachial (lateral) lymph node Central axillary lymph node Lateral (brachial) lymph node Pectoral (anterior) lymph node Posterior (subscapular) lymph node Subclavicular (apical) lymph node Subscapular (posterior) lymph node
Lymphatic, Left Lower Extremity	**Includes:** Femoral lymph node Popliteal lymph node
Lymphatic, Left Neck	**Includes:** Cervical lymph node Jugular lymph node Mastoid (postauricular) lymph node Occipital lymph node Postauricular (mastoid) lymph node Retropharyngeal lymph node Supraclavicular (Virchow's) lymph node Virchow's (supraclavicular) lymph node
Lymphatic, Left Upper Extremity	**Includes:** Cubital lymph node Deltopectoral (infraclavicular) lymph node Epitrochlear lymph node Infraclavicular (deltopectoral) lymph node Supratrochlear lymph node
Lymphatic, Mesenteric	**Includes:** Inferior mesenteric lymph node Pararectal lymph node Superior mesenteric lymph node
Lymphatic, Pelvis	**Includes:** Common iliac (subaortic) lymph node Gluteal lymph node Iliac lymph node Inferior epigastric lymph node Obturator lymph node Sacral lymph node Subaortic (common iliac) lymph node Suprainguinal lymph node

ICD-10-PCS Value	Definition
Lymphatic, Right Axillary	**Includes:** Anterior (pectoral) lymph node Apical (subclavicular) lymph node Brachial (lateral) lymph node Central axillary lymph node Lateral (brachial) lymph node Pectoral (anterior) lymph node Posterior (subscapular) lymph node Subclavicular (apical) lymph node Subscapular (posterior) lymph node
Lymphatic, Right Lower Extremity	**Includes:** Femoral lymph node Popliteal lymph node
Lymphatic, Right Neck	**Includes:** Cervical lymph node Jugular lymph node Mastoid (postauricular) lymph node Occipital lymph node Postauricular (mastoid) lymph node Retropharyngeal lymph node Right jugular trunk Right lymphatic duct Right subclavian trunk Supraclavicular (Virchow's) lymph node Virchow's (supraclavicular) lymph node
Lymphatic, Right Upper Extremity	**Includes:** Cubital lymph node Deltopectoral (infraclavicular) lymph node Epitrochlear lymph node Infraclavicular (deltopectoral) lymph node Supratrochlear lymph node
Lymphatic, Thorax	**Includes:** Intercostal lymph node Mediastinal lymph node Parasternal lymph node Paratracheal lymph node Tracheobronchial lymph node
Main Bronchus, Right	**Includes:** Bronchus intermedius Intermediate bronchus
Mandible, Left Mandible, Right	**Includes:** Alveolar process of mandible Condyloid process Mandibular notch Mental foramen
Mastoid Sinus, Left Mastoid Sinus, Right	**Includes:** Mastoid air cells
Maxilla	**Includes:** Alveolar process of maxilla
Maxillary Sinus, Left Maxillary Sinus, Right	**Includes:** Antrum of Highmore
Median Nerve	**Includes:** Anterior interosseous nerve Palmar cutaneous nerve
Mediastinum	**Includes:** Mediastinal cavity Mediastinal space
Medulla Oblongata	**Includes:** Myelencephalon
Mesentery	**Includes:** Mesoappendix Mesocolon

ICD-10-PCS Value	Definition
Metatarsal-Phalangeal Joint, Left Metatarsal-Phalangeal Joint, Right	**Includes:** Metatarsophalangeal (MTP) joint
Middle Ear, Left Middle Ear, Right	**Includes:** Oval window Tympanic cavity
Minor Salivary Gland	**Includes:** Anterior lingual gland
Mitral Valve	**Includes:** Bicuspid valve Left atrioventricular valve Mitral annulus
Nasal Bone	**Includes:** Vomer of nasal septum
Nasal Mucosa and Soft Tissue	**Includes:** Columella External naris Greater alar cartilage Internal naris Lateral nasal cartilage Lesser alar cartilage Nasal cavity Nostril
Nasal Septum	**Includes:** Quadrangular cartilage Septal cartilage Vomer bone
Nasal Turbinate	**Includes:** Inferior turbinate Middle turbinate Nasal concha Superior turbinate
Nasopharynx	**Includes:** Choana Fossa of Rosenmuller Pharyngeal recess Rhinopharynx
Neck Muscle, Left Neck Muscle, Right	**Includes:** Anterior vertebral muscle Arytenoid muscle Cricothyroid muscle Infrahyoid muscle Levator scapulae muscle Platysma muscle Scalene muscle Splenius cervicis muscle Sternocleidomastoid muscle Suprahyoid muscle Thyroarytenoid muscle
Nipple, Left Nipple, Right	**Includes:** Areola
Occipital Bone	**Includes:** Foramen magnum
Oculomotor Nerve	**Includes:** Third cranial nerve
Olfactory Nerve	**Includes:** First cranial nerve Olfactory bulb

ICD-10-PCS Value	Definition
Omentum	**Includes:** Gastrocolic ligament Gastrocolic omentum Gastrohepatic omentum Gastrophrenic ligament Gastrosplenic ligament Greater Omentum Hepatogastric ligament Lesser Omentum
Optic Nerve	**Includes:** Optic chiasma Second cranial nerve
Orbit, Left Orbit, Right	**Includes:** Bony orbit Orbital portion of ethmoid bone Orbital portion of frontal bone Orbital portion of lacrimal bone Orbital portion of maxilla Orbital portion of palatine bone Orbital portion of sphenoid bone Orbital portion of zygomatic bone
Pancreatic Duct	**Includes:** Duct of Wirsung
Pancreatic Duct, Accessory	**Includes:** Duct of Santorini
Parotid Duct, Left Parotid Duct, Right	**Includes:** Stensen's duct
Pelvic Bone, Left Pelvic Bone, Right	**Includes:** Iliac crest Ilium Ischium Pubis
Pelvic Cavity	**Includes:** Retropubic space
Penis	**Includes:** Corpus cavernosum Corpus spongiosum
Perineum Muscle	**Includes:** Bulbospongiosus muscle Cremaster muscle Deep transverse perineal muscle Ischiocavernosus muscle Levator ani muscle Superficial transverse perineal muscle
Peritoneum	**Includes:** Epiploic foramen
Peroneal Artery, Left Peroneal Artery, Right	**Includes:** Fibular artery
Peroneal Nerve	**Includes:** Common fibular nerve Common peroneal nerve External popliteal nerve Lateral sural cutaneous nerve
Pharynx	**Includes:** Base of Tongue Hypopharynx Laryngopharynx Lingual tonsil Oropharynx Piriform recess (sinus) Tongue, base of
Phrenic Nerve	**Includes:** Accessory phrenic nerve

ICD-10-PCS Value	Definition
Pituitary Gland	**Includes:** Adenohypophysis Hypophysis Neurohypophysis
Pons	**Includes:** Apneustic center Basis pontis Locus ceruleus Pneumotaxic center Pontine tegmentum Superior olivary nucleus
Popliteal Artery, Left **Popliteal Artery, Right**	**Includes:** Inferior genicular artery Middle genicular artery Superior genicular artery Sural artery Tibioperoneal trunk
Portal Vein	**Includes:** Hepatic portal vein
Prepuce	**Includes:** Foreskin Glans penis
Pudendal Nerve	**Includes:** Posterior labial nerve Posterior scrotal nerve
Pulmonary Artery, Left	**Includes:** Arterial canal (duct) Botallo's duct Pulmoaortic canal
Pulmonary Valve	**Includes:** Pulmonary annulus Pulmonic valve
Pulmonary Vein, Left	**Includes:** Left inferior pulmonary vein Left superior pulmonary vein
Pulmonary Vein, Right	**Includes:** Right inferior pulmonary vein Right superior pulmonary vein
Radial Artery, Left **Radial Artery, Right**	**Includes:** Radial recurrent artery
Radial Nerve	**Includes:** Dorsal digital nerve Musculospiral nerve Palmar cutaneous nerve Posterior interosseous nerve
Radius, Left **Radius, Right**	**Includes:** Ulnar notch
Rectum	**Includes:** Anorectal junction
Renal Artery, Left **Renal Artery, Right**	**Includes:** Inferior suprarenal artery Renal segmental artery
Renal Vein, Left	**Includes:** Left inferior phrenic vein Left ovarian vein Left second lumbar vein Left suprarenal vein Left testicular vein
Retina, Left **Retina, Right**	**Includes:** Fovea Macula Optic disc
Retroperitoneum	**Includes:** Retroperitoneal cavity Retroperitoneal space

ICD-10-PCS Value	Definition
Rib(s) Bursa and Ligament	**Includes:** Costotransverse ligament
Sacral Nerve	**Includes:** Spinal nerve, sacral
Sacral Plexus	**Includes:** Inferior gluteal nerve Posterior femoral cutaneous nerve Pudendal nerve
Sacral Sympathetic Nerve	**Includes:** Ganglion impar (ganglion of Walther) Pelvic splanchnic nerve Sacral ganglion Sacral splanchnic nerve
Sacrococcygeal Joint	**Includes:** Sacrococcygeal symphysis
Saphenous Vein, Left **Saphenous Vein, Right**	**Includes:** External pudendal vein Great(er) saphenous vein Lesser saphenous vein Small saphenous vein Superficial circumflex iliac vein Superficial epigastric vein
Scapula, Left **Scapula, Right**	**Includes:** Acromion (process) Coracoid process
Sciatic Nerve	**Includes:** Ischiatic nerve
Shoulder Bursa and Ligament, Left **Shoulder Bursa and Ligament, Right**	**Includes:** Acromioclavicular ligament Coracoacromial ligament Coracoclavicular ligament Coracohumeral ligament Costoclavicular ligament Glenohumeral ligament Interclavicular ligament Sternoclavicular ligament Subacromial bursa Transverse humeral ligament Transverse scapular ligament
Shoulder Joint, Left **Shoulder Joint, Right**	**Includes:** Glenohumeral joint Glenoid ligament (labrum)
Shoulder Muscle, Left **Shoulder Muscle, Right**	**Includes:** Deltoid muscle Infraspinatus muscle Subscapularis muscle Supraspinatus muscle Teres major muscle Teres minor muscle
Sigmoid Colon	**Includes:** Rectosigmoid junction Sigmoid flexure
Skin	**Includes:** Dermis Epidermis Sebaceous gland Sweat gland
Skin, Chest	**Includes:** Breast procedures, skin only
Sphenoid Bone	**Includes:** Greater wing Lesser wing Optic foramen Pterygoid process Sella turcica

ICD-10-PCS Value	Definition
Spinal Canal	**Includes:** Epidural space, spinal Extradural space, spinal Subarachnoid space, spinal Subdural space, spinal Vertebral canal
Spinal Meninges	**Includes:** Arachnoid mater, spinal Denticulate (dentate) ligament Dura mater, spinal Filum terminale Leptomeninges, spinal Pia mater, spinal
Spleen	**Includes:** Accessory spleen
Splenic Artery	**Includes:** Left gastroepiploic artery Pancreatic artery Short gastric artery
Splenic Vein	**Includes:** Left gastroepiploic vein Pancreatic vein
Sternum	**Includes:** Manubrium Suprasternal notch Xiphoid process
Sternum Bursa and Ligament	**Includes:** Costoxiphoid ligament Sternocostal ligament
Stomach, Pylorus	**Includes:** Pyloric antrum Pyloric canal Pyloric sphincter
Subclavian Artery, Left Subclavian Artery, Right	**Includes:** Costocervical trunk Dorsal scapular artery Internal thoracic artery
Subcutaneous Tissue and Fascia, Chest	**Includes:** Pectoral fascia
Subcutaneous Tissue and Fascia, Face	**Includes:** Masseteric fascia Orbital fascia Submandibular space
Subcutaneous Tissue and Fascia, Left Foot	**Includes:** Plantar fascia (aponeurosis)
Subcutaneous Tissue and Fascia, Left Hand	**Includes:** Palmar fascia (aponeurosis)
Subcutaneous Tissue and Fascia, Left Lower Arm	**Includes:** Antebrachial fascia Bicipital aponeurosis
Subcutaneous Tissue and Fascia, Left Neck	**Includes:** Deep cervical fascia Pretracheal fascia Prevertebral fascia
Subcutaneous Tissue and Fascia, Left Upper Arm	**Includes:** Axillary fascia Deltoid fascia Infraspinatus fascia Subscapular aponeurosis Supraspinatus fascia
Subcutaneous Tissue and Fascia, Left Upper Leg	**Includes:** Crural fascia Fascia lata Iliac fascia Iliotibial tract (band)

ICD-10-PCS Value	Definition
Subcutaneous Tissue and Fascia, Right Foot	**Includes:** Plantar fascia (aponeurosis)
Subcutaneous Tissue and Fascia, Right Hand	**Includes:** Palmar fascia (aponeurosis)
Subcutaneous Tissue and Fascia, Right Lower Arm	**Includes:** Antebrachial fascia Bicipital aponeurosis
Subcutaneous Tissue and Fascia, Right Neck	**Includes:** Deep cervical fascia Pretracheal fascia Prevertebral fascia
Subcutaneous Tissue and Fascia, Right Upper Arm	**Includes:** Axillary fascia Deltoid fascia Infraspinatus fascia Subscapular aponeurosis Supraspinatus fascia
Subcutaneous Tissue and Fascia, Right Upper Leg	**Includes:** Crural fascia Fascia lata Iliac fascia Iliotibial tract (band)
Subcutaneous Tissue and Fascia, Scalp	**Includes:** Galea aponeurotica
Subcutaneous Tissue and Fascia, Trunk	**Includes:** External oblique aponeurosis Transversalis fascia
Submaxillary Gland, Left Submaxillary Gland, Right	**Includes:** Submandibular gland
Superior Mesenteric Artery	**Includes:** Ileal artery Ileocolic artery Inferior pancreaticoduodenal artery Jejunal artery
Superior Mesenteric Vein	**Includes:** Right gastroepiploic vein
Superior Vena Cava	**Includes:** Precava
Tarsal Joint, Left Tarsal Joint, Right	**Includes:** Calcaneocuboid joint Cuboideonavicular joint Cuneonavicular joint Intercuneiform joint Subtalar (talocalcaneal) joint Talocalcaneal (subtalar) joint Talocalcaneonavicular joint
Tarsal, Left Tarsal, Right	**Includes:** Calcaneus Cuboid bone Intermediate cuneiform bone Lateral cuneiform bone Medial cuneiform bone Navicular bone Talus bone
Temporal Artery, Left Temporal Artery, Right	**Includes:** Middle temporal artery Superficial temporal artery Transverse facial artery
Temporal Bone, Left Temporal Bone, Right	**Includes:** Mastoid process Petrous part of temporal bone Tympanic part of temporal bone Zygomatic process of temporal bone

ICD-10-PCS Value	Definition
Thalamus	**Includes:** Epithalamus Geniculate nucleus Metathalamus Pulvinar
Thoracic Aorta, Ascending/Arch	**Includes:** Aortic arch Ascending aorta
Thoracic Duct	**Includes:** Left jugular trunk Left subclavian trunk
Thoracic Nerve	**Includes:** Intercostal nerve Intercostobrachial nerve Spinal nerve, thoracic Subcostal nerve
Thoracic Sympathetic Nerve	**Includes:** Cardiac plexus Esophageal plexus Greater splanchnic nerve Inferior cardiac nerve Least splanchnic nerve Lesser splanchnic nerve Middle cardiac nerve Pulmonary plexus Superior cardiac nerve Thoracic aortic plexus Thoracic ganglion
Thoracic Vertebra	**Includes:** Spinous process Transverse process Vertebral arch Vertebral body Vertebral foramen Vertebral lamina Vertebral pedicle
Thoracic Vertebral Joint	**Includes:** Costotransverse joint Costovertebral joint Thoracic facet joint
Thoracolumbar Vertebral Joint	**Includes:** Thoracolumbar facet joint
Thorax Muscle, Left Thorax Muscle, Right	**Includes:** Intercostal muscle Levatores costarum muscle Pectoralis major muscle Pectoralis minor muscle Serratus anterior muscle Subclavius muscle Subcostal muscle Transverse thoracis muscle
Thymus	**Includes:** Thymus gland
Thyroid Artery, Left Thyroid Artery, Right	**Includes:** Cricothyroid artery Hyoid artery Sternocleidomastoid artery Superior laryngeal artery Superior thyroid artery Thyrocervical trunk
Tibia, Left Tibia, Right	**Includes:** Lateral condyle of tibia Medial condyle of tibia Medial malleolus

ICD-10-PCS Value	Definition
Tibial Nerve	**Includes:** Lateral plantar nerve Medial plantar nerve Medial popliteal nerve Medial sural cutaneous nerve
Toe Nail	**Includes:** Nail bed Nail plate
Toe Phalangeal Joint, Left Toe Phalangeal Joint, Right	**Includes:** Interphalangeal (IP) joint
Tongue	**Includes:** Frenulum linguae
Tongue, Palate, Pharynx Muscle	**Includes:** Chondroglossus muscle Genioglossus muscle Hyoglossus muscle Inferior longitudinal muscle Levator veli palatini muscle Palatoglossal muscle Palatopharyngeal muscle Pharyngeal constrictor muscle Salpingopharyngeus muscle Styloglossus muscle Stylopharyngeus muscle Superior longitudinal muscle Tensor veli palatini muscle
Tonsils	**Includes:** Palatine tonsil
Trachea	**Includes:** Cricoid cartilage
Transverse Colon	**Includes:** Hepatic flexure Splenic flexure
Tricuspid Valve	**Includes:** Right atrioventricular valve Tricuspid annulus
Trigeminal Nerve	**Includes:** Fifth cranial nerve Gasserian ganglion Mandibular nerve Maxillary nerve Ophthalmic nerve Trifacial nerve
Trochlear Nerve	**Includes:** Fourth cranial nerve
Trunk Muscle, Left Trunk Muscle, Right	**Includes:** Coccygeus muscle Erector spinae muscle Interspinalis muscle Intertransversarius muscle Latissimus dorsi muscle Quadratus lumborum muscle Rhomboid major muscle Rhomboid minor muscle Serratus posterior muscle Transversospinalis muscle Trapezius muscle
Tympanic Membrane, Left Tympanic Membrane, Right	**Includes:** Pars flaccida
Ulna, Left Ulna, Right	**Includes:** Olecranon process Radial notch

ICD-10-PCS Value	Definition
Ulnar Artery, Left Ulnar Artery, Right	**Includes:** Anterior ulnar recurrent artery Common interosseous artery Posterior ulnar recurrent artery
Ulnar Nerve	**Includes:** Cubital nerve
Upper Arm Muscle, Left Upper Arm Muscle, Right	**Includes:** Biceps brachii muscle Brachialis muscle Coracobrachialis muscle Triceps brachii muscle
Upper Artery	**Includes:** Aortic intercostal artery Bronchial artery Esophageal artery Subcostal artery
Upper Eyelid, Left Upper Eyelid, Right	**Includes:** Lateral canthus Levator palpebrae superioris muscle Orbicularis oculi muscle Superior tarsal plate
Upper Femur, Left Upper Femur, Right	**Includes:** Femoral head Greater trochanter Lesser trochanter Neck of femur
Upper Leg Muscle, Left Upper Leg Muscle, Right	**Includes:** Adductor brevis muscle Adductor longus muscle Adductor magnus muscle Biceps femoris muscle Gracilis muscle Pectineus muscle Quadriceps (femoris) Rectus femoris muscle Sartorius muscle Semimembranosus muscle Semitendinosus muscle Vastus intermedius muscle Vastus lateralis muscle Vastus medialis muscle
Upper Lip	**Includes:** Frenulum labii superioris Labial gland Vermilion border
Upper Spine Bursa and Ligament	**Includes:** Interspinous ligament, thoracic Intertransverse ligament, thoracic Ligamentum flavum, thoracic Supraspinous ligament
Ureter Ureter, Left Ureter, Right Ureters, Bilateral	**Includes:** Ureteral orifice Ureterovesical orifice
Urethra	**Includes:** Bulbourethral (Cowper's) gland Cowper's (bulbourethral) gland External urethral sphincter Internal urethral sphincter Membranous urethra Penile urethra Prostatic urethra
Uterine Supporting Structure	**Includes:** Broad ligament Infundibulopelvic ligament Ovarian ligament Round ligament of uterus

ICD-10-PCS Value	Definition
Uterus	**Includes:** Fundus uteri Myometrium Perimetrium Uterine cornu
Uvula	**Includes:** Palatine uvula
Vagus Nerve	**Includes:** Anterior vagal trunk Pharyngeal plexus Pneumogastric nerve Posterior vagal trunk Pulmonary plexus Recurrent laryngeal nerve Superior laryngeal nerve Tenth cranial nerve
Vas Deferens Vas Deferens, Bilateral Vas Deferens, Left Vas Deferens, Right	**Includes:** Ductus deferens Ejaculatory duct
Ventricle, Right	**Includes:** Conus arteriosus
Ventricular Septum	**Includes:** Interventricular septum
Vertebral Artery, Left Vertebral Artery, Right	**Includes:** Anterior spinal artery Posterior spinal artery
Vertebral Vein, Left Vertebral Vein, Right	**Includes:** Deep cervical vein Suboccipital venous plexus
Vestibular Gland	**Includes:** Bartholin's (greater vestibular) gland Greater vestibular (Bartholin's) gland Paraurethral (Skene's) gland Skene's (paraurethral) gland
Vitreous, Left Vitreous, Right	**Includes:** Vitreous body
Vocal Cord, Left Vocal Cord, Right	**Includes:** Vocal fold
Vulva	**Includes:** Labia majora Labia minora
Wrist Bursa and Ligament, Left Wrist Bursa and Ligament, Right	**Includes:** Palmar ulnocarpal ligament Radial collateral carpal ligament Radiocarpal ligament Radioulnar ligament Ulnar collateral carpal ligament
Wrist Joint, Left Wrist Joint, Right	**Includes:** Distal radioulnar joint Radiocarpal joint

Device Key

Term	ICD-10-PCS Value
3f (Aortic) Bioprosthesis valve	Zooplastic Tissue in Heart and Great Vessels
AbioCor® Total Replacement Heart	Synthetic Substitute
Absolute Pro Vascular (OTW) Self-Expanding Stent System	Intraluminal Device
Acculink (RX) Carotid Stent System	Intraluminal Device
Acellular Hydrated Dermis	Nonautologous Tissue Substitute
Acetabular cup	Liner in Lower Joints
Activa PC neurostimulator	Stimulator Generator, Multiple Array for Insertion in Subcutaneous Tissue and Fascia
Activa RC neurostimulator	Stimulator Generator, Multiple Array Rechargeable for Insertion in Subcutaneous Tissue and Fascia
Activa SC neurostimulator	Stimulator Generator, Single Array for Insertion in Subcutaneous Tissue and Fascia
ACUITY™ Steerable Lead	Cardiac Lead, Pacemaker for Insertion in Heart and Great Vessels Cardiac Lead, Defibrillator for Insertion in Heart and Great Vessels
Advisa (MRI)	Pacemaker, Dual Chamber for Insertion in Subcutaneous Tissue and Fascia
AFX® Endovascular AAA System	Intraluminal Device
AMPLATZER® Muscular VSD Occluder	Synthetic Substitute
AMS 800® Urinary Control System	Artificial Sphincter in Urinary System
AneuRx® AAA Advantage®	Intraluminal Device
Annuloplasty ring	Synthetic Substitute
Articulating Spacer (Antibiotic)	Articulating Spacer in Lower Joints
Artificial anal sphincter (AAS)	Artificial Sphincter in Gastrointestinal System
Artificial bowel sphincter (neosphincter)	Artificial Sphincter in Gastrointestinal System
Artificial urinary sphincter (AUS)	Artificial Sphincter in Urinary System
Ascenda Intrathecal Catheter	Infusion Device
Assurant (Cobalt) stent	Intraluminal Device
AtriClip LAA Exclusion System	Extraluminal Device
Attain Ability® Lead	Cardiac Lead, Pacemaker for Insertion in Heart and Great Vessels Cardiac Lead, Defibrillator for Insertion in Heart and Great Vessels
Attain StarFix® (OTW) Lead	Cardiac Lead, Pacemaker for Insertion in Heart and Great Vessels Cardiac Lead, Defibrillator for Insertion in Heart and Great Vessels
Autograft	Autologous Tissue Substitute

Term	ICD-10-PCS Value
Autologous artery graft	Autologous Arterial Tissue in Heart and Great Vessels Autologous Arterial Tissue in Upper Arteries Autologous Arterial Tissue in Lower Arteries Autologous Arterial Tissue in Upper Veins Autologous Arterial Tissue in Lower Veins
Autologous vein graft	Autologous Venous Tissue in Heart and Great Vessels Autologous Venous Tissue in Upper Arteries Autologous Venous Tissue in Lower Arteries Autologous Venous Tissue in Upper Veins Autologous Venous Tissue in Lower Veins
Axial Lumbar Interbody Fusion System	Interbody Fusion Device in Lower Joints
AxiaLIF® System	Interbody Fusion Device in Lower Joints
BAK/C® Interbody Cervical Fusion System	Interbody Fusion Device in Upper Joints
Bard® Composix® (E/X)(LP) mesh	Synthetic Substitute
Bard® Composix® Kugel® patch	Synthetic Substitute
Bard® Dulex™ mesh	Synthetic Substitute
Bard® Ventralex™ hernia patch	Synthetic Substitute
Baroreflex Activation Therapy® (BAT®)	Stimulator Lead in Upper Arteries Stimulator Generator in Subcutaneous Tissue and Fascia
Berlin Heart Ventricular Assist Device	Implantable Heart Assist System in Heart and Great Vessels
Bioactive embolization coil(s)	Intraluminal Device, Bioactive in Upper Arteries
Biventricular external heart assist system	Short-term External Heart Assist System in Heart and Great Vessels
Blood glucose monitoring system	Monitoring Device
Bone anchored hearing device	Hearing Device, Bone Conduction for Insertion in Ear, Nose, Sinus Hearing Device, in Head and Facial Bones
Bone bank bone graft	Nonautologous Tissue Substitute
Bone screw (interlocking)(lag)(pedicle) (recessed)	Internal Fixation Device in Head and Facial Bones Internal Fixation Device in Upper Bones Internal Fixation Device in Lower Bones
Bovine pericardial valve	Zooplastic Tissue in Heart and Great Vessels
Bovine pericardium graft	Zooplastic Tissue in Heart and Great Vessels
Brachytherapy seeds	Radioactive Element
BRYAN® Cervical Disc System	Synthetic Substitute
BVS 5000 Ventricular Assist Device	Short-term External Heart Assist System in Heart and Great Vessels
Cardiac contractility modulation lead	Cardiac Lead in Heart and Great Vessels

Term	ICD-10-PCS Value
Cardiac event recorder	Monitoring Device
Cardiac resynchronization therapy (CRT) lead	Cardiac Lead, Pacemaker for Insertion in Heart and Great Vessels Cardiac Lead, Defibrillator for Insertion in Heart and Great Vessels
CardioMEMS® pressure sensor	Monitoring Device, Pressure Sensor for Insertion in Heart and Great Vessels
Carotid (artery) sinus (baroreceptor) lead	Stimulator Lead in Upper Arteries
Carotid WALLSTENT® Monorail® Endoprosthesis	Intraluminal Device
Centrimag® Blood Pump	Short-term External Heart Assist System in Heart and Great Vessels
Ceramic on ceramic bearing surface	Synthetic Substitute, Ceramic for Replacement in Lower Joints
Cesium-131 Collagen Implant	Radioactive Element, Cesium-131 Collagen Implant for Insertion in Central Nervous System and Cranial Nerves
CivaSheet®	Radioactive Element
Clamp and rod internal fixation system (CRIF)	Internal Fixation Device in Upper Bones Internal Fixation Device in Lower Bones
COALESCE® radiolucent interbody fusion device	Interbody Fusion Device, Radiolucent Porous in New Technology
CoAxia NeuroFlo catheter	Intraluminal Device
Cobalt/chromium head and polyethylene socket	Synthetic Substitute, Metal on Polyethylene for Replacement in Lower Joints
Cobalt/chromium head and socket	Synthetic Substitute, Metal for Replacement in Lower Joints
Cochlear implant (CI), multiple channel (electrode)	Hearing Device, Multiple Channel Cochlear Prosthesis for Insertion in Ear, Nose, Sinus
Cochlear implant (CI), single channel (electrode)	Hearing Device, Single Channel Cochlear Prosthesis for Insertion in Ear, Nose, Sinus
COGNIS® CRT-D	Cardiac Resynchronization Defibrillator Pulse Generator for Insertion in Subcutaneous Tissue and Fascia
COHERE® radiolucent interbody fusion device	Interbody Fusion Device, Radiolucent Porous in New Technology
Colonic Z-Stent®	Intraluminal Device
Complete (SE) stent	Intraluminal Device
Concerto II CRT-D	Cardiac Resynchronization Defibrillator Pulse Generator for Insertion in Subcutaneous Tissue and Fascia
CONSERVE® PLUS Total Resurfacing Hip System	Resurfacing Device in Lower Joints
Consulta CRT-D	Cardiac Resynchronization Defibrillator Pulse Generator for Insertion in Subcutaneous Tissue and Fascia
Consulta CRT-P	Cardiac Resynchronization Pacemaker Pulse Generator for Insertion in Subcutaneous Tissue and Fascia
CONTAK RENEWAL® 3 RF (HE) CRT-D	Cardiac Resynchronization Defibrillator Pulse Generator for Insertion in Subcutaneous Tissue and Fascia
Contegra Pulmonary Valved Conduit	Zooplastic Tissue in Heart and Great Vessels
Continuous Glucose Monitoring (CGM) device	Monitoring Device

Term	ICD-10-PCS Value
Cook Biodesign® Fistula Plug(s)	Nonautologous Tissue Substitute
Cook Biodesign® Hernia Graft(s)	Nonautologous Tissue Substitute
Cook Biodesign® Layered Graft(s)	Nonautologous Tissue Substitute
Cook Zenapro™ Layered Graft(s)	Nonautologous Tissue Substitute
Cook Zenith AAA Endovascular Graft	Intraluminal Device Intraluminal Device, Branched or Fenestrated, One or Two Arteries for Restriction in Lower Arteries Intraluminal Device, Branched or Fenestrated, Three or More Arteries for Restriction in Lower Arteries
CoreValve transcatheter aortic valve	Zooplastic Tissue in Heart and Great Vessels
Cormet Hip Resurfacing System	Resurfacing Device in Lower Joints
CoRoent® XL	Interbody Fusion Device in Lower Joints
Corox (OTW) Bipolar Lead	Cardiac Lead, Pacemaker for Insertion in Heart and Great Vessels Cardiac Lead, Defibrillator for Insertion in Heart and Great Vessels
Cortical strip neurostimulator lead	Neurostimulator Lead in Central Nervous System and Cranial Nerves
Cultured epidermal cell autograft	Autologous Tissue Substitute
CYPHER® Stent	Intraluminal Device, Drug-eluting in Heart and Great Vessels
Cystostomy tube	Drainage Device
DBS lead	Neurostimulator Lead in Central Nervous System and Cranial Nerves
DeBakey Left Ventricular Assist Device	Implantable Heart Assist System in Heart and Great Vessels
Deep brain neurostimulator lead	Neurostimulator Lead in Central Nervous System and Cranial Nerves
Delta frame external fixator	External Fixation Device, Hybrid for Insertion in Upper Bones External Fixation Device, Hybrid for Reposition in Upper Bones External Fixation Device, Hybrid for Insertion in Lower Bones External Fixation Device, Hybrid for Reposition in Lower Bones
Delta III Reverse shoulder prosthesis	Synthetic Substitute, Reverse Ball and Socket for Replacement in Upper Joints
Diaphragmatic pacemaker generator	Stimulator Generator in Subcutaneous Tissue and Fascia
Direct Lateral Interbody Fusion (DLIF) device	Interbody Fusion Device in Lower Joints
Driver stent (RX) (OTW)	Intraluminal Device
DuraHeart Left Ventricular Assist System	Implantable Heart Assist System in Heart and Great Vessels
Durata® Defibrillation Lead	Cardiac Lead, Defibrillator for Insertion in Heart and Great Vessels
Dynesys® Dynamic Stabilization System	Spinal Stabilization Device, Pedicle-Based for Insertion in Upper Joints Spinal Stabilization Device, Pedicle-Based for Insertion in Lower Joints
E-Luminexx™ (Biliary)(Vascular) Stent	Intraluminal Device
EDWARDS INTUITY Elite valve system	Zooplastic Tissue, Rapid Deployment Technique in New Technology

Term	ICD-10-PCS Value
Electrical bone growth stimulator (EBGS)	Bone Growth Stimulator in Head and Facial Bones Bone Growth Stimulator in Upper Bones Bone Growth Stimulator in Lower Bones
Electrical muscle stimulation (EMS) lead	Stimulator Lead in Muscles
Electronic muscle stimulator lead	Stimulator Lead in Muscles
Eluvia™ Drug-eluting Vascular Stent System	Intraluminal Device, Sustained Release Drug-eluting in New Technology Intraluminal Device, Sustained Release Drug-eluting, Two in New Technology Intraluminal Device, Sustained Release Drug-eluting, Three in New Technology Intraluminal Device, Sustained Release Drug-eluting, Four or More in New Technology
Embolization coil(s)	Intraluminal Device
Endeavor® (III)(IV) (Sprint) Zotarolimus-eluting Coronary Stent System	Intraluminal Device, Drug-eluting in Heart and Great Vessels
Endologix AFX® Endovascular AAA System	Intraluminal Device
EndoSure® sensor	Monitoring Device, Pressure Sensor for Insertion in Heart and Great Vessels
ENDOTAK RELIANCE® (G) Defibrillation Lead	Cardiac Lead, Defibrillator for Insertion in Heart and Great Vessels
Endotracheal tube (cuffed)(double-lumen)	Intraluminal Device, Endotracheal Airway in Respiratory System
Endurant® Endovascular Stent Graft	Intraluminal Device
Endurant® II AAA stent graft system	Intraluminal Device
EnRhythm	Pacemaker, Dual Chamber for Insertion in Subcutaneous Tissue and Fascia
Enterra gastric neurostimulator	Stimulator Generator, Multiple Array for Insertion in Subcutaneous Tissue and Fascia
Epic™ Stented Tissue Valve (aortic)	Zooplastic Tissue in Heart and Great Vessels
Epicel® cultured epidermal autograft	Autologous Tissue Substitute
Esophageal obturator airway (EOA)	Intraluminal Device, Airway in Gastrointestinal System
Esteem® implantable hearing system	Hearing Device in Ear, Nose, Sinus
Evera (XT)(S)(DR/VR)	Defibrillator Generator for Insertion in Subcutaneous Tissue and Fascia
Everolimus-eluting coronary stent	Intraluminal Device, Drug-eluting in Heart and Great Vessels
Ex-PRESS™ mini glaucoma shunt	Synthetic Substitute
EXCLUDER® AAA Endoprosthesis	Intraluminal Device Intraluminal Device, Branched or Fenestrated, One or Two Arteries for Restriction in Lower Arteries Intraluminal Device, Branched or Fenestrated, Three or More Arteries for Restriction in Lower Arteries
EXCLUDER® IBE Endoprosthesis	Intraluminal Device, Branched or Fenestrated, One or Two Arteries for Restriction in Lower Arteries

Term	ICD-10-PCS Value
Express® (LD) Premounted Stent System	Intraluminal Device
Express® Biliary SD Monorail® Premounted Stent System	Intraluminal Device
Express® SD Renal Monorail® Premounted Stent System	Intraluminal Device
External fixator	External Fixation Device in Head and Facial Bones External Fixation Device in Upper Bones External Fixation Device in Lower Bones External Fixation Device in Upper Joints External Fixation Device in Lower Joints
EXtreme Lateral Interbody Fusion (XLIF) device	Interbody Fusion Device in Lower Joints
Facet replacement spinal stabilization device	Spinal Stabilization Device, Facet Replacement for Insertion in Upper Joints Spinal Stabilization Device, Facet Replacement for Insertion in Lower Joints
FLAIR® Endovascular Stent Graft	Intraluminal Device
Flexible Composite Mesh	Synthetic Substitute
Flow Diverter embolization device	Intraluminal Device, Flow Diverter for Restriction in Upper Arteries
Foley catheter	Drainage Device
Formula™ Balloon-Expandable Renal Stent System	Intraluminal Device
Freestyle (Stentless) Aortic Root Bioprosthesis	Zooplastic Tissue in Heart and Great Vessels
Fusion screw (compression)(lag)(locking)	Internal Fixation Device in Upper Joints Internal Fixation Device in Lower Joints
GammaTile™	Radioactive Element, Cesium-131 Collagen Implant for Insertion in Central Nervous System and Cranial Nerves
Gastric electrical stimulation (GES) lead	Stimulator Lead in Gastrointestinal System
Gastric pacemaker lead	Stimulator Lead in Gastrointestinal System
GORE EXCLUDER® AAA Endoprosthesis	Intraluminal Device Intraluminal Device, Branched or Fenestrated, One or Two Arteries for Restriction in Lower Arteries Intraluminal Device, Branched or Fenestrated, Three or More Arteries for Restriction in Lower Arteries
GORE EXCLUDER® IBE Endoprosthesis	Intraluminal Device, Branched or Fenestrated, One or Two Arteries for Restriction in Lower Arteries
GORE TAG® Thoracic Endoprosthesis	Intraluminal Device
GORE® DUALMESH®	Synthetic Substitute
Guedel airway	Intraluminal Device, Airway in Mouth and Throat
Hancock Bioprosthesis (aortic)(mitral) valve	Zooplastic Tissue in Heart and Great Vessels
Hancock Bioprosthetic Valved Conduit	Zooplastic Tissue in Heart and Great Vessels

Term	ICD-10-PCS Value
HeartMate 3™ LVAS	Implantable Heart Assist System in Heart and Great Vessels
HeartMate II® Left Ventricular Assist Device (LVAD)	Implantable Heart Assist System in Heart and Great Vessels
HeartMate XVE® Left Ventricular Assist Device (LVAD)	Implantable Heart Assist System in Heart and Great Vessels
Herculink (RX) Elite Renal Stent System	Intraluminal Device
Hip (joint) liner	Liner in Lower Joints
Holter valve ventricular shunt	Synthetic Substitute
Ilizarov external fixator	External Fixation Device, Ring for Insertion in Upper Bones External Fixation Device, Ring for Reposition in Upper Bones External Fixation Device, Ring for Insertion in Lower Bones External Fixation Device, Ring for Reposition in Lower Bones
Ilizarov-Vecklich device	External Fixation Device, Limb Lengthening for Insertion in Upper Bones External Fixation Device, Limb Lengthening for Insertion in Lower Bones
Impella® heart pump	Short-term External Heart Assist System in Heart and Great Vessels
Implantable cardioverter-defibrillator (ICD)	Defibrillator Generator for Insertion in Subcutaneous Tissue and Fascia
Implantable drug infusion pump (anti-spasmodic) (chemotherapy)(pain)	Infusion Device, Pump in Subcutaneous Tissue and Fascia
Implantable glucose monitoring device	Monitoring Device
Implantable hemodynamic monitor (IHM)	Monitoring Device, Hemodynamic for Insertion in Subcutaneous Tissue and Fascia
Implantable hemodynamic monitoring system (IHMS)	Monitoring Device, Hemodynamic for Insertion in Subcutaneous Tissue and Fascia
Implantable Miniature Telescope™ (IMT)	Synthetic Substitute, Intraocular Telescope for Replacement in Eye
Implanted (venous)(access) port	Vascular Access Device, Totally Implantable in Subcutaneous Tissue and Fascia
InDura, intrathecal catheter (1P) (spinal)	Infusion Device
Injection reservoir, port	Vascular Access Device, Totally Implantable in Subcutaneous Tissue and Fascia
Injection reservoir, pump	Infusion Device, Pump in Subcutaneous Tissue and Fascia
Interbody fusion (spine) cage	Interbody Fusion Device in Upper Joints Interbody Fusion Device in Lower Joints
Interspinous process spinal stabilization device	Spinal Stabilization Device, Interspinous Process for Insertion in Upper Joints Spinal Stabilization Device, Interspinous Process for Insertion in Lower Joints
InterStim® Therapy lead	Neurostimulator Lead in Peripheral Nervous System

Term	ICD-10-PCS Value
InterStim® Therapy neurostimulator	Stimulator Generator, Single Array for Insertion in Subcutaneous Tissue and Fascia
Intramedullary (IM) rod (nail)	Internal Fixation Device, Intramedullary in Upper Bones Internal Fixation Device, Intramedullary in Lower Bones
Intramedullary skeletal kinetic distractor (ISKD)	Internal Fixation Device, Intramedullary in Upper Bones Internal Fixation Device, Intramedullary in Lower Bones
Intrauterine Device (IUD)	Contraceptive Device in Female Reproductive System
INTUITY Elite valve system, EDWARDS	Zooplastic Tissue, Rapid Deployment Technique in New Technology
Itrel (3)(4) neurostimulator	Stimulator Generator, Single Array for Insertion in Subcutaneous Tissue and Fascia
Joint fixation plate	Internal Fixation Device in Upper Joints Internal Fixation Device in Lower Joints
Joint liner (insert)	Liner in Lower Joints
Joint spacer (antibiotic)	Spacer in Upper Joints Spacer in Lower Joints
Kappa	Pacemaker, Dual Chamber for Insertion in Subcutaneous Tissue and Fascia
Kirschner wire (K-wire)	Internal Fixation Device in Head and Facial Bones Internal Fixation Device in Upper Bones Internal Fixation Device in Lower Bones Internal Fixation Device in Upper Joints Internal Fixation Device in Lower Joints
Knee (implant) insert	Liner in Lower Joints
Kuntscher nail	Internal Fixation Device, Intramedullary in Upper Bones Internal Fixation Device, Intramedullary in Lower Bones
LAP-BAND® adjustable gastric banding system	Extraluminal Device
LifeStent® (Flexstar)(XL) Vascular Stent System	Intraluminal Device
LIVIAN™ CRT-D	Cardiac Resynchronization Defibrillator Pulse Generator for Insertion in Subcutaneous Tissue and Fascia
Loop recorder, implantable	Monitoring Device
MAGEC® Spinal Bracing and Distraction System	Magnetically Controlled Growth Rod(s) in New Technology
Mark IV Breathing Pacemaker System	Stimulator Generator in Subcutaneous Tissue and Fascia
Maximo II DR (VR)	Defibrillator Generator for Insertion in Subcutaneous Tissue and Fascia
Maximo II DR CRT-D	Cardiac Resynchronization Defibrillator Pulse Generator for Insertion in Subcutaneous Tissue and Fascia
Medtronic Endurant® II AAA stent graft system	Intraluminal Device
Melody® transcatheter pulmonary valve	Zooplastic Tissue in Heart and Great Vessels
Metal on metal bearing surface	Synthetic Substitute, Metal for Replacement in Lower Joints
Micro-Driver stent (RX) (OTW)	Intraluminal Device

Term	ICD-10-PCS Value
MicroMed HeartAssist	Implantable Heart Assist System in Heart and Great Vessels
Micrus CERECYTE microcoil	Intraluminal Device, Bioactive in Upper Arteries
MIRODERM™ Biologic Wound Matrix	Skin Substitute, Porcine Liver Derived in New Technology
MitraClip valve repair system	Synthetic Substitute
Mitroflow® Aortic Pericardial Heart Valve	Zooplastic Tissue in Heart and Great Vessels
Mosaic Bioprosthesis (aortic) (mitral) valve	Zooplastic Tissue in Heart and Great Vessels
MULTI-LINK (VISION)(MINI-VISION)(ULTRA) Coronary Stent System	Intraluminal Device
nanoLOCK™ interbody fusion device	Interbody Fusion Device, Nanotextured Surface in New Technology
Nasopharyngeal airway (NPA)	Intraluminal Device, Airway in Ear, Nose, Sinus
Neuromuscular electrical stimulation (NEMS) lead	Stimulator Lead in Muscles
Neurostimulator generator, multiple channel	Stimulator Generator, Multiple Array for Insertion in Subcutaneous Tissue and Fascia
Neurostimulator generator, multiple channel rechargeable	Stimulator Generator, Multiple Array Rechargeable for Insertion in Subcutaneous Tissue and Fascia
Neurostimulator generator, single channel	Stimulator Generator, Single Array for Insertion in Subcutaneous Tissue and Fascia
Neurostimulator generator, single channel rechargeable	Stimulator Generator, Single Array Rechargeable for Insertion in Subcutaneous Tissue and Fascia
Neutralization plate	Internal Fixation Device in Head and Facial Bones Internal Fixation Device in Upper Bones Internal Fixation Device in Lower Bones
Nitinol framed polymer mesh	Synthetic Substitute
Non-tunneled central venous catheter	Infusion Device
Novacor Left Ventricular Assist Device	Implantable Heart Assist System in Heart and Great Vessels
Novation® Ceramic AHS® (Articulation Hip System)	Synthetic Substitute, Ceramic for Replacement in Lower Joints
Omnilink Elite Vascular Balloon Expandable Stent System	Intraluminal Device
Open Pivot Aortic Valve Graft (AVG)	Synthetic Substitute
Open Pivot (mechanical) Valve	Synthetic Substitute
Optimizer™ III implantable pulse generator	Contractility Modulation Device for Insertion in Subcutaneous Tissue and Fascia
Oropharyngeal airway (OPA)	Intraluminal Device, Airway in Mouth and Throat
Ovatio™ CRT-D	Cardiac Resynchronization Defibrillator Pulse Generator for Insertion in Subcutaneous Tissue and Fascia
OXINIUM	Synthetic Substitute, Oxidized Zirconium on Polyethylene for Replacement in Lower Joints
Paclitaxel-eluting coronary stent	Intraluminal Device, Drug-eluting in Heart and Great Vessels

Term	ICD-10-PCS Value
Paclitaxel-eluting peripheral stent	Intraluminal Device, Drug-eluting in Upper Arteries Intraluminal Device, Drug-eluting in Lower Arteries
Partially absorbable mesh	Synthetic Substitute
Pedicle-based dynamic stabilization device	Spinal Stabilization Device, Pedicle-Based for Insertion in Upper Joints Spinal Stabilization Device, Pedicle-Based for Insertion in Lower Joints
Perceval sutureless valve	Zooplastic Tissue, Rapid Deployment Technique in New Technology
Percutaneous endoscopic gastrojejunostomy (PEG/J) tube	Feeding Device in Gastrointestinal System
Percutaneous endoscopic gastrostomy (PEG) tube	Feeding Device in Gastrointestinal System
Percutaneous nephrostomy catheter	Drainage Device
Peripherally inserted central catheter (PICC)	Infusion Device
Pessary ring	Intraluminal Device, Pessary in Female Reproductive System
Phrenic nerve stimulator generator	Stimulator Generator in Subcutaneous Tissue and Fascia
Phrenic nerve stimulator lead	Diaphragmatic Pacemaker Lead in Respiratory System
PHYSIOMESH™ Flexible Composite Mesh	Synthetic Substitute
Pipeline™ (Flex) embolization device	Intraluminal Device, Flow Diverter for Restriction in Upper Arteries
Polyethylene socket	Synthetic Substitute, Polyethylene for Replacement in Lower Joints
Polymethylmethacrylate (PMMA)	Synthetic Substitute
Polypropylene mesh	Synthetic Substitute
Porcine (bioprosthetic) valve	Zooplastic Tissue in Heart and Great Vessels
PRECICE intramedullary limb lengthening system	Internal Fixation Device, Intramedullary Limb Lengthening for Insertion in Upper Bones Internal Fixation Device, Intramedullary Limb Lengthening for Insertion in Lower Bones
PRESTIGE® Cervical Disc	Synthetic Substitute
PrimeAdvanced neurostimulator (SureScan)(MRI Safe)	Stimulator Generator, Multiple Array for Insertion in Subcutaneous Tissue and Fascia
PROCEED™ Ventral Patch	Synthetic Substitute
Prodisc-C	Synthetic Substitute
Prodisc-L	Synthetic Substitute
PROLENE Polypropylene Hernia System (PHS)	Synthetic Substitute
Protecta XT CRT-D	Cardiac Resynchronization Defibrillator Pulse Generator for Insertion in Subcutaneous Tissue and Fascia
Protecta XT DR (XT VR)	Defibrillator Generator for Insertion in Subcutaneous Tissue and Fascia
Protégé® RX Carotid Stent System	Intraluminal Device
Pump reservoir	Infusion Device, Pump in Subcutaneous Tissue and Fascia
REALIZE® Adjustable Gastric Band	Extraluminal Device

Term	ICD-10-PCS Value
Rebound HRD® (Hernia Repair Device)	Synthetic Substitute
RestoreAdvanced neurostimulator (SureScan)(MRI Safe)	Stimulator Generator, Multiple Array Rechargeable for Insertion in Subcutaneous Tissue and Fascia
RestoreSensor neurostimulator (SureScan)(MRI Safe)	Stimulator Generator, Multiple Array Rechargeable for Insertion in Subcutaneous Tissue and Fascia
RestoreUltra neurostimulator (SureScan)(MRI Safe)	Stimulator Generator, Multiple Array Rechargeable for Insertion in Subcutaneous Tissue and Fascia
Reveal (LINQ)(DX)(XT)	Monitoring Device
Reverse® Shoulder Prosthesis	Synthetic Substitute, Reverse Ball and Socket for Replacement in Upper Joints
Revo MRI™ SureScan® pacemaker	Pacemaker, Dual Chamber for Insertion in Subcutaneous Tissue and Fascia
Rheos® System device	Stimulator Generator in Subcutaneous Tissue and Fascia
Rheos® System lead	Stimulator Lead in Upper Arteries
RNS System lead	Neurostimulator Lead in Central Nervous System and Cranial Nerves
RNS system neurostimulator generator	Neurostimulator Generator in Head and Facial Bones
S-ICD™ lead	Subcutaneous Defibrillator Lead in Subcutaneous Tissue and Fascia
Sacral nerve modulation (SNM) lead	Stimulator Lead in Urinary System
Sacral neuromodulation lead	Stimulator Lead in Urinary System
SAPIEN transcatheter aortic valve	Zooplastic Tissue in Heart and Great Vessels
SAVAL below-the-knee (BTK) drug-eluting stent system	Intraluminal Device, Sustained Release Drug-eluting in New Technology Intraluminal Device, Sustained Release Drug-eluting, Two in New Technology Intraluminal Device, Sustained Release Drug-eluting, Three in New Technology Intraluminal Device, Sustained Release Drug-eluting, Four or More in New Technology
Secura (DR) (VR)	Defibrillator Generator for Insertion in Subcutaneous Tissue and Fascia
Sheffield hybrid external fixator	External Fixation Device, Hybrid for Insertion in Upper Bones External Fixation Device, Hybrid for Reposition in Upper Bones External Fixation Device, Hybrid for Insertion in Lower Bones External Fixation Device, Hybrid for Reposition in Lower Bones
Sheffield ring external fixator	External Fixation Device, Ring for Insertion in Upper Bones External Fixation Device, Ring for Reposition in Upper Bones External Fixation Device, Ring for Insertion in Lower Bones External Fixation Device, Ring for Reposition in Lower Bones
Single lead pacemaker (atrium)(ventricle)	Pacemaker, Single Chamber for Insertion in Subcutaneous Tissue and Fascia

Term	ICD-10-PCS Value
Single lead rate responsive pacemaker (atrium)(ventricle)	Pacemaker, Single Chamber Rate Responsive for Insertion in Subcutaneous Tissue and Fascia
Sirolimus-eluting coronary stent	Intraluminal Device, Drug-eluting in Heart and Great Vessels
SJM Biocor® Stented Valve System	Zooplastic Tissue in Heart and Great Vessels
Spacer, Articulating (Antibiotic)	Articulating Spacer in Lower Joints
Spacer, Static (Antibiotic)	Spacer in Lower Joints
Spinal cord neurostimulator lead	Neurostimulator Lead in Central Nervous System and Cranial Nerves
Spinal growth rods, magnetically controlled	Magnetically Controlled Growth Rod(s) in New Technology
Spiration IBV™ Valve System	Intraluminal Device, Endobronchial Valve in Respiratory System
Static Spacer (Antibiotic)	Spacer in Lower Joints
Stent, intraluminal (cardiovascular)(gastrointestinal) (hepatobiliary)(urinary)	Intraluminal Device
Stented tissue valve	Zooplastic Tissue in Heart and Great Vessels
Stratos LV	Cardiac Resynchronization Pacemaker Pulse Generator for Insertion in Subcutaneous Tissue and Fascia
Subcutaneous injection reservoir, port	Vascular Access Device, Totally Implantable in Subcutaneous Tissue and Fascia
Subcutaneous injection reservoir, pump	Infusion Device, Pump in Subcutaneous Tissue and Fascia
Subdermal progesterone implant	Contraceptive Device in Subcutaneous Tissue and Fascia
Surpass Streamline™ Flow Diverter	Intraluminal Device, Flow Diverter for Restriction in Upper Arteries
Sutureless valve, Perceval	Zooplastic Tissue, Rapid Deployment Technique in New Technology
SynCardia Total Artificial Heart	Synthetic Substitute
Synchra CRT-P	Cardiac Resynchronization Pacemaker Pulse Generator for Insertion in Subcutaneous Tissue and Fascia
SyncroMed Pump	Infusion Device, Pump in Subcutaneous Tissue and Fascia
Talent® Converter	Intraluminal Device
Talent® Occluder	Intraluminal Device
Talent® Stent Graft (abdominal)(thoracic)	Intraluminal Device
TandemHeart® System	Short-term External Heart Assist System in Heart and Great Vessels
TAXUS® Liberté® Paclitaxel-eluting Coronary Stent System	Intraluminal Device, Drug-eluting in Heart and Great Vessels
Therapeutic occlusion coil(s)	Intraluminal Device
Thoracostomy tube	Drainage Device
Thoratec IVAD (Implantable Ventricular Assist Device)	Implantable Heart Assist System in Heart and Great Vessels
Thoratec Paracorporeal Ventricular Assist Device	Short-term External Heart Assist System in Heart and Great Vessels
Tibial insert	Liner in Lower Joints
Tissue bank graft	Nonautologous Tissue Substitute

Term	ICD-10-PCS Value
Tissue expander (inflatable)(injectable)	Tissue Expander in Skin and Breast Tissue Expander in Subcutaneous Tissue and Fascia
Titanium Sternal Fixation System (TSFS)	Internal Fixation Device, Rigid Plate for Insertion in Upper Bones Internal Fixation Device, Rigid Plate for Reposition in Upper Bones
Total artificial (replacement) heart	Synthetic Substitute
Tracheostomy tube	Tracheostomy Device in Respiratory System
Trifecta™ Valve (aortic)	Zooplastic Tissue in Heart and Great Vessels
Tunneled central venous catheter	Vascular Access Device, Tunneled in Subcutaneous Tissue and Fascia
Tunneled spinal (intrathecal) catheter	Infusion Device
Two lead pacemaker	Pacemaker, Dual Chamber for Insertion in Subcutaneous Tissue and Fascia
Ultraflex™ Precision Colonic Stent System	Intraluminal Device
ULTRAPRO Hernia System (UHS)	Synthetic Substitute
ULTRAPRO Partially Absorbable Lightweight Mesh	Synthetic Substitute
ULTRAPRO Plug	Synthetic Substitute
Ultrasonic osteogenic stimulator	Bone Growth Stimulator in Head and Facial Bones Bone Growth Stimulator in Upper Bones Bone Growth Stimulator in Lower Bones
Ultrasound bone healing system	Bone Growth Stimulator in Head and Facial Bones Bone Growth Stimulator in Upper Bones Bone Growth Stimulator in Lower Bones
Uniplanar external fixator	External Fixation Device, Monoplanar for Insertion in Upper Bones External Fixation Device, Monoplanar for Reposition in Upper Bones External Fixation Device, Monoplanar for Insertion in Lower Bones External Fixation Device, Monoplanar for Reposition in Lower Bones
Urinary incontinence stimulator lead	Stimulator Lead in Urinary System
Vaginal pessary	Intraluminal Device, Pessary in Female Reproductive System
Valiant Thoracic Stent Graft	Intraluminal Device

Term	ICD-10-PCS Value
Vectra® Vascular Access Graft	Vascular Access Device, Tunneled in Subcutaneous Tissue and Fascia
Ventrio™ Hernia Patch	Synthetic Substitute
Versa	Pacemaker, Dual Chamber for Insertion in Subcutaneous Tissue and Fascia
Virtuoso (II) (DR) (VR)	Defibrillator Generator for Insertion in Subcutaneous Tissue and Fascia
Viva(XT)(S)	Cardiac Resynchronization Defibrillator Pulse Generator for Insertion in Subcutaneous Tissue and Fascia
WALLSTENT® Endoprosthesis	Intraluminal Device
X-STOP® Spacer	Spinal Stabilization Device, Interspinous Process for Insertion in Upper Joints Spinal Stabilization Device, Interspinous Process for Insertion in Lower Joints
Xact Carotid Stent System	Intraluminal Device
Xenograft	Zooplastic Tissue in Heart and Great Vessels
XIENCE Everolimus Eluting Coronary Stent System	Intraluminal Device, Drug-eluting in Heart and Great Vessels
XLIF® System	Interbody Fusion Device in Lower Joints
Zenith AAA Endovascular Graft	Intraluminal Device, Branched or Fenestrated, One or Two Arteries for Restriction in Lower Arteries Intraluminal Device, Branched or Fenestrated, Three or More Arteries for Restriction in Lower Arteries Intraluminal Device
Zenith Flex® AAA Endovascular Graft	Intraluminal Device
Zenith TX2® TAA Endovascular Graft	Intraluminal Device
Zenith® Renu™ AAA Ancillary Graft	Intraluminal Device
Zilver® PTX® (paclitaxel) Drug-Eluting Peripheral Stent	Intraluminal Device, Drug-eluting in Upper Arteries Intraluminal Device, Drug-eluting in Lower Arteries
Zimmer® NexGen® LPS Mobile Bearing Knee	Synthetic Substitute
Zimmer® NexGen® LPS-Flex Mobile Knee	Synthetic Substitute
Zotarolimus-eluting coronary stent	Intraluminal Device, Drug-eluting in Heart and Great Vessels

Device Aggregation Table

This table crosswalks specific device character value definitions for specific root operations in a specific body system to the more general device character value to be used when the root operation covers a wide range of body parts and the device character represents an entire family of devices.

Specific Device	for Operation	in Body System	General Device	
Autologous Arterial Tissue (A)	All applicable	Heart and Great Vessels Lower Arteries Lower Veins Upper Arteries Upper Veins	7	Autologous Tissue Substitute
Autologous Venous Tissue (9)	All applicable	Heart and Great Vessels Lower Arteries Lower Veins Upper Arteries Upper Veins	7	Autologous Tissue Substitute
Cardiac Lead, Defibrillator (K)	Insertion	Heart and Great Vessels	M	Cardiac Lead
Cardiac Lead, Pacemaker (J)	Insertion	Heart and Great Vessels	M	Cardiac Lead
Cardiac Resynchronization Defibrillator Pulse Generator (9)	Insertion	Subcutaneous Tissue and Fascia	P	Cardiac Rhythm Related Device
Cardiac Resynchronization Pacemaker Pulse Generator (7)	Insertion	Subcutaneous Tissue and Fascia	P	Cardiac Rhythm Related Device
Contractility Modulation Device (A)	Insertion	Subcutaneous Tissue and Fascia	P	Cardiac Rhythm Related Device
Defibrillator Generator (8)	Insertion	Subcutaneous Tissue and Fascia	P	Cardiac Rhythm Related Device
Epiretinal Visual Prosthesis (5)	All applicable	Eye	J	Synthetic Substitute
External Fixation Device, Hybrid (D)	Insertion	Lower Bones Upper Bones	5	External Fixation Device
External Fixation Device, Hybrid (D)	Reposition	Lower Bones Upper Bones	5	External Fixation Device
External Fixation Device, Limb Lengthening (8)	Insertion	Lower Bones Upper Bones	5	External Fixation Device
External Fixation Device, Monoplanar (B)	Insertion	Lower Bones Upper Bones	5	External Fixation Device
External Fixation Device, Monoplanar (B)	Reposition	Lower Bones Upper Bones	5	External Fixation Device
External Fixation Device, Ring (C)	Insertion	Lower Bones Upper Bones	5	External Fixation Device
External Fixation Device, Ring (C)	Reposition	Lower Bones Upper Bones	5	External Fixation Device
Hearing Device, Bone Conduction (4)	Insertion	Ear, Nose, Sinus	S	Hearing Device
Hearing Device, Multiple Channel Cochlear Prosthesis (6)	Insertion	Ear, Nose, Sinus	S	Hearing Device
Hearing Device, Single Channel Cochlear Prosthesis (5)	Insertion	Ear, Nose, Sinus	S	Hearing Device
Internal Fixation Device, Intramedullary (6)	All applicable	Lower Bones Upper Bones	4	Internal Fixation Device
Internal Fixation Device, Intramedullary Limb Lengthening (7)	Insertion	Lower Bones Upper Bones	6	Internal Fixation Device, Intramedullary
Internal Fixation Device, Rigid Plate (Ø)	Insertion	Upper Bones	4	Internal Fixation Device
Internal Fixation Device, Rigid Plate (Ø)	Reposition	Upper Bones	4	Internal Fixation Device
Intraluminal Device, Airway (B)	All applicable	Ear, Nose, Sinus Gastrointestinal System Mouth and Throat	D	Intraluminal Device
Intraluminal Device, Bioactive (B)	All applicable	Upper Arteries	D	Intraluminal Device
Intraluminal Device, Branched or Fenestrated, One or Two Arteries (E)	Restriction	Heart and Great Vessels Lower Arteries	D	Intraluminal Device
Intraluminal Device, Branched or Fenestrated, Three or More Arteries (F)	Restriction	Heart and Great Vessels Lower Arteries	D	Intraluminal Device
Intraluminal Device, Drug-eluting (4)	All applicable	Heart and Great Vessels Lower Arteries Upper Arteries	D	Intraluminal Device
Intraluminal Device, Drug-eluting, Four or More (7)	All applicable	Heart and Great Vessels Lower Arteries Upper Arteries	D	Intraluminal Device

Specific Device	for Operation	in Body System	General Device	
Intraluminal Device, Drug-eluting, Three (6)	All applicable	Heart and Great Vessels Lower Arteries Upper Arteries	D	Intraluminal Device
Intraluminal Device, Drug-eluting, Two (5)	All applicable	Heart and Great Vessels Lower Arteries Upper Arteries	D	Intraluminal Device
Intraluminal Device, Endobronchial Valve (G)	All applicable	Respiratory System	D	Intraluminal Device
Intraluminal Device, Endotracheal Airway (E)	All applicable	Respiratory System	D	Intraluminal Device
Intraluminal Device, Flow Diverter (H)	Restriction	Upper Arteries	D	Intraluminal Device
Intraluminal Device, Four or More (G)	All applicable	Heart and Great Vessels Lower Arteries Upper Arteries	D	Intraluminal Device
Intraluminal Device, Pessary (G)	All applicable	Female Reproductive System	D	Intraluminal Device
Intraluminal Device, Radioactive (T)	All applicable	Heart and Great Vessels	D	Intraluminal Device
Intraluminal Device, Three (F)	All applicable	Heart and Great Vessels Lower Arteries Upper Arteries	D	Intraluminal Device
Intraluminal Device, Two (E)	All applicable	Heart and Great Vessels Lower Arteries Upper Arteries	D	Intraluminal Device
Monitoring Device, Hemodynamic (Ø)	Insertion	Subcutaneous Tissue and Fascia	2	Monitoring Device
Monitoring Device, Pressure Sensor (Ø)	Insertion	Heart and Great Vessels	2	Monitoring Device
Pacemaker, Dual Chamber (6)	Insertion	Subcutaneous Tissue and Fascia	P	Cardiac Rhythm Related Device
Pacemaker, Single Chamber (4)	Insertion	Subcutaneous Tissue and Fascia	P	Cardiac Rhythm Related Device
Pacemaker, Single Chamber Rate Responsive (5)	Insertion	Subcutaneous Tissue and Fascia	P	Cardiac Rhythm Related Device
Spinal Stabilization Device, Facet Replacement (D)	Insertion	Lower Joints Upper Joints	4	Internal Fixation Device
Spinal Stabilization Device, Interspinous Process (B)	Insertion	Lower Joints Upper Joints	4	Internal Fixation Device
Spinal Stabilization Device, Pedicle-Based (C)	Insertion	Lower Joints Upper Joints	4	Internal Fixation Device
Stimulator Generator, Multiple Array (D)	Insertion	Subcutaneous Tissue and Fascia	M	Stimulator Generator
Stimulator Generator, Multiple Array Rechargeable (E)	Insertion	Subcutaneous Tissue and Fascia	M	Stimulator Generator
Stimulator Generator, Single Array (B)	Insertion	Subcutaneous Tissue and Fascia	M	Stimulator Generator
Stimulator Generator, Single Array Rechargeable (C)	Insertion	Subcutaneous Tissue and Fascia	M	Stimulator Generator
Synthetic Substitute, Ceramic (3)	Replacement	Lower Joints	J	Synthetic Substitute
Synthetic Substitute, Ceramic on Polyethylene (4)	Replacement	Lower Joints	J	Synthetic Substitute
Synthetic Substitute, Intraocular Telescope (Ø)	Replacement	Eye	J	Synthetic Substitute
Synthetic Substitute, Metal (1)	Replacement	Lower Joints	J	Synthetic Substitute
Synthetic Substitute, Metal on Polyethylene (2)	Replacement	Lower Joints	J	Synthetic Substitute
Synthetic Substitute, Oxidized Zirconium on Polyethylene (6)	Replacement	Lower Joints	J	Synthetic Substitute
Synthetic Substitute, Polyethylene (Ø)	Replacement	Lower Joints	J	Synthetic Substitute
Synthetic Substitute, Reverse Ball and Socket (Ø)	Replacement	Upper Joints	J	Synthetic Substitute

ICD-10-PCS Value	Definition
Articulating Spacer in Lower Joints	**Includes:** Articulating Spacer (Antibiotic) Spacer, Articulating (Antibiotic)
Artificial Sphincter in Gastrointestinal System	**Includes:** Artificial anal sphincter (AAS) Artificial bowel sphincter (neosphincter)
Artificial Sphincter in Urinary System	**Includes:** AMS 800® Urinary Control System Artificial urinary sphincter (AUS)
Autologous Arterial Tissue in Heart and Great Vessels	**Includes:** Autologous artery graft
Autologous Arterial Tissue in Lower Arteries	**Includes:** Autologous artery graft
Autologous Arterial Tissue in Lower Veins	**Includes:** Autologous artery graft
Autologous Arterial Tissue in Upper Arteries	**Includes:** Autologous artery graft
Autologous Arterial Tissue in Upper Veins	**Includes:** Autologous artery graft
Autologous Tissue Substitute	**Includes:** Autograft Cultured epidermal cell autograft Epicel® cultured epidermal autograft
Autologous Venous Tissue in Heart and Great Vessels	**Includes:** Autologous vein graft
Autologous Venous Tissue in Lower Arteries	**Includes:** Autologous vein graft
Autologous Venous Tissue in Lower Veins	**Includes:** Autologous vein graft
Autologous Venous Tissue in Upper Arteries	**Includes:** Autologous vein graft
Autologous Venous Tissue in Upper Veins	**Includes:** Autologous vein graft
Bone Growth Stimulator in Head and Facial Bones	**Includes:** Electrical bone growth stimulator (EBGS) Ultrasonic osteogenic stimulator Ultrasound bone healing system
Bone Growth Stimulator in Lower Bones	**Includes:** Electrical bone growth stimulator (EBGS) Ultrasonic osteogenic stimulator Ultrasound bone healing system
Bone Growth Stimulator in Upper Bones	**Includes:** Electrical bone growth stimulator (EBGS) Ultrasonic osteogenic stimulator Ultrasound bone healing system
Cardiac Lead in Heart and Great Vessels	**Includes:** Cardiac contractility modulation lead

ICD-10-PCS Value	Definition
Cardiac Lead, Defibrillator for Insertion in Heart and Great Vessels	**Includes:** ACUITY™ Steerable Lead Attain Ability® lead Attain StarFix® (OTW) lead Cardiac resynchronization therapy (CRT) lead Corox (OTW) Bipolar Lead Durata® Defibrillation Lead ENDOTAK RELIANCE® (G) Defibrillation Lead
Cardiac Lead, Pacemaker for Insertion in Heart and Great Vessels	**Includes:** ACUITY™ Steerable Lead Attain Ability® lead Attain StarFix® (OTW) lead Cardiac resynchronization therapy (CRT) lead Corox (OTW) Bipolar Lead
Cardiac Resynchronization Defibrillator Pulse Generator for Insertion in Subcutaneous Tissue and Fascia	**Includes:** COGNIS® CRT-D Concerto II CRT-D Consulta CRT-D CONTAK RENEWA® 3 RF (HE) CRT-D LIVIAN™ CRT-D Maximo II DR CRT-D Ovatio™ CRT-D Protecta XT CRT-D Viva (XT)(S)
Cardiac Resynchronization Pacemaker Pulse Generator for Insertion in Subcutaneous Tissue and Fascia	**Includes:** Consulta CRT-P Stratos LV Synchra CRT-P
Contraceptive Device in Female Reproductive System	**Includes:** Intrauterine device (IUD)
Contraceptive Device in Subcutaneous Tissue and Fascia	**Includes:** Subdermal progesterone implant
Contractility Modulation Device for Insertion in Subcutaneous Tissue and Fascia	**Includes:** Optimizer™ III implantable pulse generator
Defibrillator Generator for Insertion in Subcutaneous Tissue and Fascia	**Includes:** Evera (XT)(S)(DR/VR) Implantable cardioverter-defibrillator (ICD) Maximo II DR (VR) Protecta XT DR (XT VR) Secura (DR) (VR) Virtuoso (II) (DR) (VR)
Diaphragmatic Pacemaker Lead in Respiratory System	**Includes:** Phrenic nerve stimulator lead
Drainage Device	**Includes:** Cystostomy tube Foley catheter Percutaneous nephrostomy catheter Thoracostomy tube
External Fixation Device in Head and Facial Bones	**Includes:** External fixator
External Fixation Device in Lower Bones	**Includes:** External fixator
External Fixation Device in Lower Joints	**Includes:** External fixator

ICD-10-PCS Value	Definition
External Fixation Device in Upper Bones	**Includes:** External fixator
External Fixation Device in Upper Joints	**Includes:** External fixator
External Fixation Device, Hybrid for Insertion in Lower Bones	**Includes:** Delta frame external fixator Sheffield hybrid external fixator
External Fixation Device, Hybrid for Insertion in Upper Bones	**Includes:** Delta frame external fixator Sheffield hybrid external fixator
External Fixation Device, Hybrid for Reposition in Lower Bones	**Includes:** Delta frame external fixator Sheffield hybrid external fixator
External Fixation Device, Hybrid for Reposition in Upper Bones	**Includes:** Delta frame external fixator Sheffield hybrid external fixator
External Fixation Device, Limb Lengthening for Insertion in Lower Bones	**Includes:** Ilizarov-Vecklich device
External Fixation Device, Limb Lengthening for Insertion in Upper Bones	**Includes:** Ilizarov-Vecklich device
External Fixation Device, Monoplanar for Insertion in Lower Bones	**Includes:** Uniplanar external fixator
External Fixation Device, Monoplanar for Insertion in Upper Bones	**Includes:** Uniplanar external fixator
External Fixation Device, Monoplanar for Reposition in Lower Bones	**Includes:** Uniplanar external fixator
External Fixation Device, Monoplanar for Reposition in Upper Bones	**Includes:** Uniplanar external fixator
External Fixation Device, Ring for Insertion in Lower Bones	**Includes:** Ilizarov external fixator Sheffield ring external fixator
External Fixation Device, Ring for Insertion in Upper Bones	**Includes:** Ilizarov external fixator Sheffield ring external fixator
External Fixation Device, Ring for Reposition in Lower Bones	**Includes:** Ilizarov external fixator Sheffield ring external fixator
External Fixation Device, Ring for Reposition in Upper Bones	**Includes:** Ilizarov external fixator Sheffield ring external fixator
Extraluminal Device	**Includes:** AtriClip LAA Exclusion System LAP-BAND® adjustable gastric banding system REALIZE® Adjustable Gastric Band
Feeding Device in Gastrointestinal System	**Includes:** Percutaneous endoscopic gastrojejunostomy (PEG/J) tube Percutaneous endoscopic gastrostomy (PEG) tube
Hearing Device in Ear, Nose, Sinus	**Includes:** Esteem® implantable hearing system
Hearing Device in Head and Facial Bones	**Includes:** Bone anchored hearing device

ICD-10-PCS Value	Definition
Hearing Device, Bone Conduction for Insertion in Ear, Nose, Sinus	**Includes:** Bone anchored hearing device
Hearing Device, Multiple Channel Cochlear Prosthesis for Insertion in Ear, Nose, Sinus	**Includes:** Cochlear implant (CI), multiple channel (electrode)
Hearing Device, Single Channel Cochlear Prosthesis for Insertion in Ear, Nose, Sinus	**Includes:** Cochlear implant (CI), single channel (electrode)
Implantable Heart Assist System in Heart and Great Vessels	**Includes:** Berlin Heart Ventricular Assist Device DeBakey Left Ventricular Assist Device DuraHeart Left Ventricular Assist System HeartMate 3™ LVAS HeartMate II® Left Ventricular Assist Device (LVAD) HeartMate XVE® Left Ventricular Assist Device (LVAD) MicroMed HeartAssist Novacor Left Ventricular Assist Device Thoratec IVAD (Implantable Ventricular Assist Device)
Infusion Device	**Includes:** Ascenda Intrathecal Catheter InDura, intrathecal catheter (1P) (spinal) Non-tunneled central venous catheter Peripherally inserted central catheter (PICC) Tunneled spinal (intrathecal) catheter
Infusion Device, Pump in Subcutaneous Tissue and Fascia	**Includes:** Implantable drug infusion pump (anti-spasmodic)(chemotherapy)(pain) Injection reservoir, pump Pump reservoir Subcutaneous injection reservoir, pump SynchroMed pump
Interbody Fusion Device in Lower Joints	**Includes:** Axial Lumbar Interbody Fusion System AxiaLIF® System CoRoent® XL Direct Lateral Interbody Fusion (DLIF) device EXtreme Lateral Interbody Fusion (XLIF) device Interbody fusion (spine) cage XLIF® System
Interbody Fusion Device in Upper Joints	**Includes:** BAK/C® Interbody Cervical Fusion System Interbody fusion (spine) cage
Interbody Fusion Device, Nanotextured Surface in New Technology	Includes: nanoLOCK™ interbody fusion device

ICD-10-PCS Value	Definition
Interbody Fusion Device, Radiolucent Porous in New Technology	Includes: COALESCE® radiolucent interbody fusion device COHERE® radiolucent interbody fusion device
Internal Fixation Device in Head and Facial Bones	**Includes:** Bone screw (interlocking)(lag)(pedicle) (recessed) Kirschner wire (K-wire) Neutralization plate
Internal Fixation Device in Lower Bones	**Includes:** Bone screw (interlocking)(lag)(pedicle) (recessed) Clamp and rod internal fixation system (CRIF) Kirschner wire (K-wire) Neutralization plate
Internal Fixation Device in Lower Joints	**Includes:** Fusion screw (compression)(lag)(locking) Joint fixation plate Kirschner wire (K-wire)
Internal Fixation Device in Upper Bones	**Includes:** Bone screw (interlocking)(lag)(pedicle) (recessed) Clamp and rod internal fixation system (CRIF) Kirschner wire (K-wire) Neutralization plate
Internal Fixation Device in Upper Joints	**Includes:** Fusion screw (compression)(lag)(locking) Joint fixation plate Kirschner wire (K-wire)
Internal Fixation Device, Intramedullary in Lower Bones	**Includes:** Intramedullary (IM) rod (nail) Intramedullary skeletal kinetic distractor (ISKD) Kuntscher nail
Internal Fixation Device, Intramedullary in Upper Bones	**Includes:** Intramedullary (IM) rod (nail) Intramedullary skeletal kinetic distractor (ISKD) Kuntscher nail
Internal Fixation Device Intramedullary Limb Lengthening for Insertion in Lower Bones	**Includes:** PRECICE intramedullary limb lengthening system
Internal Fixation Device Intramedullary Limb Lengthening for Insertion in Upper Bones	**Includes:** PRECICE intramedullary limb lengthening system
Internal Fixation Device, Rigid Plate for Insertion in Upper Bones	**Includes:** Titanium Sternal Fixation System (TSFS)
Internal Fixation Device, Rigid Plate for Reposition in Upper Bones	**Includes:** Titanium Sternal Fixation System (TSFS)

ICD-10-PCS Value	Definition
Intraluminal Device	**Includes:** Absolute Pro Vascular (OTW) Self-Expanding Stent System Acculink (RX) Carotid Stent System AFX® Endovascular AAA System AneuRx® AAA Advantage® Assurant (Cobalt) stent Carotid WALLSTENT® Monorail® Endoprosthesis CoAxia NeuroFlo catheter Colonic Z-Stent® Complete (SE) stent Cook Zenith AAA Endovascular Graft Driver stent (RX) (OTW) E-Luminexx™ (Biliary)(Vascular) Stent Embolization coil(s) Endologix AFX® Endovascular AAA System Endurant® Endovascular Stent Graft Endurant® II AAA stent graft system EXCLUDER® AAA Endoprosthesis Express® (LD) Premounted Stent System Express® Biliary SD Monorail® Premounted Stent System Express® SD Renal Monorail® Premounted Stent System FLAIR® Endovascular Stent Graft Formula™ Balloon-Expandable Renal Stent System GORE EXCLUDER® AAA Endoprosthesis GORE TAG® Thoracic Endoprosthesis Herculink (RX) Elite Renal Stent System LifeStent® (Flexstar)(XL) Vascular Stent System Medtronic Endurant® II AAA stent graft system Micro-Driver stent (RX) (OTW) MULTI-LINK (VISION)(MINI-VISION)(ULTRA) Coronary Stent System Omnilink Elite Vascular Balloon Expandable Stent System Protege® RX Carotid Stent System Stent, intraluminal (cardiovascular) (gastrointestinal)(hepatobiliary) (urinary) Talent® Converter Talent® Occluder Talent® Stent Graft (abdominal)(thoracic) Therapeutic occlusion coil(s) Ultraflex™ Precision Colonic Stent System Valiant Thoracic Stent Graft WALLSTENT® Endoprosthesis Xact Carotid Stent System Zenith AAA Endovascular Graft Zenith Flex® AAA Endovascular Graft Zenith TX2® TAA Endovascular Graft Zenith® Renu™ AAA Ancillary Graft
Intraluminal Device, Airway in Ear, Nose, Sinus	**Includes:** Nasopharyngeal airway (NPA)
Intraluminal Device, Airway in Gastrointestinal System	**Includes:** Esophageal obturator airway (EOA)

ICD-10-PCS Value	Definition
Intraluminal Device, Airway in Mouth and Throat	**Includes:** Guedel airway Oropharyngeal airway (OPA)
Intraluminal Device, Bioactive in Upper Arteries	**Includes:** Bioactive embolization coil(s) Micrus CERECYTE microcoil

Intraluminal Device, Branched or Fenestrated, One or Two Arteries for Restriction in Lower Arteries	**Includes:**
	Cook Zenith AAA Endovascular Graft
	EXCLUDER® AAA Endoprosthesis
	EXCLUDER® IBE Endoprosthesis
	GORE EXCLUDER® AAA
	  Endoprosthesis
	GORE EXCLUDER®IBE
	  Endoprosthesis
	Zenith AAA Endovascular Graft

Intraluminal Device, Branched or Fenestrated, Three or More Arteries for Restriction in Lower Arteries	**Includes:** Cook Zenith AAA Endovascular Graft EXCLUDER® AAA Endoprosthesis GORE EXCLUDER® AAA Endoprosthesis Zenith AAA Endovascular Graft

Intraluminal Device, Drug-eluting in Heart and Great Vessels	**Includes:**
	CYPHER® Stent
	Endeavor® (III)(IV) (Sprint)
	  Zotarolimus-eluting Coronary
	  Stent System
	Everolimus-eluting coronary stent
	Paclitaxel-eluting coronary stent
	Sirolimus-eluting coronary stent
	TAXUS® Liberte® Paclitaxel-eluting
	  Coronary Stent System
	XIENCE Everolimus Eluting Coronary
	  Stent System
	Zotarolimus-eluting coronary stent

Intraluminal Device, Drug-eluting in Lower Arteries	**Includes:** Paclitaxel-eluting peripheral stent Zilver® PTX® (paclitaxel) Drug-Eluting Peripheral Stent
Intraluminal Device, Drug-eluting in Upper Arteries	**Includes:** Paclitaxel-eluting peripheral stent Zilver® PTX® (paclitaxel) Drug-Eluting Peripheral Stent
Intraluminal Device, Endobronchial Valve in Respiratory System	**Includes:** Spiration IBV™ Valve System
Intraluminal Device, Endotracheal Airway in Respiratory System	**Includes:** Endotracheal tube (cuffed)(double-lumen)
Intraluminal Device, Flow Diverter for Restriction in Upper Arteries	**Includes:** Flow Diverter embolization device Pipeline™ (Flex) embolization device Surpass Streamline™ Flow Diverter
Intraluminal Device, Pessary in Female Reproductive System	**Includes:** Pessary ring Vaginal pessary

Intraluminal Device, Sustained Release Drug-eluting in New Technology	**Includes:**
	Eluvia™ Drug-eluting Vascular Stent
	  System
	SAVAL below-the-knee (BTK)
	  drug-eluting stent system

Intraluminal Device, Sustained Release Drug-eluting, Four or More in New Technology	**Includes:**
	Eluvia™ Drug-eluting Vascular Stent
	  System
	SAVAL below-the-knee (BTK)
	  drug-eluting stent system

ICD-10-PCS Value	Definition

Intraluminal Device, Sustained Release Drug-eluting, Three in New Technology	**Includes:**
	Eluvia™ Drug-eluting Vascular Stent
	  System
	SAVAL below-the-knee (BTK)
	  drug-eluting stent system

Intraluminal Device, Sustained Release Drug-eluting, Two in New Technology	**Includes:**
	Eluvia™ Drug-eluting Vascular Stent
	  System
	SAVAL below-the-knee (BTK)
	  drug-eluting stent system

Liner in Lower Joints	**Includes:** Acetabular cup Hip (joint) liner Joint liner (insert) Knee (implant) insert Tibial insert

Magnetically Controlled Growth Rod(s) in New Technology	**Includes:**
	MAGEC® Spinal Bracing and
	  Distraction System
	Spinal growth rods, magnetically
	  controlled

Monitoring Device	**Includes:**
	Blood glucose monitoring system
	Cardiac event recorder
	Continuous Glucose Monitoring
	  (CGM) device
	Implantable glucose monitoring
	  device
	Loop recorder, implantable
	Reveal (LINQ)(DX)(XT)

Monitoring Device, Hemodynamic for Insertion in Subcutaneous Tissue and Fascia	**Includes:**
	Implantable hemodynamic monitor
	  (IHM)
	Implantable hemodynamic
	  monitoring system (IHMS)

Monitoring Device, Pressure Sensor for Insertion in Heart and Great Vessels	**Includes:** CardioMEMS® pressure sensor EndoSure® sensor
Neurostimulator Generator in Head and Facial Bones	**Includes:** RNS system neurostimulator generator
Neurostimulator Lead in Central Nervous System and Cranial Nerves	**Includes:** Cortical strip neurostimulator lead DBS lead Deep brain neurostimulator lead RNS System lead Spinal cord neurostimulator lead
Neurostimulator Lead in Peripheral Nervous System	**Includes:** InterStim® Therapy lead
Nonautologous Tissue Substitute	**Includes:** Acellular Hydrated Dermis Bone bank bone graft Cook Biodesign® Fistula Plug(s) Cook Biodesign® Hernia Graft(s) Cook Biodesign® Layered Graft(s) Cook Zenapro™ Layered Graft(s) Tissue bank graft
Pacemaker, Dual Chamber for Insertion in Subcutaneous Tissue and Fascia	**Includes:** Advisa (MRI) EnRhythm Kappa Revo MRI™ SureScan® pacemaker Two lead pacemaker Versa

ICD-10-PCS Value	Definition
Pacemaker, Single Chamber for Insertion in Subcutaneous Tissue and Fascia	**Includes:** Single lead pacemaker (atrium)(ventricle)
Pacemaker, Single Chamber Rate Responsive for Insertion in Subcutaneous Tissue and Fascia	**Includes:** Single lead rate responsive pacemaker (atrium)(ventricle)
Radioactive Element	**Includes:** Brachytherapy seeds CivaSheet®
Radioactive Element, Cesium-131 Collagen Implant for Insertion in Central Nervous System and Cranial Nerves	**Includes:** Cesium-131 Collagen Implant GammaTile™
Resurfacing Device in Lower Joints	**Includes:** CONSERVE® PLUS Total Resurfacing Hip System Cormet Hip Resurfacing System
Short-term External Heart Assist System in Heart and Great Vessels	**Includes:** Biventricular external heart assist system BVS 5000 Ventricular Assist Device Centrimag® Blood Pump Impella® heart pump TandemHeart® System Thoratec Paracorporeal Ventricular Assist Device
Skin Substitute, Porcine Liver Derived in New Technology	**Includes:** MIRODERM™ Biologic Wound Matrix
Spacer in Lower Joints	**Includes:** Joint spacer (antibiotic) Spacer, Static (Antibiotic) Static Spacer (Antibiotic)
Spacer in Upper Joints	**Includes:** Joint spacer (antibiotic)
Spinal Stabilization Device, Facet Replacement for Insertion in Lower Joints	**Includes:** Facet replacement spinal stabilization device
Spinal Stabilization Device, Facet Replacement for Insertion in Upper Joints	**Includes:** Facet replacement spinal stabilization device
Spinal Stabilization Device, Interspinous Process for Insertion in Lower Joints	**Includes:** Interspinous process spinal stabilization device X-STOP® Spacer
Spinal Stabilization Device, Interspinous Process for Insertion in Upper Joints	**Includes:** Interspinous process spinal stabilization device X-STOP® Spacer
Spinal Stabilization Device, Pedicle-Based for Insertion in Lower Joints	**Includes:** Dynesys® Dynamic Stabilization System Pedicle-based dynamic stabilization device
Spinal Stabilization Device, Pedicle-Based for Insertion in Upper Joints	**Includes:** Dynesys® Dynamic Stabilization System Pedicle-based dynamic stabilization device

ICD-10-PCS Value	Definition
Stimulator Generator in Subcutaneous Tissue and Fascia	**Includes:** Baroreflex Activation Therapy® (BAT®) Diaphragmatic pacemaker generator Mark IV Breathing Pacemaker System Phrenic nerve stimulator generator Rheos® System device
Stimulator Generator, Multiple Array for Insertion in Subcutaneous Tissue and Fascia	**Includes:** Activa PC neurostimulator Enterra gastric neurostimulator Neurostimulator generator, multiple channel PrimeAdvanced neurostimulator (SureScan)(MRI Safe)
Stimulator Generator, Multiple Array Rechargeable for Insertion in Subcutaneous Tissue and Fascia	**Includes:** Activa RC neurostimulator Neurostimulator generator, multiple channel rechargeable RestoreAdvanced neurostimulator (SureScan)(MRI Safe) RestoreSensor neurostimulator (SureScan)(MRI Safe) RestoreUltra neurostimulator (SureScan)(MRI Safe)
Stimulator Generator, Single Array for Insertion in Subcutaneous Tissue and Fascia	**Includes:** Activa SC neurostimulator InterStim® Therapy neurostimulator Itrel (3)(4) neurostimulator Neurostimulator generator, single channel
Stimulator Generator, Single Array Rechargeable for Insertion in Subcutaneous Tissue and Fascia	**Includes:** Neurostimulator generator, single channel rechargeable
Stimulator Lead in Gastrointestinal System	**Includes:** Gastric electrical stimulation (GES) lead Gastric pacemaker lead
Stimulator Lead in Muscles	**Includes:** Electrical muscle stimulation (EMS) lead Electronic muscle stimulator lead Neuromuscular electrical stimulation (NEMS) lead
Stimulator Lead in Upper Arteries	**Includes:** Baroreflex Activation Therapy® (BAT®) Carotid (artery) sinus (baroreceptor) lead Rheos® System lead
Stimulator Lead in Urinary System	**Includes:** Sacral nerve modulation (SNM) lead Sacral neuromodulation lead Urinary incontinence stimulator lead
Subcutaneous Defibrillator Lead in Subcutaneous Tissue and Fascia	**Includes:** S-ICD™ lead

ICD-10-PCS Value	Definition
Synthetic Substitute	**Includes:** AbioCor® Total Replacement Heart AMPLATZER® Muscular VSD Occluder Annuloplasty ring Bard® Composix® (E/X) (LP) mesh Bard® Composix® Kugel® patch Bard® Dulex™ mesh Bard® Ventralex™ hernia patch BRYAN® Cervical Disc System Ex-PRESS™ mini glaucoma shunt Flexible Composite Mesh GORE® DUALMESH® Holter valve ventricular shunt MitraClip valve repair system Nitinol framed polymer mesh Open Pivot (mechanical) valve Open Pivot Aortic Valve Graft (AVG) Partially absorbable mesh PHYSIOMESH™ Flexible Composite Mesh Polymethylmethacrylate (PMMA) Polypropylene mesh PRESTIGE® Cervical Disc PROCEED™ Ventral Patch Prodisc-C Prodisc-L PROLENE Polypropylene Hernia System (PHS) Rebound HRD® (Hernia Repair Device) SynCardia Total Artificial Heart Total artificial (replacement) heart ULTRAPRO Hernia System (UHS) ULTRAPRO Partially Absorbable Lightweight Mesh ULTRAPRO Plug Ventrio™ Hernia Patch Zimmer® NexGen® LPS Mobile Bearing Knee Zimmer® NexGen® LPS-Flex Mobile Knee
Synthetic Substitute, Ceramic for Replacement in Lower Joints	**Includes:** Ceramic on ceramic bearing surface Novation® Ceramic AHS® (Articulation Hip System)
Synthetic Substitute, Intraocular Telescope for Replacement in Eye	**Includes:** Implantable Miniature Telescope™ (IMT)
Synthetic Substitute, Metal for Replacement in Lower Joints	**Includes:** Cobalt/chromium head and socket Metal on metal bearing surface
Synthetic Substitute, Metal on Polyethylene for Replacement in Lower Joints	**Includes:** Cobalt/chromium head and polyethylene socket
Synthetic Substitute, Oxidized Zirconium on Polyethylene for Replacement in Lower Joints	**Includes:** OXINIUM

ICD-10-PCS Value	Definition
Synthetic Substitute, Polyethylene for Replacement in Lower Joints	**Includes:** Polyethylene socket
Synthetic Substitute, Reverse Ball and Socket for Replacement in Upper Joints	**Includes:** Delta III Reverse shoulder prosthesis Reverse® Shoulder Prosthesis
Tissue Expander in Skin and Breast	**Includes:** Tissue expander (inflatable) (injectable)
Tissue Expander in Subcutaneous Tissue and Fascia	**Includes:** Tissue expander (inflatable) (injectable)
Tracheostomy Device in Respiratory System	**Includes:** Tracheostomy tube
Vascular Access Device, Totally Implantable in Subcutaneous Tissue and Fascia	**Includes:** Implanted (venous)(access) port Injection reservoir, port Subcutaneous injection reservoir, port
Vascular Access Device, Tunneled in Subcutaneous Tissue and Fascia	**Includes:** Tunneled central venous catheter Vectra® Vascular Access Graft
Zooplastic Tissue in Heart and Great Vessels	**Includes:** 3f (Aortic) Bioprosthesis valve Bovine pericardial valve Bovine pericardium graft Contegra Pulmonary Valved Conduit CoreValve transcatheter aortic valve Epic™ Stented Tissue Valve (aortic) Freestyle (Stentless) Aortic Root Bioprosthesis Hancock Bioprosthesis (aortic) (mitral) valve Hancock Bioprosthetic Valved Conduit Melody® transcatheter pulmonary valve Mitroflow® Aortic Pericardial Heart Valve Mosaic Bioprosthesis (aortic) (mitral) valve Porcine (bioprosthetic) valve SAPIEN transcatheter aortic valve SJM Biocor® Stented Valve System Stented tissue valve Trifecta™ Valve (aortic) Xenograft
Zooplastic Tissue, Rapid Deployment Technique in New Technology	**Includes:** EDWARDS INTUITY Elite valve system INTUITY Elite valve system, EDWARDS Perceval sutureless valve Sutureless valve, Perceval

Substance Key

This table crosswalks a specific substance, listed by trade name or synonym, to the PCS value that would be used to represent that substance in either the Administration or New Technology section. The ICD-10-PCS value may be located in either the 6th-character Substance column or the 7th-character Qualifier column depending on the section/table to which it is classified. The most specific character is listed in the table.

Trade Name or Synonym	ICD-10-PCS Value	PCS Section
AIGISRx Antibacterial Envelope	Anti-Infective Envelope (A)	Administration (3)
Andexanet Alfa, Factor Xa Inhibitor Reversal Agent	Coagulation Factor Xa, Inactivated (7)	New Technology (X)
Andexxa	Coagulation Factor Xa, Inactivated (7)	New Technology (X)
Angiotensin II	Synthetic Human Angiotensin II (H)	New technology (X)
Antibacterial Envelope (TYRX) (AIGISRx)	Anti-Infective Envelope (A)	Administration (3)
Antimicrobial envelope	Anti-Infective Envelope (A)	Administration (3)
Axicabtagene Ciloeucel	Engineered Autologous Chimeric Antigen Receptor T-cell Immunotherapy (C)	New technology (X)
AZEDRA®	Iobenguane I-131 Antineoplastic (S)	New Technology (X)
Bone morphogenetic protein 2 (BMP 2)	Recombinant Bone Morphogenetic Protein (B)	Administration (3)
CBMA (Concentrated Bone Marrow Aspirate)	Concentrated Bone Marrow Aspirate (Ø)	New technology (X)
Clolar	Clofarabine (P)	Administration (3)
Coagulation Factor Xa, (Recombinant) Inactivated	Coagulation Factor Xa, Inactivated (7)	New Technology (X)
CONTEPO™	Fosfomycin Anti-infective (K)	New Technology (X)
Defitelio	Defibrotide Sodium Anticoagulant (9)	New technology (X)
DuraGraft® Endothelial Damage Inhibitor	Endothelial Damage Inhibitor (8)	New technology (X)
ELZONRIS™	Tagraxofusp-erzs Antineoplastic (Q)	New Technology (X)
ERLEADA™	Apalutamide Antineoplastic (J)	New Technology (X)
Factor Xa Inhibitor Reversal Agent, Andexanet Alfa	Coagulation Factor Xa, Inactivated (7)	New Technology (X)
Fosfomycin injection	Fosfomycin Anti-infective (K)	New Technology (X)
GIAPREZA™	Synthetic Human Angiotensin II (H)	New Technology (X)
Human angiotensin II, synthetic	Synthetic Human Angiotensin II (H)	New technology (X)
IMI/REL	Imipenem-cilastatin-relebactam Anti-infective (U)	New Technology (X)
Iobenguane I-131, High Specific Activity (HSA)	Iobenguane I-131 Antineoplastic (S)	New Technology (X)
Jakafi®	Ruxolitinib (T)	New Technology (X)
Kcentra	4-Factor Prothrombin Complex Concentrate (B)	Administration (3)
KYMRIAH	Engineered Autologous Chimeric Antigen Receptor T-cell Immunotherapy (C)	New technology (X)
Nesiritide	Human B-type Natriuretic Peptide (H)	Administration (3)
rhBMP-2	Recombinant Bone Morphogenetic Protein (B)	Administration (3)
Seprafilm	Adhesion Barrier (5)	Administration (3)
STELARA®	Other New Technology Therapeutic Substance (F)	New technology (X)
Tisagenlecleucel	Engineered Autologous Chimeric Antigen Receptor T-cell Immunotherapy (C)	New technology (X)
Tissue Plasminogen Activator (tPA)(r- tPA)	Other Thrombolytic (7)	Administration (3)
TYRX Antibacterial Envelope	Anti-Infective Envelope (A)	Administration (3)
Ustekinumab	Other New Technology Therapeutic Substance (F)	New technology (X)
Vabomere™	Meropenem-vaborbactam Anti-infective (N)	New Technology (X)
Venclexta®	Ventoclax Antineoplastic (R)	New Technology (X)
Vistogard®	Uridine Triacetate (8)	New technology (X)
Voraxaze	Glucarpidase (Q)	Administration (3)
VYXEOS™	Cytarabine and Daunorubicin Liposome Antineoplastic (B)	New technology (X)
XOSPATA®	Gilteritinib Antineoplastic (V)	New Technology (X)
ZINPLAVA™	Bezlotoxumab Monoclonal Antibody (A)	New technology (X)
Zyvox	Oxazolidinones (8)	Administration (3)

Substance Definitions

This table crosswalks a PCS value, used in the Administration or New Technology section, to a specific substance. The specific substances are listed by trade name or synonym. The ICD-10-PCS value may be located in either the 6th-character Substance column or the 7th-character Qualifier column depending on the section/table to which it is classified.

ICD-10-PCS Value	Trade Name or Synonym	PCS Section
4-Factor Prothrombin Complex Concentrate (B)	**Includes:** Kcentra	Administration (3)
Adhesion Barrier (5)	**Includes:** Seprafilm	Administration (3)
Anti-Infective Envelope (A)	**Includes:** AIGISRx Antibacterial Envelope Antimicrobial envelope Antibacterial Envelope (TYRX) (AIGISRx) TYRX Antibacterial Envelope	Administration (3)
Apalutamide Antineoplastic (J)	**Includes:** ERLEADA™	New Technology (X)
Bezlotoxumab Monoclonal Antibody (A)	**Includes:** ZINPLAVA™	New technology (X)
Clofarabine (P)	**Includes:** Clolar	Administration (3)
Coagulation Factor Xa, Inactivated (7)	**Includes:** Andexanet Alfa, Factor Xa Inhibitor Reversal Agent Andexxa Coagulation Factor Xa, (Recombinant) Inactivated Factor Xa Inhibitor Reversal Agent, Andexanet Alfa	New Technology (X)
Concentrated Bone Marrow Aspirate (Ø)	**Includes:** CBMA (Concentrated Bone Marrow Aspirate)	New technology (X)
Cytarabine and Daunorubicin Liposome Antineoplastic (B)	**Includes:** VYXEOS™	New technology (X)
Defibrotide Sodium Anticoagulant (9)	**Includes:** Defitelio	New technology (X)
Endothelial Damage Inhibitor (8)	**Includes:** DuraGraft® Endothelial Damage Inhibitor	New technology (X)
Engineered Autologous Chimeric Antigen Receptor T-cell Immunotherapy (C)	**Includes:** Axicabtagene Ciloeucel KYMRIAH Tisagenlecleucel	New technology (X)
Fosfomycin Anti-infective (K)	**Includes:** CONTEPO™ Fosfomycin injection	New Technology (X)
Gilteritinib Antineoplastic (V)	**Includes:** XOSPATA®	New Technology (X)
Glucarpidase (Q)	**Includes:** Voraxaze	Administration (3)
Human B-type Natriuretic Peptide (H)	**Includes:** Nesiritide	Administration (3)
Imipenem-cilastatin-relebactam Anti-infective (U)	**Includes:** IMI/REL	New Technology (X)
Iobenguane I-131 Antineoplastic (S)	**Includes:** AZEDRA® Iobenguane I-131, High Specific Activity (HSA)	New Technology (X)
Meropenem-vaborbactam Anti-infective (N)	**Includes:** Vabomere™	New Technology (X)
Other New Technology Therapeutic Substance (F)	**Includes:** STELARA® Ustekinumab	New technology (X)
Other Thrombolytic (7)	**Includes:** Tissue Plasminogen Activator (tPA)(r-tPA)	Administration (3)
Oxazolidinones (8)	**Includes:** Zyvox	Administration (3)
Recombinant Bone Morphogenetic Protein (B)	**Includes:** Bone morphogenetic protein 2 (BMP 2) rhBMP-2	Administration (3)
Ruxolitinib (T)	**Includes:** Jakafi®	New Technology (X)

ICD-10-PCS Value	Trade Name or Synonym	PCS Section
Synthetic Human Angiotensin II (H)	**Includes:** Angiotensin II GIAPREZA™ Human angiotensin II, synthetic	New technology (X)
Tagraxofusp-erzs Antineoplastic (Q)	**Includes:** ELZONRIS™	New Technology (X)
Uridine Triacetate (8)	**Includes:** Vistogard®	New technology (X)
Venetoclax Antineoplastic (R)	**Includes:** Venclexta®	New Technology (X)

Appendix I: Sections B–H Character Definitions

Sections B-H (Imaging through Substance Abuse Treatment) do not include root operations. Instead, the character 3 value represents the type of procedure performed with additional details about that procedure provided by the character 4 or 5 value, when appropriate. This resource provides the specific ICD-10-PCS value and its associated definition for the character 3, character 4, and character 5 values in the ancillary sections of B-H.

Section B–Imaging

ICD-10-PCS Value (Character 3)	Definition
Computerized Tomography (CT Scan) (2)	Computer reformatted digital display of multiplanar images developed from the capture of multiple exposures of external ionizing radiation
Fluoroscopy (1)	Single plane or bi-plane real time display of an image developed from the capture of external ionizing radiation on a fluorescent screen. The image may also be stored by either digital or analog means.
Magnetic Resonance Imaging (MRI) (3)	Computer reformatted digital display of multiplanar images developed from the capture of radiofrequency signals emitted by nuclei in a body site excited within a magnetic field
Plain Radiography (Ø)	Planar display of an image developed from the capture of external ionizing radiation on photographic or photoconductive plate
Ultrasonography (4)	Real time display of images of anatomy or flow information developed from the capture of reflected and attenuated high frequency sound waves

Section C–Nuclear Medicine

ICD-10-PCS Value (Character 3)	Definition
Nonimaging Nuclear Medicine Assay (6)	Introduction of radioactive materials into the body for the study of body fluids and blood elements, by the detection of radioactive emissions
Nonimaging Nuclear Medicine Probe (5)	Introduction of radioactive materials into the body for the study of distribution and fate of certain substances by the detection of radioactive emissions; or, alternatively, measurement of absorption of radioactive emissions from an external source
Nonimaging Nuclear Medicine Uptake (4)	Introduction of radioactive materials into the body for measurements of organ function, from the detection of radioactive emissions
Planar Nuclear Medicine Imaging (1)	Introduction of radioactive materials into the body for single plane display of images developed from the capture of radioactive emissions
Positron Emission Tomographic (PET) Imaging (3)	Introduction of radioactive materials into the body for three dimensional display of images developed from the simultaneous capture, 18Ø degrees apart, of radioactive emissions
Systemic Nuclear Medicine Therapy (7)	Introduction of unsealed radioactive materials into the body for treatment
Tomographic (Tomo) Nuclear Medicine Imaging (2)	Introduction of radioactive materials into the body for three dimensional display of images developed from the capture of radioactive emissions

Section F–Physical Rehabilitation and Diagnostic Audiology

ICD-10-PCS Value (Character 3)	Definition
Activities of Daily Living Assessment (2)	Measurement of functional level for activities of daily living
Activities of Daily Living Treatment (8)	Exercise or activities to facilitate functional competence for activities of daily living
Caregiver Training (F)	Training in activities to support patient's optimal level of function
Cochlear Implant Treatment (B)	Application of techniques to improve the communication abilities of individuals with cochlear implant
Device Fitting (D)	Fitting of a device designed to facilitate or support achievement of a higher level of function
Hearing Aid Assessment (4)	Measurement of the appropriateness and/or effectiveness of a hearing device
Hearing Assessment (3)	Measurement of hearing and related functions
Hearing Treatment (9)	Application of techniques to improve, augment, or compensate for hearing and related functional impairment
Motor and/or Nerve Function Assessment (1)	Measurement of motor, nerve, and related functions
Motor Treatment (7)	Exercise or activities to increase or facilitate motor function

Continued on next page

Section F–Physical Rehabilitation and Diagnostic Audiology

Continued from previous page

ICD-10-PCS Value (Character 3)	Definition
Speech Assessment (Ø)	Measurement of speech and related functions
Speech Treatment (6)	Application of techniques to improve, augment, or compensate for speech and related functional impairment
Vestibular Assessment (5)	Measurement of the vestibular system and related functions
Vestibular Treatment (C)	Application of techniques to improve, augment, or compensate for vestibular and related functional impairment

Section F–Physical Rehabilitation and Diagnostic Audiology

ICD-10-PCS Value Qualifier (Character 5)	Definition
Acoustic Reflex Decay (J)	Measures reduction in size/strength of acoustic reflex over time Includes/Examples: Includes site of lesion test
Acoustic Reflex Patterns (G)	Defines site of lesion based upon presence/absence of acoustic reflexes with ipsilateral vs. contralateral stimulation
Acoustic Reflex Threshold (H)	Determines minimal intensity that acoustic reflex occurs with ipsilateral and/or contralateral stimulation
Aerobic Capacity and Endurance (7)	Measures autonomic responses to positional changes; perceived exertion, dyspnea or angina during activity; performance during exercise protocols; standard vital signs; and blood gas analysis or oxygen consumption
Alternate Binaural or Monaural Loudness Balance (7)	Determines auditory stimulus parameter that yields the same objective sensation Includes/Examples: Sound intensities that yield same loudness perception
Anthropometric Characteristics (B)	Measures edema, body fat composition, height, weight, length and girth
Aphasia (Assessment) (C)	Measures expressive and receptive speech and language function including reading and writing
Aphasia (Treatment) (3)	Applying techniques to improve, augment, or compensate for receptive/ expressive language impairments
Articulation/Phonology (Assessment) (9)	Measures speech production
Articulation/Phonology (Treatment) (4)	Applying techniques to correct, improve, or compensate for speech productive impairment
Assistive Listening Device (5)	Assists in use of effective and appropriate assistive listening device/system
Assistive Listening System/Device Selection (4)	Measures the effectiveness and appropriateness of assistive listening systems/devices
Assistive, Adaptive, Supportive or Protective Devices (9)	Explanation: Devices to facilitate or support achievement of a higher level of function in wheelchair mobility; bed mobility; transfer or ambulation ability; bath and showering ability; dressing; grooming; personal hygiene; play or leisure
Auditory Evoked Potentials (L)	Measures electric responses produced by the VIIIth cranial nerve and brainstem following auditory stimulation
Auditory Processing (Assessment) (Q)	Evaluates ability to receive and process auditory information and comprehension of spoken language
Auditory Processing (Treatment) (2)	Applying techniques to improve the receiving and processing of auditory information and comprehension of spoken language
Augmentative/Alternative Communication System (Assessment) (L)	Determines the appropriateness of aids, techniques, symbols, and/or strategies to augment or replace speech and enhance communication Includes/Examples: Includes the use of telephones, writing equipment, emergency equipment, and TDD
Augmentative/Alternative Communication System (Treatment) (3)	Includes/Examples: Includes augmentative communication devices and aids
Aural Rehabilitation (5)	Applying techniques to improve the communication abilities associated with hearing loss
Aural Rehabilitation Status (P)	Measures impact of a hearing loss including evaluation of receptive and expressive communication skills
Bathing/Showering (Ø)	Includes/Examples: Includes obtaining and using supplies; soaping, rinsing, and drying body parts; maintaining bathing position; and transferring to and from bathing positions

Continued on next page

Section F–Physical Rehabilitation and Diagnostic Audiology   *Continued from previous page*

ICD-10-PCS Value Qualifier (Character 5)	Definition
Bathing/Showering Techniques (Ø)	Activities to facilitate obtaining and using supplies, soaping, rinsing and drying body parts, maintaining bathing position, and transferring to and from bathing positions
Bed Mobility (Assessment) (B)	Transitional movement within bed
Bed Mobility (Treatment) (5)	Exercise or activities to facilitate transitional movements within bed
Bedside Swallowing and Oral Function (H)	Includes/Examples: Bedside swallowing includes assessment of sucking, masticating, coughing, and swallowing. Oral function includes assessment of musculature for controlled movements, structures, and functions to determine coordination and phonation.
Bekesy Audiometry (3)	Uses an instrument that provides a choice of discrete or continuously varying pure tones; choice of pulsed or continuous signal
Binaural Electroacoustic Hearing Aid Check (6)	Determines mechanical and electroacoustic function of bilateral hearing aids using hearing aid test box
Binaural Hearing Aid (Assessment) (3)	Measures the candidacy, effectiveness, and appropriateness of a hearing aid Explanation: Measures bilateral fit
Binaural Hearing Aid (Treatment) (2)	Explanation: Assists in achieving maximum understanding and performance
Bithermal, Binaural Caloric Irrigation (Ø)	Measures the rhythmic eye movements stimulated by changing the temperature of the vestibular system
Bithermal, Monaural Caloric Irrigation (1)	Measures the rhythmic eye movements stimulated by changing the temperature of the vestibular system in one ear
Brief Tone Stimuli (R)	Measures specific central auditory process
Cerumen Management (3)	Includes examination of external auditory canal and tympanic membrane and removal of cerumen from external ear canal
Cochlear Implant (Ø)	Measures candidacy for cochlear implant
Cochlear Implant Rehabilitation (Ø)	Applying techniques to improve the communication abilities of individuals with cochlear implant; includes programming the device, providing patients/families with information
Communicative/Cognitive Integration Skills (Assessment) (G)	Measures ability to use higher cortical functions Includes/Examples: Includes orientation, recognition, attention span, initiation and termination of activity, memory, sequencing, categorizing, concept formation, spatial operations, judgment, problem solving, generalization and pragmatic communication
Communicative/Cognitive Integration Skills (Treatment) (6)	Activities to facilitate the use of higher cortical functions Includes/Examples: Includes level of arousal, orientation, recognition, attention span, initiation and termination of activity, memory sequencing, judgment and problem solving, learning and generalization, and pragmatic communication
Computerized Dynamic Posturography (6)	Measures the status of the peripheral and central vestibular system and the sensory/motor component of balance; evaluates the efficacy of vestibular rehabilitation
Conditioned Play Audiometry (4)	Behavioral measures using nonspeech and speech stimuli to obtain frequency-specific and ear-specific information on auditory status from the patient Explanation: Obtains speech reception threshold by having patient point to pictures of spondaic words
Coordination/Dexterity (Assessment) (3)	Measures large and small muscle groups for controlled goal-directed movements Explanation: Dexterity includes object manipulation
Coordination/Dexterity (Treatment) (2)	Exercise or activities to facilitate gross coordination and fine coordination
Cranial Nerve Integrity (9)	Measures cranial nerve sensory and motor functions, including tastes, smell and facial expression
Dichotic Stimuli (T)	Measures specific central auditory process
Distorted Speech (S)	Measures specific central auditory process
Dix-Hallpike Dynamic (5)	Measures nystagmus following Dix-Hallpike maneuver
Dressing (1)	Includes/Examples: Includes selecting clothing and accessories, obtaining clothing from storage, dressing, fastening and adjusting clothing and shoes, and applying and removing personal devices, prosthesis or orthosis

Continued on next page

Section F–Physical Rehabilitation and Diagnostic Audiology

Continued from previous page

ICD-10-PCS Value Qualifier (Character 5)	Definition
Dressing Techniques (1)	Activities to facilitate selecting clothing and accessories, dressing and undressing, adjusting clothing and shoes, applying and removing devices, prostheses or orthoses
Dynamic Orthosis (6)	Includes/Examples: Includes customized and prefabricated splints, inhibitory casts, spinal and other braces, and protective devices; allows motion through transfer of movement from other body parts or by use of outside forces
Ear Canal Probe Microphone (1)	Real ear measures
Ear Protector Attentuation (7)	Measures ear protector fit and effectiveness
Electrocochleography (K)	Measures the VIIIth cranial nerve action potential
Environmental, Home, Work Barriers (B)	Measures current and potential barriers to optimal function, including safety hazards, access problems and home or office design
Ergonomics and Body Mechanics (C)	Ergonomic measurement of job tasks, work hardening or work conditioning needs; functional capacity; and body mechanics
Eustachian Tube Function (F)	Measures eustachian tube function and patency of eustachian tube
Evoked Otoacoustic Emissions, Diagnostic (N)	Measures auditory evoked potentials in a diagnostic format
Evoked Otoacoustic Emissions, Screening (M)	Measures auditory evoked potentials in a screening format
Facial Nerve Function (7)	Measures electrical activity of the VIIth cranial nerve (facial nerve)
Feeding/Eating (Assessment) (2)	Includes/Examples: Includes setting up food, selecting and using utensils and tableware, bringing food or drink to mouth, cleaning face, hands, and clothing, and management of alternative methods of nourishment
Feeding/Eating (Treatment) (3)	Exercise or activities to facilitate setting up food, selecting and using utensils and tableware, bringing food or drink to mouth, cleaning face, hands, and clothing, and management of alternative methods of nourishment
Filtered Speech (Ø)	Uses high or low pass filtered speech stimuli to assess central auditory processing disorders, site of lesion testing
Fluency (Assessment) (D)	Measures speech fluency or stuttering
Fluency (Treatment) (7)	Applying techniques to improve and augment fluent speech
Gait and/or Balance (D)	Measures biomechanical, arthrokinematic and other spatial and temporal characteristics of gait and balance
Gait Training/Functional Ambulation (9)	Exercise or activities to facilitate ambulation on a variety of surfaces and in a variety of environments
Grooming/Personal Hygiene (Assessment) (3)	Includes/Examples: Includes ability to obtain and use supplies in a sequential fashion, general grooming, oral hygiene, toilet hygiene, personal care devices, including care for artificial airways
Grooming/Personal Hygiene (Treatment) (2)	Activities to facilitate obtaining and using supplies in a sequential fashion: general grooming, oral hygiene, toilet hygiene, cleaning body, and personal care devices, including artificial airways
Hearing and Related Disorders Counseling (Ø)	Provides patients/families/caregivers with information, support, referrals to facilitate recovery from a communication disorder Includes/Examples: Includes strategies for psychosocial adjustment to hearing loss for clients and families/caregivers
Hearing and Related Disorders Prevention (1)	Provides patients/families/caregivers with information and support to prevent communication disorders
Hearing Screening (Ø)	Pass/refer measures designed to identify need for further audiologic assessment
Home Management (Assessment) (4)	Obtaining and maintaining personal and household possessions and environment Includes/Examples: Includes clothing care, cleaning, meal preparation and cleanup, shopping, money management, household maintenance, safety procedures, and childcare/parenting
Home Management (Treatment) (4)	Activities to facilitate obtaining and maintaining personal household possessions and environment Includes/Examples: Includes clothing care, cleaning, meal preparation and clean-up, shopping, money management, household maintenance, safety procedures, childcare/parenting

Continued on next page

Section F–Physical Rehabilitation and Diagnostic Audiology   *Continued from previous page*

ICD-10-PCS Value Qualifier (Character 5)	Definition
Instrumental Swallowing and Oral Function (J)	Measures swallowing function using instrumental diagnostic procedures Explanation: Methods include videofluoroscopy, ultrasound, manometry, endoscopy
Integumentary Integrity (1)	Includes/Examples: Includes burns, skin conditions, ecchymosis, bleeding, blisters, scar tissue, wounds and other traumas, tissue mobility, turgor and texture
Manual Therapy Techniques (7)	Techniques in which the therapist uses his/her hands to administer skilled movements Includes/Examples: Includes connective tissue massage, joint mobilization and manipulation, manual lymph drainage, manual traction, soft tissue mobilization and manipulation
Masking Patterns (W)	Measures central auditory processing status
Monaural Electroacoustic Hearing Aid Check (8)	Determines mechanical and electroacoustic function of one hearing aid using hearing aid test box
Monaural Hearing Aid (Assessment) (2)	Measures the candidacy, effectiveness, and appropriateness of a hearing aid Explanation: Measures unilateral fit
Monaural Hearing Aid (Treatment) (1)	Explanation: Assists in achieving maximum understanding and performance
Motor Function (Assessment) (4)	Measures the body's functional and versatile movement patterns Includes/Examples: Includes motor assessment scales, analysis of head, trunk and limb movement, and assessment of motor learning
Motor Function (Treatment) (3)	Exercise or activities to facilitate crossing midline, laterality, bilateral integration, praxis, neuromuscular relaxation, inhibition, facilitation, motor function and motor learning
Motor Speech (Assessment) (B)	Measures neurological motor aspects of speech production
Motor Speech (Treatment) (8)	Applying techniques to improve and augment the impaired neurological motor aspects of speech production
Muscle Performance (Assessment) (Ø)	Measures muscle strength, power and endurance using manual testing, dynamometry or computer-assisted electromechanical muscle test; functional muscle strength, power and endurance; muscle pain, tone, or soreness; or pelvic-floor musculature Explanation: Muscle endurance refers to the ability to contract a muscle repeatedly over time
Muscle Performance (Treatment) (1)	Exercise or activities to increase the capacity of a muscle to do work in terms of strength, power, and/or endurance Explanation: Muscle strength is the force exerted to overcome resistance in one maximal effort. Muscle power is work produced per unit of time, or the product of strength and speed. Muscle endurance is the ability to contract a muscle repeatedly over time.
Neuromotor Development (D)	Measures motor development, righting and equilibrium reactions, and reflex and equilibrium reactions
Non-invasive Instrumental Status (N)	Instrumental measures of oral, nasal, vocal, and velopharyngeal functions as they pertain to speech production
Nonspoken Language (Assessment) (7)	Measures nonspoken language (print, sign, symbols) for communication
Nonspoken Language (Treatment) (Ø)	Applying techniques that improve, augment, or compensate spoken communication
Oral Peripheral Mechanism (P)	Structural measures of face, jaw, lips, tongue, teeth, hard and soft palate, pharynx as related to speech production
Orofacial Myofunctional (Assessment) (K)	Measures orofacial myofunctional patterns for speech and related functions
Orofacial Myofunctional (Treatment) (9)	Applying techniques to improve, alter, or augment impaired orofacial myofunctional patterns and related speech production errors
Oscillating Tracking (3)	Measures ability to visually track
Pain (F)	Measures muscle soreness, pain and soreness with joint movement, and pain perception Includes/Examples: Includes questionnaires, graphs, symptom magnification scales or visual analog scales
Perceptual Processing (Assessment) (5)	Measures stereognosis, kinesthesia, body schema, right-left discrimination, form constancy, position in space, visual closure, figure-ground, depth perception, spatial relations and topographical orientation

Continued on next page

Section F–Physical Rehabilitation and Diagnostic Audiology

Continued from previous page

ICD-10-PCS Value Qualifier (Character 5)	Definition
Perceptual Processing (Treatment) (1)	Exercise and activities to facilitate perceptual processing Explanation: Includes stereognosis, kinesthesia, body schema, right-left discrimination, form constancy, position in space, visual closure, figure-ground, depth perception, spatial relations, and topographical orientation Includes/Examples: Includes stereognosis, kinesthesia, body schema, right-left discrimination, form constancy, position in space, visual closure, figure-ground, depth perception, spatial relations, and topographical orientation
Performance Intensity Phonetically Balanced Speech Discrimination (Q)	Measures word recognition over varying intensity levels
Postural Control (3)	Exercise or activities to increase postural alignment and control
Prosthesis (8)	Explanation: Artificial substitutes for missing body parts that augment performance or function Includes/Examples: Limb prosthesis, ocular prosthesis
Psychosocial Skills (Assessment) (6)	The ability to interact in society and to process emotions Includes/Examples: Includes psychological (values, interests, self-concept); social (role performance, social conduct, interpersonal skills, self expression); self-management (coping skills, time management, self-control)
Psychosocial Skills (Treatment) (6)	The ability to interact in society and to process emotions Includes/Examples: Includes psychological (values, interests, self-concept); social (role performance, social conduct, interpersonal skills, self expression); self-management (coping skills, time management, self-control)
Pure Tone Audiometry, Air (1)	Air-conduction pure tone threshold measures with appropriate masking
Pure Tone Audiometry, Air and Bone (2)	Air-conduction and bone-conduction pure tone threshold measures with appropriate masking
Pure Tone Stenger (C)	Measures unilateral nonorganic hearing loss based on simultaneous presentation of pure tones of differing volume
Range of Motion and Joint Integrity (5)	Measures quantity, quality, grade, and classification of joint movement and/or mobility Explanation: Range of Motion is the space, distance or angle through which movement occurs at a joint or series of joints. Joint integrity is the conformance of joints to expected anatomic, biomechanical and kinematic norms.
Range of Motion and Joint Mobility (Ø)	Exercise or activities to increase muscle length and joint mobility
Receptive/Expressive Language (Assessment) (8)	Measures receptive and expressive language
Receptive/Expressive Language (Treatment) (B)	Applying techniques to improve and augment receptive/expressive language
Reflex Integrity (G)	Measures the presence, absence, or exaggeration of developmentally appropriate, pathologic or normal reflexes
Select Picture Audiometry (5)	Establishes hearing threshold levels for speech using pictures
Sensorineural Acuity Level (4)	Measures sensorineural acuity masking presented via bone conduction
Sensory Aids (5)	Determines the appropriateness of a sensory prosthetic device, other than a hearing aid or assistive listening system/device
Sensory Awareness/ Processing/ Integrity (6)	Includes/Examples: Includes light touch, pressure, temperature, pain, sharp/dull, proprioception, vestibular, visual, auditory, gustatory, and olfactory
Short Increment Sensitivity Index (9)	Measures the ear's ability to detect small intensity changes; site of lesion test requiring a behavioral response
Sinusoidal Vertical Axis Rotational (4)	Measures nystagmus following rotation
Somatosensory Evoked Potentials (9)	Measures neural activity from sites throughout the body
Speech/Language Screening (6)	Identifies need for further speech and/or language evaluation
Speech Threshold (1)	Measures minimal intensity needed to repeat spondaic words

Continued on next page

Section F–Physical Rehabilitation and Diagnostic Audiology   *Continued from previous page*

ICD-10-PCS Value Qualifier (Character 5)	Definition
Speech-Language Pathology and Related Disorders Counseling (1)	Provides patients/families with information, support, referrals to facilitate recovery from a communication disorder
Speech-Language Pathology and Related Disorders Prevention (2)	Applying techniques to avoid or minimize onset and/or development of a communication disorder
Speech/Word Recognition (2)	Measures ability to repeat/identify single syllable words; scores given as a percentage; includes word recognition/speech discrimination
Staggered Spondaic Word (3)	Measures central auditory processing site of lesion based upon dichotic presentation of spondaic words
Static Orthosis (7)	Includes/Examples: Includes customized and prefabricated splints, inhibitory casts, spinal and other braces, and protective devices; has no moving parts, maintains joint(s) in desired position
Stenger (B)	Measures unilateral nonorganic hearing loss based on simultaneous presentation of signals of differing volume
Swallowing Dysfunction (D)	Activities to improve swallowing function in coordination with respiratory function Includes/Examples: Includes function and coordination of sucking, mastication, coughing, swallowing
Synthetic Sentence Identification (5)	Measures central auditory dysfunction using identification of third order approximations of sentences and competing messages
Temporal Ordering of Stimuli (V)	Measures specific central auditory process
Therapeutic Exercise (6)	Exercise or activities to facilitate sensory awareness, sensory processing, sensory integration, balance training, conditioning, reconditioning Includes/Examples: Includes developmental activities, breathing exercises, aerobic endurance activities, aquatic exercises, stretching and ventilatory muscle training
Tinnitus Masker (Assessment) (7)	Determines candidacy for tinnitus masker
Tinnitus Masker (Treatment) (Ø)	Explanation: Used to verify physical fit, acoustic appropriateness, and benefit; assists in achieving maximum benefit
Tone Decay (8)	Measures decrease in hearing sensitivity to a tone; site of lesion test requiring a behavioral response
Transfer (C)	Transitional movement from one surface to another
Transfer Training (8)	Exercise or activities to facilitate movement from one surface to another
Tympanometry (D)	Measures the integrity of the middle ear; measures ease at which sound flows through the tympanic membrane while air pressure against the membrane is varied
Unithermal Binaural Screen (2)	Measures the rhythmic eye movements stimulated by changing the temperature of the vestibular system in both ears using warm water, screening format
Ventilation/Respiration/Circulation (G)	Measures ventilatory muscle strength, power and endurance, pulmonary function and ventilatory mechanics Includes/Examples: Includes ability to clear airway, activities that aggravate or relieve edema, pain, dyspnea or other symptoms, chest wall mobility, cardiopulmonary response to performance of ADL and IAD, cough and sputum, standard vital signs
Vestibular (Ø)	Applying techniques to compensate for balance disorders; includes habituation, exercise therapy, and balance retraining
Visual Motor Integration (Assessment) (2)	Coordinating the interaction of information from the eyes with body movement during activity
Visual Motor Integration (Treatment) (2)	Exercise or activities to facilitate coordinating the interaction of information from eyes with body movement during activity
Visual Reinforcement Audiometry (6)	Behavioral measures using nonspeech and speech stimuli to obtain frequency/ear-specific information on auditory status Includes/Examples: Includes a conditioned response of looking toward a visual reinforcer (e.g., lights, animated toy) every time auditory stimuli are heard
Vocational Activities and Functional Community or Work Reintegration Skills (Assessment) (H)	Measures environmental, home, work (job/school/play) barriers that keep patients from functioning optimally in their environment Includes/Examples: Includes assessment of vocational skills and interests, environment of work (job/school/play), injury potential and injury prevention or reduction, ergonomic stressors, transportation skills, and ability to access and use community resources

Continued on next page

Section F–Physical Rehabilitation and Diagnostic Audiology

Continued from previous page

ICD-10-PCS Value Qualifier (Character 5)	Definition
Vocational Activities and Functional Community or Work Reintegration Skills (Treatment) (7)	Activities to facilitate vocational exploration, body mechanics training, job acquisition, and environmental or work (job/school/play) task adaptation Includes/Examples: Includes injury prevention and reduction, ergonomic stressor reduction, job coaching and simulation, work hardening and conditioning, driving training, transportation skills, and use of community resources
Voice (Assessment) (F)	Measures vocal structure, function and production
Voice (Treatment) (C)	Applying techniques to improve voice and vocal function
Voice Prosthetic (Assessment) (M)	Determines the appropriateness of voice prosthetic/adaptive device to enhance or facilitate communication
Voice Prosthetic (Treatment) (4)	Includes/Examples: Includes electrolarynx, and other assistive, adaptive, supportive devices
Wheelchair Mobility (Assessment) (F)	Measures fit and functional abilities within wheelchair in a variety of environments
Wheelchair Mobility (Treatment) (4)	Management, maintenance and controlled operation of a wheelchair, scooter or other device, in and on a variety of surfaces and environments
Wound Management (5)	Includes/Examples: Includes non-selective and selective debridement (enzymes, autolysis, sharp debridement), dressings (wound coverings, hydrogel, vacuum-assisted closure), topical agents, etc.

Section G–Mental Health

ICD-10-PCS Value (Character 3)	Definition
Biofeedback (C)	Provision of information from the monitoring and regulating of physiological processes in conjunction with cognitive-behavioral techniques to improve patient functioning or well-being Includes/Examples: Includes EEG, blood pressure, skin temperature or peripheral blood flow, ECG, electrooculogram, EMG, respirometry or capnometry, GSR/EDR, perineometry to monitor/regulate bowel/bladder activity, electrogastrogram to monitor/regulate gastric motility
Counseling (6)	The application of psychological methods to treat an individual with normal developmental issues and psychological problems in order to increase function, improve well-being, alleviate distress, maladjustment or resolve crises
Crisis Intervention (2)	Treatment of a traumatized, acutely disturbed or distressed individual for the purpose of short-term stabilization Includes/Examples: Includes defusing, debriefing, counseling, psychotherapy and/or coordination of care with other providers or agencies
Electroconvulsive Therapy (B)	The application of controlled electrical voltages to treat a mental health disorder Includes/Examples: Includes appropriate sedation and other preparation of the individual
Family Psychotherapy (7)	Treatment that includes one or more family members of an individual with a mental health disorder by behavioral, cognitive, psychoanalytic, psychodynamic or psychophysiological means to improve functioning or well-being Explanation: Remediation of emotional or behavioral problems presented by one or more family members in cases where psychotherapy with more than one family member is indicated
Group Psychotherapy (H)	Treatment of two or more individuals with a mental health disorder by behavioral, cognitive, psychoanalytic, psychodynamic or psychophysiological means to improve functioning or well-being
Hypnosis (F)	Induction of a state of heightened suggestibility by auditory, visual and tactile techniques to elicit an emotional or behavioral response
Individual Psychotherapy (5)	Treatment of an individual with a mental health disorder by behavioral, cognitive, psychoanalytic, psychodynamic or psychophysiological means to improve functioning or well-being
Light Therapy (J)	Application of specialized light treatments to improve functioning or well-being
Medication Management (3)	Monitoring and adjusting the use of medications for the treatment of a mental health disorder
Narcosynthesis (G)	Administration of intravenous barbiturates in order to release suppressed or repressed thoughts
Psychological Tests (1)	The administration and interpretation of standardized psychological tests and measurement instruments for the assessment of psychological function

Continued on next page

Section G–Mental Health

ICD-10-PCS Value Qualifier (Character 4)	Definition
Behavioral (1)	Primarily to modify behavior Includes/Examples: Includes modeling and role playing, positive reinforcement of target behaviors, response cost, and training of self-management skills
Cognitive (2)	Primarily to correct cognitive distortions and errors
Cognitive-Behavioral (8)	Combining cognitive and behavioral treatment strategies to improve functioning Explanation: Maladaptive responses are examined to determine how cognitions relate to behavior patterns in response to an event. Uses learning principles and information-processing models.
Developmental (Ø)	Age-normed developmental status of cognitive, social and adaptive behavior skills
Intellectual and Psychoeducational (2)	Intellectual abilities, academic achievement and learning capabilities (including behaviors and emotional factors affecting learning)
Interactive (Ø)	Uses primarily physical aids and other forms of non-oral interaction with a patient who is physically, psychologically or developmentally unable to use ordinary language for communication Includes/Examples: Includes the use of toys in symbolic play
Interpersonal (3)	Helps an individual make changes in interpersonal behaviors to reduce psychological dysfunction Includes/Examples: Includes exploratory techniques, encouragement of affective expression, clarification of patient statements, analysis of communication patterns, use of therapy relationship and behavior change techniques
Neurobehavioral and Cognitive Status (4)	Includes neurobehavioral status exam, interview(s), and observation for the clinical assessment of thinking, reasoning and judgment, acquired knowledge, attention, memory, visual spatial abilities, language functions, and planning
Neuropsychological (3)	Thinking, reasoning and judgment, acquired knowledge, attention, memory, visual spatial abilities, language functions, planning
Personality and Behavioral (1)	Mood, emotion, behavior, social functioning, psychopathological conditions, personality traits and characteristics
Psychoanalysis (4)	Methods of obtaining a detailed account of past and present mental and emotional experiences to determine the source and eliminate or diminish the undesirable effects of unconscious conflicts Explanation: Accomplished by making the individual aware of their existence, origin, and inappropriate expression in emotions and behavior
Psychodynamic (5)	Exploration of past and present emotional experiences to understand motives and drives using insight-oriented techniques to reduce the undesirable effects of internal conflicts on emotions and behavior Explanation: Techniques include empathetic listening, clarifying self-defeating behavior patterns, and exploring adaptive alternatives
Psychophysiological (9)	Monitoring and alteration of physiological processes to help the individual associate physiological reactions combined with cognitive and behavioral strategies to gain improved control of these processes to help the individual cope more effectively
Supportive (6)	Formation of therapeutic relationship primarily for providing emotional support to prevent further deterioration in functioning during periods of particular stress Explanation: Often used in conjunction with other therapeutic approaches
Vocational (1)	Exploration of vocational interests, aptitudes and required adaptive behavior skills to develop and carry out a plan for achieving a successful vocational placement Includes/Examples: Includes enhancing work related adjustment and/or pursuing viable options in training education or preparation

Section H - Substance Abuse Treatment

ICD-10-PCS Value (Character 3)	Definition
Detoxification Services (2)	Detoxification from alcohol and/or drugs Explanation: Not a treatment modality, but helps the patient stabilize physically and psychologically until the body becomes free of drugs and the effects of alcohol
Family Counseling (6)	The application of psychological methods that includes one or more family members to treat an individual with addictive behavior Explanation: Provides support and education for family members of addicted individuals. Family member participation is seen as a critical area of substance abuse treatment.
Group Counseling (4)	The application of psychological methods to treat two or more individuals with addictive behavior Explanation: Provides structured group counseling sessions and healing power through the connection with others
Individual Counseling (3)	The application of psychological methods to treat an individual with addictive behavior Explanation: Comprised of several different techniques, which apply various strategies to address drug addiction
Individual Psychotherapy (5)	Treatment of an individual with addictive behavior by behavioral, cognitive, psychoanalytic, psychodynamic or psychophysiological means
Medication Management (8)	Monitoring and adjusting the use of replacement medications for the treatment of addiction
Pharmacotherapy (9)	The use of replacement medications for the treatment of addiction

Appendix J: Hospital Acquired Conditions

Hospital-acquired conditions (HACs) are conditions considered reasonably preventable through the application of evidence-based guidelines. Although it is the ICD-10-CM code that drives a HAC designation, in some cases a specific ICD-10-PCS code must also be present before that ICD-10-CM code can be considered a HAC. For example, the yellow color bar identifies ØJH63XZ as a HAC in the tabular section of this manual. In the annotation box below table ØJH it is noted that when the ICD-10-CM code J95.811 is reported as a secondary diagnosis, not present on admission, AND ØJH63XZ is also reported during that same admission, J95.811 would be considered a hospital-acquired condition. This resource provides all 14 HAC categories, as well as the specific ICD-10-CM codes and, when applicable, the specific ICD-10-PCS codes applicable to each category.

Note: The resource used to compile this list is the fiscal 2019 ICD-10 MS-DRG Definitions Manual Files v36. The most current version, v37, of ICD-10 MS-DRG Definitions Manual was not available at the time this book was printed. For the most current files related to IPPS please refer to the following: https://www.cms.gov/Medicare/Medicare-Fee-for-Service-Payment/AcuteInpatientPPS/IPPS-Regulations-and-Notices.html.

HAC 01: Foreign Object Retained After Surgery

Secondary diagnosis not POA:

T81.500A
T81.501A
T81.502A
T81.503A
T81.504A
T81.505A
T81.506A
T81.507A
T81.508A
T81.509A
T81.510A
T81.511A
T81.512A
T81.513A
T81.514A
T81.515A
T81.516A
T81.517A
T81.518A
T81.519A
T81.520A
T81.521A
T81.522A
T81.523A
T81.524A
T81.525A
T81.526A
T81.527A
T81.528A
T81.529A
T81.530A
T81.531A
T81.532A
T81.533A
T81.534A
T81.535A
T81.536A
T81.537A
T81.538A
T81.539A
T81.590A
T81.591A
T81.592A
T81.593A
T81.594A
T81.595A
T81.596A
T81.597A
T81.598A
T81.599A
T81.60XA
T81.61XA
T81.69XA

HAC 02: Air Embolism

Secondary diagnosis not POA:

T80.0XXA

HAC 03: Blood Incompatibility

Secondary diagnosis not POA:

T80.30XA
T80.310A
T80.311A
T80.319A
T80.39XA

HAC 04: Stage III and IV Pressure Ulcers

Secondary diagnosis not POA:

L89.003
L89.004
L89.013
L89.014
L89.023
L89.024
L89.103
L89.104
L89.113
L89.114
L89.123
L89.124
L89.133
L89.134
L89.143
L89.144
L89.153
L89.154
L89.203
L89.204
L89.213
L89.214
L89.223
L89.224
L89.303
L89.304
L89.313
L89.314
L89.323
L89.324
L89.43
L89.44
L89.503
L89.504
L89.513
L89.514
L89.523
L89.524
L89.603
L89.604
L89.613
L89.614
L89.623
L89.624
L89.813
L89.814
L89.893
L89.894
L89.93
L89.94

HAC 05: Falls and Trauma

Secondary diagnosis not POA:

M99.10
M99.11
M99.18
S02.0XXA
S02.0XXB
S02.101A
S02.101B
S02.102A
S02.102B
S02.109A
S02.109B
S02.110A
S02.110B
S02.111A
S02.111B
S02.112A
S02.112B
S02.113A
S02.113B
S02.118A
S02.118B
S02.119A
S02.119B
S02.11AA
S02.11AB
S02.11BA
S02.11BB
S02.11CA
S02.11CB
S02.11DA
S02.11DB
S02.11EA
S02.11EB
S02.11FA
S02.11FB
S02.11GA
S02.11GB
S02.11HA
S02.11HB
S02.19XA
S02.19XB
S02.2XXB
S02.30XA
S02.30XB

S02.31XA
S02.31XB
S02.32XA
S02.32XB
S02.400A
S02.400B
S02.401A
S02.401B
S02.402A
S02.402B
S02.40AA
S02.40AB
S02.40BA
S02.40BB
S02.40CA
S02.40CB
S02.40DA
S02.40DB
S02.40EA
S02.40EB
S02.40FA
S02.40FB
S02.411A
S02.411B
S02.412A
S02.412B
S02.413A
S02.413B
S02.42XA
S02.42XB
S02.600A
S02.600B
S02.601A
S02.601B
S02.602A
S02.602B
S02.609A
S02.609B
S02.610A
S02.610B
S02.611A
S02.611B
S02.612A
S02.612B
S02.620A
S02.620B
S02.621A
S02.621B
S02.622A
S02.622B
S02.630A
S02.630B
S02.631A
S02.631B
S02.632A
S02.632B
S02.640A
S02.640B
S02.641A

S02.641B
S02.642A
S02.642B
S02.650A
S02.650B
S02.651A
S02.651B
S02.652A
S02.652B
S02.66XA
S02.66XB
S02.670A
S02.670B
S02.671A
S02.671B
S02.672A
S02.672B
S02.69XA
S02.69XB
S02.80XA
S02.80XB
S02.81XA
S02.81XB
S02.82XA
S02.82XB
S02.91XA
S02.91XB
S02.92XA
S02.92XB
S06.0X1A
S06.0X9A
S06.1X1A
S06.1X2A
S06.1X3A
S06.1X4A
S06.1X5A
S06.1X6A
S06.1X7A
S06.1X8A
S06.1X9A
S06.2X1A
S06.2X2A
S06.2X3A
S06.2X4A
S06.2X5A
S06.2X6A
S06.2X7A
S06.2X8A
S06.2X9A
S06.301A
S06.302A
S06.303A
S06.304A
S06.305A
S06.306A
S06.307A
S06.308A
S06.309A
S06.310A

S06.311A
S06.312A
S06.313A
S06.314A
S06.315A
S06.316A
S06.317A
S06.318A
S06.319A
S06.320A
S06.321A
S06.322A
S06.323A
S06.324A
S06.325A
S06.326A
S06.327A
S06.328A
S06.329A
S06.330A
S06.331A
S06.332A
S06.333A
S06.334A
S06.335A
S06.336A
S06.337A
S06.338A
S06.339A
S06.340A
S06.341A
S06.342A
S06.343A
S06.344A
S06.345A
S06.346A
S06.347A
S06.348A
S06.349A
S06.350A
S06.351A
S06.352A
S06.353A
S06.354A
S06.355A
S06.356A
S06.357A
S06.358A
S06.359A
S06.360A
S06.361A
S06.362A
S06.363A
S06.364A
S06.365A
S06.366A
S06.367A
S06.368A
S06.369A

HAC 05: Falls and Trauma (continued)

S06.370A	S06.897A	S12.251A	S12.691A	S22.011B	S22.089B
S06.371A	S06.898A	S12.251B	S12.691B	S22.012A	S22.20XA
S06.372A	S06.899A	S12.290A	S12.8XXA	S22.012B	S22.20XB
S06.373A	S06.9X1A	S12.290B	S12.9XXA	S22.018A	S22.21XA
S06.374A	S06.9X2A	S12.291A	S13.0XXA	S22.018B	S22.21XB
S06.375A	S06.9X3A	S12.291B	S13.100A	S22.019A	S22.22XA
S06.376A	S06.9X4A	S12.300A	S13.101A	S22.019B	S22.22XB
S06.377A	S06.9X5A	S12.300B	S13.110A	S22.020A	S22.23XA
S06.378A	S06.9X6A	S12.301A	S13.111A	S22.020B	S22.23XB
S06.379A	S06.9X7A	S12.301B	S13.120A	S22.021A	S22.24XA
S06.380A	S06.9X8A	S12.330A	S13.121A	S22.021B	S22.24XB
S06.381A	S06.9X9A	S12.330B	S13.130A	S22.022A	S22.31XA
S06.382A	S07.0XXA	S12.331A	S13.131A	S22.022B	S22.31XB
S06.383A	S07.1XXA	S12.331B	S13.140A	S22.028A	S22.32XA
S06.384A	S07.8XXA	S12.34XA	S13.141A	S22.028B	S22.32XB
S06.385A	S07.9XXA	S12.34XB	S13.150A	S22.029A	S22.39XA
S06.386A	S12.000A	S12.350A	S13.151A	S22.029B	S22.39XB
S06.387A	S12.000B	S12.350B	S13.160A	S22.030A	S22.41XA
S06.388A	S12.001A	S12.351A	S13.161A	S22.030B	S22.41XB
S06.389A	S12.001B	S12.351B	S13.170A	S22.031A	S22.42XA
S06.4X0A	S12.01XA	S12.390A	S13.171A	S22.031B	S22.42XB
S06.4X1A	S12.01XB	S12.390B	S13.180A	S22.032A	S22.43XA
S06.4X2A	S12.02XA	S12.391A	S13.181A	S22.032B	S22.43XB
S06.4X3A	S12.02XB	S12.391B	S13.20XA	S22.038A	S22.49XA
S06.4X4A	S12.030A	S12.400A	S13.29XA	S22.038B	S22.49XB
S06.4X5A	S12.030B	S12.400B	S14.101A	S22.039A	S22.5XXA
S06.4X6A	S12.031A	S12.401A	S14.102A	S22.039B	S22.5XXB
S06.4X7A	S12.031B	S12.401B	S14.103A	S22.040A	S22.9XXA
S06.4X8A	S12.040A	S12.430A	S14.104A	S22.040B	S22.9XXB
S06.4X9A	S12.040B	S12.430B	S14.105A	S22.041A	S24.101A
S06.5X0A	S12.041A	S12.431A	S14.106A	S22.041B	S24.102A
S06.5X1A	S12.041B	S12.431B	S14.107A	S22.042A	S24.103A
S06.5X2A	S12.090A	S12.44XA	S14.111A	S22.042B	S24.104A
S06.5X3A	S12.090B	S12.44XB	S14.112A	S22.048A	S24.111A
S06.5X4A	S12.091A	S12.450A	S14.113A	S22.048B	S24.112A
S06.5X5A	S12.091B	S12.450B	S14.114A	S22.049A	S24.113A
S06.5X6A	S12.100A	S12.451A	S14.115A	S22.049B	S24.114A
S06.5X7A	S12.100B	S12.451B	S14.116A	S22.050A	S24.131A
S06.5X8A	S12.101A	S12.490A	S14.117A	S22.050B	S24.132A
S06.5X9A	S12.101B	S12.490B	S14.121A	S22.051A	S24.133A
S06.6X0A	S12.110A	S12.491A	S14.122A	S22.051B	S24.134A
S06.6X1A	S12.110B	S12.491B	S14.123A	S22.052A	S24.151A
S06.6X2A	S12.111A	S12.500A	S14.124A	S22.052B	S24.152A
S06.6X3A	S12.111B	S12.500B	S14.125A	S22.058A	S24.153A
S06.6X4A	S12.112A	S12.501A	S14.126A	S22.058B	S24.154A
S06.6X5A	S12.112B	S12.501B	S14.127A	S22.059A	S32.000A
S06.6X6A	S12.120A	S12.530A	S14.131A	S22.059B	S32.000B
S06.6X7A	S12.120B	S12.530B	S14.132A	S22.060A	S32.001A
S06.6X8A	S12.121A	S12.531A	S14.133A	S22.060B	S32.001B
S06.6X9A	S12.121B	S12.531B	S14.134A	S22.061A	S32.002A
S06.811A	S12.130A	S12.54XA	S14.135A	S22.061B	S32.002B
S06.812A	S12.130B	S12.54XB	S14.136A	S22.062A	S32.008A
S06.813A	S12.131A	S12.550A	S14.137A	S22.062B	S32.008B
S06.814A	S12.131B	S12.550B	S14.151A	S22.068A	S32.009A
S06.815A	S12.14XA	S12.551A	S14.152A	S22.068B	S32.009B
S06.816A	S12.14XB	S12.551B	S14.153A	S22.069A	S32.010A
S06.817A	S12.150A	S12.590A	S14.154A	S22.069B	S32.010B
S06.818A	S12.150B	S12.590B	S14.155A	S22.070A	S32.011A
S06.819A	S12.151A	S12.591A	S14.156A	S22.070B	S32.011B
S06.821A	S12.151B	S12.591B	S14.157A	S22.071A	S32.012A
S06.822A	S12.190A	S12.600A	S17.0XXA	S22.071B	S32.012B
S06.823A	S12.190B	S12.600B	S17.8XXA	S22.072A	S32.018A
S06.824A	S12.191A	S12.601A	S17.9XXA	S22.072B	S32.018B
S06.825A	S12.191B	S12.601B	S22.000A	S22.078A	S32.019A
S06.826A	S12.200A	S12.630A	S22.000B	S22.078B	S32.019B
S06.827A	S12.200B	S12.630B	S22.001A	S22.079A	S32.020A
S06.828A	S12.201A	S12.631A	S22.001B	S22.079B	S32.020B
S06.829A	S12.201B	S12.631B	S22.002A	S22.080A	S32.021A
S06.891A	S12.230A	S12.64XA	S22.002B	S22.080B	S32.021B
S06.892A	S12.230B	S12.64XB	S22.008A	S22.081A	S32.022A
S06.893A	S12.231A	S12.650A	S22.008B	S22.081B	S32.022B
S06.894A	S12.231B	S12.650B	S22.009A	S22.082A	S32.028A
S06.895A	S12.24XA	S12.651A	S22.009B	S22.082B	S32.028B
S06.896A	S12.24XB	S12.651B	S22.010A	S22.088A	S32.029A
	S12.250A	S12.690A	S22.010B	S22.088B	S32.029B
	S12.250B	S12.690B	S22.011A	S22.089A	S32.030A

HAC 05: Falls and Trauma (continued)

S32.030B	S32.311B	S32.453B	S32.612B	S42.113B	S42.252B
S32.031A	S32.312A	S32.454A	S32.613A	S42.114B	S42.253A
S32.031B	S32.312B	S32.454B	S32.613B	S42.115B	S42.253B
S32.032A	S32.313A	S32.455A	S32.614A	S42.116B	S42.254A
S32.032B	S32.313B	S32.455B	S32.614B	S42.121B	S42.254B
S32.038A	S32.314A	S32.456A	S32.615A	S42.122B	S42.255A
S32.038B	S32.314B	S32.456B	S32.615B	S42.123B	S42.255B
S32.039A	S32.315A	S32.461A	S32.616A	S42.124B	S42.256A
S32.039B	S32.315B	S32.461B	S32.616B	S42.125B	S42.256B
S32.040A	S32.316A	S32.462A	S32.691A	S42.126B	S42.261A
S32.040B	S32.316B	S32.462B	S32.691B	S42.131B	S42.261B
S32.041A	S32.391A	S32.463A	S32.692A	S42.132B	S42.262A
S32.041B	S32.391B	S32.463B	S32.692B	S42.133B	S42.262B
S32.042A	S32.392A	S32.464A	S32.699A	S42.134B	S42.263A
S32.042B	S32.392B	S32.464B	S32.699B	S42.135B	S42.263B
S32.048A	S32.399A	S32.465A	S32.810A	S42.136B	S42.264A
S32.048B	S32.399B	S32.465B	S32.810B	S42.141B	S42.264B
S32.049A	S32.401A	S32.466A	S32.811A	S42.142B	S42.265A
S32.049B	S32.401B	S32.466B	S32.811B	S42.143B	S42.265B
S32.050A	S32.402A	S32.471A	S32.82XA	S42.144B	S42.266A
S32.050B	S32.402B	S32.471B	S32.82XB	S42.145B	S42.266B
S32.051A	S32.409A	S32.472A	S32.89XA	S42.146B	S42.271A
S32.051B	S32.409B	S32.472B	S32.89XB	S42.151B	S42.272A
S32.052A	S32.411A	S32.473A	S32.9XXA	S42.152B	S42.279A
S32.052B	S32.411B	S32.473B	S32.9XXB	S42.153B	S42.291A
S32.058A	S32.412A	S32.474A	S34.101A	S42.154B	S42.291B
S32.058B	S32.412B	S32.474B	S34.102A	S42.155B	S42.292A
S32.059A	S32.413A	S32.475A	S34.103A	S42.156B	S42.292B
S32.059B	S32.413B	S32.475B	S34.104A	S42.191B	S42.293A
S32.10XA	S32.414A	S32.476A	S34.105A	S42.192B	S42.293B
S32.10XB	S32.414B	S32.476B	S34.109A	S42.199B	S42.294A
S32.110A	S32.415A	S32.481A	S34.111A	S42.201A	S42.294B
S32.110B	S32.415B	S32.481B	S34.112A	S42.201B	S42.295A
S32.111A	S32.416A	S32.482A	S34.113A	S42.202A	S42.295B
S32.111B	S32.416B	S32.482B	S34.114A	S42.202B	S42.296A
S32.112A	S32.421A	S32.483A	S34.115A	S42.209A	S42.296B
S32.112B	S32.421B	S32.483B	S34.119A	S42.209B	S42.301A
S32.119A	S32.422A	S32.484A	S34.121A	S42.211A	S42.301B
S32.119B	S32.422B	S32.484B	S34.122A	S42.211B	S42.302A
S32.120A	S32.423A	S32.485A	S34.123A	S42.212A	S42.302B
S32.120B	S32.423B	S32.485B	S34.124A	S42.212B	S42.309A
S32.121A	S32.424A	S32.486A	S34.125A	S42.213A	S42.309B
S32.121B	S32.424B	S32.486B	S34.129A	S42.213B	S42.311A
S32.122A	S32.425A	S32.491A	S34.131A	S42.214A	S42.312A
S32.122B	S32.425B	S32.491B	S34.132A	S42.214B	S42.319A
S32.129A	S32.426A	S32.492A	S34.139A	S42.215A	S42.321A
S32.129B	S32.426B	S32.492B	S34.3XXA	S42.215B	S42.321B
S32.130A	S32.431A	S32.499A	S42.001B	S42.216A	S42.322A
S32.130B	S32.431B	S32.499B	S42.002B	S42.216B	S42.322B
S32.131A	S32.432A	S32.501A	S42.009B	S42.221A	S42.323A
S32.131B	S32.432B	S32.501B	S42.011B	S42.221B	S42.323B
S32.132A	S32.433A	S32.502A	S42.012B	S42.222A	S42.324A
S32.132B	S32.433B	S32.502B	S42.013B	S42.222B	S42.324B
S32.139A	S32.434A	S32.509A	S42.014B	S42.223A	S42.325A
S32.139B	S32.434B	S32.509B	S42.015B	S42.223B	S42.325B
S32.14XA	S32.435A	S32.511A	S42.016B	S42.224A	S42.326A
S32.14XB	S32.435B	S32.511B	S42.017B	S42.224B	S42.326B
S32.15XA	S32.436A	S32.512A	S42.018B	S42.225A	S42.331A
S32.15XB	S32.436B	S32.512B	S42.019B	S42.225B	S42.331B
S32.16XA	S32.441A	S32.519A	S42.021B	S42.226A	S42.332A
S32.16XB	S32.441B	S32.519B	S42.022B	S42.226B	S42.332B
S32.17XA	S32.442A	S32.591A	S42.023B	S42.231A	S42.333A
S32.17XB	S32.442B	S32.591B	S42.024B	S42.231B	S42.333B
S32.19XA	S32.443A	S32.592A	S42.025B	S42.232A	S42.334A
S32.19XB	S32.443B	S32.592B	S42.026B	S42.232B	S42.334B
S32.2XXA	S32.444A	S32.599A	S42.031B	S42.239A	S42.335A
S32.2XXB	S32.444B	S32.599B	S42.032B	S42.239B	S42.335B
S32.301A	S32.445A	S32.601A	S42.033B	S42.241A	S42.336A
S32.301B	S32.445B	S32.601B	S42.034B	S42.241B	S42.336B
S32.302A	S32.446A	S32.602A	S42.035B	S42.242A	S42.341A
S32.302B	S32.446B	S32.602B	S42.036B	S42.242B	S42.341B
S32.309A	S32.451A	S32.609A	S42.101B	S42.249A	S42.342A
S32.309B	S32.451B	S32.609B	S42.102B	S42.249B	S42.342B
S32.311A	S32.452A	S32.611A	S42.109B	S42.251A	S42.343A
	S32.452B	S32.611B	S42.111B	S42.251B	S42.343B
	S32.453A	S32.612A	S42.112B	S42.252A	S42.344A

HAC 05: Falls and Trauma (continued)

S42.344B	S42.435B	S42.92XA	S52.026C	S52.209A	S52.256B
S42.345A	S42.436A	S42.92XB	S52.031B	S52.209B	S52.256C
S42.345B	S42.436B	S43.201A	S52.031C	S52.209C	S52.261A
S42.346A	S42.441A	S43.202A	S52.032B	S52.211A	S52.261B
S42.346B	S42.441B	S43.203A	S52.032C	S52.212A	S52.261C
S42.351A	S42.442A	S43.204A	S52.033B	S52.219A	S52.262A
S42.351B	S42.442B	S43.205A	S52.033C	S52.221A	S52.262B
S42.352A	S42.443A	S43.206A	S52.034B	S52.221B	S52.262C
S42.352B	S42.443B	S43.211A	S52.034C	S52.221C	S52.263A
S42.353A	S42.444A	S43.212A	S52.035B	S52.222A	S52.263B
S42.353B	S42.444B	S43.213A	S52.035C	S52.222B	S52.263C
S42.354A	S42.445A	S43.214A	S52.036B	S52.222C	S52.264A
S42.354B	S42.445B	S43.215A	S52.036C	S52.223A	S52.264B
S42.355A	S42.446A	S43.216A	S52.041B	S52.223B	S52.264C
S42.355B	S42.446B	S43.221A	S52.041C	S52.223C	S52.265A
S42.356A	S42.447A	S43.222A	S52.042B	S52.224A	S52.265B
S42.356B	S42.447B	S43.223A	S52.042C	S52.224B	S52.265C
S42.361A	S42.448A	S43.224A	S52.043B	S52.224C	S52.266A
S42.361B	S42.448B	S43.225A	S52.043C	S52.225A	S52.266B
S42.362A	S42.449A	S43.226A	S52.044B	S52.225B	S52.266C
S42.362B	S42.449B	S49.001A	S52.044C	S52.225C	S52.271B
S42.363A	S42.451A	S49.002A	S52.045B	S52.226A	S52.271C
S42.363B	S42.451B	S49.009A	S52.045C	S52.226B	S52.272B
S42.364A	S42.452A	S49.011A	S52.046B	S52.226C	S52.272C
S42.364B	S42.452B	S49.012A	S52.046C	S52.231A	S52.279B
S42.365A	S42.453A	S49.019A	S52.091B	S52.231B	S52.279C
S42.365B	S42.453B	S49.021A	S52.091C	S52.231C	S52.281A
S42.366A	S42.454A	S49.022A	S52.092B	S52.232A	S52.281B
S42.366B	S42.454B	S49.029A	S52.092C	S52.232B	S52.281C
S42.391A	S42.455A	S49.031A	S52.099B	S52.232C	S52.282A
S42.391B	S42.455B	S49.032A	S52.099C	S52.233A	S52.282B
S42.392A	S42.456A	S49.039A	S52.101B	S52.233B	S52.282C
S42.392B	S42.456B	S49.041A	S52.101C	S52.233C	S52.283A
S42.399A	S42.461A	S49.042A	S52.102B	S52.234A	S52.283B
S42.399B	S42.461B	S49.049A	S52.102C	S52.234B	S52.283C
S42.401A	S42.462A	S49.091A	S52.109B	S52.234C	S52.291A
S42.401B	S42.462B	S49.092A	S52.109C	S52.235A	S52.291B
S42.402A	S42.463A	S49.099A	S52.111A	S52.235B	S52.291C
S42.402B	S42.463B	S49.101A	S52.112A	S52.235C	S52.292A
S42.409A	S42.464A	S49.102A	S52.119A	S52.236A	S52.292B
S42.409B	S42.464B	S49.109A	S52.121B	S52.236B	S52.292C
S42.411A	S42.465A	S49.111A	S52.121C	S52.236C	S52.299A
S42.411B	S42.465B	S49.112A	S52.122B	S52.241A	S52.299B
S42.412A	S42.466A	S49.119A	S52.122C	S52.241B	S52.299C
S42.412B	S42.466B	S49.121A	S52.123B	S52.241C	S52.301A
S42.413A	S42.471A	S49.122A	S52.123C	S52.242A	S52.301B
S42.413B	S42.471B	S49.129A	S52.124B	S52.242B	S52.301C
S42.414A	S42.472A	S49.131A	S52.124C	S52.242C	S52.302A
S42.414B	S42.472B	S49.132A	S52.125B	S52.243A	S52.302B
S42.415A	S42.473A	S49.139A	S52.125C	S52.243B	S52.302C
S42.415B	S42.473B	S49.141A	S52.126B	S52.243C	S52.309A
S42.416A	S42.474A	S49.142A	S52.126C	S52.244A	S52.309B
S42.416B	S42.474B	S49.149A	S52.131B	S52.244B	S52.309C
S42.421A	S42.475A	S49.191A	S52.131C	S52.244C	S52.311A
S42.421B	S42.475B	S49.192A	S52.132B	S52.245A	S52.312A
S42.422A	S42.476A	S49.199A	S52.132C	S52.245B	S52.319A
S42.422B	S42.476B	S52.001B	S52.133B	S52.245C	S52.321A
S42.423A	S42.481A	S52.001C	S52.133C	S52.246A	S52.321B
S42.423B	S42.482A	S52.002B	S52.134B	S52.246B	S52.321C
S42.424A	S42.489A	S52.002C	S52.134C	S52.246C	S52.322A
S42.424B	S42.491A	S52.009B	S52.135B	S52.251A	S52.322B
S42.425A	S42.491B	S52.009C	S52.135C	S52.251B	S52.322C
S42.425B	S42.492A	S52.011A	S52.136B	S52.251C	S52.323A
S42.426A	S42.492B	S52.012A	S52.136C	S52.252A	S52.323B
S42.426B	S42.493A	S52.019A	S52.181B	S52.252B	S52.323C
S42.431A	S42.493B	S52.021B	S52.181C	S52.252C	S52.324A
S42.431B	S42.494A	S52.021C	S52.182B	S52.253A	S52.324B
S42.432A	S42.494B	S52.022B	S52.182C	S52.253B	S52.324C
S42.432B	S42.495A	S52.022C	S52.189B	S52.253C	S52.325A
S42.433A	S42.495B	S52.023B	S52.189C	S52.254A	S52.325B
S42.433B	S42.496A	S52.023C	S52.201A	S52.254B	S52.325C
S42.434A	S42.496B	S52.024B	S52.201B	S52.254C	S52.326A
S42.434B	S42.90XA	S52.024C	S52.201C	S52.255A	S52.326B
S42.435A	S42.90XB	S52.025B	S52.202A	S52.255B	S52.331A
	S42.91XA	S52.025C	S52.202B	S52.255C	S52.331B
	S42.91XB	S52.026B	S52.202C	S52.256A	

HAC 05: Falls and Trauma (continued)

S52.331C	S52.372B	S52.552C	S52.92XA	S62.132B	S62.308B
S52.332A	S52.372C	S52.559A	S52.92XB	S62.133B	S62.309B
S52.332B	S52.379A	S52.559B	S52.92XC	S62.134B	S62.310B
S52.332C	S52.379B	S52.559C	S59.001A	S62.135B	S62.311B
S52.333A	S52.379C	S52.561A	S59.002A	S62.136B	S62.312B
S52.333B	S52.381A	S52.561B	S59.009A	S62.141B	S62.313B
S52.333C	S52.381B	S52.561C	S59.011A	S62.142B	S62.314B
S52.334A	S52.381C	S52.562A	S59.012A	S62.143B	S62.315B
S52.334B	S52.382A	S52.562B	S59.019A	S62.144B	S62.316B
S52.334C	S52.382B	S52.562C	S59.021A	S62.145B	S62.317B
S52.335A	S52.382C	S52.569A	S59.022A	S62.146B	S62.318B
S52.335B	S52.389A	S52.569B	S59.029A	S62.151B	S62.319B
S52.335C	S52.389B	S52.569C	S59.031A	S62.152B	S62.320B
S52.336A	S52.389C	S52.571A	S59.032A	S62.153B	S62.321B
S52.336B	S52.391A	S52.571B	S59.039A	S62.154B	S62.322B
S52.336C	S52.391B	S52.571C	S59.041A	S62.155B	S62.323B
S52.341A	S52.391C	S52.572A	S59.042A	S62.156B	S62.324B
S52.341B	S52.392A	S52.572B	S59.049A	S62.161B	S62.325B
S52.341C	S52.392B	S52.572C	S59.091A	S62.162B	S62.326B
S52.342A	S52.392C	S52.579A	S59.092A	S62.163B	S62.327B
S52.342B	S52.399A	S52.579B	S59.099A	S62.164B	S62.328B
S52.342C	S52.399B	S52.579C	S59.201A	S62.165B	S62.329B
S52.343A	S52.399C	S52.591A	S59.202A	S62.166B	S62.330B
S52.343B	S52.501A	S52.591B	S59.209A	S62.171B	S62.331B
S52.343C	S52.501B	S52.591C	S59.211A	S62.172B	S62.332B
S52.344A	S52.501C	S52.592A	S59.212A	S62.173B	S62.333B
S52.344B	S52.502A	S52.592B	S59.219A	S62.174B	S62.334B
S52.344C	S52.502B	S52.592C	S59.221A	S62.175B	S62.335B
S52.345A	S52.502C	S52.599A	S59.222A	S62.176B	S62.336B
S52.345B	S52.509A	S52.599B	S59.229A	S62.181B	S62.337B
S52.345C	S52.509B	S52.599C	S59.231A	S62.182B	S62.338B
S52.346A	S52.509C	S52.601A	S59.232A	S62.183B	S62.339B
S52.346B	S52.511A	S52.601B	S59.239A	S62.184B	S62.340B
S52.346C	S52.511B	S52.601C	S59.241A	S62.185B	S62.341B
S52.351A	S52.511C	S52.602A	S59.242A	S62.186B	S62.342B
S52.351B	S52.512A	S52.602B	S59.249A	S62.201B	S62.343B
S52.351C	S52.512B	S52.602C	S59.291A	S62.202B	S62.344B
S52.352A	S52.512C	S52.609A	S59.292A	S62.209B	S62.345B
S52.352B	S52.513A	S52.609B	S59.299A	S62.211B	S62.346B
S52.352C	S52.513B	S52.609C	S62.001B	S62.212B	S62.347B
S52.353A	S52.513C	S52.611A	S62.002B	S62.213B	S62.348B
S52.353B	S52.514A	S52.611B	S62.009B	S62.221B	S62.349B
S52.353C	S52.514B	S52.611C	S62.011B	S62.222B	S62.350B
S52.354A	S52.514C	S52.612A	S62.012B	S62.223B	S62.351B
S52.354B	S52.515A	S52.612B	S62.013B	S62.224B	S62.352B
S52.354C	S52.515B	S52.612C	S62.014B	S62.225B	S62.353B
S52.355A	S52.515C	S52.613A	S62.015B	S62.226B	S62.354B
S52.355B	S52.516A	S52.613B	S62.016B	S62.231B	S62.355B
S52.355C	S52.516B	S52.613C	S62.021B	S62.232B	S62.356B
S52.356A	S52.516C	S52.614A	S62.022B	S62.233B	S62.357B
S52.356B	S52.521A	S52.614B	S62.023B	S62.234B	S62.358B
S52.356C	S52.522A	S52.614C	S62.024B	S62.235B	S62.359B
S52.361A	S52.529A	S52.615A	S62.025B	S62.236B	S62.360B
S52.361B	S52.531A	S52.615B	S62.026B	S62.241B	S62.361B
S52.361C	S52.531B	S52.615C	S62.031B	S62.242B	S62.362B
S52.362A	S52.531C	S52.616A	S62.032B	S62.243B	S62.363B
S52.362B	S52.532A	S52.616B	S62.033B	S62.244B	S62.364B
S52.362C	S52.532B	S52.616C	S62.034B	S62.245B	S62.365B
S52.363A	S52.532C	S52.621A	S62.035B	S62.246B	S62.366B
S52.363B	S52.539A	S52.622A	S62.036B	S62.251B	S62.367B
S52.363C	S52.539B	S52.629A	S62.101B	S62.252B	S62.368B
S52.364A	S52.539C	S52.691A	S62.102B	S62.253B	S62.369B
S52.364B	S52.541A	S52.691B	S62.109B	S62.254B	S62.390B
S52.364C	S52.541B	S52.691C	S62.111B	S62.255B	S62.391B
S52.365A	S52.541C	S52.692A	S62.112B	S62.256B	S62.392B
S52.365B	S52.542A	S52.692B	S62.113B	S62.291B	S62.393B
S52.365C	S52.542B	S52.692C	S62.114B	S62.292B	S62.394B
S52.366A	S52.542C	S52.699A	S62.115B	S62.299B	S62.395B
S52.366B	S52.549A	S52.699B	S62.116B	S62.300B	S62.396B
S52.366C	S52.549B	S52.699C	S62.121B	S62.301B	S62.397B
S52.371A	S52.549C	S52.90XA	S62.122B	S62.302B	S62.398B
S52.371B	S52.551A	S52.90XB	S62.123B	S62.303B	S62.399B
S52.371C	S52.551B	S52.90XC	S62.124B	S62.304B	S62.501B
S52.372A	S52.551C	S52.91XA	S62.125B	S62.305B	S62.502B
	S52.552A	S52.91XB	S62.126B	S62.306B	S62.509B
	S52.552B	S52.91XC	S62.131B	S62.307B	S62.511B

HAC 05: Falls and Trauma (continued)

S62.512B	S62.663B	S72.045A	S72.123B	S72.321C	S72.363A
S62.513B	S62.664B	S72.045B	S72.123C	S72.322A	S72.363B
S62.514B	S62.665B	S72.045C	S72.124A	S72.322B	S72.363C
S62.515B	S62.666B	S72.046A	S72.124B	S72.322C	S72.364A
S62.516B	S62.667B	S72.046B	S72.124C	S72.323A	S72.364B
S62.521B	S62.668B	S72.046C	S72.125A	S72.323B	S72.364C
S62.522B	S62.669B	S72.051A	S72.125B	S72.323C	S72.365A
S62.523B	S62.90XB	S72.051B	S72.125C	S72.324A	S72.365B
S62.524B	S62.91XB	S72.051C	S72.126A	S72.324B	S72.365C
S62.525B	S62.92XB	S72.052A	S72.126B	S72.324C	S72.366A
S62.526B	S72.001A	S72.052B	S72.126C	S72.325A	S72.366B
S62.600B	S72.001B	S72.052C	S72.131A	S72.325B	S72.366C
S62.601B	S72.001C	S72.059A	S72.131B	S72.325C	S72.391A
S62.602B	S72.002A	S72.059B	S72.131C	S72.326A	S72.391B
S62.603B	S72.002B	S72.059C	S72.132A	S72.326B	S72.391C
S62.604B	S72.002C	S72.061A	S72.132B	S72.326C	S72.392A
S62.605B	S72.009A	S72.061B	S72.132C	S72.331A	S72.392B
S62.606B	S72.009B	S72.061C	S72.133A	S72.331B	S72.392C
S62.607B	S72.009C	S72.062A	S72.133B	S72.331C	S72.399A
S62.608B	S72.011A	S72.062B	S72.133C	S72.332A	S72.399B
S62.609B	S72.011B	S72.062C	S72.134A	S72.332B	S72.399C
S62.610B	S72.011C	S72.063A	S72.134B	S72.332C	S72.401A
S62.611B	S72.012A	S72.063B	S72.134C	S72.333A	S72.401B
S62.612B	S72.012B	S72.063C	S72.135A	S72.333B	S72.401C
S62.613B	S72.012C	S72.064A	S72.135B	S72.333C	S72.402A
S62.614B	S72.019A	S72.064B	S72.135C	S72.334A	S72.402B
S62.615B	S72.019B	S72.064C	S72.136A	S72.334B	S72.402C
S62.616B	S72.019C	S72.065A	S72.136B	S72.334C	S72.409A
S62.617B	S72.021A	S72.065B	S72.136C	S72.335A	S72.409B
S62.618B	S72.021B	S72.065C	S72.141A	S72.335B	S72.409C
S62.619B	S72.021C	S72.066A	S72.141B	S72.335C	S72.411A
S62.620B	S72.022A	S72.066B	S72.141C	S72.336A	S72.411B
S62.621B	S72.022B	S72.066C	S72.142A	S72.336B	S72.411C
S62.622B	S72.022C	S72.091A	S72.142B	S72.336C	S72.412A
S62.623B	S72.023A	S72.091B	S72.142C	S72.341A	S72.412B
S62.624B	S72.023B	S72.091C	S72.143A	S72.341B	S72.412C
S62.625B	S72.023C	S72.092A	S72.143B	S72.341C	S72.413A
S62.626B	S72.024A	S72.092B	S72.143C	S72.342A	S72.413B
S62.627B	S72.024B	S72.092C	S72.144A	S72.342B	S72.413C
S62.628B	S72.024C	S72.099A	S72.144B	S72.342C	S72.414A
S62.629B	S72.025A	S72.099B	S72.144C	S72.343A	S72.414B
S62.630B	S72.025B	S72.099C	S72.145A	S72.343B	S72.414C
S62.631B	S72.025C	S72.101A	S72.145B	S72.343C	S72.415A
S62.632B	S72.026A	S72.101B	S72.145C	S72.344A	S72.415B
S62.633B	S72.026B	S72.101C	S72.146A	S72.344B	S72.415C
S62.634B	S72.026C	S72.102A	S72.146B	S72.344C	S72.416A
S62.635B	S72.031A	S72.102B	S72.146C	S72.345A	S72.416B
S62.636B	S72.031B	S72.102C	S72.21XA	S72.345B	S72.416C
S62.637B	S72.031C	S72.109A	S72.21XB	S72.345C	S72.421A
S62.638B	S72.032A	S72.109B	S72.21XC	S72.346A	S72.421B
S62.639B	S72.032B	S72.109C	S72.22XA	S72.346B	S72.421C
S62.640B	S72.032C	S72.111A	S72.22XB	S72.346C	S72.422A
S62.641B	S72.033A	S72.111B	S72.22XC	S72.351A	S72.422B
S62.642B	S72.033B	S72.111C	S72.23XA	S72.351B	S72.422C
S62.643B	S72.033C	S72.112A	S72.23XB	S72.351C	S72.423A
S62.644B	S72.034A	S72.112B	S72.23XC	S72.352A	S72.423B
S62.645B	S72.034B	S72.112C	S72.24XA	S72.352B	S72.423C
S62.646B	S72.034C	S72.113A	S72.24XB	S72.352C	S72.424A
S62.647B	S72.035A	S72.113B	S72.24XC	S72.353A	S72.424B
S62.648B	S72.035B	S72.113C	S72.25XA	S72.353B	S72.424C
S62.649B	S72.035C	S72.114A	S72.25XB	S72.353C	S72.425A
S62.650B	S72.036A	S72.114B	S72.25XC	S72.354A	S72.425B
S62.651B	S72.036B	S72.114C	S72.26XA	S72.354B	S72.425C
S62.652B	S72.036C	S72.115A	S72.26XB	S72.354C	S72.426A
S62.653B	S72.041A	S72.115B	S72.26XC	S72.355A	S72.426B
S62.654B	S72.041B	S72.115C	S72.301A	S72.355B	S72.426C
S62.655B	S72.041C	S72.116A	S72.301B	S72.355C	S72.431A
S62.656B	S72.042A	S72.116B	S72.301C	S72.356A	S72.431B
S62.657B	S72.042B	S72.116C	S72.302A	S72.356B	S72.431C
S62.658B	S72.042C	S72.121A	S72.302B	S72.356C	S72.432A
S62.659B	S72.043A	S72.121B	S72.302C	S72.361A	S72.432B
S62.660B	S72.043B	S72.121C	S72.309A	S72.361B	S72.432C
S62.661B	S72.043C	S72.122A	S72.309B	S72.361C	S72.433A
S62.662B	S72.044A	S72.122B	S72.309C	S72.362A	S72.433B
	S72.044B	S72.122C	S72.321A	S72.362B	S72.433C
	S72.044C	S72.123A	S72.321B	S72.362C	S72.434A

HAC 05: Falls and Trauma (continued)

S72.434B	S72.8X1A	S79.142A	S82.043C	S82.135A	S82.225B
S72.434C	S72.8X1B	S79.149A	S82.044A	S82.135B	S82.225C
S72.435A	S72.8X1C	S79.191A	S82.044B	S82.135C	S82.226A
S72.435B	S72.8X2A	S79.192A	S82.044C	S82.136A	S82.226B
S72.435C	S72.8X2B	S79.199A	S82.045A	S82.136B	S82.226C
S72.436A	S72.8X2C	S82.001A	S82.045B	S82.136C	S82.231A
S72.436B	S72.8X9A	S82.001B	S82.045C	S82.141A	S82.231B
S72.436C	S72.8X9B	S82.001C	S82.046A	S82.141B	S82.231C
S72.441A	S72.8X9C	S82.002A	S82.046B	S82.141C	S82.232A
S72.441B	S72.90XA	S82.002B	S82.046C	S82.142A	S82.232B
S72.441C	S72.90XB	S82.002C	S82.091A	S82.142B	S82.232C
S72.442A	S72.90XC	S82.009A	S82.091B	S82.142C	S82.233A
S72.442B	S72.91XA	S82.009B	S82.091C	S82.143A	S82.233B
S72.442C	S72.91XB	S82.009C	S82.092A	S82.143B	S82.233C
S72.443A	S72.91XC	S82.011A	S82.092B	S82.143C	S82.234A
S72.443B	S72.92XA	S82.011B	S82.092C	S82.144A	S82.234B
S72.443C	S72.92XB	S82.011C	S82.099A	S82.144B	S82.234C
S72.444A	S72.92XC	S82.012A	S82.099B	S82.144C	S82.235A
S72.444B	S73.001A	S82.012B	S82.099C	S82.145A	S82.235B
S72.444C	S73.002A	S82.012C	S82.101A	S82.145B	S82.235C
S72.445A	S73.003A	S82.013A	S82.101B	S82.145C	S82.236A
S72.445B	S73.004A	S82.013B	S82.101C	S82.146A	S82.236B
S72.445C	S73.005A	S82.013C	S82.102A	S82.146B	S82.236C
S72.446A	S73.006A	S82.014A	S82.102B	S82.146C	S82.241A
S72.446B	S73.011A	S82.014B	S82.102C	S82.151A	S82.241B
S72.446C	S73.012A	S82.014C	S82.109A	S82.151B	S82.241C
S72.451A	S73.013A	S82.015A	S82.109B	S82.151C	S82.242A
S72.451B	S73.014A	S82.015B	S82.109C	S82.152A	S82.242B
S72.451C	S73.015A	S82.015C	S82.111A	S82.152B	S82.242C
S72.452A	S73.016A	S82.016A	S82.111B	S82.152C	S82.243A
S72.452B	S73.021A	S82.016B	S82.111C	S82.153A	S82.243B
S72.452C	S73.022A	S82.016C	S82.112A	S82.153B	S82.243C
S72.453A	S73.023A	S82.021A	S82.112B	S82.153C	S82.244A
S72.453B	S73.024A	S82.021B	S82.112C	S82.154A	S82.244B
S72.453C	S73.025A	S82.021C	S82.113A	S82.154B	S82.244C
S72.454A	S73.026A	S82.022A	S82.113B	S82.154C	S82.245A
S72.454B	S73.031A	S82.022B	S82.113C	S82.155A	S82.245B
S72.454C	S73.032A	S82.022C	S82.114A	S82.155B	S82.245C
S72.455A	S73.033A	S82.023A	S82.114B	S82.155C	S82.246A
S72.455B	S73.034A	S82.023B	S82.114C	S82.156A	S82.246B
S72.455C	S73.035A	S82.023C	S82.115A	S82.156B	S82.246C
S72.456A	S73.036A	S82.024A	S82.115B	S82.156C	S82.251A
S72.456B	S73.041A	S82.024B	S82.115C	S82.161A	S82.251B
S72.456C	S73.042A	S82.024C	S82.116A	S82.162A	S82.251C
S72.461A	S73.043A	S82.025A	S82.116B	S82.169A	S82.252A
S72.461B	S73.044A	S82.025B	S82.116C	S82.191A	S82.252B
S72.461C	S73.045A	S82.025C	S82.121A	S82.191B	S82.252C
S72.462A	S73.046A	S82.026A	S82.121B	S82.191C	S82.253A
S72.462B	S77.00XA	S82.026B	S82.121C	S82.192A	S82.253B
S72.462C	S77.01XA	S82.026C	S82.122A	S82.192B	S82.253C
S72.463A	S77.02XA	S82.031A	S82.122B	S82.192C	S82.254A
S72.463B	S77.10XA	S82.031B	S82.122C	S82.199A	S82.254B
S72.463C	S77.11XA	S82.031C	S82.123A	S82.199B	S82.254C
S72.464A	S77.12XA	S82.032A	S82.123B	S82.199C	S82.255A-
S72.464B	S79.001A	S82.032B	S82.123C	S82.201A	S82.255B
S72.464C	S79.002A	S82.032C	S82.124A	S82.201B	S82.255C
S72.465A	S79.009A	S82.033A	S82.124B	S82.201C	S82.256A
S72.465B	S79.011A	S82.033B	S82.124C	S82.202A	S82.256B
S72.465C	S79.012A	S82.033C	S82.125A	S82.202B	S82.256C
S72.466A	S79.019A	S82.034A	S82.125B	S82.202C	S82.261A
S72.466B	S79.091A	S82.034B	S82.125C	S82.209A	S82.261B
S72.466C	S79.092A	S82.034C	S82.126A	S82.209B	S82.261C
S72.471A	S79.099A	S82.035A	S82.126B	S82.209C	S82.262A
S72.472A	S79.101A	S82.035B	S82.126C	S82.221A	S82.262B
S72.479A	S79.102A	S82.035C	S82.131A	S82.221B	S82.262C
S72.491A	S79.109A	S82.036A	S82.131B	S82.221C	S82.263A
S72.491B	S79.111A	S82.036B	S82.131C	S82.222A	S82.263B
S72.491C	S79.112A	S82.036C	S82.132A	S82.222B	S82.263C
S72.492A	S79.119A	S82.041A	S82.132B	S82.222C	S82.264A
S72.492B	S79.121A	S82.041B	S82.132C	S82.223A	S82.264B
S72.492C	S79.122A	S82.041C	S82.133A	S82.223B	S82.264C
S72.499A	S79.129A	S82.042A	S82.133B	S82.223C	S82.265A
S72.499B	S79.131A	S82.042B	S82.133C	S82.224A	S82.265B
S72.499C	S79.132A	S82.042C	S82.134A	S82.224B	S82.265C
	S79.139A	S82.043A	S82.134B	S82.224C	S82.266A
	S79.141A	S82.043B	S82.134C	S82.225A	S82.266B

HAC 05: Falls and Trauma (continued)

S82.266C	S82.454C	S82.856C	S92.041B	S92.242B	T21.34XA
S82.291A	S82.455B	S82.861B	S92.042B	S92.243B	T21.35XA
S82.291B	S82.455C	S82.861C	S92.043B	S92.244B	T21.36XA
S82.291C	S82.456B	S82.862B	S92.044B	S92.245B	T21.37XA
S82.292A	S82.456C	S82.862C	S92.045B	S92.246B	T21.39XA
S82.292B	S82.461B	S82.863B	S92.046B	S92.251B	T21.70XA
S82.292C	S82.461C	S82.863C	S92.051B	S92.252B	T21.71XA
S82.299A	S82.462B	S82.864B	S92.052B	S92.253B	T21.72XA
S82.299B	S82.462C	S82.864C	S92.053B	S92.254B	T21.73XA
S82.299C	S82.463B	S82.865B	S92.054B	S92.255B	T21.74XA
S82.301B	S82.463C	S82.865C	S92.055B	S92.256B	T21.75XA
S82.301C	S82.464B	S82.866B	S92.056B	S92.301B	T21.76XA
S82.302B	S82.464C	S82.866C	S92.061B	S92.302B	T21.77XA
S82.302C	S82.465B	S82.871B	S92.062B	S92.309B	T21.79XA
S82.309B	S82.465C	S82.871C	S92.063B	S92.311B	T22.30XA
S82.309C	S82.466B	S82.872B	S92.064B	S92.312B	T22.311A
S82.311A	S82.466C	S82.872C	S92.065B	S92.313B	T22.312A
S82.312A	S82.491B	S82.873B	S92.066B	S92.314B	T22.319A
S82.319A	S82.491C	S82.873C	S92.101B	S92.315B	T22.321A
S82.391B	S82.492B	S82.874B	S92.102B	S92.316B	T22.322A
S82.391C	S82.492C	S82.874C	S92.109B	S92.321B	T22.329A
S82.392B	S82.499B	S82.875B	S92.111B	S92.322B	T22.331A
S82.392C	S82.499C	S82.875C	S92.112B	S92.323B	T22.332A
S82.399B	S82.51XB	S82.876B	S92.113B	S92.324B	T22.339A
S82.399C	S82.51XC	S82.876C	S92.114B	S92.325B	T22.341A
S82.401B	S82.52XB	S82.891B	S92.115B	S92.326B	T22.342A
S82.401C	S82.52XC	S82.891C	S92.116B	S92.331B	T22.349A
S82.402B	S82.53XB	S82.892B	S92.121B	S92.332B	T22.351A
S82.402C	S82.53XC	S82.892C	S92.122B	S92.333B	T22.352A
S82.409B	S82.54XB	S82.899B	S92.123B	S92.334B	T22.359A
S82.409C	S82.54XC	S82.899C	S92.124B	S92.335B	T22.361A
S82.421B	S82.55XB	S82.90XB	S92.125B	S92.336B	T22.362A
S82.421C	S82.55XC	S82.90XC	S92.126B	S92.341B	T22.369A
S82.422B	S82.56XB	S82.91XB	S92.131B	S92.342B	T22.391A
S82.422C	S82.56XC	S82.91XC	S92.132B	S92.343B	T22.392A
S82.423B	S82.61XB	S82.92XB	S92.133B	S92.344B	T22.399A
S82.423C	S82.61XC	S82.92XC	S92.134B	S92.345B	T22.70XA
S82.424B	S82.62XB	S89.001A	S92.135B	S92.346B	T22.711A
S82.424C	S82.62XC	S89.002A	S92.136B	S92.351B	T22.712A
S82.425B	S82.63XB	S89.009A	S92.141B	S92.352B	T22.719A
S82.425C	S82.63XC	S89.011A	S92.142B	S92.353B	T22.721A
S82.426B	S82.64XB	S89.012A	S92.143B	S92.354B	T22.722A
S82.426C	S82.64XC	S89.019A	S92.144B	S92.355B	T22.729A
S82.431B	S82.65XB	S89.021A	S92.145B	S92.356B	T22.731A
S82.431C	S82.65XC	S89.022A	S92.146B	S92.811B	T22.732A
S82.432B	S82.66XB	S89.029A	S92.151B	S92.812B	T22.739A
S82.432C	S82.66XC	S89.031A	S92.152B	S92.819B	T22.741A
S82.433B	S82.831B	S89.032A	S92.153B	S92.901B	T22.742A
S82.433C	S82.831C	S89.039A	S92.154B	S92.902B	T22.749A
S82.434B	S82.832B	S89.041A	S92.155B	S92.909B	T22.751A
S82.434C	S82.832C	S89.042A	S92.156B	T20.30XA	T22.752A
S82.435B	S82.839B	S89.049A	S92.191B	T20.311A	T22.759A
S82.435C	S82.839C	S89.091A	S92.192B	T20.312A	T22.761A
S82.436B	S82.841B	S89.092A	S92.199B	T20.319A	T22.762A
S82.436C	S82.841C	S89.099A	S92.201B	T20.32XA	T22.769A
S82.441B	S82.842B	S92.001B	S92.202B	T20.33XA	T22.791A
S82.441C	S82.842C	S92.002B	S92.209B	T20.34XA	T22.792A
S82.442B	S82.843B	S92.009B	S92.211B	T20.35XA	T22.799A
S82.442C	S82.843C	S92.011B	S92.212B	T20.36XA	T23.301A
S82.443B	S82.844B	S92.012B	S92.213B	T20.37XA	T23.302A
S82.443C	S82.844C	S92.013B	S92.214B	T20.39XA	T23.309A
S82.444B	S82.845B	S92.014B	S92.215B	T20.70XA	T23.311A
S82.444C	S82.845C	S92.015B	S92.216B	T20.711A	T23.312A
S82.445B	S82.846B	S92.016B	S92.221B	T20.712A	T23.319A
S82.445C	S82.846C	S92.021B	S92.222B	T20.719A	T23.321A
S82.446B	S82.851B	S92.022B	S92.223B	T20.72XA	T23.322A
S82.446C	S82.851C	S92.023B	S92.224B	T20.73XA	T23.329A
S82.451B	S82.852B	S92.024B	S92.225B	T20.74XA	T23.331A
S82.451C	S82.852C	S92.025B	S92.226B	T20.75XA	T23.332A
S82.452B	S82.853B	S92.026B	S92.231B	T20.76XA	T23.339A
S82.452C	S82.853C	S92.031B	S92.232B	T20.77XA	T23.341A
S82.453B	S82.854B	S92.032B	S92.233B	T20.79XA	T23.342A
S82.453C	S82.854C	S92.033B	S92.234B	T21.30XA	T23.349A
S82.454B	S82.855B	S92.034B	S92.235B	T21.31XA	T23.351A
	S82.855C	S92.035B	S92.236B	T21.32XA	T23.352A
	S82.856B	S92.036B	S92.241B	T21.33XA	T23.359A

HAC 05: Falls and Trauma (continued)

T23.361A
T23.362A
T23.369A
T23.371A
T23.372A
T23.379A
T23.391A
T23.392A
T23.399A
T23.701A
T23.702A
T23.709A
T23.711A
T23.712A
T23.719A
T23.721A
T23.722A
T23.729A
T23.731A
T23.732A
T23.739A
T23.741A
T23.742A
T23.749A
T23.751A
T23.752A
T23.759A
T23.761A
T23.762A
T23.769A
T23.771A
T23.772A
T23.779A
T23.791A
T23.792A
T23.799A
T24.301A
T24.302A
T24.309A
T24.311A
T24.312A
T24.319A
T24.321A
T24.322A
T24.329A
T24.331A
T24.332A
T24.339A
T24.391A
T24.392A
T24.399A
T24.701A
T24.702A
T24.709A
T24.711A
T24.712A
T24.719A
T24.721A
T24.722A

T24.729A
T24.731A
T24.732A
T24.739A
T24.791A
T24.792A
T24.799A
T25.311A
T25.312A
T25.319A
T25.321A
T25.322A
T25.329A
T25.331A
T25.332A
T25.339A
T25.391A
T25.392A
T25.399A
T25.711A
T25.712A
T25.719A
T25.721A
T25.722A
T25.729A
T25.731A
T25.732A
T25.739A
T25.791A
T25.792A
T25.799A
T26.20XA
T26.21XA
T26.22XA
T26.70XA
T26.71XA
T26.72XA
T27.0XXA
T27.1XXA
T27.2XXA
T27.3XXA
T27.4XXA
T27.5XXA
T27.6XXA
T27.7XXA
T28.1XXA
T28.2XXA
T28.6XXA
T28.7XXA
T31.10
T31.11
T31.20
T31.21
T31.22
T31.30
T31.31
T31.32
T31.33
T31.40
T31.41
T31.42
T31.43

T31.44
T31.50
T31.51
T31.52
T31.53
T31.54
T31.55
T31.60
T31.61
T31.62
T31.63
T31.64
T31.65
T31.66
T31.70
T31.71
T31.72
T31.73
T31.74
T31.75
T31.76
T31.77
T31.80
T31.81
T31.82
T31.83
T31.84
T31.85
T31.86
T31.87
T31.88
T31.90
T31.91
T31.92
T31.93
T31.94
T31.95
T31.96
T31.97
T31.98
T31.99
T32.10
T32.11
T32.20
T32.21
T32.22
T32.30
T32.31
T32.32
T32.33
T32.40
T32.41
T32.42
T32.43
T32.44
T32.50
T32.51
T32.52
T32.53
T32.54
T32.55
T32.60

T32.61
T32.62
T32.63
T32.64
T32.65
T32.66
T32.70
T32.71
T32.72
T32.73
T32.74
T32.75
T32.76
T32.77
T32.80
T32.81
T32.82
T32.83
T32.84
T32.85
T32.86
T32.87
T32.88
T32.90
T32.91
T32.92
T32.93
T32.94
T32.95
T32.96
T32.97
T32.98
T32.99
T33.011A
T33.012A
T33.019A
T33.02XA
T33.09XA
T33.1XXA
T33.2XXA
T33.3XXA
T33.40XA
T33.41XA
T33.42XA
T33.511A
T33.512A
T33.519A
T33.521A
T33.522A
T33.529A
T33.531A
T33.532A
T33.539A
T33.60XA
T33.61XA
T33.62XA
T33.70XA
T33.71XA
T33.72XA
T33.811A
T33.812A
T33.819A

T33.821A
T33.822A
T33.829A
T33.831A
T33.832A
T33.839A
T33.90XA
T33.99XA
T34.011A
T34.012A
T34.019A
T34.02XA
T34.09XA
T34.1XXA
T34.2XXA
T34.3XXA
T34.40XA
T34.41XA
T34.42XA
T34.511A
T34.512A
T34.519A
T34.521A
T34.522A
T34.529A
T34.531A
T34.532A
T34.539A
T34.60XA
T34.61XA
T34.62XA
T34.70XA
T34.71XA
T34.72XA
T34.811A
T34.812A
T34.819A
T34.821A
T34.822A
T34.829A
T34.831A
T34.832A
T34.839A
T34.90XA
T34.99XA
T67.0XXA
T69.021A
T69.022A
T69.029A
T70.3XXA
T71.111A
T71.112A
T71.113A
T71.114A
T71.121A
T71.122A
T71.123A
T71.124A
T71.131A
T71.132A
T71.133A
T71.134A

T71.141A
T71.143A
T71.144A
T71.151A
T71.152A
T71.153A
T71.154A
T71.161A
T71.162A
T71.163A
T71.164A
T71.191A
T71.192A
T71.193A
T71.194A
T71.20XA
T71.21XA
T71.29XA
T71.9XXA
T75.1XXA

HAC 06: Catheter Associated Urinary Tract Infection (UTI)

Secondary diagnosis not POA:

T83.511A
T83.518A

With or Without

Secondary diagnosis (also not POA) of:

B37.41
B37.49
N10
N11.9
N12
N13.6
N15.1
N28.84
N28.85
N28.86
N30.00
N30.01
N34.0
N39.0

HAC 07: Vascular Catheter Associated Infection

Secondary diagnosis not POA:

T80.211A
T80.212A
T80.218A
T80.219A

HAC 08: Surgical Site Infection of Mediastinitis After Coronary Bypass Graft (CABG) Procedures

Secondary diagnosis not POA:

J98.51

J98.59

AND

Any of the following procedures:

0210083 Bypass Coronary Artery, One Artery from Coronary Artery with Zooplastic Tissue, Open Approach

0210088 Bypass Coronary Artery, One Artery from Right Internal Mammary with Zooplastic Tissue, Open Approach

0210089 Bypass Coronary Artery, One Artery from Left Internal Mammary with Zooplastic Tissue, Open Approach

021008C Bypass Coronary Artery, One Artery from Thoracic Artery with Zooplastic Tissue, Open Approach

021008F Bypass Coronary Artery, One Artery from Abdominal Artery with Zooplastic Tissue, Open Approach

021008W Bypass Coronary Artery, One Artery from Aorta with Zooplastic Tissue, Open Approach

0210093 Bypass Coronary Artery, One Artery from Coronary Artery with Autologous Venous Tissue, Open Approach

0210098 Bypass Coronary Artery, One Artery from Right Internal Mammary with Autologous Venous Tissue, Open Approach

0210099 Bypass Coronary Artery, One Artery from Left Internal Mammary with Autologous Venous Tissue, Open Approach

021009C Bypass Coronary Artery, One Artery from Thoracic Artery with Autologous Venous Tissue, Open Approach

021009F Bypass Coronary Artery, One Artery from Abdominal Artery with Autologous Venous Tissue, Open Approach

021009W Bypass Coronary Artery, One Artery from Aorta with Autologous Venous Tissue, Open Approach

02100A3 Bypass Coronary Artery, One Artery from Coronary Artery with Autologous Arterial Tissue, Open Approach

02100A8 Bypass Coronary Artery, One Artery from Right Internal Mammary with Autologous Arterial Tissue, Open Approach

02100A9 Bypass Coronary Artery, One Artery from Left Internal Mammary with Autologous Arterial Tissue, Open Approach

02100AC Bypass Coronary Artery, One Artery from Thoracic Artery with Autologous Arterial Tissue, Open Approach

02100AF Bypass Coronary Artery, One Artery from Abdominal Artery with Autologous Arterial Tissue, Open Approach

02100AW Bypass Coronary Artery, One Artery from Aorta with Autologous Arterial Tissue, Open Approach

02100J3 Bypass Coronary Artery, One Artery from Coronary Artery with Synthetic Substitute, Open Approach

02100J8 Bypass Coronary Artery, One Artery from Right Internal Mammary with Synthetic Substitute, Open Approach

02100J9 Bypass Coronary Artery, One Artery from Left Internal Mammary with Synthetic Substitute, Open Approach

02100JC Bypass Coronary Artery, One Artery from Thoracic Artery with Synthetic Substitute, Open Approach

02100JF Bypass Coronary Artery, One Artery from Abdominal Artery with Synthetic Substitute, Open Approach

02100JW Bypass Coronary Artery, One Artery from Aorta with Synthetic Substitute, Open Approach

02100K3 Bypass Coronary Artery, One Artery from Coronary Artery with Nonautologous Tissue Substitute, Open Approach

02100K8 Bypass Coronary Artery, One Artery from Right Internal Mammary with Nonautologous Tissue Substitute, Open Approach

02100K9 Bypass Coronary Artery, One Artery from Left Internal Mammary with Nonautologous Tissue Substitute, Open Approach

02100KC Bypass Coronary Artery, One Artery from Thoracic Artery with Nonautologous Tissue Substitute, Open Approach

02100KF Bypass Coronary Artery, One Artery from Abdominal Artery with Nonautologous Tissue Substitute, Open Approach

02100KW Bypass Coronary Artery, One Artery from Aorta with Nonautologous Tissue Substitute, Open Approach

02100Z3 Bypass Coronary Artery, One Artery from Coronary Artery, Open Approach

02100Z8 Bypass Coronary Artery, One Artery from Right Internal Mammary, Open Approach

02100Z9 Bypass Coronary Artery, One Artery from Left Internal Mammary, Open Approach

02100ZC Bypass Coronary Artery, One Artery from Thoracic Artery, Open Approach

02100ZF Bypass Coronary Artery, One Artery from Abdominal Artery, Open Approach

0210483 Bypass Coronary Artery, One Artery from Coronary Artery with Zooplastic Tissue, Percutaneous Endoscopic Approach

0210488 Bypass Coronary Artery, One Artery from Right Internal Mammary with Zooplastic Tissue, Percutaneous Endoscopic Approach

0210489 Bypass Coronary Artery, One Artery from Left Internal Mammary with Zooplastic Tissue, Percutaneous Endoscopic Approach

021048C Bypass Coronary Artery, One Artery from Thoracic Artery with Zooplastic Tissue, Percutaneous Endoscopic Approach

021048F Bypass Coronary Artery, One Artery from Abdominal Artery with Zooplastic Tissue, Percutaneous Endoscopic Approach

021048W Bypass Coronary Artery, One Artery from Aorta with Zooplastic Tissue, Percutaneous Endoscopic Approach

0210493 Bypass Coronary Artery, One Artery from Coronary Artery with Autologous Venous Tissue, Percutaneous Endoscopic Approach

0210498 Bypass Coronary Artery, One Artery from Right Internal Mammary with Autologous Venous Tissue, Percutaneous Endoscopic Approach

0210499 Bypass Coronary Artery, One Artery from Left Internal Mammary with Autologous Venous Tissue, Percutaneous Endoscopic Approach

021049C Bypass Coronary Artery, One Artery from Thoracic Artery with Autologous Venous Tissue, Percutaneous Endoscopic Approach

021049F Bypass Coronary Artery, One Artery from Abdominal Artery with Autologous Venous Tissue, Percutaneous Endoscopic Approach

021049W Bypass Coronary Artery, One Artery from Aorta with Autologous Venous Tissue, Percutaneous Endoscopic Approach

02104A3 Bypass Coronary Artery, One Artery from Coronary Artery with Autologous Arterial Tissue, Percutaneous Endoscopic Approach

02104A8 Bypass Coronary Artery, One Artery from Right Internal Mammary with Autologous Arterial Tissue, Percutaneous Endoscopic Approach

02104A9 Bypass Coronary Artery, One Artery from Left Internal Mammary with Autologous Arterial Tissue, Percutaneous Endoscopic Approach

02104AC Bypass Coronary Artery, One Artery from Thoracic Artery with Autologous Arterial Tissue, Percutaneous Endoscopic Approach

02104AF Bypass Coronary Artery, One Artery from Abdominal Artery with Autologous Arterial Tissue, Percutaneous Endoscopic Approach

02104AW Bypass Coronary Artery, One Artery from Aorta with Autologous Arterial Tissue, Percutaneous Endoscopic Approach

02104J3 Bypass Coronary Artery, One Artery from Coronary Artery with Synthetic Substitute, Percutaneous Endoscopic Approach

02104J8 Bypass Coronary Artery, One Artery from Right Internal Mammary with Synthetic Substitute, Percutaneous Endoscopic Approach

02104J9 Bypass Coronary Artery, One Artery from Left Internal Mammary with Synthetic Substitute, Percutaneous Endoscopic Approach

02104JC Bypass Coronary Artery, One Artery from Thoracic Artery with Synthetic Substitute, Percutaneous Endoscopic Approach

02104JF Bypass Coronary Artery, One Artery from Abdominal Artery with Synthetic Substitute, Percutaneous Endoscopic Approach

02104JW Bypass Coronary Artery, One Artery from Aorta with Synthetic Substitute, Percutaneous Endoscopic Approach

02104K3 Bypass Coronary Artery, One Artery from Coronary Artery with Nonautologous Tissue Substitute, Percutaneous Endoscopic Approach

02104K8 Bypass Coronary Artery, One Artery from Right Internal Mammary with Nonautologous Tissue Substitute, Percutaneous Endoscopic Approach

02104K9 Bypass Coronary Artery, One Artery from Left Internal Mammary with Nonautologous Tissue Substitute, Percutaneous Endoscopic Approach

02104KC Bypass Coronary Artery, One Artery from Thoracic Artery with Nonautologous Tissue Substitute, Percutaneous Endoscopic Approach

HAC 08: Surgical Artery Infection of Mediastinitis After Coronary Bypass Graft (CABG) Procedures (continued)

02104KF   Bypass Coronary Artery, One Artery from Abdominal Artery with Nonautologous Tissue Substitute, Percutaneous Endoscopic Approach

02104KW   Bypass Coronary Artery, One Artery from Aorta with Nonautologous Tissue Substitute, Percutaneous Endoscopic Approach

02104Z3   Bypass Coronary Artery, One Artery from Coronary Artery, Percutaneous Endoscopic Approach

02104Z8   Bypass Coronary Artery, One Artery from Right Internal Mammary, Percutaneous Endoscopic Approach

02104Z9   Bypass Coronary Artery, One Artery from Left Internal Mammary, Percutaneous Endoscopic Approach

02104ZC   Bypass Coronary Artery, One Artery from Thoracic Artery, Percutaneous Endoscopic Approach

02104ZF   Bypass Coronary Artery, One Artery from Abdominal Artery, Percutaneous Endoscopic Approach

0211083   Bypass Coronary Artery, Two Arteries from Coronary Artery with Zooplastic Tissue, Open Approach

0211088   Bypass Coronary Artery, Two Arteries from Right Internal Mammary with Zooplastic Tissue, Open Approach

0211089   Bypass Coronary Artery, Two Arteries from Left Internal Mammary with Zooplastic Tissue, Open Approach

021108C   Bypass Coronary Artery, Two Arteries from Thoracic Artery with Zooplastic Tissue, Open Approach

021108F   Bypass Coronary Artery, Two Arteries from Abdominal Artery with Zooplastic Tissue, Open Approach

021108W   Bypass Coronary Artery, Two Arteries from Aorta with Zooplastic Tissue, Open Approach

0211093   Bypass Coronary Artery, Two Arteries from Coronary Artery with Autologous Venous Tissue, Open Approach

0211098   Bypass Coronary Artery, Two Arteries from Right Internal Mammary with Autologous Venous Tissue, Open Approach

0211099   Bypass Coronary Artery, Two Arteries from Left Internal Mammary with Autologous Venous Tissue, Open Approach

021109C   Bypass Coronary Artery, Two Arteries from Thoracic Artery with Autologous Venous Tissue, Open Approach

021109F   Bypass Coronary Artery, Two Arteries from Abdominal Artery with Autologous Venous Tissue, Open Approach

021109W   Bypass Coronary Artery, Two Arteries from Aorta with Autologous Venous Tissue, Open Approach

02110A3   Bypass Coronary Artery, Two Arteries from Coronary Artery with Autologous Arterial Tissue, Open Approach

02110A8   Bypass Coronary Artery, Two Arteries from Right Internal Mammary with Autologous Arterial Tissue, Open Approach

02110A9   Bypass Coronary Artery, Two Arteries from Left Internal Mammary with Autologous Arterial Tissue, Open Approach

02110AC   Bypass Coronary Artery, Two Arteries from Thoracic Artery with Autologous Arterial Tissue, Open Approach

02110AF   Bypass Coronary Artery, Two Arteries from Abdominal Artery with Autologous Arterial Tissue, Open Approach

02110AW   Bypass Coronary Artery, Two Arteries from Aorta with Autologous Arterial Tissue, Open Approach

02110J3   Bypass Coronary Artery, Two Arteries from Coronary Artery with Synthetic Substitute, Open Approach

02110J8   Bypass Coronary Artery, Two Arteries from Right Internal Mammary with Synthetic Substitute, Open Approach

02110J9   Bypass Coronary Artery, Two Arteries from Left Internal Mammary with Synthetic Substitute, Open Approach

02110JC   Bypass Coronary Artery, Two Arteries from Thoracic Artery with Synthetic Substitute, Open Approach

02110JF   Bypass Coronary Artery, Two Arteries from Abdominal Artery with Synthetic Substitute, Open Approach

02110JW   Bypass Coronary Artery, Two Arteries from Aorta with Synthetic Substitute, Open Approach

02110K3   Bypass Coronary Artery, Two Arteries from Coronary Artery with Nonautologous Tissue Substitute, Open Approach

02110K8   Bypass Coronary Artery, Two Arteries from Right Internal Mammary with Nonautologous Tissue Substitute, Open Approach

02110K9   Bypass Coronary Artery, Two Arteries from Left Internal Mammary with Nonautologous Tissue Substitute, Open Approach

02110KC   Bypass Coronary Artery, Two Arteries from Thoracic Artery with Nonautologous Tissue Substitute, Open Approach

02110KF   Bypass Coronary Artery, Two Arteries from Abdominal Artery with Nonautologous Tissue Substitute, Open Approach

02110KW   Bypass Coronary Artery, Two Arteries from Aorta with Nonautologous Tissue Substitute, Open Approach

02110Z3   Bypass Coronary Artery, Two Arteries from Coronary Artery, Open Approach

02110Z8   Bypass Coronary Artery, Two Arteries from Right Internal Mammary, Open Approach

02110Z9   Bypass Coronary Artery, Two Arteries from Left Internal Mammary, Open Approach

02110ZC   Bypass Coronary Artery, Two Arteries from Thoracic Artery, Open Approach

02110ZF   Bypass Coronary Artery, Two Arteries from Abdominal Artery, Open Approach

0211483   Bypass Coronary Artery, Two Arteries from Coronary Artery with Zooplastic Tissue, Percutaneous Endoscopic Approach

0211488   Bypass Coronary Artery, Two Arteries from Right Internal Mammary with Zooplastic Tissue, Percutaneous Endoscopic Approach

0211489   Bypass Coronary Artery, Two Arteries from Left Internal Mammary with Zooplastic Tissue, Percutaneous Endoscopic Approach

021148C   Bypass Coronary Artery, Two Arteries from Thoracic Artery with Zooplastic Tissue, Percutaneous Endoscopic Approach

021148F   Bypass Coronary Artery, Two Arteries from Abdominal Artery with Zooplastic Tissue, Percutaneous Endoscopic Approach

021148W   Bypass Coronary Artery, Two Arteries from Aorta with Zooplastic Tissue, Percutaneous Endoscopic Approach

0211493   Bypass Coronary Artery, Two Arteries from Coronary Artery with Autologous Venous Tissue, Percutaneous Endoscopic Approach

0211498   Bypass Coronary Artery, Two Arteries from Right Internal Mammary with Autologous Venous Tissue, Percutaneous Endoscopic Approach

0211499   Bypass Coronary Artery, Two Arteries from Left Internal Mammary with Autologous Venous Tissue, Percutaneous Endoscopic Approach

021149C   Bypass Coronary Artery, Two Arteries from Thoracic Artery with Autologous Venous Tissue, Percutaneous Endoscopic Approach

021149F   Bypass Coronary Artery, Two Arteries from Abdominal Artery with Autologous Venous Tissue, Percutaneous Endoscopic Approach

021149W   Bypass Coronary Artery, Two Arteries from Aorta with Autologous Venous Tissue, Percutaneous Endoscopic Approach

02114A3   Bypass Coronary Artery, Two Arteries from Coronary Artery with Autologous Arterial Tissue, Percutaneous Endoscopic Approach

02114A8   Bypass Coronary Artery, Two Arteries from Right Internal Mammary with Autologous Arterial Tissue, Percutaneous Endoscopic Approach

02114A9   Bypass Coronary Artery, Two Arteries from Left Internal Mammary with Autologous Arterial Tissue, Percutaneous Endoscopic Approach

02114AC   Bypass Coronary Artery, Two Arteries from Thoracic Artery with Autologous Arterial Tissue, Percutaneous Endoscopic Approach

02114AF   Bypass Coronary Artery, Two Arteries from Abdominal Artery with Autologous Arterial Tissue, Percutaneous Endoscopic Approach

02114AW   Bypass Coronary Artery, Two Arteries from Aorta with Autologous Arterial Tissue, Percutaneous Endoscopic Approach

02114J3   Bypass Coronary Artery, Two Arteries from Coronary Artery with Synthetic Substitute, Percutaneous Endoscopic Approach

02114J8   Bypass Coronary Artery, Two Arteries from Right Internal Mammary with Synthetic Substitute, Percutaneous Endoscopic Approach

02114J9   Bypass Coronary Artery, Two Arteries from Left Internal Mammary with Synthetic Substitute, Percutaneous Endoscopic Approach

02114JC   Bypass Coronary Artery, Two Arteries from Thoracic Artery with Synthetic Substitute, Percutaneous Endoscopic Approach

HAC 08: Surgical Site Infection of Mediastinitis After Coronary Bypass Graft (CABG) Procedures (continued)

Ø2114JF   Bypass Coronary Artery, Two Arteries from Abdominal Artery with Synthetic Substitute, Percutaneous Endoscopic Approach

Ø2114JW   Bypass Coronary Artery, Two Arteries from Aorta with Synthetic Substitute, Percutaneous Endoscopic Approach

Ø2114K3   Bypass Coronary Artery, Two Arteries from Coronary Artery with Nonautologous Tissue Substitute, Percutaneous Endoscopic Approach

Ø2114K8   Bypass Coronary Artery, Two Arteries from Right Internal Mammary with Nonautologous Tissue Substitute, Percutaneous Endoscopic Approach

Ø2114K9   Bypass Coronary Artery, Two Arteries from Left Internal Mammary with Nonautologous Tissue Substitute, Percutaneous Endoscopic Approach

Ø2114KC   Bypass Coronary Artery, Two Arteries from Thoracic Artery with Nonautologous Tissue Substitute, Percutaneous Endoscopic Approach

Ø2114KF   Bypass Coronary Artery, Two Arteries from Abdominal Artery with Nonautologous Tissue Substitute, Percutaneous Endoscopic Approach

Ø2114KW   Bypass Coronary Artery, Two Arteries from Aorta with Nonautologous Tissue Substitute, Percutaneous Endoscopic Approach

Ø2114Z3   Bypass Coronary Artery, Two Arteries from Coronary Artery, Percutaneous Endoscopic Approach

Ø2114Z8   Bypass Coronary Artery, Two Arteries from Right Internal Mammary, Percutaneous Endoscopic Approach

Ø2114Z9   Bypass Coronary Artery, Two Arteries from Left Internal Mammary, Percutaneous Endoscopic Approach

Ø2114ZC   Bypass Coronary Artery, Two Arteries from Thoracic Artery, Percutaneous Endoscopic Approach

Ø2114ZF   Bypass Coronary Artery, Two Arteries from Abdominal Artery, Percutaneous Endoscopic Approach

Ø212Ø83   Bypass Coronary Artery, Three Arteries from Coronary Artery with Zooplastic Tissue, Open Approach

Ø212Ø88   Bypass Coronary Artery, Three Arteries from Right Internal Mammary with Zooplastic Tissue, Open Approach

Ø212Ø89   Bypass Coronary Artery, Three Arteries from Left Internal Mammary with Zooplastic Tissue, Open Approach

Ø212Ø8C   Bypass Coronary Artery, Three Arteries from Thoracic Artery with Zooplastic Tissue, Open Approach

Ø212Ø8F   Bypass Coronary Artery, Three Arteries from Abdominal Artery with Zooplastic Tissue, Open Approach

Ø212Ø8W   Bypass Coronary Artery, Three Arteries from Aorta with Zooplastic Tissue, Open Approach

Ø212Ø93   Bypass Coronary Artery, Three Arteries from Coronary Artery with Autologous Venous Tissue, Open Approach

Ø212Ø98   Bypass Coronary Artery, Three Arteries from Right Internal Mammary with Autologous Venous Tissue, Open Approach

Ø212Ø99   Bypass Coronary Artery, Three Arteries from Left Internal Mammary with Autologous Venous Tissue, Open Approach

Ø212Ø9C   Bypass Coronary Artery, Three Arteries from Thoracic Artery with Autologous Venous Tissue, Open Approach

Ø212Ø9F   Bypass Coronary Artery, Three Arteries from Abdominal Artery with Autologous Venous Tissue, Open Approach

Ø212Ø9W   Bypass Coronary Artery, Three Arteries from Aorta with Autologous Venous Tissue, Open Approach

Ø212ØA3   Bypass Coronary Artery, Three Arteries from Coronary Artery with Autologous Arterial Tissue, Open Approach

Ø212ØA8   Bypass Coronary Artery, Three Arteries from Right Internal Mammary with Autologous Arterial Tissue, Open Approach

Ø212ØA9   Bypass Coronary Artery, Three Arteries from Left Internal Mammary with Autologous Arterial Tissue, Open Approach

Ø212ØAC   Bypass Coronary Artery, Three Arteries from Thoracic Artery with Autologous Arterial Tissue, Open Approach

Ø212ØAF   Bypass Coronary Artery, Three Arteries from Abdominal Artery with Autologous Arterial Tissue, Open Approach

Ø212ØAW   Bypass Coronary Artery, Three Arteries from Aorta with Autologous Arterial Tissue, Open Approach

Ø212ØJ3   Bypass Coronary Artery, Three Arteries from Coronary Artery with Synthetic Substitute, Open Approach

Ø212ØJ8   Bypass Coronary Artery, Three Arteries from Right Internal Mammary with Synthetic Substitute, Open Approach

Ø212ØJ9   Bypass Coronary Artery, Three Arteries from Left Internal Mammary with Synthetic Substitute, Open Approach

Ø212ØJC   Bypass Coronary Artery, Three Arteries from Thoracic Artery with Synthetic Substitute, Open Approach

Ø212ØJF   Bypass Coronary Artery, Three Arteries from Abdominal Artery with Synthetic Substitute, Open Approach

Ø212ØJW   Bypass Coronary Artery, Three Arteries from Aorta with Synthetic Substitute, Open Approach

Ø212ØK3   Bypass Coronary Artery, Three Arteries from Coronary Artery with Nonautologous Tissue Substitute, Open Approach

Ø212ØK8   Bypass Coronary Artery, Three Arteries from Right Internal Mammary with Nonautologous Tissue Substitute, Open Approach

Ø212ØK9   Bypass Coronary Artery, Three Arteries from Left Internal Mammary with Nonautologous Tissue Substitute, Open Approach

Ø212ØKC   Bypass Coronary Artery, Three Arteries from Thoracic Artery with Nonautologous Tissue Substitute, Open Approach

Ø212ØKF   Bypass Coronary Artery, Three Arteries from Abdominal Artery with Nonautologous Tissue Substitute, Open Approach

Ø212ØKW   Bypass Coronary Artery, Three Arteries from Aorta with Nonautologous Tissue Substitute, Open Approach

Ø212ØZ3   Bypass Coronary Artery, Three Arteries from Coronary Artery, Open Approach

Ø212ØZ8   Bypass Coronary Artery, Three Arteries from Right Internal Mammary, Open Approach

Ø212ØZ9   Bypass Coronary Artery, Three Arteries from Left Internal Mammary, Open Approach

Ø212ØZC   Bypass Coronary Artery, Three Arteries from Thoracic Artery, Open Approach

Ø212ØZF   Bypass Coronary Artery, Three Arteries from Abdominal Artery, Open Approach

Ø212483   Bypass Coronary Artery, Three Arteries from Coronary Artery with Zooplastic Tissue, Percutaneous Endoscopic Approach

Ø212488   Bypass Coronary Artery, Three Arteries from Right Internal Mammary with Zooplastic Tissue, Percutaneous Endoscopic Approach

Ø212489   Bypass Coronary Artery, Three Arteries from Left Internal Mammary with Zooplastic Tissue, Percutaneous Endoscopic Approach

Ø21248C   Bypass Coronary Artery, Three Arteries from Thoracic Artery with Zooplastic Tissue, Percutaneous Endoscopic Approach

Ø21248F   Bypass Coronary Artery, Three Arteries from Abdominal Artery with Zooplastic Tissue, Percutaneous Endoscopic Approach

Ø21248W   Bypass Coronary Artery, Three Arteries from Aorta with Zooplastic Tissue, Percutaneous Endoscopic Approach

Ø212493   Bypass Coronary Artery, Three Arteries from Coronary Artery with Autologous Venous Tissue, Percutaneous Endoscopic Approach

Ø212498   Bypass Coronary Artery, Three Arteries from Right Internal Mammary with Autologous Venous Tissue, Percutaneous Endoscopic Approach

Ø212499   Bypass Coronary Artery, Three Arteries from Left Internal Mammary with Autologous Venous Tissue, Percutaneous Endoscopic Approach

Ø21249C   Bypass Coronary Artery, Three Arteries from Thoracic Artery with Autologous Venous Tissue, Percutaneous Endoscopic Approach

Ø21249F   Bypass Coronary Artery, Three Arteries from Abdominal Artery with Autologous Venous Tissue, Percutaneous Endoscopic Approach

Ø21249W   Bypass Coronary Artery, Three Arteries from Aorta with Autologous Venous Tissue, Percutaneous Endoscopic Approach

Ø2124A3   Bypass Coronary Artery, Three Arteries from Coronary Artery with Autologous Arterial Tissue, Percutaneous Endoscopic Approach

Ø2124A8   Bypass Coronary Artery, Three Arteries from Right Internal Mammary with Autologous Arterial Tissue, Percutaneous Endoscopic Approach

Ø2124A9   Bypass Coronary Artery, Three Arteries from Left Internal Mammary with Autologous Arterial Tissue, Percutaneous Endoscopic Approach

Ø2124AC   Bypass Coronary Artery, Three Arteries from Thoracic Artery with Autologous Arterial Tissue, Percutaneous Endoscopic Approach

HAC 08: Surgical Site Infection of Mediastinitis After Coronary Bypass Graft (CABG) Procedures (continued)

02124AF   Bypass Coronary Artery, Three Arteries from Abdominal Artery with Autologous Arterial Tissue, Percutaneous Endoscopic Approach

02124AW   Bypass Coronary Artery, Three Arteries from Aorta with Autologous Arterial Tissue, Percutaneous Endoscopic Approach

02124J3   Bypass Coronary Artery, Three Arteries from Coronary Artery with Synthetic Substitute, Percutaneous Endoscopic Approach

02124J8   Bypass Coronary Artery, Three Arteries from Right Internal Mammary with Synthetic Substitute, Percutaneous Endoscopic Approach

02124J9   Bypass Coronary Artery, Three Arteries from Left Internal Mammary with Synthetic Substitute, Percutaneous Endoscopic Approach

02124JC   Bypass Coronary Artery, Three Arteries from Thoracic Artery with Synthetic Substitute, Percutaneous Endoscopic Approach

02124JF   Bypass Coronary Artery, Three Arteries from Abdominal Artery with Synthetic Substitute, Percutaneous Endoscopic Approach

02124JW   Bypass Coronary Artery, Three Arteries from Aorta with Synthetic Substitute, Percutaneous Endoscopic Approach

02124K3   Bypass Coronary Artery, Three Arteries from Coronary Artery with Nonautologous Tissue Substitute, Percutaneous Endoscopic Approach

02124K8   Bypass Coronary Artery, Three Arteries from Right Internal Mammary with Nonautologous Tissue Substitute, Percutaneous Endoscopic Approach

02124K9   Bypass Coronary Artery, Three Arteries from Left Internal Mammary with Nonautologous Tissue Substitute, Percutaneous Endoscopic Approach

02124KC   Bypass Coronary Artery, Three Arteries from Thoracic Artery with Nonautologous Tissue Substitute, Percutaneous Endoscopic Approach

02124KF   Bypass Coronary Artery, Three Arteries from Abdominal Artery with Nonautologous Tissue Substitute, Percutaneous Endoscopic Approach

02124KW   Bypass Coronary Artery, Three Arteries from Aorta with Nonautologous Tissue Substitute, Percutaneous Endoscopic Approach

02124Z3   Bypass Coronary Artery, Three Arteries from Coronary Artery, Percutaneous Endoscopic Approach

02124Z8   Bypass Coronary Artery, Three Arteries from Right Internal Mammary, Percutaneous Endoscopic Approach

02124Z9   Bypass Coronary Artery, Three Arteries from Left Internal Mammary, Percutaneous Endoscopic Approach

02124ZC   Bypass Coronary Artery, Three Arteries from Thoracic Artery, Percutaneous Endoscopic Approach

02124ZF   Bypass Coronary Artery, Three Arteries from Abdominal Artery, Percutaneous Endoscopic Approach

0213083   Bypass Coronary Artery, Four or More Arteries from Coronary Artery with Zooplastic Tissue, Open Approach

0213088   Bypass Coronary Artery, Four or More Arteries from Right Internal Mammary with Zooplastic Tissue, Open Approach

0213089   Bypass Coronary Artery, Four or More Arteries from Left Internal Mammary with Zooplastic Tissue, Open Approach

021308C   Bypass Coronary Artery, Four or More Arteries from Thoracic Artery with Zooplastic Tissue, Open Approach

021308F   Bypass Coronary Artery, Four or More Arteries from Abdominal Artery with Zooplastic Tissue, Open Approach

021308W   Bypass Coronary Artery, Four or More Arteries from Aorta with Zooplastic Tissue, Open Approach

0213093   Bypass Coronary Artery, Four or More Arteries from Coronary Artery with Autologous Venous Tissue, Open Approach

0213098   Bypass Coronary Artery, Four or More Arteries from Right Internal Mammary with Autologous Venous Tissue, Open Approach

0213099   Bypass Coronary Artery, Four or More Arteries from Left Internal Mammary with Autologous Venous Tissue, Open Approach

021309C   Bypass Coronary Artery, Four or More Arteries from Thoracic Artery with Autologous Venous Tissue, Open Approach

021309F   Bypass Coronary Artery, Four or More Arteries from Abdominal Artery with Autologous Venous Tissue, Open Approach

021309W   Bypass Coronary Artery, Four or More Arteries from Aorta with Autologous Venous Tissue, Open Approach

02130A3   Bypass Coronary Artery, Four or More Arteries from Coronary Artery with Autologous Arterial Tissue, Open Approach

02130A8   Bypass Coronary Artery, Four or More Arteries from Right Internal Mammary with Autologous Arterial Tissue, Open Approach

02130A9   Bypass Coronary Artery, Four or More Arteries from Left Internal Mammary with Autologous Arterial Tissue, Open Approach

02130AC   Bypass Coronary Artery, Four or More Arteries from Thoracic Artery with Autologous Arterial Tissue, Open Approach

02130AF   Bypass Coronary Artery, Four or More Arteries from Abdominal Artery with Autologous Arterial Tissue, Open Approach

02130AW   Bypass Coronary Artery, Four or More Arteries from Aorta with Autologous Arterial Tissue, Open Approach

02130J3   Bypass Coronary Artery, Four or More Arteries from Coronary Artery with Synthetic Substitute, Open Approach

02130J8   Bypass Coronary Artery, Four or More Arteries from Right Internal Mammary with Synthetic Substitute, Open Approach

02130J9   Bypass Coronary Artery, Four or More Arteries from Left Internal Mammary with Synthetic Substitute, Open Approach

02130JC   Bypass Coronary Artery, Four or More Arteries from Thoracic Artery with Synthetic Substitute, Open Approach

02130JF   Bypass Coronary Artery, Four or More Arteries from Abdominal Artery with Synthetic Substitute, Open Approach

02130JW   Bypass Coronary Artery, Four or More Arteries from Aorta with Synthetic Substitute, Open Approach

02130K3   Bypass Coronary Artery, Four or More Arteries from Coronary Artery with Nonautologous Tissue Substitute, Open Approach

02130K8   Bypass Coronary Artery, Four or More Arteries from Right Internal Mammary with Nonautologous Tissue Substitute, Open Approach

02130K9   Bypass Coronary Artery, Four or More Arteries from Left Internal Mammary with Nonautologous Tissue Substitute, Open Approach

02130KC   Bypass Coronary Artery, Four or More Arteries from Thoracic Artery with Nonautologous Tissue Substitute, Open Approach

02130KF   Bypass Coronary Artery, Four or More Arteries from Abdominal Artery with Nonautologous Tissue Substitute, Open Approach

02130KW   Bypass Coronary Artery, Four or More Arteries from Aorta with Nonautologous Tissue Substitute, Open Approach

02130Z3   Bypass Coronary Artery, Four or More Arteries from Coronary Artery, Open Approach

02130Z8   Bypass Coronary Artery, Four or More Arteries from Right Internal Mammary, Open Approach

02130Z9   Bypass Coronary Artery, Four or More Arteries from Left Internal Mammary, Open Approach

02130ZC   Bypass Coronary Artery, Four or More Arteries from Thoracic Artery, Open Approach

02130ZF   Bypass Coronary Artery, Four or More Arteries from Abdominal Artery, Open Approach

0213483   Bypass Coronary Artery, Four or More Arteries from Coronary Artery with Zooplastic Tissue, Percutaneous Endoscopic Approach

0213488   Bypass Coronary Artery, Four or More Arteries from Right Internal Mammary with Zooplastic Tissue, Percutaneous Endoscopic Approach

0213489   Bypass Coronary Artery, Four or More Arteries from Left Internal Mammary with Zooplastic Tissue, Percutaneous Endoscopic Approach

021348C   Bypass Coronary Artery, Four or More Arteries from Thoracic Artery with Zooplastic Tissue, Percutaneous Endoscopic Approach

021348F   Bypass Coronary Artery, Four or More Arteries from Abdominal Artery with Zooplastic Tissue, Percutaneous Endoscopic Approach

021348W   Bypass Coronary Artery, Four or More Arteries from Aorta with Zooplastic Tissue, Percutaneous Endoscopic Approach

0213493   Bypass Coronary Artery, Four or More Arteries from Coronary Artery with Autologous Venous Tissue, Percutaneous Endoscopic Approach

0213498   Bypass Coronary Artery, Four or More Arteries from Right Internal Mammary with Autologous Venous Tissue, Percutaneous Endoscopic Approach

HAC 08: Surgical Site Infection of Mediastinitis After Coronary Bypass Graft (CABG) Procedures (continued)

0213499 Bypass Coronary Artery, Four or More Arteries from Left Internal Mammary with Autologous Venous Tissue, Percutaneous Endoscopic Approach

021349C Bypass Coronary Artery, Four or More Arteries from Thoracic Artery with Autologous Venous Tissue, Percutaneous Endoscopic Approach

021349F Bypass Coronary Artery, Four or More Arteries from Abdominal Artery with Autologous Venous Tissue, Percutaneous Endoscopic Approach

021349W Bypass Coronary Artery, Four or More Arteries from Aorta with Autologous Venous Tissue, Percutaneous Endoscopic Approach

02134A3 Bypass Coronary Artery, Four or More Arteries from Coronary Artery with Autologous Arterial Tissue, Percutaneous Endoscopic Approach

02134A8 Bypass Coronary Artery, Four or More Arteries from Right Internal Mammary with Autologous Arterial Tissue, Percutaneous Endoscopic Approach

02134A9 Bypass Coronary Artery, Four or More Arteries from Left Internal Mammary with Autologous Arterial Tissue, Percutaneous Endoscopic Approach

02134AC Bypass Coronary Artery, Four or More Arteries from Thoracic Artery with Autologous Arterial Tissue, Percutaneous Endoscopic Approach

02134AF Bypass Coronary Artery, Four or More Arteries from Abdominal Artery with Autologous Arterial Tissue, Percutaneous Endoscopic Approach

02134AW Bypass Coronary Artery, Four or More Arteries from Aorta with Autologous Arterial Tissue, Percutaneous Endoscopic Approach

02134J3 Bypass Coronary Artery, Four or More Arteries from Coronary Artery with Synthetic Substitute, Percutaneous Endoscopic Approach

02134J8 Bypass Coronary Artery, Four or More Arteries from Right Internal Mammary with Synthetic Substitute, Percutaneous Endoscopic Approach

02134J9 Bypass Coronary Artery, Four or More Arteries from Left Internal Mammary with Synthetic Substitute, Percutaneous Endoscopic Approach

02134JC Bypass Coronary Artery, Four or More Arteries from Thoracic Artery with Synthetic Substitute, Percutaneous Endoscopic Approach

02134JF Bypass Coronary Artery, Four or More Arteries from Abdominal Artery with Synthetic Substitute, Percutaneous Endoscopic Approach

02134JW Bypass Coronary Artery, Four or More Arteries from Aorta with Synthetic Substitute, Percutaneous Endoscopic Approach

02134K3 Bypass Coronary Artery, Four or More Arteries from Coronary Artery with Nonautologous Tissue Substitute, Percutaneous Endoscopic Approach

02134K8 Bypass Coronary Artery, Four or More Arteries from Right Internal Mammary with Nonautologous Tissue Substitute, Percutaneous Endoscopic Approach

02134K9 Bypass Coronary Artery, Four or More Arteries from Left Internal Mammary with Nonautologous Tissue Substitute, Percutaneous Endoscopic Approach

02134KC Bypass Coronary Artery, Four or More Arteries from Thoracic Artery with Nonautologous Tissue Substitute, Percutaneous Endoscopic Approach

02134KF Bypass Coronary Artery, Four or More Arteries from Abdominal Artery with Nonautologous Tissue Substitute, Percutaneous Endoscopic Approach

02134KW Bypass Coronary Artery, Four or More Arteries from Aorta with Nonautologous Tissue Substitute, Percutaneous Endoscopic Approach

02134Z3 Bypass Coronary Artery, Four or More Arteries from Coronary Artery, Percutaneous Endoscopic Approach

02134Z8 Bypass Coronary Artery, Four or More Arteries from Right Internal Mammary, Percutaneous Endoscopic Approach

02134Z9 Bypass Coronary Artery, Four or More Arteries from Left Internal Mammary, Percutaneous Endoscopic Approach

02134ZC Bypass Coronary Artery, Four or More Arteries from Thoracic Artery, Percutaneous Endoscopic Approach

02134ZF Bypass Coronary Artery, Four or More Arteries from Abdominal Artery, Percutaneous Endoscopic Approach

HAC 09: Manifestations of Poor Glycemic Control

Secondary diagnosis not POA:

E08.00
E08.01
E08.10
E09.00
E09.01
E09.10
E10.10
E11.00
E11.01
E13.00
E13.01
E13.10
E15

HAC 10: Deep Vein Thrombosis (DVT) or Pulmonary Embolism (PE) with Total Knee or Hip Replacement

Secondary diagnosis not POA:

I26.02
I26.09
I26.92
I26.99
I82.401
I82.402
I82.403
I82.409
I82.411
I82.412
I82.413
I82.419
I82.421
I82.422
I82.423
I82.429
I82.431
I82.432
I82.433
I82.439
I82.441
I82.442
I82.443
I82.449
I82.491

I82.492
I82.493
I82.499
I82.4Y1
I82.4Y2
I82.4Y3
I82.4Y9
I82.4Z1
I82.4Z2
I82.4Z3
I82.4Z9

AND

Any of the following procedures:

0SR9019 Replacement of Right Hip Joint with Metal Synthetic Substitute, Cemented, Open Approach

0SR901A Replacement of Right Hip Joint with Metal Synthetic Substitute, Uncemented, Open Approach

0SR901Z Replacement of Right Hip Joint with Metal Synthetic Substitute, Open Approach

0SR9029 Replacement of Right Hip Joint with Metal on Polyethylene Synthetic Substitute, Cemented, Open Approach

0SR902A Replacement of Right Hip Joint with Metal on Polyethylene Synthetic Substitute, Uncemented, Open Approach

0SR902Z Replacement of Right Hip Joint with Metal on Polyethylene Synthetic Substitute, Open Approach

0SR9039 Replacement of Right Hip Joint with Ceramic Synthetic Substitute, Cemented, Open Approach

0SR903A Replacement of Right Hip Joint with Ceramic Synthetic Substitute, Uncemented, Open Approach

0SR903Z Replacement of Right Hip Joint with Ceramic Synthetic Substitute, Open Approach

0SR9049 Replacement of Right Hip Joint with Ceramic on Polyethylene Synthetic Substitute, Cemented, Open Approach

0SR904A Replacement of Right Hip Joint with Ceramic on Polyethylene Synthetic Substitute, Uncemented, Open Approach

0SR904Z Replacement of Right Hip Joint with Ceramic on Polyethylene Synthetic Substitute, Open Approach

0SR9069 Replacement of Right Hip Joint with Oxidized Zirconium on Polyethylene Synthetic Substitute, Cemented, Open Approach

0SR906A Replacement of Right Hip Joint with Oxidized Zirconium on Polyethylene Synthetic Substitute, Uncemented, Open Approach

0SR906Z Replacement of Right Hip Joint with Oxidized Zirconium on Polyethylene Synthetic Substitute, Open Approach

0SR907Z Replacement of Right Hip Joint with Autologous Tissue Substitute, Open Approach

0SR90EZ Replacement of Right Hip Joint with Articulating Spacer, Open Approach

0SR90J9 Replacement of Right Hip Joint with Synthetic Substitute, Cemented, Open Approach

0SR90JA Replacement of Right Hip Joint with Synthetic Substitute, Uncemented, Open Approach

0SR90JZ Replacement of Right Hip Joint with Synthetic Substitute, Open Approach

HAC 10: Deep Vein Thrombosis (DVT) or Pulmonary Embolism (PE) with Total Knee or Hip Replacement (continued)

ØSR9ØKZ Replacement of Right Hip Joint with Nonautologous Tissue Substitute, Open Approach

ØSRAØØ9 Replacement of Right Hip Joint, Acetabular Surface with Polyethylene Synthetic Substitute, Cemented, Open Approach

ØSRAØØA Replacement of Right Hip Joint, Acetabular Surface with Polyethylene Synthetic Substitute, Uncemented, Open Approach

ØSRAØØZ Replacement of Right Hip Joint, Acetabular Surface with Polyethylene Synthetic Substitute, Open Approach

ØSRAØ19 Replacement of Right Hip Joint, Acetabular Surface with Metal Synthetic Substitute, Cemented, Open Approach

ØSRAØ1A Replacement of Right Hip Joint, Acetabular Surface with Metal Synthetic Substitute, Uncemented, Open Approach

ØSRAØ1Z Replacement of Right Hip Joint, Acetabular Surface with Metal Synthetic Substitute, Open Approach

ØSRAØ39 Replacement of Right Hip Joint, Acetabular Surface with Ceramic Synthetic Substitute, Cemented, Open Approach

ØSRAØ3A Replacement of Right Hip Joint, Acetabular Surface with Ceramic Synthetic Substitute, Uncemented, Open Approach

ØSRAØ3Z Replacement of Right Hip Joint, Acetabular Surface with Ceramic Synthetic Substitute, Open Approach

ØSRAØ7Z Replacement of Right Hip Joint, Acetabular Surface with Autologous Tissue Substitute, Open Approach

ØSRAØJ9 Replacement of Right Hip Joint, Acetabular Surface with Synthetic Substitute, Cemented, Open Approach

ØSRAØJA Replacement of Right Hip Joint, Acetabular Surface with Synthetic Substitute, Uncemented, Open Approach

ØSRAØJZ Replacement of Right Hip Joint, Acetabular Surface with Synthetic Substitute, Open Approach

ØSRAØKZ Replacement of Right Hip Joint, Acetabular Surface with Nonautologous Tissue Substitute, Open Approach

ØSRBØ19 Replacement of Left Hip Joint with Metal Synthetic Substitute, Cemented, Open Approach

ØSRBØ1A Replacement of Left Hip Joint with Metal Synthetic Substitute, Uncemented, Open Approach

ØSRBØ1Z Replacement of Left Hip Joint with Metal Synthetic Substitute, Open Approach

ØSRBØ29 Replacement of Left Hip Joint with Metal on Polyethylene Synthetic Substitute, Cemented, Open Approach

ØSRBØ2A Replacement of Left Hip Joint with Metal on Polyethylene Synthetic Substitute, Uncemented, Open Approach

ØSRBØ2Z Replacement of Left Hip Joint with Metal on Polyethylene Synthetic Substitute, Open Approach

ØSRBØ39 Replacement of Left Hip Joint with Ceramic Synthetic Substitute, Cemented, Open Approach

ØSRBØ3A Replacement of Left Hip Joint with Ceramic Synthetic Substitute, Uncemented, Open Approach

ØSRBØ3Z Replacement of Left Hip Joint with Ceramic Synthetic Substitute, Open Approach

ØSRBØ49 Replacement of Left Hip Joint with Ceramic on Polyethylene Synthetic Substitute, Cemented, Open Approach

ØSRBØ4A Replacement of Left Hip Joint with Ceramic on Polyethylene Synthetic Substitute, Uncemented, Open Approach

ØSRBØ4Z Replacement of Left Hip Joint with Ceramic on Polyethylene Synthetic Substitute, Open Approach

ØSRBØ69 Replacement of Left Hip Joint with Oxidized Zirconium on Polyethylene Synthetic Substitute, Cemented, Open Approach

ØSRBØ6A Replacement of Left Hip Joint with Oxidized Zirconium on Polyethylene Synthetic Substitute, Uncemented, Open Approach

ØSRBØ6Z Replacement of Left Hip Joint with Oxidized Zirconium on Polyethylene Synthetic Substitute, Open Approach

ØSRBØ7Z Replacement of Left Hip Joint with Autologous Tissue Substitute, Open Approach

ØSRBØEZ Replacement of Left Hip Joint with Articulating Spacer, Open Approach

ØSRBØJ9 Replacement of Left Hip Joint with Synthetic Substitute, Cemented, Open Approach

ØSRBØJA Replacement of Left Hip Joint with Synthetic Substitute, Uncemented, Open Approach

ØSRBØJZ Replacement of Left Hip Joint with Synthetic Substitute, Open Approach

ØSRBØKZ Replacement of Left Hip Joint with Nonautologous Tissue Substitute, Open Approach

ØSRCØ69 Replacement of Right Knee Joint with Oxidized Zirconium on Polyethylene Synthetic Substitute, Cemented, Open Approach

ØSRCØ6A Replacement of Right Knee Joint with Oxidized Zirconium on Polyethylene Synthetic Substitute, Uncemented, Open Approach

ØSRCØ6Z Replacement of Right Knee Joint with Oxidized Zirconium on Polyethylene Synthetic Substitute, Open Approach

ØSRCØ7Z Replacement of Right Knee Joint with Autologous Tissue Substitute, Open Approach

ØSRCØEZ Replacement of Right Knee Joint with Articulating Spacer, Open Approach

ØSRCØJ9 Replacement of Right Knee Joint with Synthetic Substitute, Cemented, Open Approach

ØSRCØJA Replacement of Right Knee Joint with Synthetic Substitute, Uncemented, Open Approach

ØSRCØJZ Replacement of Right Knee Joint with Synthetic Substitute, Open Approach

ØSRCØKZ Replacement of Right Knee Joint with Nonautologous Tissue Substitute, Open Approach

ØSRCØL9 Replacement of Right Knee Joint with Medial Unicondylar Synthetic Substitute, Cemented, Open Approach

ØSRCØLA Replacement of Right Knee Joint with Medial Unicondylar Synthetic Substitute, Uncemented, Open Approach

ØSRCØLZ Replacement of Right Knee Joint with Medial Unicondylar Synthetic Substitute, Open Approach

ØSRCØM9 Replacement of Right Knee Joint with Lateral Unicondylar Synthetic Substitute, Cemented, Open Approach

ØSRCØMA Replacement of Right Knee Joint with Lateral Unicondylar Synthetic Substitute, Uncemented, Open Approach

ØSRCØMZ Replacement of Right Knee Joint with Lateral Unicondylar Synthetic Substitute, Open Approach

ØSRCØN9 Replacement of Right Knee Joint with Patellofemoral Synthetic Substitute, Cemented, Open Approach

ØSRCØNA Replacement of Right Knee Joint with Patellofemoral Synthetic Substitute, Uncemented, Open Approach

ØSRCØNZ Replacement of Right Knee Joint with Patellofemoral Synthetic Substitute, Open Approach

ØSRDØ69 Replacement of Left Knee Joint with Oxidized Zirconium on Polyethylene Synthetic Substitute, Cemented, Open Approach

ØSRDØ6A Replacement of Left Knee Joint with Oxidized Zirconium on Polyethylene Synthetic Substitute, Uncemented, Open Approach

ØSRDØ6Z Replacement of Left Knee Joint with Oxidized Zirconium on Polyethylene Synthetic Substitute, Open Approach

ØSRDØ7Z Replacement of Left Knee Joint with Autologous Tissue Substitute, Open Approach

ØSRDØEZ Replacement of Left Knee Joint with Articulating Spacer, Open Approach

ØSRDØJ9 Replacement of Left Knee Joint with Synthetic Substitute, Cemented, Open Approach

ØSRDØJA Replacement of Left Knee Joint with Synthetic Substitute, Uncemented, Open Approach

ØSRDØJZ Replacement of Left Knee Joint with Synthetic Substitute, Open Approach

ØSRDØKZ Replacement of Left Knee Joint with Nonautologous Tissue Substitute, Open Approach

ØSRDØL9 Replacement of Left Knee Joint with Medial Unicondylar Synthetic Substitute, Cemented, Open Approach

ØSRDØLA Replacement of Left Knee Joint with Medial Unicondylar Synthetic Substitute, Uncemented, Open Approach

ØSRDØLZ Replacement of Left Knee Joint with Medial Unicondylar Synthetic Substitute, Open Approach

ØSRDØM9 Replacement of Left Knee Joint with Lateral Unicondylar Synthetic Substitute, Cemented, Open Approach

ØSRDØMA Replacement of Left Knee Joint with Lateral Unicondylar Synthetic Substitute, Uncemented, Open Approach

ØSRDØMZ Replacement of Left Knee Joint with Lateral Unicondylar Synthetic Substitute, Open Approach

ØSRDØN9 Replacement of Left Knee Joint with Patellofemoral Synthetic Substitute, Cemented, Open Approach

HAC 10: Deep Vein Thrombosis (DVT) or Pulmonary Embolism (PE) with Total Knee or Hip Replacement (continued)

ØSRDØNA Replacement of Left Knee Joint with Patellofemoral Synthetic Substitute, Uncemented, Open Approach

ØSRDØNZ Replacement of Left Knee Joint with Patellofemoral Synthetic Substitute, Open Approach

ØSRE009 Replacement of Left Hip Joint, Acetabular Surface with Polyethylene Synthetic Substitute, Cemented, Open Approach

ØSRE00A Replacement of Left Hip Joint, Acetabular Surface with Polyethylene Synthetic Substitute, Uncemented, Open Approach

ØSRE00Z Replacement of Left Hip Joint, Acetabular Surface with Polyethylene Synthetic Substitute, Open Approach

ØSRE019 Replacement of Left Hip Joint, Acetabular Surface with Metal Synthetic Substitute, Cemented, Open Approach

ØSRE01A Replacement of Left Hip Joint, Acetabular Surface with Metal Synthetic Substitute, Uncemented, Open Approach

ØSRE01Z Replacement of Left Hip Joint, Acetabular Surface with Metal Synthetic Substitute, Open Approach

ØSRE039 Replacement of Left Hip Joint, Acetabular Surface with Ceramic Synthetic Substitute, Cemented, Open Approach

ØSRE03A Replacement of Left Hip Joint, Acetabular Surface with Ceramic Synthetic Substitute, Uncemented, Open Approach

ØSRE03Z Replacement of Left Hip Joint, Acetabular Surface with Ceramic Synthetic Substitute, Open Approach

ØSRE07Z Replacement of Left Hip Joint, Acetabular Surface with Autologous Tissue Substitute, Open Approach

ØSRE0J9 Replacement of Left Hip Joint, Acetabular Surface with Synthetic Substitute, Cemented, Open Approach

ØSRE0JA Replacement of Left Hip Joint, Acetabular Surface with Synthetic Substitute, Uncemented, Open Approach

ØSRE0JZ Replacement of Left Hip Joint, Acetabular Surface with Synthetic Substitute, Open Approach

ØSRE0KZ Replacement of Left Hip Joint, Acetabular Surface with Nonautologous Tissue Substitute, Open Approach

ØSRR019 Replacement of Right Hip Joint, Femoral Surface with Metal Synthetic Substitute, Cemented, Open Approach

ØSRR01A Replacement of Right Hip Joint, Femoral Surface with Metal Synthetic Substitute, Uncemented, Open Approach

ØSRR01Z Replacement of Right Hip Joint, Femoral Surface with Metal Synthetic Substitute, Open Approach

ØSRR039 Replacement of Right Hip Joint, Femoral Surface with Ceramic Synthetic Substitute, Cemented, Open Approach

ØSRR03A Replacement of Right Hip Joint, Femoral Surface with Ceramic Synthetic Substitute, Uncemented, Open Approach

ØSRR03Z Replacement of Right Hip Joint, Femoral Surface with Ceramic Synthetic Substitute, Open Approach

ØSRR07Z Replacement of Right Hip Joint, Femoral Surface with Autologous Tissue Substitute, Open Approach

ØSRR0J9 Replacement of Right Hip Joint, Femoral Surface with Synthetic Substitute, Cemented, Open Approach

ØSRR0JA Replacement of Right Hip Joint, Femoral Surface with Synthetic Substitute, Uncemented, Open Approach

ØSRR0JZ Replacement of Right Hip Joint, Femoral Surface with Synthetic Substitute, Open Approach

ØSRR0KZ Replacement of Right Hip Joint, Femoral Surface with Nonautologous Tissue Substitute, Open Approach

ØSRS019 Replacement of Left Hip Joint, Femoral Surface with Metal Synthetic Substitute, Cemented, Open Approach

ØSRS01A Replacement of Left Hip Joint, Femoral Surface with Metal Synthetic Substitute, Uncemented, Open Approach

ØSRS01Z Replacement of Left Hip Joint, Femoral Surface with Metal Synthetic Substitute, Open Approach

ØSRS039 Replacement of Left Hip Joint, Femoral Surface with Ceramic Synthetic Substitute, Cemented, Open Approach

ØSRS03A Replacement of Left Hip Joint, Femoral Surface with Ceramic Synthetic Substitute, Uncemented, Open Approach

ØSRS03Z Replacement of Left Hip Joint, Femoral Surface with Ceramic Synthetic Substitute, Open Approach

ØSRS07Z Replacement of Left Hip Joint, Femoral Surface with Autologous Tissue Substitute, Open Approach

ØSRS0J9 Replacement of Left Hip Joint, Femoral Surface with Synthetic Substitute, Cemented, Open Approach

ØSRS0JA Replacement of Left Hip Joint, Femoral Surface with Synthetic Substitute, Uncemented, Open Approach

ØSRS0JZ Replacement of Left Hip Joint, Femoral Surface with Synthetic Substitute, Open Approach

ØSRS0KZ Replacement of Left Hip Joint, Femoral Surface with Nonautologous Tissue Substitute, Open Approach

ØSRT07Z Replacement of Right Knee Joint, Femoral Surface with Autologous Tissue Substitute, Open Approach

ØSRT0J9 Replacement of Right Knee Joint, Femoral Surface with Synthetic Substitute, Cemented, Open Approach

ØSRT0JA Replacement of Right Knee Joint, Femoral Surface with Synthetic Substitute, Uncemented, Open Approach

ØSRT0JZ Replacement of Right Knee Joint, Femoral Surface with Synthetic Substitute, Open Approach

ØSRT0KZ Replacement of Right Knee Joint, Femoral Surface with Nonautologous Tissue Substitute, Open Approach

ØSRU07Z Replacement of Left Knee Joint, Femoral Surface with Autologous Tissue Substitute, Open Approach

ØSRU0J9 Replacement of Left Knee Joint, Femoral Surface with Synthetic Substitute, Cemented, Open Approach

ØSRU0JA Replacement of Left Knee Joint, Femoral Surface with Synthetic Substitute, Uncemented, Open Approach

ØSRU0JZ Replacement of Left Knee Joint, Femoral Surface with Synthetic Substitute, Open Approach

ØSRU0KZ Replacement of Left Knee Joint, Femoral Surface with Nonautologous Tissue Substitute, Open Approach

ØSRV07Z Replacement of Right Knee Joint, Tibial Surface with Autologous Tissue Substitute, Open Approach

ØSRV0J9 Replacement of Right Knee Joint, Tibial Surface with Synthetic Substitute, Cemented, Open Approach

ØSRV0JA Replacement of Right Knee Joint, Tibial Surface with Synthetic Substitute, Uncemented, Open Approach

ØSRV0JZ Replacement of Right Knee Joint, Tibial Surface with Synthetic Substitute, Open Approach

ØSRV0KZ Replacement of Right Knee Joint, Tibial Surface with Nonautologous Tissue Substitute, Open Approach

ØSRW07Z Replacement of Left Knee Joint, Tibial Surface with Autologous Tissue Substitute, Open Approach

ØSRW0J9 Replacement of Left Knee Joint, Tibial Surface with Synthetic Substitute, Cemented, Open Approach

ØSRW0JA Replacement of Left Knee Joint, Tibial Surface with Synthetic Substitute, Uncemented, Open Approach

ØSRW0JZ Replacement of Left Knee Joint, Tibial Surface with Synthetic Substitute, Open Approach

ØSRW0KZ Replacement of Left Knee Joint, Tibial Surface with Nonautologous Tissue Substitute, Open Approach

ØSU90BZ Supplement Right Hip Joint with Resurfacing Device, Open Approach

ØSUA0BZ Supplement Right Hip Joint, Acetabular Surface with Resurfacing Device, Open Approach

ØSUB0BZ Supplement Left Hip Joint with Resurfacing Device, Open Approach

ØSUE0BZ Supplement Left Hip Joint, Acetabular Surface with Resurfacing Device, Open Approach

ØSUR0BZ Supplement Right Hip Joint, Femoral Surface with Resurfacing Device, Open Approach

ØSUS0BZ Supplement Left Hip Joint, Femoral Surface with Resurfacing Device, Open Approach

HAC 11: Surgical Site Infection-Bariatric Surgery

Principal diagnosis of:
E66.01

AND

Secondary diagnosis not POA:
K68.11
K95.01
K95.81
T81.40XA
T81.41XA
T81.42XA
T81.43XA
T81.44XA
T81.49XA

AND

Any of the following procedures:

ØD16079 Bypass Stomach to Duodenum with Autologous Tissue Substitute, Open Approach

ØD1607A Bypass Stomach to Jejunum with Autologous Tissue Substitute, Open Approach

HAC 11: Surgical Site Infection-Bariatric Surgery (continued)

ØD16Ø7B Bypass Stomach to Ileum with Autologous Tissue Substitute, Open Approach

ØD16Ø7L Bypass Stomach to Transverse Colon with Autologous Tissue Substitute, Open Approach

ØD16ØJ9 Bypass Stomach to Duodenum with Synthetic Substitute, Open Approach

ØD16ØJA Bypass Stomach to Jejunum with Synthetic Substitute, Open Approach

ØD16ØJB Bypass Stomach to Ileum with Synthetic Substitute, Open Approach

ØD16ØJL Bypass Stomach to Transverse Colon with Synthetic Substitute, Open Approach

ØD16ØK9 Bypass Stomach to Duodenum with Nonautologous Tissue Substitute, Open Approach

ØD16ØKA Bypass Stomach to Jejunum with Nonautologous Tissue Substitute, Open Approach

ØD16ØKB Bypass Stomach to Ileum with Nonautologous Tissue Substitute, Open Approach

ØD16ØKL Bypass Stomach to Transverse Colon with Nonautologous Tissue Substitute, Open Approach

ØD16ØZ9 Bypass Stomach to Duodenum, Open Approach

ØD16ØZA Bypass Stomach to Jejunum, Open Approach

ØD16ØZB Bypass Stomach to Ileum, Open Approach

ØD16ØZL Bypass Stomach to Transverse Colon, Open Approach

ØD16479 Bypass Stomach to Duodenum with Autologous Tissue Substitute, Percutaneous Endoscopic Approach

ØD1647A Bypass Stomach to Jejunum with Autologous Tissue Substitute, Percutaneous Endoscopic Approach

ØD1647B Bypass Stomach to Ileum with Autologous Tissue Substitute, Percutaneous Endoscopic Approach

ØD1647L Bypass Stomach to Transverse Colon with Autologous Tissue Substitute, Percutaneous Endoscopic Approach

ØD164J9 Bypass Stomach to Duodenum with Synthetic Substitute, Percutaneous Endoscopic Approach

ØD164JA Bypass Stomach to Jejunum with Synthetic Substitute, Percutaneous Endoscopic Approach

ØD164JB Bypass Stomach to Ileum with Synthetic Substitute, Percutaneous Endoscopic Approach

ØD164JL Bypass Stomach to Transverse Colon with Synthetic Substitute, Percutaneous Endoscopic Approach

ØD164K9 Bypass Stomach to Duodenum with Nonautologous Tissue Substitute, Percutaneous Endoscopic Approach

ØD164KA Bypass Stomach to Jejunum with Nonautologous Tissue Substitute, Percutaneous Endoscopic Approach

ØD164KB Bypass Stomach to Ileum with Nonautologous Tissue Substitute, Percutaneous Endoscopic Approach

ØD164KL Bypass Stomach to Transverse Colon with Nonautologous Tissue Substitute, Percutaneous Endoscopic Approach

ØD164Z9 Bypass Stomach to Duodenum, Percutaneous Endoscopic Approach

ØD164ZA Bypass Stomach to Jejunum, Percutaneous Endoscopic Approach

ØD164ZB Bypass Stomach to Ileum, Percutaneous Endoscopic Approach

ØD164ZL Bypass Stomach to Transverse Colon, Percutaneous Endoscopic Approach

ØD16879 Bypass Stomach to Duodenum with Autologous Tissue Substitute, Via Natural or Artificial Opening Endoscopic

ØD1687A Bypass Stomach to Jejunum with Autologous Tissue Substitute, Via Natural or Artificial Opening Endoscopic

ØD1687B Bypass Stomach to Ileum with Autologous Tissue Substitute, Via Natural or Artificial Opening Endoscopic

ØD1687L Bypass Stomach to Transverse Colon with Autologous Tissue Substitute, Via Natural or Artificial Opening Endoscopic

ØD168J9 Bypass Stomach to Duodenum with Synthetic Substitute, Via Natural or Artificial Opening Endoscopic

ØD168JA Bypass Stomach to Jejunum with Synthetic Substitute, Via Natural or Artificial Opening Endoscopic

ØD168JB Bypass Stomach to Ileum with Synthetic Substitute, Via Natural or Artificial Opening Endoscopic

ØD168JL Bypass Stomach to Transverse Colon with Synthetic Substitute, Via Natural or Artificial Opening Endoscopic

ØD168K9 Bypass Stomach to Duodenum with Nonautologous Tissue Substitute, Via Natural or Artificial Opening Endoscopic

ØD168KA Bypass Stomach to Jejunum with Nonautologous Tissue Substitute, Via Natural or Artificial Opening Endoscopic

ØD168KB Bypass Stomach to Ileum with Nonautologous Tissue Substitute, Via Natural or Artificial Opening Endoscopic

ØD168KL Bypass Stomach to Transverse Colon with Nonautologous Tissue Substitute, Via Natural or Artificial Opening Endoscopic

ØD168Z9 Bypass Stomach to Duodenum, Via Natural or Artificial Opening Endoscopic

ØD168ZA Bypass Stomach to Jejunum, Via Natural or Artificial Opening Endoscopic

ØD168ZB Bypass Stomach to Ileum, Via Natural or Artificial Opening Endoscopic

ØD168ZL Bypass Stomach to Transverse Colon, Via Natural or Artificial Opening Endoscopic

ØDV64CZ Restriction of Stomach with Extraluminal Device, Percutaneous Endoscopic Approach

HAC 12: Surgical Site Infection-Certain Orthopedic Procedures of the Spine, Shoulder, and Elbow

Secondary diagnosis not POA:

K68.11
T81.4ØXA
T81.41XA
T81.42XA
T81.43XA
T81.44XA
T81.49XA
T84.6ØXA
T84.61ØA
T84.611A
T84.612A
T84.613A
T84.614A
T84.615A
T84.619A
T84.63XA
T84.69XA

T84.7XXA

AND

Any of the following procedures:

ØRG0070 Fusion of Occipital-cervical Joint with Autologous Tissue Substitute, Anterior Approach, Anterior Column, Open Approach

ØRG0071 Fusion of Occipital-cervical Joint with Autologous Tissue Substitute, Posterior Approach, Posterior Column, Open Approach

ØRG007J Fusion of Occipital-cervical Joint with Autologous Tissue Substitute, Posterior Approach, Anterior Column, Open Approach

ØRG00A0 Fusion of Occipital-cervical Joint with Interbody Fusion Device, Anterior Approach, Anterior Column, Open Approach

ØRG00AJ Fusion of Occipital-cervical Joint with Interbody Fusion Device, Posterior Approach, Anterior Column, Open Approach

ØRG00J0 Fusion of Occipital-cervical Joint with Synthetic Substitute, Anterior Approach, Anterior Column, Open Approach

ØRG00J1 Fusion of Occipital-cervical Joint with Synthetic Substitute, Posterior Approach, Posterior Column, Open Approach

ØRG00JJ Fusion of Occipital-cervical Joint with Synthetic Substitute, Posterior Approach, Anterior Column, Open Approach

ØRG00K0 Fusion of Occipital-cervical Joint with Nonautologous Tissue Substitute, Anterior Approach, Anterior Column, Open Approach

ØRG00K1 Fusion of Occipital-cervical Joint with Nonautologous Tissue Substitute, Posterior Approach, Posterior Column, Open Approach

ØRG00KJ Fusion of Occipital-cervical Joint with Nonautologous Tissue Substitute, Posterior Approach, Anterior Column, Open Approach

ØRG0370 Fusion of Occipital-cervical Joint with Autologous Tissue Substitute, Anterior Approach, Anterior Column, Percutaneous Approach

ØRG0371 Fusion of Occipital-cervical Joint with Autologous Tissue Substitute, Posterior Approach, Posterior Column, Percutaneous Approach

ØRG037J Fusion of Occipital-cervical Joint with Autologous Tissue Substitute, Posterior Approach, Anterior Column, Percutaneous Approach

ØRG03A0 Fusion of Occipital-cervical Joint with Interbody Fusion Device, Anterior Approach, Anterior Column, Percutaneous Approach

ØRG03AJ Fusion of Occipital-cervical Joint with Interbody Fusion Device, Posterior Approach, Anterior Column, Percutaneous Approach

ØRG03J0 Fusion of Occipital-cervical Joint with Synthetic Substitute, Anterior Approach, Anterior Column, Percutaneous Approach

ØRG03J1 Fusion of Occipital-cervical Joint with Synthetic Substitute, Posterior Approach, Posterior Column, Percutaneous Approach

HAC 12: Surgical Site Infection-Certain Orthopedic Procedures of the Spine, Shoulder, and Elbow (continued)

ØRGØ3JJ Fusion of Occipital-cervical Joint with Synthetic Substitute, Posterior Approach, Anterior Column, Percutaneous Approach

ØRGØ3KØ Fusion of Occipital-cervical Joint with Nonautologous Tissue Substitute, Anterior Approach, Anterior Column, Percutaneous Approach

ØRGØ3K1 Fusion of Occipital-cervical Joint with Nonautologous Tissue Substitute, Posterior Approach, Posterior Column, Percutaneous Approach

ØRGØ3KJ Fusion of Occipital-cervical Joint with Nonautologous Tissue Substitute, Posterior Approach, Anterior Column, Percutaneous Approach

ØRGØ47Ø Fusion of Occipital-cervical Joint with Autologous Tissue Substitute, Anterior Approach, Anterior Column, Percutaneous Endoscopic Approach

ØRGØ471 Fusion of Occipital-cervical Joint with Autologous Tissue Substitute, Posterior Approach, Posterior Column, Percutaneous Endoscopic Approach

ØRGØ47J Fusion of Occipital-cervical Joint with Autologous Tissue Substitute, Posterior Approach, Anterior Column, Percutaneous Endoscopic Approach

ØRGØ4AØ Fusion of Occipital-cervical Joint with Interbody Fusion Device, Anterior Approach, Anterior Column, Percutaneous Endoscopic Approach

ØRGØ4AJ Fusion of Occipital-cervical Joint with Interbody Fusion Device, Posterior Approach, Anterior Column, Percutaneous Endoscopic Approach

ØRGØ4JØ Fusion of Occipital-cervical Joint with Synthetic Substitute, Anterior Approach, Anterior Column, Percutaneous Endoscopic Approach

ØRGØ4J1 Fusion of Occipital-cervical Joint with Synthetic Substitute, Posterior Approach, Posterior Column, Percutaneous Endoscopic Approach

ØRGØ4JJ Fusion of Occipital-cervical Joint with Synthetic Substitute, Posterior Approach, Anterior Column, Percutaneous Endoscopic Approach

ØRGØ4KØ Fusion of Occipital-cervical Joint with Nonautologous Tissue Substitute, Anterior Approach, Anterior Column, Percutaneous Endoscopic Approach

ØRGØ4K1 Fusion of Occipital-cervical Joint with Nonautologous Tissue Substitute, Posterior Approach, Posterior Column, Percutaneous Endoscopic Approach

ØRGØ4KJ Fusion of Occipital-cervical Joint with Nonautologous Tissue Substitute, Posterior Approach, Anterior Column, Percutaneous Endoscopic Approach

ØRG1Ø7Ø Fusion of Cervical Vertebral Joint with Autologous Tissue Substitute, Anterior Approach, Anterior Column, Open Approach

ØRG1Ø71 Fusion of Cervical Vertebral Joint with Autologous Tissue Substitute, Posterior Approach, Posterior Column, Open Approach

ØRG1Ø7J Fusion of Cervical Vertebral Joint with Autologous Tissue Substitute, Posterior Approach, Anterior Column, Open Approach

ØRG1ØAØ Fusion of Cervical Vertebral Joint with Interbody Fusion Device, Anterior Approach, Anterior Column, Open Approach

ØRG1ØAJ Fusion of Cervical Vertebral Joint with Interbody Fusion Device, Posterior Approach, Anterior Column, Open Approach

ØRG1ØJØ Fusion of Cervical Vertebral Joint with Synthetic Substitute, Anterior Approach, Anterior Column, Open Approach

ØRG1ØJ1 Fusion of Cervical Vertebral Joint with Synthetic Substitute, Posterior Approach, Posterior Column, Open Approach

ØRG1ØJJ Fusion of Cervical Vertebral Joint with Synthetic Substitute, Posterior Approach, Anterior Column, Open Approach

ØRG1ØKØ Fusion of Cervical Vertebral Joint with Nonautologous Tissue Substitute, Anterior Approach, Anterior Column, Open Approach

ØRG1ØK1 Fusion of Cervical Vertebral Joint with Nonautologous Tissue Substitute, Posterior Approach, Posterior Column, Open Approach

ØRG1ØKJ Fusion of Cervical Vertebral Joint with Nonautologous Tissue Substitute, Posterior Approach, Anterior Column, Open Approach

ØRG137Ø Fusion of Cervical Vertebral Joint with Autologous Tissue Substitute, Anterior Approach, Anterior Column, Percutaneous Approach

ØRG1371 Fusion of Cervical Vertebral Joint with Autologous Tissue Substitute, Posterior Approach, Posterior Column, Percutaneous Approach

ØRG137J Fusion of Cervical Vertebral Joint with Autologous Tissue Substitute, Posterior Approach, Anterior Column, Percutaneous Approach

ØRG13AØ Fusion of Cervical Vertebral Joint with Interbody Fusion Device, Anterior Approach, Anterior Column, Percutaneous Approach

ØRG13AJ Fusion of Cervical Vertebral Joint with Interbody Fusion Device, Posterior Approach, Anterior Column, Percutaneous Approach

ØRG13JØ Fusion of Cervical Vertebral Joint with Synthetic Substitute, Anterior Approach, Anterior Column, Percutaneous Approach

ØRG13J1 Fusion of Cervical Vertebral Joint with Synthetic Substitute, Posterior Approach, Posterior Column, Percutaneous Approach

ØRG13JJ Fusion of Cervical Vertebral Joint with Synthetic Substitute, Posterior Approach, Anterior Column, Percutaneous Approach

ØRG13KØ Fusion of Cervical Vertebral Joint with Nonautologous Tissue Substitute, Anterior Approach, Anterior Column, Percutaneous Approach

ØRG13K1 Fusion of Cervical Vertebral Joint with Nonautologous Tissue Substitute, Posterior Approach, Posterior Column, Percutaneous Approach

ØRG13KJ Fusion of Cervical Vertebral Joint with Nonautologous Tissue Substitute, Posterior Approach, Anterior Column, Percutaneous Approach

ØRG147Ø Fusion of Cervical Vertebral Joint with Autologous Tissue Substitute, Anterior Approach, Anterior Column, Percutaneous Endoscopic Approach

ØRG1471 Fusion of Cervical Vertebral Joint with Autologous Tissue Substitute, Posterior Approach, Posterior Column, Percutaneous Endoscopic Approach

ØRG147J Fusion of Cervical Vertebral Joint with Autologous Tissue Substitute, Posterior Approach, Anterior Column, Percutaneous Endoscopic Approach

ØRG14AØ Fusion of Cervical Vertebral Joint with Interbody Fusion Device, Anterior Approach, Anterior Column, Percutaneous Endoscopic Approach

ØRG14AJ Fusion of Cervical Vertebral Joint with Interbody Fusion Device, Posterior Approach, Anterior Column, Percutaneous Endoscopic Approach

ØRG14JØ Fusion of Cervical Vertebral Joint with Synthetic Substitute, Anterior Approach, Anterior Column, Percutaneous Endoscopic Approach

ØRG14J1 Fusion of Cervical Vertebral Joint with Synthetic Substitute, Posterior Approach, Posterior Column, Percutaneous Endoscopic Approach

ØRG14JJ Fusion of Cervical Vertebral Joint with Synthetic Substitute, Posterior Approach, Anterior Column, Percutaneous Endoscopic Approach

ØRG14KØ Fusion of Cervical Vertebral Joint with Nonautologous Tissue Substitute, Anterior Approach, Anterior Column, Percutaneous Endoscopic Approach

ØRG14K1 Fusion of Cervical Vertebral Joint with Nonautologous Tissue Substitute, Posterior Approach, Posterior Column, Percutaneous Endoscopic Approach

ØRG14KJ Fusion of Cervical Vertebral Joint with Nonautologous Tissue Substitute, Posterior Approach, Anterior Column, Percutaneous Endoscopic Approach

ØRG2Ø7Ø Fusion of 2 or more Cervical Vertebral Joints with Autologous Tissue Substitute, Anterior Approach, Anterior Column, Open Approach

ØRG2Ø71 Fusion of 2 or more Cervical Vertebral Joints with Autologous Tissue Substitute, Posterior Approach, Posterior Column, Open Approach

ØRG2Ø7J Fusion of 2 or more Cervical Vertebral Joints with Autologous Tissue Substitute, Posterior Approach, Anterior Column, Open Approach

ØRG2ØAØ Fusion of 2 or more Cervical Vertebral Joints with Interbody Fusion Device, Anterior Approach, Anterior Column, Open Approach

ØRG2ØAJ Fusion of 2 or more Cervical Vertebral Joints with Interbody Fusion Device, Posterior Approach, Anterior Column, Open Approach

ØRG2ØJØ Fusion of 2 or more Cervical Vertebral Joints with Synthetic Substitute, Anterior Approach, Anterior Column, Open Approach

ØRG2ØJ1 Fusion of 2 or more Cervical Vertebral Joints with Synthetic Substitute, Posterior Approach, Posterior Column, Open Approach

ØRG2ØJJ Fusion of 2 or more Cervical Vertebral Joints with Synthetic Substitute, Posterior Approach, Anterior Column, Open Approach

HAC 12: Surgical Site Infection–Certain Orthopedic Procedures of the Spine, Shoulder, and Elbow (continued)

ØRG20KØ   Fusion of 2 or more Cervical Vertebral Joints with Nonautologous Tissue Substitute, Anterior Approach, Anterior Column, Open Approach

ØRG20K1   Fusion of 2 or more Cervical Vertebral Joints with Nonautologous Tissue Substitute, Posterior Approach, Posterior Column, Open Approach

ØRG20KJ   Fusion of 2 or more Cervical Vertebral Joints with Nonautologous Tissue Substitute, Posterior Approach, Anterior Column, Open Approach

ØRG237Ø   Fusion of 2 or more Cervical Vertebral Joints with Autologous Tissue Substitute, Anterior Approach, Anterior Column, Percutaneous Approach

ØRG2371   Fusion of 2 or more Cervical Vertebral Joints with Autologous Tissue Substitute, Posterior Approach, Posterior Column, Percutaneous Approach

ØRG237J   Fusion of 2 or more Cervical Vertebral Joints with Autologous Tissue Substitute, Posterior Approach, Anterior Column, Percutaneous Approach

ØRG23AØ   Fusion of 2 or more Cervical Vertebral Joints with Interbody Fusion Device, Anterior Approach, Anterior Column, Percutaneous Approach

ØRG23AJ   Fusion of 2 or more Cervical Vertebral Joints with Interbody Fusion Device, Posterior Approach, Anterior Column, Percutaneous Approach

ØRG23JØ   Fusion of 2 or more Cervical Vertebral Joints with Synthetic Substitute, Anterior Approach, Anterior Column, Percutaneous Approach

ØRG23J1   Fusion of 2 or more Cervical Vertebral Joints with Synthetic Substitute, Posterior Approach, Posterior Column, Percutaneous Approach

ØRG23JJ   Fusion of 2 or more Cervical Vertebral Joints with Synthetic Substitute, Posterior Approach, Anterior Column, Percutaneous Approach

ØRG23KØ   Fusion of 2 or more Cervical Vertebral Joints with Nonautologous Tissue Substitute, Anterior Approach, Anterior Column, Percutaneous Approach

ØRG23K1   Fusion of 2 or more Cervical Vertebral Joints with Nonautologous Tissue Substitute, Posterior Approach, Posterior Column, Percutaneous Approach

ØRG23KJ   Fusion of 2 or more Cervical Vertebral Joints with Nonautologous Tissue Substitute, Posterior Approach, Anterior Column, Percutaneous Approach

ØRG247Ø   Fusion of 2 or more Cervical Vertebral Joints with Autologous Tissue Substitute, Anterior Approach, Anterior Column, Percutaneous Endoscopic Approach

ØRG2471   Fusion of 2 or more Cervical Vertebral Joints with Autologous Tissue Substitute, Posterior Approach, Posterior Column, Percutaneous Endoscopic Approach

ØRG247J   Fusion of 2 or more Cervical Vertebral Joints with Autologous Tissue Substitute, Posterior Approach, Anterior Column, Percutaneous Endoscopic Approach

ØRG24AØ   Fusion of 2 or more Cervical Vertebral Joints with Interbody Fusion Device, Anterior Approach, Anterior Column, Percutaneous Endoscopic Approach

ØRG24AJ   Fusion of 2 or more Cervical Vertebral Joints with Interbody Fusion Device, Posterior Approach, Anterior Column, Percutaneous Endoscopic Approach

ØRG24JØ   Fusion of 2 or more Cervical Vertebral Joints with Synthetic Substitute, Anterior Approach, Anterior Column, Percutaneous Endoscopic Approach

ØRG24J1   Fusion of 2 or more Cervical Vertebral Joints with Synthetic Substitute, Posterior Approach, Posterior Column, Percutaneous Endoscopic Approach

ØRG24JJ   Fusion of 2 or more Cervical Vertebral Joints with Synthetic Substitute, Posterior Approach, Anterior Column, Percutaneous Endoscopic Approach

ØRG24KØ   Fusion of 2 or more Cervical Vertebral Joints with Nonautologous Tissue Substitute, Anterior Approach, Anterior Column, Percutaneous Endoscopic Approach

ØRG24K1   Fusion of 2 or more Cervical Vertebral Joints with Nonautologous Tissue Substitute, Posterior Approach, Posterior Column, Percutaneous Endoscopic Approach

ØRG24KJ   Fusion of 2 or more Cervical Vertebral Joints with Nonautologous Tissue Substitute, Posterior Approach, Anterior Column, Percutaneous Endoscopic Approach

ØRG4Ø7Ø   Fusion of Cervicothoracic Vertebral Joint with Autologous Tissue Substitute, Anterior Approach, Anterior Column, Open Approach

ØRG4Ø71   Fusion of Cervicothoracic Vertebral Joint with Autologous Tissue Substitute, Posterior Approach, Posterior Column, Open Approach

ØRG4Ø7J   Fusion of Cervicothoracic Vertebral Joint with Autologous Tissue Substitute, Posterior Approach, Anterior Column, Open Approach

ØRG4ØAØ   Fusion of Cervicothoracic Vertebral Joint with Interbody Fusion Device, Anterior Approach, Anterior Column, Open Approach

ØRG4ØAJ   Fusion of Cervicothoracic Vertebral Joint with Interbody Fusion Device, Posterior Approach, Anterior Column, Open Approach

ØRG4ØJØ   Fusion of Cervicothoracic Vertebral Joint with Synthetic Substitute, Anterior Approach, Anterior Column, Open Approach

ØRG4ØJ1   Fusion of Cervicothoracic Vertebral Joint with Synthetic Substitute, Posterior Approach, Posterior Column, Open Approach

ØRG4ØJJ   Fusion of Cervicothoracic Vertebral Joint with Synthetic Substitute, Posterior Approach, Anterior Column, Open Approach

ØRG4ØKØ   Fusion of Cervicothoracic Vertebral Joint with Nonautologous Tissue Substitute, Anterior Approach, Anterior Column, Open Approach

ØRG4ØK1   Fusion of Cervicothoracic Vertebral Joint with Nonautologous Tissue Substitute, Posterior Approach, Posterior Column, Open Approach

ØRG4ØKJ   Fusion of Cervicothoracic Vertebral Joint with Nonautologous Tissue Substitute, Posterior Approach, Anterior Column, Open Approach

ØRG437Ø   Fusion of Cervicothoracic Vertebral Joint with Autologous Tissue Substitute, Anterior Approach, Anterior Column, Percutaneous Approach

ØRG4371   Fusion of Cervicothoracic Vertebral Joint with Autologous Tissue Substitute, Posterior Approach, Posterior Column, Percutaneous Approach

ØRG437J   Fusion of Cervicothoracic Vertebral Joint with Autologous Tissue Substitute, Posterior Approach, Anterior Column, Percutaneous Approach

ØRG43AØ   Fusion of Cervicothoracic Vertebral Joint with Interbody Fusion Device, Anterior Approach, Anterior Column, Percutaneous Approach

ØRG43AJ   Fusion of Cervicothoracic Vertebral Joint with Interbody Fusion Device, Posterior Approach, Anterior Column, Percutaneous Approach

ØRG43JØ   Fusion of Cervicothoracic Vertebral Joint with Synthetic Substitute, Anterior Approach, Anterior Column, Percutaneous Approach

ØRG43J1   Fusion of Cervicothoracic Vertebral Joint with Synthetic Substitute, Posterior Approach, Posterior Column, Percutaneous Approach

ØRG43JJ   Fusion of Cervicothoracic Vertebral Joint with Synthetic Substitute, Posterior Approach, Anterior Column, Percutaneous Approach

ØRG43KØ   Fusion of Cervicothoracic Vertebral Joint with Nonautologous Tissue Substitute, Anterior Approach, Anterior Column, Percutaneous Approach

ØRG43K1   Fusion of Cervicothoracic Vertebral Joint with Nonautologous Tissue Substitute, Posterior Approach, Posterior Column, Percutaneous Approach

ØRG43KJ   Fusion of Cervicothoracic Vertebral Joint with Nonautologous Tissue Substitute, Posterior Approach, Anterior Column, Percutaneous Approach

ØRG447Ø   Fusion of Cervicothoracic Vertebral Joint with Autologous Tissue Substitute, Anterior Approach, Anterior Column, Percutaneous Endoscopic Approach

ØRG4471   Fusion of Cervicothoracic Vertebral Joint with Autologous Tissue Substitute, Posterior Approach, Posterior Column, Percutaneous Endoscopic Approach

ØRG447J   Fusion of Cervicothoracic Vertebral Joint with Autologous Tissue Substitute, Posterior Approach, Anterior Column, Percutaneous Endoscopic Approach

ØRG44AØ   Fusion of Cervicothoracic Vertebral Joint with Interbody Fusion Device, Anterior Approach, Anterior Column, Percutaneous Endoscopic Approach

ØRG44AJ   Fusion of Cervicothoracic Vertebral Joint with Interbody Fusion Device, Posterior Approach, Anterior Column, Percutaneous Endoscopic Approach

ØRG44JØ   Fusion of Cervicothoracic Vertebral Joint with Synthetic Substitute, Anterior Approach, Anterior Column, Percutaneous Endoscopic Approach

ØRG44J1   Fusion of Cervicothoracic Vertebral Joint with Synthetic Substitute, Posterior Approach, Posterior Column, Percutaneous Endoscopic Approach

HAC 12: Surgical Site Infection–Certain Orthopedic Procedures of the Spine, Shoulder, and Elbow (continued)

ØRG44JJ   Fusion of Cervicothoracic Vertebral Joint with Synthetic Substitute, Posterior Approach, Anterior Column, Percutaneous Endoscopic Approach

ØRG44KØ   Fusion of Cervicothoracic Vertebral Joint with Nonautologous Tissue Substitute, Anterior Approach, Anterior Column, Percutaneous Endoscopic Approach

ØRG44K1   Fusion of Cervicothoracic Vertebral Joint with Nonautologous Tissue Substitute, Posterior Approach, Posterior Column, Percutaneous Endoscopic Approach

ØRG44KJ   Fusion of Cervicothoracic Vertebral Joint with Nonautologous Tissue Substitute, Posterior Approach, Anterior Column, Percutaneous Endoscopic Approach

ØRG6070   Fusion of Thoracic Vertebral Joint with Autologous Tissue Substitute, Anterior Approach, Anterior Column, Open Approach

ØRG6071   Fusion of Thoracic Vertebral Joint with Autologous Tissue Substitute, Posterior Approach, Posterior Column, Open Approach

ØRG607J   Fusion of Thoracic Vertebral Joint with Autologous Tissue Substitute, Posterior Approach, Anterior Column, Open Approach

ØRG60AØ   Fusion of Thoracic Vertebral Joint with Interbody Fusion Device, Anterior Approach, Anterior Column, Open Approach

ØRG60AJ   Fusion of Thoracic Vertebral Joint with Interbody Fusion Device, Posterior Approach, Anterior Column, Open Approach

ØRG60JØ   Fusion of Thoracic Vertebral Joint with Synthetic Substitute, Anterior Approach, Anterior Column, Open Approach

ØRG60J1   Fusion of Thoracic Vertebral Joint with Synthetic Substitute, Posterior Approach, Posterior Column, Open Approach

ØRG60JJ   Fusion of Thoracic Vertebral Joint with Synthetic Substitute, Posterior Approach, Anterior Column, Open Approach

ØRG60KØ   Fusion of Thoracic Vertebral Joint with Nonautologous Tissue Substitute, Anterior Approach, Anterior Column, Open Approach

ØRG60K1   Fusion of Thoracic Vertebral Joint with Nonautologous Tissue Substitute, Posterior Approach, Posterior Column, Open Approach

ØRG60KJ   Fusion of Thoracic Vertebral Joint with Nonautologous Tissue Substitute, Posterior Approach, Anterior Column, Open Approach

ØRG6370   Fusion of Thoracic Vertebral Joint with Autologous Tissue Substitute, Anterior Approach, Anterior Column, Percutaneous Approach

ØRG6371   Fusion of Thoracic Vertebral Joint with Autologous Tissue Substitute, Posterior Approach, Posterior Column, Percutaneous Approach

ØRG637J   Fusion of Thoracic Vertebral Joint with Autologous Tissue Substitute, Posterior Approach, Anterior Column, Percutaneous Approach

ØRG63AØ   Fusion of Thoracic Vertebral Joint with Interbody Fusion Device, Anterior Approach, Anterior Column, Percutaneous Approach

ØRG63AJ   Fusion of Thoracic Vertebral Joint with Interbody Fusion Device, Posterior Approach, Anterior Column, Percutaneous Approach

ØRG63JØ   Fusion of Thoracic Vertebral Joint with Synthetic Substitute, Anterior Approach, Anterior Column, Percutaneous Approach

ØRG63J1   Fusion of Thoracic Vertebral Joint with Synthetic Substitute, Posterior Approach, Posterior Column, Percutaneous Approach

ØRG63JJ   Fusion of Thoracic Vertebral Joint with Synthetic Substitute, Posterior Approach, Anterior Column, Percutaneous Approach

ØRG63KØ   Fusion of Thoracic Vertebral Joint with Nonautologous Tissue Substitute, Anterior Approach, Anterior Column, Percutaneous Approach

ØRG63K1   Fusion of Thoracic Vertebral Joint with Nonautologous Tissue Substitute, Posterior Approach, Posterior Column, Percutaneous Approach

ØRG63KJ   Fusion of Thoracic Vertebral Joint with Nonautologous Tissue Substitute, Posterior Approach, Anterior Column, Percutaneous Approach

ØRG6470   Fusion of Thoracic Vertebral Joint with Autologous Tissue Substitute, Anterior Approach, Anterior Column, Percutaneous Endoscopic Approach

ØRG6471   Fusion of Thoracic Vertebral Joint with Autologous Tissue Substitute, Posterior Approach, Posterior Column, Percutaneous Endoscopic Approach

ØRG647J   Fusion of Thoracic Vertebral Joint with Autologous Tissue Substitute, Posterior Approach, Anterior Column, Percutaneous Endoscopic Approach

ØRG64AØ   Fusion of Thoracic Vertebral Joint with Interbody Fusion Device, Anterior Approach, Anterior Column, Percutaneous Endoscopic Approach

ØRG64AJ   Fusion of Thoracic Vertebral Joint with Interbody Fusion Device, Posterior Approach, Anterior Column, Percutaneous Endoscopic Approach

ØRG64JØ   Fusion of Thoracic Vertebral Joint with Synthetic Substitute, Anterior Approach, Anterior Column, Percutaneous Endoscopic Approach

ØRG64J1   Fusion of Thoracic Vertebral Joint with Synthetic Substitute, Posterior Approach, Posterior Column, Percutaneous Endoscopic Approach

ØRG64JJ   Fusion of Thoracic Vertebral Joint with Synthetic Substitute, Posterior Approach, Anterior Column, Percutaneous Endoscopic Approach

ØRG64KØ   Fusion of Thoracic Vertebral Joint with Nonautologous Tissue Substitute, Anterior Approach, Anterior Column, Percutaneous Endoscopic Approach

ØRG64K1   Fusion of Thoracic Vertebral Joint with Nonautologous Tissue Substitute, Posterior Approach, Posterior Column, Percutaneous Endoscopic Approach

ØRG64KJ   Fusion of Thoracic Vertebral Joint with Nonautologous Tissue Substitute, Posterior Approach, Anterior Column, Percutaneous Endoscopic Approach

ØRG7070   Fusion of 2 to 7 Thoracic Vertebral Joints with Autologous Tissue Substitute, Anterior Approach, Anterior Column, Open Approach

ØRG7071   Fusion of 2 to 7 Thoracic Vertebral Joints with Autologous Tissue Substitute, Posterior Approach, Posterior Column, Open Approach

ØRG707J   Fusion of 2 to 7 Thoracic Vertebral Joints with Autologous Tissue Substitute, Posterior Approach, Anterior Column, Open Approach

ØRG70AØ   Fusion of 2 to 7 Thoracic Vertebral Joints with Interbody Fusion Device, Anterior Approach, Anterior Column, Open Approach

ØRG70AJ   Fusion of 2 to 7 Thoracic Vertebral Joints with Interbody Fusion Device, Posterior Approach, Anterior Column, Open Approach

ØRG70JØ   Fusion of 2 to 7 Thoracic Vertebral Joints with Synthetic Substitute, Anterior Approach, Anterior Column, Open Approach

ØRG70J1   Fusion of 2 to 7 Thoracic Vertebral Joints with Synthetic Substitute, Posterior Approach, Posterior Column, Open Approach

ØRG70JJ   Fusion of 2 to 7 Thoracic Vertebral Joints with Synthetic Substitute, Posterior Approach, Anterior Column, Open Approach

ØRG70KØ   Fusion of 2 to 7 Thoracic Vertebral Joints with Nonautologous Tissue Substitute, Anterior Approach, Anterior Column, Open Approach

ØRG70K1   Fusion of 2 to 7 Thoracic Vertebral Joints with Nonautologous Tissue Substitute, Posterior Approach, Posterior Column, Open Approach

ØRG70KJ   Fusion of 2 to 7 Thoracic Vertebral Joints with Nonautologous Tissue Substitute, Posterior Approach, Anterior Column, Open Approach

ØRG7370   Fusion of 2 to 7 Thoracic Vertebral Joints with Autologous Tissue Substitute, Anterior Approach, Anterior Column, Percutaneous Approach

ØRG7371   Fusion of 2 to 7 Thoracic Vertebral Joints with Autologous Tissue Substitute, Posterior Approach, Posterior Column, Percutaneous Approach

ØRG737J   Fusion of 2 to 7 Thoracic Vertebral Joints with Autologous Tissue Substitute, Posterior Approach, Anterior Column, Percutaneous Approach

ØRG73AØ   Fusion of 2 to 7 Thoracic Vertebral Joints with Interbody Fusion Device, Anterior Approach, Anterior Column, Percutaneous Approach

ØRG73AJ   Fusion of 2 to 7 Thoracic Vertebral Joints with Interbody Fusion Device, Posterior Approach, Anterior Column, Percutaneous Approach

ØRG73JØ   Fusion of 2 to 7 Thoracic Vertebral Joints with Synthetic Substitute, Anterior Approach, Anterior Column, Percutaneous Approach

ØRG73J1   Fusion of 2 to 7 Thoracic Vertebral Joints with Synthetic Substitute, Posterior Approach, Posterior Column, Percutaneous Approach

ØRG73JJ   Fusion of 2 to 7 Thoracic Vertebral Joints with Synthetic Substitute, Posterior Approach, Anterior Column, Percutaneous Approach

HAC 12: Surgical Site Infection-Certain Orthopedic Procedures of the Spine, Shoulder, and Elbow (continued)

ØRG73KØ Fusion of 2 to 7 Thoracic Vertebral Joints with Nonautologous Tissue Substitute, Anterior Approach, Anterior Column, Percutaneous Approach

ØRG73K1 Fusion of 2 to 7 Thoracic Vertebral Joints with Nonautologous Tissue Substitute, Posterior Approach, Posterior Column, Percutaneous Approach

ØRG73KJ Fusion of 2 to 7 Thoracic Vertebral Joints with Nonautologous Tissue Substitute, Posterior Approach, Anterior Column, Percutaneous Approach

ØRG747Ø Fusion of 2 to 7 Thoracic Vertebral Joints with Autologous Tissue Substitute, Anterior Approach, Anterior Column, Percutaneous Endoscopic Approach

ØRG7471 Fusion of 2 to 7 Thoracic Vertebral Joints with Autologous Tissue Substitute, Posterior Approach, Posterior Column, Percutaneous Endoscopic Approach

ØRG747J Fusion of 2 to 7 Thoracic Vertebral Joints with Autologous Tissue Substitute, Posterior Approach, Anterior Column, Percutaneous Endoscopic Approach

ØRG74AØ Fusion of 2 to 7 Thoracic Vertebral Joints with Interbody Fusion Device, Anterior Approach, Anterior Column, Percutaneous Endoscopic Approach

ØRG74AJ Fusion of 2 to 7 Thoracic Vertebral Joints with Interbody Fusion Device, Posterior Approach, Anterior Column, Percutaneous Endoscopic Approach

ØRG74JØ Fusion of 2 to 7 Thoracic Vertebral Joints with Synthetic Substitute, Anterior Approach, Anterior Column, Percutaneous Endoscopic Approach

ØRG74J1 Fusion of 2 to 7 Thoracic Vertebral Joints with Synthetic Substitute, Posterior Approach, Posterior Column, Percutaneous Endoscopic Approach

ØRG74JJ Fusion of 2 to 7 Thoracic Vertebral Joints with Synthetic Substitute, Posterior Approach, Anterior Column, Percutaneous Endoscopic Approach

ØRG74KØ Fusion of 2 to 7 Thoracic Vertebral Joints with Nonautologous Tissue Substitute, Anterior Approach, Anterior Column, Percutaneous Endoscopic Approach

ØRG74K1 Fusion of 2 to 7 Thoracic Vertebral Joints with Nonautologous Tissue Substitute, Posterior Approach, Posterior Column, Percutaneous Endoscopic Approach

ØRG74KJ Fusion of 2 to 7 Thoracic Vertebral Joints with Nonautologous Tissue Substitute, Posterior Approach, Anterior Column, Percutaneous Endoscopic Approach

ØRG807Ø Fusion of 8 or More Thoracic Vertebral Joints with Autologous Tissue Substitute, Anterior Approach, Anterior Column, Open Approach

ØRG8071 Fusion of 8 or More Thoracic Vertebral Joints with Autologous Tissue Substitute, Posterior Approach, Posterior Column, Open Approach

ØRG807J Fusion of 8 or More Thoracic Vertebral Joints with Autologous Tissue Substitute, Posterior Approach, Anterior Column, Open Approach

ØRG80AØ Fusion of 8 or More Thoracic Vertebral Joints with Interbody Fusion Device, Anterior Approach, Anterior Column, Open Approach

ØRG80AJ Fusion of 8 or More Thoracic Vertebral Joints with Interbody Fusion Device, Posterior Approach, Anterior Column, Open Approach

ØRG80JØ Fusion of 8 or More Thoracic Vertebral Joints with Synthetic Substitute, Anterior Approach, Anterior Column, Open Approach

ØRG80J1 Fusion of 8 or More Thoracic Vertebral Joints with Synthetic Substitute, Posterior Approach, Posterior Column, Open Approach

ØRG80JJ Fusion of 8 or More Thoracic Vertebral Joints with Synthetic Substitute, Posterior Approach, Anterior Column, Open Approach

ØRG80KØ Fusion of 8 or More Thoracic Vertebral Joints with Nonautologous Tissue Substitute, Anterior Approach, Anterior Column, Open Approach

ØRG80K1 Fusion of 8 or More Thoracic Vertebral Joints with Nonautologous Tissue Substitute, Posterior Approach, Posterior Column, Open Approach

ØRG80KJ Fusion of 8 or More Thoracic Vertebral Joints with Nonautologous Tissue Substitute, Posterior Approach, Anterior Column, Open Approach

ØRG837Ø Fusion of 8 or More Thoracic Vertebral Joints with Autologous Tissue Substitute, Anterior Approach, Anterior Column, Percutaneous Approach

ØRG8371 Fusion of 8 or More Thoracic Vertebral Joints with Autologous Tissue Substitute, Posterior Approach, Posterior Column, Percutaneous Approach

ØRG837J Fusion of 8 or More Thoracic Vertebral Joints with Autologous Tissue Substitute, Posterior Approach, Anterior Column, Percutaneous Approach

ØRG83AØ Fusion of 8 or More Thoracic Vertebral Joints with Interbody Fusion Device, Anterior Approach, Anterior Column, Percutaneous Approach

ØRG83AJ Fusion of 8 or More Thoracic Vertebral Joints with Interbody Fusion Device, Posterior Approach, Anterior Column, Percutaneous Approach

ØRG83JØ Fusion of 8 or More Thoracic Vertebral Joints with Synthetic Substitute, Anterior Approach, Anterior Column, Percutaneous Approach

ØRG83J1 Fusion of 8 or More Thoracic Vertebral Joints with Synthetic Substitute, Posterior Approach, Posterior Column, Percutaneous Approach

ØRG83JJ Fusion of 8 or More Thoracic Vertebral Joints with Synthetic Substitute, Posterior Approach, Anterior Column, Percutaneous Approach

ØRG83KØ Fusion of 8 or More Thoracic Vertebral Joints with Nonautologous Tissue Substitute, Anterior Approach, Anterior Column, Percutaneous Approach

ØRG83K1 Fusion of 8 or More Thoracic Vertebral Joints with Nonautologous Tissue Substitute, Posterior Approach, Posterior Column, Percutaneous Approach

ØRG83KJ Fusion of 8 or More Thoracic Vertebral Joints with Nonautologous Tissue Substitute, Posterior Approach, Anterior Column, Percutaneous Approach

ØRG847Ø Fusion of 8 or More Thoracic Vertebral Joints with Autologous Tissue Substitute, Anterior Approach, Anterior Column, Percutaneous Endoscopic Approach

ØRG8471 Fusion of 8 or More Thoracic Vertebral Joints with Autologous Tissue Substitute, Posterior Approach, Posterior Column, Percutaneous Endoscopic Approach

ØRG847J Fusion of 8 or More Thoracic Vertebral Joints with Autologous Tissue Substitute, Posterior Approach, Anterior Column, Percutaneous Endoscopic Approach

ØRG84AØ Fusion of 8 or More Thoracic Vertebral Joints with Interbody Fusion Device, Anterior Approach, Anterior Column, Percutaneous Endoscopic Approach

ØRG84AJ Fusion of 8 or More Thoracic Vertebral Joints with Interbody Fusion Device, Posterior Approach, Anterior Column, Percutaneous Endoscopic Approach

ØRG84JØ Fusion of 8 or More Thoracic Vertebral Joints with Synthetic Substitute, Anterior Approach, Anterior Column, Percutaneous Endoscopic Approach

ØRG84J1 Fusion of 8 or More Thoracic Vertebral Joints with Synthetic Substitute, Posterior Approach, Posterior Column, Percutaneous Endoscopic Approach

ØRG84JJ Fusion of 8 or More Thoracic Vertebral Joints with Synthetic Substitute, Posterior Approach, Anterior Column, Percutaneous Endoscopic Approach

ØRG84KØ Fusion of 8 or More Thoracic Vertebral Joints with Nonautologous Tissue Substitute, Anterior Approach, Anterior Column, Percutaneous Endoscopic Approach

ØRG84K1 Fusion of 8 or More Thoracic Vertebral Joints with Nonautologous Tissue Substitute, Posterior Approach, Posterior Column, Percutaneous Endoscopic Approach

ØRG84KJ Fusion of 8 or More Thoracic Vertebral Joints with Nonautologous Tissue Substitute, Posterior Approach, Anterior Column, Percutaneous Endoscopic Approach

ØRGAØ7Ø Fusion of Thoracolumbar Vertebral Joint with Autologous Tissue Substitute, Anterior Approach, Anterior Column, Open Approach

ØRGAØ71 Fusion of Thoracolumbar Vertebral Joint with Autologous Tissue Substitute, Posterior Approach, Posterior Column, Open Approach

ØRGAØ7J Fusion of Thoracolumbar Vertebral Joint with Autologous Tissue Substitute, Posterior Approach, Anterior Column, Open Approach

ØRGAØAØ Fusion of Thoracolumbar Vertebral Joint with Interbody Fusion Device, Anterior Approach, Anterior Column, Open Approach

ØRGAØAJ Fusion of Thoracolumbar Vertebral Joint with Interbody Fusion Device, Posterior Approach, Anterior Column, Open Approach

ØRGAØJØ Fusion of Thoracolumbar Vertebral Joint with Synthetic Substitute, Anterior Approach, Anterior Column, Open Approach

HAC 12: Surgical Site Infection-Certain Orthopedic Procedures of the Spine, Shoulder, and Elbow (continued)

ØRGAØJ1 Fusion of Thoracolumbar Vertebral Joint with Synthetic Substitute, Posterior Approach, Posterior Column, Open Approach

ØRGAØJJ Fusion of Thoracolumbar Vertebral Joint with Synthetic Substitute, Posterior Approach, Anterior Column, Open Approach

ØRGAØKØ Fusion of Thoracolumbar Vertebral Joint with Nonautologous Tissue Substitute, Anterior Approach, Anterior Column, Open Approach

ØRGAØK1 Fusion of Thoracolumbar Vertebral Joint with Nonautologous Tissue Substitute, Posterior Approach, Posterior Column, Open Approach

ØRGAØKJ Fusion of Thoracolumbar Vertebral Joint with Nonautologous Tissue Substitute, Posterior Approach, Anterior Column, Open Approach

ØRGA37Ø Fusion of Thoracolumbar Vertebral Joint with Autologous Tissue Substitute, Anterior Approach, Anterior Column, Percutaneous Approach

ØRGA371 Fusion of Thoracolumbar Vertebral Joint with Autologous Tissue Substitute, Posterior Approach, Posterior Column, Percutaneous Approach

ØRGA37J Fusion of Thoracolumbar Vertebral Joint with Autologous Tissue Substitute, Posterior Approach, Anterior Column, Percutaneous Approach

ØRGA3AØ Fusion of Thoracolumbar Vertebral Joint with Interbody Fusion Device, Anterior Approach, Anterior Column, Percutaneous Approach

ØRGA3AJ Fusion of Thoracolumbar Vertebral Joint with Interbody Fusion Device, Posterior Approach, Anterior Column, Percutaneous Approach

ØRGA3JØ Fusion of Thoracolumbar Vertebral Joint with Synthetic Substitute, Anterior Approach, Anterior Column, Percutaneous Approach

ØRGA3J1 Fusion of Thoracolumbar Vertebral Joint with Synthetic Substitute, Posterior Approach, Posterior Column, Percutaneous Approach

ØRGA3JJ Fusion of Thoracolumbar Vertebral Joint with Synthetic Substitute, Posterior Approach, Anterior Column, Percutaneous Approach

ØRGA3KØ Fusion of Thoracolumbar Vertebral Joint with Nonautologous Tissue Substitute, Anterior Approach, Anterior Column, Percutaneous Approach

ØRGA3K1 Fusion of Thoracolumbar Vertebral Joint with Nonautologous Tissue Substitute, Posterior Approach, Posterior Column, Percutaneous Approach

ØRGA3KJ Fusion of Thoracolumbar Vertebral Joint with Nonautologous Tissue Substitute, Posterior Approach, Anterior Column, Percutaneous Approach

ØRGA47Ø Fusion of Thoracolumbar Vertebral Joint with Autologous Tissue Substitute, Anterior Approach, Anterior Column, Percutaneous Endoscopic Approach

ØRGA471 Fusion of Thoracolumbar Vertebral Joint with Autologous Tissue Substitute, Posterior Approach, Posterior Column, Percutaneous Endoscopic Approach

ØRGA47J Fusion of Thoracolumbar Vertebral Joint with Autologous Tissue Substitute, Posterior Approach, Anterior Column, Percutaneous Endoscopic Approach

ØRGA4AØ Fusion of Thoracolumbar Vertebral Joint with Interbody Fusion Device, Anterior Approach, Anterior Column, Percutaneous Endoscopic Approach

ØRGA4AJ Fusion of Thoracolumbar Vertebral Joint with Interbody Fusion Device, Posterior Approach, Anterior Column, Percutaneous Endoscopic Approach

ØRGA4JØ Fusion of Thoracolumbar Vertebral Joint with Synthetic Substitute, Anterior Approach, Anterior Column, Percutaneous Endoscopic Approach

ØRGA4J1 Fusion of Thoracolumbar Vertebral Joint with Synthetic Substitute, Posterior Approach, Posterior Column, Percutaneous Endoscopic Approach

ØRGA4JJ Fusion of Thoracolumbar Vertebral Joint with Synthetic Substitute, Posterior Approach, Anterior Column, Percutaneous Endoscopic Approach

ØRGA4KØ Fusion of Thoracolumbar Vertebral Joint with Nonautologous Tissue Substitute, Anterior Approach, Anterior Column, Percutaneous Endoscopic Approach

ØRGA4K1 Fusion of Thoracolumbar Vertebral Joint with Nonautologous Tissue Substitute, Posterior Approach, Posterior Column, Percutaneous Endoscopic Approach

ØRGA4KJ Fusion of Thoracolumbar Vertebral Joint with Nonautologous Tissue Substitute, Posterior Approach, Anterior Column, Percutaneous Endoscopic Approach

ØRGEØ4Z Fusion of Right Sternoclavicular Joint with Internal Fixation Device, Open Approach

ØRGEØ7Z Fusion of Right Sternoclavicular Joint with Autologous Tissue Substitute, Open Approach

ØRGEØJZ Fusion of Right Sternoclavicular Joint with Synthetic Substitute, Open Approach

ØRGEØKZ Fusion of Right Sternoclavicular Joint with Nonautologous Tissue Substitute, Open Approach

ØRGE34Z Fusion of Right Sternoclavicular Joint with Internal Fixation Device, Percutaneous Approach

ØRGE37Z Fusion of Right Sternoclavicular Joint with Autologous Tissue Substitute, Percutaneous Approach

ØRGE3JZ Fusion of Right Sternoclavicular Joint with Synthetic Substitute, Percutaneous Approach

ØRGE3KZ Fusion of Right Sternoclavicular Joint with Nonautologous Tissue Substitute, Percutaneous Approach

ØRGE44Z Fusion of Right Sternoclavicular Joint with Internal Fixation Device, Percutaneous Endoscopic Approach

ØRGE47Z Fusion of Right Sternoclavicular Joint with Autologous Tissue Substitute, Percutaneous Endoscopic Approach

ØRGE4JZ Fusion of Right Sternoclavicular Joint with Synthetic Substitute, Percutaneous Endoscopic Approach

ØRGE4KZ Fusion of Right Sternoclavicular Joint with Nonautologous Tissue Substitute, Percutaneous Endoscopic Approach

ØRGFØ4Z Fusion of Left Sternoclavicular Joint with Internal Fixation Device, Open Approach

ØRGFØ7Z Fusion of Left Sternoclavicular Joint with Autologous Tissue Substitute, Open Approach

ØRGFØJZ Fusion of Left Sternoclavicular Joint with Synthetic Substitute, Open Approach

ØRGFØKZ Fusion of Left Sternoclavicular Joint with Nonautologous Tissue Substitute, Open Approach

ØRGF34Z Fusion of Left Sternoclavicular Joint with Internal Fixation Device, Percutaneous Approach

ØRGF37Z Fusion of Left Sternoclavicular Joint with Autologous Tissue Substitute, Percutaneous Approach

ØRGF3JZ Fusion of Left Sternoclavicular Joint with Synthetic Substitute, Percutaneous Approach

ØRGF3KZ Fusion of Left Sternoclavicular Joint with Nonautologous Tissue Substitute, Percutaneous Approach

ØRGF44Z Fusion of Left Sternoclavicular Joint with Internal Fixation Device, Percutaneous Endoscopic Approach

ØRGF47Z Fusion of Left Sternoclavicular Joint with Autologous Tissue Substitute, Percutaneous Endoscopic Approach

ØRGF4JZ Fusion of Left Sternoclavicular Joint with Synthetic Substitute, Percutaneous Endoscopic Approach

ØRGF4KZ Fusion of Left Sternoclavicular Joint with Nonautologous Tissue Substitute, Percutaneous Endoscopic Approach

ØRGGØ4Z Fusion of Right Acromioclavicular Joint with Internal Fixation Device, Open Approach

ØRGGØ7Z Fusion of Right Acromioclavicular Joint with Autologous Tissue Substitute, Open Approach

ØRGGØJZ Fusion of Right Acromioclavicular Joint with Synthetic Substitute, Open Approach

ØRGGØKZ Fusion of Right Acromioclavicular Joint with Nonautologous Tissue Substitute, Open Approach

ØRGG34Z Fusion of Right Acromioclavicular Joint with Internal Fixation Device, Percutaneous Approach

ØRGG37Z Fusion of Right Acromioclavicular Joint with Autologous Tissue Substitute, Percutaneous Approach

ØRGG3JZ Fusion of Right Acromioclavicular Joint with Synthetic Substitute, Percutaneous Approach

ØRGG3KZ Fusion of Right Acromioclavicular Joint with Nonautologous Tissue Substitute, Percutaneous Approach

ØRGG44Z Fusion of Right Acromioclavicular Joint with Internal Fixation Device, Percutaneous Endoscopic Approach

ØRGG47Z Fusion of Right Acromioclavicular Joint with Autologous Tissue Substitute, Percutaneous Endoscopic Approach

ØRGG4JZ Fusion of Right Acromioclavicular Joint with Synthetic Substitute, Percutaneous Endoscopic Approach

ØRGG4KZ Fusion of Right Acromioclavicular Joint with Nonautologous Tissue Substitute, Percutaneous Endoscopic Approach

ØRGHØ4Z Fusion of Left Acromioclavicular Joint with Internal Fixation Device, Open Approach

ØRGHØ7Z Fusion of Left Acromioclavicular Joint with Autologous Tissue Substitute, Open Approach

HAC 12: Surgical Site Infection-Certain Orthopedic Procedures of the Spine, Shoulder, and Elbow (continued)

ØRGHØJZ   Fusion of Left Acromioclavicular Joint with Synthetic Substitute, Open Approach

ØRGHØKZ   Fusion of Left Acromioclavicular Joint with Nonautologous Tissue Substitute, Open Approach

ØRGH34Z   Fusion of Left Acromioclavicular Joint with Internal Fixation Device, Percutaneous Approach

ØRGH37Z   Fusion of Left Acromioclavicular Joint with Autologous Tissue Substitute, Percutaneous Approach

ØRGH3JZ   Fusion of Left Acromioclavicular Joint with Synthetic Substitute, Percutaneous Approach

ØRGH3KZ   Fusion of Left Acromioclavicular Joint with Nonautologous Tissue Substitute, Percutaneous Approach

ØRGH44Z   Fusion of Left Acromioclavicular Joint with Internal Fixation Device, Percutaneous Endoscopic Approach

ØRGH47Z   Fusion of Left Acromioclavicular Joint with Autologous Tissue Substitute, Percutaneous Endoscopic Approach

ØRGH4JZ   Fusion of Left Acromioclavicular Joint with Synthetic Substitute, Percutaneous Endoscopic Approach

ØRGH4KZ   Fusion of Left Acromioclavicular Joint with Nonautologous Tissue Substitute, Percutaneous Endoscopic Approach

ØRGJ04Z   Fusion of Right Shoulder Joint with Internal Fixation Device, Open Approach

ØRGJ07Z   Fusion of Right Shoulder Joint with Autologous Tissue Substitute, Open Approach

ØRGJ0JZ   Fusion of Right Shoulder Joint with Synthetic Substitute, Open Approach

ØRGJ0KZ   Fusion of Right Shoulder Joint with Nonautologous Tissue Substitute, Open Approach

ØRGJ34Z   Fusion of Right Shoulder Joint with Internal Fixation Device, Percutaneous Approach

ØRGJ37Z   Fusion of Right Shoulder Joint with Autologous Tissue Substitute, Percutaneous Approach

ØRGJ3JZ   Fusion of Right Shoulder Joint with Synthetic Substitute, Percutaneous Approach

ØRGJ3KZ   Fusion of Right Shoulder Joint with Nonautologous Tissue Substitute, Percutaneous Approach

ØRGJ44Z   Fusion of Right Shoulder Joint with Internal Fixation Device, Percutaneous Endoscopic Approach

ØRGJ47Z   Fusion of Right Shoulder Joint with Autologous Tissue Substitute, Percutaneous Endoscopic Approach

ØRGJ4JZ   Fusion of Right Shoulder Joint with Synthetic Substitute, Percutaneous Endoscopic Approach

ØRGJ4KZ   Fusion of Right Shoulder Joint with Nonautologous Tissue Substitute, Percutaneous Endoscopic Approach

ØRGK04Z   Fusion of Left Shoulder Joint with Internal Fixation Device, Open Approach

ØRGK07Z   Fusion of Left Shoulder Joint with Autologous Tissue Substitute, Open Approach

ØRGK0JZ   Fusion of Left Shoulder Joint with Synthetic Substitute, Open Approach

ØRGK0KZ   Fusion of Left Shoulder Joint with Nonautologous Tissue Substitute, Open Approach

ØRGK34Z   Fusion of Left Shoulder Joint with Internal Fixation Device, Percutaneous Approach

ØRGK37Z   Fusion of Left Shoulder Joint with Autologous Tissue Substitute, Percutaneous Approach

ØRGK3JZ   Fusion of Left Shoulder Joint with Synthetic Substitute, Percutaneous Approach

ØRGK3KZ   Fusion of Left Shoulder Joint with Nonautologous Tissue Substitute, Percutaneous Approach

ØRGK44Z   Fusion of Left Shoulder Joint with Internal Fixation Device, Percutaneous Endoscopic Approach

ØRGK47Z   Fusion of Left Shoulder Joint with Autologous Tissue Substitute, Percutaneous Endoscopic Approach

ØRGK4JZ   Fusion of Left Shoulder Joint with Synthetic Substitute, Percutaneous Endoscopic Approach

ØRGK4KZ   Fusion of Left Shoulder Joint with Nonautologous Tissue Substitute, Percutaneous Endoscopic Approach

ØRGL04Z   Fusion of Right Elbow Joint with Internal Fixation Device, Open Approach

ØRGL05Z   Fusion of Right Elbow Joint with External Fixation Device, Open Approach

ØRGL07Z   Fusion of Right Elbow Joint with Autologous Tissue Substitute, Open Approach

ØRGL0JZ   Fusion of Right Elbow Joint with Synthetic Substitute, Open Approach

ØRGL0KZ   Fusion of Right Elbow Joint with Nonautologous Tissue Substitute, Open Approach

ØRGL34Z   Fusion of Right Elbow Joint with Internal Fixation Device, Percutaneous Approach

ØRGL35Z   Fusion of Right Elbow Joint with External Fixation Device, Percutaneous Approach

ØRGL37Z   Fusion of Right Elbow Joint with Autologous Tissue Substitute, Percutaneous Approach

ØRGL3JZ   Fusion of Right Elbow Joint with Synthetic Substitute, Percutaneous Approach

ØRGL3KZ   Fusion of Right Elbow Joint with Nonautologous Tissue Substitute, Percutaneous Approach

ØRGL44Z   Fusion of Right Elbow Joint with Internal Fixation Device, Percutaneous Endoscopic Approach

ØRGL45Z   Fusion of Right Elbow Joint with External Fixation Device, Percutaneous Endoscopic Approach

ØRGL47Z   Fusion of Right Elbow Joint with Autologous Tissue Substitute, Percutaneous Endoscopic Approach

ØRGL4JZ   Fusion of Right Elbow Joint with Synthetic Substitute, Percutaneous Endoscopic Approach

ØRGL4KZ   Fusion of Right Elbow Joint with Nonautologous Tissue Substitute, Percutaneous Endoscopic Approach

ØRGM04Z   Fusion of Left Elbow Joint with Internal Fixation Device, Open Approach

ØRGM05Z   Fusion of Left Elbow Joint with External Fixation Device, Open Approach

ØRGM07Z   Fusion of Left Elbow Joint with Autologous Tissue Substitute, Open Approach

ØRGM0JZ   Fusion of Left Elbow Joint with Synthetic Substitute, Open Approach

ØRGM0KZ   Fusion of Left Elbow Joint with Nonautologous Tissue Substitute, Open Approach

ØRGM34Z   Fusion of Left Elbow Joint with Internal Fixation Device, Percutaneous Approach

ØRGM35Z   Fusion of Left Elbow Joint with External Fixation Device, Percutaneous Approach

ØRGM37Z   Fusion of Left Elbow Joint with Autologous Tissue Substitute, Percutaneous Approach

ØRGM3JZ   Fusion of Left Elbow Joint with Synthetic Substitute, Percutaneous Approach

ØRGM3KZ   Fusion of Left Elbow Joint with Nonautologous Tissue Substitute, Percutaneous Approach

ØRGM44Z   Fusion of Left Elbow Joint with Internal Fixation Device, Percutaneous Endoscopic Approach

ØRGM45Z   Fusion of Left Elbow Joint with External Fixation Device, Percutaneous Endoscopic Approach

ØRGM47Z   Fusion of Left Elbow Joint with Autologous Tissue Substitute, Percutaneous Endoscopic Approach

ØRGM4JZ   Fusion of Left Elbow Joint with Synthetic Substitute, Percutaneous Endoscopic Approach

ØRGM4KZ   Fusion of Left Elbow Joint with Nonautologous Tissue Substitute, Percutaneous Endoscopic Approach

ØRQE0ZZ   Repair Right Sternoclavicular Joint, Open Approach

ØRQE3ZZ   Repair Right Sternoclavicular Joint, Percutaneous Approach

ØRQE4ZZ   Repair Right Sternoclavicular Joint, Percutaneous Endoscopic Approach

ØRQEXZZ   Repair Right Sternoclavicular Joint, External Approach

ØRQF0ZZ   Repair Left Sternoclavicular Joint, Open Approach

ØRQF3ZZ   Repair Left Sternoclavicular Joint, Percutaneous Approach

ØRQF4ZZ   Repair Left Sternoclavicular Joint, Percutaneous Endoscopic Approach

ØRQFXZZ   Repair Left Sternoclavicular Joint, External Approach

ØRQG0ZZ   Repair Right Acromioclavicular Joint, Open Approach

ØRQG3ZZ   Repair Right Acromioclavicular Joint, Percutaneous Approach

ØRQG4ZZ   Repair Right Acromioclavicular Joint, Percutaneous Endoscopic Approach

ØRQGXZZ   Repair Right Acromioclavicular Joint, External Approach

ØRQH0ZZ   Repair Left Acromioclavicular Joint, Open Approach

ØRQH3ZZ   Repair Left Acromioclavicular Joint, Percutaneous Approach

ØRQH4ZZ   Repair Left Acromioclavicular Joint, Percutaneous Endoscopic Approach

ØRQHXZZ   Repair Left Acromioclavicular Joint, External Approach

ØRQJ0ZZ   Repair Right Shoulder Joint, Open Approach

ØRQJ3ZZ   Repair Right Shoulder Joint, Percutaneous Approach

ØRQJ4ZZ   Repair Right Shoulder Joint, Percutaneous Endoscopic Approach

ØRQJXZZ   Repair Right Shoulder Joint, External Approach

ØRQK0ZZ   Repair Left Shoulder Joint, Open Approach

ØRQK3ZZ   Repair Left Shoulder Joint, Percutaneous Approach

HAC 12: Surgical Site Infection-Certain Orthopedic Procedures of the Spine, Shoulder, and Elbow (continued)

ØRQK4ZZ Repair Left Shoulder Joint, Percutaneous Endoscopic Approach

ØRQKXZZ Repair Left Shoulder Joint, External Approach

ØRQLØZZ Repair Right Elbow Joint, Open Approach

ØRQL3ZZ Repair Right Elbow Joint, Percutaneous Approach

ØRQL4ZZ Repair Right Elbow Joint, Percutaneous Endoscopic Approach

ØRQLXZZ Repair Right Elbow Joint, External Approach

ØRQMØZZ Repair Left Elbow Joint, Open Approach

ØRQM3ZZ Repair Left Elbow Joint, Percutaneous Approach

ØRQM4ZZ Repair Left Elbow Joint, Percutaneous Endoscopic Approach

ØRQMXZZ Repair Left Elbow Joint, External Approach

ØRUEØ7Z Supplement Right Sternoclavicular Joint with Autologous Tissue Substitute, Open Approach

ØRUEØJZ Supplement Right Sternoclavicular Joint with Synthetic Substitute, Open Approach

ØRUEØKZ Supplement Right Sternoclavicular Joint with Nonautologous Tissue Substitute, Open Approach

ØRUE37Z Supplement Right Sternoclavicular Joint with Autologous Tissue Substitute, Percutaneous Approach

ØRUE3JZ Supplement Right Sternoclavicular Joint with Synthetic Substitute, Percutaneous Approach

ØRUE3KZ Supplement Right Sternoclavicular Joint with Nonautologous Tissue Substitute, Percutaneous Approach

ØRUE47Z Supplement Right Sternoclavicular Joint with Autologous Tissue Substitute, Percutaneous Endoscopic Approach

ØRUE4JZ Supplement Right Sternoclavicular Joint with Synthetic Substitute, Percutaneous Endoscopic Approach

ØRUE4KZ Supplement Right Sternoclavicular Joint with Nonautologous Tissue Substitute, Percutaneous Endoscopic Approach

ØRUFØ7Z Supplement Left Sternoclavicular Joint with Autologous Tissue Substitute, Open Approach

ØRUFØJZ Supplement Left Sternoclavicular Joint with Synthetic Substitute, Open Approach

ØRUFØKZ Supplement Left Sternoclavicular Joint with Nonautologous Tissue Substitute, Open Approach

ØRUF37Z Supplement Left Sternoclavicular Joint with Autologous Tissue Substitute, Percutaneous Approach

ØRUF3JZ Supplement Left Sternoclavicular Joint with Synthetic Substitute, Percutaneous Approach

ØRUF3KZ Supplement Left Sternoclavicular Joint with Nonautologous Tissue Substitute, Percutaneous Approach

ØRUF47Z Supplement Left Sternoclavicular Joint with Autologous Tissue Substitute, Percutaneous Endoscopic Approach

ØRUF4JZ Supplement Left Sternoclavicular Joint with Synthetic Substitute, Percutaneous Endoscopic Approach

ØRUF4KZ Supplement Left Sternoclavicular Joint with Nonautologous Tissue Substitute, Percutaneous Endoscopic Approach

ØRUGØ7Z Supplement Right Acromioclavicular Joint with Autologous Tissue Substitute, Open Approach

ØRUGØJZ Supplement Right Acromioclavicular Joint with Synthetic Substitute, Open Approach

ØRUGØKZ Supplement Right Acromioclavicular Joint with Nonautologous Tissue Substitute, Open Approach

ØRUG37Z Supplement Right Acromioclavicular Joint with Autologous Tissue Substitute, Percutaneous Approach

ØRUG3JZ Supplement Right Acromioclavicular Joint with Synthetic Substitute, Percutaneous Approach

ØRUG3KZ Supplement Right Acromioclavicular Joint with Nonautologous Tissue Substitute, Percutaneous Approach

ØRUG47Z Supplement Right Acromioclavicular Joint with Autologous Tissue Substitute, Percutaneous Endoscopic Approach

ØRUG4JZ Supplement Right Acromioclavicular Joint with Synthetic Substitute, Percutaneous Endoscopic Approach

ØRUG4KZ Supplement Right Acromioclavicular Joint with Nonautologous Tissue Substitute, Percutaneous Endoscopic Approach

ØRUHØ7Z Supplement Left Acromioclavicular Joint with Autologous Tissue Substitute, Open Approach

ØRUHØJZ Supplement Left Acromioclavicular Joint with Synthetic Substitute, Open Approach

ØRUHØKZ Supplement Left Acromioclavicular Joint with Nonautologous Tissue Substitute, Open Approach

ØRUH37Z Supplement Left Acromioclavicular Joint with Autologous Tissue Substitute, Percutaneous Approach

ØRUH3JZ Supplement Left Acromioclavicular Joint with Synthetic Substitute, Percutaneous Approach

ØRUH3KZ Supplement Left Acromioclavicular Joint with Nonautologous Tissue Substitute, Percutaneous Approach

ØRUH47Z Supplement Left Acromioclavicular Joint with Autologous Tissue Substitute, Percutaneous Endoscopic Approach

ØRUH4JZ Supplement Left Acromioclavicular Joint with Synthetic Substitute, Percutaneous Endoscopic Approach

ØRUH4KZ Supplement Left Acromioclavicular Joint with Nonautologous Tissue Substitute, Percutaneous Endoscopic Approach

ØRUJØ7Z Supplement Right Shoulder Joint with Autologous Tissue Substitute, Open Approach

ØRUJØJZ Supplement Right Shoulder Joint with Synthetic Substitute, Open Approach

ØRUJØKZ Supplement Right Shoulder Joint with Nonautologous Tissue Substitute, Open Approach

ØRUJ37Z Supplement Right Shoulder Joint with Autologous Tissue Substitute, Percutaneous Approach

ØRUJ3JZ Supplement Right Shoulder Joint with Synthetic Substitute, Percutaneous Approach

ØRUJ3KZ Supplement Right Shoulder Joint with Nonautologous Tissue Substitute, Percutaneous Approach

ØRUJ47Z Supplement Right Shoulder Joint with Autologous Tissue Substitute, Percutaneous Endoscopic Approach

ØRUJ4JZ Supplement Right Shoulder Joint with Synthetic Substitute, Percutaneous Endoscopic Approach

ØRUJ4KZ Supplement Right Shoulder Joint with Nonautologous Tissue Substitute, Percutaneous Endoscopic Approach

ØRUKØ7Z Supplement Left Shoulder Joint with Autologous Tissue Substitute, Open Approach

ØRUKØJZ Supplement Left Shoulder Joint with Synthetic Substitute, Open Approach

ØRUKØKZ Supplement Left Shoulder Joint with Nonautologous Tissue Substitute, Open Approach

ØRUK37Z Supplement Left Shoulder Joint with Autologous Tissue Substitute, Percutaneous Approach

ØRUK3JZ Supplement Left Shoulder Joint with Synthetic Substitute, Percutaneous Approach

ØRUK3KZ Supplement Left Shoulder Joint with Nonautologous Tissue Substitute, Percutaneous Approach

ØRUK47Z Supplement Left Shoulder Joint with Autologous Tissue Substitute, Percutaneous Endoscopic Approach

ØRUK4JZ Supplement Left Shoulder Joint with Synthetic Substitute, Percutaneous Endoscopic Approach

ØRUK4KZ Supplement Left Shoulder Joint with Nonautologous Tissue Substitute, Percutaneous Endoscopic Approach

ØRULØ7Z Supplement Right Elbow Joint with Autologous Tissue Substitute, Open Approach

ØRULØJZ Supplement Right Elbow Joint with Synthetic Substitute, Open Approach

ØRULØKZ Supplement Right Elbow Joint with Nonautologous Tissue Substitute, Open Approach

ØRUL37Z Supplement Right Elbow Joint with Autologous Tissue Substitute, Percutaneous Approach

ØRUL3JZ Supplement Right Elbow Joint with Synthetic Substitute, Percutaneous Approach

ØRUL3KZ Supplement Right Elbow Joint with Nonautologous Tissue Substitute, Percutaneous Approach

ØRUL47Z Supplement Right Elbow Joint with Autologous Tissue Substitute, Percutaneous Endoscopic Approach

ØRUL4JZ Supplement Right Elbow Joint with Synthetic Substitute, Percutaneous Endoscopic Approach

ØRUL4KZ Supplement Right Elbow Joint with Nonautologous Tissue Substitute, Percutaneous Endoscopic Approach

ØRUMØ7Z Supplement Left Elbow Joint with Autologous Tissue Substitute, Open Approach

ØRUMØJZ Supplement Left Elbow Joint with Synthetic Substitute, Open Approach

ØRUMØKZ Supplement Left Elbow Joint with Nonautologous Tissue Substitute, Open Approach

ØRUM37Z Supplement Left Elbow Joint with Autologous Tissue Substitute, Percutaneous Approach

ØRUM3JZ Supplement Left Elbow Joint with Synthetic Substitute, Percutaneous Approach

ØRUM3KZ Supplement Left Elbow Joint with Nonautologous Tissue Substitute, Percutaneous Approach

HAC 12: Surgical Site Infection-Certain Orthopedic Procedures of the Spine, Shoulder, and Elbow (continued)

ØRUM47Z Supplement Left Elbow Joint with Autologous Tissue Substitute, Percutaneous Endoscopic Approach

ØRUM4JZ Supplement Left Elbow Joint with Synthetic Substitute, Percutaneous Endoscopic Approach

ØRUM4KZ Supplement Left Elbow Joint with Nonautologous Tissue Substitute, Percutaneous Endoscopic Approach

ØSG0070 Fusion of Lumbar Vertebral Joint with Autologous Tissue Substitute, Anterior Approach, Anterior Column, Open Approach

ØSG0071 Fusion of Lumbar Vertebral Joint with Autologous Tissue Substitute, Posterior Approach, Posterior Column, Open Approach

ØSG007J Fusion of Lumbar Vertebral Joint with Autologous Tissue Substitute, Posterior Approach, Anterior Column, Open Approach

ØSG00A0 Fusion of Lumbar Vertebral Joint with Interbody Fusion Device, Anterior Approach, Anterior Column, Open Approach

ØSG00AJ Fusion of Lumbar Vertebral Joint with Interbody Fusion Device, Posterior Approach, Anterior Column, Open Approach

ØSG00J0 Fusion of Lumbar Vertebral Joint with Synthetic Substitute, Anterior Approach, Anterior Column, Open Approach

ØSG00J1 Fusion of Lumbar Vertebral Joint with Synthetic Substitute, Posterior Approach, Posterior Column, Open Approach

ØSG00JJ Fusion of Lumbar Vertebral Joint with Synthetic Substitute, Posterior Approach, Anterior Column, Open Approach

ØSG00K0 Fusion of Lumbar Vertebral Joint with Nonautologous Tissue Substitute, Anterior Approach, Anterior Column, Open Approach

HAC G00K1 Fusion of Lumbar Vertebral Joint with Nonautologous Tissue Substitute, Posterior Approach, Posterior Column, Open Approach

ØSG00KJ Fusion of Lumbar Vertebral Joint with Nonautologous Tissue Substitute, Posterior Approach, Anterior Column, Open Approach

ØSG0370 Fusion of Lumbar Vertebral Joint with Autologous Tissue Substitute, Anterior Approach, Anterior Column, Percutaneous Approach

ØSG0371 Fusion of Lumbar Vertebral Joint with Autologous Tissue Substitute, Posterior Approach, Posterior Column, Percutaneous Approach

ØSG037J Fusion of Lumbar Vertebral Joint with Autologous Tissue Substitute, Posterior Approach, Anterior Column, Percutaneous Approach

ØSG03A0 Fusion of Lumbar Vertebral Joint with Interbody Fusion Device, Anterior Approach, Anterior Column, Percutaneous Approach

ØSG03AJ Fusion of Lumbar Vertebral Joint with Interbody Fusion Device, Posterior Approach, Anterior Column, Percutaneous Approach

ØSG03J0 Fusion of Lumbar Vertebral Joint with Synthetic Substitute, Anterior Approach, Anterior Column, Percutaneous Approach

ØSG03J1 Fusion of Lumbar Vertebral Joint with Synthetic Substitute, Posterior Approach, Posterior Column, Percutaneous Approach

ØSG03JJ Fusion of Lumbar Vertebral Joint with Synthetic Substitute, Posterior Approach, Anterior Column, Percutaneous Approach

ØSG03K0 Fusion of Lumbar Vertebral Joint with Nonautologous Tissue Substitute, Anterior Approach, Anterior Column, Percutaneous Approach

ØSG03K1 Fusion of Lumbar Vertebral Joint with Nonautologous Tissue Substitute, Posterior Approach, Posterior Column, Percutaneous Approach

ØSG03KJ Fusion of Lumbar Vertebral Joint with Nonautologous Tissue Substitute, Posterior Approach, Anterior Column, Percutaneous Approach

ØSG0470 Fusion of Lumbar Vertebral Joint with Autologous Tissue Substitute, Anterior Approach, Anterior Column, Percutaneous Endoscopic Approach

ØSG0471 Fusion of Lumbar Vertebral Joint with Autologous Tissue Substitute, Posterior Approach, Posterior Column, Percutaneous Endoscopic Approach

ØSG047J Fusion of Lumbar Vertebral Joint with Autologous Tissue Substitute, Posterior Approach, Anterior Column, Percutaneous Endoscopic Approach

ØSG04A0 Fusion of Lumbar Vertebral Joint with Interbody Fusion Device, Anterior Approach, Anterior Column, Percutaneous Endoscopic Approach

ØSG04AJ Fusion of Lumbar Vertebral Joint with Interbody Fusion Device, Posterior Approach, Anterior Column, Percutaneous Endoscopic Approach

ØSG04J0 Fusion of Lumbar Vertebral Joint with Synthetic Substitute, Anterior Approach, Anterior Column, Percutaneous Endoscopic Approach

ØSG04J1 Fusion of Lumbar Vertebral Joint with Synthetic Substitute, Posterior Approach, Posterior Column, Percutaneous Endoscopic Approach

ØSG04JJ Fusion of Lumbar Vertebral Joint with Synthetic Substitute, Posterior Approach, Anterior Column, Percutaneous Endoscopic Approach

ØSG04K0 Fusion of Lumbar Vertebral Joint with Nonautologous Tissue Substitute, Anterior Approach, Anterior Column, Percutaneous Endoscopic Approach

ØSG04K1 Fusion of Lumbar Vertebral Joint with Nonautologous Tissue Substitute, Posterior Approach, Posterior Column, Percutaneous Endoscopic Approach

ØSG04KJ Fusion of Lumbar Vertebral Joint with Nonautologous Tissue Substitute, Posterior Approach, Anterior Column, Percutaneous Endoscopic Approach

ØSG1070 Fusion of 2 or More Lumbar Vertebral Joints with Autologous Tissue Substitute, Anterior Approach, Anterior Column, Open Approach

ØSG1071 Fusion of 2 or More Lumbar Vertebral Joints with Autologous Tissue Substitute, Posterior Approach, Posterior Column, Open Approach

ØSG107J Fusion of 2 or More Lumbar Vertebral Joints with Autologous Tissue Substitute, Posterior Approach, Anterior Column, Open Approach

ØSG10A0 Fusion of 2 or More Lumbar Vertebral Joints with Interbody Fusion Device, Anterior Approach, Anterior Column, Open Approach

ØSG10AJ Fusion of 2 or More Lumbar Vertebral Joints with Interbody Fusion Device, Posterior Approach, Anterior Column, Open Approach

ØSG10J0 Fusion of 2 or More Lumbar Vertebral Joints with Synthetic Substitute, Anterior Approach, Anterior Column, Open Approach

ØSG10J1 Fusion of 2 or More Lumbar Vertebral Joints with Synthetic Substitute, Posterior Approach, Posterior Column, Open Approach

ØSG10JJ Fusion of 2 or More Lumbar Vertebral Joints with Synthetic Substitute, Posterior Approach, Anterior Column, Open Approach

ØSG10K0 Fusion of 2 or More Lumbar Vertebral Joints with Nonautologous Tissue Substitute, Anterior Approach, Anterior Column, Open Approach

ØSG10K1 Fusion of 2 or More Lumbar Vertebral Joints with Nonautologous Tissue Substitute, Posterior Approach, Posterior Column, Open Approach

ØSG10KJ Fusion of 2 or More Lumbar Vertebral Joints with Nonautologous Tissue Substitute, Posterior Approach, Anterior Column, Open Approach

ØSG1370 Fusion of 2 or More Lumbar Vertebral Joints with Autologous Tissue Substitute, Anterior Approach, Anterior Column, Percutaneous Approach

ØSG1371 Fusion of 2 or More Lumbar Vertebral Joints with Autologous Tissue Substitute, Posterior Approach, Posterior Column, Percutaneous Approach

ØSG137J Fusion of 2 or More Lumbar Vertebral Joints with Autologous Tissue Substitute, Posterior Approach, Anterior Column, Percutaneous Approach

ØSG13A0 Fusion of 2 or More Lumbar Vertebral Joints with Interbody Fusion Device, Anterior Approach, Anterior Column, Percutaneous Approach

ØSG13AJ Fusion of 2 or More Lumbar Vertebral Joints with Interbody Fusion Device, Posterior Approach, Anterior Column, Percutaneous Approach

ØSG13J0 Fusion of 2 or More Lumbar Vertebral Joints with Synthetic Substitute, Anterior Approach, Anterior Column, Percutaneous Approach

ØSG13J1 Fusion of 2 or More Lumbar Vertebral Joints with Synthetic Substitute, Posterior Approach, Posterior Column, Percutaneous Approach

ØSG13JJ Fusion of 2 or More Lumbar Vertebral Joints with Synthetic Substitute, Posterior Approach, Anterior Column, Percutaneous Approach

ØSG13K0 Fusion of 2 or More Lumbar Vertebral Joints with Nonautologous Tissue Substitute, Anterior Approach, Anterior Column, Percutaneous Approach

HAC 12: Surgical Site Infection–Certain Orthopedic Procedures of the Spine, Shoulder, and Elbow (continued)

0SG13K1 Fusion of 2 or More Lumbar Vertebral Joints with Nonautologous Tissue Substitute, Posterior Approach, Posterior Column, Percutaneous Approach

0SG13KJ Fusion of 2 or More Lumbar Vertebral Joints with Nonautologous Tissue Substitute, Posterior Approach, Anterior Column, Percutaneous Approach

0SG1470 Fusion of 2 or More Lumbar Vertebral Joints with Autologous Tissue Substitute, Anterior Approach, Anterior Column, Percutaneous Endoscopic Approach

0SG1471 Fusion of 2 or More Lumbar Vertebral Joints with Autologous Tissue Substitute, Posterior Approach, Posterior Column, Percutaneous Endoscopic Approach

0SG147J Fusion of 2 or More Lumbar Vertebral Joints with Autologous Tissue Substitute, Posterior Approach, Anterior Column, Percutaneous Endoscopic Approach

0SG14A0 Fusion of 2 or More Lumbar Vertebral Joints with Interbody Fusion Device, Anterior Approach, Anterior Column, Percutaneous Endoscopic Approach

0SG14AJ Fusion of 2 or More Lumbar Vertebral Joints with Interbody Fusion Device, Posterior Approach, Anterior Column, Percutaneous Endoscopic Approach

0SG14J0 Fusion of 2 or More Lumbar Vertebral Joints with Synthetic Substitute, Anterior Approach, Anterior Column, Percutaneous Endoscopic Approach

0SG14J1 Fusion of 2 or More Lumbar Vertebral Joints with Synthetic Substitute, Posterior Approach, Posterior Column, Percutaneous Endoscopic Approach

0SG14JJ Fusion of 2 or More Lumbar Vertebral Joints with Synthetic Substitute, Posterior Approach, Anterior Column, Percutaneous Endoscopic Approach

0SG14K0 Fusion of 2 or More Lumbar Vertebral Joints with Nonautologous Tissue Substitute, Anterior Approach, Anterior Column, Percutaneous Endoscopic Approach

0SG14K1 Fusion of 2 or More Lumbar Vertebral Joints with Nonautologous Tissue Substitute, Posterior Approach, Posterior Column, Percutaneous Endoscopic Approach

0SG14KJ Fusion of 2 or More Lumbar Vertebral Joints with Nonautologous Tissue Substitute, Posterior Approach, Anterior Column, Percutaneous Endoscopic Approach

0SG3070 Fusion of Lumbosacral Joint with Autologous Tissue Substitute, Anterior Approach, Anterior Column, Open Approach

0SG3071 Fusion of Lumbosacral Joint with Autologous Tissue Substitute, Posterior Approach, Posterior Column, Open Approach

0SG307J Fusion of Lumbosacral Joint with Autologous Tissue Substitute, Posterior Approach, Anterior Column, Open Approach

0SG30A0 Fusion of Lumbosacral Joint with Interbody Fusion Device, Anterior Approach, Anterior Column, Open Approach

0SG30AJ Fusion of Lumbosacral Joint with Interbody Fusion Device, Posterior Approach, Anterior Column, Open Approach

0SG30J0 Fusion of Lumbosacral Joint with Synthetic Substitute, Anterior Approach, Anterior Column, Open Approach

0SG30J1 Fusion of Lumbosacral Joint with Synthetic Substitute, Posterior Approach, Posterior Column, Open Approach

0SG30JJ Fusion of Lumbosacral Joint with Synthetic Substitute, Posterior Approach, Anterior Column, Open Approach

0SG30K0 Fusion of Lumbosacral Joint with Nonautologous Tissue Substitute, Anterior Approach, Anterior Column, Open Approach

0SG30K1 Fusion of Lumbosacral Joint with Nonautologous Tissue Substitute, Posterior Approach, Posterior Column, Open Approach

0SG30KJ Fusion of Lumbosacral Joint with Nonautologous Tissue Substitute, Posterior Approach, Anterior Column, Open Approach

0SG3370 Fusion of Lumbosacral Joint with Autologous Tissue Substitute, Anterior Approach, Anterior Column, Percutaneous Approach

0SG3371 Fusion of Lumbosacral Joint with Autologous Tissue Substitute, Posterior Approach, Posterior Column, Percutaneous Approach

0SG337J Fusion of Lumbosacral Joint with Autologous Tissue Substitute, Posterior Approach, Anterior Column, Percutaneous Approach

0SG33A0 Fusion of Lumbosacral Joint with Interbody Fusion Device, Anterior Approach, Anterior Column, Percutaneous Approach

0SG33AJ Fusion of Lumbosacral Joint with Interbody Fusion Device, Posterior Approach, Anterior Column, Percutaneous Approach

0SG33J0 Fusion of Lumbosacral Joint with Synthetic Substitute, Anterior Approach, Anterior Column, Percutaneous Approach

0SG33J1 Fusion of Lumbosacral Joint with Synthetic Substitute, Posterior Approach, Posterior Column, Percutaneous Approach

0SG33JJ Fusion of Lumbosacral Joint with Synthetic Substitute, Posterior Approach, Anterior Column, Percutaneous Approach

0SG33K0 Fusion of Lumbosacral Joint with Nonautologous Tissue Substitute, Anterior Approach, Anterior Column, Percutaneous Approach

0SG33K1 Fusion of Lumbosacral Joint with Nonautologous Tissue Substitute, Posterior Approach, Posterior Column, Percutaneous Approach

0SG33KJ Fusion of Lumbosacral Joint with Nonautologous Tissue Substitute, Posterior Approach, Anterior Column, Percutaneous Approach

0SG3470 Fusion of Lumbosacral Joint with Autologous Tissue Substitute, Anterior Approach, Anterior Column, Percutaneous Endoscopic Approach

0SG3471 Fusion of Lumbosacral Joint with Autologous Tissue Substitute, Posterior Approach, Posterior Column, Percutaneous Endoscopic Approach

0SG347J Fusion of Lumbosacral Joint with Autologous Tissue Substitute, Posterior Approach, Anterior Column, Percutaneous Endoscopic Approach

0SG34A0 Fusion of Lumbosacral Joint with Interbody Fusion Device, Anterior Approach, Anterior Column, Percutaneous Endoscopic Approach

0SG34AJ Fusion of Lumbosacral Joint with Interbody Fusion Device, Posterior Approach, Anterior Column, Percutaneous Endoscopic Approach

0SG34J0 Fusion of Lumbosacral Joint with Synthetic Substitute, Anterior Approach, Anterior Column, Percutaneous Endoscopic Approach

0SG34J1 Fusion of Lumbosacral Joint with Synthetic Substitute, Posterior Approach, Posterior Column, Percutaneous Endoscopic Approach

0SG34JJ Fusion of Lumbosacral Joint with Synthetic Substitute, Posterior Approach, Anterior Column, Percutaneous Endoscopic Approach

0SG34K0 Fusion of Lumbosacral Joint with Nonautologous Tissue Substitute, Anterior Approach, Anterior Column, Percutaneous Endoscopic Approach

0SG34K1 Fusion of Lumbosacral Joint with Nonautologous Tissue Substitute, Posterior Approach, Posterior Column, Percutaneous Endoscopic Approach

0SG34KJ Fusion of Lumbosacral Joint with Nonautologous Tissue Substitute, Posterior Approach, Anterior Column, Percutaneous Endoscopic Approach

0SG704Z Fusion of Right Sacroiliac Joint with Internal Fixation Device, Open Approach

0SG707Z Fusion of Right Sacroiliac Joint with Autologous Tissue Substitute, Open Approach

0SG70JZ Fusion of Right Sacroiliac Joint with Synthetic Substitute, Open Approach

0SG70KZ Fusion of Right Sacroiliac Joint with Nonautologous Tissue Substitute, Open Approach

0SG734Z Fusion of Right Sacroiliac Joint with Internal Fixation Device, Percutaneous Approach

0SG737Z Fusion of Right Sacroiliac Joint with Autologous Tissue Substitute, Percutaneous Approach

0SG73JZ Fusion of Right Sacroiliac Joint with Synthetic Substitute, Percutaneous Approach

0SG73KZ Fusion of Right Sacroiliac Joint with Nonautologous Tissue Substitute, Percutaneous Approach

0SG744Z Fusion of Right Sacroiliac Joint with Internal Fixation Device, Percutaneous Endoscopic Approach

0SG747Z Fusion of Right Sacroiliac Joint with Autologous Tissue Substitute, Percutaneous Endoscopic Approach

0SG74JZ Fusion of Right Sacroiliac Joint with Synthetic Substitute, Percutaneous Endoscopic Approach

HAC 12: Surgical Site Infection-Certain Orthopedic Procedures of the Spine, Shoulder, and Elbow (continued)

ØSG74KZ Fusion of Right Sacroiliac Joint with Nonautologous Tissue Substitute, Percutaneous Endoscopic Approach

ØSG8Ø4Z Fusion of Left Sacroiliac Joint with Internal Fixation Device, Open Approach

ØSG8Ø7Z Fusion of Left Sacroiliac Joint with Autologous Tissue Substitute, Open Approach

ØSG8ØJZ Fusion of Left Sacroiliac Joint with Synthetic Substitute, Open Approach

ØSG8ØKZ Fusion of Left Sacroiliac Joint with Nonautologous Tissue Substitute, Open Approach

ØSG834Z Fusion of Left Sacroiliac Joint with Internal Fixation Device, Percutaneous Approach

ØSG837Z Fusion of Left Sacroiliac Joint with Autologous Tissue Substitute, Percutaneous Approach

ØSG83JZ Fusion of Left Sacroiliac Joint with Synthetic Substitute, Percutaneous Approach

ØSG83KZ Fusion of Left Sacroiliac Joint with Nonautologous Tissue Substitute, Percutaneous Approach

ØSG844Z Fusion of Left Sacroiliac Joint with Internal Fixation Device, Percutaneous Endoscopic Approach

ØSG847Z Fusion of Left Sacroiliac Joint with Autologous Tissue Substitute, Percutaneous Endoscopic Approach

ØSG84JZ Fusion of Left Sacroiliac Joint with Synthetic Substitute, Percutaneous Endoscopic Approach

ØSG84KZ Fusion of Left Sacroiliac Joint with Nonautologous Tissue Substitute, Percutaneous Endoscopic Approach

XRGØØ92 Fusion of Occipital-cervical Joint using Nanotextured Surface Interbody Fusion Device, Open Approach, New Technology Group 2

XRGØØF3 Fusion of Occipital-cervical Joint using Radiolucent Porous Interbody Fusion Device, Open Approach, New Technology Group 3

XRG1Ø92 Fusion of Cervical Vertebral Joint using Nanotextured Surface Interbody Fusion Device, Open Approach, New Technology Group 2

XRG1ØF3 Fusion of Cervical Vertebral Joint using Radiolucent Porous Interbody Fusion Device, Open Approach, New Technology Group 3

XRG2Ø92 Fusion of 2 or more Cervical Vertebral Joints using Nanotextured Surface Interbody Fusion Device, Open Approach, New Technology Group 2

XRG2ØF3 Fusion of 2 or more Cervical Vertebral Joints using Radiolucent Porous Interbody Fusion Device, Open Approach, New Technology Group 3

XRG4Ø92 Fusion of Cervicothoracic Vertebral Joint using Nanotextured Surface Interbody Fusion Device, Open Approach, New Technology Group 2

XRG4ØF3 Fusion of Cervicothoracic Vertebral Joint using Radiolucent Porous Interbody Fusion Device, Open Approach, New Technology Group 3

XRG6Ø92 Fusion of Thoracic Vertebral Joint using Nanotextured Surface Interbody Fusion Device, Open Approach, New Technology Group 2

XRG6ØF3 Fusion of Thoracic Vertebral Joint using Radiolucent Porous Interbody Fusion Device, Open Approach, New Technology Group 3

XRG7Ø92 Fusion of 2 to 7 Thoracic Vertebral Joints using Nanotextured Surface Interbody Fusion Device, Open Approach, New Technology Group 2

XRG7ØF3 Fusion of 2 to 7 Thoracic Vertebral Joints using Radiolucent Porous Interbody Fusion Device, Open Approach, New Technology Group 3

XRG8Ø92 Fusion of 8 or more Thoracic Vertebral Joints using Nanotextured Surface Interbody Fusion Device, Open Approach, New Technology Group 2

XRG8ØF3 Fusion of 8 or more Thoracic Vertebral Joints using Radiolucent Porous Interbody Fusion Device, Open Approach, New Technology Group 3

XRGAØ92 Fusion of Thoracolumbar Vertebral Joint using Nanotextured Surface Interbody Fusion Device, Open Approach, New Technology Group 2

XRGAØF3 Fusion of Thoracolumbar Vertebral Joint using Radiolucent Porous Interbody Fusion Device, Open Approach, New Technology Group 3

XRGBØ92 Fusion of Lumbar Vertebral Joint using Nanotextured Surface Interbody Fusion Device, Open Approach, New Technology Group 2

XRGBØF3 Fusion of Lumbar Vertebral Joint using Radiolucent Porous Interbody Fusion Device, Open Approach, New Technology Group 3

XRGCØ92 Fusion of 2 or more Lumbar Vertebral Joints using Nanotextured Surface Interbody Fusion Device, Open Approach, New Technology Group 2

XRGCØF3 Fusion of 2 or more Lumbar Vertebral Joints using Radiolucent Porous Interbody Fusion Device, Open Approach, New Technology Group 3

XRGDØ92 Fusion of Lumbosacral Joint using Nanotextured Surface Interbody Fusion Device, Open Approach, New Technology Group 2

XRGDØF3 Fusion of Lumbosacral Joint using Radiolucent Porous Interbody Fusion Device, Open Approach, New Technology Group 3

HAC 13: Surgical Site Infection (SSI) Following Cardiac Implantable Electronic Device (CIED) Procedures

Secondary diagnosis not POA:

K68.11
T81.4ØXA
T81.41XA
T81.42XA
T81.43XA
T81.44XA
T81.49XA
T82.6XXA
T82.7XXA

AND

Any of the following procedures:

Ø2H43JZ Insertion of Pacemaker Lead into Coronary Vein, Percutaneous Approach

Ø2H43KZ Insertion of Defibrillator Lead into Coronary Vein, Percutaneous Approach

Ø2H43MZ Insertion of Cardiac Lead into Coronary Vein, Percutaneous Approach

Ø2H63JZ Insertion of Pacemaker Lead into Right Atrium, Percutaneous Approach

Ø2H63MZ Insertion of Cardiac Lead into Right Atrium, Percutaneous Approach

Ø2H73JZ Insertion of Pacemaker Lead into Left Atrium, Percutaneous Approach

Ø2H73MZ Insertion of Cardiac Lead into Left Atrium, Percutaneous Approach

Ø2HK3JZ Insertion of Pacemaker Lead into Right Ventricle, Percutaneous Approach

Ø2HL3JZ Insertion of Pacemaker Lead into Left Ventricle, Percutaneous Approach

Ø2HNØJZ Insertion of Pacemaker Lead into Pericardium, Open Approach

Ø2HNØMZ Insertion of Cardiac Lead into Pericardium, Open Approach

Ø2HN3JZ Insertion of Pacemaker Lead into Pericardium, Percutaneous Approach

Ø2HN3MZ Insertion of Cardiac Lead into Pericardium, Percutaneous Approach

Ø2HN4JZ Insertion of Pacemaker Lead into Pericardium, Percutaneous Endoscopic Approach

Ø2HN4MZ Insertion of Cardiac Lead into Pericardium, Percutaneous Endoscopic Approach

Ø2PAØMZ Removal of Cardiac Lead from Heart, Open Approach

Ø2PA3MZ Removal of Cardiac Lead from Heart, Percutaneous Approach

Ø2PA4MZ Removal of Cardiac Lead from Heart, Percutaneous Endoscopic Approach

Ø2PAXMZ Removal of Cardiac Lead from Heart, External Approach

Ø2WAØMZ Revision of Cardiac Lead in Heart, Open Approach

Ø2WA3MZ Revision of Cardiac Lead in Heart, Percutaneous Approach

Ø2WA4MZ Revision of Cardiac Lead in Heart, Percutaneous Endoscopic Approach

ØJH6Ø4Z Insertion of Pacemaker, Single Chamber into Chest Subcutaneous Tissue and Fascia, Open Approach

ØJH6Ø5Z Insertion of Pacemaker, Single Chamber Rate Responsive into Chest Subcutaneous Tissue and Fascia, Open Approach

ØJH6Ø6Z Insertion of Pacemaker, Dual Chamber into Chest Subcutaneous Tissue and Fascia, Open Approach

ØJH6Ø7Z Insertion of Cardiac Resynchronization Pacemaker Pulse Generator into Chest Subcutaneous Tissue and Fascia, Open Approach

ØJH6Ø8Z Insertion of Defibrillator Generator into Chest Subcutaneous Tissue and Fascia, Open Approach

ØJH6Ø9Z Insertion of Cardiac Resynchronization Defibrillator Pulse Generator into Chest Subcutaneous Tissue and Fascia, Open Approach

ØJH6ØPZ Insertion of Cardiac Rhythm Related Device into Chest Subcutaneous Tissue and Fascia, Open Approach

ØJH634Z Insertion of Pacemaker, Single Chamber into Chest Subcutaneous Tissue and Fascia, Percutaneous Approach

ØJH635Z Insertion of Pacemaker, Single Chamber Rate Responsive into Chest Subcutaneous Tissue and Fascia, Percutaneous Approach

ØJH636Z Insertion of Pacemaker, Dual Chamber into Chest Subcutaneous Tissue and Fascia, Percutaneous Approach

ØJH637Z Insertion of Cardiac Resynchronization Pacemaker Pulse Generator into Chest Subcutaneous Tissue and Fascia, Percutaneous Approach

HAC 13: Surgical Site Infection (SSI) Following Cardiac Implantable Electronic Device (CIED) Procedures (continued)

ØJH638Z Insertion of Defibrillator Generator into Chest Subcutaneous Tissue and Fascia, Percutaneous Approach

ØJH639Z Insertion of Cardiac Resynchronization Defibrillator Pulse Generator into Chest Subcutaneous Tissue and Fascia, Percutaneous Approach

ØJH63PZ Insertion of Cardiac Rhythm Related Device into Chest Subcutaneous Tissue and Fascia, Percutaneous Approach

ØJH804Z Insertion of Pacemaker, Single Chamber into Abdomen Subcutaneous Tissue and Fascia, Open Approach

ØJH805Z Insertion of Pacemaker, Single Chamber Rate Responsive into Abdomen Subcutaneous Tissue and Fascia, Open Approach

ØJH806Z Insertion of Pacemaker, Dual Chamber into Abdomen Subcutaneous Tissue and Fascia, Open Approach

ØJH807Z Insertion of Cardiac Resynchronization Pacemaker Pulse Generator into Abdomen Subcutaneous Tissue and Fascia, Open Approach

ØJH808Z Insertion of Defibrillator Generator into Abdomen Subcutaneous Tissue and Fascia, Open Approach

ØJH809Z Insertion of Cardiac Resynchronization Defibrillator Pulse Generator into Abdomen Subcutaneous Tissue and Fascia, Open Approach

ØJH80PZ Insertion of Cardiac Rhythm Related Device into Abdomen Subcutaneous Tissue and Fascia, Open Approach

ØJH834Z Insertion of Pacemaker, Single Chamber into Abdomen Subcutaneous Tissue and Fascia, Percutaneous Approach

ØJH835Z Insertion of Pacemaker, Single Chamber Rate Responsive into Abdomen Subcutaneous Tissue and Fascia, Percutaneous Approach

ØJH836Z Insertion of Pacemaker, Dual Chamber into Abdomen Subcutaneous Tissue and Fascia, Percutaneous Approach

ØJH837Z Insertion of Cardiac Resynchronization Pacemaker Pulse Generator into Abdomen Subcutaneous Tissue and Fascia, Percutaneous Approach

ØJH838Z Insertion of Defibrillator Generator into Abdomen Subcutaneous Tissue and Fascia, Percutaneous Approach

ØJH839Z Insertion of Cardiac Resynchronization Defibrillator Pulse Generator into Abdomen Subcutaneous Tissue and Fascia, Percutaneous Approach

ØJH83PZ Insertion of Cardiac Rhythm Related Device into Abdomen Subcutaneous Tissue and Fascia, Percutaneous Approach

ØJPTØPZ Removal of Cardiac Rhythm Related Device from Trunk Subcutaneous Tissue and Fascia, Open Approach

ØJPT3PZ Removal of Cardiac Rhythm Related Device from Trunk Subcutaneous Tissue and Fascia, Percutaneous Approach

ØJWTØPZ Revision of Cardiac Rhythm Related Device in Trunk Subcutaneous Tissue and Fascia, Open Approach

ØJWT3PZ Revision of Cardiac Rhythm Related Device in Trunk Subcutaneous Tissue and Fascia, Percutaneous Approach

HAC 14: Iatrogenic Pneumothorax with Venous Catheterization

Secondary diagnosis not POA:
J95.811

AND

Any of the following procedures:

02H633Z Insertion of Infusion Device into Right Atrium, Percutaneous Approach

02HK33Z Insertion of Infusion Device into Right Ventricle, Percutaneous Approach

02HS33Z Insertion of Infusion Device into Right Pulmonary Vein, Percutaneous Approach

02HS43Z Insertion of Infusion Device into Right Pulmonary Vein, Percutaneous Endoscopic Approach

02HT33Z Insertion of Infusion Device into Left Pulmonary Vein, Percutaneous Approach

02HT43Z Insertion of Infusion Device into Left Pulmonary Vein, Percutaneous Endoscopic Approach

02HV33Z Insertion of Infusion Device into Superior Vena Cava, Percutaneous Approach

02HV43Z Insertion of Infusion Device into Superior Vena Cava, Percutaneous Endoscopic Approach

05H033Z Insertion of Infusion Device into Azygos Vein, Percutaneous Approach

05H043Z Insertion of Infusion Device into Azygos Vein, Percutaneous Endoscopic Approach

05H133Z Insertion of Infusion Device into Hemiazygos Vein, Percutaneous Approach

05H143Z Insertion of Infusion Device into Hemiazygos Vein, Percutaneous Endoscopic Approach

05H333Z Insertion of Infusion Device into Right Innominate Vein, Percutaneous Approach

05H343Z Insertion of Infusion Device into Right Innominate Vein, Percutaneous Endoscopic Approach

05H433Z Insertion of Infusion Device into Left Innominate Vein, Percutaneous Approach

05H443Z Insertion of Infusion Device into Left Innominate Vein, Percutaneous Endoscopic Approach

05H533Z Insertion of Infusion Device into Right Subclavian Vein, Percutaneous Approach

05H543Z Insertion of Infusion Device into Right Subclavian Vein, Percutaneous Endoscopic Approach

05H633Z Insertion of Infusion Device into Left Subclavian Vein, Percutaneous Approach

05H643Z Insertion of Infusion Device into Left Subclavian Vein, Percutaneous Endoscopic Approach

05HM33Z Insertion of Infusion Device into Right Internal Jugular Vein, Percutaneous Approach

05HN33Z Insertion of Infusion Device into Left Internal Jugular Vein, Percutaneous Approach

05HP33Z Insertion of Infusion Device into Right External Jugular Vein, Percutaneous Approach

05HQ33Z Insertion of Infusion Device into Left External Jugular Vein, Percutaneous Approach

ØJH63XZ Insertion of Vascular Access Device into Chest Subcutaneous Tissue and Fascia, Percutaneous Approach

Appendix K: Coding Exercises and Answers

Using the ICD-10-PCS tables construct the code that accurately represents the procedure performed.

Medical Surgical Section

Procedure	Code
1. Excision of malignant melanoma from skin of right ear	
2. Laparoscopy with excision of endometrial implant from left ovary	
3. Percutaneous needle core biopsy of right kidney	
4. EGD with gastric biopsy	
5. Open endarterectomy of left common carotid artery	
6. Excision of basal cell carcinoma of lower lip	
7. Open excision of tail of pancreas	
8. Percutaneous biopsy of right gastrocnemius muscle	
9. Sigmoidoscopy with sigmoid polypectomy	
10. Open excision of lesion from right Achilles tendon	
11. Open resection of cecum	
12. Total excision of pituitary gland, open	
13. Explantation of left failed kidney, open	
14. Open left axillary total lymphadenectomy	
15. Laparoscopic-assisted vaginal hysterectomy	
16. Right total mastectomy, open	
17. Open resection of papillary muscle	
18. Total retropubic prostatectomy, open	
19. Laparoscopic cholecystectomy	
20. Endoscopic bilateral total maxillary sinusectomy	
21. Amputation at right elbow level	
22. Right below-knee amputation, proximal tibia/fibula	
23. Fifth ray carpometacarpal joint amputation, left hand	
24. Right leg and hip amputation through ischium	
25. DIP joint amputation of right thumb	
26. Right wrist joint amputation	
27. Trans-metatarsal amputation of foot at left big toe	
28. Mid-shaft amputation, right humerus	
29. Left fourth toe amputation, mid-proximal phalanx	
30. Right above-knee amputation, distal femur	
31. Cryotherapy of wart on left hand	
32. Percutaneous radiofrequency ablation of right vocal cord lesion	
33. Left heart catheterization with laser destruction of arrhythmogenic focus, A-V node	
34. Cautery of nosebleed	
35. Transurethral endoscopic laser ablation of prostate	
36. Percutaneous cautery of oozing varicose vein, left calf	

Procedure	Code
37. Laparoscopy with destruction of endometriosis, bilateral ovaries	
38. Laser coagulation of right retinal vessel hemorrhage, percutaneous	
39. Thoracoscopic pleurodesis, left side	
40. Percutaneous insertion of Greenfield IVC filter	
41. Forceps total mouth extraction, upper and lower teeth	
42. Removal of left thumbnail	
43. Extraction of right intraocular lens without replacement, percutaneous	
44. Laparoscopy with needle aspiration of ova for in vitro fertilization	
45. Nonexcisional debridement of skin ulcer, right foot	
46. Open stripping of abdominal fascia, right side	
47. Hysteroscopy with D&C, diagnostic	
48. Liposuction for medical purposes, left upper arm	
49. Removal of tattered right ear drum fragments with tweezers	
50. Microincisional phlebectomy of spider veins, right lower leg	
51. Routine Foley catheter placement	
52. Incision and drainage of external anal abscess	
53. Percutaneous drainage of ascites	
54. Laparoscopy with left ovarian cystotomy and drainage	
55. Laparotomy and drain placement for liver abscess, right lobe	
56. Right knee arthrotomy with drain placement	
57. Thoracentesis of left pleural effusion	
58. Phlebotomy of left median cubital vein for polycythemia vera	
59. Percutaneous chest tube placement for right pneumothorax	
60. Endoscopic drainage of left ethmoid sinus	
61. External ventricular CSF drainage catheter placement via burr hole	
62. Removal of foreign body, right cornea	
63. Percutaneous mechanical thrombectomy, left brachial artery	
64. Esophagogastroscopy with removal of bezoar from stomach	
65. Foreign body removal, skin of left thumb	
66. Transurethral cystoscopy with removal of bladder stone	
67. Forceps removal of foreign body in right nostril	
68. Laparoscopy with excision of old suture from mesentery	
69. Incision and removal of right lacrimal duct stone	
70. Nonincisional removal of intraluminal foreign body from vagina	
71. Right common carotid endarterectomy, open	
72. Open excision of retained sliver, subcutaneous tissue of left foot	
73. Extracorporeal shockwave lithotripsy (ESWL), bilateral ureters	

Procedure	Code	Procedure	Code
74. Endoscopic retrograde cholangiopancreatography (ERCP) with lithotripsy of common bile duct stone		111. Bilateral TRAM pedicle flap reconstruction status post mastectomy, muscle only, open	
75. Thoracotomy with crushing of pericardial calcifications		112. Skin transfer flap closure of complex open wound, left lower back	
76. Transurethral cystoscopy with fragmentation of bladder calculus		113. Open fracture reduction, right tibia	
77. Hysteroscopy with intraluminal lithotripsy of left fallopian tube calcification		114. Laparoscopy with gastropexy for malrotation	
78. Division of right foot tendon, percutaneous		115. Left knee arthroscopy with reposition of anterior cruciate ligament	
79. Left heart catheterization with division of bundle of HIS		116. Open transposition of ulnar nerve	
80. Open osteotomy of capitate, left hand		117. Closed reduction with percutaneous internal fixation of right femoral neck fracture	
81. EGD with esophagotomy of esophagogastric junction		118. Trans-vaginal intraluminal cervical cerclage	
82. Sacral rhizotomy for pain control, percutaneous		119. Cervical cerclage using Shirodkar technique	
83. Laparotomy with exploration and adhesiolysis of right ureter		120. Thoracotomy with banding of left pulmonary artery using extraluminal device	
84. Incision of scar contracture, right elbow		121. Restriction of thoracic duct with intraluminal stent, percutaneous	
85. Frenulotomy for treatment of tongue-tie syndrome		122. Craniotomy with clipping of cerebral aneurysm	
86. Right shoulder arthroscopy with coracoacromial ligament release		123. Nonincisional, transnasal placement of restrictive stent in right lacrimal duct	
87. Mitral valvulotomy for release of fused leaflets, open approach		124. Catheter-based temporary restriction of blood flow in abdominal aorta for treatment of cerebral ischemia	
88. Percutaneous left Achilles tendon release		125. Percutaneous ligation of esophageal vein	
89. Laparoscopy with lysis of peritoneal adhesions		126. Percutaneous embolization of left internal carotid-cavernous fistula	
90. Manual rupture of right shoulder joint adhesions under general anesthesia		127. Laparoscopy with bilateral occlusion of fallopian tubes using Hulka extraluminal clips	
91. Open posterior tarsal tunnel release		128. Open suture ligation of failed AV graft, left brachial artery	
92. Laparoscopy with freeing of left ovary and fallopian tube		129. Percutaneous embolization of vascular supply, intracranial meningioma	
93. Liver transplant with donor matched liver		130. Percutaneous embolization of right uterine artery, using coils	
94. Orthotopic heart transplant using porcine heart		131. Open occlusion of left atrial appendage, using extraluminal pressure clips	
95. Right lung transplant, open, using organ donor match		132. Percutaneous suture exclusion of left atrial appendage, via femoral artery access	
96. Transplant of large intestine, organ donor match		133. ERCP with balloon dilation of common bile duct	
97. Left kidney/pancreas organ bank transplant		134. PTCA of two coronary arteries, LAD with stent placement, RCA with no stent	
98. Replantation of avulsed scalp		135. Cystoscopy with intraluminal dilation of bladder neck stricture	
99. Reattachment of severed right ear		136. Open dilation of old anastomosis, left femoral artery	
100. Reattachment of traumatic left gastrocnemius avulsion, open		137. Dilation of upper esophageal stricture, direct visualization, with Bougie sound	
101. Closed replantation of three avulsed teeth, lower jaw		138. PTA of right brachial artery stenosis	
102. Reattachment of severed left hand		139. Transnasal dilation and stent placement in right lacrimal duct	
103. Right open palmaris longus tendon transfer		140. Hysteroscopy with balloon dilation of bilateral fallopian tubes	
104. Endoscopic radial to median nerve transfer		141. Tracheoscopy with intraluminal dilation of tracheal stenosis	
105. Fasciocutaneous flap closure of left thigh, open		142. Cystoscopy with dilation of left ureteral stricture, with stent placement	
106. Transfer left index finger to left thumb position, open		143. Open gastric bypass with Roux-en-Y limb to jejunum	
107. Percutaneous fascia transfer to fill defect, right neck		144. Right temporal artery to intracranial artery bypass using Gore-Tex graft, open	
108. Trigeminal to facial nerve transfer, percutaneous endoscopic			
109. Endoscopic left leg flexor hallucis longus tendon transfer			
110. Right scalp advancement flap to right temple			

Procedure	Code
145. Tracheostomy formation with tracheostomy tube placement, percutaneous	
146. PICVA (percutaneous in situ coronary venous arterialization) of single coronary artery	
147. Open left femoral-popliteal artery bypass using cadaver vein graft	
148. Shunting of intrathecal cerebrospinal fluid to peritoneal cavity using synthetic shunt	
149. Colostomy formation, open, transverse colon to abdominal wall	
150. Open urinary diversion, left ureter, using ileal conduit to skin	
151. CABG of LAD using pedicled left internal mammary artery, open off-bypass	
152. Open pleuroperitoneal shunt, right pleural cavity, using synthetic device	
153. Percutaneous placement of ventriculoperitoneal shunt for treatment of hydrocephalus	
154. End-of-life replacement of spinal neurostimulator generator, multiple array, in lower abdomen	
155. Percutaneous insertion of spinal neurostimulator lead, lumbar spinal cord	
156. Percutaneous replacement of broken pacemaker lead in left atrium	
157. Open placement of dual chamber pacemaker generator in chest wall	
158. Percutaneous placement of venous central line in right internal jugular, with tip in superior vena cava	
159. Open insertion of multiple channel cochlear implant, left ear	
160. Percutaneous placement of Swan-Ganz catheter in pulmonary trunk	
161. Bronchoscopy with insertion of Low Dose, Pd-103 brachytherapy seeds, right main bronchus	
162. Open insertion of interspinous process device into lumbar vertebral joint	
163. Open placement of bone growth stimulator, left femoral shaft	
164. Cystoscopy with placement of brachytherapy seeds in prostate gland	
165. Percutaneous insertion of Greenfield IVC filter	
166. Full-thickness skin graft to right lower arm, autograft (do not code graft harvest for this exercise)	
167. Excision of necrosed left femoral head with bone bank bone graft to fill the defect, open	
168. Penetrating keratoplasty of right cornea with donor matched cornea, percutaneous approach	
169. Excision of abdominal aorta with Gore-Tex graft replacement, open	
170. Total right knee arthroplasty with insertion of total knee prosthesis	
171. Tenonectomy with graft to right ankle using cadaver graft, open	
172. Mitral valve replacement using porcine valve, open	
173. Percutaneous phacoemulsification of right eye cataract with prosthetic lens insertion	

Procedure	Code
174. Transcatheter replacement of pulmonary valve using of bovine jugular vein valve	
175. Total left hip replacement using ceramic on ceramic prosthesis, without bone cement	
176. Aortic valve annuloplasty using ring, open	
177. Laparoscopic repair of left inguinal hernia with marlex plug	
178. Autograft nerve graft to right median nerve, percutaneous endoscopic (do not code graft harvest for this exercise)	
179. Exchange of liner in femoral component of previous left hip replacement, open approach	
180. Anterior colporrhaphy with polypropylene mesh reinforcement, open approach	
181. Implantation of CorCap cardiac support device, open approach	
182. Abdominal wall herniorrhaphy, open, using synthetic mesh	
183. Tendon graft to strengthen injured left shoulder using autograft, open (do not code graft harvest for this exercise)	
184. Onlay lamellar keratoplasty of left cornea using autograft, external approach	
185. Resurfacing procedure on right femoral head, open approach	
186. Exchange of drainage tube from right hip joint	
187. Tracheostomy tube exchange	
188. Change chest tube for left pneumothorax	
189. Exchange of cerebral ventriculostomy drainage tube	
190. Foley urinary catheter exchange	
191. Open removal of lumbar sympathetic neurostimulator lead	
192. Nonincisional removal of Swan-Ganz catheter from right pulmonary artery	
193. Laparotomy with removal of pancreatic drain	
194. Extubation, endotracheal tube	
195. Nonincisional PEG tube removal	
196. Transvaginal removal of brachytherapy seeds	
197. Transvaginal removal of extraluminal cervical cerclage	
198. Incision with removal of K-wire fixation, right first metatarsal	
199. Cystoscopy with retrieval of left ureteral stent	
200. Removal of nasogastric drainage tube for decompression	
201. Removal of external fixator, left radial fracture	
202. Trimming and reanastomosis of stenosed femorofemoral synthetic bypass graft, open	
203. Open revision of right hip replacement, with readjustment of prosthesis	
204. Adjustment of position, pacemaker lead in left ventricle, percutaneous	
205. External repositioning of Foley catheter to bladder	
206. Taking out loose screw and putting larger screw in fracture repair plate, left tibia	
207. Revision of totally implantable VAD port placement in chest wall, causing patient discomfort, open	
208. Thoracotomy with exploration of right pleural cavity	

Procedure	Code
209. Diagnostic laryngoscopy	
210. Exploratory arthrotomy of left knee	
211. Colposcopy with diagnostic hysteroscopy	
212. Digital rectal exam	
213. Diagnostic arthroscopy of right shoulder	
214. Endoscopy of maxillary sinus	
215. Laparotomy with palpation of liver	
216. Transurethral diagnostic cystoscopy	
217. Colonoscopy, discontinued at sigmoid colon	
218. Percutaneous mapping of basal ganglia	
219. Heart catheterization with cardiac mapping	
220. Intraoperative whole brain mapping via craniotomy	
221. Mapping of left cerebral hemisphere, percutaneous endoscopic	
222. Intraoperative cardiac mapping during open heart surgery	
223. Hysteroscopy with cautery of post-hysterectomy oozing and evacuation of clot	
224. Open exploration and ligation of post-op arterial bleeder, left forearm	
225. Control of post-operative retroperitoneal bleeding via laparotomy	
226. Reopening of thoracotomy site with drainage and control of post-op hemopericardium	
227. Arthroscopy with drainage of hemarthrosis at previous operative site, right knee	
228. Radiocarpal fusion of left hand with internal fixation, open	
229. Posterior approach spinal fusion at L1-L3 level with BAK cage interbody fusion device, open	
230. Intercarpal fusion of right hand with bone bank bone graft, open	
231. Sacrococcygeal fusion with bone graft from same operative site, open	
232. Interphalangeal fusion of left great toe, percutaneous pin fixation	
233. Suture repair of left radial nerve laceration	
234. Laparotomy with suture repair of blunt force duodenal laceration	
235. Perineoplasty with repair of old obstetric laceration, open	
236. Suture repair of right biceps tendon (upper arm) laceration, open	
237. Closure of abdominal wall stab wound	
238. Cosmetic face lift, open, no other information available	
239. Bilateral breast augmentation with silicone implants, open	
240. Cosmetic rhinoplasty with septal reduction and tip elevation using local tissue graft, open	
241. Abdominoplasty (tummy tuck), open	
242. Liposuction of bilateral thighs	
243. Creation of penis in female patient using tissue bank donor graft	
244. Creation of vagina in male patient using synthetic material	
245. Laparoscopic vertical (sleeve) gastrectomy	
246. Left uterine artery embolization with intraluminal biosphere injection	

Obstetrics

Procedure	Code
1. Abortion by dilation and evacuation following laminaria insertion	
2. Manually assisted spontaneous abortion	
3. Abortion by abortifacient insertion	
4. Bimanual pregnancy examination	
5. Extraperitoneal C-section, low transverse incision	
6. Fetal spinal tap, percutaneous	
7. Fetal kidney transplant, laparoscopic	
8. Open in utero repair of congenital diaphragmatic hernia	
9. Laparoscopy with total excision of tubal pregnancy	
10. Transvaginal removal of fetal monitoring electrode	

Placement

Procedure	Code
1. Placement of packing material, right ear	
2. Mechanical traction of entire left leg	
3. Removal of splint, right shoulder	
4. Placement of neck brace	
5. Change of vaginal packing	
6. Packing of wound, chest wall	
7. Sterile dressing placement to left groin region	
8. Removal of packing material from pharynx	
9. Placement of intermittent pneumatic compression device, covering entire right arm	
10. Exchange of pressure dressing to left thigh	

Administration

Procedure	Code
1. Peritoneal dialysis via indwelling catheter	
2. Transvaginal artificial insemination	
3. Infusion of total parenteral nutrition via central venous catheter	
4. Esophagogastroscopy with Botox injection into esophageal sphincter	
5. Percutaneous irrigation of knee joint	
6. Systemic infusion of recombinant tissue plasminogen activator (r-tPA) via peripheral venous catheter	
7. Transabdominal in vitro fertilization, implantation of donor ovum	
8. Autologous bone marrow transplant via central venous line	
9. Implantation of anti-microbial envelope with cardiac defibrillator placement, open	
10. Sclerotherapy of brachial plexus lesion, alcohol injection	
11. Percutaneous peripheral vein injection, glucarpidase	
12. Introduction of anti-infective envelope into subcutaneous tissue, open	

Measurement and Monitoring

Procedure	Code
1. Cardiac stress test, single measurement	
2. EGD with biliary flow measurement	
3. Right and left heart cardiac catheterization with bilateral sampling and pressure measurements	
4. Temperature monitoring, rectal	
5. Peripheral venous pulse, external, single measurement	
6. Holter monitoring	
7. Respiratory rate, external, single measurement	
8. Fetal heart rate monitoring, transvaginal	
9. Visual mobility test, single measurement	
10. Left ventricular cardiac output monitoring from pulmonary artery wedge (Swan-Ganz) catheter	
11. Olfactory acuity test, single measurement	

Extracorporeal or Systemic Assistance and Performance

Procedure	Code
1. Intermittent mechanical ventilation, 16 hours	
2. Liver dialysis, single encounter	
3. Cardiac countershock with successful conversion to sinus rhythm	
4. IPPB (intermittent positive pressure breathing) for mobilization of secretions, 22 hours	
5. Renal dialysis, 12 hours	
6. IABP (intra-aortic balloon pump) continuous	
7. Intra-operative cardiac pacing, continuous	
8. ECMO (extracorporeal membrane oxygenation), central	
9. Controlled mechanical ventilation (CMV), 45 hours	
10. Pulsatile compression boot with intermittent inflation	

Extracorporeal or Systemic Therapies

Procedure	Code
1. Donor thrombocytapheresis, single encounter	
2. Bili-lite phototherapy, series treatment	
3. Whole body hypothermia, single treatment	
4. Circulatory phototherapy, single encounter	
5. Shock wave therapy of plantar fascia, single treatment	
6. Antigen-free air conditioning, series treatment	
7. TMS (transcranial magnetic stimulation), series treatment	
8. Therapeutic ultrasound of peripheral vessels, single treatment	
9. Plasmapheresis, series treatment	
10. Extracorporeal electromagnetic stimulation (EMS) for urinary incontinence, single treatment	

Osteopathic

Procedure	Code
1. Isotonic muscle energy treatment of right leg	
2. Low velocity-high amplitude osteopathic treatment of head	
3. Lymphatic pump osteopathic treatment of left axilla	
4. Indirect osteopathic treatment of sacrum	
5. Articulatory osteopathic treatment of cervical region	

Other Procedures

Procedure	Code
1. Near infrared spectroscopy of leg vessels	
2. CT computer assisted sinus surgery	
3. Suture removal, abdominal wall	
4. Isolation after infectious disease exposure	
5. Robotic assisted open prostatectomy	
6. In vitro fertilization	

Chiropractic

Procedure	Code
1. Chiropractic treatment of lumbar region using long lever specific contact	
2. Chiropractic manipulation of abdominal region, indirect visceral	
3. Chiropractic extra-articular treatment of hip region	
4. Chiropractic treatment of sacrum using long and short lever specific contact	
5. Mechanically-assisted chiropractic manipulation of head	

Imaging

Procedure	Code
1. Noncontrast CT of abdomen and pelvis	
2. Intravascular ultrasound, left subclavian artery	
3. Fluoroscopic guidance for insertion of central venous catheter in SVC, low osmolar contrast	

Procedure	Code
4. Chest x-ray, AP/PA and lateral views	
5. Endoluminal ultrasound of gallbladder and bile ducts	
6. MRI of thyroid gland, contrast unspecified	
7. Esophageal videofluoroscopy study with oral barium contrast	
8. Portable x-ray study of right radius/ulna shaft, standard series	
9. Routine fetal ultrasound, second trimester twin gestation	
10. CT scan of bilateral lungs, high osmolar contrast with densitometry	
11. Fluoroscopic guidance for percutaneous transluminal angioplasty (PTA) of left common femoral artery, low osmolar contrast	

Nuclear Medicine

Procedure	Code
1. Tomo scan of right and left heart, unspecified radiopharmaceutical, qualitative gated rest	
2. Technetium pentetate assay of kidneys, ureters, and bladder	
3. Uniplanar scan of spine using technetium oxidronate, with first-pass study	
4. Thallous chloride tomographic scan of bilateral breasts	
5. PET scan of myocardium using rubidium	
6. Gallium citrate scan of head and neck, single plane imaging	
7. Xenon gas nonimaging probe of brain	
8. Upper GI scan, radiopharmaceutical unspecified, for gastric emptying	
9. Carbon 11 PET scan of brain with quantification	
10. Iodinated albumin nuclear medicine assay, blood plasma volume study	

Radiation Therapy

Procedure	Code
1. Plaque radiation of left eye, single port	
2. 8 MeV photon beam radiation to brain	
3. IORT of colon, 3 ports	
4. HDR brachytherapy of prostate using low dose palladium-103	
5. Electron radiation treatment of right breast, with custom device	
6. Hyperthermia oncology treatment of pelvic region	
7. Contact radiation of tongue	
8. Heavy particle radiation treatment of pancreas, four risk sites	
9. LDR brachytherapy to spinal cord using iodine	
10. Whole body Phosphorus 32 administration with risk to hematopoetic system	

Physical Rehabilitation and Diagnostic Audiology

Procedure	Code
1. Bekesy assessment using audiometer	
2. Individual fitting of left eye prosthesis	

Procedure	Code
3. Physical therapy for range of motion and mobility, patient right hip, no special equipment	
4. Bedside swallow assessment using assessment kit	
5. Caregiver training in airway clearance techniques	
6. Application of short arm cast in rehabilitation setting	
7. Verbal assessment of patient's pain level	
8. Caregiver training in communication skills using manual communication board	
9. Group musculoskeletal balance training exercises, whole body, no special equipment	
10. Individual therapy for auditory processing using tape recorder	

Mental Health

Procedure	Code
1. Cognitive-behavioral psychotherapy, individual	
2. Narcosynthesis	
3. Light therapy	
4. ECT (electroconvulsive therapy), unilateral, multiple seizure	
5. Crisis intervention	
6. Neuropsychological testing	
7. Hypnosis	
8. Developmental testing	
9. Vocational counseling	
10. Family psychotherapy	

Substance Abuse Treatment

Procedure	Code
1. Naltrexone treatment for drug dependency	
2. Substance abuse treatment family counseling	
3. Medication monitoring of patient on methadone maintenance	
4. Individual interpersonal psychotherapy for drug abuse	
5. Patient in for alcohol detoxification treatment	
6. Group motivational counseling	
7. Individual 12-step psychotherapy for substance abuse	
8. Post-test infectious disease counseling for IV drug abuser	
9. Psychodynamic psychotherapy for drug dependent patient	
10. Group cognitive-behavioral counseling for substance abuse	

New Technology

Procedure	Code
1. Infusion of ceftazidime via peripheral venous catheter	

Answers to Coding Exercises

Medical Surgical Section

Procedure	Code
1. Excision of malignant melanoma from skin of right ear	0HB2XZZ
2. Laparoscopy with excision of endometrial implant from left ovary	0UB14ZZ
3. Percutaneous needle core biopsy of right kidney	0TB03ZX
4. EGD with gastric biopsy	0DB68ZX
5. Open endarterectomy of left common carotid artery	03CJ0ZZ
6. Excision of basal cell carcinoma of lower lip	0CB1XZZ
7. Open excision of tail of pancreas	0FBG0ZZ
8. Percutaneous biopsy of right gastrocnemius muscle	0KBS3ZX
9. Sigmoidoscopy with sigmoid polypectomy	0DBN8ZZ
10. Open excision of lesion from right Achilles tendon	0LBN0ZZ
11. Open resection of cecum	0DTH0ZZ
12. Total excision of pituitary gland, open	0GT00ZZ
13. Explantation of left failed kidney, open	0TT10ZZ
14. Open left axillary total lymphadenectomy	07T60ZZ (RESECTION is coded for cutting out a chain of lymph nodes.)
15. Laparoscopic-assisted vaginal hysterectomy	0UT9FZZ
16. Right total mastectomy, open	0HTT0ZZ
17. Open resection of papillary muscle	02TD0ZZ (The papillary muscle refers to the heart and is found in the *Heart and Great Vessels* body system.)
18. Total retropubic prostatectomy, open	0VT00ZZ
19. Laparoscopic cholecystectomy	0FT44ZZ
20. Endoscopic bilateral total maxillary sinusectomy	09TQ8ZZ, 09TR8ZZ
21. Amputation at right elbow level	0X6B0ZZ
22. Right below-knee amputation, proximal tibia/fibula	0Y6H0Z1 (The qualifier *High* here means the portion of the tib/fib closest to the knee.)
23. Fifth ray carpometacarpal joint amputation, left hand	0X6K0Z8 (A *complete* ray amputation is through the carpometacarpal joint.)
24. Right leg and hip amputation through ischium	0Y620ZZ (The *Hindquarter* body part includes amputation along any part of the hip bone.)
25. DIP joint amputation of right thumb	0X6L0Z3 (The qualifier *low* here means through the distal interphalangeal joint.)
26. Right wrist joint amputation	0X6J0Z0 (Amputation at the wrist joint is actually complete amputation of the hand.)
27. Trans-metatarsal amputation of foot at left big toe	0Y6N0Z9 (A *partial* amputation is through the shaft of the metatarsal bone.)
28. Mid-shaft amputation, right humerus	0X680Z2

Procedure	Code
29. Left fourth toe amputation, mid-proximal phalanx	0Y6W0Z1 (The qualifier *High* here means anywhere along the proximal phalanx.)
30. Right above-knee amputation, distal femur	0Y6C0Z3
31. Cryotherapy of wart on left hand	0H5GXZZ
32. Percutaneous radiofrequency ablation of right vocal cord lesion	0C5T3ZZ
33. Left heart catheterization with laser destruction of arrhythmogenic focus, A-V node	02583ZZ
34. Cautery of nosebleed	095KXZZ
35. Transurethral endoscopic laser ablation of prostate	0V508ZZ
36. Percutaneous cautery of oozing varicose vein, left calf	065Y3ZZ
37. Laparoscopy with destruction of endometriosis, bilateral ovaries	0U524ZZ
38. Laser coagulation of right retinal vessel hemorrhage, percutaneous	085G3ZZ (The *Retinal Vessel* body-part values are in the *Eye* body system.)
39. Thoracoscopic pleurodesis, left side	0B5P4ZZ
40. Percutaneous insertion of Greenfield IVC filter	06H03DZ
41. Forceps total mouth extraction, upper and lower teeth	0CDWXZ2, 0CDXXZ2
42. Removal of left thumbnail	0HDQXZZ (No separate body-part value is given for thumbnail, so this is coded to *Fingernail*.)
43. Extraction of right intraocular lens without replacement, percutaneous	08DJ3ZZ
44. Laparoscopy with needle aspiration of ova for in vitro fertilization	0UDN4ZZ
45. Nonexcisional debridement of skin ulcer, right foot	0HDMXZZ
46. Open stripping of abdominal fascia, right side	0JD80ZZ
47. Hysteroscopy with D&C, diagnostic	0UDB8ZX
48. Liposuction for medical purposes, left upper arm	0JDF3ZZ (The *Percutaneous* approach is inherent in the liposuction technique.)
49. Removal of tattered right ear drum fragments with tweezers	09D77ZZ
50. Microincisional phlebectomy of spider veins, right lower leg	06DY3ZZ
51. Routine Foley catheter placement	0T9B70Z
52. Incision and drainage of external anal abscess	0D9QXZZ
53. Percutaneous drainage of ascites	0W9G3ZZ (This is drainage of the cavity and not the peritoneal membrane itself.)
54. Laparoscopy with left ovarian cystotomy and drainage	0U914ZZ
55. Laparotomy and drain placement for liver abscess, right lobe	0F9100Z
56. Right knee arthrotomy with drain placement	0S9C00Z
57. Thoracentesis of left pleural effusion	0W9B3ZZ (This is drainage of the pleural cavity)
58. Phlebotomy of left median cubital vein for polycythemia vera	059C3ZZ (The median cubital vein is a branch of the basilic vein)

Procedure	Code
59. Percutaneous chest tube placement for right pneumothorax	ØW9930Z
60. Endoscopic drainage of left ethmoid sinus	Ø99V4ZZ
61. External ventricular CSF drainage catheter placement via burr hole	ØØ9630Z
62. Removal of foreign body, right cornea	Ø8C8XZZ
63. Percutaneous mechanical thrombectomy, left brachial artery	Ø3C83ZZ
64. Esophagogastroscopy with removal of bezoar from stomach	ØDC68ZZ
65. Foreign body removal, skin of left thumb	ØHCGXZZ (There is no specific value for thumb skin, so the procedure is coded to *Hand*.)
66. Transurethral cystoscopy with removal of bladder stone	ØTCB8ZZ
67. Forceps removal of foreign body in right nostril	Ø9CKXZZ (Nostril is coded to *Nasal mucosa and soft tissue* body-part value.)
68. Laparoscopy with excision of old suture from mesentery	ØDCV4ZZ
69. Incision and removal of right lacrimal duct stone	Ø8CXØZZ
70. Nonincisional removal of intraluminal foreign body from vagina	ØUCG7ZZ (The approach *External* is also a possibility. It is assumed here that since the patient went to the doctor to have the object removed, that it was not in the vaginal orifice.)
71. Right common carotid endarterectomy, open	Ø3CHØZZ
72. Open excision of retained sliver, subcutaneous tissue of left foot	ØJCRØZZ
73. Extracorporeal shockwave lithotripsy (ESWL), bilateral ureters	ØTF6XZZ, ØTF7XZZ (The *Bilateral Ureter* body-part value is not available for the root operation FRAGMENTATION, so the procedures are coded separately.)
74. Endoscopic retrograde cholangiopancreatography (ERCP) with lithotripsy of common bile duct stone	ØFF98ZZ (ERCP is performed through the mouth to the biliary system via the duodenum, so the approach value is *Via Natural or Artificial Opening Endoscopic*.)
75. Thoracotomy with crushing of pericardial calcifications	Ø2FNØZZ
76. Transurethral cystoscopy with fragmentation of bladder calculus	ØTFB8ZZ
77. Hysteroscopy with intraluminal lithotripsy of left fallopian tube calcification	ØUF68ZZ
78. Division of right foot tendon, percutaneous	ØL8V3ZZ
79. Left heart catheterization with division of bundle of HIS	Ø2883ZZ
80. Open osteotomy of capitate, left hand	ØP8NØZZ (The capitate is one of the carpal bones of the hand.)
81. EGD with esophagotomy of esophagogastric junction	ØD948ZZ
82. Sacral rhizotomy for pain control, percutaneous	Ø18R3ZZ
83. Laparotomy with exploration and adhesiolysis of right ureter	ØTN6ØZZ

Procedure	Code
84. Incision of scar contracture, right elbow	ØHNDXZZ (The skin of the elbow region is coded to *Lower Arm*.)
85. Frenulotomy for treatment of tongue-tie syndrome	ØCN7XZZ (The frenulum is coded to the body-part value *Tongue*.)
86. Right shoulder arthroscopy with coracoacromial ligament release	ØMN14ZZ
87. Mitral valvulotomy for release of fused leaflets, open approach	Ø2NGØZZ
88. Percutaneous left Achilles tendon release	ØLNP3ZZ
89. Laparoscopy with lysis of peritoneal adhesions	ØDNW4ZZ
90. Manual rupture of right shoulder joint adhesions under general anesthesia	ØRNJXZZ
91. Open posterior tarsal tunnel release	Ø1NGØZZ (The nerve released in the posterior tarsal tunnel is the tibial nerve.)
92. Laparoscopy with freeing of left ovary and fallopian tube	ØUN14ZZ, ØUN64ZZ
93. Liver transplant with donor matched liver	ØFYØØZØ
94. Orthotopic heart transplant using porcine heart	Ø2YAØZ2 (The donor heart comes from an animal [pig], so the qualifier value is *Zooplastic*.)
95. Right lung transplant, open, using organ donor match	ØBYKØZØ
96. Transplant of large intestine, organ donor match	ØDYEØZØ
97. Left kidney/pancreas organ bank transplant	ØFYGØZØ, ØTY1ØZØ
98. Replantation of avulsed scalp	ØHMØXZZ
99. Reattachment of severed right ear	Ø9MØXZZ
100. Reattachment of traumatic left gastrocnemius avulsion, open	ØKMTØZZ
101. Closed replantation of three avulsed teeth, lower jaw	ØCMXXZ1
102. Reattachment of severed left hand	ØXMKØZZ
103. Right open palmaris longus tendon transfer	ØLX5ØZZ
104. Endoscopic radial to median nerve transfer	Ø1X64Z5
105. Fasciocutaneous flap closure of left thigh, open	ØJXMØZC (The qualifier identifies the body layers in addition to fascia included in the procedure.)
106. Transfer left index finger to left thumb position, open	ØXXPØZM
107. Percutaneous fascia transfer to fill defect, right neck	ØJX43ZZ
108. Trigeminal to facial nerve transfer, percutaneous endoscopic	ØØXK4ZM
109. Endoscopic left leg flexor hallucis longus tendon transfer	ØLXP4ZZ
110. Right scalp advancement flap to right temple	ØHXØXZZ
111. Bilateral TRAM pedicle flap reconstruction status post mastectomy, muscle only, open	ØKXKØZ6, ØKXLØZ6 (The transverse rectus abdominus muscle (TRAM) flap is coded for each flap developed.)
112. Skin transfer flap closure of complex open wound, left lower back	ØHX6XZZ
113. Open fracture reduction, right tibia	ØQSGØZZ
114. Laparoscopy with gastropexy for malrotation	ØDS64ZZ
115. Left knee arthroscopy with reposition of anterior cruciate ligament	ØMSP4ZZ

Procedure	Code
116. Open transposition of ulnar nerve	01S40ZZ
117. Closed reduction with percutaneous internal fixation of right femoral neck fracture	0QS634Z
118. Trans-vaginal intraluminal cervical cerclage	0UVC7DZ
119. Cervical cerclage using Shirodkar technique	0UVC7ZZ
120. Thoracotomy with banding of left pulmonary artery using extraluminal device	02VR0CZ
121. Restriction of thoracic duct with intraluminal stent, percutaneous	07VK3DZ
122. Craniotomy with clipping of cerebral aneurysm	03VG0CZ (The clip is placed lengthwise on the outside wall of the widened portion of the vessel.)
123. Nonincisional, transnasal placement of restrictive stent in right lacrimal duct	08VX7DZ
124. Catheter-based temporary restriction of blood flow in abdominal aorta for treatment of cerebral ischemia	04V03DJ
125. Percutaneous ligation of esophageal vein	06L33ZZ
126. Percutaneous embolization of left internal carotid-cavernous fistula	03LL3DZ
127. Laparoscopy with bilateral occlusion of fallopian tubes using Hulka extraluminal clips	0UL74CZ
128. Open suture ligation of failed AV graft, left brachial artery	03L80ZZ
129. Percutaneous embolization of vascular supply, intracranial meningioma	03LG3DZ
130. Percutaneous embolization of right uterine artery, using coils	04LE3DT
131. Open occlusion of left atrial appendage, using extraluminal pressure clips	02L70CK
132. Percutaneous suture exclusion of left atrial appendage, via femoral artery access	02L73ZK
133. ERCP with balloon dilation of common bile duct	0F798ZZ
134. PTCA of two coronary arteries, LAD with stent placement, RCA with no stent	02703DZ, 02703ZZ (A separate procedure is coded for each artery dilated, since the device value differs for each artery.)
135. Cystoscopy with intraluminal dilation of bladder neck stricture	0T7C8ZZ
136. Open dilation of old anastomosis, left femoral artery	047L0ZZ
137. Dilation of upper esophageal stricture, direct visualization, with Bougie sound	0D717ZZ
138. PTA of right brachial artery stenosis	03773ZZ
139. Transnasal dilation and stent placement in right lacrimal duct	087X7DZ
140. Hysteroscopy with balloon dilation of bilateral fallopian tubes	0U778ZZ
141. Tracheoscopy with intraluminal dilation of tracheal stenosis	0B718ZZ
142. Cystoscopy with dilation of left ureteral stricture, with stent placement	0T778DZ
143. Open gastric bypass with Roux-en-Y limb to jejunum	0D160ZA
144. Right temporal artery to intracranial artery bypass using Gore-Tex graft, open	031S0JG
145. Tracheostomy formation with tracheostomy tube placement, percutaneous	0B113F4
146. PICVA (percutaneous in situ coronary venous arterialization) of single coronary artery	02103D4

Procedure	Code
147. Open left femoral-popliteal artery bypass using cadaver vein graft	041L0KL
148. Shunting of intrathecal cerebrospinal fluid to peritoneal cavity using synthetic shunt	00160J6
149. Colostomy formation, open, transverse colon to abdominal wall	0D1L0Z4
150. Open urinary diversion, left ureter, using ileal conduit to skin	0T170ZC
151. CABG of LAD using pedicled left internal mammary artery, open off-bypass	02100Z9
152. Open pleuroperitoneal shunt, right pleural cavity, using synthetic device	0W190JG
153. Percutaneous placement of ventriculoperitoneal shunt for treatment of hydrocephalus	00163J6
154. End-of-life replacement of spinal neurostimulator generator, multiple array, in lower abdomen	0JH80DZ (Taking out of the old generator is coded separately to the root operation *Removal*)
155. Percutaneous insertion of spinal neurostimulator lead, lumbar spinal cord	00HV3MZ
156. Percutaneous replacement of broken pacemaker lead in left atrium	02H73JZ (Taking out the broken pacemaker lead is coded separately to the root operation *Removal*.)
157. Open placement of dual chamber pacemaker generator in chest wall	0JH606Z
158. Percutaneous placement of venous central line in right internal jugular, with tip in superior vena cava	02HV33Z
159. Open insertion of multiple channel cochlear implant, left ear	09HE06Z
160. Percutaneous placement of Swan-Ganz catheter in pulmonary trunk	02HP32Z (The Swan-Ganz catheter is coded to the device value *Monitoring Device* because it monitors pulmonary artery output.)
161. Bronchoscopy with insertion of Low Dose Pd-103 brachytherapy seeds, right main bronchus	0BH081Z, DB11BBZ
162. Open insertion of interspinous process device into lumbar vertebral joint	0SH00BZ
163. Open placement of bone growth stimulator, left femoral shaft	0QHY0MZ
164. Cystoscopy with placement of brachytherapy seeds in prostate gland	0VH081Z
165. Percutaneous insertion of Greenfield IVC filter	06H03DZ
166. Full-thickness skin graft to right lower arm, autograft (do not code graft harvest for this exercise)	0HRDX73
167. Excision of necrosed left femoral head with bone bank bone graft to fill the defect, open	0QR70KZ
168. Penetrating keratoplasty of right cornea with donor matched cornea, percutaneous approach	08R83KZ
169. Excision of abdominal aorta with Gore-Tex graft replacement, open	04R00JZ
170. Total right knee arthroplasty with insertion of total knee prosthesis	0SRC0JZ
171. Tenonectomy with graft to right ankle using cadaver graft, open	0LRS0KZ
172. Mitral valve replacement using porcine valve, open	02RG08Z
173. Percutaneous phacoemulsification of right eye cataract with prosthetic lens insertion	08RJ3JZ

Procedure	Code
174. Transcatheter replacement of pulmonary valve using of bovine jugular vein valve	02RH38Z
175. Total left hip replacement using ceramic on ceramic prosthesis, without bone cement	0SRB03A
176. Aortic valve annuloplasty using ring, open	02UF0JZ
177. Laparoscopic repair of left inguinal hernia with marlex plug	0YU64JZ
178. Autograft nerve graft to right median nerve, percutaneous endoscopic (do not code graft harvest for this exercise)	01U547Z
179. Exchange of liner in femoral component of previous left hip replacement, open approach	0SUS09Z (Taking out of the old liner is coded separately to the root operation *Removal*)
180. Anterior colporrhaphy with polypropylene mesh reinforcement, open approach	0JUC0JZ
181. Implantation of CorCap cardiac support device, open approach	02UA0JZ
182. Abdominal wall herniorrhaphy, open, using synthetic mesh	0WUF0JZ
183. Tendon graft to strengthen injured left shoulder using autograft, open (do not code graft harvest for this exercise)	0LU207Z
184. Onlay lamellar keratoplasty of left cornea using autograft, external approach	08U9X7Z
185. Resurfacing procedure on right femoral head, open approach	0SUR0BZ
186. Exchange of drainage tube from right hip joint	0S2YX0Z
187. Tracheostomy tube exchange	0B21XFZ
188. Change chest tube for left pneumothorax	0W2BX0Z
189. Exchange of cerebral ventriculostomy drainage tube	0020X0Z
190. Foley urinary catheter exchange	0T2BX0Z (This is coded to *Drainage Device* because urine is being drained.)
191. Open removal of lumbar sympathetic neurostimulator lead	01PY0MZ
192. Nonincisional removal of Swan-Ganz catheter from right pulmonary artery	02PYX2Z
193. Laparotomy with removal of pancreatic drain	0FPG00Z
194. Extubation, endotracheal tube	0BP1XDZ
195. Nonincisional PEG tube removal	0DP6XUZ
196. Transvaginal removal of brachytherapy seeds	0UPH71Z
197. Transvaginal removal of extraluminal cervical cerclage	0UPD7CZ
198. Incision with removal of K-wire fixation, right first metatarsal	0QPN04Z
199. Cystoscopy with retrieval of left ureteral stent	0TP98DZ
200. Removal of nasogastric drainage tube for decompression	0DP6X0Z
201. Removal of external fixator, left radial fracture	0PPJX5Z
202. Trimming and reanastomosis of stenosed femorofemoral synthetic bypass graft, open	04WY0JZ
203. Open revision of right hip replacement, with readjustment of prosthesis	0SW90JZ
204. Adjustment of position, pacemaker lead in left ventricle, percutaneous	02WA3MZ
205. External repositioning of Foley catheter to bladder	0TWBX0Z
206. Taking out loose screw and putting larger screw in fracture repair plate, left tibia	0QWH04Z
207. Revision of totally implantable VAD port placement in chest wall, causing patient discomfort, open	0JWT0WZ

Procedure	Code
208. Thoracotomy with exploration of right pleural cavity	0WJ90ZZ
209. Diagnostic laryngoscopy	0CJS8ZZ
210. Exploratory arthrotomy of left knee	0SJD0ZZ
211. Colposcopy with diagnostic hysteroscopy	0UJD8ZZ
212. Digital rectal exam	0DJD7ZZ
213. Diagnostic arthroscopy of right shoulder	0RJJ4ZZ
214. Endoscopy of maxillary sinus	09JY4ZZ
215. Laparotomy with palpation of liver	0FJ00ZZ
216. Transurethral diagnostic cystoscopy	0TJB8ZZ
217. Colonoscopy, discontinued at sigmoid colon	0DJD8ZZ
218. Percutaneous mapping of basal ganglia	00K83ZZ
219. Heart catheterization with cardiac mapping	02K83ZZ
220. Intraoperative whole brain mapping via craniotomy	00K00ZZ
221. Mapping of left cerebral hemisphere, percutaneous endoscopic	00K74ZZ
222. Intraoperative cardiac mapping during open heart surgery	02K80ZZ
223. Hysteroscopy with cautery of post-hysterectomy oozing and evacuation of clot	0W3R8ZZ
224. Open exploration and ligation of post-op arterial bleeder, left forearm	0X3F0ZZ
225. Control of post-operative retroperitoneal bleeding via laparotomy	0W3H0ZZ
226. Reopening of thoracotomy site with drainage and control of post-op hemopericardium	0W3D0ZZ
227. Arthroscopy with drainage of hemarthrosis at previous operative site, right knee	0Y3F4ZZ
228. Radiocarpal fusion of left hand with internal fixation, open	0RGP04Z
229. Posterior approach spinal fusion at L1-L3 level with BAK cage interbody fusion device, open	0SG10AJ
230. Intercarpal fusion of right hand with bone bank bone graft, open	0RGQ0KZ
231. Sacrococcygeal fusion with bone graft from same operative site, open	0SG507Z
232. Interphalangeal fusion of left great toe, percutaneous pin fixation	0SGQ34Z
233. Suture repair of left radial nerve laceration	01Q60ZZ (The approach value is *Open*, though the surgical exposure may have been created by the wound itself.)
234. Laparotomy with suture repair of blunt force duodenal laceration	0DQ90ZZ
235. Perineoplasty with repair of old obstetric laceration, open	0WQN0ZZ
236. Suture repair of right biceps tendon (upper arm) laceration, open	0LQ30ZZ
237. Closure of abdominal wall stab wound	0WQF0ZZ
238. Cosmetic face lift, open, no other information available	0W020ZZ
239. Bilateral breast augmentation with silicone implants, open	0H0V0JZ
240. Cosmetic rhinoplasty with septal reduction and tip elevation using local tissue graft, open	090K07Z
241. Abdominoplasty (tummy tuck), open	0W0F0ZZ
242. Liposuction of bilateral thighs	0J0L3ZZ, 0J0M3ZZ
243. Creation of penis in female patient using tissue bank donor graft	0W4N0K1
244. Creation of vagina in male patient using synthetic material	0W4M0J0

Procedure	Code
245. Laparoscopic vertical (sleeve) gastrectomy	0DB64Z3
246. Left uterine artery embolization with intraluminal biosphere injection	04LF3DU

Obstetrics

Procedure	Code
1. Abortion by dilation and evacuation following laminaria insertion	10A07ZW
2. Manually assisted spontaneous abortion	10E0XZZ (Since the pregnancy was not artificially terminated, this is coded to *Delivery* because it captures the procedure objective. The fact that it was an abortion will be identified in the diagnosis code.)
3. Abortion by abortifacient insertion	10A07ZX
4. Bimanual pregnancy examination	10J07ZZ
5. Extraperitoneal C-section, low transverse incision	10D00Z1
6. Fetal spinal tap, percutaneous	10903ZA
7. Fetal kidney transplant, laparoscopic	10Y04ZS
8. Open in utero repair of congenital diaphragmatic hernia	10Q00ZK (Diaphragm is classified to the *Respiratory* body system in the *Medical and Surgical* section.)
9. Laparoscopy with total excision of tubal pregnancy	10T24ZZ
10. Transvaginal removal of fetal monitoring electrode	10P073Z

Placement

Procedure	Code
1. Placement of packing material, right ear	2Y42X5Z
2. Mechanical traction of entire left leg	2W6MX0Z
3. Removal of splint, right shoulder	2W5AX1Z
4. Placement of neck brace	2W32X3Z
5. Change of vaginal packing	2Y04X5Z
6. Packing of wound, chest wall	2W44X5Z
7. Sterile dressing placement to left groin region	2W27X4Z
8. Removal of packing material from pharynx	2Y50X5Z
9. Placement of intermittent pneumatic compression device, covering entire right arm	2W18X7Z
10. Exchange of pressure dressing to left thigh	2W0PX6Z

Administration

Procedure	Code
1. Peritoneal dialysis via indwelling catheter	3E1M39Z
2. Transvaginal artificial insemination	3E0P7LZ
3. Infusion of total parenteral nutrition via central venous catheter	3E0436Z
4. Esophagogastroscopy with Botox injection into esophageal sphincter	3E0G8GC (Botulinum toxin is a paralyzing agent with temporary effects; it does not sclerose or destroy the nerve.)
5. Percutaneous irrigation of knee joint	3E1U38Z
6. Systemic infusion of recombinant tissue plasminogen activator (r-tPA) via peripheral venous catheter	3E03317
7. Transabdominal in vitro fertilization, implantation of donor ovum	3E0P3Q1
8. Autologous bone marrow transplant via central venous line	30243G0
9. Implantation of anti-microbial envelope with cardiac defibrillator placement, open	3E0102A
10. Sclerotherapy of brachial plexus lesion, alcohol injection	3E0T3TZ
11. Percutaneous peripheral vein injection, glucarpidase	3E033GQ
12. Introduction of anti-infective envelope into subcutaneous tissue, open	3E0102A

Measurement and Monitoring

Procedure	Code
1. Cardiac stress test, single measurement	4A02XM4
2. EGD with biliary flow measurement	4A0C85Z
3. Right and left heart cardiac catheterization with bilateral sampling and pressure measurements	4A023N8
4. Temperature monitoring, rectal	4A1Z7KZ
5. Peripheral venous pulse, external, single measurement	4A04XJ1
6. Holter monitoring	4A12X45
7. Respiratory rate, external, single measurement	4A09XCZ
8. Fetal heart rate monitoring, transvaginal	4A1H7CZ
9. Visual mobility test, single measurement	4A07X7Z
10. Left ventricular cardiac output monitoring from pulmonary artery wedge (Swan-Ganz) catheter	4A1239Z
11. Olfactory acuity test, single measurement	4A08X0Z

Extracorporeal or Systemic Assistance and Performance

	Procedure	Code
1.	Intermittent mechanical ventilation, 16 hours	5A1935Z
2.	Liver dialysis, single encounter	5A1C00Z
3.	Cardiac countershock with successful conversion to sinus rhythm	5A2204Z
4.	IPPB (intermittent positive pressure breathing) for mobilization of secretions, 22 hours	5A09358
5.	Renal dialysis, 12 hours	5A1D80Z
6.	IABP (intra-aortic balloon pump) continuous	5A02210
7.	Intra-operative cardiac pacing, continuous	5A1223Z
8.	ECMO (extracorporeal membrane oxygenation), central	5A1522F
9.	Controlled mechanical ventilation (CMV), 45 hours	5A1945Z
10.	Pulsatile compression boot with intermittent inflation	5A02115 (This is coded to the function value *Cardiac Output*, because the purpose of such compression devices is to return blood to the heart faster.)

Extracorporeal or Systemic Therapies

	Procedure	Code
1.	Donor thrombocytapheresis, single encounter	6A550Z2
2.	Bili-lite phototherapy, series treatment	6A601ZZ
3.	Whole body hypothermia, single treatment	6A4Z0ZZ
4.	Circulatory phototherapy, single encounter	6A650ZZ
5.	Shock wave therapy of plantar fascia, single treatment	6A930ZZ
6.	Antigen-free air conditioning, series treatment	6A0Z1ZZ
7.	TMS (transcranial magnetic stimulation), series treatment	6A221ZZ
8.	Therapeutic ultrasound of peripheral vessels, single treatment	6A750Z6
9.	Plasmapheresis, series treatment	6A551Z3
10.	Extracorporeal electromagnetic stimulation (EMS) for urinary incontinence, single treatment	6A210ZZ

Osteopathic

	Procedure	Code
1.	Isotonic muscle energy treatment of right leg	7W06X8Z
2.	Low velocity-high amplitude osteopathic treatment of head	7W00X5Z
3.	Lymphatic pump osteopathic treatment of left axilla	7W07X6Z
4.	Indirect osteopathic treatment of sacrum	7W04X4Z
5.	Articulatory osteopathic treatment of cervical region	7W01X0Z

Other Procedures

	Procedure	Code
1.	Near infrared spectroscopy of leg vessels	8E023DZ
2.	CT computer assisted sinus surgery	8E09XBG (The primary procedure is coded separately.)
3.	Suture removal, abdominal wall	8E0WXY8
4.	Isolation after infectious disease exposure	8E0ZXY6
5.	Robotic assisted open prostatectomy	8E0W0CZ (The primary procedure is coded separately.)
6.	In vitro fertilization	8E0ZXY1

Chiropractic

	Procedure	Code
1.	Chiropractic treatment of lumbar region using long lever specific contact	9WB3XGZ
2.	Chiropractic manipulation of abdominal region, indirect visceral	9WB9XCZ
3.	Chiropractic extra-articular treatment of hip region	9WB6XDZ
4.	Chiropractic treatment of sacrum using long and short lever specific contact	9WB4XJZ
5.	Mechanically-assisted chiropractic manipulation of head	9WB0XKZ

Imaging

	Procedure	Code
1.	Noncontrast CT of abdomen and pelvis	BW21ZZZ
2.	Intravascular ultrasound, left subclavian artery	B342ZZ3
3.	Fluoroscopic guidance for insertion of central venous catheter in SVC, low osmolar contrast	B5181ZA
4.	Chest x-ray, AP/PA and lateral views	BW03ZZZ
5.	Endoluminal ultrasound of gallbladder and bile ducts	BF43ZZZ
6.	MRI of thyroid gland, contrast unspecified	BG34YZZ
7.	Esophageal videofluoroscopy study with oral barium contrast	BD11YZZ
8.	Portable x-ray study of right radius/ulna shaft, standard series	BP0JZZZ
9.	Routine fetal ultrasound, second trimester twin gestation	BY4DZZZ
10.	CT scan of bilateral lungs, high osmolar contrast with densitometry	BB240ZZ
11.	Fluoroscopic guidance for percutaneous transluminal angioplasty (PTA) of left common femoral artery, low osmolar contrast	B41G1ZZ

Nuclear Medicine

Procedure	Code
1. Tomo scan of right and left heart, unspecified radiopharmaceutical, qualitative gated rest	C226YZZ
2. Technetium pentetate assay of kidneys, ureters, and bladder	CT631ZZ
3. Uniplanar scan of spine using technetium oxidronate, with first-pass study	CP151ZZ
4. Thallous chloride tomographic scan of bilateral breasts	CH22SZZ
5. PET scan of myocardium using rubidium	C23GQZZ
6. Gallium citrate scan of head and neck, single plane imaging	CW1BLZZ
7. Xenon gas nonimaging probe of brain	C050VZZ
8. Upper GI scan, radiopharmaceutical unspecified, for gastric emptying	CD15YZZ
9. Carbon 11 PET scan of brain with quantification	C030BZZ
10. Iodinated albumin nuclear medicine assay, blood plasma volume study	C763HZZ

Radiation Therapy

Procedure	Code
1. Plaque radiation of left eye, single port	D8Y0FZZ
2. 8 MeV photon beam radiation to brain	D0011ZZ
3. IORT of colon, 3 ports	DDY5CZZ
4. HDR brachytherapy of prostate using low dose palladium-103	DV10BBZ
5. Electron radiation treatment of right breast, with custom device	DM013ZZ
6. Hyperthermia oncology treatment of pelvic region	DWY68ZZ
7. Contact radiation of tongue	D9Y57ZZ
8. Heavy particle radiation treatment of pancreas, four risk sites	DF034ZZ
9. LDR brachytherapy to spinal cord using iodine	D016B9Z
10. Whole body Phosphorus 32 administration with risk to hematopoetic system	DWY5GFZ

Physical Rehabilitation and Diagnostic Audiology

Procedure	Code
1. Bekesy assessment using audiometer	F13Z31Z
2. Individual fitting of left eye prosthesis	F0DZ8UZ
3. Physical therapy for range of motion and mobility, patient right hip, no special equipment	F07L0ZZ
4. Bedside swallow assessment using assessment kit	F00ZHYZ
5. Caregiver training in airway clearance techniques	F0FZ8ZZ
6. Application of short arm cast in rehabilitation setting	F0DZ7EZ (Inhibitory cast is listed in the equipment reference table under E, *Orthosis*.)
7. Verbal assessment of patient's pain level	F02ZFZZ

Procedure	Code
8. Caregiver training in communication skills using manual communication board	F0FZJMZ (Manual communication board is listed in the equipment reference table under M, *Augmentative/ Alternative Communication*.)
9. Group musculoskeletal balance training exercises, whole body, no special equipment	F07M6ZZ (Balance training is included in the motor treatment reference table under *Therapeutic Exercise*.)
10. Individual therapy for auditory processing using tape recorder	F09Z2KZ (Tape recorder is listed in the equipment reference table under *Audiovisual Equipment*.)

Mental Health

Procedure	Code
1. Cognitive-behavioral psychotherapy, individual	GZ58ZZZ
2. Narcosynthesis	GZGZZZZ
3. Light therapy	GZJZZZZ
4. ECT (electroconvulsive therapy), unilateral, multiple seizure	GZB1ZZZ
5. Crisis intervention	GZ2ZZZZ
6. Neuropsychological testing	GZ13ZZZ
7. Hypnosis	GZFZZZZ
8. Developmental testing	GZ10ZZZ
9. Vocational counseling	GZ61ZZZ
10. Family psychotherapy	GZ72ZZZ

Substance Abuse Treatment

Procedure	Code
1. Naltrexone treatment for drug dependency	HZ94ZZZ
2. Substance abuse treatment family counseling	HZ63ZZZ
3. Medication monitoring of patient on methadone maintenance	HZ81ZZZ
4. Individual interpersonal psychotherapy for drug abuse	HZ54ZZZ
5. Patient in for alcohol detoxification treatment	HZ2ZZZZ
6. Group motivational counseling	HZ47ZZZ
7. Individual 12-step psychotherapy for substance abuse	HZ53ZZZ
8. Post-test infectious disease counseling for IV drug abuser	HZ3CZZZ
9. Psychodynamic psychotherapy for drug dependent patient	HZ5CZZZ
10. Group cognitive-behavioral counseling for substance abuse	HZ42ZZZ

New Technology

Procedure	Code
1. Infusion of ceftazidime via peripheral venous catheter	XW03321

Appendix L: Procedure Combination Tables

The tables below were developed to help simplify the relationship between ICD-10-PCS coding and MS-DRG assignment. The Centers for Medicare & Medicaid Services (CMS) has identified in the MS-DRG v36 Definitions Manual certain procedure combinations that must occur in order to assign a specific MS-DRG. There are many factors influencing MS-DRG assignment, including principal and secondary diagnoses, MCC or CC use, sex of the patient, and discharge status. These tables should be used only as a guide.

DRG 001-002 Heart Transplant or Implant of Heart Assist System

Heart Transplant
Replacement of Right and Left Ventricle 02RK0JZ and 02RL0JZ

Insertion With Removal of Heart Assist System

Type of Heart Assist System	Code as appropriate Insertion by approach	Code also as appropriate Removal of Heart Assist System by approach
Biventricular External	02HA[0,3,4]RS	02PA[0,3,4]RZ
External	02HA[0,4]RZ	02PA[0,3,4]RZ

Revision With Removal of Heart Assist System

Type of Heart Assist System	Code as appropriate Revision by approach	Code also as appropriate Removal of Heart Assist System by approach
Implantable	02WA[0,3,4]QZ	02PA[0,3,4]RZ
External	02WA[0,3,4]RZ	02PA[0,3,4]RZ

DRG 008 Simultaneous Pancreas/Kidney Transplant

Transplanted Body Part Laterality	Code Transplant as appropriate by tissue type			Code also Pancreas Transplant as appropriate by tissue type		
	Allogeneic	Syngeneic	Zooplastic	Allogeneic	Syngeneic	Zooplastic
Kidney, Right	0TY00Z0	0TY00Z1	0TY00Z2	0FYG0Z0	0FYG0Z1	0FYG0Z2
Kidney, Left	0TY10Z0	0TY10Z1	0TY10Z2	0FYG0Z0	0FYG0Z1	0FYG0Z2

DRG 023-027 Craniotomy

Site of Neurostimulator Lead	Code as appropriate Insertion of Lead by approach	Code also as appropriate Insertion of Device by type and subcutaneous site						
		Neuro-stimulator Generator	Stimulator Multiple Array Code as appropriate by approach			Stimulator Multiple Array, Rechargeable Code as appropriate by approach		
		Skull	Chest	Back	Abdomen	Chest	Back	Abdomen
Brain	00H0[0,3,4]MZ	0NH00NZ	0JH6[0,3]DZ	0JH7[0,3]DZ	0JH8[0,3]DZ	0JH6[0,3]EZ	0JH7[0,3]EZ	0JH8[0,3]EZ
Cerebral Ventricle	00H6[0,3,4]MZ	0NH00NZ	0JH6[0,3]DZ	0JH7[0,3]DZ	0JH8[0,3]DZ	0JH6[0,3]EZ	0JH7[0,3]EZ	0JH8[0,3]EZ

DRG 028-030 Spinal Procedures

Generator Type	Insertion of Generator by Site			Code also as appropriate Insertion of Neurostimulator Lead by approach	
	Chest	Abdomen	Back	Spinal Canal	Spinal Cord
Single Array	0JH6[0,3]BZ	0JH8[0,3]BZ	0JH7[0,3]BZ	00HU[0,3,4]MZ	00HV[0,3,4]MZ
Single Array, Rechargeable	0JH6[0,3]CZ	0JH8[0,3]CZ	0JH7[0,3]CZ	00HU[0,3,4]MZ	00HV[0,3,4]MZ
Multiple Array	0JH6[0,3]DZ	0JH8[0,3]DZ	0JH7[0,3]DZ	00HU[0,3,4]MZ	00HV[0,3,4]MZ
Multiple Array, Rechargable	0JH6[0,3]EZ	—	0JH7[0,3]EZ	00HU[0,3,4]MZ	00HV[0,3,4]MZ
Multiple Array, Rechargable	—	0JH8[0,3]EZ	—	00HU[0,3,4]MZ	00HV[0,3,4]MZ

DRG 040-042 Peripheral and Cranial Nerve and Other Nervous System Procedures

Insertion of Neurostimulator Lead With Device

Site of Neurostimulator Lead	Code as appropriate Insertion by approach	Code also as appropriate Insertion of Device by type and subcutaneous site					
		Stimulator Single Array Code as appropriate by approach			Stimulator Single Array, Rechargeable Code as appropriate by approach		
		Chest	Back	Abdomen	Chest	Back	Abdomen
Cranial Nerve	00HE[0,3,4]MZ	0JH6[0,3]BZ	0JH7[0,3]BZ	0JH8[0,3]BZ	0JH6[0,3]CZ	0JH7[0,3]CZ	0JH8[0,3]CZ
Peripheral Nerve	01HY[0,3,4]MZ	0JH6[0,3]BZ	0JH7[0,3]BZ	0JH8[0,3]BZ	0JH6[0,3]CZ	0JH7[0,3]CZ	0JH8[0,3]CZ
Stomach	0DH6[0,3,4]MZ	0JH6[0,3]BZ	0JH7[0,3]BZ	0JH8[0,3]BZ	0JH6[0,3]CZ	0JH7[0,3]CZ	0JH8[0,3]CZ
Azygos vein	05H0[0,3,4]MZ	0JH6[0,3]BZ	0JH7[0,S]BZ	0JH8[0,3]BZ	0JH6[0,3]CZ	0JH7[0,S]CZ	0JH8[0,3]CZ
Innominate Vein, Right	05H3[0,3,4]MZ	0JH6[0,3]BZ	0JH7[0,S]BZ	0JH8[0,3]BZ	0JH6[0,3]CZ	0JH7[0,S]CZ	0JH8[0,3]CZ
Innominate Vein, Left	05H4[0,3,4]MZ	0JH6[0,3]BZ	0JH7[0,S]BZ	0JH8[0,3]BZ	0JH6[0,3]CZ	0JH7[0,S]CZ	0JH8[0,3]CZ
		Stimulator Multiple Array Code as appropriate by approach			Stimulator Multiple Array, Rechargeable Code as appropriate by approach		
		Chest	Back	Abdomen	Chest	Back	Abdomen
Cranial Nerve	00HE[0,3,4]MZ	0JH6[0,3]DZ	0JH7[0,3]DZ	0JH8[0,3]DZ	0JH6[0,3]EZ	0JH7[0,3]EZ	0JH8[0,3]EZ
Peripheral Nerve	01HY[0,3,4]MZ	0JH6[0,3]DZ	0JH7[0,3]DZ	0JH8[0,3]DZ	0JH6[0,3]EZ	0JH7[0,3]EZ	0JH8[0,3]EZ
Stomach	0DH6[0,3,4]MZ	0JH6[0,3]DZ	0JH7[0,3]DZ	0JH8[0,3]DZ	0JH6[0,3]EZ	0JH7[0,3]EZ	0JH8[0,3]EZ
Azygos vein	05H0[0,3,4]MZ	0JH6[0,3]DZ	0JH7[0,S]DZ	0JH8[0,3]DZ	0JH6[0,3]EZ	0JH7[0,S]EZ	0JH8[0,3]EZ
Innominate Vein, Right	05H3[0,3,4]MZ	0JH6[0,3]DZ	0JH7[0,S]DZ	0JH8[0,3]DZ	0JH6[0,3]EZ	0JH7[0,S]EZ	0JH8[0,3]EZ
Innominate Vein, Left	05H4[0,3,4]MZ	0JH6[0,3]DZ	0JH7[0,S]DZ	0JH8[0,3]DZ	0JH6[0,3]EZ	0JH7[0,S]EZ	0JH8[0,3]EZ

DRG 222-227 Cardiac Defibrillator Implant

Insertion of Generator With Insertion of Lead(s) into Coronary Vein, Atrium or Ventricle

Generator Type	Insertion of Generator by Site		Code also as appropriate Insertion of Leads by site				
	Chest	Abdomen	Coronary Vein	Atrium		Ventricle	
				Right	Left	Right	Left
Defibrillator	0JH6[0,3]8Z	0JH8[0,3]8Z	02H4[0,4]KZ	02H6[0,3,4]KZ	02H7[0,3,4]KZ	02HK[0,3,4]KZ	02HL[0,3,4]KZ
Cardiac Resynch Defibrillator Pulse Generator	0JH6[0,3]9Z	0JH8[0,3]9Z	02H4[0,3,4]KZ or 02H43[J,M]Z	02H6[0,3,4]KZ	02H7[0,3,4]KZ	02HK[0,3,4]KZ	02HL[0,3,4]KZ
Contractility Modulation Device	0JH6[0,3]AZ	0JH8[0,3]AZ	—	—	—	—	02HL[0,3,4]MZ

Insertion of Generator with Insertion of Lead(s) into Pericardium

Generator Type	Insertion of Generator by Site		Code also as appropriate Insertion of Leads by Type		
	Chest	Abdomen	Pericardium		
			Pacemaker	Defibrillator	Cardiac
Defibrillator	0JH6[0,3]8Z	0JH8[0,3]8Z	02HN[0,3,4]JZ	02HN[0,3,4]KZ	02HN[0,3,4]MZ
Cardiac Resynch Defibrillator Pulse Generator	0JH6[0,3]9Z	0JH8[0,3]9Z	02HN[0,3,4]JZ	02HN[0,3,4]KZ	02HN[0,3,4]MZ

DRG 242-244 Permanent Cardiac Pacemaker Implant

Insertion of Generator and Lead(s) Only

Generator Type	Insertion of Generator by Site		Code also as appropriate Insertion of Leads by site					
	Chest	Abdomen	Coronary Vein	Atrium		Ventricle		Pericardium
				Right	Left	Right	Left	
Single Chamber	ØJH6[0,3]4Z	ØJH8[0,3]4Z	02H4[0,3,4][J,M]Z	02H6[0,3,4][J,M]Z	02H7[0,3,4][J,M]Z	02HK[0,3,4][J,M]Z	02HL[0,3,4][J,M]Z	02HN[0,3,4][J,M]Z
Single Chamber RR	ØJH6[0,3]5Z	ØJH8[0,3]5Z	02H4[0,3,4][J,M]Z	02H6[0,3,4][J,M]Z	02H7[0,3,4][J,M]Z	02HK[0,3,4][J,M]Z	02HL[0,3,4][J,M]Z	02HN[0,3,4][J,M]Z
Dual Chamber	ØJH6[0,3]6Z	ØJH8[0,3]6Z	02H4[0,3,4][J,M]Z	02H6[0,3,4][J,M]Z	02H7[0,3,4][J,M]Z	02HK[0,3,4][J,M]Z	02HL[0,3,4][J,M]Z	02HN[0,3,4][J,M]Z
Cardiac Resynch Pulse Generator	ØJH6[0,3]7Z	ØJH8[0,3]7Z	02H4[0,3,4][J,M]Z	02H6[0,3,4][J,M]Z	02H7[0,3,4][J,M]Z	02HK[0,3,4][J,M]Z	02HL[0,3,4][J,M]Z	02HN[0,3,4][J,M]Z
Cardiac Rhythm Related	ØJH6[0,3]PZ	ØJH8[0,3]PZ	02H4[0,3,4][J,M]Z	02H6[0,3,4][J,M]Z	02H7[0,3,4][J,M]Z	02HK[0,3,4][J,M]Z	02HL[0,3,4][J,M]Z	02HN[0,3,4][J,M]Z

DRG 326-328 Stomach, Esophageal and Duodenal Procedures

Site	Resection by Open Approach	Code also as appropriate Resection of Pancreas by Open Approach
Duodenum	ØDT90ZZ	ØFTG0ZZ

DRG 344-346 Minor Small and Large Bowel Procedures

Site	Repair by Open Approach	Code also as appropriate Repair by external approach of Abdominal Wall Stoma
Small Intestine	ØDQ80ZZ	ØWQFXZ2
Duodenum	ØDQ90ZZ	ØWQFXZ2
Jejunum	ØDQA0ZZ	ØWQFXZ2
Ileum	ØDQB0ZZ	ØWQFXZ2
Large Intestine	ØDQE0ZZ	ØWQFXZ2
Large Intestine, Right	ØDQF0ZZ	ØWQFXZ2
Large Intestine, Left	ØDQG0ZZ	ØWQFXZ2
Cecum	ØDQH0ZZ	ØWQFXZ2
Ascending Colon	ØDQK0ZZ	ØWQFXZ2
Transverse Colon	ØDQL0ZZ	ØWQFXZ2
Descending Colon	ØDQM0ZZ	ØWQFXZ2
Sigmoid Colon	ØDQN0ZZ	ØWQFXZ2

DRG 456-458 Spinal Fusion Except Cervical with Spinal Curvature/Malignancy/ Infection or Extensive Fusions

Fusion of Thoracic and Lumbar Vertebra, Anterior Column

2 to 7 Thoracic Vertebra		Code also 2 or more Lumbar Vertebra	
ØRG[0,3,4][7,A,J,K]0	XRG70F3	ØSG1[0,3,4][7,A,J,K]0	XRGC0F3

Fusion of Thoracic and Lumbar Vertebra, Posterior Column

2 to 7 Thoracic Vertebra			Code also 2 or more Lumbar Vertebra		
Posterior Approach	Anterior Approach	New Technology	Posterior Approach	Anterior Approach	New Technology
ØRG7[0,3,4][7,J,K]1	ØRG7[0,3,4][7,A,J,K]J	XRG7092 XRG70F3	ØSG1[0,3,4][7,J,K]1	ØSG1[0,3,4][7,A,J,K]J	XRGC092 XRGC0F3

DRG 466-468 Revision of Hip or Knee Replacement

Open Removal of Hip Joint Spacer, Liner, or Resurfacing Device With Supplement of Liner

Body Part	Removal Spacer/Liner/Resurfacing Device	Code also as appropriate Supplement of Body Part by Site		
		Joint	Acetabular Surface	Femoral Surface
Hip, RT	ØSP90[8,9,B,E]Z	ØSU909Z	ØSUAØ9Z	ØSURØ9Z
Hip, LT	ØSPBØ[8,9,B,E]Z	ØSUBØ9Z	ØSUEØ9Z	ØSUSØ9Z

Open Removal of Hip Joint Spacer, Liner, Resurfacing Device, or Synthetic Substitute With Replacement

Body Part	Removal Spacer/Liner/Resurfacing Device/Synthetic Substitute	Code also as appropriate Replacement of Body Part by Device Type						
		Polyethylene	Metal	Metal on Poly	Ceramic	Ceramic on Poly	Oxidized Zirc on Poly	Synth Subst
Hip, RT	ØSP90[8,9,B,E,J]Z	—	ØSR901[9,A,Z]	ØSR902[9,A,Z]	ØSR903[9,A,Z]	ØSR904[9,A,Z]	ØSR906[9,A,Z]	ØSR90J[9,A,Z]
Hip, LT	ØSPBØ[8,9,B,E,J]Z	—	ØSRBØ1[9,A,Z]	ØSRBØ2[9,A,Z]	ØSRBØ3[9,A,Z]	ØSRBØ4[9,A,Z]	ØSRBØ6[9,A,Z]	ØSRBØJ[9,A,Z]
Acetabular Surface, RT	ØSP90[8,9,B,J]Z	ØSRAØØ[9,A,Z]	ØSRAØ1[9,A,Z]	—	ØSRAØ3[9,A,Z]	—	—	ØSRAØJ[9,A,Z]
Acetabular Surface, LT	ØSPBØ[8,9,B,J]Z	ØSREØØ[9,A,Z]	ØSREØ1[9,A,Z]	—	ØSREØ3[9,A,Z]	—	—	ØSREØJ[9,A,Z]
Femoral Surface, RT	ØSP90[8,9,B,J]Z	—	ØSRRØ1[9,A,Z]	—	ØSRRØ3[9,A,Z]	—	—	ØSRRØJ[9,A,Z]
Femoral Surface, LT	ØSPBØ[8,9,B,J]Z	—	ØSRSØ1[9,A,Z]	—	ØSRSØ3[9,A,Z]	—	—	ØSRSØJ[9,A,Z]

Percutaneous Endoscopic Removal of Hip Joint Spacer or Synthetic Substitute With Supplement of Liner

Body Part	Removal Spacer/Synthetic Substitute	Code also as appropriate Supplement of Body Part by Site		
		Joint	Acetabular Surface	Femoral Surface
Hip, RT	ØSP94[8,J]Z	ØSU909Z	ØSUAØ9Z	ØSURØ9Z
Hip, LT	ØSPB4[8,J]Z	ØSUBØ9Z	ØSUEØ9Z	ØSUSØ9Z

Percutaneous Endoscopic Removal of Hip Joint Spacer or Synthetic Substitute With Replacement

Body Part	Removal Spacer/Synthetic Substitute	Code also as appropriate Replacement of Body Part by Device Type						
		Polyethylene	Metal	Metal on Poly	Ceramic	Ceramic on Poly	Oxidized Zircon Poly	Synth Subst
Hip, RT	ØSP94[8,J]Z	-	ØSR901[9,A,Z]	ØSR902[9,A,Z]	ØSR903[9,A,Z]	ØSR904[9,A,Z]	ØSR906[9,A,Z]	ØSR90J[9,A,Z]
Hip, LT	ØSPB4[8,J]Z	-	ØSRBØ1[9,A,Z]	ØSRBØ2[9,A,Z]	ØSRBØ3[9,A,Z]	ØSRBØ4[9,A,Z]	ØSRBØ6[9,A,Z]	ØSRBØJ[9,A,Z]
Acetabular Surface, RT	ØSP94[8,J]Z	ØSRAØØ[9,A,Z]	ØSRAØ1[9,A,Z]	-	ØSRAØ3[9,A,Z]	-		ØSRAØJ[9,A,Z]
Acetabular Surface, LT	ØSPB4[8,J]Z	ØSREØØ[9,A,Z]	ØSREØ1[9,A,Z]	-	ØSREØ3[9,A,Z]	-		ØSREØJ[9,A,Z]
Femoral Surface, RT	ØSP94[8,J]Z	-	ØSRRØ1[9,A,Z]		ØSRRØ3[9,A,Z]	-		ØSRRØJ[9,A,Z]
Femoral Surface, LT	ØSPB4[8,J]Z	-	ØSRSØ1[9,A,Z]		ØSRSØ3[9,A,Z]	-		ØSRSØJ[9,A,Z]

Removal of Hip Joint Surface With Hip Joint Replacement

Body Part	Removal of Spacer/Liner/Resurfacing Device/Synthetic Substitute	Code also as appropriate Replacement of Hip Joint					
		Metal	Metal on Poly	Ceramic	Ceramic on Poly	Oxidized Zircon Poly	Synth Subst
Acetabular Surface, RT	ØSPA[Ø,4]JZ	ØSR901[9,A,Z]	ØSR902[9,A,Z]	ØSR903[9,A,Z]	ØSR904[9,A,Z]	ØSR906[9,A,Z]	ØSR90J[9,A,Z]
Acetabular Surface, LT	ØSPE[Ø,4]JZ	ØSRBØ1[9,A,Z]	ØSRBØ2[9,A,Z]	ØSRBØ3[9,A,Z]	ØSRBØ4[9,A,Z]	ØSRBØ6[9,A,Z]	ØSRBØJ[9,A,Z]
Femoral Surface, RT	ØSPR[Ø,4]JZ	ØSR901[9,A,Z]	ØSR902[9,A,Z]	ØSR903[9,A,Z]	ØSR904[9,A,Z]	ØSR906[9,A,Z]	ØSR90J[9,A,Z]
Femoral Surface, LT	ØSPS[Ø,4]JZ	ØSRBØ1[9,A,Z]	ØSRBØ2[9,A,Z]	ØSRBØ3[9,A,Z]	ØSRBØ4[9,A,Z]	ØSRBØ6[9,A,Z]	ØSRBØJ[9,A,Z]

DRG 466-468 Revision of Hip or Knee Replacement *(Continued)*

Removal of Hip Joint Surface with Replacement with New Joint Acetabular Surface

Body Part	Removal of Spacer/Liner/Resurfacing Device/Synthetic Substitute	Code also as appropriate Replacement of Acetabular Surface			
		Polyethylene	**Metal**	**Ceramic**	**Synth Subst**
Acetabular Surface, RT	ØSPA[Ø,4]JZ	ØSRAØØ[9,A,Z]	ØSRAØ1[9,A,Z]	ØSRAØ3[9,A,Z]	ØSRAØJ[9,A,Z]
Acetabular Surface, LT	ØSPE[Ø,4]JZ	ØSREØØ[9,A,Z]	ØSREØ1[9,A,Z]	ØSREØ3[9,A,Z]	ØSREØJ[9,A,Z]
Femoral Surface, RT	ØSPR[Ø,4]JZ	ØSRAØØ[9,A,Z]	ØSRAØ1[9,A,Z]	ØSRAØ3[9,A,Z]	ØSRAØJ[9,A,Z]
Femoral Surface, LT	ØSPS[Ø,4]JZ	ØSREØØ[9,A,Z]	ØSREØ1[9,A,Z]	ØSREØ3[9,A,Z]	ØSREØJ[9,A,Z]

Removal of Hip Joint Surface With Replacement with New Joint Femoral Surface

Body Part	Removal of Spacer/Liner/Resurfacing Device/Synthetic Substitute	Code also as appropriate Replacement of Femoral Surface		
		Metal	**Ceramic**	**Synth Subst**
Acetabular Surface, RT	ØSPA[Ø,4]JZ	ØSRRØ1[9,A,Z]	ØSRRØ3[9,A,Z]	ØSRRØJ[9,A,Z]
Acetabular Surface, LT	ØSPE[Ø,4]JZ	ØSRSØ1[9,A,Z]	ØSRSØ3[9,A,Z]	ØSRSØJ[9,A,Z]
Femoral Surface, RT	ØSPR[Ø,4]JZ	ØSRRØ1[9,A,Z]	ØSRRØ3[9,A,Z]	ØSRRØJ[9,A,Z]
Femoral Surface, LT	ØSPS[Ø,4]JZ	ØSRSØ1[9,A,Z]	ØSRSØ3[9,A,Z]	ØSRSØJ[9,A,Z]

Percutaneous Endoscopic Removal of Hip Joint Surface With Supplement of Liner

Body Part	Removal of Spacer/Liner/Resurfacing Device/Synthetic Substitute	Code also as appropriate Body Part by Site		
		Joint	**Acetabular Surface**	**Femoral Surface**
Acetabular Surface, RT	ØSPA4JZ	ØSU9Ø9Z	ØSUAØ9Z	ØSURØ9Z
Acetabular Surface, LT	ØSPE4JZ	ØSUBØ9Z	ØSUEØ9Z	ØSUSØ9Z
Femoral Surface, RT	ØSPR4JZ	ØSU9Ø9Z	ØSUAØ9Z	ØSURØ9Z
Femoral Surface, LT	ØSPS4JZ	ØSUBØ9Z	ØSUEØ9Z	ØSUSØ9Z

Removal of Knee Joint, Liner, With Replacement

Body Part	Removal of Liner	Code also as appropriate Replacement of Body Part				
		Synthetic Substitute	**Oxidized Zircon Poly**	**Femoral Surface**	**Tibial Surface**	**Articulating Spacer**
Knee, RT	ØSPC09Z	ØSRCØJ[9,A,Z]	ØSRCØ6[9,A,Z]	ØSRTØJ[9,A,Z]	ØSRVØJ[9,A,Z]	ØSRCØEZ
Knee, LT	ØSPD09Z	ØSRDØJ[9,A,Z]	ØSRDØ6[9,A,Z]	ØSRUØJ[9,A,Z]	ØSRWØJ[9,A,Z]	ØSRDØEZ

Removal of Knee Joint, Spacer, With Replacement

Body Part	Removal of Spacer	Code also as appropriate Replacement of Body Part				
		Synthetic Substitute	**Oxidized Zircon Poly**	**Femoral Surface**	**Tibial Surface**	**Articulating Spacer**
Knee, RT	ØSPC[Ø,3,4]8Z	ØSRCØJ[9,A,Z]	ØSRCØ6[9,A,Z]	ØSRTØJ[9,A,Z]	ØSRVØJ[9,A,Z]	ØSRCØEZ
Knee, LT	ØSPD[Ø,3,4]8Z	ØSRDØJ[9,A,Z]	ØSRDØ6[9,A,Z]	ØSRUØJ[9,A,Z]	ØSRWØJ[9,A,Z]	ØSRDØEZ

Removal of Knee Joint, Synthetic Substitute, With Replacement

Body Part	Removal of Synthetic Substitute	Code also as appropriate Replacement of Body Part						
		Synthetic Substitute	**Oxidized Zircon Poly**	**Unicondylar**	**Patellofemoral**	**Femoral Surface**	**Tibial Surface**	**Articulating Spacer**
Knee, RT	ØSPC09Z	ØSRCØJ[9,A,Z]	ØSRCØ6[9,A,Z]	ØSRCØ[L,M][9,A,Z]	ØSRCØN[9,A,Z]	ØSRTØJ[9,A,Z]	ØSRVØJ[9,A]	ØSRCØEZ
Knee, LT	ØSPD09Z	ØSRDØJ[9,A,Z]	ØSRDØ6[9,A,Z]	ØSRDØ[L,M][9,A,Z]	ØSRDØN[9,A,Z]	ØSRUØJ[9,A,Z]	ØSRWØJ[9,A]	ØSRDØEZ

DRG 466-468 Revision of Hip or Knee Replacement *(Continued)*

Open Removal of Knee Joint, Patellar Surface, With Replacement

Body Part	Removal of Patellar Surface	Code also as appropriate Replacement of Body Part					
		Synthetic Substitute	Oxidized Zirc on Poly	Patellofemoral	Femoral Surface	Tibial Surface	Articulating Spacer
Knee, RT	ØSPCØJZ	ØSRCØJ[9,A,Z]	ØSRCØ6[9,A,Z]	ØSRCØN[9,A,Z]	ØSRTØJ[9,A,Z]	ØSRVØJ[9,A]	ØSRCØEZ
Knee, LT	ØSPDØJZ	ØSRDØJ[9,A,Z]	ØSRDØ6[9,A,Z]	ØSRDØN[9,A,Z]	ØSRUØJ[9,A,Z]	ØSRWØJ[9,A]	ØSRDØEZ

Percutaneous Endoscopic Removal of Knee Joint, Patellar Surface, With Replacement

Body Part	Removal of Patellar Surface	Code also as appropriate Replacement of Body Part					
		Synthetic Substitute	Oxidized Zircon Poly	Patellofemoral	Femoral Surface	Tibial Surface	Articulating Spacer
Knee, RT	ØSPC4JC	ØSRCØJ[9,A,Z]	ØSRCØ6[9,A,Z]	ØSRCØN[9,A,Z]	ØSRTØJ[9,A,Z]	ØSRVØJ[9,A,Z]	ØSRCØEZ
Knee, LT	ØSPD4JC	ØSRDØJ[9,A,Z]	ØSRDØ6[9,A,Z]	ØSRDØN[9,A,Z]	ØSRUØJ[9,A,Z]	ØSRWØJ[9,A,Z]	ØSRDØEZ

Open Removal of Knee Joint, Synthetic Substitute, With Replacement

Body Part	Removal of Synthetic Substitute	Code also as appropriate Replacement of Body Part					
		Synthetic Substitute	Oxidized Zircon Poly	Femoral Surface	Tibial Surface	Articulating Spacer
Femoral Surface, RT	ØSPTØJZ	ØSRCØJ[9,A,Z]	ØSRCØ6[9,A,Z]	ØSRTØJ[9,A,Z]	ØSRVØJ[9,A,Z]	ØSRCØEZ
Femoral Surface, LT	ØSPUØJZ	ØSRDØJ[9,A,Z]	ØSRDØ6[9,A,Z]	ØSRUØJ[9,A,Z]	ØSRWØJ[9,A,Z]	ØSRDØEZ
Tibial Surface, RT	ØSPVØJZ	ØSRCØJ[9,A,Z]	ØSRCØ6[9,A,Z]	ØSRTØJ[9,A,Z]	ØSRVØJ[9,A,Z]	ØSRCØEZ
Tibial Surface, LT	ØSPWØJZ	ØSRDØJ[9,A,Z]	ØSRDØ6[9,A,Z]	ØSRUØJ[9,A,Z]	ØSRWØJ[9,A,Z]	ØSRDØEZ

Percutaneous Endoscopic Removal of Knee Joint, Synthetic Substitute, With Replacement

Body Part	Removal of Synthetic Substitute	Code also as appropriate Replacement of Body Part					
		Synthetic Substitute	Oxidized Zircon Poly	Femoral	Tibial	Articulating Spacer
Femoral Surface, RT	ØSPT4JZ	ØSRCØJ[9,A,Z]	ØSRCØ6[9,A,Z]	ØSRTØJ[9,A]	ØSRVØJ[9,A]	ØSRCØEZ
Femoral Surface, LT	ØSPU4JZ	ØSRDØJ[9,A,Z]	ØSRDØ6[9,A,Z]	ØSRUØJ[9,A]	ØSRWØJ[9,A,Z]	ØSRDØEZ
Tibial Surface, RT	ØSPV4JZ	ØSRCØJ[9,A,Z]	ØSRCØ6[9,A,Z]	ØSRTØJ[9,A]	ØSRVØJ[9,A]	ØSRCØEZ
Tibial Surface, LT	ØSPW4JZ	ØSRDØJ[9,A,Z]	ØSRDØ6[9,A,Z]	ØSRUØJ[9,A]	ØSRWØJ[9,A,Z]	ØSRDØEZ

DRG 485-489 Knee Procedures

Joint	Removal of Liner by open approach	Code also as appropriate Supplement of Tibial Surface by Site
Knee, RT	ØSPCØ9Z	ØSUVØ9Z
Knee, LT	ØSPDØ9Z	ØSUWØ9Z

DRG 515-517 Other Musculoskeletal System and Connective Tissue Procedures

Site	Reposition of Vertebra by percutaneous approach	Code also as appropriate Supplement With Synthetic Substitute by Percutaneous Approach at site of Repositioned Vertebra
Cervical	ØPS33ZZ	ØPU33JZ
Coccyx	ØQSS3ZZ	ØQUS3JZ
Lumbar	ØQSØ3ZZ	ØQUØ3JZ
Sacrum	ØQS13ZZ	ØQU13JZ
Thoracic	ØPS43ZZ	ØPU43JZ

DRG 518-520 Back and Neck Procedures, Except Spinal Fusion, or Disc Devices/Neurostimulators

Generator Type	Insertion of Generator by Site			Code also as appropriate Insertion Neurostimulator Lead by approach and Site	
	Chest	Abdomen	Back	Spinal Canal	Spinal Cord
Single Array	0JH6[0,3]BZ	0JH8[0,3]BZ	0JH7[0,3]BZ	00HU[0,3,4]MZ	00HV[0,3,4]MZ
Single Array, Rechargeable	0JH6[0,3]CZ	0JH8[0,3]CZ	0JH7[0,3]CZ	00HU[0,3,4]MZ	00HV[0,3,4]MZ
Multiple Array	0JH6[0,3]DZ	0JH8[0,3]DZ	0JH7[0,3]DZ	00HU[0,3,4]MZ	00HV[0,3,4]MZ
Multiple Array, Rechargable	0JH6[0,3]EZ	—	0JH7[0,3]EZ	00HU[0,3,4]MZ	00HV[0,3,4]MZ
Multiple Array, Rechargable	—	0JH8[0,3]EZ	—	00HU[0,3,4]MZ	00HV[0,3,4]MZ

DRG 582-583 Mastectomy for Malignancy

Site	Resection by Open approach	Code also as appropriate Resection of Lymph Nodes by Open approach by site			Code also as appropriate Resection of Thorax Muscle by Open approach	
		Axillary	Internal Mammary	Thorax	Right	Left
Breast, Right	0HTT0ZZ	07T50ZZ	07T80ZZ	07T70ZZ	0KTH0ZZ	—
Breast, Left	0HTU0ZZ	07T60ZZ	07T90ZZ	07T70ZZ	—	0KTJ0ZZ
Breast, Bilateral	0HTV0ZZ	07T50ZZ and 07T60ZZ	07T80ZZ and 07T90ZZ	07T70ZZ	0KTH0ZZ	0KTJ0ZZ

DRG 584-585 Breast Biopsy, Local Excision and Other Breast procedures

Resection of Breast With Resection of Lymph Nodes and Thorax Muscle

Site	Resection by Open approach	Code also as appropriate Resection of Lymph Nodes by Open approach by site			Code also as appropriate Resection of Thorax Muscle by Open approach	
		Axillary	Internal Mammary	Thorax	Right	Left
Breast, Right	0HTT0ZZ	07T50ZZ	07T80ZZ	07T70ZZ	0KTH0ZZ	—
Breast, Left	0HTU0ZZ	07T60ZZ	07T90ZZ	07T70ZZ	—	0KTJ0ZZ
Breast, Bilateral	0HTV0ZZ	07T50ZZ and 07T60ZZ	07T80ZZ and 07T90ZZ	07T70ZZ	0KTH0ZZ	0KTJ0ZZ

Replacement of Breast Tissue

Site	Replacement by Percutaneous approach with Autologous Tissue	Code also as appropriate Extraction of Subcutaneous Tissue by Percutaneous approach					
		Abdomen	Back	Buttock	Chest	Leg, Upper, Right	Leg, Upper, Left
Breast, Right	0HRT37Z	0JD83ZZ	0JD73ZZ	0JD93ZZ	0JD63ZZ	0JDL3ZZ	0JDM3ZZ
Breast, Left	0HRU37Z	0JD83ZZ	0JD73ZZ	0JD93ZZ	0JD63ZZ	0JDL3ZZ	0JDM3ZZ
Breast, Bilateral	0HRV37Z	0JD83ZZ	0JD73ZZ	0JD93ZZ	0JD63ZZ	0JDL3ZZ	0JDM3ZZ

DRG 628–630 Other Endocrine, Nutritional and Metabolic Procedures

Open Removal of Hip Joint Spacer, Liner, Resurfacing Device, or Synthetic Substitute With Replacement

Body Part	Removal Spacer/ Liner/Resurfacing Device/Synthetic Substitute	Code also as appropriate Replacement of Body Part by Device Type					
		Polyethylene	Metal	Metal on Poly	Ceramic	Ceramic on Poly	Synth Subst
Hip, RT	ØSP90[8,9,B,J]Z	—	ØSR901[9,A,Z]	ØSR902[9,A,Z]	ØSR903[9,A,Z]	ØSR904[9,A,Z]	ØSR90J[9,A,Z]
Hip, LT	ØSPBØ[8,9,B,J]Z	—	ØSRBØ1[9,A,Z]	ØSRBØ2[9,A,Z]	ØSRBØ3[9,A,Z]	ØSRBØ4[9,A,Z]	ØSRBØJ[9,A,Z]
Acetabular Surface, RT	ØSP90[8,9,B,J]Z	ØSRAØØ[9,A,Z]	ØSRAØ1[9,A,Z]	—	ØSRAØ3[9,A,Z]	—	ØSRAØJ[9,A,Z]
Acetabular Surface, LT	ØSPBØ[8,9,B,J]Z	ØSREØØ[9,A,Z]	ØSREØ1[9,A,Z]	—	ØSREØ3[9,A,Z]	—	ØSREØJ[9,A,Z]
Femoral Surface, RT	ØSP90[8,9,B,J]Z	—	ØSRRØ1[9,A,Z]	—	ØSRRØ3[9,A,Z]	—	ØSRRØJ[9,A,Z]
Femoral Surface, LT	ØSPBØ[8,9,B,J]Z	—	ØSRSØ1[9,A,Z]	—	ØSRSØ3[9,A,Z]	—	ØSRSØJ[9,A,Z]

Open Removal of Hip Joint Spacer, Liner, or Resurfacing Device With Supplement of Liner

Body Part	Removal Spacer/Liner/ Resurfacing Device	Code also as appropriate Supplement of Body Part		
		Joint	Acetabular Surface	Femoral Surface
Hip, RT	ØSP90[8,9,B]Z	ØSU909Z	ØSUAØ9Z	ØSURØ9Z
Hip, LT	ØSPBØ[8,9,B]Z	ØSUBØ9Z	ØSUEØ9Z	ØSUSØ9Z

Percutaneous Endoscopic Removal of Hip Joint Spacer or Synthetic Substitute With Replacement

Body Part	Removal Spacer/Synthetic Substitute	Code also as appropriate Replacement of Body Part by Device Type					
		Polyethylene	Metal	Metal on Poly	Ceramic	Ceramic on Poly	Synth Subst
Hip, RT	ØSP94[8,J]Z	—	ØSR901[9,A,Z]	ØSR902[9,A,Z]	ØSR903[9,A,Z]	ØSR904[9,A,Z]	ØSR90J[9,A,Z]
Hip, LT	ØSPB4[8,J]Z	—	ØSRBØ1[9,A,Z]	ØSRBØ2[9,A,Z]	ØSRBØ3[9,A,Z]	ØSRBØ4[9,A,Z]	ØSRBØJ[9,A,Z]
Acetabular Surface, RT	ØSP94[8,J]Z	ØSRAØØ[9,A,Z]	ØSRAØ1[9,A,Z]	—	ØSRAØ3[9,A,Z]	—	ØSRAØJ[9,A,Z]
Acetabular Surface, LT	ØSPB4[8,J]Z	ØSREØØ[9,A,Z]	ØSREØ1[9,A,Z]	—	ØSREØ3[9,A,Z]	—	ØSREØJ[9,A,Z]
Femoral Surface, RT	ØSP94[8,J]Z	—	ØSRRØ1[9,A,Z]	—	ØSRRØ3[9,A,Z]	—	ØSRRØJ[9,A,Z]
Femoral Surface, LT	ØSPB4[8,J]Z	—	ØSRSØ1[9,A,Z]	—	ØSRSØ3[9,A,Z]	—	ØSRSØJ[9,A,Z]

Percutaneous Endoscopic Removal of Hip Joint Spacer or Synthetic Substitute With Supplement of Liner

Body Part	Removal Spacer/Synthetic Substitute	Code also as appropriate Supplement of Body Part by Site		
		Joint	Acetabular Surface	Femoral Surface
Hip, RT	ØSP94[8,J]Z	ØSU909Z	ØSUAØ9Z	ØSURØ9Z
Hip, LT	ØSPB4[8,J]Z	ØSUBØ9Z	ØSUEØ9Z	ØSUSØ9Z

Removal of Hip Joint Surface with Replacement with New Joint Acetabular Surface

Body Part	Removal of Spacer/ Liner/Resurfacing Device/Synthetic Substitute	Code also as appropriate Replacement of Acetabular Surface			
		Polyethylene	Metal	Ceramic	Synth Subst
Acetabular Surface, RT	ØSPA[Ø,4]JZ	ØSRAØØ[9,A,Z]	ØSRAØ1[9,A,Z]	ØSRAØ3[9,A,Z]	ØSRAØJ[9,A,Z]
Acetabular Surface, LT	ØSPE[Ø,4]JZ	ØSREØØ[9,A,Z]	ØSREØ1[9,A,Z]	ØSREØ3[9,A,Z]	ØSREØJ[9,A,Z]
Femoral Surface, RT	ØSPR[Ø,4]JZ	ØSRAØØ[9,A,Z]	ØSRAØ1[9,A,Z]	ØSRAØ3[9,A,Z]	ØSRAØJ[9,A,Z]
Femoral Surface, LT	ØSPS[Ø,4]JZ	ØSREØØ[9,A,Z]	ØSREØ1[9,A,Z]	ØSREØ3[9,A,Z]	ØSREØJ[9,A,Z]

DRG 628-630 Other Endocrine, Nutritional and Metabolic Procedures (Continued)

Removal of Hip Joint Surface With Replacement with New Joint Femoral Surface

Body Part	Removal of Spacer/ Liner/Resurfacing Device/Synthetic Substitute	Code also as appropriate Replacement of Femoral Surface		
		Metal	Ceramic	Synth Subst
Acetabular Surface, RT	ØSPA[Ø,4]JZ	ØSRRØ1[9,A,Z]	ØSRRØ3[9,A,Z]	ØSRRØJ[9,A,Z]
Acetabular Surface, LT	ØSPE[Ø,4]JZ	ØSRSØ1[9,A,Z]	ØSRSØ3[9,A,Z]	ØSRSØJ[9,A,Z]
Femoral Surface, RT	ØSPR[Ø,4]JZ	ØSRRØ1[9,A,Z]	ØSRRØ3[9,A,Z]	ØSRRØJ[9,A,Z]
Femoral Surface, LT	ØSPS[Ø,4]JZ	ØSRSØ1[9,A,Z]	ØSRSØ3[9,A,Z]	ØSRSØJ[9,A,Z]

Percutaneous Endoscopic Removal of Hip Joint Surface With Supplement of Liner

Body Part	Removal of Spacer/ Liner/Resurfacing Device/Synthetic Substitute	Code also as appropriate Body Part by Site		
		Joint	Acetabular Surface	Femoral Surface
Acetabular Surface, RT	ØSPA4JZ	ØSU9Ø9Z	ØSUAØ9Z	ØSURØ9Z
Acetabular Surface, LT	ØSPE4JZ	ØSUBØ9Z	ØSUEØ9Z	ØSUSØ9Z
Femoral Surface, RT	ØSPR4JZ	ØSU9Ø9Z	ØSUAØ9Z	ØSURØ9Z
Femoral Surface, LT	ØSPS4JZ	ØSUBØ9Z	ØSUEØ9Z	ØSUSØ9Z

Removal of Knee Joint, Liner, With Replacement

Body Part	Removal of Liner	Code also as appropriate Replacement of Body Part					
		Synthetic Substitute	Medial Unicondylar	Lateral Unicondylar	Patellofemoral	Femoral Surface	Tibial Surface
Knee, RT	ØSPCØ9Z	ØSRCØJ[9,A,Z]	ØSRCØL[9,A,Z]	ØSRCØM[9,A,Z]	ØSRCØN[9,A,Z]	ØSRTØJ[9,A,Z]	ØSRVØJ[9,A]
Knee, LT	ØSPDØ9Z	ØSRDØJ[9,A,Z]	ØSRDØL[9,A,Z]	ØSRDØM[9,A,Z]	ØSRDØN[9,A,Z]	ØSRUØJ[9,A,Z]	ØSRWØJ[9,A]

Removal of Knee Joint, Patellar Surface, With Replacement

Body Part	Removal of Patellar Surface	Code also as appropriate Replacement of Body Part	
		Femoral Surface	Tibial Surface
Knee, RT	ØSPC[Ø,4]JC	ØSRTØJ[9,A]	ØSRVØJ[9,A]
Knee, LT	ØSPD[Ø,4]JC	ØSRUØJ[9,A]	ØSRWØJ[9,A,Z]

Removal of Knee Joint, Synthetic Substitute, With Replacement

Body Part	Removal of Synthetic Substitute				Code also as appropriate Replacement of Body Part	
	Synthetic Substitute	Medial Unicondylar	Lateral Unicondylar	Patellofemoral	Femoral Surface	Tibial Surface
Knee, RT	ØSPC[Ø,4]JZ	ØSPC[Ø,4]LZ	ØSPC[Ø,4]MZ	ØSPC[Ø,4]NZ	ØSRTØJ[9,A]	ØSRVØJ[9,A]
Knee, LT	ØSPD[Ø,4]JZ	ØSPD[Ø,4]LZ	ØSPD[Ø,4]MZ	ØSPD[Ø,4]NZ	ØSRUØJ[9,A]	ØSRWØJ[9,A,Z]
Femoral Surface, RT	ØSPT[Ø,4]JZ	—	—	—	ØSRTØJ[9,A]	ØSRVØJ[9,A]
Femoral Surface, LT	ØSPU[Ø,4]JZ	—	—	—	ØSRUØJ[9,A]	ØSRWØJ[9,A,Z]
Tibial Surface, RT	ØSPV[Ø,4]JZ	—	—	—	ØSRTØJ[9,A]	ØSRVØJ[9,A]
Tibial Surface, LT	ØSPW[Ø,4]JZ	—	—	—	ØSRUØJ[9,A]	ØSRWØJ[9,A,Z]

DRG 662-664 Minor Bladder Procedure

Repair of Bladder	Code also as appropriate Repair of Abdominal Wall	
	with Stoma	without Stoma
ØTQB[Ø,3,4]ZZ	ØWQFXZ2	ØWQFXZZ

DRG 665-667 Prostatectomy

Site	Resection by approach				Code also as appropriate Resection of Seminal Vesicles, Bilateral by approach	
	Open	Percutaneous Endoscopic	Via Natural or Artificial Opening	Via Natural or Artificial Opening Endoscopic	Open	Percutaneous Endoscopic
Prostate	ØVT00ZZ	ØVT04ZZ	ØVT07ZZ	ØVT08ZZ	ØVT30ZZ	ØVT34ZZ

DRG 707-708 Major Male Pelvic Procedures

Site	Resection by approach				Code also as appropriate Resection of Seminal Vesicles, Bilateral by approach	
	Open	Percutaneous Endoscopic	Via Natural or Artificial Opening	Via Natural or Artificial Opening Endoscopic	Open	Percutaneous Endoscopic
Prostate	ØVT00ZZ	ØVT04ZZ	ØVT07ZZ	ØVT08ZZ	ØVT30ZZ	ØVT34ZZ

DRG 734-735 Pelvic Evisceration, Radical Hysterectomy and Radical Vulvectomy

Pelvic Evisceration

			Resection by Site			
Bladder	Cervix	Fallopian Tubes, Bilateral	Ovaries, Bilateral	Urethra	Uterus	Vagina
ØTTBØZZ	ØUTCØZZ	ØUT70ZZ	ØUT20ZZ	ØTTDØZZ	ØUT90ZZ	ØUTGØZZ

Radical Hysterectomy

Approach	Resection by Site		
	Cervix	Uterus	Uterine Support Structure
Vaginal	ØUTC[7,8]ZZ	ØUT9[7,8]ZZ	ØUT4[7,8]ZZ
Abdominal, Endoscopic	ØUTC4ZZ	ØUT9[4,F]ZZ	ØUT44ZZ
Abdominal, Open	ØUTCØZZ	ØUT90ZZ	ØUT40ZZ

Radical Vulvectomy

Resection by Site	Code also as appropriate Excision of Inguinal Lymph Nodes by Approach	
Vulva	Right	Left
ØUTM[0,X]ZZ	07BH[0,4]ZZ	07BJ[0,4]ZZ

Non-OR procedure combinations

Note: The following table identifies procedure combinations that are considered Non-OR even though one or more procedures of the combination are considered valid DRG OR procedures

Insertion With Removal of Intraluminal Device

Code as appropriate Insertion of Intraluminal Device into Hepatobiliary Duct	Code also as appropriate Removal of Intraluminal Device by Approach and Site			
	Via Natural or Artificial Opening		External	
	Hepatobiliary Duct	Pancreatic Duct	Hepatobiliary Duct	Pancreatic Duct
ØFHB7DZ	ØFPB[7,8]DZ	ØFPD[7,8]DZ	ØFPBXDZ	ØFPDXDZ

Notes

Notes

Notes

Notes